M000286414

AACN Essentials of Progressive Care Nursing
Third Edition

Suzanne M. Burns, MSN, RRT, ACNP, CCRN, FAAN, FCCM, FAANP
Professor Emeritus, School of Nursing
University of Virginia
Consultant, Critical and Progressive Care and Clinical Nursing Research
Charlottesville, Virginia

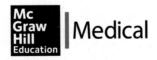
Medical

New York   Chicago   San Francisco   Athens   London   Madrid   Mexico City
Milan   New Delhi   Singapore   Sydney   Toronto

Barbas

AACN Essentials of Progressive Care Nursing, Third Edition

Copyright © 2014, 2010, 2006 by The McGraw-Hill Companies, Inc. All rights reserved. Printed in China. Except as permitted under the United States Copyright Act of 1976, no part of this publication may be reproduced or distributed in any form or by any means, or stored in a data base or retrieval system, without the prior written permission of the publisher.

1 2 3 4 5 6 7 8 9 0   QVS/QVS   19 18 17 16 15 14

ISBN 978-0-07-182292-3
MHID 0-07-182292-5

NOTICE

Medicine is an ever-changing science. As new research and clinical experience broaden our knowledge, changes in treatment and drug therapy are required. The authors and the publisher of this work have checked with sources believed to be reliable in their efforts to provide information that is complete and generally in accord with the standards accepted at the time of publication. However, in view of the possibility of human error or changes in medical sciences, neither the authors nor the publisher nor any other party who has been involved in the preparation or publication of this work warrants that the information contained herein is in every respect accurate or complete, and they disclaim all responsibility for any errors or omissions or for the results obtained from use of the information contained in this work. Readers are encouraged to confirm the information contained herein with other sources. For example and in particular, readers are advised to check the product information sheet included in the package of each drug they plan to administer to be certain that the information contained in this work is accurate and that changes have not been made in the recommended dose or in the contraindications for administration. This recommendation is of particular importance in connection with new or infrequently used drugs.

This book was set in Minion Pro by Cenveo® Publisher Services.
The editors were Andrew Moyer and Christie Naglieri.
The production supervisor was Richard Ruzycka.
Project management was provided by Vastavikta Sharma, Cenveo Publisher Services.
Quad Graphics Versailles was printer and binder.

This book is printed on acid-free paper.

AACN essentials of progressive care nursing / [edited by] Suzanne M. Burns. —Third edition.
     p. ; cm.
   Essentials of progressive care nursing
   Includes bibliographical references and index.
   ISBN-13: 978-0-07-182292-3 (pbk. : alk. paper)
   ISBN-10: 0-07-182292-5 (pbk. : alk. paper)
   I. Burns, Suzanne M., editor of compilation.   II. American Association of Critical-Care Nurses.   III.
     Title: Essentials of progressive care nursing.
   [DNLM: 1. Critical Illness—nursing.   2. Critical Care—methods.   3. Progressive Patient Care—
     methods. WY 154]
   RT120.I5
   616.02′8—dc23
                                                                        2013044514

McGraw-Hill Education books are available at special quantity discounts to use as premiums and sales promotions or for use in corporate training programs. To contact a representative, please visit the Contact Us pages at www.mhprofessional.com.

*To my progressive care nursing colleagues around the world
whose wonderful work and efforts ensure the safe passage of patients
through the progressive care environment. Special thanks to Marianne Chulay, RN, PhD, FAAN, my dear friend and colleague,
for her many contributions and mentoring during the development of the first two editions of the* Essentials of Critical Care
Nursing *and the* Essentials of Progressive Care Nursing *books. Her inspiration, drive, and thoughtful approach to the books
continue to be an inspiration to me and the authors with whom she worked.*

Contents

Contents in Detail

Acknowledgments

Special thanks to those who made contributions to the previous editions of both the *Essentials of Critical Care Nursing* and the *Essentials of Progressive Care Nursing.*

To Cathie Guzzetta, RN, PhD, FAAN and Barbara Dossey, RN, MS, FAAN for their early work in creating the *Handbook of Critical Care Nursing* which preceded the *Essentials of Critical Care Nursing* and the *Essentials of Progressive Care Nursing* books.

To Marianne Chulay, RN, PhD, FAAN, my dear friend and colleague, for her many contributions and mentoring during the development of the first two editions of the *Essentials of Critical Care Nursing* and the *Essentials of Progressive Care Nursing* books. Her inspiration, drive, and thoughtful approach to the books continue to be an inspiration to me and the authors with whom she worked.

Thank you to the many authors for their past contributions:

Tom Ahrens, RNS, DNS, CCNS, FAAN (Chapter 4 and key reference materials)

Sue Simmons-Alling, RN, MSN (Chapter 2)

Suzanne M. Burns, RN, MSN, RRT ACNP, CCRN, FAAN, FCCM, FAANP (Chapters 4, 5, 11)

Deb Byram, RN, MS (Chapter 1)

Karen Carlson, RN, MN (Chapter 15)

Joan Michiko, Ching RN, MN, CPHQ (Chapter 6)

Marianne Chulay, RN, PhD, FAAN: (Chapter 10, and the key reference materials)

Maria Connolly, RN, DNSc (Chapters 5, 10)

Dorrie Fontaine, RN, DNSc, FAAN (Chapter 17)

Bradi Granger, RN, PhD (Chapter 9)

Anne Marie Gregoire, RN, MSN, CRNP (Chapter 19)

Joanne Krumberger, RN, MSN, CHE, FAAN (Chapters 14, 16)

Sally Miller, RN, PhD, APN, FAANP (Chapter 14)

Carol A. Rauen, RN, MS, CCNS, CCRN, PCCN (Chapter 17)

Juanita Reigle, RN, MSN, ACNP (Chapter 8)

Anita Sherer, RN, MSN (Chapter 2)

Jamie Sinks, RN, MS (Chapter 17)

Greg Susla, Pharm D, FCCM (Chapters 7 and key reference materials)

Debbie Tribett, RN, MS, CS, LNP (Chapter 13)

Debra Lynn-McHale Wiegand, RN, PhD, CS (Chapter 19)

Lorie Wild, RN, PhD (Chapter 6)

Susan Woods, PhD, RN (Chapters 3, 18)

Marlene Yates, RN, MSN (Chapter 2)

Contibutors

Earnest Alexander, PharmD, FCCM
Assistant Director, Clinical Pharmacy Services
Program Director, PGY2 Critical Care Residency
Department of Pharmacy Services
Tampa General Hospital
Tampa, Florida
Chapter 7: Pharmacology
Chapter 22: Pharmacology Tables

Deborah A. Andris, MSN, APNP
Nurse Practitioner
Division of Colorectal Surgery
Medical College of Wisconsin
Milwaukee, Wisconsin
Chapter 14: Gastrointestinal System

Yvonne D'Arcy, MS, CRNP, CNS
Pain Management and Palliative Care Nurse Practitioner
Suburban Hospital-Johns Hopkins Medicine
Bethesda, Maryland
Chapter 6: Pain and Sedation Management

Suzanne M. Burns, RN, MSN, RRT, ACNP, CCRN, FAAN,
    FCCM, FAANP
Professor Emeritus, School of Nursing
University of Virginia
Consultant, Critical and Progressive Care and Clinical
    Nursing Research
Charlottesville, Virginia
Chapter 6: Pain and Sedation Management
Chapter 21: Normal Values Table
Chapter 23: Advanced Cardiac Life Support Algorithms

Sarah Delgado, RN, MSN, ACNP
Chronic Care Nurse Practitioner
PIH Health Physicians
Whittier, California
Chapter 8: Ethical and Legal Considerations

Diane K. Dressler, MSN, RN, CCRN
Clinical Assistant Professor
Marquette University College of Nursing
Milwaukee, Wisconsin
Chapter 13: Hematologic and Immune Systems

Carol Hinkle, MSN, RN-BC
Brookwoood Medical Center
Birmingham, Alabama
Chapter 15: Renal System

Benjamin W. Hughes, RN, MSN, MS, CCRN
Director
Trauma Institute and Cardiopulmonary Services
University of Louisville Hospital
Louisville, Kentucky
Chapter 17: Trauma

Carol Jacobson, RN, MN
Director, Quality Education Services & Partner
Cardiovascular Nursing Education Associates
Clinical Faculty
University of Washington School of Nursing
Seattle, Washington
*Chapter 3: Interpretation and Management of Basic Cardiac
    Rhythms*
Chapter 18: Advanced ECG Concepts
*Chapter 24: Cardiac Rhythms, ECG Characteristics, and
    Treatment Guide*

Robert E. St. John, MSN, RN, RRT
Covidien
Care Area Manager–US Patient Monitoring
Respiratory and Monitoring Solutions
Boulder, Colorado
Chapter 5: Airway and Ventilatory Management

Christine Kessler, MN, CNS, ANP, BC-ADM
Nurse Practitioner, Diabetes Institute
Department of Endocrinology and Metabolic Medicine
Walter Reed Army Medical Center
Washington, DC
Chapter 16: Endocrine System

Ruth M. Kleinpell, PhD, RN-CS, FAAN, FCCM, FAANP, ACNP, CCRN
Director, Center for Clinical Research and Scholarship
Rush University Medical Center
Professor, Rush University College of Nursing
Nurse Practitioner, Our Lady of the Resurrection
  Medical Center
Chicago, Illinois
Chapter 11: Multisystem Problems

Joe Krenitsky, MS, RD
Nutrition Support Specialist
Digestive Health Center of Excellence
Department of Nutrition Services
University of Virginia Health System
Charlottesvillle, Virginia
Chapter 14: Gastrointestinal System

Elizabeth Krzywda, MSN, APNP
Nurse Practitioner
Pancreaticobiliary Surgery Program
Medical College of Wisconsin
Milwaukee, Wisconsin
Chapter 14: Gastrointestinal System

Barbara Leeper, MN, RN-BC, CNS-MS, CCRN, FAHA
Clinical Nurse Specialist
Cardiovascular Services
Baylor University Medical Center
Dallas, Texas
Chapter 9: Cardiovascular System
Chapter 19: Advanced Cardiovascular Concepts

Dea Mahanes, RN, MSN, CCRN, CNRN, CCNS
Advanced Practice Nurse 3
Clinical Nurse Specialist
Nerancy Neuro ICU
University of Virginia Health System
Charlottesvillle, Virginia
Chapter 12: Neurologic System
Chapter 20: Advanced Neurologic Concepts

Leanna R. Miller, RN, MN, CCRN-CMC, PCCN-CSC, CEN, CNRN, CMSRN, NP
Instructor
Western Kentucky University
Bowling Green, Kentucky
*Chapter 4: Interpretation and Management of Basic
  Cardiac Rhythms*

Carol Rees Parrish, MS, RD
Nutrition Support Specialist
Digestive Health Center of Excellence
Department of Nutrition Services
University of Virginia Health System
Charlottesvillle, Virginia
Chapter 14: Gastrointestinal System

Maureen A. Seckel, APN, ACNS, BC, CCNS, CCRN
Clinical Nurse Specialist Medical Pulmonary Critical Care
Christiana Care Health System
Newark, Delaware
Chapter 5: Airway and Ventilatory Management
Chapter 10: Respiratory System

Mary Fran Tracy, PhD, RN, CCNS, FAAN
Critical Care Clinical Nurse Specialist
University of Minnesota Medical Center, Fairview
Minneapolis, Minnesota
*Chapter 1: Assessment of Progressive Care Patients and
  Their Families*
*Chapter 2: Planning Care for Progressive Care Patients and
  Their Families*

Allen C. Wolfe, Jr., MSN, RN, CFRN, CCRN, CMTE
Clinical Education Director/Clinical Specialist
Air Methods Corporation
Community Based Services
Denver, Colorado
Chapter 17: Trauma

Reviewers

John M. Allen, PharmD, BCPS
Assistant Clinical Professor
Auburn University
Harrison School of Pharmacy
Mobile, Alabama

Richard Arbour, MSN, RN, CCRN, CNRN, CCNS, FAAN
Advanced Practice Nurse; Clinical Faculty
La Salle University
Holy Family University
Philadelphia, Pennsylvania

Cheri S. Blevins, MSN RN CCRN CCNS
APN-2 Clinical Nurse Specialist
Medical ICU
University of Virginia Health System
Charlottesville, Virginia

Shawn Cosper, MSN, RN
Education Consultant-Critical Care
Education Department
Brookwood Medical Center
Birmingham, Alabama

Sarah Jane White Craig, MSN, RN, CCNS, CCRN
Clinical Nurse Specialist
Postoperative Thoracic-Cardiovascular Surgery Service
University of Virginia Health System
Charlottesville, Virginia

Tina Cronin, APRN, CCNS, CCRN, CNRN
Director Nursing Education, Practice
Novant Health Greater Charlotte Market
Charlotte, North Carolina

Linda DeStefano, CNS, NP, FCCM
Clinical Nurse Specialist, Critical Care Services
Saddleback Memorial Medical Center
Laguna Hills, California

Beth Epstein, PhD, RN
Associate Professor
University of Virginia School of Nursing
Faculty Affiliate University of Virginia Center for Biomedical Ethics and Humanities
University of Virginia
Charlottesville, Virginia

John J. Gallagher, MSN, RN, CCNS, CCRN, RRT
Trauma Program Manager
Division of Traumatology, Surgical Critical Care and Emergency Surgery
Hospital of the University of Pennsylvania
Philadelphia, Pennsylvania

Tonja Hartjes, DNP, ACNP/FNP-BC, CCRN-CSC
Associate Clinical Professor
University of Florida, College of Nursing
Adult Gerontology and Acute Care ARNP Program and Cardiothoracic Surgery ARNP Shands UF
Gainesville, Florida

Barbara S. Jacobs, MSN, RN-BC, CCRN, CENP
Senior Director/Chief Nurse Officer
Suburban Hospital/Johns Hopkins Medicine
Bethesda, Maryland

Katherine Johnson, MS, CNRN
Neuro CNS
Queens Medical Center
Honolulu, Hawaii

Victoria A. Kark, RN, MSN, CCRN,CCNS, CSC
Clinical Nurse Specialist
Surgical Intensive Care Unit
Walter Reed National Military Medical Center
Bethesda, Maryland

Deborah Klein, MSN, RN, ACNS-BC, CCRN, CHFN, FAHA
Clinical Nurse Specialist Coronary ICU, Heart Failure ICU, and Cardiac Short Stay/PACU
Cleveland Clinic
Cleveland, Ohio

Julie Painter, RN, MSN, OCN
Community Health Network
Oncology Clinical Nurse Specialist
Indianapolis, Indiana

Carol A. Rauen, RN, MS, CCNS, CCRN, PCCN, CEN
Independent Clinical Nurse Specialist and Education Consultant
Kill Devil Hills, North Carolina

Christine Schulman, MS, RN, CNS, CCRN
Critical Care CNS
Legacy Health
Portland, Oregon

Michelle VanDemark, MSN, RN, ANP-BC, CNRN, CCSN
Neurocritical Care Nurse Practitioner
Sanford Medical Center
Sioux Falls, South Dakota

Michelle A. Weber, RN, MSN, ACNP-BC
Nurse Practitioner
Division of General Surgery
Medical College of Wisconsin
Milwaukee, Wisconsin

Brian Widmar, PhD, RN, ACNP-BC, CCRN
Assistant Professor of Nursing
Vanderbilt University School of Nursing
Nashville, Tennessee

Susan L. Woods, PhD, RN, FAAN
Professor Emerita
Department of Biobehavioral Nursing and Health Systems
School of Nursing
University of Washington
Seattle, Washington

Amanda Zomp, PharmD, BCPS
Critical Care Clinical Pharmacist
University of Virginia Medical Center
Charlottesville, Virginia

Preface

Progressive care nursing is a complex, challenging area of nursing practice, where clinical expertise is developed over time by integrating progressive care knowledge, clinical skills, and caring practices. This textbook, the first to specifically address the educational needs of the new progressive care practitioner, succinctly presents essential information about how best to safely and competently care for acutely ill patients and their families.

As it has since the first edition, the American Association of Critical-Care Nurses reaffirms this book's value to the AACN community and especially to clinicians at the point of care. The title continues to carry AACN's name, as it has since the first edition.

AACN Essentials of Progressive Care Nursing provides essential information on the care of adult acutely ill patients and families. The book recognizes the learner's need to assimilate foundational knowledge before attempting to master more complex progressive care nursing concepts. Written by nationally acknowledged clinical experts in critical and acute care nursing, this textbook sets the standard for progressive care nursing education.

AACN Essentials of Progressive Care Nursing:

- Succinctly presents essential information for the safe and competent care of progressive care patients and their families, building on the clinician's significant medical-surgical nursing knowledge base, avoiding repetition of previously acquired information
- Stages the introduction of advanced concepts in progressive care nursing after essential concepts have been mastered
- Provides clinicians with clinically relevant tools and guides to use as they care for progressive care patients and families

The AACN Essentials of Progressive Care Nursing is divided into four parts:

- *Part I: The Essentials* presents essential information that clinicians must understand to provide safe, competent nursing care to the majority of progressive care patients, regardless of their underlying medical diagnoses. This part includes content on essential concepts of assessment, diagnosis, planning, and interventions common to progressive care patients and families; interpretation and management of cardiac rhythms; hemodynamic monitoring; airway and ventilatory management; pain and sedation management; pharmacology; and ethical and legal considerations. Chapters in Part I present content in enough depth to ensure that essential information is available for the new progressive care clinician to develop competence, while sequencing pathological conditions in Part II and advanced content in a later part of the book (Part III).
- *Part II: Pathologic Conditions* covers pathologic conditions and management strategies commonly encountered in progressive care, closely paralleling the blueprint for the PCCN certification examination. Chapters in this part are organized by body systems and selected progressive care conditions (cardiovascular, respiratory, multisystem, neurologic, hematologic and immune, gastrointestinal, renal, endocrine, and trauma).
- *Part III: Advanced Concepts in Caring for the Progressive Care Patient* presents advanced progressive care concepts or pathologic conditions that are more complex and represent expert level information. Specific advanced chapter content includes ECG concepts, cardiovascular concepts, and neurologic concepts.
- *Part IV: Key Reference Information* contains reference information that clinicians will find helpful in the clinical area (normal laboratory and diagnostic values; algorithms for advanced cardiac life support; and summary tables of progressive care drugs and cardiac rhythms). Content is presented primarily in table format for quick reference.

Each chapter in Part I, II, and III, begins with "Knowledge Competencies" that can be used to guide informal or formal teaching and to gauge the learner's progress. In addition, each of the chapters provide "Essential Content Case" studies that focus on key information presented in the chapters in order to assist clinicians in understanding the chapter content and how to best assess and manage conditions and problems encountered in progressive care. The case studies also are designed to enhance the learners understanding of the magnitude of the pathologic problems/conditions and their impact on patients and families. Questions and answers are provided for each case so the learner may test his/her knowledge of the essential content.

I believe that there is no greater way to protect our patients than to ensure that an educated clinician cares for them. Safe passage in progressive care is ensured by competent, skilled, knowledgeable, and caring clinicians. I sincerely believe that this textbook will help you make it so!

Suzi Burns

THE ESSENTIALS | I

Assessment of Progressive Care Patients and Their Families

1

Mary Fran Tracy

KNOWLEDGE COMPETENCIES

1. Discuss the importance of a consistent and systematic approach to assessment of progressive care patients and their families.
2. Identify the assessment priorities for different stages of an acute illness:
   - Prearrival assessment
   - Arrival quick check

- Comprehensive initial assessment
- Ongoing assessment
3. Describe how the assessment is altered based on the patient's clinical status.

The assessment of acutely ill patients and their families is an essential competency for progressive care practitioners. Information obtained from an assessment identifies the immediate and future needs of the patient and family so a plan of care can be initiated to address or resolve these needs.

Traditional approaches to patient assessment include a complete evaluation of the patient's history and a comprehensive physical examination of all body systems. This approach is ideal, though progressive care clinicians must balance the need to gather data while simultaneously prioritizing and providing care to acutely ill patients who may either be improving or decompensating. Traditional approaches and techniques for assessment must be modified in progressive care to balance the need for information, while considering the acute nature of the patient and family's situation.

This chapter outlines an assessment approach that recognizes the dynamic nature of an acute illness. This approach emphasizes the collection of assessment data in a phased or staged manner consistent with patient care priorities. The components of the assessment can be used as a generic template for assessing most progressive care patients and families. The assessment can then be individualized by adding more specific assessment requirements depending on the specific patient diagnosis. These specific components of the assessment are identified in subsequent chapters.

Crucial to developing competence in assessing progressive care patients and their families is a consistent and systematic approach to assessments. Without this approach, it would be easy to miss subtle signs or details that may identify an actual or potential problem and also indicate a patient's changing status. Assessments should focus first on the patient, then on the technology. The patient needs to be the focal point of the progressive care practitioner's attention, with technology augmenting the information obtained from the direct assessment.

There are two standard approaches to assessing patients—the head-to-toe approach and the body systems approach. Most progressive care nurses use a combination—a systems approach applied in a top-to-bottom manner. The admission and ongoing assessment sections of this chapter are presented with this combined approach in mind.

ASSESSMENT FRAMEWORK

Assessing the progressive care patient and family begins from the moment the nurse is made aware of the pending admission or transfer of the patient and continues until transitioning to the next phase of care. The assessment process can be viewed as four distinct stages: (1) prearrival, (2) arrival quick check ("just the basics"), (3) comprehensive initial assessment, and (4) ongoing assessment.

Prearrival Assessment

Patients admitted to a progressive care unit may be transitioning from a more intensive level of care, as they become more stable and improve in condition. Conversely, they may be transferred from a lower level of care, as their physiologic status may be deteriorating. In either case, the progressive care patient has the potential to have a rapid change in status. A prearrival assessment begins the moment the information is received about the upcoming admission of the patient to the progressive care unit. This notification comes from the initial healthcare team contact. The contact may be a transfer from another facility or a transfer from other areas within the hospital such as the emergency room, operating room, the intensive care unit (ICU), or medical/surgical nursing unit. The prearrival assessment paints the initial picture of the patient and allows the progressive care nurse to begin anticipating the patient's physiologic and psychological needs. This assessment also allows the progressive care nurse to determine the appropriate resources that are needed to care for the patient. The information received in the prearrival phase is crucial because it allows the progressive care nurse to adequately prepare the environment to meet the specialized needs of the patient and family.

Arrival Quick Check

An arrival quick check assessment is obtained immediately upon arrival and is based on assessing the parameters represented by the ABCDE acronym (Table 1-1). The arrival quick check assessment is a quick overview of the adequacy of ventilation and perfusion to ensure early intervention for any life-threatening situations. The arrival quick check is a high-level view of the patient, but is essential because it validates that basic cardiac and respiratory function is sufficient, and can be used as a baseline for potential future changes in a condition.

Comprehensive Initial Assessment

A comprehensive assessment is performed as soon as possible, with the timing dictated by the degree of physiologic stability and emergent treatment needs of the patient. If the patient is being admitted directly to the progressive care unit from outside the hospital, the comprehensive assessment is

TABLE 1-1. ABCDE ACRONYM

Airway
Breathing
Circulation, Cerebral perfusion, and Chief complaint
Drugs and Diagnostic tests
Equipment

an in-depth assessment of the past medical and social history and a complete physical examination of each body system. If the patient is being transferred to the progressive care unit from another area in the hospital, the comprehensive assessment includes a review of the admission assessment data and comparison to the current assessment of the patient. The comprehensive assessment is vital to successful outcomes because it provides the nurse invaluable insight into proactive interventions that may be needed.

Ongoing Assessment

After the baseline comprehensive assessment is completed, ongoing assessments—an abbreviated version of the comprehensive assessment—are performed at varying intervals. The assessment parameters outlined in this section are usually completed for all patients, in addition to other ongoing assessment requirements related to the patient's specific condition, treatments, and response to therapy.

Patient Safety Considerations in Admission Assessments

Admission of an acutely ill patient can be a chaotic event with multiple disciplines involved in many activities. It is at this time, however, that health-care providers must be particularly cognizant of accurate assessments and data gathering to ensure the patient is cared for safely with appropriate interventions. Obtaining inaccurate information on admission can lead to ongoing errors that may not be easily rectified or discovered and lead to poor patient outcomes.

Obtaining information from an acutely ill patient may be difficult, if possible at all. If the patient is unable to supply information, other sources must be utilized such as family members, electronic health records (EHRs), past medical records, transport records, or information from the patient's belongings. Of particular importance at admission is obtaining accurate patient identification, as well as past medical history including any known allergies. Current medication regimens are extremely helpful if feasible, as they can provide clues to the patient's medical condition and perhaps contributing factors to the current condition.

With the increasing use of EHRs, there are improving opportunities for timely access to past and current medical history information of patients. Healthcare providers may have access to both inpatient and outpatient records within the same healthcare system, assisting them to quickly identify the patient's most recent medication regimen and laboratory and diagnostic results. In addition, many healthcare systems within the same geographic locations are working together to make available intersystem access to medical records of patients being treated at multiple healthcare institutions. This is particularly beneficial when patients are unable to articulate imperative medical information including advance directives, allergies, and next of kin.

Careful physical assessment on admission to the progressive care unit is pivotal for providing prevention and/or early treatment for complications associated with the illness.

Of particular importance is the assessment of risk for pressure ulcer formation, alteration in mental status, and/or falls. Risks associated with accurate patient identification never lessen, particularly as these relate to interventions such as performing invasive procedures, medication administration, blood administration, and obtaining laboratory tests. Nurses need to be cognizant of safety issues as treatment begins as well; for example, accurate programming of pumps infusing high-risk medications is essential. It is imperative that nurses use all safety equipment available to them such as pre-programmed drug libraries in infusion pumps and bar coding technology. Healthcare providers must also ensure the safety of invasive procedures that may be performed emergently.

PREARRIVAL ASSESSMENT: BEFORE THE ACTION BEGINS

A prearrival assessment begins when information is received about the pending arrival of the patient. The prearrival report, although abbreviated, provides key information about the chief complaint, diagnosis, or reason for admission, pertinent history details, and physiologic stability of the patient (Table 1-2). It also contains the gender and age of the patient and information on the presence of invasive tubes and lines, medications being administered, other

TABLE 1-2. SUMMARY OF PREARRIVAL AND ARRIVAL QUICK CHECK ASSESSMENTS

Prearrival Assessment
• Abbreviated report on patient (age, gender, chief complaint, diagnosis, allergies pertinent history, physiologic status, invasive devices, equipment, and status of laboratory/diagnostic tests)
• Complete room setup, including verification of proper equipment functioning
Admission Quick Check Assessment
• General appearance (consciousness)
• Airway: Patency Position of artificial airway (if present) such as tracheostomy
• Breathing: Quantity and quality of respirations (rate, depth, pattern, symmetry, effort, use of accessory muscles) Breath sounds Presence of spontaneous breathing
• Circulation and Cerebral Perfusion: ECG (rate, rhythm, and presence of ectopy) Blood pressure Peripheral pulses and capillary refill Skin color, temperature, moisture Presence of bleeding Level of consciousness, responsiveness
• Chief Complaint: Primary body system Associated symptoms
• Drugs and Diagnostic Tests: Drugs prior to admission (prescribed, over-the-counter, illicit) Current medications Review diagnostic test results
• Equipment: Patency of vascular and drainage systems Appropriate functioning and labeling of all equipment connected to patient

TABLE 1-3. EQUIPMENT FOR STANDARD ROOM SETUP

• Bedside ECG or telemetry monitoring and invasive pressure monitor with appropriate cables
• ECG electrodes
• Blood pressure cuff
• Pulse oximetry
• Suction gauges and canister setup
• Suction catheters
• Bag valve mask device
• Oxygen flow meter, appropriate tubing, and appropriate oxygen delivery device
• IV poles and infusion pumps
• Bedside supply cart that contains such things as alcohol swabs, nonsterile gloves, syringes, chux, and dressing supplies
• Admission kit that usually contains bath basin and general hygiene supplies (if direct admission)
• Admission and progressive care paper and/or electronic documentation forms

ongoing treatments, and pending or completed laboratory or diagnostic tests. It is also important to consider the potential isolation requirements for the patient (eg, neutropenic precautions or special respiratory isolation). Being prepared for isolation needs prevents potentially serious exposures to the patient, roommates, or the healthcare providers. This information assists the clinician in anticipating the patient's physiologic and emotional needs prior to admission or transfer and in ensuring that the bedside environment is set up to provide all monitoring, supply, and equipment needs prior to the patient's arrival.

Many progressive care units have a standard room setup, guided by the major diagnosis-related groups of patients each unit receives. The standard monitoring and equipment list for each unit varies; however, there are certain common requirements (Table 1-3). The standard room setup is modified for each admission to accommodate patient-specific needs (eg, additional equipment, intravenous [IV] fluids, medications). Proper functioning of all bedside equipment should be verified prior to the patient's arrival.

It is also important to prepare the medical records forms, which usually consist of paper flow sheets or computerized data entry system to record vital signs, intake and output, medication administration, patient care activities, and patient assessment. The prearrival report may suggest pending procedures, necessitating the organization of appropriate supplies at the bedside. Having the room prepared and all equipment available facilitates a rapid, smooth, and safe admission of the patient.

ARRIVAL QUICK CHECK ASSESSMENT

From the moment the patient arrives in the progressive care unit setting, his or her general appearance is immediately observed and assessment of ABCDEs is quickly performed (see Table 1-1). The seriousness of the problem(s) is determined so any urgent needs can be addressed first. The patient is connected to the appropriate monitoring and support equipment, medications being administered are verified,

ESSENTIAL CONTENT CASE

Prearrival Assessment

The charge nurse notifies Sue that she will be receiving a 26-year-old man from the ICU who was involved in a serious car accident 14 days ago. The ICU nurse caring for the patient has called to give Sue a report following the hospital's standardized report format.

Case Question 1: What basic information will Sue want to know from the pre-arrival communication with the ICU nurse?

Case Question 2: What patient issues are likely to need immediate assessment and/or intervention on arrival to the progressive care unit in order to ensure the appropriate equipment is set up in the room?

Case Question 3: What information should be included in the more formal handoff between the ICU nurse and Sue after the patient is settled in his room in the Progressive Care Unit?

Answers

1. Patient name/age, type and date of accident, extent of accident injuries, pertinent medical history, allergies, vital signs and significant assessment information, placement of lines and tubes, medications being administered, significant laboratory results, anticipated plan for care and discharge plan, presence of family, and any other special instructions.

   The patient suffered a closed head injury and chest trauma with collapsed left lung. The patient had been intubated and placed on a mechanical ventilator. The patient had developed pneumonia when in the ICU and though he now exhibited stable oxygenation, a tracheostomy was required to manage copious secretions. He had now been weaned off the ventilator and was requiring 30% Fio_2. A central line with a central venous pressure (CVP) setup and a left chest tube to water seal were in place. Sue questions the critical care nurse regarding whether the patient has been agitated, his level of consciousness (LOC) and neuro deficits, if a Foley catheter or nasogastric tube is present, and whether the family has been notified of the transfer to the progressive care unit.

2. Vital signs, neurologic status, the tracheostomy and oxygen requirements of the patient, medications are appropriately infusing and whether the patient is agitated or experiencing extensive pain.

   Sue goes to check the patient's room prior to admission and begins to do a mental check of what will be needed. "The patient has a tracheostomy so I'll connect the AMBU bag to the oxygen source, check for suction catheters, and make sure the suction systems are working. The pulse oximetry is ready to use. I'll also ensure the telemetry pack has fully charged batteries and have the ECG electrodes ready to apply. The CVP line flush system and transducer are also ready to be connected. The IV infusion devices are set up. This patient has an altered LOC, which means frequent neuro checks. I have my pen light handy. The computer in the room is on and ready for me to begin documentation. I think I'm ready."

3. Using an SBAR format, the ICU nurse can give more detailed information about the injuries from the car accident, the patient's complete medical history as known, reiteration of known allergies, a system by system assessment review, significant diagnostic test results, confirmation of all invasive lines and equipment settings, the anticipated plan for ongoing assessments, interventions, and discharge planning, and any pertinent family information. Sue should also have an opportunity to ask any clarifying questions she might have.

and essential laboratory and diagnostic tests are ordered. Simultaneously with the ABCDE assessment, the patient's nurse must validate that the patient is appropriately identified through a hospital wristband, personal identification, or family identification. In addition, the patient's allergy status is verified, including the type of reaction that occurs and what, if any, treatment is used to alleviate the allergic response.

There may be other healthcare professionals present to receive the patient and assist with arrival tasks. The progressive care nurse, however, is the leader of the receiving team. While assuming the primary responsibility for assessing the ABCDEs, the progressive care nurse directs the team in completing delegated tasks, such as changing over to the unit equipment or attaching monitoring cables. Without a leader of the receiving team, care can be fragmented and vital assessment clues overlooked.

The progressive care nurse rapidly assesses the ABCDEs in the sequence outlined in this section. If any aspect of this preliminary assessment deviates from normal, interventions are immediately initiated to address the problem before continuing with the arrival quick check assessment. Additionally, regardless of whether the patient appears to be conscious or not, it is important to talk to him or her throughout this admission process regarding what is occurring with each interaction and intervention.

Airway and Breathing

Patency of the patient's airway is verified by having the patient speak, watching the patient's chest rise or fall, or both. If the airway is compromised, verify that the head has been positioned properly to prevent the tongue from occluding the airway. Inspect the upper airway for the presence of blood, vomitus, and foreign objects before inserting an oral airway if one is needed. If the patient already has an artificial airway, such as a cricothyrotomy or tracheostomy, ensure that the airway is secured properly. Note the position of the tracheostomy and size marking to assist future comparisons for proper placement. Suctioning of the upper airway, either through the oral cavity or artificial airway, may be required to ensure that the airway is free from secretions. Note the amount, color, and consistency of secretions removed.

Note the rate, depth, pattern, and symmetry of breathing; the effort it is taking to breathe; the use of accessory muscles; and, if mechanically ventilated, whether breathing is in synchrony with the ventilator. Observe for nonverbal signs of respiratory distress such as restlessness, anxiety, or change in mental status. Auscultate the chest for presence of bilateral breath sounds, quality of breath sounds, and bilateral chest expansion. Optimally, both anterior and posterior breath sounds are auscultated, but during this arrival quick check assessment, time generally dictates that just the anterior chest is assessed. If noninvasive oxygen saturation monitoring is available, observe and quickly analyze the values.

If chest tubes are present, note whether they are pleural or mediastinal chest tubes. Ensure that they are connected to suction, if appropriate, and are not clamped or kinked. Assess whether they are functioning properly (eg, airleak, fluid fluctuation with respirations) and the amount and character of the drainage.

Circulation and Cerebral Perfusion

Assess circulation by quickly palpating a pulse and viewing the electrocardiogram (ECG) and monitor for the heart rate, rhythm, and presence of ectopy if ECG monitoring is ordered. Obtain blood pressure and temperature. Assess peripheral perfusion by evaluating the color, temperature, and moisture of the skin along with capillary refill. Based on the prearrival report and reason for admission, there may be a need to inspect the body for any signs of blood loss and determine if active bleeding is occurring.

Evaluating cerebral perfusion in the arrival quick check assessment is focused on determining the functional integrity of the brain as a whole, which is done by rapidly evaluating the gross LOC. Evaluate whether the patient is alert and aware of his or her surroundings, whether it takes a verbal or painful stimulus to obtain a response, or whether the patient is unresponsive. Observing the response of the patient during movement from the stretcher to the progressive care unit bed can supply additional information about the LOC. Note whether the patient's eyes are open and watching the events around him or her; for example, does the patient follow simple commands such as "Place your hands on your chest" or "Slide your hips over"? If the patient is unable to talk because of trauma or the presence of an artificial airway, note whether his or her head nods appropriately to questions.

Chief Complaint

Optimally, the description of the chief complaint is obtained from the patient, but this may not be realistic. The patient may be unable to respond or may not speak English. Data may need to be gathered from family, friends, or bystanders, or from the completed admission database if the patient has been transferred from another area in the hospital. If the patient or family cannot speak English, an approved hospital translator should be contacted to help with the interview and subsequent evaluations and communication. It is not advised to use family or friends to translate for a non-English speaking patient for reasons such as protection of the patient's privacy, the likelihood that family will not understand appropriate medical terminology for translation, and to avoid well-intentioned but potential bias in translating back and forth for the patient.

In the absence of a history source, practitioners must depend exclusively on the physical findings (eg, presence of medication patches, permanent pacemaker, or old surgery scars), knowledge of pathophysiology, and access to prior paper or electronic medical records to identify the potential causes of the admission.

Assessment of the chief complaint focuses on determining the body systems involved and the extent of associated symptoms. Additional questions explore the time of onset, precipitating factors, and severity. Although the arrival quick check phase is focused on obtaining a quick overview of the key life-sustaining systems, a more in-depth assessment of a particular system may need to be done at this time; for example, in the prearrival case study scenario presented, completion of the ABCDEs is followed quickly by more extensive assessment of both the nervous and respiratory systems.

Drugs and Diagnostic Tests

Information about infusing medications and diagnostic tests is integrated into the priority of the arrival quick check. If IV access is not already present, it should be immediately obtained and intake and output records started. If IV medications are presently being infused, check the drug(s) and verify the correct infusion of the desired dosage and rate.

Determine the latest results of any diagnostic tests already performed. Augment basic screening tests (Table 1-4) with additional tests appropriate to the underlying diagnosis, chief complaint, transfer status, and recent procedures. Review any available laboratory or diagnostic data for abnormalities or indications of potential problems that may develop. The abnormal laboratory and diagnostic data for specific pathologic conditions will be covered in subsequent chapters.

Equipment

Quickly evaluate all vascular and drainage tubes for location and patency, and connect them to appropriate monitoring or suction devices. Note the amount, color, consistency, and odor of drainage secretions. Verify the appropriate functioning of all equipment attached to the patient and label as required. While connecting the monitoring and care equipment, it is important for the nurse to continue assessing the patient's respiratory and cardiovascular status until it is clear

TABLE 1-4. COMMON DIAGNOSTIC TESTS OBTAINED DURING ARRIVAL QUICK CHECK ASSESSMENT

Serum electrolytes
Glucose
Complete blood count with platelets
Coagulation studies
Chest x-ray
ECG

that all equipment are functioning appropriately and can be relied on to transmit accurate patient data.

The arrival quick check assessment is accomplished in a matter of a few minutes. After completion of the ABCDEs assessment, the comprehensive assessment begins. If at any phase during the arrival quick check a component of the ABCDEs has not been stabilized and controlled, energy is focused first on resolving the abnormality before proceeding to the comprehensive admission assessment.

After the arrival, quick check assessment is complete, and if the patient requires no urgent intervention, there may now be time for a more thorough report from the healthcare providers transferring the patient to the progressive care unit. It is important to note that handoffs with transitions of care are possible intervals when safety gaps may occur. Omission of pertinent information or miscommunication at this critical juncture can result in patient care errors. Use of a standardized handoff format—such as the "SBAR" format which includes communication of the **S**ituation, **B**ackground, **A**ssessment, and **R**ecommendations—can minimize the potential for miscommunication. Use the handoff as an opportunity to confirm your observations such as dosage of infusing medications, abnormalities found on the quick check assessment, and any potential inconsistencies noted between your assessment and the prearrival report. It is easier to clarify questions while the transporters are still present, if possible.

This may also be an opportunity for introductory interactions with family members or friends, if present. Introduce yourself, offer reassurance, and confirm the intention to give the patient the best care possible (Table 1-5). If feasible, allow them to stay with the patient in the room during the arrival process. If this is not possible, give them an approximate time frame when they can expect to receive an update from you on the patient's condition. Have another member of the healthcare team escort them to the appropriate waiting area.

COMPREHENSIVE INITIAL ASSESSMENT

Comprehensive assessments determine the physiologic and psychosocial baseline so that future changes can be compared to determine whether the status is improving or deteriorating.

TABLE 1-5.   EVIDENCE-BASED PRACTICE: FAMILY NEEDS ASSESSMENT

Quick Assessment
- Offer realistic hope
- Give honest answers and information
- Give reassurance

Comprehensive Assessment
- Use open-ended communication and assess their communication style
- Assess family members' level of anxiety
- Assess perceptions of the situation (knowledge, comprehension, expectations of staff, expected outcome)
- Assess family roles and dynamics (cultural and religious practices, values, spokesperson)
- Assess coping mechanisms and resources (what do they use, social network and support)

The comprehensive assessment also defines the patient's pre-event health status, determining problems or limitations that may impact patient status during this admission as well as potential issues for future transitioning of care. The content presented in this section is a template to screen for abnormalities or determine the extent of injury or disease. Any abnormal findings or changes from baseline warrant a more in-depth evaluation of the pertinent system.

The comprehensive assessment includes the patient's medical and brief social history, and physical examination of each body system. The comprehensive assessment of the progressive care patient is similar to admission assessments for medical-surgical patients. This section describes only those aspects of the assessment that are unique to progressive care patients or require more extensive information than is obtained from a medical-surgical patient. The entire assessment process is summarized in Tables 1-6 and 1-7.

Changing demographics of progressive care units indicate that an increasing proportion of patients are elderly,

TABLE 1-6.   SUMMARY OF COMPREHENSIVE INITIAL ASSESSMENT REQUIREMENTS

Past Medical History
- Medical conditions, surgical procedures
- Psychiatric/emotional problems
- Hospitalizations
- Medications (prescription, over-the-counter, illicit drugs) and time of last medication dose
- Allergies
- Review of body systems (see Table 1-7)

Social History
- Age, gender
- Ethnic origin
- Height, weight
- Highest educational level completed
- Occupation
- Marital status
- Primary family members/significant others/decision makers
- Religious affiliation
- Advance Directive and Durable Power of Attorney for Health Care
- Substance use (alcohol, drugs, caffeine, tobacco)
- Domestic Abuse or Vulnerable Adult Screen

Psychosocial Assessment
- General communication
- Coping styles
- Anxiety and stress
- Expectations of progressive care unit
- Current stresses
- Family needs

Spirituality
- Faith/spiritual preference
- Healing practices

Physical Assessment
- Nervous system
- Cardiovascular system
- Respiratory system
- Renal system
- Gastrointestinal system
- Endocrine, hematologic, and immune systems
- Integumentary system

TABLE 1-7. SUGGESTED QUESTIONS FOR REVIEW OF PAST HISTORY CATEGORIZED BY BODY SYSTEM

Body System	History Questions
Nervous	• Have you ever had a seizure? • Have you ever fainted, blacked out, or had delirium tremens (DTs)? • Do you ever have numbness, tingling, or weakness in any part of your body? • Do you have any difficulty with your hearing, vision, or speech? • Has your daily activity level changed due to your present condition? • Do you require any assistive devices such as canes?
Cardiovascular	• Have you experienced any heart problems or disease such as heart attacks or strokes? • Do you have any problems with extreme fatigue? • Do you have an irregular heart rhythm? • Do you have high blood pressure? • Do you have a pacemaker or an implanted defibrillator?
Respiratory	• Do you ever experience shortness of breath? • Do you have any pain associated with breathing? • Do you have a persistent cough? Is it productive? • Have you had any exposure to environmental agents that might affect the lungs? • Do you have sleep apnea?
Renal	• Have you had any change in frequency of urination? • Do you have any burning, pain, discharge, or difficulty when you urinate? • Have you had blood in your urine?
Gastrointestinal	• Has there been any recent weight loss or gain? • Have you had any change in appetite? • Do you have any problems with nausea or vomiting? • How often do you have a bowel movement and has there been a change in the normal pattern? Do you have blood in your stools? • Do you have dentures? • Do you have any food allergies?
Integumentary	• Do you have any problems with your skin?
Endocrine	• Do you have any problems with bleeding?
Hematologic	• Do you have problems with chronic infections?
Immunologic	• Have you recently been exposed to a contagious illness?
Psychosocial	• Do you have any physical conditions, which make communication difficult (hearing loss, visual disturbances, language barriers, etc)? • How do you best learn? Do you need information repeated several times and/or require information in advance of teaching sessions? • What are the ways you cope with stress, crises, or pain? • Who are the important people in your family or network? • Who do you want to make decisions with you, or for you? • Have you had any previous experiences with acute illness? • Have you ever been abused? • Have you ever experienced trouble with anxiety, irritability, being confused, mood swings, or suicidal attempts? • What are the cultural practices, religious influences, and values that are important to you or your family? • What are family members' perceptions and expectations of the progressive care staff and the setting?
Spiritual	• What is your faith or spiritual preference? • What practices help you heal or deal with stress? • Would you like to see a chaplain, priest, or other spiritual guide?

requiring assessments to incorporate the effects of aging. Although assessment of the aging adult does not differ significantly from the younger adult, understanding how aging alters the physiologic and psychological status of the patient is important. Key physiologic changes pertinent to the progressive care elderly adult are summarized in Table 1-8. Additional emphasis must also be placed on the past medical history because the aging adult frequently has multiple coexisting illnesses and is taking several prescriptive and over-the-counter medications. Social history must address issues related to home environment, support systems, and self-care abilities. The interpretation of clinical findings in the elderly must also take into consideration the fact that the coexistence of several disease processes and the diminished reserves of most body systems often result in more rapid physiologic deterioration than in younger adults.

Past Medical History

If the patient is being directly admitted to the progressive care unit, it is important to determine prior medical and surgical conditions, hospitalization, medications, and symptoms besides the primary event that brought the patient to the hospital (see Table 1-7). In reviewing medication use, ensure assessment of over-the-counter medication use as well as any herbal or alternative supplements. For every positive symptom response, additional questions should be asked to explore the characteristics of that symptom (Table 1-9). If the patient is a transfer from another area in the hospital, review the admission assessment information, and clarify as needed with the patient and family. Be aware of opportunities for health teaching and transition planning needs for discharge to home or to a rehabilitation facility.

Social History

Inquire about the use and abuse of caffeine, alcohol, tobacco, and other substances. Because the use of these agents can have major implications for the progressive care patient, questions are aimed at determining the frequency, amount, and duration of use. Honest information regarding alcohol and substance abuse, however, may not be always forthcoming. Alcohol use is common in all age groups. Phrasing questions about alcohol use by acknowledging this fact may be helpful in obtaining an accurate answer (eg, "How much alcohol do you drink?" vs "Do you drink alcohol and how much?"). Family or friends might provide additional information that might assist in assessing these parameters. The information revealed during the social history can often be verified during the physical assessment through the presence of signs such as needle track marks, nicotine stains on teeth and fingers, or the smell of alcohol on the breath.

Patients should also be asked about physical and emotional safety in their home environment in order to uncover potential domestic or elder abuse. It is best if patients can be assessed for vulnerability when they are alone to prevent placing them in a position of answering in front of family

TABLE 1-8. PHYSIOLOGIC EFFECTS OF AGING

Body System	Effects
Nervous	Diminished hearing and vision, short-term memory loss, altered motor coordination, decreased muscle tone and strength, slower response to verbal and motor stimuli, decreased ability to synthesize new information, increased sensitivity to altered temperature states, increased sensitivity to sedation (confusion or agitation), decreased alertness levels
Cardiovascular	Increased effects of atherosclerosis of vessels and heart valves, decreased stroke volume with resulting decreased cardiac output, decreased myocardial compliance, increased workload of heart, diminished peripheral pulses
Respiratory	Decreased compliance and elasticity, decreased vital capacity, increased residual volume, less effective cough, decreased response to hypercapnia
Renal	Decreased glomerular filtration rate, increased risk of fluid and electrolyte imbalances
Gastrointestinal	Increased presence of dentition problems, decreased intestinal mobility, decreased hepatic metabolism, increased risk of altered nutritional states
Endocrine, hematologic, and immunologic	Increased incidence of diabetes, thyroid disorders, and anemia; decreased antibody response and cellular immunity
Integumentary	Decreased skin turgor, increased capillary fragility and bruising, decreased elasticity
Miscellaneous	Altered pharmacokinetics and pharmacodynamics, decreased range of motion of joints and extremities
Psychosocial	Difficulty falling asleep and fragmented sleep patterns, increased incidence of depression and anxiety, cognitive impairment disorders, difficulty with change

members or friends who may be abusive. Ask questions such as "Is anyone hurting you?" or "Do you feel safe at home?" in a non-threatening manner. Any suspicion of abuse or vulnerability should result in a consultation with social work to determine additional assessments.

Physical Assessment by Body System

The physical assessment section is presented in the sequence in which the combined system, head-to-toe approach, is followed. Although content is presented as separate components, generally the history questions are integrated into the physical assessment. The physical assessment section uses the techniques of inspection, auscultation, and palpation. Although percussion is a common technique in physical examinations, it is infrequently used in progressive care patients.

Pain assessment is generally linked to each body system rather than considered as a separate system category; for example, if the patient has chest pain, assessment and

TABLE 1-9. IDENTIFICATION OF SYMPTOM CHARACTERISTICS

Characteristic	Sample Questions
Onset	How and under what circumstances did it begin? Was the onset sudden or gradual? Did it progress?
Location	Where is it? Does it stay in the same place or does it radiate or move around?
Frequency	How often does it occur?
Quality	Is it dull, sharp, burning, throbbing, and so on?
Intensity	Rank pain on a scale (numeric, word description, FACES, FLACC)
Quantity	How long does it last?
Setting	What are you doing when it happens?
Associated findings	Are there other signs and symptoms that occur when this happens?
Aggravating and Alleviating factors	What things make it worse? What things make it better?

documentation of that pain is incorporated into the cardiovascular assessment. Rather than have general pain assessment questions repeated under each system assessment, they are presented here.

Pain and discomfort are clues that alert both the patient and the progressive care nurse that something is wrong and needs prompt attention. Pain assessment includes differentiating acute from chronic pain, determining related physiologic symptoms, and investigating the patient's perceptions and emotional reactions to the pain. Explore the qualities and characteristics of the pain by using the questions listed in Table 1-9. Pain is a subjective assessment, and progressive care practitioners sometimes struggle with applying their own values when attempting to evaluate the patient's pain. To resolve this dilemma, use the patient's own words and descriptions of the pain whenever possible and use a patient-preferred pain scale (see Chapter 6, Pain and Sedation Management) to evaluate pain levels objectively and consistently.

Nervous System

The nervous system is the master computer of all systems and is divided into the central and peripheral nervous systems. With the exception of the peripheral nervous system's cranial nerves, almost all attention in the acutely ill patient is focused on evaluating the central nervous system (CNS). The physiologic and psychological impact of an acute illness, in addition to pharmacologic interventions, frequently alters CNS functioning. The single most important indicator of cerebral functioning is the LOC.

Assess pupils for size, shape, symmetry, and reactivity to direct light. When interpreting the implication of altered pupil size, remember that certain medications such as atropine, morphine, or illicit drugs may affect pupil size. Baseline pupil assessment is important even in patients without a neurologic diagnosis because some individuals have unequal or unreactive pupils normally. If pupils are not checked as a baseline, a later check of pupils during an acute event could inappropriately attribute pupil abnormalities to a pathophysiologic event.

Level of consciousness and pupil assessment are followed by motor function assessment of the upper and lower extremities for symmetry and quality of strength. Traditional motor strength exercises include having the patient squeeze the nurse's hands and plantar flexing and dorsiflexing of the patient's feet. If the patient cannot follow commands, an estimate of strength and quality of movements can be inferred by observing activities such as pulling against restraints or thrashing around. If the patient has no voluntary movement or is unresponsive, check the gag reflex.

If head trauma is involved or suspected, check for signs of fluid leakage around the nose or ears, differentiating between cerebral spinal fluid and blood (see Chapter 12, Neurologic System). Complete cranial nerve assessment is rarely warranted, with specific cranial nerve evaluation based on the injury or diagnosis; for example, extraocular movements are routinely assessed in patients with facial trauma. Sensory testing is a baseline standard for spinal cord injuries, extremity trauma, and epidural analgesia.

Now, it is a good time to assess mental status if the patient is responsive. Assess orientation to person, place, and time. Ask the patient to state their understanding of what is happening. As you ask the questions, observe for eye contact, pressured or muted speech, and rate of speech. Rate of speech is usually consistent with the patient's psychomotor status. Underlying cognitive impairments such as dementia and developmental delays are typically exacerbated during an acute illness due to physiologic changes, medications, and environmental changes. It may be necessary to ascertain baseline level of functioning from the family.

It is also important to assess patients for the risk of a fall. With the goal of increasing the mobility and independence of progressive care patients, it is imperative that the nurse understand the fall risk for each individual patient and implement interventions to minimize the potential for a fall.

Laboratory data pertinent to the nervous system include serum and urine electrolytes and osmolarity and urinary specific gravity. Drug toxicology and alcohol levels may be evaluated to rule out potential sources of altered LOC.

Cardiovascular System

The cardiovascular system assessment is directed at evaluating central and peripheral perfusion. Revalidate your admission quick check assessment of the blood pressure, heart rate, and rhythm. If the patient is being monitored, assess the ECG for T-wave abnormalities and ST-segment changes and determine the PR, QRS, and QT intervals and the QTc measurements. Note any abnormalities or indications of myocardial damage, electrical conduction problems, and electrolyte imbalances. Note the pulse pressure. If treatment decisions will be based on the cuff pressure, blood pressure is taken in both arms. If an arterial pressure line is in place, compare the arterial line pressure to the cuff pressure. In either case,

TABLE 1-10. EDEMA RATING SCALE

Following the application and removal of firm digital pressure against the tissue, the edema is evaluated for one of the following responses:
- 0   No depression in tissue
- +1 Small depression in tissue, disappearing in < 1 second
- +2 Depression in tissue disappears in < 1-2 seconds
- +3 Depression in tissue disappears in < 2-3 seconds
- +4 Depression in tissue disappears in ≥ 4 seconds

if a 10- to 15-mm Hg difference exists, a decision must be made as to which pressure is the most accurate and will be followed for future treatment decisions. If a different method is used inconsistently, changes in blood pressure might be inappropriately attributed to physiologic changes rather than anatomic differences.

Note the color and temperature of the skin, with particular emphasis on lips, mucous membranes, and distal extremities. Also evaluate nail color and capillary refill. Inspect for the presence of edema, particularly in the dependent parts of the body such as feet, ankles, and sacrum. If edema is present, rate the quality of edema by using a 0 to +4 scale (Table 1-10).

Auscultate heart sounds for S_1 and S_2 quality, intensity, and pitch, and for the presence of extra heart sounds, murmurs, clicks, or rubs. Listen to one sound at a time, consistently progressing through the key anatomic landmarks of the heart each time. Note whether there are any changes with respiration or patient position.

Palpate the peripheral pulses for amplitude and quality, using the 0 to +4 scale (Table 1-11). Check bilateral pulses simultaneously, except the carotid, comparing each pulse to its partner. If the pulse is difficult to palpate, an ultrasound (Doppler) device should be used. To facilitate finding a weak pulse for subsequent assessments, mark the location of the pulse with an indelible pen. It is also helpful to compare quality of the pulses to the ECG to evaluate the perfusion of heartbeats.

Electrolyte levels, complete blood counts (CBCs), coagulation studies, and lipid profiles are common laboratory tests evaluated for abnormalities of the cardiovascular system. Cardiac enzyme levels (troponin, creatine kinase MB, β-natriuretic peptide) are obtained for any complaint of chest pain or suspected chest trauma. Drug levels of commonly used cardiovascular medications, such as digoxin, may be warranted for certain types of arrhythmias. A 12-lead ECG may be evaluated, either due to the chief reason for admission (eg, with complaints of chest pain, irregular rhythms, or suspected myocardial bruising from trauma) or as a baseline for future comparison if needed.

TABLE 1-11. PERIPHERAL PULSE RATING SCALE

- 0   Absent pulse
- +1 Palpable but thready; easily obliterated with light pressure
- +2 Normal; cannot obliterate with light pressure
- +3 Full
- +4 Full and bounding

Note the type, size, and location of IV catheters, and verify their patency. If continuous infusions of medications such as antiarrhythmics are being administered, ensure that they are being infused into an appropriately sized vessel and are compatible with any piggybacked IV solution.

Verify all monitoring system alarm parameters as active with appropriate limits set. Note the size and location of invasive monitoring lines such as arterial and central venous catheters. Confirm that the appropriate flush solution is hanging and that the correct amount of pressure is applied to the flush solution bag. Level the invasive line to the appropriate anatomic landmark and zero the monitor as needed. Interpret hemodynamic pressure readings against normals and with respect to the patient's underlying pathophysiology. Assess waveforms to determine the quality of the waveform (eg, dampened or hyperresonant) and whether the waveform appropriately matches the expected characteristics for the anatomic placement of the invasive catheter (see Chapter 4, Hemodynamic Monitoring); for example, a right ventricular waveform for a CVP line indicates a problem with the position of the central venous line that needs to be corrected. Evaluate all cardiovascular devices that are in place as feasible, such as a pacemaker, or any ventricular assist device. Verify and document equipment settings, appropriate function of the device, and the patient response to that device function.

Respiratory System

Oxygenation and ventilation are the focal basis of respiratory assessment parameters. Reassess the rate and rhythm of respirations and the symmetry of chest wall movement. If the patient has a productive cough or secretions are suctioned from an artificial airway, note the color, consistency, and amount of secretions. Evaluate whether the trachea is midline or shifted. Inspect the thoracic cavity for shape, anterior-posterior diameter, and structural deformities (eg, kyphosis or scoliosis). Palpate for equal chest excursion, presence of crepitus, and any areas of tenderness or fractures. If the patient is receiving supplemental oxygen, verify the mode of delivery and percentage of oxygen against physician orders.

Auscultate all lobes anteriorly and posteriorly for bilateral breath sounds to determine the presence of air movement and the presence of adventitious sounds such as crackles or wheezes. Note the quality and depth of respirations, and the length and pitch of the inspiratory and expiratory phases.

Arterial blood gases (ABGs) may be used to assess for interpretation of oxygenation, ventilatory status, and acid-base balance. Hemoglobin and hematocrit values are interpreted for impact on oxygenation and fluid balance. If the patient's condition warrants, the oxygen saturation values may be continuously monitored.

If the patient is connected to a mechanical ventilator, verify the ventilatory mode, tidal volume, respiratory rate, positive end expiratory pressure, and percentage of oxygen against prescribed settings. Observe whether the patient has spontaneous breaths, noting both the rate and average tidal volume of each breath. Note the amount of pressure required to ventilate the patient for later comparisons to determine changes in pulmonary compliance. If the patient has a tracheostomy, note the size and type of tube in place and the location to assist future comparisons for proper placement. If the patient is on biphasic positive airway pressure (BiPAP), note and verify the pressure settings against ordered parameters. Also assess the patient's tolerance to the full face or nasal mask. Patients frequently exhibit anxiety with BiPAP and have difficulty tolerating the feeling of the mask.

If chest tubes are present, assess the area around the insertion site for crepitus. Note the amount and color of drainage and whether an air leak is present. Verify whether the chest tube drainage system is an underwater seal or is connected to suction.

Renal System

Urinary characteristics and electrolyte status are the major parameters used to evaluate the function of the kidneys. In conjunction with the cardiovascular system, the renal system's impact on fluid volume status is also assessed.

Some progressive care patients have a Foley catheter in place to initially evaluate urinary output every 2 to 4 hours. Note the amount and color of the urine and, if warranted, obtain a sample to assess for the abnormal presence of glucose, protein, and blood. Inspect the genitalia for inflammation, swelling, ulcers, and drainage. If suprapubic tubes or a ureterostomy are present, note the position as well as the amount and characteristics of the drainage. Observe whether any drainage is leaking around the drainage tube.

In addition to the urinalysis, serum electrolyte levels, blood urea nitrogen, creatinine, and urinary and serum osmolarity are common diagnostic tests used to evaluate kidney function.

Gastrointestinal System

The key factors when reviewing the gastrointestinal system are the nutritional and fluid status. Inspect the abdomen for overall symmetry, noting whether the contour is flat, round, protuberant, or distended. Note the presence of discoloration or striae. Nutritional status is evaluated by looking at the patient's weight and muscle tone, the condition of the oral mucosa, and laboratory values such as serum albumin and transferrin.

Auscultation of bowel sounds should be done in all four quadrants in a clockwise order, noting the frequency and presence or absence of sounds. Bowel sounds are usually rated as absent, hypoactive, normal, or hyperactive. Before noting absent bowel sounds, a quadrant should be listened to for at least 60 to 90 seconds. Characteristics and frequency of the sounds are noted. After listening for the presence of normal sounds, determine whether any adventitious bowel sounds such as friction rubs, bruits, or hums are present.

Light palpation of the abdomen helps determine areas of fluid, rigidity, tenderness, pain, and guarding or rebound tenderness. Remember to auscultate before palpating because palpation may change the frequency and character of the patient's peristaltic sounds.

Assess any drainage tube for location and function, and for the characteristics of any drainage. Validate the proper placement of the nasogastric (NG) tube. Ensure patency of any feeding tube or percutaneously placed gastric tubes. Check placement and assess for any drainage or leaking around the tubes. Check emesis and stool for occult blood as appropriate. Evaluate ostomies for location, color of the stoma, and the type of drainage.

Endocrine, Hematologic, and Immune Systems

The endocrine, hematologic, and immune systems often are overlooked when assessing progressive care patients. The assessment parameters used to evaluate these systems are included under other system assessments, but it is important to consider these systems consciously when reviewing these parameters. Assessing the endocrine, hematologic, and immune systems is based on a thorough understanding of the primary function of each of the hormones, blood cells, or immune components of each of the respective systems.

Assessing the specific functions of the endocrine system's hormones is challenging because much of the symptomatology related to the hypo- or hypersecretion of the hormones can be found with other systems' problems. The patient's history may help differentiate the source, but any abnormal assessment findings detected with regard to fluid balance, metabolic rate, altered LOC, color and temperature of the skin, electrolytes, glucose, and acid-base balance require the progressive care nurse to consider the potential involvement of the endocrine system; for example, are the signs and symptoms of hypervolemia related to cardiac insufficiency or excessive amounts of antidiuretic hormone? Serum blood tests for specific hormone levels may be required to rule out involvement of the endocrine system.

Assessment parameters specific to the hematologic system include laboratory evaluation of the red blood cells (RBCs) and coagulation studies. Diminished RBCs may affect the oxygen-carrying capacity of the blood as evidenced by pallor, cyanosis, light-headedness, tachypnea, and tachycardia. Insufficient clotting factors are evidenced by bruising, oozing of blood from puncture sites or mucous membranes, or overt bleeding.

The immune system's primary function of fighting infection is assessed by evaluating the white cell and differential counts from the CBC, and assessing puncture sites and mucous membranes for oozing drainage and inflamed, reddened areas. Spiking or persistent low-grade temperatures often are indicative of underlying infections. It is important to keep in mind, however, that many progressive care patients have impaired immune systems and the normal response to infection, such as white pus around an insertion site or elevated temperature and WBC, may not be evident.

Integumentary System

The skin is the first line of defense against infection so assessment parameters are focused on evaluating the intactness of the skin. Assessing the skin can be undertaken while performing other system assessments; for example, while listening to breath sounds or bowel sounds, the condition of the thoracic cavity or abdominal skin can be observed, respectively. It is important that a thorough head to toe, anterior, posterior, and between skin folds assessment is performed on admission to the progressive care unit to identify any pre-existing skin issues that need to be immediately addressed as well as to establish a baseline skin assessment.

Inspect the skin for overall integrity, color, temperature, and turgor. Note the presence of rashes, striae, discoloration, scars, or lesions. For any abrasions, lesions, pressure ulcers, or wounds, note the size, depth, and presence or absence of drainage. Consider use of a skin integrity risk assessment tool to determine immediate interventions that may be needed to prevent further skin integrity breakdown.

Psychosocial Assessment

The rapid physiologic and psychological changes associated with acute illnesses, coupled with pharmacologic and biological treatments, can profoundly affect behavior. Patients may suffer from illnesses that have psychological responses that are predictable, and, if untreated, may threaten recovery or life. To avoid making assumptions about how a patient feels about his or her care, there is no substitute for asking the patient directly or asking a collateral informant, such as the family or significant other.

General Communication

Factors that affect communication include culture, developmental stage, physical condition, stress, perception, neurocognitive deficits, emotional state, and language skills. The nature of an acute illness coupled with pharmacologic and airway technologies can interfere with patients' usual methods of communication. It is essential to determine pre-illness communication abilities as well as methods and styles to ensure optimal communication with the progressive care patient and family. The inability of some progressive care patients to communicate verbally necessitates that progressive care practitioners become expert at assessing nonverbal clues to determine important information from, and needs of, patients. Important assessment data are gained by observation of body gestures, facial expressions, eye movements, involuntary movements, and changes in physiologic parameters, particularly heart rate, blood pressure, and respiratory rate. Often, these nonverbal behaviors may be more reflective of patients' actual feelings, particularly if they are denying symptoms and attempting to be the "good patient" by not complaining.

Anxiety and Stress

Anxiety is both psychologically and physiologically exhausting. Being in a prolonged state of arousal is hard work and uses adaptive reserves needed for recovery. The progressive care environment can be stressful, full of constant auditory and tactile stimuli, and may contribute to a patient's anxiety level. The progressive care setting may force isolation from social supports, dependency, loss of control, trust in unknown care providers, helplessness, and an inability to solve problems. Restlessness, distractibility, hyperventilation, and unrealistic demands for attention are warning signs of escalating anxiety.

Medications such as interferon, corticosteroids, angiotensin-converting enzyme inhibitors, and vasopressors can induce anxiety. Abrupt withdrawal from benzodiazepines, caffeine, nicotine, and narcotics as well as akathisia from phenothiazines may mimic anxiety. Additional etiologic variables associated with anxiety include pain, sleep loss, delirium, hypoxia, ventilator synchronization or weaning, fear of death, loss of control, high-technology equipment, and a dehumanizing setting. Admission to or repeated transfers to the progressive care unit may also induce anxiety.

Coping Styles

Individuals cope with an acute illness in different ways and their pre-illness coping style, personality traits, or temperament will assist you in anticipating coping styles in the progressive care setting. Include the patient's family when assessing previous resources, coping skills, or defense mechanisms that strengthen adaptation or problem-solving resolution. For instance, some patients want to be informed of everything that is happening with them in the progressive care unit. Providing information reduces their anxiety and gives them a sense of control. Other patients prefer to have others receive information about them and make decisions for them. Giving them detailed information only exacerbates their level of anxiety and diminishes their ability to cope. It is most important to understand the meaning assigned to the event by the patient and family and the purpose the coping defense serves. Does the coping resource fit with the event and meet the patient's and family's need?

This may also be the time to conduct a brief assessment of the spiritual beliefs and needs of the patient and how those assist them in their coping. Minimally, patients should be asked if they have a faith or spiritual preference and wish to see a chaplain, priest, or other spiritual guide. However, patients should also be asked about spiritual and cultural healing practices that are important to them to determine whether those can possibly be maintained during their progressive care unit stay.

Patients express their coping styles in a variety of ways. Persons who are stoic by personality or culture usually present as the good patient. Assess for behaviors of not wanting to bother the busy staff or not admitting pain because family or others are nearby. Some patients express their anxiety and stress through manipulative behavior. Progressive care nurses must understand that patients' and families' impulsivity, deception, low tolerance for frustration, unreliability, superficial charm, splitting among the provider team, and general avoidance of rules or limits are modes of interacting and coping and attempts to feel safe. Still other patients may withdraw and actually request use of sedatives and sleeping medications to blunt the stimuli and stress of the environment.

Fear has an identifiable source and an important role in the ability of the patient to cope. Treatments, procedures, pain, and separation are common objects of fear. The dying process elicits specific fears, such as fear of the unknown, loneliness, loss of body, loss of self-control, suffering, pain, loss of identity, and loss of everyone loved by the patient. The family, as well as the patient, experiences the grieving process, which includes the phases of denial, shock, anger, bargaining, depression, and acceptance.

Family Needs

The concept of family is not simple today and extends beyond the nuclear family to any loving, supportive person regardless of social and legal boundaries. Ideally the patient should be asked who they identify as family, who should receive information about patient status, and who should make decisions for the patient if he or she becomes unable to make decisions for self. This may also be an opportune time to ask whether they have an advance directive, a physician order for life sustaining treatment (POLST) on file, or if they have discussed their wishes with any family members or friends. Progressive care practitioners need to be flexible around traditional legal boundaries of next of kin so that communication is extended to, and sought from, surrogate decision makers and whomever the patient designates.

Families can have a positive impact on the patient's ability to cope with and recover from an acute illness. Each family system is unique and varies by culture, values, religion, previous experience with crisis, socioeconomic status, psychological integrity, role expectations, communication patterns, health beliefs, and ages. It is important to assess the family's needs and resources to develop interventions that will optimize family impact on the patient and their interactions with the healthcare team. Areas for family needs assessments are outlined in Table 1-5.

Unit Orientation

The progressive care nurse must take the time to educate the patient (if alert) and family about the specialized progressive care unit environment. This orientation should include a simple explanation of the equipment being used in the care of the patient, visitation policies, the routines of the unit, and how the patient can communicate needs to the unit staff. Additionally, the family should be given the unit telephone number and the names of the nurse manager as well as the nurse caring for the patient in case problems or concerns arise during the progressive care unit stay.

Referrals

After completing the comprehensive assessment, analyze the information gathered for the need to make referrals to other healthcare providers and resources (Table 1-12). With length of stay and appropriate resource management a continual challenge, it is important to start referrals as soon as possible

TABLE 1-12. EXAMPLES OF POTENTIAL REFERRALS NEEDED FOR PROGRESSIVE CARE PATIENTS

Referral	Resources Needed
Social work	• Financial needs/resources for patient and/or family • Coping resources for patient and/or family
Nutrition	• Nutritional status at risk and in need of in-depth nutritional assessment • Altered nutritional status on admission
Therapies	• Physical therapy for maintaining or improving physical flexibility and strength • Occupational therapy for assistive devices • Speech therapy for assessment of ability to swallow or communication needs
Pastoral care	• Spiritual guidance for patient and/or family • Coping resources for patient and/or family
Enterostomal nursing	• Stoma assessment and needs • In-depth skin integrity needs
Ethics committee	• Decisions involving significant ethical complexity • Decisions involving disagreements over care between care providers or between care providers and patient/family
Care coordinator	• Anticipate transition needs throughout and post hospitalization

to maintain continuity of care and avoid worsening decline of status. Assess whether any ancillary service referrals may have already been initiated in the ICU or medical-surgical unit and ensure those services are aware of the transfer in order to avoid any gaps in coverage.

Transition/Discharge Planning

It is important that transition and/or discharge planning starts on arrival of the patient to the progressive care unit. Length of stays continues to decrease for patients in progressive care, creating a challenge for progressive care nurses to assess the appropriate transition location for the progressive care patient adequately. Educational and logistical processes need to be put into place in a timely manner so as to avoid any delays in patient progress and recovery. This necessitates early and active involvement by all appropriate healthcare team members to ensure smooth transitioning.

ONGOING ASSESSMENT

After the arrival quick check and comprehensive assessments are completed, all subsequent assessments are used to determine trends, evaluate response to therapy, and identify new potential problems or changes from the comprehensive baseline assessment. Ongoing assessments become more focused, and the frequency is driven by the stability of the patient; however, routine periodic assessments are the norm; for example, ongoing assessments can occur every 1 to 2 hours for patients who are exhibiting changes in physiological status to every 2 to 4 hours for stable patients. Additional assessments should be made when any of the following situations occur:

- When caregivers change
- Before and after any major procedural intervention, such as chest tube insertion
- Before and after transport out of the progressive care unit for diagnostic procedures or other events
- Deterioration in physiologic or mental status
- Initiation of any new therapy

As with the arrival quick check, the ongoing assessment section is offered as a generic template that can be used as a basis for all patients (Table 1-13). More in-depth

TABLE 1-13. ONGOING ASSESSMENT TEMPLATE

Body System	Assessment Parameters
Nervous	• LOC • Pupils • Motor strength of extremities
Cardiovascular	• Blood pressure • Heart rate and rhythm • Heart sounds • Capillary refill • Peripheral pulses • Patency of IVs • Verification of IV solutions and medications • Hemodynamic pressures and waveforms
Respiratory	• Respiratory rate and rhythm • Breath sounds • Color and amount of secretions • Noninvasive technology information (eg, pulse oximetry) • Mechanical ventilatory parameters • Arterial and venous blood gases
Renal	• Intake and output • Color and amount of urinary output • BUN/creatinine values
Gastrointestinal	• Bowel sounds • Contour of abdomen • Position of drainage tubes • Color and amount of secretions • Bilirubin and albumin values
Endocrine, hematologic, and immunologic	• Fluid balance • Electrolyte and glucose values • CBC and coagulation values • Temperature • WBC with differential count
Integumentary	• Color and temperature of skin • Intactness of skin • Areas of redness
Pain/discomfort	• Assessed in each system • Response to interventions
Psychosocial	• Mental status and behavioral responses • Reaction to acute illness experience (eg, stress, anxiety, coping, mood) • Presence of cognitive impairments (dementia, delirium), depression, or demoralization • Family functioning and needs • Ability to communicate needs and participate in care • Sleep patterns

and system-specific assessment parameters are added based on the patient's diagnosis and pathophysiologic problems.

SELECTED BIBLIOGRAPHY

Progressive Care Assessment

American Association of Critical-Care Nurses. *Core Curriculum for Progressive Care Nursing.* St. Louis, MO: Elsevier Saunders; 2010.

American Association of Critical-Care Nurses Progressive Care Task Force. Progressive care fact sheet. 2009. Available at www.aacn.org/WD/Practice/Docs/ProgressiveCareFactSheet.pdf. Accessed February 15, 2013.

Bickley LS, Szilagyi PG. Bates' Guide to Physical Examination and History Taking. 11th ed. Philadelphia, PA: Lippincott Williams & Wilkins; 2013.

Gorman LM, Sultan DF. Psychosocial Nursing for General Patient Care, 3rd ed. Philadelphia, PA: FA Davis Co; 2008.

Stacy KM. Progressive care units: different but the same. *Crit Care Nurs.* 2011;31(3):77-83.

Evidence-Based Practice

American Association of Critical-Care Nurses. *Protocols for Practice: Creating a Healing Environment.* 2nd ed. Aliso Viejo, CA: AACN; 2007.

American College of Critical Care Medicine. Guidelines on admission and discharge for adult intermediate care units. *Crit Care Med.* 1998;26(3):607-610.

Gephart SM. The art of effective handoffs. What is the evidence? *Adv Neonatal Care.* 2012;12(1):37-39.

Hilligoss B, Cohen MD. The unappreciated challenges of between-unit handoffs: negotiating and coordinating across boundaries. *Ann Emerg Med.* 2013;61(1):15-160.

Maxwell KE, Stuenkel D, Saylor C. Needs of family members of critically ill patients: a comparison of nurse and family perceptions. *Heart Lung.* 2007;36(5):367-376.

Murphy TH, Labonte P, Klock M, Houser L. Falls prevention for elders in acute care: an evidence-based nursing practice initiative. *Crit Care Nurs Q.* 2008;31(1):33-39.

Sendelbach S, Guthrie PF, Schoenfelder DP. Acute confusion/delirium. Identification, assessment, treatment, and prevention. *J Gerontol Nurs.* 2009;35(11):11-18.

Staggers N, Blaz JW. Research on nursing handoffs for medical and surgical settings: an integrative review. *J Adv Nurs.* 2013;69(2):247-262.

Tescher AN, Branda ME, OByrne TJ, Naessens JM. All at-risk patients are not created equal. Analysis of Braden pressure ulcer risk scores to identify specific risks. *J Wound Ostomy Continence Nurs.* 2012;39(3):282-291.

Verhaeghe S, Defloor T, Van Zuuren F, Duijnstee M, Grypdonck M. The needs and experiences of family members of adult patients in an intensive care unit: a review of the literature. *J Clin Nurs.* 2005;14:501-509.

Planning Care for Progressive Care Patients and Their Families

Mary Fran Tracy

KNOWLEDGE COMPETENCIES

1. Discuss the importance of a multidisciplinary plan of care for optimizing clinical outcomes.

2. Describe interventions for prevention of common complications in progressive care patients:
   - Deep venous thrombosis
   - Infection
   - Sleep pattern disturbances
   - Skin breakdown

3. Discuss interventions to maintain psychosocial integrity and minimize anxiety for the progressive care patient and family members.

4. Describe interventions to promote family-focused care, and patient and family education.

5. Identify necessary equipment and personnel required to safely transport the progressive care patient within the hospital.

6. Describe transfer-related complications and preventive measures to be taken before and during patient transport.

It is important to be mindful of the unique needs of patients and their families as they transition from the intensive care or medical-surgical environment to a progressive care environment. Because lengths of stay in progressive care are typically short, preparation for the next anticipated level of care is initiated on arrival to the progressive care unit. Patient and family education is key to preparing for transitioning or potential discharge to home. While it is difficult to ensure all education is done during this short length of stay (LOS), it is important to evaluate educational needs and start a good knowledge foundation. It is also important to recognize anxiety that the patient may experience due to the change of level of care. If the patient is transferring from critical care to progressive care, the patient and family may feel nervous at the perceived decrease in level of nursing vigilance and technology. This can create questions on the part of the patient and family as to whether staff will be available to respond quickly to patient needs and changes in condition. Conversely, if a patient is transferred to the progressive care unit from a medical-surgical area because of declining physiologic status,

anxiety on the part of the patient and family is related to the uncertainty of the patient condition. In either case, it is important to reassure the patient and family that the progressive care nurses have the skills and equipment needed to monitor and meet the needs of the patient.

The achievement of optimal clinical outcomes in the progressive care patient requires a coordinated approach to care delivery by multidisciplinary team members. Experts in nutrition, respiratory therapy, progressive care nursing and medicine, psychiatry, and social work, as well as other disciplines, must work collaboratively to effectively and efficiently provide optimal care.

The use of a multidisciplinary plan of care is a useful approach to facilitate the coordination of a patient's care by the multidisciplinary team and optimize clinical outcomes. These multidisciplinary plans of care are increasingly being used to replace individual, discipline-specific plans of care. Each clinical condition presented in this text discusses the management of patient needs or problems with an integrated, multidisciplinary approach.

The following section provides an overview of multidisciplinary plans of care and their benefits. In addition, this chapter discusses common patient management approaches to needs or problems during acute illnesses that are not diagnosis specific, but common to a majority of progressive care patients, such as sleep deprivation, skin breakdown, and patient and family education. Additional discussion of these needs or problems is also presented in other chapters related to specific disease management.

MULTIDISCIPLINARY PLAN OF CARE

A multidisciplinary plan of care is a set of expectations for the major components of care a patient should receive during the hospitalization to manage a specific medical or surgical problem. Other types of plans include clinical pathways, interdisciplinary care plans, and care maps. The multidisciplinary plan of care expands the concept of a medical or nursing care plan and provides an interdisciplinary, comprehensive blueprint for patient care. The result is a diagnosis-specific plan of care that focuses the entire care team on expected patient outcomes.

The multidisciplinary plan of care outlines what tests, medications, care, and treatments are needed to discharge the patient in a timely manner with all patient outcomes met. Multidisciplinary plans of care have a variety of benefits to both patients and the hospital system:

- Improved patient outcomes (survival rates, morbidity)
- Increased quality and continuity of care
- Improved communication and collaboration
- Identification of hospital system problems
- Coordination of necessary services and reduced duplication
- Prioritization of activities
- Reduced LOS and healthcare costs

Multidisciplinary plans of care are developed by a team of individuals who closely interact with a specific patient population. It is this process of multiple disciplines communicating and collaborating around the needs of the patient that creates benefits for the patients. Representatives of disciplines commonly involved in pathway development include physicians, nurses, respiratory therapists, physical therapists, social workers, and dieticians. The format for the multidisciplinary plans of care typically includes the following categories:

- Discharge outcomes
- Patient goals (eg, pain control, activity level, absence of complications)
- Assessment and evaluation
- Consultations
- Tests
- Medications
- Nutrition
- Activity
- Education
- Discharge planning

The suggested activities within each of these categories may be divided into daily activities or grouped into phases of the hospitalization (eg, preoperative, intraoperative, and postoperative phases). All staff members who use the path require education as to the specifics of the pathway. This team approach in development and utilization optimizes communication, collaboration, coordination, and commitment to the pathway process.

With the increasing use of electronic health records, multidisciplinary plans of care or pathways are evolving into many different forms as institutions transition from paper to electronic formats. Some electronic formats mimic the paper version. Other institutions may incorporate pieces of the pathway into varied electronic flow sheets (eg, orders, assessments, interventions, education, outcomes, specific plans of care). Regardless of the specific format, multidisciplinary plans of care are used by a wide range of disciplines. Each individual who assesses and implements various aspects of the multidisciplinary plan of care is accountable for documenting that care in the approved format. Specific items of the pathway can then be evaluated and tracked to determine if the items are met, not met, or are not applicable. Items on the plan of care that are not completed typically are termed variances, which are deviations from the expected activities or goals outlined. Events outlined on the plans of care that occur early are termed positive variances. Negative variances are those planned events that are not accomplished on time. Negative variances typically include items not completed due to the patient's condition, hospital system problems (diagnostic studies or therapeutic interventions not completed within the optimal time frame), or lack of orders. Assessing patient progression on the pathway helps caregivers to have an overall picture of patient recovery as compared to the goals and can be helpful in early recognition and resolution of problems. It is important to remember that individual discipline documentation on the plan of care or pathway does not preclude the need for ongoing, direct communication between disciplines in order to facilitate optimal patient care and achievement of goals.

PLANNING CARE THROUGH STAFFING CONSIDERATIONS

Planning care for individual acutely ill patients begins with ensuring each nurse caring for a patient has the corresponding competencies and skills to meet the patient's needs. The American Association of Critical-Care Nurses has developed the AACN Synergy Model for Patient Care to delineate core patient characteristics and needs that drive the core competencies of nurses required to care for patients and families (Table 2-1). All eight competencies identified in the Synergy Model are essential for the progressive care nurse's practice, though the extent to which any particular competency is needed on a daily basis depends on the patient's needs at that

TABLE 2-1. CORE PATIENT CHARACTERISTICS AND NURSE COMPETENCIES AS DEFINED IN THE SYNERGY MODEL

Patient Characteristics	Description
Resiliency	The capacity to return to a restorative level of functioning using compensatory/coping mechanisms
Vulnerability	Susceptibility to actual or potential stressors that may adversely affect patient outcomes
Stability	The ability to maintain a steady-state equilibrium
Complexity	The intricate entanglement of two or more systems
Resource Availability	Extent of resources (technical, fiscal, personal, psychological, and social) the patient/family bring to the situation
Participation in Care	Extent to which patient/family engages in aspects of care
Participation in Decision Making	Extent to which patient/family engages in decision making
Predictability	Characteristic that allows one to expect a certain course of events or course of illness

Nurse Competencies	Description
Clinical Judgment	Clinical reasoning (clinical decision making, critical thinking, and global understanding of situation) coupled with nursing skills (formal and informal experiential knowledge and evidence-based practice)
Advocacy and Moral Agency	Working on another's behalf and representing concerns of patients/families and nursing staff
Caring Practices	Activities that create a compassionate, supportive, and therapeutic environment
Collaboration	Working with others in a way that promotes each person's contributions toward achieving optimal patient/family goals
Systems Thinking	Body of knowledge that allows the nurse to manage environment and system resources for patients, families, and staff
Response to Diversity	Sensitivity to recognize, appreciate, and incorporate differences into provision of care
Facilitation of Learning	Ability to facilitate learning for patients, families, and staff
Clinical Inquiry	Ongoing process of questioning and evaluating practice and providing informed practice

Data from American Association of Critical-Care Nurses. The AACN Synergy Model for Patient Care. Aliso Viejo, CA: AACN. Available at: http://www.aacn.org/WD/Certifications/Content/synmodel.content?menu=Certification. Accessed February 18, 2013.

point in time. When making patient staffing assignments, the charge nurse or nurse manager should assess the priority needs of the patient and assign a nurse who has the proficiencies to meet those patient needs. By matching the competencies of the nurse with the needs of the patient, synergy occurs resulting in optimal patient outcomes.

PATIENT SAFETY CONSIDERATIONS IN PLANNING CARE

Progressive care units are high-technology, high-intervention environments with multiple providers. It is an ongoing challenge for nurses to be ever thoughtful of minimizing the safety risks inherent in such an environment. Progressive care units are constantly working to improve ways to optimize care and minimize risks to patients.

As the nurse develops an ongoing plan of care, he or she must incorporate safety initiatives into that care. Conditions of acutely ill patients can change quickly, so ongoing awareness and vigilance is the key even when the patient appears to be stable or improving. The progressive care unit environment itself can contain safety issues. Inappropriate use of medical gas equipment or ventilator settings, electrical safety with invasive lines, certain types of restraints, bedside rails, and cords and tubings lying on the floor may all be hazardous to the acutely ill patient. In addition, with so many healthcare providers involved in the care of each patient, it is imperative that communication remains accurate and timely. Use of a standardized handoff communication tool is a fundamental step in preventing errors related to poor communication among healthcare providers.

ESSENTIAL CONTENT CASE:

Synergy between Patient Characteristics and Nurse Competencies

MG is an 83-year-old woman with a history of coronary heart disease and metastatic breast cancer who is transferred to the progressive care unit with shortness of breath. Her respiratory status is continuing to worsen and CPAP is initiated though the physician is evaluating MG for the potential for intubation and sedation. In addition, MG is experiencing episodes of tachycardia. It has been determined the shortness of breath is due to a large, pleural effusion. MG is widowed with three children who are very supportive but all live at least 5 hours away and are unclear about their mother's wishes regarding ongoing aggressive medical treatment.

Case Question 1: Based on the Synergy Model (see Table 2-1), what four priority patient characteristics would the charge nurse consider in making a nurse assignment for MG?

Case Question 2: The charge nurse assigns Rebecca to care for MG. What particular skills will Rebecca use in caring for MG during the upcoming shift?

Answers
1. MG's priority characteristics include instability, minimally resilient, vulnerable and currently unable to fully participate in decision-making.
2. Clinical judgment, advocacy and moral agency, and caring practices.

Finally, as described in more detail under section "Prevention of Common Complications," many common complications can be prevented by patient safety initiatives such as preventing ventilator-acquired pneumonia, blood stream infections, and urinary tract infections. In addition to meticulous care of patients, it is advisable for the healthcare team to have daily discussions on rounds as to whether the invasive lines and catheters need to remain in place. Removing these pieces of equipment as soon as clinically appropriate is the first step in preventing complications from occurring.

PREVENTION OF COMMON COMPLICATIONS

The development of an acute illness, regardless of its cause, predisposes the patient to a number of physiologic and psychological complications. A major focus when providing care to progressive care patients is the prevention of complications associated with acute illness. The following content overviews some of the most common complications.

Physiologic Instability

Ongoing assessments and monitoring of progressive care patients (see Table 1-13) are key to early identification of physiologic changes and to ensuring that the patient is progressing to the identified transition goals. It is important for the nurse to use critical thinking skills throughout the provision of care to accurately analyze patient changes.

After each assessment, the data obtained should be looked at in totality as they relate to the status of the patient. When an assessment changes in one body system, rarely does it remain an isolated issue, but rather it frequently either impacts or is a result of changes in other systems. Only by analyzing the entire patient assessment can the nurse see what is truly happening with the patient and anticipate interventions and responses.

When you assume care of the patient, define what goals the patient should achieve by the end of the shift, either as identified by the plan of care or by your assessment. This provides opportunities to evaluate care over a period of time. It prevents a narrow focus on the completion of individual tasks and interventions rather than the overall progression of the patient toward various goals. In addition, it is key to anticipate the potential patient responses to interventions. For instance, have you noticed that you need to increase the insulin infusion in response to higher glucose levels every morning around 10.00 AM? When looking at the whole picture, you may realize that the patient is receiving several medications in the early morning that are being given in a dextrose diluent. Recognition of this pattern helps you to stabilize swings in blood glucose.

Deep Venous Thrombosis

Progressive care patients are at increased risk of deep venous thrombosis (DVT) due to their underlying condition and immobility. Routine interventions can prevent this potentially devastating complication from occurring. There is increasing evidence to support early and progressive mobility of patients to decrease the risk of DVTs in addition to improving respiratory function and muscle strength. It takes a team effort to fully implement early mobility protocols, including nurses, physical therapists, respiratory therapists, and physicians. Increased mobility is emphasized as soon as the patient is stable. Even transferring the patient from the bed to the chair changes positioning of extremities and improves circulation. Additionally, use of sequential compression devices assists in enhancing lower extremity circulation. Avoid placing intravenous (IV) access in the groin site or lower limbs as this impedes mobility and potentially blood flow, and can thus increase DVT risk. Ensure adequate hydration. Many patients may also be placed on low-dose heparin or enoxaparin protocols as a preventative measure.

Hospital-Acquired Infections

Progressive care patients are especially vulnerable to infection during their stay in the progressive care unit. It is estimated that 20% to 60% of progressive care patients acquire some type of infection. In general, hospital-acquired infections because of the high use of multiple invasive devices and the frequent presence of debilitating underlying diseases are a risk in the progressive care unit. Hospital-acquired infections increase the patient's LOS and hospitalization costs, and can markedly increase mortality rates depending on the type and severity of the infection and the underlying disease. Although urinary tract infections are the most common hospital-acquired infections in the progressive care setting, hospital-acquired pneumonias are the second most common infection and the most common cause of mortality from infections. Details of specific risk factors and control measures for the prevention of hospital-acquired pneumonias are presented in Chapter 10 (Respiratory System). Other frequent infections include bloodstream and surgical site infections. It is imperative for progressive care practitioners to understand the processes that contribute to these potentially lethal infections and their roles in preventing these untoward events.

Prevention

Standard precautions, sometimes referred to as *universal precautions* or *body substance isolation*, refer to the basic precautions that are to be used on all patients, regardless of their diagnosis. The general premise of standard precautions is that all body fluids have the potential to transmit any number of infectious diseases, both bacterial and viral. Certain basic principles must be followed to prevent direct and indirect transmission of these organisms. Nonsterile examination gloves should be worn when performing venipuncture, touching nonintact skin or mucous membranes of the patient or for touching any moist body fluid. This includes urine, stool, saliva, emesis, sputum, blood, and any type of drainage. Other personal protective equipment, such as face shields and protective gowns, should be worn whenever

TABLE 2-2. ISOLATION CATEGORIES AND RELATED INFECTION EXAMPLES

Isolation Categories	Infection Examples When Used
Standard precautions	Used with care of all patients
Airborne precautions	Tuberculosis, measles (rubeola), varicella
Droplet precautions	*Neisseria meningitidis, Haemophilus influenzae,* pertussis, mumps
Contact precautions	Vancomycin-resistant enterococcus (VRE), methicillin-resistant *Staphylococcus aureus* (MRSA), *Clostridium difficile,* scabies, impetigo, varicella

there is a risk of splashing body fluids into the face or onto clothing. This protects not only the healthcare worker, but also prevents any contamination that may be transmitted between patients via the caregiver. Specific control measures are aimed at specific routes of transmission. See Table 2-2 for examples of isolation precaution categories and the types of infections for which they are instituted.

Other interventions to prevent nosocomial infections are similar regardless of the site. Maintaining glycemic control in both diabetic and nondiabetic patients may help decrease the patient's risk for developing an infection. Invasive lines or tubes should never remain in place longer than absolutely necessary and never simply for staff convenience. Avoid breaks in systems such as urinary drainage systems and IV lines. Use of aseptic technique is essential if breaks into these systems are necessary. Hand washing before and after any manipulation of invasive lines is essential.

The current recommendation from the United States Centers for Disease Control and Prevention (CDC) is that peripheral IV lines remain in place no longer than 72 to 96 hours. There is no standard recommendation for routine removal of central venous catheters when required for prolonged periods. If the patient begins to show signs of sepsis that could be catheter-related, these catheters should be removed. More important than the length of time the catheter is in place is how carefully the catheter was inserted and cared for while in place. All catheters that have been placed in an emergency situation should be replaced as soon as possible or within 48 hours. Dressings should be kept dry and intact and changed at the first signs of becoming damp, soiled, or loosened. IV tubing should be changed no more frequently than every 72 hours, with the exception of tubing for blood, blood products, or lipid-based products, each of which has specific criteria for how often the tubing should be changed.

Strategies to prevent hospital-acquired pneumonia in progressive care patients include the following for patients at high risk of aspiration, which is the primary risk factor: maintain the head of the bed at greater than or equal to 30°, assess residual volumes during enteral feeding and adjust feeding rates accordingly, and wash hands before and after contact with patient secretions or respiratory equipment (refer to chapters 5 and 14 for specific content related to these recommendations).

One of the most important defenses to preventing infection, though, is hand washing. Hand washing is defined by the CDC as vigorous rubbing together of lathered hands for 15 seconds followed by a thorough rinsing under a stream of running water. Particular attention should be paid around rings and under fingernails. It is best to keep natural fingernails well trimmed and unpolished. Cracked nail polish is a good place for microorganisms to hide.

Artificial fingernails should not be worn in any healthcare setting because they are virtually impossible to clean without a nailbrush and vigorous scrubbing. Hand washing should be performed prior to donning examination gloves to carry out patient care activities and after removing examination gloves. Washing should occur any time bare hands become contaminated with any wet body fluid and should be done before the body fluid dries. Once it dries, microorganisms begin to colonize the skin, making it more difficult to remove them. Use of alcohol-based waterless cleansers is convenient and effective when no visible soiling or contamination has occurred.

Dry, cracked skin, a long-standing problem associated with hand washing, has new significance with the emergence of blood-borne pathogens. Frequent hand washing, especially with antimicrobial soap, can lead to extremely dry skin. The frequent use of latex examination gloves has been associated with increased sensitivities and allergies, causing even more skin breakdown. All of this skin breakdown can put the healthcare provider at risk for blood-borne pathogen transmission, as well as for colonization or infection with bacteria. Attention to skin care is extremely important for the progressive care practitioner who is using antimicrobial soap and latex gloves frequently. Lotions and emollients should be used to prevent skin breakdown. If skin breakdown does occur, the employee health nurse should be consulted for possible treatment or work restriction until the condition resolves.

Skin Breakdown

Skin breakdown is a major risk with progressive care patients due to immobility, poor nutrition, invasive lines, surgical sites, poor circulation, edema, and incontinence issues. Skin can become fragile and easily tear. Pressure ulcers can start to occur in as little as 2 hours. Healthy people constantly reposition themselves, even in their sleep, to relieve areas of pressure. Progressive care patients who cannot reposition themselves rely on caregivers to assist them. Pay particular attention to pressure points that are most prone to developing breakdown, namely, heels, elbows, coccyx, and occiput. When receiving progressive care patients following prolonged surgical procedures, ask the perioperative providers about the patient's positioning during the procedure. This will help determine the need for close monitoring of the related pressure points for early indication of tissue injury. Also be cognizant of equipment that may contribute to breakdown, such as drainage tubes and even bed rails, if patients are positioned in constant contact with them. As the patient's condition changes, so does the risk of developing a pressure ulcer. Assessing the patient's risk routinely with a risk assessment tool alerts the caregiver to increasing or decreasing risk and therefore potential changes in interventions.

There are many simple interventions to maintain skin integrity: reposition the patient minimally every 2 hours, particularly if they are not spontaneously moving; use pressure-reduction mattresses for patients at high risk of breakdown; elevate heels off the bed using pillows placed under the calves or heel protectors; consider elbow pads; avoid long periods of sitting in a chair without repositioning; inflatable cushions (donuts) should never be used for either the sacrum or the head because they can actually cause increases in pressure on surrounding skin surfaces; and use a skin care protocol with ointment barriers for patients experiencing incontinence to prevent skin irritation and tissue breakdown.

Sleep Pattern Disturbance

Progressive care patients are at risk for altered sleep patterns. Sleep is a problem for patients for many reasons, not the least of which are the pain and anxiety of an acute illness within an environment that is inundated with the multiple activities of healthcare providers. Table 2-3 identifies the many reasons for patients to experience sleep deprivation. The priority of sleep in the hierarchy of patient needs is often perceived to be low by clinicians. This contradicts patients' own statements about the progressive care experience. Patients complain about lack of sleep as a major stressor along with the discomfort of unrelieved pain. The vicious cycle of undertreated

pain, anxiety, and sleeplessness continues unless clinicians intervene to break the cycle with simple but essential interventions individualized to each patient.

Noise, lights, and frequent patient interruptions are common in many progressive care settings, with staff able to tune out the disturbances after they have worked in the setting for even a short period of time. Subjecting patients to these environmental stimuli and interruptions to rest/sleep can quickly lead to sleep deprivation. Psychological changes in sleep deprivation include confusion, irritability, and agitation. Physiologic changes include depressed immune and respiratory systems and a decreased pain threshold. Patients may already be sleep-deprived when they are transferred from a critical care unit to the progressive care setting. The progressive care unit routine can help start to reestablish a healing sleep pattern.

Enhancing patients' sleep potential in the progressive care setting involves knowledge of how the environment affects the patient and where to target interventions to best promote sleep and rest. A nighttime sleep protocol where patients are closely monitored but untouched from 1 to 5 AM is an excellent example of eliminating the hourly disturbances that may have been occurring in the ICU. Encouraging blocks of time for sleep and careful assessment of the quantity and quality of sleep are important to patient well-being. The middle-of-the-night bath should not be a standard of care for any patient. Table 2-4 details basic recommendations for sleep assessment, protecting or shielding the patient from the environment, and modifying the internal and external environments of the patient. When these activities are incorporated into standard practice routines, progressive care patients receive optimal opportunity to achieve sleep.

Psychosocial Impact

Basic Tenets

Keys to maintaining psychological integrity during an acute illness include keeping stressors at a minimum; encouraging family participation in care; promoting a proper sleep-wake cycle; encouraging communication, questions, and honest and positive feedback; empowering the patient to participate in decisions as appropriate; providing patient and family education about unit expectations and rules, procedures, medications, and the patient's physical condition; ensuring pain relief and comfort; and providing continuity of care providers. It is also important to have the patient's usual sensory

TABLE 2-3. FACTORS CONTRIBUTING TO SLEEP DISTURBANCES IN PROGRESSIVE CARE

Illness
- Metabolic changes
- Underlying diseases (eg, cardiovascular disease, chronic obstructive pulmonary disease [COPD])
- Pain
- Anxiety, fear
- Delirium

Medications
- Beta-blockers
- Bronchodilators
- Benzodiazepines
- Narcotics

Environment
- Noise
- Staff conversations
- Television/radio
- Equipment alarms
- Frequent care interruptions
- Lighting
- Lack of usual bedtime routine
- Room temperature
- Uncomfortable sleep surface

TABLE 2-4. EVIDENCE-BASED PRACTICE: SLEEP PROMOTION IN PROGRESSIVE CARE

- Assess patient's usual sleep patterns
- Minimize effects of underlying disease process as much as possible (eg, reduce fever, eliminate pain, minimize metabolic disturbances)
- Avoid medications that disturb sleep patterns
- Mimic patients' usual bedtime routine as much as possible
- Minimize environmental impact on sleep as much as possible
- Utilize complementary and alternative therapies to promote sleep as appropriate

and physical aids available, such as glasses, hearing aids, and dentures, as they may help prevent confusion. Encourage the family to bring something familiar or personal from home, such as a family or pet picture.

Delirium

Delirium is evidenced by disorientation, confusion, perceptual disturbances, restlessness, distractibility, and sleep-wake cycle disturbances. Any prior LOS in an ICU may have already resulted in, or put a patient at risk for, development of confusion. Causes of confusion are usually multifactorial and include metabolic disturbances, polypharmacy, immobility, infections (particularly urinary tract and upper respiratory infections), dehydration, electrolyte imbalances, sensory impairment, and environmental challenges. Treatment of delirium is a challenge and therefore prevention is ideal.

Delirium is most common in postsurgical and elderly patients and is the most common cause of disruptive behavior in progressive care. It is not unusual for providers to suspect delirium when acutely ill patients are confused and restless, however in reality there are several different subtypes of delirium: hyperactive (restlessness, agitation, irritability, aggression); hypoactive (slow response to verbal stimuli, psychomotor slowing); and mixed delirium (both hyperactive and hypoactive behaviors). Assessment of delirium should be routine in the progressive care unit, and there are several valid and reliable tools that can be used to identify delirium.

Often mislabeled as psychosis, delirium is not psychosis. Sensory overload is a common risk factor that contributes to delirium in the acutely ill. Medications that may also play a role in instigating delirium include prochlorperazine, diphenhydramine, famotidine, benzodiazepines, opioids, and antiarrhythmic medications.

Medication for managing delirious behavior is best reserved for those cases in which behavioral interventions have failed. Sedative-hypnotics and anxiolytics may have precipitated the delirium and can exacerbate the sleep-wake cycle disturbances causing more confusion. The agitated patient may require low-dose neuroleptics or short-acting benzodiazepines. Restraints are discouraged because they tend to increase agitation.

External stimulation should be minimized and a quiet, restful, well-lit room maintained during the day. Consistency in care providers is also important. Repeating orientation cues minimizes fear and confusion; for example, "Good morning Bill, my name is Sue. It's Monday morning in April and you are in the hospital. I'm a nurse and will stay here with you." Background noise from a television or radio often increases anxiety as the patient has trouble processing the noise and content. Explain all procedures and tests concretely. Introduce one idea at a time, slowly, and have the patient repeat the information. Repeat and reinforce as often as needed.

If the patient demonstrates a paranoid element in his or her delirium, avoid confrontation and remain at a safe distance. Accept bizarre statements calmly, with a nod, but without agreement. Explain to the family that the behaviors are symptoms that will most likely resolve with time, resumption of normal sleep patterns, and medication. Delirious patients usually remember the events, thoughts, conversations, and provider responses that occur during delirium. The recovered patients may be embarrassed and feel guilty if they were combative during their illness.

Depression

Depression occurring with a medical illness affects the long-term recovery outcomes by lengthening the course of the illness, and increasing morbidity and mortality. Risk factors that predispose for depression with medical disorders include social isolation, recent loss, pessimism, financial pressures, history of mood disorder, alcohol or substance abuse/withdrawal, previous suicide attempts, and pain. Many patients arrive in the hospital with a history of treatment for depression which can be exacerbated by a critical illness crisis. It is important that healthcare providers don't forget to maintain the patient's psychiatric medication regimen if at all possible in order to avoid worsening of the patient's psychological status.

Educating the patient and family about the temporary nature of most depressions during acute illness assists in providing reassurance that this is not an unusual phenomenon. Severe depressive symptoms often respond to pharmacologic intervention, so a psychiatric consultation may be warranted. Keep in mind that it may take several weeks for antidepressants to reach their full effectiveness. If you suspect a person is depressed, ask directly. Allow the patient to initiate conversation. If negative distortions about illness and treatment are communicated, it is appropriate to correct, clarify, and reassure with realistic information to promote a more hopeful outcome. Consistency in care providers promotes trust in an ongoing relationship and enhances recovery.

A patient who has attempted suicide or is suicidal can be frightening to hospital staff. Staff members are often uncertain of what to say when the patient says, "I want to kill myself … my life no longer has meaning." Do not avoid asking if the person is feeling suicidal; you do not promote suicidal thoughts by asking the question. Many times the communication of feeling suicidal is a cover for wanting to discuss fear, pain, or loneliness. A psychiatric referral is recommended in these situations for further evaluation and intervention.

Anxiety

Medical disorders can cause anxiety and panic-like symptoms, which are distressing to the patient and family and may exacerbate the medical condition. Treatment of the underlying medical condition may decrease the concomitant anxiety. Both pharmacologic and nonpharmacologic interventions can be helpful in managing anxiety during acute illness. Pharmacologic agents for anxiety are discussed in Chapter 6 (Pain and Sedation Management) and Chapter 7 (Pharmacology). Goals of pharmacologic therapy are to titrate the drug dose so that the patient can remain cognizant and interactive with staff, family, and environment; to complement pain control; and to assist in promoting sleep. There are also a variety of nonpharmacologic interventions to decrease or control anxiety:

- Breathing techniques: These techniques target somatic symptoms and include deep and slow abdominal breathing patterns. It is important to demonstrate and do the breathing with patients, as their heightened anxiety decreases their attention span. Practicing this technique may decrease anxiety and assist the patient through difficult procedures.
- Muscle relaxation: Reduce psychomotor tension with muscle relaxation. Again, the patient will most likely be unable to cue himself or herself, so this is an excellent opportunity for the family to participate as the cuing partner. Cuing might be, "The mattress under your head, elbow, heel, and back feels heavy against your body, press harder, and then try to drift away from the mattress as you relax." Commercial relaxation tapes are available but are not as useful as the cuing by a familiar voice.
- Imagery: Interventions targeting cognition, such as imagery techniques, depend on the patient's capacity for attention, memory, and processing. Visualization imagery involves recalling a pleasurable, relaxing situation; for example, a hot bath, lying on a warm beach, listening to waves, or hearing birds sing. Guided imagery and hypnosis are additional therapies, but require some competency to be effective; thus, a referral is suggested. Patients who practice meditation as an alternative for stress control should be encouraged to continue, but the environment may need modification to optimize the effects.
- Preparatory information: Providing the patient and family with preparatory information is extremely helpful in controlling anxiety. Allowing the patient and family to control some aspects of the illness process, even if only minor aspects of care, can be anxiolytic.
- Distraction techniques: Distraction techniques can also interrupt the anxiety cycle. Methods for distracting can be listening to familiar music or humorous tapes, watching videos, or counting backward from 200 by 2 rapidly.
- Use of previous coping methods: Identify how the patient and family have dealt with stress and anxiety in the past and suggest that approach if feasible. Supporting previous coping techniques may well be adaptive.

PATIENT AND FAMILY EDUCATION

Patient and family education in the progressive care environment is essential to providing information regarding diagnosis, prognosis, treatments, and procedures. In addition, education

provides patients and family members a mechanism by which fears and concerns can be put in perspective and confronted so that they can become active members in the decisions made about care.

Providing patient and family education in acute care is challenging; multiple barriers (eg, environmental factors, patient stability, patient and family anxiety) must be overcome or adapted to provide this essential intervention. The importance of education, coupled with the barriers common in progressive care, necessitates that education be a continuous ongoing process engaged in by all members of the team.

Education in the progressive care setting is most often done informally, though some patients may be able to tolerate limited sessions in a classroom setting. Education of the patient and family can often be subtle, occurring with each interaction between the patient, family, and members of the healthcare team. Education may also now be more direct, particularly in relation to self-care or managing equipment at home.

Assessment of Learning Readiness

Assessment of the patient's and family's learning needs should focus primarily on learning readiness. *Learning readiness* refers to that moment in time when the learner is able to comprehend and synthesize the shared information. Without learning readiness, teaching may not be useful. Questions to assess learning readiness are listed in Table 2-5.

Strategies to Address Patient and Family Education

Prior to teaching, the information gathered in the assessment is prioritized and organized into a format that is meaningful to the learner (Table 2-6). Next, the outcome of the teaching is established along with appropriate content, and then a decision should be made about how to share the information.

TABLE 2-5. ASSESSMENT OF LEARNING READINESS

Generic Principles
• Do the patient and the family have questions about the diagnosis, prognosis, treatments, or procedures?
• What do the patient and the family desire to learn about?
• What is the knowledge level of the individuals being taught? What do they already know about the issues that will be taught?
• What is their current situation (condition and environment) and have they had any prior experience in a similar situation?
• Do the patient or the family have any communication barriers (eg, language, illiteracy, culture, listening/comprehension deficits)?

Special Considerations in Progressive Care
• Does the patient's condition allow you to assess this information from them (eg, physiologic/psychological stability)?
• Is the patient's support system/family/significant other available or ready to receive this information?
• What environmental factors (including time) present as barriers in the progressive care unit?
• Are there other members of the healthcare team who may possess vital assessment information?

TABLE 2-6. PRINCIPLES FOR TEACHING PLANS

Generic Principles
• Establish the outcome of the teaching.
• Determine what content needs to be taught, given the assessment.
• Identify what support systems are in place to support your educational efforts (eg, unit leadership, education department, standardized teaching plans, teaching materials such as pamphlets, brochures, videos).
• Familiarize yourself with the content and teaching materials.
• Contact resources to clarify and provide consistency in information and to also provide additional educational support and follow-up.
• Determine the most appropriate teaching strategy (video, written materials, discussion) and to whom (patient or family) it should be directed.

Special Considerations in Progressive Care
• Plan the teaching strategy *carefully*. Patients and families in the progressive care environment are stressed and an overload of information adds to their stress. When planning education, consider content and amount based on the assessment of the patient, nature, and severity of the patient's illness, availability of significant others, and existing environmental barriers.

The next step is to teach the patient, family, and significant others (Table 2-7). Although this phase often appears to be the easiest, it is actually the most difficult. It is crucial during the communication of the content, regardless of the type of communication vehicle used (video, pamphlet, discussion), to listen carefully to the needs expressed by the learner and to provide clear and precise responses to those needs.

Outcome Measurement

Following educational interventions, it is essential to determine if the educational outcomes have been achieved (Table 2-8). Even if the outcome appears to have been achieved, it is not unusual that the learners may not retain all the information.

TABLE 2-7. PRINCIPLES FOR EDUCATIONAL SESSIONS

Generic Principles
• Consider the time needed to convey both the information and support system availability.
• Consider the situation the patient is currently experiencing. Postponement may need to be considered.
• Be aware of the amount of content and the patient's and the family's ability to process the information.
• Be sensitive in the delivery of the information. Make sure it is conveyed at a level that the patient and the family can understand.
• Refer to and involve resources as appropriate.
• Convey accurate and precise information. Make sure this information is consistent with previous information given to the patient.
• Listen carefully and solicit feedback during the session to guide the discussion and clarify any potential misinterpretations.

Special Considerations in Progressive Care
• Keep the time frame and content as set. Education must be episodic due to the nature of the patient's condition and the environment.
• Provide repetition of the information. Stress and the progressive care environment can alter comprehension; for this reason repetition is necessary.
• More details will need to be given as the patient's condition improves and transitioning to the next level of care occurs. Return demonstrations may be required for self-care activities.

TABLE 2-8. PRINCIPLES FOR EDUCATIONAL OUTCOME MONITORING

Generic Principles
• Measure the outcome. Was the outcome met? Was the outcome unmet?
• Communicate the outcome verbally and in a written format to other members of the healthcare team.
• Provide necessary follow-up and reinforcement of the teaching.
• Make referrals that may have been identified in or as a result of patient and family education.
• Evaluate the teaching process for barriers or problems, and then address those areas and be aware of these for future interactions.

Special Considerations in Progressive Care
• Recognize that repetition of information is the rule, not the exception. Be prepared to repeat information previously given, many times if necessary.

Patients and families experience a great deal of stress while in the acute care environment; reinforcement is often necessary and should be anticipated.

FAMILY-FOCUSED CARE

There is a strong evidence base to support that family presence and involvement in the progressive care unit aids in the recovery of progressive care patients. Family members can help patients cope, reduce anxiety, and provide a resource for the patient. Families, however, also need support in maintaining their strength and having needs met to be able to function as a positive influence for the patient rather than having a negative impact.

Developing a partnership with the family and a trusting relationship is in everyone's best interest so that optimal functioning can occur. Research shows that there can frequently be disagreement between the nurse and family perspectives about the type or priorities of family needs. Therefore, it is important to discuss family needs and perceptions directly with each family and tailor interventions based on those needs (Table 2-9).

TABLE 2-9. EVIDENCE-BASED PRACTICE: FAMILY INTERVENTIONS

Planning
• Determine what the family sees as priority needs.

Interventions
• Determine spokesperson and contact person.
• Establish optimum methods to contact and communicate with family.
• Make referrals for support services as appropriate.
• Provide information according to family needs.
• Include family in direct care.
• Provide a comfortable environment.

Evaluation
• Evaluate achievement of meeting family needs through multiple methods (eg, feedback, satisfaction surveys, care conferences, follow-up after discharge).

Data from Leske JS. Interventions to decrease family anxiety. Crit Care Nurse. 2002;22: 61-65.

Research has consistently identified five major areas of family needs (receiving assurance, remaining near the patient, receiving information, being comfortable, and having support available). These and the importance of unrestricted family visitation are addressed next.

Receiving Assurance

Family members need reassurance that the best possible care is being given to the patient. This instills confidence and a sense of security for the family. It can also assist in either maintaining hope or can be helpful in redefining hope to a more realistic image when appropriate.

Remaining Near the Patient

Family members need to have consistent access to their loved one. Of primary importance to the family is the unit visiting policy. Specifics to be discussed include the number of visitors allowed at one time, age restrictions, visiting times if not flexible or open, and how to gain access to the unit (Table 2-10). There is increasing evidence to support the presence of a family member with the patient during invasive procedures, as well as during cardiopulmonary resuscitation (CPR). Although this practice may still be controversial, family members have reported a sense of relief and gratitude at being able to remain close to the patient. It is recommended that written policies be developed through an interdisciplinary approach prior to implementing family presence at CPR or procedures.

Receiving Information

Communication with the patient and family should be open and honest. Clinicians should keep promises (be thoughtful about what you promise), describe expectations, not contract for secrets or elicit care provider preferences, should apologize for inconveniences and mistakes, and maintain confidentiality. Concise, simplistic explanations without medical jargon or alphabet shorthand facilitate understanding. Contact interpreters, as appropriate, when language barriers exist.

Evaluate your communication by asking the patient and family for their understanding of the message you sent and its content and intent. When conflict occurs, find a private place for discussion. Avoid taking the confrontation personally. Ask yourself what the issue is and what needs to occur to reach resolution. If too much emotion is present, agree to address the issue at a later time, if possible.

It is helpful to establish a communication tree so that one family member is designated to be called if there are changes in the patient's condition. Establish a time for that person to call the unit for updates. Reassure them you are there to help or refer them to other system supports. Unit expectations and rules can be conveyed in a pamphlet for the family to refer to over time. Content that is helpful includes orientation about the philosophy of care; routines such as shift changes and physician rounds; the varied roles of personnel who work with patients; and comfort information such as food services, bathrooms, waiting areas, chapel services, transportation, and lodging. Clarify what they see and hear. Mobilize resources and include them in patient care and problem solving, as appropriate. Some progressive care units invite family members to medical rounds for the discussion of their loved ones. Adequate communication can decrease anxiety, increase a sense of control, and assist in improving decision making by families.

Being Comfortable

There should be space available in or near the progressive care unit to meet comfort needs of the family. This should include comfortable furniture, access to phones and restrooms, and assistance with finding overnight accommodations. Encourage the family to admit when they are overwhelmed, take breaks, go to meals, rest, sleep, take care of themselves, and not to abandon members at home. Helping the family with basic comfort needs helps decrease their distress and maintain their reserves and coping mechanisms. This improves their ability to be a valuable resource for the patient.

Having Support Available

Utilize all potential resources in meeting family needs. Relying on nurses to fulfill all family needs while they are also trying to care for a progressive care patient can create tension and frustration. Assess the family for their own resources that can be maximized. Utilize hospital referrals that can assist in family support such as chaplains, social workers, and child-family life departments.

Family Visitation

There is an abundance of evidence demonstrating that unrestricted access of the patient's support network (family, significant others, trusted friends) can be beneficial to the patient by providing emotional and social support; conveying the patient's wishes when he or she is unable to speak for self, improving communication, and improving patient and family satisfaction. However, many hospitals continue to have policies that restrict visitation. There are certainly individual circumstances where open visiting can be ill-advised due to medical, therapeutic, or safety considerations (eg disruptive behavior, infectious disease concerns, patient privacy, or per patient request). On admission to the progressive care unit, the patient should be asked to identify their "family" and their

TABLE 2-10. EVIDENCE-BASED PRACTICE: FAMILY VISITATION IN PROGRESSIVE CARE

- Establish ways for families to have access to the patient (eg, open visitation, contract visitation, unit phone numbers).
- Ask patients their preferences related to visiting.
- Promote access to patients with consistent unit policies and procedures with options for individualization.
- Prepare families for visit.
- Model interaction with patient.
- Give information about the patient's condition, equipment, and technology being used.
- Monitor the response of the patient and family to visitation.

visiting preferences, and care providers should partner with the patient and family to accommodate those preferences while meeting safety, privacy, and decision-making needs.

For the family, the progressive care setting symbolizes a variety of hopes, fears, and beliefs that range from hope of a cure to end-of-life care. A family-focused approach can promote coping and cohesion among family members and minimize the isolation and anxiety for patients. Anticipating family needs, focusing on the present, fostering open communication, and providing information are vital to promoting psychological integrity for families. By using the event of hospitalization as a point of access, progressive care clinicians assume a major role in primary prevention and assisting families to cope positively with crisis and grow from the experience.

TRANSPORTING THE PROGRESSIVE CARE PATIENT

Preventing common complications and maintaining physiologic and psychosocial stability is a challenge even when in the controlled environment of the progressive care unit. It is even more challenging when the need for transporting the progressive care patient to other areas of the hospital is necessary for diagnostic and therapeutic purposes. The decision to transport the progressive care patient out of the well-controlled environment of the progressive care unit elicits a variety of responses from clinicians. It's not uncommon to hear phrases like these: "What if something happens en route?" "Who will take care of my other patients while I'm gone?" Responses like these underscore the clinician's understanding of the risks involved in transporting progressive care patients.

Transporting a progressive care patient involves more than putting the patient on a stretcher and rolling him or her down the hall. Safe patient transport requires thoughtful planning, organization, and interdisciplinary communication and cooperation. The goal during transport is to maintain the same level of care, regardless of the location in the hospital. The transfer of progressive care patients always involves some degree of risk to the patient. The decision to transfer, therefore, should be based on an assessment of the potential benefits of transfer and be weighed against the potential risks.

The reason for moving a progressive care patient is typically the need for care, technology, or specialists not available in the progressive care unit. Whenever feasible, diagnostic testing or simple procedures should be performed at the patient's bedside within the progressive care unit. If the diagnostic test or procedural intervention under consideration is unlikely to alter management or outcome of the patient, then the risk of transfer may outweigh the benefit. It is imperative that every member of the healthcare team assists in clarifying what, if any, benefit may be derived from transport.

Assessment of Risk for Complications

Prior to initiating transport, a patient's risk for development of complications during transport should be systematically

TABLE 2-11. POTENTIAL COMPLICATIONS DURING TRANSPORT

Pulmonary
- Hyperventilation
- Hypoventilation
- Airway obstruction
- Aspiration
- Recurrent pneumothorax
- Arterial blood gas changes

Cardiovascular
- Hypotension
- Hypertension
- Arrhythmias
- Decreased tissue perfusion
- Cardiac ischemia
- Peripheral ischemia

Neurologic
- Increased intracranial pressure
- Cerebral hypoxia
- Cerebral hypercarbia
- Paralysis

Gastrointestinal
- Nausea
- Vomiting

Pain

assessed. The switching of technologies in the progressive care unit to portable devices may lead to undesired physiologic changes. In addition, complications may arise from environmental conditions outside the progressive care unit that are difficult to control, such as body temperature fluctuations or inadvertent movement of invasive devices (eg, tracheostomies, chest tubes, IV devices). Common complications associated with transportation are summarized in Table 2-11.

Pulmonary Complications

Maintaining adequate ventilation and oxygenation during transport is a challenge. Patients who are not intubated prior to their transfer are at risk for developing airway compromise. This is particularly a problem in patients with decreased levels of consciousness. Continuous monitoring of airway patency is critical to ensure rapid implementation of airway strategies, if necessary.

Hypoventilation or hyperventilation can result in pH changes, which may lead to deficits in tissue perfusion and oxygenation. Therefore, respiratory and nursing personnel who are properly trained in the mechanisms of unique ventilatory requirements need to provide ventilation during transport. Patients requiring continuous bilevel positive airway pressure (BiPAP) or high-flow oxygen may experience changes in respiratory status during transport. The percentage of inspired oxygen (Fio_2) may need to be increased during transport. Increasing the Fio_2 for any patient requiring transfer may help avoid other complications from hypoxia. Ensuring the appropriate portable equipment to maintain adequate oxygenation may be complex but imperative. The patient's special respiratory equipment may also be transported to the destination so that he or she can be placed back on the equipment during the procedure.

Cardiovascular Complications

Whether related to their underlying disease processes or the anxiety of being taken out of a controlled environment, the potential for cardiovascular complications exists in all patients being transported. These complications include hypotension, hypertension, arrhythmias, tachycardia, ischemia, and acute pulmonary edema. Many of these complications can be avoided by adequate patient preparation with pharmacologic agents to maintain hemodynamic stability and manage pain and anxiety. Continuous infusions should be carefully maintained during transport, with special attention given to IV lines during movement of the patient from one surface to another. Additional emergency equipment may need to be taken on the transport such as hand pumps for patients on ventricular assist devices.

Neurologic Complications

The potential for respiratory and cardiovascular changes during transport increases the risk for cerebral hypoxia, hypercarbia, and intracranial pressure (ICP) changes. Patients with high baseline ICP may require additional interventions to stabilize cerebral perfusion and oxygenation prior to transport (eg, hyperventilation, increased partial pressure of oxygen in arterial blood [PaO_2], blood pressure control). In addition, patients with suspected cranial or vertebral fractures are at high risk for neurologic damage during repositioning from bed to transport carts or diagnostic tables. Proper immobilization of the spine is imperative in these situations, as is the avoidance of unnecessary repositioning of the patient. Positioning the head in the midline position with the head of the bed elevated, when not contraindicated, may decrease the risk of increases in ICP.

Gastrointestinal Complications

Gastrointestinal (GI) complications may include nausea or vomiting, which can threaten the patient's airway, as well as cause discomfort. Premedicating patients at risk for GI upset with an H_2-blocker, proton pump inhibitor or an antiemetic as appropriate may be helpful. For patients with large volume nasogastric (NG) drainage, preparations to continue NG drainage during transportation or in the destination location may be necessary.

Pain

The level of pain experienced by the patient is likely to be increased during transport. Many of the diagnostic tests and therapeutic interventions in other hospital departments are uncomfortable or painful. Anxiety associated with transport may also increase the level of pain. Additional analgesic or anxiolytic agents, or both may be required to ensure adequate pain and anxiety management during the transport process. Keeping the patient and family members well informed is also helpful in decreasing anxiety levels.

TABLE 2-12. TRANSPORT PERSONNEL AND EQUIPMENT REQUIREMENTS

Personnel
- Patients whose conditions are unstable, or are at risk for instability, or who require a specific type of monitoring should be accompanied by staff competent in managing the instability and in interpreting and intervening appropriately, based on the monitoring data.
- Additional personnel may include a respiratory therapist, registered nurse, transport aide, or physician.

Equipment
The following minimal equipment should be available:
- Cardiac monitor/defibrillator.
- Airway management equipment and resuscitation bag of proper size and fit for the patient.
- Oxygen source of ample volume to support the patient's needs for the projected time out of the progressive care unit, with an additional 30-minute reserve.
- Standard resuscitation drugs: epinephrine, atropine, amiodarone.
- Blood pressure cuff (sphygmomanometer) and stethoscope.
- Ample supply of the IV fluids and continuous drip medications (regulated by battery-operated infusion pumps) being administered to the patient.
- Additional medications to provide the patient's scheduled intermittent medication doses and to meet anticipated needs (eg, sedation) with appropriate orders to allow their administration if a physician is not present.
- Resuscitation cart and suction equipment need not accompany each patient being transferred, but such equipment should be stationed in areas used by acutely ill patients and be readily available (within 4 minutes) by a predetermined mechanism for emergencies that may occur en route.

Data from Day D. Keeping patients safe during intrahospital transport. Crit Care Nurse. 2010; 20(4): 18-32.

Level of Care Required During Transport

During transport, there should be no interruption in the monitoring or maintenance of the patient's vital functions. The equipment used during transport as well as the skill level of accompanying personnel must be equivalent with the interventions required or anticipated for the patient while in the progressive care unit (Table 2-12). Intermittent and continuous monitoring of physiologic status (eg, cardiac rhythm, blood pressure, oxygenation, ventilation) should continue during transport and while the patient is away from the progressive care unit (Table 2-13).

Questions that need to be answered to prepare for transfer include the following:

- What is the current level of care (equipment, personnel)?
- What will be needed during the transfer or at the destination to maintain that level of care?

TABLE 2-13. MONITORING DURING TRANSFER

- If technologically possible, patients being transferred should receive the same physiologic monitoring (eg, ECG, BP, SpO_2, vital signs; continuous or intermittent) during transfer that they were receiving in the progressive care unit.
- In addition, selected patients, based on clinical status, may benefit from continuous measurement of blood pressure and intermittent measurement of CVP.

Data from Day D. Keeping patients safe during intrahospital transport. Crit Care Nurse. 2010; 20(4): 18-32.

TABLE 2-14. PRETRANSFER COORDINATION AND COMMUNICATION

- Physician-to-physician and/or nurse-to-nurse communication regarding the patient's condition and treatment preceding and following the transfer should be documented in the medical record when the management of the patient will be assumed by a different team while the patient is away from the progressive care unit.
- The area to which the patient is being transferred (x-ray, operating room, nuclear medicine, etc) must confirm that it is ready to receive the patient and immediately begin the procedure or test for which the patient is being transferred.
- Ancillary services (eg, security, respiratory therapy, escort) must be notified as to the timing of the transfer and the equipment and support needed.
- Documentation in the medical record must include the indication for transfer, the patient's status during transfer and whether the patient is expected to return to the progressive care unit.

Data from Day D. Keeping patients safe during intrahospital transport. Crit Care Nurse. 2010; 20(4): 18-32.

- What additional therapeutic interventions may be required before or during transport (eg, pain and sedation medications or titration of infusions)?
- Do I have all the necessary equipment needed in the event of an emergency during the transport?

If you are unsure what capabilities exist at the destination, call the receiving area in advance to ask about their support capabilities; for example, are there adequate outlets to plug in electrical equipment rather than continuing to use battery power, do they have capability for high levels of suction pressure if needed, or what specialty instructions need to be followed in magnetic resonance imaging? Will they be ready to take the patient immediately into the procedure with no waiting?

Preparation

Before transfer, the plan of care for the patient during and after transfer should be coordinated to ensure continuity of care and availability of appropriate resources (Table 2-14). The receiving units should be contacted to confirm that all preparations for the patient's arrival have been completed.

ESSENTIAL CONTENT CASE

Risk Factors During Transport

Mr. W, a 45-year-old man, was involved in a motor vehicle accident when he fell asleep on his way home from work. He was not wearing a seat belt, and there were no air bags in the car. His injuries included chest contusions and broken ribs from the steering wheel and lacerations of his scalp from the windshield. He had been treated in the ICU for 7 days with the insertion of a chest tube to relieve his left pneumothorax and mechanical ventilation for 6 days. He had been transferred to the progressive care unit 24 hours previously. Mr. W was assigned to one of the progressive care nurses, Nancy, who had three other patients. One of these patients was recovering from repair of an abdominal aortic aneurysm 2 days ago, the second

patient was recovering from a large anterior myocardial infarction suffered after a total hip replacement, and the third patient was being discharged to home that day after a 3-day stay for an exacerbation of heart failure. Mr. W was now complaining of a new onset of shortness of breath and was requiring 50% Fio_2 per face mask for slowly falling oxygen saturations. A chest computed tomography (CT) had been ordered for him.

Case Question 1: Which of Mr. W's physiologic systems or clinical states are at particular risk of compromise during the transport for his CT scan?

Case Question 2: Why is Nancy concerned about the possibility of Mr. W experiencing pain and anxiety during the transport?

Answers

1. Respiratory, cardiovascular, pain, anxiety Nancy was aware of the possible complications he might experience during transport—respiratory, cardiovascular, or safety compromises. Possible respiratory complications included upper airway obstruction, respiratory depression, hypoxia, or hypercarbia, especially in a patient who has head and chest trauma and whose oxygenation is already compromised. Cardiovascular risks included hypotension, tachycardia due to cardiac tamponade, and decreased tissue perfusion because of decreased cardiac output and increased tissue oxygen demand during the transfer. Acute pain may occur or be exacerbated as a result of increased anxiety, patient movement and positioning, and hard surfaces during transport as well as potential manipulation/movement of invasive devices such as chest tubes. Nancy noted that anxiety from both the activity of transfer and from the uncertainty of Mr. W's future could certainly result in adverse physiologic changes during transport.

2. In addition to Nancy's goal to keep Mr. W comfortable while under her care, she also recognizes that increasing pain and anxiety can result in an increasing respiratory rate, heart rate, and blood pressure. All of these physiologic changes can exacerbate his worsening respiratory status and increased oxygen demands. It is important that the potential for these complications be minimized, particularly when Mr. W is being transported to the Imaging Department where it would be more challenging to address any physiologic decompensation or emergency situations.

    Anticipating complications, Nancy planned ahead. She asked the respiratory therapist to gather the appropriate oxygen equipment and accompany Nancy on the transport. With his respiratory status stable for the time being, Mr. W could be safely medicated with small dosages for pain and anxiety, and ultimately decrease his oxygen demand.

Communication, both written and verbal, between team members should delineate the current status of the patient, management priorities, and the process to follow in the event of untoward events (eg, unexpected hemodynamic instability or airway problems).

After you have assessed the patient's risk for transport complications, the patient should be prepared for transfer, both physically and mentally. As you are organizing the equipment and monitors, explain the transfer process to the patient and family. The explanation should include a description of the sensations the patient may expect, how long the procedure should last, and the role of individual members of the transport team. It is important to allay any patient or family anxiety by identifying current caregivers who will accompany the patient during transport. The availability of emergency equipment and drugs and how communication is handled during transportation also may be information that will reassure the patient and family.

Transport

Once preparations are complete, the actual transfer can begin. Ensure that the portable equipment has adequate battery life to last well beyond the anticipated transfer time in case of unanticipated delays. Connect each of the portable monitoring devices prior to disconnection from the bedside equipment, if possible. This enables a comparison of vital sign values with the portable equipment.

Once vital sign measurement equipment and noninvasive oxygenation monitors are in place and values verified, disconnect the patient from the bedside oxygen source and begin portable oxygenation. Assess for clinical signs and symptoms of respiratory distress and changes in ventilation and oxygenation. It may be easier to transfer the patient on the bed if it will fit in elevators and spaces in the receiving area. Check IV lines, pressure lines, monitor cables, NG tubes, chest tubes, urinary catheters, or drains of any sort to ensure proper placement during transport and to guard against accidental removal during transport.

Is there oxygen available in CT? Is there suction equipment in the CT suite? When would Imaging be ready to receive Mr. W?

Nancy gathered the portable equipment and connected it to Mr. W. This included a cardiac monitor, a blood pressure monitor, and a pulse oximeter. Intravenous lines were organized so that only essential infusions were transported with Mr. W. Other concerns that Nancy considered included: How long will the equipment batteries last? Will the water seal for the chest tube hang on the bed? Will he need suctioning? What medications does Mr. W need while he is off the progressive care unit? Does he need something for pain or his next dose of antibiotic? Will he need new IV fluids while he is gone? If he is able, does he understand the procedure that he's going to have? Where is his family? Do they know what is going on?

Fortunately for Nancy, one battery-operated machine was able to monitor pressures, cardiac rhythm, and pulse oximetry. The respiratory therapist brought high-flow oxygen equipment on the transport in case it was needed during the CT scan. The chest tube drain fit over the rail around the bed, maintaining the water seal without suction. The urinary catheter also had a special hook allowing it to hang safely on the side of the bed.

Mr. W was understandably anxious about what was going on, as was his wife.

2. Nancy talked to both of them about what to expect during the transport, as well as in the CT suite. She explained how long the procedure should last, and where Mrs. W's wife could wait while the procedure was in progress. She assured them that a nurse would be with Mr. W throughout the entire procedure and that any pain or discomfort would be adequately treated. She allowed Mr. W's wife to stay with her husband as long as possible during the transfer.

ESSENTIAL CONTENT CASE

Preparing for Transport

Having recognized and addressed Mr. W's risk factors, his nurse, Nancy, organized the team for the transport of Mr. W to CT scan, making sure another nurse was able to care for her other patients while she was off the unit. He needed a respiratory therapist during the transport. Other members of the transport team included two transporters to help manage the equipment, open doors, and hold elevators.

Case Question 1: Nancy decided to contact the Imaging Department prior to transporting Mr. W. What types of questions should she ask of the radiology nurse?

Case Question 2: What information could Nancy provide to Mr. W and his wife to allay some of their concerns?

Answers
1. Examples of questions that Nancy asked for clarification: Is there a nurse in the CT suite who can care for Mr. W once he arrives there? How long should she expect him to be gone from the progressive care unit? Are there electrical outlets for all the equipment in CT?

During transport, the progressive care nurse is responsible for continuous assessment of cardiopulmonary status (ie, electrocardiograph, blood pressures, respiration, oxygenation) and interventions as required to ensure stability. Throughout the time away from the progressive care environment, it is imperative that vigilant monitoring occurs regarding the patient's response not only to the transport, but also to the procedure or therapeutic intervention. Alterations in drug administration, particularly analgesics, sedatives, and vasoactive drugs, are frequently needed during the time away from the progressive care unit to maintain physiologic stability. Documentation of assessment findings, interventions, and the patient's responses should continue throughout the transport process.

Following return to the progressive care unit, monitoring systems and interventions are reestablished and the patient is completely reassessed. Often, some adjustment in pharmacologic therapy or oxygen support is required following transport. Allowing for some uninterrupted time for the family to be at the patient's bedside and for patient rest is another important priority following return to the unit. Documentation of the patient's overall response to the transport situation should be included in the medical record.

Interfacility Transfers

Interfacility patient transfers, although similar to transfers within a hospital, can be more challenging. The biggest differences between the two are the isolation of the patient in the transfer vehicle, limited equipment and personnel, and a high complication rate due to longer transport periods and inability to control environmental conditions (eg, temperature, atmospheric pressure, sudden movements), which may cause physiologic instability.

The primary consideration in interfacility transfer is maintaining the same level of care provided in the progressive care unit. Accordingly, the mode of transfer should be selected with this in mind. The resources available in the sending facility must be made as portable as possible and must accompany the patient; for example, ventricular assist devices must be continued without interruption. This requirement often challenges progressive care practitioners' skills and abilities, as well as the equipment resources necessary to ensure a safe transport.

TRANSITIONING TO THE NEXT STAGE OF CARE

Planning for transitioning of the patient to the next stage of care (eg, transfer from progressive care to rehabilitation) should begin soon after the patient is admitted to the progressive care unit. It involves assessing minimally where and with whom the patient lives, what external resources were being used prior to admission, and what resources are anticipated to be required on transfer out of the progressive care unit. Complex patients require extensive preplanning in achieving a successful transition. As the patient stabilizes and improves, the thought of leaving the progressive care unit can be frightening as it is perceived as moving to a level of care where there are fewer staff to monitor the patient. Reinforce the positive aspect of planning for the transition in that it is a sign that the patient is improving and making progress.

If the patient is transferring to another institution, such as an acute or subacute rehabilitation facility, consider having the family visit the facility prior to transfer. This gives them an opportunity to meet the new caregivers, ask any questions they may have, and be a positive influence to alleviate anxiety the patient may be experiencing about the transfer.

If the transfer is internal to another patient care unit and the patient's care is complex, consider working with the receiving unit staff in advance to inform them of the anticipated plan of care and any patient preferences. Identify a primary nurse in advance from the receiving unit, if possible, who may be able to take the time to meet the patient before

the transfer. Clinical nurse specialists or nurse managers may also be able to meet the patient and family, describe the receiving unit, and act as a resource after the transfer, again giving a sense of control to the patient and family.

SUPPORTING PATIENTS AND THEIR FAMILIES DURING THE DYING PROCESS

Transitioning of care also includes planning care for the patient who is dying. Caring for the dying patient and his or her family can be the most rewarding challenge. The use of advance directives provides a means for the acutely ill patient to communicate wishes regarding end-of-life issues. A dialogue with the patient about end-of-life care is an appropriate avenue for discussing values and beliefs associated with dying and living. Hopefully, discussions prior to a traumatic event or progressive care admission have occurred so the patient is empowered to institute stopping or continuing life-support measures and has designated a surrogate decision maker. If advance directives are in place, then advocating for those wishes and promoting comfort are primary responsibilities of clinicians. If previous discussions have not taken place, as with an unexpected traumatic accident, then requesting system resources to assist the family while you attend to the patient's critical needs is appropriate. Providing for clergy to assist with spiritual needs and rituals also can help the family to cope with the crisis.

It is important to have an awareness of your own philosophical feelings about death when caring for dying persons. Be genuine in your care, touch, and presence, and do not feel compelled to talk. Take your cue from the patient. Crying or laughing with the patient and family is an acknowledgment of humanness—an existential relationship and a rare gift in a unique encounter.

SELECTED BIBLIOGRAPHY

Family Interventions/Visitation

Agard AS, Lomberg K. Flexible family visitation in the intensive care unit: nurses' decision making. *J Clin Nurs.* 2010;20:1106-1114.

American Association of Critical-Care Nurses. AACN practice alert. Family presence: visitation in the adult ICU. 2011. Available at http://www.aacn.org/WD/practice/docs/practicealerts/family-visitation-adult-icu-practicealer. Accessed February 18, 2013.

American Association of Critical-Care Nurses. The AACN Synergy Model for patient care. Aliso Viejo, CA: AACN. Available at http://www.aacn.org/WD/Certifications/Content/synmodel.content?menu=Certification. Accessed February 18, 2103.

DeCourcey M, Russell AC, Keister KJ. Animal-assisted therapy. Evaluation and implementation of a complementary therapy to improve the psychological and physiological health of critically ill patients. *Dimens Crit Care Nurs.* 2010;29(5):211-214.

Duran DR, Oman KS, Abel JJ, Koziell VM, Szymanski D. Attitudes toward and beliefs about family presence: a survey of healthcare providers, patients' families, and patients. *Am J Crit Care.* 2007;16(3):270-282.

Hoghaug G, Fagermoen MS. Lerdal A. The visitor's regard of their need for support, comfort, information, proximity, and assurance in the intensive care unit. *Inten and Crit Care Nurs.* 2012;28(6):263-268.

Obringer K, Hilgenberg C, Booker K. Needs of adult family members of intensive care unit patients. *J Clin Nurs.* 2012;21(11-12):1651-1658.

Whitcomb J, Roy D, Blackman VS. Evidence-based practice in a military intensive care unit family visitation. *Nurs Res.* 2010; 59(1):S32-S39.

Infection Control

Center for Disease Control and Prevention. Improving surveillance for ventilator-associated events in adults. Overview and proposed new definition algorithm. Available at www.cdc.gov/nhsn/PDFs/vae/CDC_VAE_CommunicationSummary-for-compliance_20120313.pdf. Accessed February 18, 2013.

Bennett JV, Brockmann PS, eds. *Hospital Infections.* 5th ed. Philadelphia, PA: Lippincott Williams & Wilkins; 2007.

Gould CV, Umscheid CA, Argawal RK, et al. Guideline for prevention of catheter-related urinary tract infections, 2009. Available at http://www.cdc.gov/hicpac/cauti/001_cauti.html. Accessed February 18, 2013.

O'Grady NP, Alexander M, Burns LA, et al. Guidelines for the prevention of intravascular catheter-related infections, 2011. Available at http://www.cdc.gov/hicpac/BSI/BSI=guidelines-2100.html. Accessed February 18, 2013.

Siegel JD, Rhinehart E, Jackson M, et al. Management of multi-drug-resistant organisms in healthcare settings, 2006. Available at http://www.cdc.gov/hicpac/mdro/mdro_0.html. Accessed February 18, 2103.

Wenzel RP, ed. *Prevention and Control of Nosocomial Infections.* 4th ed. Baltimore, MD: Williams & Wilkins; 2002.

Patient and Family Education

Rankin SH, Stallings KD, London E. *Patient Education in Health and Illness.* 5th ed. Philadelphia, PA: Lippincott Williams & Wilkins; 2005.

Redman BK. *The Practice of Patient Education.* 10th ed. St. Louis, MO: Mosby-Elsevier; 2006.

Psychological Problems

Gorman LM, Sultan DF. *Psychosocial Nursing for General Patient Care.* Philadelphia, PA: FA Davis Co; 2008.

ICU Delirium and Cognitive Impairment Study Group. Vanderbilt University. http://www.icudelirium.org/. Accessed June 1, 2009.

Neufeld KJ, Bienvenu OJ, Rosenberg PB, et al. The Johns Hopkins Delirium Consortium: a model for collaborating across disciplines and departments for delirium prevention and treatment. *JAGS.* 2011;59:S244-S248.

Olson T. Delirium in the intensive care unit: role of the critical care nurse in early detection and treatment. *Dynamics.* 2012; 23(4):32-36.

Sendelbach S, Guthrie PF, Schoenfelder DP. Acute confusion/delirium. Identification, assessment, treatment, and prevention. *J Gerontol Nurs.* 2009;35(11):11-18.

Sleep Deprivation

Friese RS. Sleep and recovery from critical illness and injury: a review of theory, current practice, and future directions. *Crit Care Med.* 2008;36(3):697-705.

Jones C, Dawson D. Eye masks and earplugs improve patient's perception of sleep. *Crit Care Nurs.* 2012;17(5):247-254.

Patel M, Chipman J, Carlin BW, Shade D. Sleep in the intensive care unit setting. *Crit Care Nurse Q.* 2008;31(4):309-320.

Transport of Critically Ill Patients

Day D. Keeping patients safe during intrahospital transport. *Crit Care Nurs.* 2010;30(4):18-32.

Warren J, Fromm RE, Orr RA, et al. Guidelines for the inter- and intrahospital transport of critically ill patients. *Crit Care Med.* 2004;32:256-262.

Evidence-Based Practice

Agency for Healthcare Research and Quality. Preventing pressure ulcers in hospitals: a toolkit for improving quality of care. Available at www. ahrq.gov/research/ltc/pressureulcertoolkit/putool3a.html. Accessed February 18, 2103.

American Association of Critical-Care Nurses. AACN practice alert. Ventilator associated pneumonia. Aliso Viejo, CA: AACN. Available at http://www.aacn.org/WD/Practice/ Docs/PracticeAlerts/ventilator%20Associated%20Pneumonia%201-2008.pdf. Accessed February 18, 2013.

American Association of Critical-Care Nurses. *Protocols for Practice: Creating Healing Environments.* 2nd ed. Aliso Viejo, CA: AACN; 2007.

Barr J, Fraser GL, Puntillo K, et al. Clinical practice guidelines for the management of pain, agitation, and delirium in the intensive care unit. *Crit Care Med.* 2013;41(1):263-306.

Geerts WH, Bergqvist D, Piolo GF, et al. Prevention of venous thromboembolism. 8th ed. *CHEST.* 2008;133(suppl 6):381S-453S.

Sedwick MB, Lance-Smith M, Reeder SJ, Nardi J. Using evidence-based practice to prevent ventilator-associated pneumonia. *Crit Care Nurse.* 2012;32(4):41-50.

Wound, Ostomy, and Continence Nurses Society. *Guidelines for Prevention and Management of Pressure Ulcers.* Glenview, IL: WOCN; 2010.

INTERPRETATION AND MANAGEMENT OF BASIC CARDIAC RHYTHMS

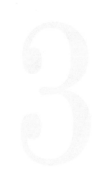

Carol Jacobson

KNOWLEDGE COMPETENCIES

1. Correctly identify key elements of electrocardiogram (ECG) waveforms, complexes, and intervals:
   • P wave
   • QRS complex
   • T wave
   • ST segment
   • PR interval
   • QT interval
   • RR interval
   • Rate (atrial and ventricular)

2. Compare and contrast the etiology, ECG characteristics, and management of common cardiac rhythms and conduction abnormalities:
   • Sinus node rhythms
   • Atrial rhythms
   • Junctional rhythms
   • Ventricular rhythms
   • AV blocks

3. Describe the indications for, and use of, temporary pacemakers, defibrillation, and cardioversion for the treatment of serious cardiac arrhythmias.

Continuous monitoring of cardiac rhythm in the critically or acutely ill patient is an important aspect of cardiovascular assessment. Frequent analysis of electrocardiogram (ECG) rate and rhythm provides for early identification and treatment of alternations in cardiac rhythm, as well as abnormal conditions in other body systems. This chapter presents a review of basic cardiac electrophysiology and information essential to the identification and treatment of common cardiac arrhythmias. Advanced cardiac arrhythmias, and 12-lead ECG interpretation, are described in Chapter 18, Advanced ECG Concepts.

BASIC ELECTROPHYSIOLOGY

The electrical impulse of the heart is the stimulus for cardiac contraction. The cardiac conduction system is responsible for the initiation of the electrical impulse and its sequential spread through the atria, atrioventricular (AV) junction, and ventricles. The conduction system of the heart consists of the following structures (Figure 3-1):

Sinus node: The sinus node is a small group of cells in the upper right atrium that functions as the normal pacemaker of the heart because it has the highest rate of automaticity of all potential pacemaker sites. The sinus node normally depolarizes at a regular rate of 60 to 100 times/min.

Atrioventricular (AV) node: The AV node is a small group of cells in the low right atrium near the tricuspid valve. The AV node has three main functions:

1. Its major job is to slow conduction of the impulse from the atria to the ventricles to allow time for the atria to contract and empty their blood into the ventricles.
2. Its rate of automaticity is 40 to 60 beats/min and can function as a backup pacemaker if the sinus node fails.
3. It screens out rapid atrial impulses to protect the ventricles from dangerously fast rates when the atrial rate is very rapid.

Bundle of His: The bundle of His is a short bundle of fibers at the bottom of the AV node leading to the bundle

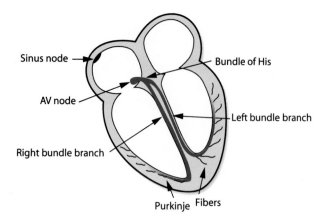

Figure 3-1. The conduction system of the heart.

branches. Conduction velocity accelerates in the bundle of His and the impulse is transmitted to both bundle branches.

Bundle branches: The bundle branches are bundles of fibers that rapidly conduct the impulse into the right and left ventricles. The *right bundle branch* travels along the right side of the interventricular septum and carries the impulse into the right ventricle. The *left bundle branch* has two main divisions: the anterior fascicle and the posterior fascicle, which carry the impulse into the left ventricle.

Purkinje fibers: The Purkinje fibers are hairlike fibers that spread out from the bundle branches along the endocardial

surface of both ventricles and rapidly conduct the impulse to the ventricular muscle cells. Cells in the Purkinje system have automaticity at a rate of 20 to 40 beats/min and can function as a backup pacemaker if all other pacemakers fail.

The electrical impulse normally begins in the sinus node and spreads through both atria in an inferior and leftward direction, resulting in depolarization of the atrial muscle. When the impulse reaches the AV node, its conduction velocity is slowed before it continues into the ventricles. When the impulse emerges from the AV node, it travels rapidly through the bundle of His and down the right and left bundle branches into the Purkinje network of both ventricles, and results in depolarization of the ventricular muscle. The spread of this wave of depolarization through the heart produces the classic surface ECG, which can be recorded by an electrocardiograph (ECG machine) or monitored continuously on a bedside cardiac monitor.

ECG WAVEFORMS, COMPLEXES, AND INTERVALS

The ECG waveforms, complexes, and intervals are illustrated in Figure 3-2.

P Wave

The P wave represents atrial muscle depolarization. It is normally 2.5 mm or less in height and 0.11 second or less in duration. P waves can be upright, inverted, or biphasic

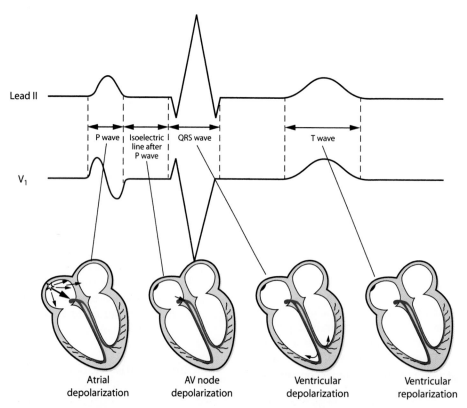

Figure 3-2. Electrocardiographic waves, complexes, and intervals in leads II and V₁.

depending on how the electrical impulse conducts through the atria and on which lead it is being recorded.

QRS Complex

The QRS complex represents ventricular muscle depolarization. A Q wave is an initial negative deflection from baseline. An R wave is the first positive deflection from baseline. An S wave is a negative deflection that follows an R wave. The shape of the QRS complex depends on the lead being recorded and the ventricular activation sequence; not all leads record all waves of the QRS complex. Regardless of the shape of the complex, ventricular depolarization waves are called QRS complexes (Figure 3-3). The width of the QRS complex represents intraventricular conduction time and is measured from the point at which it first leaves the baseline to the point at which the last wave ends. Normal QRS width is 0.04 to 0.10 second in an adult. When describing the shape of the QRS complex in writing, a capital letter is used when the voltage of a wave is 5 mm or more, and a lower case letter is used for smaller waves, as in Figure 3-3.

T Wave

The T wave represents ventricular muscle repolarization. It follows the QRS complex and is normally in the same direction as the QRS complex. T waves can be upright, flat, or inverted depending on many things, including the presence of myocardial ischemia, electrolyte levels, drug effect, myocardial disease, and the lead being recorded.

U Wave

The U wave is a small, rounded wave that sometimes follows the T wave and is thought to be due to repolarization of the M-cells (mid-myocardial cells) in the ventricles. U waves should be positive, especially when the T wave is positive. Large U waves can be seen when repolarization is abnormally prolonged, with hypokalemia, or with certain drugs.

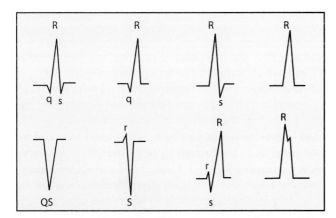

Figure 3-3. Examples of different configurations of QRS complexes. (*Jacobson C, Marzlin K, Webner C. Cardiovascular Nursing Practice: A Comprehensive Resource Manual and Study Guide for Clinical Nurses. Burien, WA: Cardiovascular Nursing Education Associates; 2007.*)

PR Interval

The PR interval is measured from the beginning of the P wave to the beginning of the QRS complex and represents the time required for the impulse to travel through the atria, AV junction, and to the Purkinje system. The normal PR interval in adults is 0.12 to 0.20 second. The PR segment extends from the end of the P wave to the beginning of the QRS complex.

ST Segment

The ST segment represents early ventricular repolarization. It begins at the end of the QRS complex (J point) and extends to the beginning of the T wave. The J point is where the QRS complex ends and the ST segment begins. The ST segment should be at the isoelectric line.

QT Interval

The QT interval measures the duration of ventricular depolarization and repolarization and varies with age, gender, and heart rate. The QT interval is measured from the beginning of the QRS complex to the end of the T wave. Because heart rate greatly affects the length of the QT interval, the QT interval must be corrected to a heart rate of 60 beats/min (QTc). This correction is usually done using the Bazett formula:

QTc = measured QT interval divided by the square root of the RR interval (all measurements in seconds)

The QTc should not exceed 0.45 second in men and 0.46 second in women.

BASIC ELECTROCARDIOGRAPHY

The ECG is a graphic record of the electrical activity of the heart. The spread of the electrical impulse through the heart produces weak electrical currents that can be detected and amplified by the ECG machine and recorded on calibrated graph paper. These amplified signals form the ECG tracing, consisting of the waveforms and intervals described previously, that are inscribed onto grid paper. The grid on the paper consists of a series of small and large boxes, both horizontal and vertical; horizontal boxes measure time, and vertical boxes measure voltage (Figure 3-4). On the horizontal axis, each small box is equal to 0.04 second, and each large box is equal to 0.20 second. On the vertical axis, each small box measures 1 mm and is equal to 0.1 mV; each large box measures 5 mm and is equal to 0.5 mV. In addition to the grid, most ECG papers place a vertical line in the top margin at 3-second intervals or place a mark at 1-second intervals.

CARDIAC MONITORING

Cardiac monitoring provides continuous observation of the patient's heart rate and rhythm and is a routine nursing procedure in all types of critical care and telemetry units as well

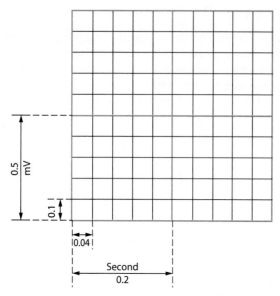

Figure 3-4. Time and voltage lines on ECG paper at standard paper speed of 25 mm/s. Horizontal axis measures time: each small box = 0.04 second, one large box = 0.20 second. Vertical axis measures voltage and also represents mm of ST segment deviation: each small box = 0.1 mV or 1 mm, one large box = 0.5 mV or 5 mm. (*Gilmore SB, Woods SL. Electrocardiography and vectorcardiography. In: Woods SL, Froelicher ES, Motzer SU, eds. Cardiac Nursing. 3rd ed. Philadelphia, PA: JB Lippincott; 1995:291.*)

as in emergency departments, postanesthesia recovery units, and many operating rooms. Cardiac monitoring has also become common in areas where patients receive treatments or procedures requiring conscious sedation or where the administration of certain medications could result in cardiac arrhythmias. The goals of cardiac monitoring can range from simple heart rate and basic rhythm monitoring to sophisticated arrhythmia diagnosis and ST-segment monitoring for cardiac ischemia detection. Cardiac monitoring can be done using a 3-wire, 5-wire, or 10-wire cable, which connects the patient to the cardiac monitor or portable telemetry box.

The choice of monitoring lead is based on the goals of monitoring in a particular patient population and by the patient's clinical situation. Because arrhythmias are the most common complication of ischemic heart disease and myocardial infarction (MI), monitoring for arrhythmia diagnosis is a priority in these patients. Although many arrhythmias can be recognized in any lead, research consistently shows that leads V_1 and V_6, or their bipolar equivalents MCL_1 and MCL_6, are the best leads for differentiating wide QRS rhythms (Table 3-1). The QRS morphologies displayed in these leads are useful in differentiating ventricular tachycardia (VT) from supraventricular tachycardia with aberrant intraventricular conduction and for recognizing right and left bundle branch block (see Chapter 18, Advanced ECG Concepts).

Correct placement of monitoring electrodes is critical to obtaining accurate information from any monitoring lead. Most currently available bedside monitors utilize either a 3-wire or a 5-wire monitoring cable. A 5-wire system offers several advantages over the 3-wire system (Table 3-2). With

TABLE 3-1. EVIDENCE-BASED PRACTICE: BEDSIDE CARDIAC MONITORING FOR ARRHYTHMIA DETECTION

Electrode Application

- Make sure skin is clean and dry before applying monitoring electrodes.
- Place arm electrodes on shoulder (front, top, or back) as close as possible to where arm joins torso.
- Place leg electrodes below the rib cage or on hips.
- Place V_1 electrode at the fourth intercostal space at right sternal border.
- Place V_6 electrode at the left midaxillary line at the V_4 level.
- Replace electrodes every 48 hours or more often if skin irritation occurs.
- Mark electrode position with indelible ink to ensure consistent lead placement.

Lead Selection

- Use lead V_1 as the primary arrhythmia monitoring lead whenever possible.
- Use lead V_6 if lead V_1 is not available.
- If using a 3-wire system, use MCL_1 as the primary lead and MCL_6 as the second choice lead.

Alarm Limits

- Set heart rate alarms as appropriate for patient's current heart rate and clinical condition.
- Never turn heart rate alarms off while patient's rhythm is being monitored.
- Set alarm limits on other parameters if using a computerized arrhythmia monitoring system.

Documentation

- Document the monitoring lead on every rhythm strip.
- Document heart rate, PR interval, QRS width, QT interval with every shift and with any significant rhythm change.
- Document rhythm strip with every significant rhythm change:
  – Onset and termination of tachycardias.
  – Symptomatic bradycardias or tachycardias.
  – Conversion into or out of atrial flutter or atrial fibrillation.
  – All rhythms requiring immediate treatment.
- Place rhythm strips flat on page (avoid folding or winding strips into chart).

Transporting Monitored Patients

- Continue cardiac monitoring using a portable, battery-operated monitor-defibrillator if patient is required to leave a monitored unit for diagnostic or therapeutic procedures.
- Monitored patients must be accompanied by a health-care provider skilled in ECG interpretation and defibrillation during transport.

Data from Jacobson (2010); Drew, Califf, Funk, et al (2004); and the American Association of Critical Care Nurses (2006).

a 5-wire system, it is possible to monitor more than one lead at a time and it is possible to monitor a true unipolar V_1 lead, which is superior to its bipolar equivalent MCL_1 in differentiating wide QRS rhythms. With a 5-wire system, all 12 standard ECG leads can be obtained by selecting the desired lead on the bedside monitor and moving the one chest lead to the appropriate spot on the thorax to record the precordial leads V_1 through V_6 (see Chapter 18, Advanced ECG Concepts). Figure 3-5 illustrates correct lead placement for a 5-wire system. Arm electrodes are placed on the shoulders as close as possible to where the arms join the torso. Placing the arm electrodes on the posterior shoulder keeps the anterior chest area clear for defibrillation paddles if needed, and avoids irritating the skin in the subclavicular area where an intravenous (IV) catheter might need to be placed.

TABLE 3-2. ADVANTAGES OF COMMON MONITORING LEADS

Lead	Advantages
Preferred Monitoring Leads	
V_1 and V_6 (or MCL_1 and MCL_6 if using a 3-wire system)	Differentiate between right and left bundle branch block
	Morphology clues to differentiate between ventricular beats and supraventricular beats with aberrant conduction
	Differentiate between right and left ventricular ectopy
	Differentiate between right and left ventricular pacing
	Usually shows well-formed P waves
	Placement of electrodes keeps apex clear for auscultation or defibrillation
Other Monitoring Leads	
Lead II	Usually shows well-formed P waves
	Often best lead for identification of atrial flutter waves
	Usually has tall, upright QRS complex on which to synchronize machine for cardioversion
	Allows identification of retrograde P waves
Lead III or aVF	Assists in diagnosis of hemiblock
	Allows identification of retrograde P waves
	Allows identification of atrial flutter waves
	Best limb leads for ST-segment monitoring
Lewis lead (negative electrode at second right intercostal space, positive electrode at fourth right intercostal space)	Often best lead to identify P waves

Leg electrodes are placed at the level of the lowest ribs on the thorax or on the hips. The desired V or precordial lead is obtained by placing the chest electrode at the appropriate location on the chest and selecting "V" on the bedside monitor. To monitor in V_1, place the chest electrode in the fourth intercostal space at the right sternal border. To monitor in V_6, place the chest electrode at the left midaxillary line at the V_4 level (V_4 level is fifth intercostal space, midclavicular line).

When using a 3-wire monitoring system with electrodes placed in their conventional locations on the right and left

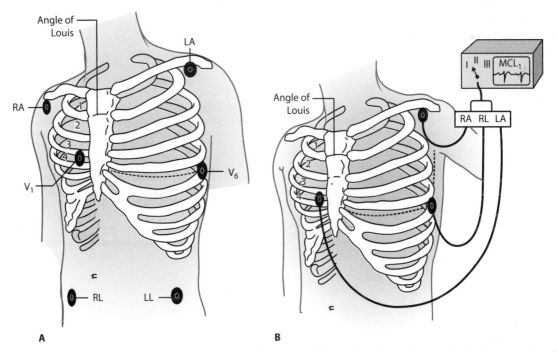

Figure 3-5. (A) Correct electrode placement for using a 5-wire monitoring cable. Right and left arm electrodes are placed on the shoulders and right and left leg electrodes are placed low on the thorax or on the hips. With the arm and leg electrodes placed as illustrated, leads I, II, III, aVR, aVL, and aVF can be obtained by selecting the desired lead on the bedside monitor. To obtain lead V_1 place the chest lead in the fourth intercostal space at the right sternal border and select "V" on the bedside monitor. To obtain lead V_6, place the chest lead at the level of V_4 in the left midaxillary line and select "V" on the bedside monitor. **(B)** Correct lead placement for obtaining MCL_1 and MCL_6 using a 3-wire lead system. Place the right arm electrode on the left shoulder; the left arm electrode in the fourth intercostal space at the right sternal border; and the left leg electrode at the level of V_4 in the left midaxillary line. To monitor in MCL_1, select lead I on the bedside monitor. To monitor in MCL_6, select lead II on the bedside monitor. (*Adapted from Drew BJ. Bedside electrocardiogram monitoring.* AACN Clin Issues Crit Care Nurs. *1993;4:26, 28.*)

shoulders and on the left hip or low thorax, leads I, II, or III can be monitored by selecting the desired lead on the bedside monitor. It is not possible to obtain a true unipolar V_1 or V_6 lead with a 3-wire system. In this case, the bipolar equivalents MCL_1 and MCL_6 can be used as substitutes for V_1 and V_6 but to obtain them requires placing electrodes in unconventional places. Figure 3-5 shows electrode placement for a 3-wire system that allows the user to monitor either MCL_1 or MCL_6. Place the right arm electrode on the left shoulder, the left arm electrode at the V_1 position (fourth intercostal space at the right sternal border), and the left leg electrode in the V_6 position (fifth intercostal space at the left midaxillary line). With electrodes in this position, select "lead I" on the monitor to obtain MCL_1 and switch to lead II on the monitor to record MCL_6.

The electrode sites on the skin should be clean, dry, and relatively flat. Shave hair, if present, and clean the skin with alcohol to remove any oils. Mildly abrade the skin with a gauze or abrading pad supplied on electrode packaging to improve transmission of the ECG signal. Apply the pregelled electrodes to the chest in the appropriate locations. Set the heart rate alarm limits based on the patient's clinical situation and current heart rate. Bedside monitoring systems have default alarms that adjust the high- and low-rate limits based on the learned heart rate. Electrodes are changed often enough to prevent skin breakdown and provide artifact-free tracings.

DETERMINATION OF THE HEART RATE

Heart rate can be obtained from the ECG strip by several methods. The first, and most accurate if the rhythm is regular, is to count the number of small boxes (one small box = 0.04 second) between two R waves, and then divide that number into 1500. There are 1500 boxes of 0.04-second interval in a 1-minute strip (Figure 3-6A). Another method is to count the number of large boxes (one large box = 0.20 second) between two R waves, and then divide that number into 300 or use a standardized table (Table 3-3).

The third method for computing heart rate, especially useful when the rhythm is irregular, is to count the number of RR intervals in 6 seconds and multiply that number by 10. The ECG paper is usually marked at 3-second intervals (15 large boxes horizontally) by a vertical line at the top of the paper (Figure 3-6B). The RR intervals are counted, not the QRS complexes, to avoid overestimating the heart rate.

Any of these three methods can also be used to calculate the atrial rate by using P waves instead of R waves.

DETERMINATION OF CARDIAC RHYTHM

Correct determination of the cardiac rhythm requires a systematic evaluation of the ECG. The following steps are used to determine the cardiac rhythm:

1. Calculate the atrial (P wave) rate.
2. Calculate the ventricular (QRS complex) rate.
3. Determine the regularity and shape of the P waves.
4. Determine the regularity, shape, and width of the QRS complexes.
5. Measure the PR interval.
6. Interpret the arrhythmia as described later.

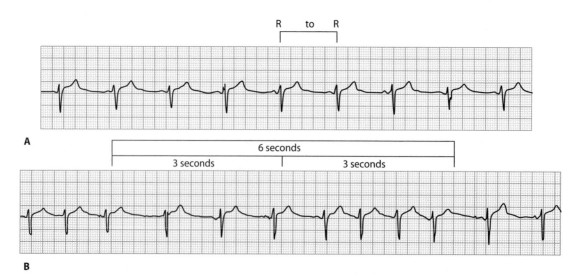

Figure 3-6. **(A)** Heart rate determination for a regular rhythm using little boxes between two R waves. One RR interval is marked at the top of the ECG paper. There are 25 little boxes between these two R waves. There are 1500 little boxes in a 60-second strip. By dividing 1500 by 25, one calculates a heart rate of 60 beats/min. Heart rate can also be determined for a regular rhythm counting large boxes between R waves. There are five large boxes between R waves. There are 300 large boxes in a 60-second strip. By dividing 300 by 5, one calculates a heart rate of 60 beats/min. **(B)** Heart rate determination for a regular or irregular rhythm using the number of RR intervals in a 6-second strip and multiplying by 10. There are seven RR intervals in this example. Multiplying by 10 gives a heart rate of 70 beats/min. (*Gilmore SB, Woods SL. Electrocardiography and vectorcardiography. In: Woods SL, Froelicher ES, Motzer SU, eds. Cardiac Nursing. 3rd ed. Philadelphia, PA: JB Lippincott; 1995:295.*)

TABLE 3-3. HEART RATE DETERMINATION USING THE ELECTROCARDIOGRAM LARGE BOXES

Number of Large Boxes Between R Waves	Heart Rate (beats/min)
1	300
2	150
3	100
4	75
5	60
6	50
7	40
8	38
9	33
10	30

COMMON ARRHYTHMIAS

An *arrhythmia* is any cardiac rhythm that is not normal sinus rhythm. An arrhythmia may result from altered impulse formation or altered impulse conduction. The term *ectopic* refers to any beat or rhythm that arises from a location other than the sinus node. Ectopic beats can arise in the atria, AV junction, or ventricles. Arrhythmias are named by the place where they originate and by their rate. Arrhythmias are grouped as rhythms originating:

1. in the sinus node.
2. in the atria.
3. in the AV junction.
4. in the ventricle.
5. AV blocks

The etiology, ECG characteristics, and treatment of the basic cardiac arrhythmias are presented here and summarized in Chapter 26, Cardiac Rhythms, ECG Characteristics, and Treatment Guide.

RHYTHMS ORIGINATING IN THE SINUS NODE

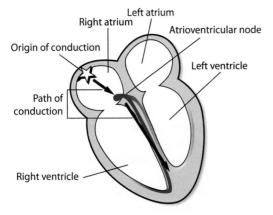

Figure 3-7. Rhythms originating in the sinus node.

Normal Sinus Rhythm

ECG Characteristics

- *Rate:* 60 to 100 beats/min.
- *Rhythm:* Regular.
- *P waves:* Precede every QRS complex; consistent in shape.
- *PR interval:* 0.12 to 0.20 second.
- *QRS complex:* 0.04 to 0.10 second.
- *Conduction:* Normal through atria, AV node, bundle branches, and ventricles.
- *Example of normal sinus rhythm:* Figure 3-8.

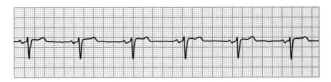

Figure 3-8. Normal sinus rhythm.

Sinus Bradycardia

All aspects of sinus bradycardia are the same as normal sinus rhythm except the rate is slower. It can be a normal finding in athletes and during sleep. Sinus bradycardia may be a response to vagal stimulation, such as carotid sinus massage, ocular pressure, or vomiting. Sinus bradycardia can be caused by inferior MI, myxedema, obstructive jaundice, uremia, increased intracranial pressure, glaucoma, anorexia nervosa, and sick sinus syndrome. Sinus bradycardia can be a response to several medications, including digitalis, beta-blockers, and some calcium channel blockers.

ECG Characteristics

- *Rate:* Less than 60 beats/min.
- *Rhythm:* Regular.
- *P waves:* Precede every QRS; consistent in shape.
- *PR interval:* Usually normal (0.12-0.20 second).
- *QRS complex:* Usually normal (0.04-0.10 second).
- *Conduction:* Normal through atria, AV node, bundle branches, and ventricles.
- *Example of sinus bradycardia:* Figure 3-9.

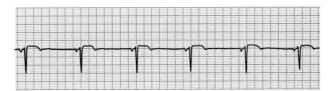

Figure 3-9. Sinus bradycardia.

Treatment

Treatment of sinus bradycardia is not required unless the patient is symptomatic. If the arrhythmia is accompanied by hypotension, confusion, diaphoresis, chest pain, or other signs of hemodynamic compromise or by ventricular ectopy, 0.5 mg of atropine IV is the treatment of choice. Attempts are made to decrease vagal stimulation. If the arrhythmia is due to medications, they are held until their need has been reevaluated. Temporary or permanent pacing may be necessary.

Sinus Tachycardia

Sinus tachycardia is a sinus rhythm at a rate greater than 100 beats/min. Sinus tachycardia is a normal response to exercise and emotion. Sinus tachycardia that persists at rest usually indicates some underlying problem, such as fever, acute blood loss, shock, pain, anxiety, heart failure, hypermetabolic states, or anemia. Sinus tachycardia is a normal physiologic response to a decrease in cardiac output; cardiac output is the product of heart rate and stroke volume. Sinus tachycardia can be caused by the following medications: atropine, isoproterenol, epinephrine, dopamine, dobutamine, norepinephrine, nitroprusside, and caffeine.

ECG Characteristics

- *Rate:* Greater than 100 beats/min.
- *Rhythm:* Regular.
- *P waves:* Precede every QRS; consistent in shape; may be buried in the preceding T wave.
- *PR interval:* Usually normal; may be difficult to measure if P waves are buried in T waves.
- *QRS complex:* Usually normal.
- *Conduction:* Normal through atria, AV node, bundle branches, and ventricles.
- *Example of sinus tachycardia:* Figure 3-10.

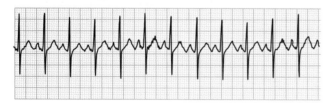

Figure 3-10. Sinus tachycardia.

Treatment

Treatment of sinus tachycardia is directed at the underlying cause. This arrhythmia is a physiologic response to a decrease in cardiac output, and it should never be ignored, especially in the cardiac patient. Because the ventricles fill with blood and the coronary arteries perfuse during diastole, persistent tachycardia can cause decreased stroke volume, decreased cardiac output, and decreased coronary perfusion secondary to the decreased diastolic time that occurs with rapid heart rates. Carotid sinus pressure may slow the heart rate temporarily and thereby help in ruling out other arrhythmias.

Sinus Arrhythmia

Sinus arrhythmia occurs when the sinus node discharges irregularly. It occurs frequently as a normal phenomenon and is commonly associated with the phases of respiration. During inspiration, the sinus node fires faster; during expiration, it slows. Digitalis toxicity may also cause this arrhythmia. Sinus arrhythmia looks like normal sinus rhythm except for the sinus irregularity.

ECG Characteristics

- *Rate:* 60 to 100 beats/min.
- *Rhythm:* Irregular; phasic increase and decrease in rate, which may or may not be related to respiration.
- *P waves:* Precede every QRS complex; consistent in shape.
- *PR interval:* Usually normal.
- *QRS complex:* Usually normal.
- *Conduction:* Normal through atria, AV node, bundle branches, and ventricles.
- *Example of sinus arrhythmia:* Figure 3-11.

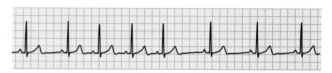

Figure 3-11. Sinus arrhythmia.

Treatment

Treatment of sinus arrhythmia usually is not necessary. If the arrhythmia is thought to be because of digitalis toxicity, then digitalis is held. Atropine increases the rate and eliminates the irregularity.

Sinus Arrest

Sinus arrest occurs when sinus node firing is depressed and impulses are not formed when expected. The result is an absent P wave at the expected time. The QRS complex is also missing, unless there is escape of a junctional or ventricular impulse. If only one sinus impulse fails to form, this is usually called a *sinus pause.* If more than one sinus impulse in a row fails to form, this is termed a *sinus arrest.* Because the sinus node is not forming impulses regularly as expected, the PP interval in sinus arrest is not an exact multiple of the sinus cycle. Causes of sinus arrest include vagal stimulation, carotid sinus sensitivity, and MI interrupting the blood supply to the sinus node. Drugs such as digitalis, beta-blockers, and calcium channel blockers can also cause sinus arrest.

ECG Characteristics

- *Rate:* Usually within normal range but may be in the bradycardia range.
- *Rhythm:* Irregular due to absence of sinus node discharge.
- *P waves:* Present when sinus node is firing and absent during periods of sinus arrest. When present, they precede every QRS complex and are consistent in shape.

- *PR interval:* Usually normal when P waves are present.
- *QRS complex:* Usually normal when sinus node is functioning and absent during periods of sinus arrest, unless escape beats occur.
- *Conduction:* Normal through atria, AV node, bundle branches, and ventricles when sinus node is firing. When the sinus node fails to form impulses, there is no conduction through the atria.
- *Example of sinus arrest:* Figure 3-12.

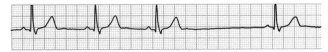

Figure 3-12. Sinus arrest.

Treatment

Treatment of sinus arrest is aimed at the underlying cause. Drugs that are thought to be responsible are discontinued and vagal stimulation is minimized. If periods of sinus arrest are frequent and cause hemodynamic compromise, 0.5 mg of atropine IV may increase the rate. Pacemaker therapy may be necessary if other forms of management fail to increase the rate to acceptable levels.

ARRHYTHMIAS ORIGINATING IN THE ATRIA

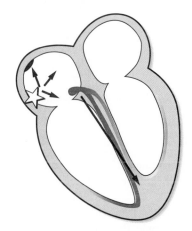

Figure 3-13. Arrhythmias originating in the atria.

Premature Atrial Complexes

A premature atrial complex (PAC) occurs when an irritable focus in the atria fires before the next sinus node impulse is due to fire. PACs can be caused by caffeine, alcohol, nicotine, heart failure (HF), pulmonary disease, interruption of atrial blood supply by myocardial ischemia or infarction, anxiety, and hypermetabolic states. PACs can also occur in normal hearts.

ECG Characteristics

- *Rate:* Usually within normal range.
- *Rhythm:* Usually regular except when PACs occur, resulting in early beats. PACs usually have a noncompensatory pause (interval between the complex preceding and that following the PAC is less than two normal RR intervals) because premature depolarization of the atria by the PAC usually causes premature depolarization of the sinus node as well, thus causing the sinus node to "reset" itself.
- *P waves:* Precede every QRS complex. The configuration of the premature P wave differs from that of the sinus P waves because the premature impulse originates in a different part of the atria, with atrial depolarization occurring in a different pattern. Very early P waves may be buried in the preceding T wave.
- *PR interval:* May be normal or long depending on the prematurity of the beat; very early PACs may find the AV junction still partially refractory and unable to conduct at a normal rate, resulting in a prolonged PR interval.
- *QRS complex:* May be normal, aberrant (wide) or absent, depending on the prematurity of the beat. If the ventricles have repolarized completely, they will be able to conduct the early impulse normally, resulting in a normal QRS. If the PAC occurs during the relative refractory period of the AV node, bundle branches or ventricles, the impulse will conduct aberrantly and the QRS will be wide. If the PAC occurs very early during the complete refractory period of the AV node, bundle branches or ventricles, the impulse will not conduct to the ventricles and the QRS will be absent.
- *Conduction:* PACs travel through the atria differently from sinus impulses because they originate from a different spot; conduction through the AV node, bundle branches, and ventricles is usually normal unless the PAC is very early.
- *Example of PAC:* Figure 3-14A, B.

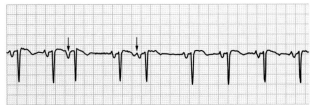

A

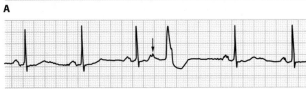

B

Figure 3-14. (A) PAC conducted normally in the ventricle. **(B)** PAC conducted aberrantly in the ventricle.

Treatment

Treatment of PACs usually is not necessary because they do not cause hemodynamic compromise. Frequent PACs may precede more serious arrhythmias such as atrial fibrillation. Treatment is directed at the cause. Drugs such as beta-blockers, disopyramide, procainamide, flecainide, and propafenone can be used to suppress atrial activity, but this is rarely necessary.

Wandering Atrial Pacemaker

Wandering atrial pacemaker (WAP) refers to rhythms that exhibit varying P-wave morphology as the site of impulse formation shifts from the sinus node to various sites in the atria or into the AV junction. This occurs when two (usually sinus and junctional) or more supraventricular pacemakers compete with each other for control of the heart. Because the rates of these competing pacemakers are almost identical, it is common to have atrial fusion occur as the atria are activated by more than one wave of depolarization at a time, resulting in varying P-wave morphology. Wandering atrial pacemaker can be due to increased vagal tone that slows the sinus pacemaker or to enhanced automaticity in atrial or junctional pacemaker cells, causing them to compete with the sinus node for control.

ECG Characteristics

- *Rate:* 60 to 100 beats/min. If the rate is faster than 100 beats/min, it is called *multifocal atrial tachycardia* (MAT).
- *Rhythm:* May be slightly irregular.
- *P waves:* Varying shapes (upright, flat, inverted, notched) as impulses originate in different parts of the atria or junction. At least three different P-wave shapes should be seen.
- *PR interval:* May vary depending on proximity of the pacemaker to the AV node.
- *QRS complex:* Usually normal.
- *Conduction:* Conduction through the atria varies as they are depolarized from different spots. Conduction through the bundle branches and ventricles is usually normal.
- *Example of WAP:* Figure 3-15.

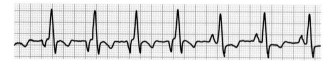

Figure 3-15. Wandering atrial pacemaker.

Treatment

Treatment of WAP usually is not necessary. If slow heart rates lead to symptoms, atropine can be given. Treatment of MAT is directed toward eliminating the cause, including hypoxia and electrolyte imbalances. Antiarrhythmic therapy is often ineffective. Beta-blockers, verapamil, flecainide, amiodarone, and magnesium may be successful.

Atrial Tachycardia

Atrial tachycardia (AT) is a rapid atrial rhythm occurring at a rate of 120 to 250 beats/min and can be due to abnormal automaticity or to reentry within the atrium (Figure 3-16). When the arrhythmia abruptly starts and terminates, it is called *paroxysmal atrial tachycardia*. Rapid atrial rate can be caused by emotions, caffeine, tobacco, alcohol, fatigue, or sympathomimetic drugs. Whenever the atrial rate is rapid, the AV node begins to block some of the impulses attempting to travel through it to protect the ventricles from excessively rapid rates. In normal healthy hearts, the AV node can usually conduct each atrial impulse up to rates of about 180 to 200 beats/min. In patients with cardiac disease or who are on AV nodal blocking drugs such as digitalis, beta blockers or calcium channel blockers, the AV node may not be able to conduct each impulse and AT with block occurs. Atrial tachycardia with block may indicate digitalis toxicity.

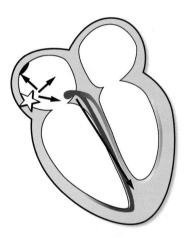

Figure 3-16. Atrial tachycardia.

ECG Characteristics

- *Rate:* Atrial rate is 120 to 250 beats/min.
- *Rhythm:* Regular unless there is variable block at the AV node.
- *P waves:* Differ in shape from sinus P waves because they are ectopic. Precede each QRS complex but may be hidden in preceding T wave. When block is present, more than one P wave will appear before each QRS complex.
- *PR interval:* May be shorter than normal but often difficult to measure because of hidden P waves.
- *QRS complex:* Usually normal but may be wide if aberrant conduction is present.
- *Conduction:* Usually normal through the AV node and into the ventricles. In atrial tachycardia with block, some atrial impulses do not conduct into the ventricles. Aberrant ventricular conduction may

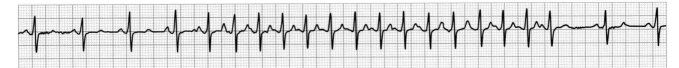

Figure 3-17. Atrial tachycardia.

occur if atrial impulses are conducted into the ventricles while the bundle branches or ventricles are still partially refractory.

- *Example of atrial tachycardia:* Figure 3-17.

Treatment

Treatment of AT is directed at eliminating the cause, if possible, controlling the ventricular rate, and reestablishing sinus rhythm. If the patient is hemodynamically unstable due to a rapid AT, cardioversion can be attempted, although automatic ATs usually do not respond to cardioversion. Some ATs may terminate with IV adenosine, but more often IV verapamil or diltiazem, or an IV beta-blocker, is used for acute therapy to slow the ventricular rate, and they may occasionally terminate the AT. Other drugs that can be tried to suppress AT are procainamide, flecainide, propafenone, amiodarone, or sotalol. Catheter ablation is a class I recommendation for preventing recurrent AT. See Table 3-4 for class I recommendations for management of AT.

Atrial Flutter

In atrial flutter (Figure 3-18) the atria are depolarized at rates of 250 to 350 times/min. Classic or typical atrial flutter is due to a fixed reentry circuit in the right atrium around which the impulse circulates in a counterclockwise direction, resulting in negative flutter waves in leads II and III and an atrial rate between 250 and 350 beats/min (most commonly 300 beats/min). At such rapid atrial rates, the AV node usually blocks at least half of the impulses to protect the ventricles from excessive rates. Causes of atrial flutter include rheumatic heart disease, atherosclerotic heart disease, thyrotoxicosis, heart failure, and myocardial ischemia or infarction. Because the

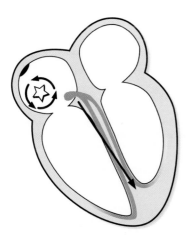

Figure 3-18. Atrial flutter.

ventricular rate in atrial flutter can be quite fast, symptoms associated with decreased cardiac output can occur. Mural thrombi may form in the atria due to the fact that there is no strong atrial contraction, and blood stasis occurs, leading to a risk of systemic or pulmonary emboli.

ECG Characteristics

- *Rate:* Atrial rate varies between 250 and 350 beats/min, most commonly 300. Ventricular rate varies depending on the amount of block at the AV node. New onset atrial flutter usually has a ventricular rate around 150 beats/min, and rarely 300 beats/min if 1:1 conduction occurs to the ventricles. With AV nodal blocking drug therapy, the ventricular rate is usually in the normal range, commonly around 75 beats/min.
- *Rhythm:* Atrial rhythm is regular. Ventricular rhythm may be regular or irregular because of varying AV block.
- *F waves:* F waves (flutter waves) are seen, characterized by a very regular, "sawtooth" pattern. One F wave is usually hidden in the QRS complex, and when 2:1 conduction occurs, F waves may not be readily apparent.
- *FR interval (flutter wave to the beginning of the QRS complex):* May be consistent or may vary.
- *QRS complex:* Usually normal; aberration can occur.
- *Conduction:* Usually normal through the AV node and ventricles.
- *Example of atrial flutter:* Figure 3-19A, B.

Treatment

The immediate goal of treatment depends on the hemodynamic consequences of the arrhythmia. Ventricular rate control is the priority if cardiac output is markedly compromised due to rapid ventricular rates. Electrical (direct current) cardioversion may be necessary as an immediate treatment, especially if 1:1 conduction occurs. IV calcium channel blockers (verapamil or diltiazem) or beta-blockers can be used for ventricular rate control. Conversion to sinus rhythm can be accomplished by electrical cardioversion, drug therapy, or overdrive atrial pacing. Drug therapy for atrial flutter is the same as that for atrial fibrillation and is discussed in the next section on atrial fibrillation. Drugs that slow the atrial rate, like flecainide or propafenone, should not be used unless the ventricular rate has been controlled with an AV nodal blocking agent (a calcium channel blocker, beta-blocker, or digitalis). The danger of giving these drugs alone is that the atrial rate may decrease from 300 beats/min to a slower rate, making it possible for the AV node to conduct each impulse and resulting in even faster ventricular rates (Table 3-4).

TABLE 3-4. GUIDELINES FOR MANAGEMENT OF SUPRAVENTRICULAR ARRHYTHMIAS (CLASS I RECOMMENDATIONS ONLY)

Acute Management of Hemodynamically Stable and Regular Tachycardia

Narrow QRS (SVT) and SVT with BBB
1. Vagal maneuvers (Valsalva, CSM) (level B)
2. Adenosine (level A)
3. Verapamil, diltiazem (level A)

Preexcited SVT/AF
1. Flecainide (level B)
2. Ibutilide (level B)
3. Procainamide (level B)
4. Electrical cardioversion (level C)

Wide QRS Tachycardia of Unknown Origin
1. Procainamide (level B)
2. Sotalol (level B)
3. Amiodarone (level B)
4. Electrical cardioversion (level B)

Wide QRS Tachycardia of Unknown Origin in Patients with Poor LV Function
1. Amiodarone (level B)
2. Lidocaine (level B)
3. Electrical cardioversion (level B)

Long-Term Treatment of Recurrent AVNRT
1. Catheter ablation (level B)
2. Verapamil for recurrent symptomatic AVNRT (level B)
3. Diltiazem or beta-blockers for recurrent symptomatic AVNRT (level C)

Infrequent, well-tolerated episodes of AVNRT
1. Vagal maneuvers (level B)
2. Pill-in-the-pocket (single dose oral diltiazem plus propranolol) (level B)
3. Verapamil, diltiazem, beta-blockers, catheter ablation (level B)

Focal and Nonparoxysmal Junctional Tachycardia Syndromes

There are no class I recommendations for focal junctional tachycardia.
Nonparoxysmal junctional tachycardia
1. Reverse digitalis toxicity (level C)
2. Correct hypokalemia (level C)
3. Treat myocardial ischemia (level C)

Long-Term Therapy of Accessory Pathway-Mediated Arrhythmias

1. Catheter ablation for WPW syndrome (preexcitation and symptomatic arrhythmias) that are well tolerated; or with AF and rapid conduction or poorly tolerated CMT (level B)
2. Vagal maneuvers for single or infrequent episodes (level B)
3. Pill-in-the-pocket (verapamil, diltiazem, beta-blockers) for single or infrequent episodes with no pre-excitation (level B)
CONTRAINDICATED: verapamil, diltiazem, digoxin when preexcitation is present.

Treatment of Focal Atrial Tachycardia

Acute Treatment
1. Electrical cardioversion if hemodynamically unstable (level B)
2. Beta-blockers, verapamil, diltiazem for rate control (in absence of digitalis therapy) (level C)
Prophylactic Therapy
1. Catheter ablation for recurrent symptomatic or incessant AT (level B)
2. Beta-blockers, verapamil, diltiazem (level C)
Level of Evidence Definitions
Level A: Data derived from multiple randomized clinical trials or meta-analyses.
Level B: Data derived from a single randomized trial or nonrandomized studies.
Level C: Only consensus opinion of experts, case studies, or standard-of-care.

Source: *Blomstrom-Lundqvist, C, Scheinman, MM, Aliot, EM, Alpert, JS, Calkins, H, Camm, JA, et al. ACC/AHA/ESC Guidelines for the Management of Patients with Supraventricular Arrhythmias - Executive Summary. A Report of the American College of Cardiology/American Heart Association Task Force on Practice Guidelines and the European Society of Cardiology Committee for Practice Guidelines (Writing Committee to Develop Guidelines for the Management of Patients With Supraventricular Arrhythmias). Circulation, 2003, 108,* 1871-1909.

Abbreviations used in this table: AT: atrial tachycardia; AVNRT: atrioventricular nodal reentry tachycardia; BBB: bundle branch block; CMT: circus movement tachycardia; LV: left ventricular; SVT: supraventricular tachycardia.

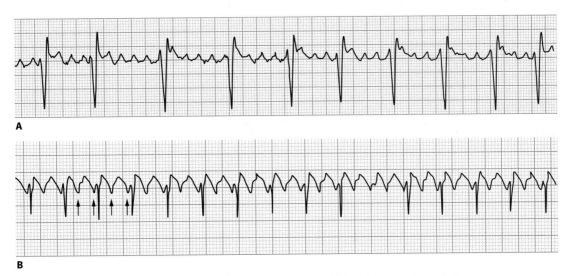

Figure 3-19. (A) Atrial flutter with 4:1 and 5:1 conduction. **(B)** Atrial flutter with 2:1 conduction.

Atrial Fibrillation

Atrial fibrillation (AF) is an extremely rapid and disorganized pattern of depolarization in the atria, and is the most common arrhythmia seen in clinical practice (Figure 3-20). Atrial fibrillation commonly occurs in the presence of atherosclerotic or rheumatic heart disease, thyroid disease, HF, cardiomyopathy, valve disease, pulmonary disease, MI, congenital heart disease, and after cardiac surgery. Atrial fibrillation is classified into three categories: *paroxysmal*, episodes that last < 7 days and often < 24 hours; *persistent*, episodes that last > 7 days and often require electrical or pharmacological cardioversion; and *permanent*, longstanding AF that is usually present for more than a year and has failed cardioversion or in which cardioversion is considered futile. The term *recurrent* is used when the patient has two or more episodes of AF, and the term *lone AF* is used when AF occurs in the absence of cardiac disease or any other known cause (usually in people < 60 years of age). Nonvalvular AF occurs in patients without mitral valve disease, prosthetic valve, or history of valve surgery.

Atrial fibrillation has several adverse consequences that require prompt recognition and treatment in order to prevent complications:

1. Decreased cardiac output due to loss of atrial kick, rapid ventricular rate, and irregular ventricular rhythm. Cardiac output is dependent on adequate ventricular filling, and the loss of atrial contraction and the rapid ventricular rate that commonly occurs in AF contribute to reduced ventricular filling.
2. Tachycardia-induced cardiomyopathy can occur whenever the ventricular rate is rapid for a prolonged period of time. This is more common in asymptomatic patients who are unaware that they are in AF.
3. Thromboembolism because of formation of clots in the fibrillating atria, usually in the left atrial appendage. Stroke is the most common and potentially devastating embolic event, but pulmonary embolus and embolization to any other part of the body can also occur.

ECG Characteristics

- *Rate:* Atrial rate is 400 to 600 beats/min or faster. Ventricular rate varies depending on the amount of block at the AV node. In new AF, the ventricular response is usually quite rapid, 160 to 200 beats/min; in treated atrial fibrillation, the ventricular rate is controlled in the normal range of 60 to 100 beats/min.
- *Rhythm:* Irregular; one of the distinguishing features of AF is the marked irregularity of the ventricular response.
- *F waves:* Not present; atrial activity is chaotic with no formed atrial impulses visible; irregular F waves are often seen, and vary in size from coarse to very fine.
- *PR interval:* Not measurable; there are no P waves.

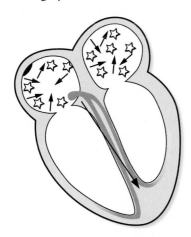

Figure 3-20. Atrial fibrillation.

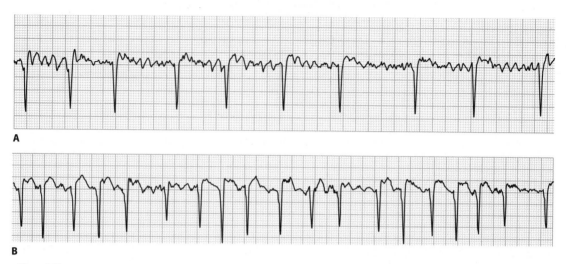

Figure 3-21. **(A)** Atrial fibrillation with a controlled ventricular response. **(B)** Atrial fibrillation with an uncontrolled ventricular response.

- *QRS complex:* Usually normal; aberration is common.
- *Conduction:* Conduction within the atria is disorganized and follows a very irregular pattern. Most of the atrial impulses are blocked within the AV junction. Those impulses that are conducted through the AV junction are usually conducted normally through the ventricles. If an atrial impulse reaches the bundle branch system during its refractory period, aberrant intraventricular conduction can occur.
- *Example of atrial fibrillation:* Figure 3-21 A, B.

Pharmacological Treatment of Atrial Fibrillation

Treatment of AF is directed toward eliminating the cause, controlling ventricular rate, restoring and maintaining sinus rhythm, and preventing thromboembolism. The American College of Cardiology, American Heart Association, European Society of Cardiology, and the Heart Rhythm Society have collaborated to publish guidelines for the management of AF. The American Heart Association and American Stroke Association released a science advisory on oral antithrombotic drugs for the prevention of stroke in nonvalvular atrial fibrillation in 2011. See Table 3-5 for the guidelines class I recommendations for management of AF.

Ventricular rate control is aimed at improving hemodynamics and relieving symptoms. New onset AF often results in a very rapid ventricular rate that can be mildly to moderately symptomatic or cause extreme hemodynamic instability. Patients with Wolff-Parkinson-White (WPW) syndrome have an accessory pathway that can conduct atrial fibrillation impulses directly into the ventricle via the accessory pathway, resulting in an extremely rapid ventricular rate that can cause ventricular fibrillation and sudden cardiac death (see Chapter 18). In the unstable patient, ventricular rate control is a priority, and electrical cardioversion may be necessary if the patient is hemodynamically unstable because of rapid ventricular rate. Intravenous calcium channel blockers

(eg, diltiazem, verapamil) and beta-blockers are commonly used in the acute situation for ventricular rate control but should be used with caution in the presence of heart failure or hypotension and are contraindicated if WPW is present. Beta-blockers, calcium channel blockers, and digitalis can be used orally for long-term rate control.

Rhythm control is restoration of sinus rhythm using pharmacologic or electrical cardioversion, and maintenance of sinus rhythm using antiarrhythmic drugs. Antiarrhythmic drugs with a class I recommendation for pharmacological cardioversion of AF are flecainide, dofetilide, propafenone, and ibutilide; amiodarone is a class IIa recommendation. Drug therapy is most effective in restoring sinus rhythm when started within 7 days of AF onset. There are no drugs with a class I recommendation for maintenance of sinus rhythm, but several antiarrhythmics can be effective, including amiodarone, dofetilide, dronedarone, flecainide, propafenone, and sotalol. Oral beta-blocker therapy is often used to try to prevent postoperative AF in patients undergoing cardiac surgery. Refer to specific drug guidelines for patient selection criteria.

Preventing thromboembolism is a goal in all patients with AF regardless of rhythm or rate control strategy. Antithrombotic therapy is recommended for all patients with AF, except those with lone AF or those with contraindications. The risk of stroke must be weighed against the risk of bleeding when considering drug therapy for thromboembolism prevention. The CHADS2 risk index is commonly used to assess stroke risk in AF patients: C = congestive heart failure, H = hypertension, A = age > 75 years, D = diabetes, and S = history of stroke or TIA. CHADS2 assigns 2 points for a history of stroke or TIA and 1 point for each of the other risk factors. Oral anticoagulation with warfarin to maintain INR between 2.0 and 3.0 (target INR = 2.5) is the usual recommendation for patients with a CHADS2 score of 2 or higher. Aspirin or aspirin with clopidogrel is an alternative in low

TABLE 3-5. GUIDELINES FOR MANAGEMENT OF ATRIAL FIBRILLATION AND ATRIAL FLUTTER (CLASS I RECOMMENDATIONS ONLY)

Pharmacological Rate Control During Atrial Fibrillation

1. Control of rate using either a beta-blocker or nondihydropyridine CCB (in most cases) for patients with persistent or permanent AF. (level B)
2. Administration of AV nodal blocking agents is recommended to achieve rate control in patients who develop postoperative AF. (level B)
3. In the absence of preexcitation, IV administration of beta-blockers (esmolol, metoprolol, or propranolol) or nondihydropyridine CCBs (verapamil, diltiazem) to slow ventricular response to AF in the acute setting, exercising caution in patients with hypotension or HF. (level B)
4. IV administration of digoxin or amiodarone to control heart rate in patients with AF and HF who do not have an accessory pathway. (level B)
5. Oral digoxin is effective to control heart rate at rest and is indicated for patients with HF, LV dysfunction, or for sedentary individuals. (level C)
6. IV amiodarone is recommended to slow a rapid ventricular response to AF and improve LV function in patients with acute MI. (level C)
7. IV beta-blockers and nondihydropyridine CCBs are recommended to slow a rapid ventricular response to AF in patients with acute MI who do not have clinical LV dysfunction, bronchospasm, or AV block. (level C)

Preventing Thromboembolism

1. Antithrombotic therapy is recommended for all patients with AF except those with lone AF or contraindications. (level A)
2. For patients without mechanical heart valves at high risk of stroke (prior stroke, TIA, or systemic embolism; rheumatic mitral stenosis), chronic oral anticoagulant therapy with a vitamin K antagonist is recommended in a dose to achieve the target INR of 2.0 to 3.0 unless contraindicated. (level A)
3. Anticoagulation with a vitamin K antagonist is recommended for patients with more than one moderate risk factor (age $\geq$ 75, hypertension, HF, LVEF < 35%, diabetes). (level A)
4. INR should be determined at least weekly during initiation of therapy with a vitamin K antagonist and monthly when anticoagulation is stable. (level A)
5. Dabigatran is useful as an alternative to warfarin for the prevention of stroke and systemic thromboembolism in patients with paroxysmal to permanent AF and risk factors for stroke or systemic embolization who do not have a prosthetic heart valve or hemodynamically significant valve disease, severe renal failure (CrCl <15 mL/min), or advanced liver disease (impaired baseline clotting function). (level B)
6. Aspirin 81-325 mg daily is an alternative to vitamin K antagonists in low-risk patients or those with contraindications to anticoagulation. (level A)
7. For patients with mechanical heart valves, the target intensity of anticoagulation should be based on the type of prosthesis, maintaining an INR of at least 2.5. (level B)
8. For patients with AF of $\geq$ 48 hours duration, or when the duration is unknown, anticoagulation (INR 2.0 to 3.0) is recommended for at least 3 weeks prior to and 4 weeks after cardioversion (electrical or pharmacological). (level B)
9. For patients with AF of more than 48 hours duration requiring immediate cardioversion, heparin should be administered concurrently (unless contraindicated) by an initial IV bolus followed by a continuous infusion in a dose adjusted to prolong the aPTT to 1.5 to 2 times the reference control value. Oral anticoagulation (INR 2.0 to 3.0) should be given for at least 4 weeks after cardioversion. Limited data support SQ administration of LMWH in this indication. (level C)
10. For patients with AF of less than 48 hours duration and hemodynamic instability (angina, MI, shock, or pulmonary edema), cardioversion should be performed immediately without delay for prior anticoagulation. (level C)

Cardioversion of Atrial Fibrillation

1. Administration of flecainide, dofetilide, propafenone, or ibutilide is recommended for pharmacological cardioversion. (level A)
2. Immediate electrical (direct-current) cardioversion is recommended for patients with AF involving preexcitation when very rapid tachycardia or hemodynamic instability occurs. (level B)
3. When a rapid ventricular response does not respond promptly to pharmacological measures in patients with MI, symptomatic hypotension, angina, or HF, immediate R-wave synchronized cardioversion is recommended. (level C)
4. Electrical cardioversion is recommended in patients without hemodynamic instability when symptoms of AF are unacceptable to the patient. In case of early relapse of AF after cardioversion, repeated electrical cardioversion attempts may be made following administration of antiarrhythmic medication. (level C)
5. Electrical cardioversion is recommended for patients with acute MI and severe hemodynamic compromise, intractable ischemia, or inadequate rate control with drugs. (level C)

Maintenance of Sinus Rhythm

1. An oral beta-blocker to prevent postoperative AF is recommended for patients undergoing cardiac surgery (unless contraindicated). (level A)
2. Before initiating antiarrhythmic drug therapy, treatment of precipitating or reversible causes of AF is recommended. (level C)

There are no class I recommendations for pharmacologic maintenance of sinus rhythm. See the guidelines for recommendations for maintenance of sinus rhythm.

Level of Evidence Definitions

Level A: Data derived from multiple randomized clinical trials or meta-analyses.
Level B: Data derived from a single randomized trial or nonrandomized studies.
Level C: Only consensus opinion of experts, case studies, or standard-of-care.

Source: *Data from Fuster V, Ryden LE, Cannom DS, et al. 2011 ACCF/AHA/HRS focused updates incorporated into the ACC/AHA/ESC 2006 guidelines for the management of patients with atrial fibrillation: a report of the American College of Cardiology Foundation/American Heart Association Task Force on Practice Guidelines. Circulation. 2011;123:e269–e367. Wann LS, Curtis AB, Ellenbogen KA, et al. 2011 ACCF/AHA/HRS focused update on the management of patients with atrial fibrillation (update on dabigatran): a report of the American College of Cardiology Foundation/American Heart Association Task Force on Practice Guidelines. Circulation. 2011; 123:1144–1150.*

Abbreviations used in this table: AF: atrial fibrillation; aPTT: activated partial thromboplastin time; CCB: calcium channel blocker; HF: heart failure; INR: international normalized ratio; LMWH: low molecular weight heparin; LV: left ventricular; MI: myocardial infarction; TIA: transient ischemic attack.

risk patients or those with contraindications. Dabigatran, rivaroxaban, and apixaban are three new oral drugs recently approved by the FDA for stroke prevention in patients with nonvalvular AF. Table 3-5 contains class I recommendations for thromboembolism prevention in patients with AF or atrial flutter.

Nonpharmacological Management of Atrial Fibrillation

Radiofrequency (RF) catheter ablation and surgical management of AF include AV node ablation, pulmonary vein ablation, surgical or ablation Maze procedures, and occlusion or surgical removal of the left atrial appendage. These procedures are briefly described here.

ESSENTIAL CONTENT CASE

Atrial Arrhythmia and Cardioversion

You are caring for a patient who was admitted for an elective cardioversion. She was seen in her physician's office this morning for complaints of SOB and palpitations that had started around 7 AM. She has a history of hypertension and diabetes but no previous cardiac history. In the office, her ECG showed atrial fibrillation with a ventricular response between 120 and 130 beats/minute. Previous ECGs had all shown normal sinus rhythm, and since her symptoms were new and time of onset was just a few hours ago, her physician elected to treat her with cardioversion. Her BP is 136/74 and she is breathing comfortably at this time. You place her on the bedside cardiac monitor in lead V1.

Case Question 1. What are the diagnostic features of AF that you expect to see on the monitor?
Figure 3-22A shows her rhythm strip:

Case Question 2. Is her admitting diagnosis of AF correct?

Case Question 3. What other treatments besides electrical cardioversion would be appropriate for managing this rhythm?
You gather the equipment and supplies needed for the cardioversion. The cardiologist arrives and an anesthesiologist is present to sedate the patient. The cardiologist asks you to deliver a 100 joule shock after the patient is asleep.

Case Question 4. What safety considerations are necessary before delivering the cardioversion shock?
The shock is delivered and Figure 3-22B shows the postshock rhythm.

Case Question 5. What is the rhythm?

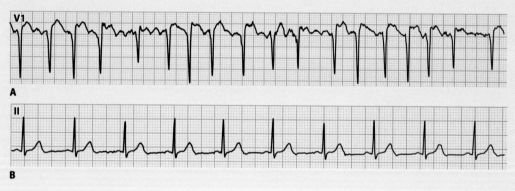

Figure 3-22.

Answers
1. Atrial fibrillation is characterized by the presence of "fibrillation" waves instead of organized P waves, and an irregularly irregular ventricular response.
2. Yes. This is a typical example of AF.
3. The first goal of treatment for AF is ventricular rate control. AV nodal blocking agents such as a beta-blocker or calcium channel blocker (ie, verapamil or diltiazem) are used for rate control. Antiarrhythmics such as flecainide, dofetilide, propafenone, ibutilide or amiodarone can be used for pharmacological conversion of atrial fibrillation to sinus rhythm. Patients with persistent AF are on chronic therapy with a rate control drug and oral anticoagulation.

4. Every member of the team participating in the procedure should be involved in assuring patient safety. The patient should be monitored with non-invasive BP monitoring and pulse oximetry. Airway management supplies, emergency drugs, and sedation reversal agent should be present at the bedside. The patient should be adequately sedated prior to shock delivery. The defibrillator must be synchronized on the QRS complex to avoid delivering the shock on the T wave, which could cause ventricular fibrillation. Prior to shock delivery, the operator should assure that no one is touching the patient or the bed.
5. This is normal sinus rhythm, indicating a successful cardioversion.

Radiofrequency AV node ablation is the most common nonpharmacologic method of rate control in AF and is usually done only when drug therapy for rate control is ineffective or not tolerated. RF energy is directed at the AV node to heat the tissue and destroy its ability to conduct impulses to the ventricle. This procedure results in complete AV block and requires a ventricular pacemaker implant to maintain an adequate ventricular rate. AV node ablation does not stop atrial fibrillation; therefore, patients must be chronically anticoagulated to prevent stroke.

Radiofrequency ablation of AF trigger sites in the pulmonary veins or atria is the mainstay of ablation therapy for AF. The most common site of AF triggers is the first 2-4 cm inside the pulmonary veins leading into the left atrium, although triggers can be present in multiple sites within both atria. The most successful procedures are segmental ostial pulmonary vein isolation (PVI) and circumferential PVI. In segmental ostial PVI, specific sites of electrical conduction in the ostia of the pulmonary veins are ablated. In circumferential PVI, continuous ablation lesions encircle the ostia of all four pulmonary veins, usually in two pairs (ie, one circle of lesions around the left pulmonary veins and another circle around the right pulmonary veins). These ablation lesions completely isolate the pulmonary veins from the atrial myocardium and prevent conduction from trigger sites in to the atria.

The Cox-Maze III procedure involves creation of multiple incisions within both atria using the "cut and sew" technique during cardiac surgery. The incisions create scars in the atria that direct the impulse from the sinus node to the AV node through both atria in an orderly fashion and prevent reentry of impulses that could lead to AF. Similar scars can be created using bipolar RF ablation clamps (Cox-Maze IV procedure), which still requires cardiac surgery and cardiopulmonary bypass. Catheter-based RF ablation procedures create the lesions from the endocardial approach and are done percutaneously in the electrophysiology laboratory rather than requiring surgery.

Left atrial appendage (LAA) amputation is done along with surgical Cox-Maze procedures as well as with mitral valve procedures to reduce the likelihood of thromboembolism, since most clots develop in the LAA during AF. Left atrial appendage occlusion devices can be inserted via the right femoral vein and into the LAA through a trans-septal approach and expanded within the LAA to seal it from the rest of the atrium, thus trapping clots and preventing them from embolizing.

Supraventricular Tachycardia (SVT)

A supraventricular tachycardia by definition is any rhythm at a rate faster than 100 beats/min that originates above the ventricle or utilizes the atria or AV junction as part of the circuit that maintains the tachycardia. Technically, this can include sinus tachycardia, AT, atrial flutter, atrial fibrillation, and junctional tachycardia. However, the term SVT is meant to be used to describe a regular, narrow QRS tachycardia in which the exact mechanism cannot be determined from the surface ECG. If P waves or atrial activity such a fibrillation or flutter waves can be clearly seen, then the mechanism can usually be identified. Occasionally in AT the P waves are hidden in preceding T waves and in that case use of the term SVT is appropriate.

The two most common arrhythmias for which the term SVT is appropriate are AV nodal reentry tachycardia (AVNRT) and circus movement tachycardia (CMT) that occurs when an accessory pathway is present, such as in WPW. Another term used to describe CMT is AV reentry tachycardia (AVRT) but CMT is used here to prevent confusion between these two common arrhythmias. The mechanisms of these SVTs are described in detail in Chapter 18, Advanced Arrhythmia Interpretation. ECG characteristics of both SVTs are very similar and described here.

ECG Characteristics

- *Rate*: 140-250 beats/minute.
- *Rhythm*: Regular.
- *P waves*: Usually not visible. In AVNRT, the P wave is hidden in the QRS or barely peeking out at the end of the QRS. In CMT, the P wave is usually present in the ST segment, but is often not visible.
- *PR interval*: Not measurable, since P waves are usually not visible.
- *QRS complex*: Usually normal.
- *Conduction:* In AVNRT, the impulse travels in a small circuit that includes the AV node as one limb of the circuit and a slower conducting pathway just outside the AV node as the second limb of the circuit. The impulse depolarizes the atria in a retrograde direction at the same time as it depolarizes the ventricles through the normal His-Purkinje system, resulting in a regular narrow QRS tachycardia. In CMT, the impulse follows a reentry circuit that includes the atria, AV node, ventricles, and accessory pathway. The most common type of CMT is called orthodromic CMT, in which the impulse travels from atria to ventricles through the normal AV node and His-Purkinje system, then back to the atria from the ventricles through the accessory pathway. This results in a regular, narrow QRS tachycardia because the ventricles are depolarized via the normal conduction system. If the circuit reverses direction and the ventricles depolarize through conduction down the accessory pathway, this is called antidromic CMT, and the resulting tachycardia has a wide QRS complex.
- Example of SVT: See Figure 3-23 A, B.

Treatment

These SVTs are usually well tolerated and often paroxysmal in nature. If the ventricular rate is very rapid and sustained, symptoms such as palpitations, dizziness, or syncope can occur.

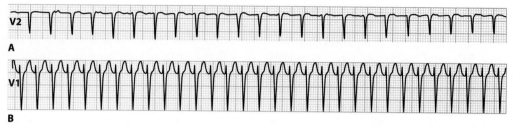

Figure 3-23. **(A)** SVT at a rate of 190 beats/min found to be AVNRT at electrophysiology study. **(B)** SVT at a rate of 214 found to be CMT at electrophysiology study.

Vagal maneuvers such as carotid sinus massage, Valsalva's maneuver, gagging or coughing, drinking ice water, or putting the face in ice water may be effective in terminating the tachycardia. Adenosine (6 mg given rapidly IV, may repeat with 12 mg if necessary) is the most effective drug to terminate the tachycardia. Drugs that slow AV conduction, like calcium channel blockers (diltiazem, verapamil) or beta-blockers, can terminate tachycardia and can be used long term to prevent recurrences. Synchronized cardioversion can be used if drugs are contraindicated or fail to terminate tachycardia. Radiofrequency ablation offers a cure for AVNRT and CMT. See Table 3-4 for class I recommendations for management of supraventricular tachycardias.

ARRHYTHMIAS ORIGINATING IN THE ATRIOVENTRICULAR JUNCTION

Cells surrounding the AV node in the AV junction are capable of initiating impulses and controlling the heart rhythm (Figure 3-24). Junctional beats and junctional rhythms can appear in any of three ways on the ECG depending on the location of the junctional pacemaker and the speed of conduction of the impulse into the atria and ventricles:

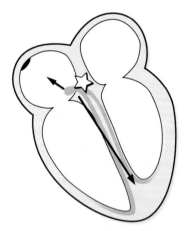

Figure 3-24. Arrhythmias originating in the AV junction.

- When a junctional focus fires, the wave of depolarization spreads backward (retrograde) into the atria as well as forward (antegrade) into the ventricles. If the impulse arrives in the atria before it arrives in the ventricles, the ECG shows a P wave (usually inverted because the atria are depolarizing from bottom to top) followed immediately by a QRS complex as the

impulse reaches the ventricles. In this case the PR interval is very short, usually 0.10 second or less.
- If the junctional impulse reaches both the atria and the ventricles at the same time, only a QRS is seen on the ECG because the ventricles are much larger than the atria and only ventricular depolarization will be seen, even though the atria are also depolarizing.
- If the junctional impulse reaches the ventricles before it reaches the atria, the QRS precedes the P wave on the ECG. Again, the P wave is usually inverted because of retrograde atrial depolarization, and the RP interval (distance from the beginning of the QRS to the beginning of the following P wave) is short.

Premature Junctional Complexes

Premature junctional complexes (PJCs) are due to an irritable focus in the AV junction. Irritability can be because of coronary heart disease or MI disrupting blood flow to the AV junction, nicotine, caffeine, emotions, or drugs such as digitalis.

ECG Characteristics

- *Rate:* 60 to 100 beats/min or whatever the rate of the basic rhythm.
- *Rhythm:* Regular except for occurrence of premature beats.
- *P waves:* May occur before, during, or after the QRS complex of the premature beat and are usually inverted.
- *PR interval:* Short, usually 0.10 second or less when P waves precede the QRS.
- *QRS complex:* Usually normal but may be aberrant if the PJC occurs very early and conducts into the ventricles during the refractory period of a bundle branch.
- *Conduction:* Retrograde through the atria; usually normal through the ventricles.
- *Example of a PJC:* Figure 3-25.

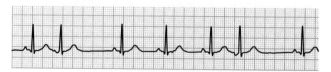

Figure 3-25. Premature junctional complexes.

Treatment

Treatment is not necessary for PJCs.

Junctional Rhythm, Accelerated Junctional Rhythm, and Junctional Tachycardia

Junctional rhythms can occur if the sinus node rate falls below the rate of the AV junctional pacemakers or when atrial conduction through the AV junction has been disrupted. Junctional rhythms commonly occur from digitalis toxicity or following inferior MI owing to disruption of blood supply to the sinus node and the AV junction. These rhythms are classified according to their rate. Junctional rhythm usually occurs at a rate of 40 to 60 beats/min, accelerated junctional rhythm occurs at a rate of 60 to 100 beats/min, and junctional tachycardia occurs at a rate of 100 to 250 beats/min.

ECG Characteristics

- *Rate:* Junctional rhythm, 40 to 60 beats/min; accelerated junctional rhythm, 60 to 100 beats/min; junctional tachycardia, 100 to 250 beats/min.
- *Rhythm:* Regular.
- *P waves:* May precede or follow QRS.
- *PR interval:* Short, 0.10 second or less.
- *QRS complex:* Usually normal.
- *Conduction:* Retrograde through the atria; normal through the ventricles.
- *Example of junctional rhythm and accelerated junctional rhythm:* Figure 3-26A, B.

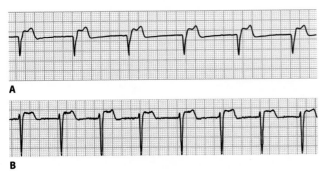

A

B

Figure 3-26. **(A)** Junctional rhythm. **(B)** Accelerated junctional rhythm.

Treatment

Treatment of junctional rhythm rarely is required unless the rate is too slow or too fast to maintain adequate cardiac output. If the rate is slow, atropine is given to increase the sinus rate and override the junctional focus or to increase the rate of firing of the junctional pacemaker. If the rate is fast, drugs such as verapamil, propranolol, or beta-blockers may be effective in slowing the rate or terminating the arrhythmia. Because digitalis toxicity is a common cause of junctional rhythms, the drug should be held.

ARRHYTHMIAS ORIGINATING IN THE VENTRICLES

Ventricular arrhythmias originate in the ventricular muscle or Purkinje system and are considered to be more dangerous than other arrhythmias because of their potential to initiate VT and severely decrease cardiac output (Figure 3-27). However, as with any arrhythmia, ventricular rate is a key determinant of how well a patient can tolerate a ventricular rhythm. Ventricular rhythms can range in severity from mild, well-tolerated rhythms to pulseless rhythms leading to sudden cardiac death.

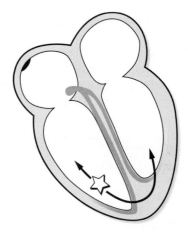

Figure 3-27. Arrhythmias originating in the ventricles.

Premature Ventricular Complexes

Premature ventricular complexes (PVCs) are caused by premature depolarization of cells in the ventricular myocardium or Purkinje system or to reentry in the ventricles. PVCs can be caused by hypoxia, myocardial ischemia, hypokalemia, acidosis, exercise, increased levels of circulating catecholamines, digitalis toxicity, caffeine, and alcohol, among other causes. PVCs increase with aging and are more common in people with coronary disease, valve disease, hypertension, cardiomyopathy, and other forms of heart disease. PVCs are not dangerous in people with normal hearts but are associated with higher mortality rates in patients with structural heart disease or acute MI, especially if left ventricular function is reduced. PVCs are considered potentially malignant when they occur more frequently than 10 per hour or are repetitive (occur in pairs, triplets, or more than three in a row) in patients with coronary disease, previous MI, cardiomyopathy, and reduced ejection fraction.

ECG Characteristics

- *Rate:* 60 to 100 beats/min or the rate of the basic rhythm.
- *Rhythm:* Irregular because of the early beats.
- *P waves:* Not related to the PVCs. Sinus rhythm is usually not interrupted by the premature beats, so sinus P waves can often be seen occurring regularly throughout the rhythm. P waves may occasionally

follow PVCs due to retrograde conduction from the ventricle backward through the atria. These P waves are inverted.

- *PR interval:* Not present before most PVCs. If a P wave happens, by coincidence, to precede a PVC, the PR interval is short.
- *QRS complex:* Wide and bizarre; greater than 0.10 second in duration. These may vary in morphology (size, shape) if they originate from more than one focus in the ventricles (multifocal PVCs).
- *Conduction:* Impulses originating in the ventricles conduct through the ventricles from muscle cell to muscle cell rather than through Purkinje fibers, resulting in wide QRS complexes. Some PVCs may conduct retrograde into the atria, resulting in inverted P waves following the PVC. When the sinus rhythm is undisturbed by PVCs, the atria depolarize normally.
- *Example of PVCs:* Figure 3-28A, B.

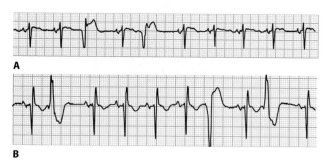

Figure 3-28. Premature ventricular complexes.

Treatment

The significance of PVCs depends on the clinical setting in which they occur. Many people have chronic PVCs that do not need to be treated, and most of these people are asymptomatic. There is no evidence that suppression of PVCs reduces mortality, especially in patients with no structural heart disease. If PVCs cause bothersome palpitations, patients are told to avoid caffeine, tobacco, other stimulants, and try stress reduction techniques. Low-dose beta-blockers may reduce PVC frequency and the perception of palpitations and can be used for symptom relief. In the setting of an acute MI or myocardial ischemia, PVCs may be precursors of more dangerous ventricular arrhythmias, especially when they occur near the apex of the T wave (R on T PVCs). Unless PVCs result in hemodynamic instability or symptomatic VT, most providers elect not to treat them. If PVCs are to be treated, IV lidocaine or amiodarone are the drugs usually used. Procainamide can also be used IV for acute control. Beta-blockers are often effective in suppressing repetitive PVCs and have become the drugs of choice for treating post-MI PVCs that are symptomatic. Several anti-arrhythmic drugs are effective in reducing the frequency of PVCs but are not recommended due to the risk of proarrhythmia and their association with sudden cardiac death in patients with structural heart disease.

Ventricular Rhythm and Accelerated Ventricular Rhythm

Ventricular rhythm occurs when an ectopic focus in the ventricle fires at a rate less than 50 beats/min. This rhythm occurs as an escape rhythm when the sinus node and junctional tissue fail to fire or fail to conduct their impulses to the ventricle. Accelerated ventricular rhythm occurs when an ectopic focus in the ventricles fires at a rate of 50 to 100 beats/min. The causes of this accelerated ventricular rhythm are similar to those of VT, but accelerated ventricular rhythm commonly occurs in the presence of inferior MI when the rate of the sinus node slows below the rate of the latent ventricular pacemaker. Accelerated ventricular rhythm is a common arrhythmia after thrombolytic therapy, when reperfusion of the damaged myocardium occurs.

ECG Characteristics

- *Rate:* Less than 50 beats/min for ventricular rhythm and 50 to 100 beats/min for accelerated ventricular rhythm.
- *Rhythm:* Usually regular.
- *P waves:* May be seen but at a slower rate than the ventricular focus, with dissociation from the QRS complex.
- *PR interval:* Not measured.
- *QRS complex:* Wide and bizarre.
- *Conduction:* If sinus rhythm is the basic rhythm, atrial conduction is normal. Impulses originating in the ventricles conduct via muscle cell-to-cell conduction, resulting in the wide QRS complex.
- *Example of escape ventricular rhythm and accelerated ventricular rhythm:* Figure 3-29 A, B.

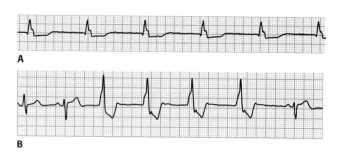

Figure 3-29. (A) Escape ventricular rhythm. **(B)** Accelerated ventricular rhythm.

Treatment

The treatment of accelerated ventricular rhythm depends on its cause and how well it is tolerated by the patient. This arrhythmia alone is usually not harmful because the ventricular rate is within normal limits and usually adequate to maintain cardiac output. Suppressive therapy is rarely used because abolishing the ventricular rhythm may leave an even less desirable heart rate. If the patient is symptomatic because of the loss of atrial kick, atropine can be used to increase the rate of the sinus node and overdrive the ventricular rhythm.

If the ventricular rhythm is an escape rhythm, then treatment is directed toward increasing the rate of the escape rhythm or pacing the heart temporarily. Usually, accelerated ventricular rhythm is transient and benign and does not require treatment.

Ventricular Tachycardia

Ventricular tachycardia (VT) is a rapid ventricular rhythm at a rate greater than 100 beats/min. VT can be classified according to: (1) duration, *nonsustained* (lasts less than 30 seconds), *sustained* (lasts longer than 30 seconds), or *incessant* (VT present most of the time); and (2) morphology (ECG appearance of QRS complexes), *monomorphic* (QRS complexes have the same shape during tachycardia), *polymorphic* (QRS complexes vary randomly in shape), or *bidirectional* (alternating upright and negative QRS complexes during tachycardia). Polymorphic VT that occurs in the presence of a long QT interval is called *torsades de pointes* (meaning "twisting of the points"). The most common cause of VT is coronary artery disease, including acute ischemia, acute MI, and prior MI. Other causes include cardiomyopathy, valvular heart disease, congenital heart disease, arrhythmogenic right ventricular dysplasia, cardiac tumors, cardiac surgery, and the proarrhythmic effects of many drugs. See Chapter 18 for more information on ventricular tachycardias and the differential diagnosis of wide QRS tachycardias.

ECG Characteristics

- *Rate:* Ventricular rate is faster than 100 beats/min.
- *Rhythm:* Monomorphic VT is usually regular, polymorphic VT can be irregular.
- *P waves:* Dissociated from QRS complexes. If sinus rhythm is the underlying basic rhythm, they are regular. P waves may be seen but are not related to QRS complexes. P waves are often buried within QRS complexes.
- *PR interval:* Not measurable because of dissociation of P waves from QRS complexes.
- *QRS complex:* Usually 0.12 second or more in duration.
- *Conduction:* Impulse originates in one ventricle and spreads via muscle cell-to-cell conduction through both ventricles. There may be retrograde conduction through the atria, but more often the sinus node continues to fire regularly and depolarize the atria normally.
- *Example of VT:* Figure 3-30.

Treatment

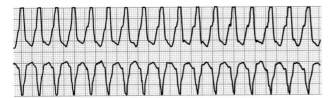

Figure 3-30. Monomorphic ventricular tachycardia.

Immediate treatment of VT depends on how well the rhythm is tolerated by the patient. The two main determinants of patient tolerance of any tachycardia are ventricular rate and underlying left ventricular function. VT can be an emergency if cardiac output is severely decreased because of a very rapid rate or poor left ventricular function.

Hemodynamically unstable VT is treated with synchronized cardioversion. If VT is pulseless then immediate defibrillation is required. VT that is hemodynamically stable can be treated with drug therapy. Amiodarone is often the drug of choice but lidocaine or procainamide can also be used. Drugs used to treat VT on a long-term basis include amiodarone, sotalol, and beta-blockers. Some VTs can be treated with radiofrequency catheter ablation to abolish the ectopic focus. The implantable cardioverter defibrillator is frequently used for recurrent VT in patients with reduced ejection fractions or drug refractory VT. See Table 3-6 for class I recommendations for management of ventricular arrhythmias.

TABLE 3-6. GUIDELINES FOR MANAGEMENT OF VENTRICULAR ARRHYTHMIAS (CLASS I RECOMMENDATIONS ONLY)

Sustained Monomorphic Ventricular Tachycardia
1. Wide QRS tachycardia should be presumed to be VT if the diagnosis is unclear (level C).
2. Electrical cardioversion with sedation is recommended with hemodynamically unstable sustained monomorphic VT (level C).
Contraindicated: Calcium channel blockers (verapamil, diltiazem) should not be used to terminate wide QRS tachycardia of unknown origin, especially with history of myocardial dysfunction.

Polymorphic Ventricular Tachycardia
1. Electrical cardioversion with sedation is recommended for sustained PVT with hemodynamic compromise (level B).
2. IV beta-blockers are useful if ischemia is suspected or cannot be excluded (level B).
3. IV amiodarone is useful for recurrent PVT in the absence of QT prolongation (congenital or acquired) (level C).
4. Urgent angiography and revascularization should be considered with PVT when myocardial ischemia cannot be excluded (level C).

Torsades de Pointes
1. Withdrawal of any offending drugs and correction of electrolyte abnormalities are recommended for TdP (level A).
2. Acute and long-term pacing is recommended for TdP due to heart block and symptomatic bradycardia (level A).

Incessant Ventricular Tachycardia
1. Revascularization and beta blockade followed by IV antiarrhythmic drugs such as procainamide or amiodarone are recommended for recurrent or incessant PVT (level B).

Level of Evidence Definitions
Level A: Data derived from multiple randomized clinical trials or meta-analyses.
Level B: Data derived from a single randomized trial or nonrandomized studies.
Level C: Only consensus opinion of experts, case studies, or standard of care.

Source: *Data from Zipes DP, Camm JA, Borggrefe M et al. ACC/AHA/ESC 2006 Guidelines for Management of Patients With Ventricular Arrhythmias and the Prevention of Sudden Cardiac Death: executive summary: a report of the American College of Cardiology/American Heart Association Task Force and the European Society of Cardiology Committee for Practice Guidelines (Writing Committee to Revise the 2001 Guidelines for the Management of Patients with Atrial Fibrillation). Circulation. 2006;114:1088-1132. Abbreviations: PVT, polymorphic ventricular tachycardia; TdP, torsades de pointes; VT, ventricular tachycardia.*

Ventricular Fibrillation

Ventricular fibrillation (VF) is rapid, ineffective quivering of the ventricles and is fatal without immediate treatment (Figure 3-31). Electrical activity originates in the ventricles and spreads in a chaotic, irregular pattern throughout both ventricles. There is no cardiac output or palpable pulse with VF.

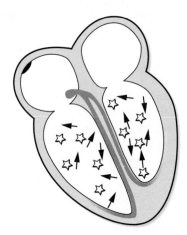

Figure 3-31. Ventricular fibrillation.

ECG Characteristics

- *Rate:* Rapid, uncoordinated, ineffective.
- *Rhythm:* Chaotic, irregular.
- *P waves:* None seen.
- *PR interval:* None.
- *QRS complex:* No formed QRS complexes seen; rapid, irregular undulations without any specific pattern.
- *Conduction:* Multiple ectopic foci firing simultaneously in ventricles and depolarizing them irregularly and without any organized pattern. Ventricles are not contracting.
- *Example of ventricular fibrillation:* Figure 3-32.

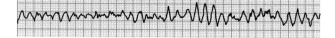

Figure 3-32. Ventricular fibrillation.

Treatment

Ventricular fibrillation requires immediate defibrillation. Synchronized cardioversion is not possible because there are no formed QRS complexes on which to synchronize the shock. Cardiopulmonary resuscitation (CPR) must be performed until a defibrillator is available, and then defibrillation at 200 J (biphasic defibrillation) or 360 J (monophasic defibrillation) is recommended followed by CPR and drug therapy. Antiarrhythmic agents such as lidocaine, amiodarone, or magnesium are commonly used in an effort to convert VF. Once the rhythm has converted, maintenance therapy with IV antiarrhythmic agents is continued. Beta-blockers and amiodarone appear to be the most effective agents for long-term drug therapy options. The implantable

cardioverter defibrillator has become the standard of care for survivors of VF that occurs in the absence of acute ischemia.

Ventricular Asystole

Ventricular asystole is the absence of any ventricular rhythm: no QRS complex, no pulse, and no cardiac output (Figure 3-33). Ventricular asystole is always fatal unless the cause can be identified and treated immediately. If atrial activity is still present the term ventricular standstill is used.

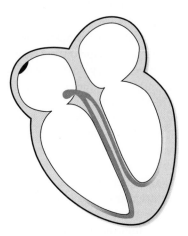

Figure 3-33. Ventricular asystole.

ECG Characteristics

- *Rate:* None.
- *Rhythm:* None.
- *P waves:* May be present if the sinus node is functioning.
- *PR interval:* None.
- *QRS complex:* None.
- *Conduction:* Atrial conduction may be normal if the sinus node is functioning. There is no conduction into the ventricles.
- *Example of ventricular asystole:* Figure 3-34.

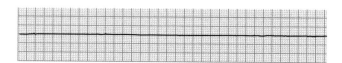

Figure 3-34. Ventricular asystole.

Treatment

Cardiopulmonary resuscitation must be initiated immediately if the patient is to survive. IV epinephrine and vasopressin are the only drugs currently recommended for treating asystole. The cause of asystole should be determined and treated as rapidly as possible to improve the chance of survival. Asystole has a very poor prognosis despite the best resuscitation efforts because it usually represents extensive myocardial ischemia or severe underlying metabolic problems. Pacing and atropine are no longer recommended for treatment for asystole.

ATRIOVENTRICULAR BLOCKS

The term *atrioventricular block* is used to describe arrhythmias in which there is delayed or failed conduction of supraventricular impulses into the ventricles. AV blocks have been classified according to location of the block and severity of the conduction abnormality.

First-Degree Atrioventricular Block

First-degree AV block is defined as prolonged AV conduction time of supraventricular impulses into the ventricles (Figure 3-35). This delay usually occurs in the AV node, and all impulses conduct to the ventricles, but with delayed conduction times. First-degree AV block can be due to coronary heart disease, rheumatic heart disease, or administration of digitalis, beta-blockers, or calcium channel blockers. First-degree AV block can be normal in people with slow heart rates or high vagal tone.

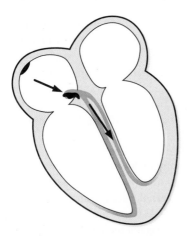

Figure 3-35. First-degree AV block.

ECG Characteristics

- *Rate:* Can occur at any sinus rate, usually 60 to 100 beats/min.
- *Rhythm:* Regular.
- *P waves:* Normal; precede every QRS complex.
- *PR interval:* Prolonged above 0.20 second.
- *QRS complex:* Usually normal.
- *Conduction:* Normal through the atria, delayed through the AV node, and normal through the ventricles.
- *Example of first-degree AV block:* Figure 3-36.

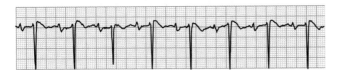

Figure 3-36. First-degree AV block.

Treatment

Treatment of first-degree AV block is usually not required, but the rhythm should be observed for progression to more severe block.

Second-Degree Atrioventricular Block

Second-degree AV block occurs when one atrial impulse at a time fails to be conducted to the ventricles. Second-degree AV block can be divided into two distinct categories: type I block, occurring in the AV node, and type II block, occurring below the AV node in the bundle of His or bundle-branch system (Figure 3-37).

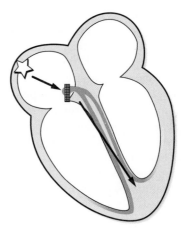

Figure 3-37. Type I second-degree AV block.

Type I Second-Degree Atrioventricular Block

Type I second-degree AV block, often referred to as *Wenckebach block,* is a progressive increase in conduction times of consecutive atrial impulses into the ventricles until one impulse fails to conduct, or is "dropped." The PR intervals gradually lengthen until one P wave fails to conduct and is not followed by a QRS complex, resulting in a pause, after which the cycle repeats itself. This type of block is commonly associated with inferior MI, coronary heart disease, aortic valve disease, mitral valve prolapse, atrial septal defects, and administration of digitalis, beta-blockers, or calcium channel blockers.

ECG Characteristics

- *Rate:* Can occur at any sinus or atrial rate.
- *Rhythm:* Irregular. Overall appearance of the rhythm demonstrates "group beating."
- *P waves:* Normal. Some P waves are not conducted to the ventricles, but only one at a time fails to conduct to the ventricle.
- *PR interval:* Gradually lengthens on consecutive beats. The PR interval preceding the pause is longer than that following the pause (unless 2:1 conduction is present).
- *QRS complex:* Usually normal unless there is associated bundle branch block.

- *Conduction:* Normal through the atria; progressively delayed through the AV node until an impulse fails to conduct. Ventricular conduction is normal. Conduction ratios can vary, with ratios as low as 2:1 (every other P wave is blocked) up to high ratios such as 15:14 (every 15th P wave is blocked).
- *Example of second-degree AV block type I:* Figure 3-38.

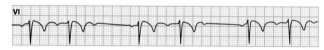

Figure 3-38. Second-degree AV block, type I.

Treatment

Treatment of type I second-degree AV block depends on the conduction ratio, the resulting ventricular rate, and the patient's tolerance for the rhythm. If ventricular rates are slow enough to decrease cardiac output, the treatment is atropine to increase the sinus rate and speed conduction through the AV node. At higher conduction ratios where the ventricular rate is within a normal range, no treatment is necessary. If the block is due to digitalis, calcium channel blockers, or beta-blockers, those drugs are held. This type of block is usually temporary and benign, and seldom requires pacing, although temporary pacing may be needed when the ventricular rate is slow.

Type II Second-Degree Atrioventricular Block

Type II second-degree AV block is sudden failure of conduction of an atrial impulse to the ventricles without progressive increases in conduction time of consecutive P waves (Figure 3-39). Type II block occurs below the AV node and is usually associated with bundle branch block; therefore, the

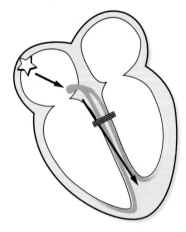

Figure 3-39. Type II second-degree AV block.

dropped beats are usually a manifestation of bilateral bundle branch block. This form of block appears on the ECG much the same as type I block except that there is no progressive increase in PR intervals before the blocked beats and the QRS is almost always wide. Type II block is less common than type I block, but is a more serious form of block. It occurs in rheumatic heart disease, coronary heart disease, primary disease of the conduction system, and in the presence of acute anterior MI. Type II block is more dangerous than type I because of a higher incidence of associated symptoms and progression to complete AV block.

ECG Characteristics

- *Rate:* Can occur at any basic rate.
- *Rhythm:* Irregular due to blocked beats.
- *P waves:* Usually regular and precede each QRS. Periodically a P wave is not followed by a QRS complex.
- *PR interval:* Constant before conducted beats. The PR interval preceding the pause is the same as that following the pause.
- *QRS complex:* Usually wide because of associated bundle branch block.
- *Conduction:* Normal through the atria and through the AV node but intermittently blocked in the bundle branch system and fails to reach the ventricles. Conduction through the ventricles is abnormally slow due to associated bundle branch block. Conduction ratios can vary from 2:1 to only occasional blocked beats.
- *Example of second-degree AV block type II:* Figure 3-40.

Treatment

Treatment usually includes pacemaker therapy because this type of block is often permanent and progresses to complete block. External pacing can be used for treatment of symptomatic type II block until transvenous pacing can be initiated. Atropine is not recommended because it may result in further slowing of ventricular rate by increasing the number of impulses conducting through the AV node and bombarding the diseased bundles with more impulses than they can handle, resulting in further conduction failure.

High-Grade Atrioventricular Block

High-grade (or advanced) AV block is present when two or more consecutive atrial impulses are blocked when the atrial rate is reasonable (less than 135 beats/min) and conduction fails because of the block itself and not because of interference from an escape pacemaker. High-grade AV block may be type I, occurring in the AV node, or type II, occurring below the AV node. The importance of high-grade block depends

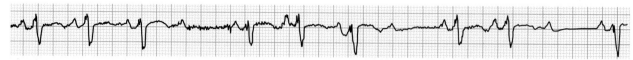

Figure 3-40. Second-degree AV block, type II.

on the conduction ratio and the resulting ventricular rate. Because ventricular rates tend to be slow, this arrhythmia is frequently symptomatic and requires treatment.

ECG Characteristics

- *Rate:* Atrial rate less than 135 beats/min.
- *Rhythm:* Regular or irregular, depending on conduction pattern.
- *P waves:* Normal. Present before every conducted QRS, but several P waves may not be followed by QRS complexes.
- *PR interval:* Constant before conducted beats. May be normal or prolonged.
- *QRS complex:* Usually normal in type I block and wide in type II block.
- *Conduction:* Normal through the atria. Two or more consecutive atrial impulses fail to conduct to the ventricles. Ventricular conduction is normal in type I block and abnormally slow in type II block.
- *Example of high-grade AV block:* Figure 3-41.

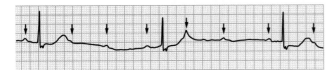

Figure 3-41. High-grade AV block.

Treatment

Treatment of high-grade block is necessary if the patient is symptomatic. Atropine can be given and is generally more effective in type I block. An external pacemaker may be required until transvenous pacing can be initiated, and permanent pacing is often necessary in type II high-grade block.

Third-Degree Atrioventricular Block (Complete Block)

Third-degree AV block is complete failure of conduction of all atrial impulses to the ventricles (Figure 3-42). In third-degree AV block, there is complete AV dissociation; the atria are usually under the control of the sinus node, although complete block can occur with any atrial arrhythmia; and either a junctional or ventricular pacemaker controls the ventricles. The ventricular rate is usually less than 45 beats/min; a faster rate could indicate an accelerated junctional or ventricular rhythm that interferes with conduction from the atria into the ventricles by causing physiologic refractoriness in the conduction system, thus causing a physiologic failure of conduction that must be differentiated from the abnormal conduction system function of complete AV block. Causes of complete AV block include coronary heart disease, MI, Lev disease, Lenègre disease, cardiac surgery, congenital heart disease, and drugs that slow AV conduction such as digitalis, beta-blockers, and calcium channel blockers.

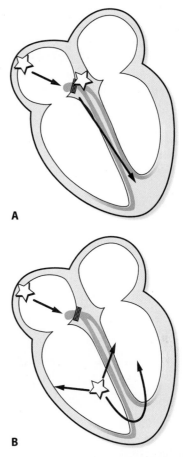

A

B

Figure 3-42. Third-degree AV block (complete block). **(A)** Third-degree AV block with junctional escape pacemaker. **(B)** Third-degree AV block with ventricular escape pacemaker. (*Gilmore SB, Woods SL. Electrocardiography and vector-cardiography. In: Woods SL, Froelicher ES, Motzer SU, eds.* Cardiac Nursing. *3rd ed. Philadelphia, PA: JB Lippincott; 1995:291.*)

ECG Characteristics

- *Rate:* Atrial rate is usually normal. Ventricular rate is less than 45 beats/min.
- *Rhythm:* Regular.
- *P waves:* Normal but dissociated from QRS complexes.
- *PR interval:* No consistent PR intervals because there is no relationship between P waves and QRS complexes.
- *QRS complex:* Normal if ventricles are controlled by a junctional pacemaker. Wide if controlled by a ventricular pacemaker.
- *Conduction:* Normal through the atria. All impulses are blocked at the AV node or in the bundle branches, so there is no conduction to the ventricles. Conduction through the ventricles is normal if a junctional escape rhythm occurs, and abnormally slow if a ventricular escape rhythm occurs.
- *Examples of third-degree AV block:* Figure 3-44A,B.

Treatment

Third-degree AV block can occur without significant symptoms if it occurs gradually and the heart has time to compensate

ESSENTIAL CONTENT CASE

Heart Block and Epicardial Pacemaker

You are caring for a patient who had an aortic valve replacement yesterday. He has been extubated, he has a mediastinal chest tube, and two ventricular epicardial pacing leads are in place and coiled under a dressing. He is in sinus rhythm at a rate in the 80s, BP is 146/80, RR is 16 and he is breathing comfortably. The monitor alarm sounds and when you enter the room he is pale and complaining of dizziness but no chest pain. This is what you now see on the monitor:

Figure 3-43A

Case Question 1. What is his rhythm?
He is dizzy and his BP is 92/60.

Case Question 2. What can you do to treat this arrhythmia?

Case Question 3. Describe how to initiate epicardial ventricular pacing.
You connect the pacing leads to a temporary pulse generator and set the rate at 70 beats/min.
This is the rhythm:

Figure 3-43 B

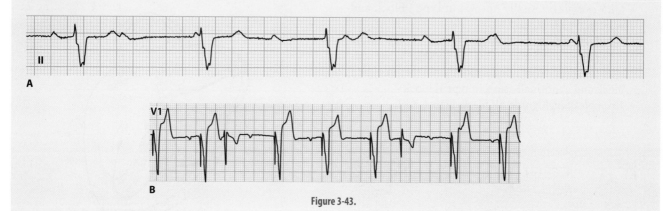

Figure 3-43.

Case Question 4. What is this rhythm?

Case Question 5. Evaluate pacemaker function in terms of ventricular capture and ventricular sensing.

Answers

1. This rhythm is third degree AV block with a ventricular pacemaker at a rate of about 40 beats/minute.
2. Third degree AV block is best treated with pacing. Atropine may speed up the rate of the sinus rhythm but it doesn't improve conduction in complete heart block. Since this patient has ventricular epicardial pacing leads in place, the best treatment is to initiate temporary ventricular pacing.

3. To initiate ventricular epicardial pacing with two ventricular leads present, connect one epicardial lead to the negative terminal of the temporary pacemaker pulse generator and connect the other lead to the positive terminal of the pacemaker. Set the desired rate, output, and sensitivity and turn the pacemaker on.
4. Ventricular paced rhythm at a rate of 70 beats/min. Sinus P waves are present and two of them are conducted to the ventricles.
5. Capture is good: every ventricular pacing spike is followed by a wide QRS complex. Sensing is also good: the two conducted beats are sensed and the pacemaker inhibits its output appropriately.

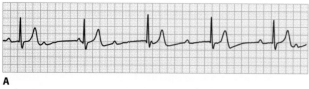

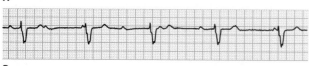

Figure 3-44. **(A)** Third-degree AV block with a junctional escape pacemaker at a rate of about 36 beats/min. **(B)** Third-degree AV block with a ventricular escape pacemaker at a rate of about 40 beats/min.

for the slow ventricular rate. If it occurs suddenly in the presence of acute MI, its significance depends on the resulting ventricular rate and the patient's tolerance. Treatment of complete heart block with symptoms of decreased cardiac output includes external pacing until transvenous pacing can be initiated. Atropine can be given but is not usually effective in restoring conduction.

TEMPORARY PACING

Indications

If the heart fails to generate or conduct impulses to the ventricle, the myocardium can be electrically stimulated using a cardiac pacemaker. A cardiac pacemaker has two components: a pulse generator and a pacing electrode or lead. Temporary cardiac pacing is indicated in any situation in which bradycardia results in symptoms of decreased cerebral perfusion or hemodynamic compromise and does not respond to drug therapy. Signs and symptoms of hemodynamic instability are hypotension, change in mental status, angina, or pulmonary edema. Temporary pacing is also used to terminate some rapid reentrant tachycardias by briefly pacing the heart at a faster rate than the existing rate. When pacing is stopped, the sinus node may resume control of the rhythm if the tachycardia has been terminated. This type of pacing is termed *overdrive pacing* to distinguish it from pacing for bradycardic conditions.

Temporary cardiac pacing is accomplished by transvenous, epicardial, or external pacing methods. If continued cardiac pacing is required, insertion of permanent pacemakers is done electively. The following section presents an overview of temporary ventricular pacing principles. A more detailed explanation of pacemaker functions is covered in Chapter 18, Advanced ECG Concepts.

Transvenous Pacing

Transvenous pacing is usually done by percutaneous puncture of the internal jugular, subclavian, antecubital, or femoral vein and advancing a pacing lead into the apex of the right ventricle so that the tip of the pacing lead contacts the wall of the ventricle (Figure 3-45A). The transvenous pacing lead

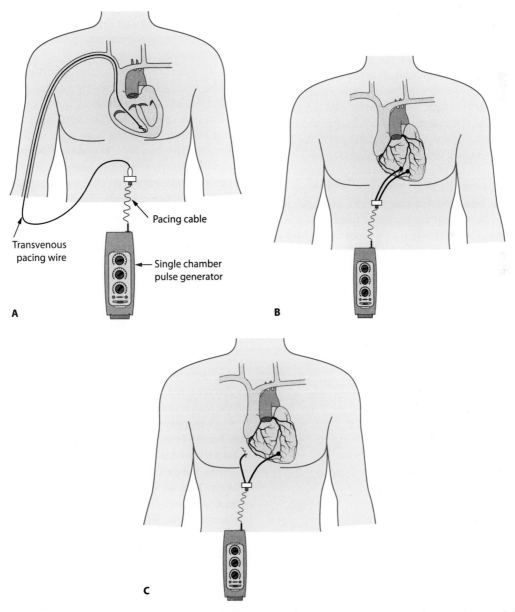

Figure 3-45. Temporary single chamber ventricular pacing. **(A)** Transvenous pacing with pacing lead in apex of right ventricle. **(B)** Bipolar epicardial pacing with two epicardial wires on ventricle. **(C)** Unipolar epicardial pacing with one wire on ventricle and one ground wire in mediastinum.

is attached to an external pulse generator that is kept either on the patient or at the bedside. Transvenous pacing is usually necessary only for a few days until the rhythm returns to normal or a permanent pacemaker is inserted.

Epicardial Pacing

Epicardial pacing is done through electrodes placed on the atria or ventricles during cardiac surgery. The pacing electrode end of the lead is looped through or loosely sutured to the epicardial surface of the atria or ventricles and the other end is pulled through the chest wall, sutured to the skin, and attached to an external pulse generator (Figure 3-45B,C). A ground wire is often placed subcutaneously in the chest wall and pulled through with the other leads. The number and placement of leads varies with the surgeon.

Components of a Pacing System

The basic components of a cardiac pacing system are the pulse generator and the pacing lead. The *pulse generator* contains the power source (battery) and all of the electronic circuitry that controls pacemaker function. A temporary pulse generator is a box that is kept at the bedside and is usually powered by a regular 9-V battery. It has controls on the front that allow the operator to set pacing rate, strength of the pacing stimulus (output), and sensitivity settings (Figure 3-46).

The *pacing lead* is an insulated wire used to transmit the electrical current from the pulse generator to the myocardium. A unipolar lead contains a single wire and a bipolar lead contains two wires that are insulated from each other. In a unipolar lead, the electrode is an exposed metal tip at the end of the lead that contacts the myocardium and serves

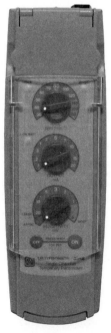

Figure 3-46. Temporary pacemaker pulse generator. (*Medtronic, Inc., Minneapolis, MN.*)

as the negative pole of the pacing circuit. In a bipolar lead, the end of the lead is a metal tip that contacts myocardium and serves as the negative pole, and the positive pole is an exposed metal ring located a few millimeters proximal to the distal tip.

Basics of Pacemaker Operation

Electrical current flows in a closed-loop circuit between two pieces of metal (poles). For current to flow, there must be conductive material (ie, a lead, muscle, or conductive solution) between the two poles. In the heart, the pacing lead, cardiac muscle, and body tissues serve as conducting material for the flow of electrical current in the pacing system. The pacing circuit consists of the pacemaker pulse generator (the power source), the conducting lead (pacing lead), and the myocardium. The electrical stimulus travels from the pulse generator through the pacing lead to the myocardium, through the myocardium, and back to the pulse generator, thus completing the circuit.

Temporary transvenous pacing is done using a bipolar pacing lead with its tip in the apex of the RV (see Figure 3-45A). Epicardial pacing can be done with either bipolar or unipolar leads. The term *bipolar* means that both of the poles in the pacing system are in or on the heart (see Figure 3-45B). In a bipolar system, the pulse generator initiates the electrical impulse and delivers it out the negative terminal of the pacemaker to the pacing lead. The impulse travels down the lead to the distal electrode (negative pole or cathode) that is in contact with myocardium. As the impulse reaches the tip, it travels through the myocardium and returns to the positive pole (or anode) of the system, completing the circuit. In a transvenous bipolar system, the positive pole is the proximal ring located a few millimeters proximal to the distal tip. The circuit over which the electrical impulse travels in a bipolar system is small because the two poles are located close together on the lead. This results in a small pacing spike on the ECG as the pacing stimulus travels between the two poles. If the stimulus is strong enough to depolarize the myocardium, the pacing spike is immediately followed by a P wave if the lead is in the atrium, or a wide QRS complex if the lead is in the ventricle.

A unipolar system has only one of the two poles in or on the heart (see Figure 3-45C). In a temporary unipolar epicardial pacing system, a ground lead placed in the subcutaneous tissue in the mediastinum serves as the second pole. Unipolar pacemakers work the same way as bipolar systems, but the circuit over which the impulse travels is larger because of the greater distance between the two poles. This results in a large pacing spike on the ECG as the impulse travels between the two poles.

Capture and Sensing

The two main functions of a pacing system are capture and sensing. *Capture* means that a pacing stimulus results in depolarization of the chamber being paced (Figure 3-47A).

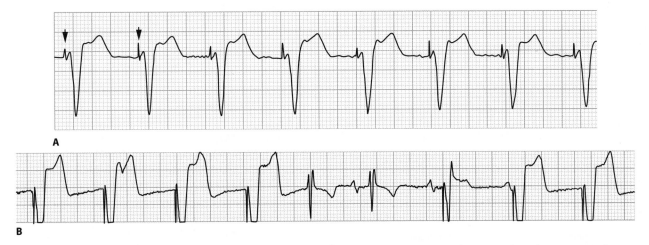

Figure 3-47. **(A)** Ventricular pacing with 100% capture. Arrows show pacing spikes, each one followed by a wide QRS complex indicating ventricular capture. **(B)** Rhythm strip of a ventricular pacemaker in the demand mode. There is appropriate sensing of intrinsic QRS complexes and appropriate pacing with ventricular capture when the intrinsic QRS complexes fall below the preset rate of the pacemaker. The seventh beat is fusion between the intrinsic QRS and the paced beat, a normal phenomenon in ventricular pacing.

Capture is determined by the strength of the stimulus, which is measured in milliamperes (mA), the amount of time the stimulus is applied to the heart (pulse width), and by contact of the pacing electrode with the myocardium. Capture cannot occur unless the distal tip of the pacing lead is in contact with healthy myocardium that is capable of responding to the stimulus. Pacing in infarcted tissue usually prevents capture. Similarly, if the catheter is floating in the cavity of the ventricle and not in direct contact with myocardium, capture will not occur. In temporary pacing, the output dial on the face of the pulse generator controls stimulus strength, and can be set and changed easily by the operator. Temporary pulse generators usually are capable of delivering a stimulus of 0.1 to 20 mA.

Sensing means that the pacemaker is able to detect the presence of intrinsic cardiac activity (Figure 3-47B). The sensing circuit controls how sensitive the pacemaker is to intrinsic cardiac depolarizations. Intrinsic activity is measured in millivolts (mV), and the higher the number, the larger the intrinsic signal; for example, a 10-mV QRS complex is larger than a 2-mV QRS. When pacemaker sensitivity needs to be increased to make the pacemaker "see" smaller signals, the sensitivity number must be decreased; for example, a sensitivity of 2 mV is more sensitive than one of 5 mV.

A fence analogy may help to explain sensitivity. Think of sensitivity as a fence standing between the pacemaker and what it wants to see, the ventricle; for example, if there is a 10-ft-high fence (or a 10-mV sensitivity) between the two, the pacemaker may not see what the ventricle is doing. To make the pacemaker able to see, the fence needs to be lowered. Lowering the fence to 2 ft would probably enable the pacemaker to see the ventricle. Changing the sensitivity from 10 to 2 mV is like lowering the fence—the pacemaker becomes more sensitive and is able to "see" intrinsic activity more easily. Thus, to increase the sensitivity of a pacemaker, the millivolt number (fence) must be decreased.

Asynchronous (Fixed-Rate) Pacing Mode

A pacemaker programmed to an asynchronous mode paces at the programmed rate regardless of intrinsic cardiac activity. This can result in competition between the pacemaker and the heart's own electrical activity. Asynchronous pacing in the ventricle is unsafe because of the potential for pacing stimuli to fall in the vulnerable period of repolarization and cause VF.

Demand Mode

The term *demand* means that the pacemaker paces only when the heart fails to depolarize on its own, that is, the pacemaker fires only "on demand." In demand mode, the pacemaker's sensing circuit is capable of sensing intrinsic cardiac activity and inhibiting pacer output when intrinsic activity is present. Sensing takes place between the two poles of the pacemaker. A bipolar system senses over a small area because the poles are close together, and this can result in "undersensing" of intrinsic signals. A unipolar system senses over a large area because the poles are far apart, and this can result in "oversensing." A unipolar system is more likely to sense myopotentials caused by muscle movement and inappropriately inhibit pacemaker output, potentially resulting in periods of asystole if the patient has no underlying cardiac rhythm. The demand mode should always be used for ventricular pacing to avoid the possibility of VF.

A paced ventricular beat begins with a pacing spike, which indicates that an electrical stimulus was released by the pacemaker (Figure 3-48). If the pacing stimulus is strong enough to depolarize the ventricle, the spike is followed by a wide QRS complex and a T wave that is oriented in the opposite direction of the QRS complex. Figure 3-47A illustrates ventricular pacing with 100% capture.

Figure 3-47B is the ECG of a ventricular pacemaker that is functioning correctly in the demand mode. The pacemaker generates an impulse when it senses that the heart rate has

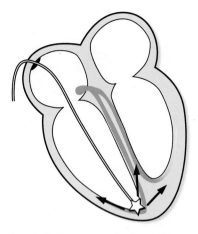

Figure 3-48. Temporary pacing lead in RV apex.

decreased below the set pacing rate. Therefore, the pacemaker senses the intrinsic cardiac rhythm of the patient and only generates an impulse when the rate falls below the preset pacing rate. Refer Chapter 18, Advanced ECG Concepts, for more detailed information on single and dual chamber pacing.

Initiating Transvenous Ventricular Pacing

Temporary transvenous pacing leads are bipolar and have two tails, one marked "positive" or "proximal" and the other marked "negative" or "distal," that are connected to the pulse generator. To initiate ventricular pacing using a transvenous lead (see Figure 3-45A):

1. Connect the negative terminal of the pulse generator to the distal end of the pacing lead.
2. Connect the positive terminal of the pulse generator to the proximal end of the pacing lead.
3. Set the rate at 70 to 80 beats/min or as ordered by physician.
4. Set the output at 5 mA, then determine stimulation threshold and set two to three times higher.
5. Set the sensitivity at 2 mV and adjust according to sensitivity threshold.

Initiating Epicardial Pacing

To initiate bipolar ventricular pacing (two leads on the ventricle; see Figure 3-45B):

1. Connect the negative terminal of the pulse generator to one of the ventricular leads.
2. Connect the positive terminal of the pulse generator to the other ventricular lead.
3. Set the rate at 70 to 80 beats/min or as ordered.
4. Set the output at 5 mA, then determine stimulation threshold and set two to three times higher.
5. Set the sensitivity at 2 mV and adjust according to sensitivity threshold.

To initiate unipolar ventricular pacing (one lead on the ventricle; see Figure 3-45C):

1. Connect the negative terminal of the pulse generator to the ventricular lead.
2. Connect the positive terminal of the pulse generator to the ground lead.
3. Set the rate at 70 to 80 beats/min or as ordered by physician.
4. Set the output at 5 mA, then determine stimulation threshold and set two to three times higher.
5. Set the sensitivity at 2 mV and adjust according to sensitivity threshold. See Chapter 18, Advanced ECG Concepts, for information on how to obtain capture and sensing thresholds.

External (Transcutaneous) Pacemakers

The emergent nature of many bradycardic rhythms requires immediate temporary pacing. Because transvenous catheter placement is difficult to accomplish quickly, external pacing is the preferred method for rapid, easy initiation of cardiac pacing in emergent situations until a transvenous pacemaker can be inserted. External pacing is done through large-surface adhesive electrodes attached to the anterior and posterior chest wall and connected to an external pacing unit (Figure 3-49). The pacing current passes through skin and chest wall structures to reach the heart; therefore, large energies are required to achieve capture. Sedation and analgesia are usually needed to minimize the discomfort felt by the patient during pacing. Transcutaneous pacing spikes are usually very large, often distorting the QRS complex. The presence of a pulse with every pacing spike confirms ventricular capture.

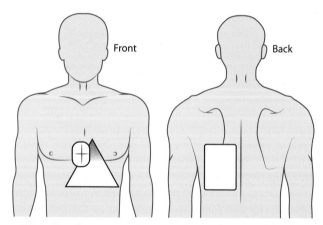

Figure 3-49. External pacemaker with pacing electrode pads on anterior and posterior chest and back.

DEFIBRILLATION AND CARDIOVERSION

Defibrillation

Defibrillation is the therapeutic delivery of electrical energy to the myocardium to terminate life-threatening ventricular arrhythmias (VF and pulseless VT). The defibrillating shock

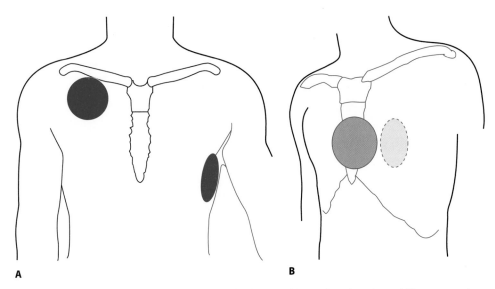

Figure 3-50. Paddle or adhesive pad placement for external defibrillation via **(A)** anterolateral position and **(B)** anteroposterior position.

depolarizes all cells in the heart simultaneously, stopping all electrical activity and allowing the sinus node to resume its function as the normal pacemaker of the heart. Early defibrillation is the only treatment for VF or pulseless VT and should not be delayed for any reason when a defibrillator is available. If a defibrillator is not immediately available, CPR should be started until a defibrillator arrives.

Defibrillation is done externally using two paddles or adhesive pads applied to the skin in the anterolateral position (Figure 3-50A). One paddle or pad is placed under the right clavicle to the right of the sternum and the other paddle or pad is placed to the left of the cardiac apex. If paddles are used, place conductive gel pads on the patient's skin, then place paddles on the gel pads using 25 lb of pressure to decrease transthoracic impedance and protect the skin from burns. Avoid placing paddles over medication patches or over pacemaker or implantable cardioverter defibrillator (ICD) pulse generators.

Advanced Cardiac Life Support (ACLS) guidelines recommend an initial energy of 360 J with a monophasic defibrillator and the manufacturer's recommended energy level for biphasic defibrillators. If the manufacturer's suggested energy level is not known, a 200-J shock is recommended. Make sure no one is touching the patient, the bed, or anything attached to the patient when the shock is delivered; call "all clear" and visually verify before delivering the shock. Depress the discharge button to release the energy. If using paddles, depress both discharge buttons (one on each paddle) simultaneously. The shock is delivered immediately when buttons are pushed (Figure 3-50A). Immediately resume CPR for 2 minutes before rhythm and pulse check (this may be modified in a monitored situation where ECG and hemodynamic monitoring is available).

Automatic External Defibrillators

An automatic external defibrillator (AED) is a device that incorporates a rhythm-analysis system and a shock advisory system for use by trained laypeople or medical personnel in treating victims of sudden cardiac death. The American Heart Association recommends that AEDs should be available in selected areas where large gatherings of people occur and where immediate access to emergency care may be limited, such as on airplanes, in airports, sports stadiums, health and fitness facilities, and so on. It is well known that early defibrillation is the key to survival in patients experiencing VF or pulseless VT. Any delay in the delivery of the first shock, including delays related to waiting for the arrival of trained medical personnel and equipment, can decrease the chance of survival. The availability of an AED in public areas can prevent unnecessary delays in treatment and improve survival in victims of sudden cardiac death.

Operation of an AED is quite simple and can be performed by laypeople. Instructions for use are printed on the machines and voice commands also guide the operator in using the AED. Adhesive pads are placed in the standard defibrillation position on the chest (see Figure 3-50A), the machine is turned on, and the rhythm analysis system analyzes the patient's rhythm. If the rhythm analysis system detects a shockable rhythm, such as VF or rapid VT, a voice advises the operator to shock the patient. Delivery of the shock is a simple maneuver that only involves pushing a button. The operator is advised to "stand clear" prior to delivering the shock. After a shock is delivered, the system prompts the operator to resume CPR. After 2 minutes of CPR it prompts the operator to stop CPR while it reanalyzes the rhythm.

Cardioversion

Cardioversion is the delivery of electrical energy that is synchronized to the QRS complex so that the energy is delivered during ventricular depolarization in order to avoid the T wave and the vulnerable period of ventricular repolarization. The delivery of electrical energy near the T wave can lead to

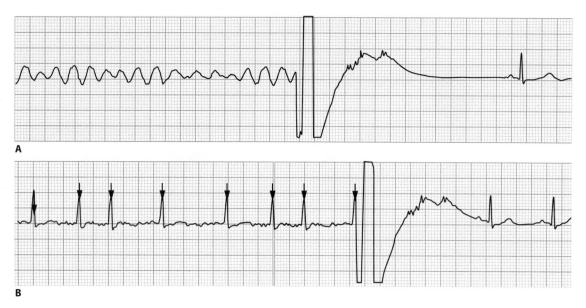

Figure 3-51. **(A)** Defibrillation of VF to sinus rhythm. **(B)** Cardioversion of atrial fibrillation to sinus rhythm. Note the synchronization mark on the QRS.

ventricular fibrillation. Synchronized cardioversion is used to terminate both supraventricular and ventricular tachycardias and is usually an elective procedure, although it should be performed urgently if the patient is hemodynamically unstable. Cardioversion can be performed via anterolateral electrode placement (see Figure 3-50A) or via anteroposterior (AP) electrode placement (see Figure 3-50B). Anteroposterior placement is preferred because less energy is required and the success rate is higher when energy travels through the short axis of the chest. Either paddles or hands-free adhesive pads can be used.

Sedation is required for cardioversion since the patient is usually awake and alert and able to feel the pain caused by the procedure. Sedation can be accomplished with drugs like midazolam (Versed), methohexital (Brevital Sodium), propofol, or others at the discretion of the physician; or an anesthesiologist may be used to administer deep sedation. Because sedation is used, an emergency cart, emergency drugs (lidocaine, epinephrine, amiodarone, atropine), sedation-reversal agent, O_2-delivery equipment, and suction equipment should be immediately available; and an O_2 saturation monitor and noninvasive blood pressure (BP) monitoring should be done continuously during the procedure and until the patient is completely awake and recovered.

Initial energy level for cardioversion is typically 50 to 100 J and varies with different arrhythmias. If the first shock is unsuccessful, energy level is increased for subsequent shocks. The machine must be synchronized to the QRS complex for cardioversion. Most machines put a bright dot or similar marker on the QRS complex when in the "synch" mode (Figure 3-51B). The machine will not discharge its energy until it sees the synch marker. Make sure to visually verify that the synch marker is actually on the QRS complex and not on a tall T wave. When delivering energy during cardioversion, push and hold the discharge button until

the energy is delivered; the synchronized machine will not discharge until it sees a QRS complex. When the energy is released, the machine automatically returns to the asynchronous mode, so if subsequent shocks are needed the machine must be resynchronized.

SELECTED BIBLIOGRAPHY

Brenyo, AJ, Aktas, MK. Non-pharmacologic management of atrial fibrillation. *Am J Cardiol.* 2011;108:317-325.

Calkins, H. Supraventricular tachycardia: atrioventricular nodal reentry and Wolff-Parkinson-White syndrome. In Fuster V, Walsh RA, Harrington RA. eds. *Hurst's The Heart.* 13th ed. New York: McGraw Hill. 2011: 987-1005.

Jacobson, C. Arrhythmias and conduction disturbances. In Woods SL, Froelicher ES, Motzer SU, Bridges EJ. eds. *Cardiac Nursing.* 6th ed. Philadelphia: Lippincott Williams & Wilkins. 2010: 333-387.

Jacobson, C. Gerity, D. Pacemakers and implantable difibrillators. In Woods SL, Froelicher ES, Motzer SU, Bridges EJ. eds. *Cardiac Nursing.* 6th ed. Philadelphia: Lippincott Williams & Wilkins. 2010: 655-704.

Jacobson C, Marzlin K, Webner C. *Cardiovascular Nursing Practice: A Comprehensive Resource Manual and Study Guide for Clinical Nurses.* Burien, WA: Cardiovascular Nursing Education Associates. 2007.

Kenny, T. *The Nuts and Bolts of Cardiac Pacing.* Malden, MA: Blackwell Futura. 2005.

Kerber, RE. Indications and techniques of electrical defibrillation and cardioversion. In Fuster V, Walsh RA, Harrington RA. eds. *Hurst's The Heart.* 13th ed. New York: McGraw Hill. 2011: 1088-1093.

Link, MS, Atkins, DL, Passman, RS, et al. Electrical therapies: automated external defibrillators, defibrillation, cardioversion, and pacing: 2010 American Heart Association Guidelines for Cardiopulmonary Resuscitation and Emergency Cardiovascular Care. *Circulation.* 2010:122(suppl 3), Part 6, S706–S719.

Olgin, J, Zipes, DP. Specific arrhythmias: diagnosis and treatment. In Bonow RO, Mann DL, Zipes DP, Libby P. eds. *Braunwald's Heart Disease—A Textbook of Cardiovascular Medicine*. 9th ed. Philadelphia: Elsevier. 2011: 771-824.

Prystowsky, EN, Padanilam, BJ, Waldo, AL. Atrial fibrillation, atrial flutter, and atrial tachycardia. In Fuster V, Walsh RA, Harrington RA. eds. *Hurst's The Heart*. 13th ed. New York: McGraw Hill. 2011: 963-986.

Pugazhendhi, V, Ellenbogen, KA. Bradyarrhythmias and pacemakers. In Fuster V, Walsh RA, Harrington RA. eds. *Hurst's The Heart*. 13th ed. New York: McGraw Hill. 2011: 1025-1057.

Rho, RW, Page, RL. Ventricular arrhythmias. In Fuster V, Walsh RA, Harrington RA. eds. *Hurst's The Heart*. 13th ed. New York: McGraw Hill. 2011: 1006-1024.

Evidence-Based Practice

Advanced Cardiovascular Life Support Provider Manual. Dallas, TX: American Heart Association. 2011.

Blomstrom-Lundqvist C, Scheinman MM, Aliot EM, et al. ACC/AHA/ESC Guidelines for the Management of Patients with Supraventricular Arrhythmias - Executive Summary. A Report of the American College of Cardiology/American Heart Association Task Force on Practice Guidelines and the European Society of Cardiology Committee for Practice Guidelines (Writing Committee to Develop Guidelines for the Management of Patients With Supraventricular Arrhythmias). Circulation. 2003:108;1871-1909.

Bourgault, A. (2008). AACN Practice Alert: Dysrhythmia Monitoring. Aliso Viejo, CA: American Association of Critical Care Nurses. http://www.aacn.org

Drew, BJ, Califf, RM, Funk, M, et al. Practice standards for electrocardiographic monitoring in hospital settings. *Circulation*. 2004:110;2721-2746.

Furie, KL, Goldstein, LB, Albers, GW, et al. Oral antithrombotic agents for the prevention of stroke in nonvalvular atrial fibrillation: a science advisory for healthcare professionals from the American Heart Association/American Stroke Association. *Stroke*, 2012:43;3442-3453.

Fuster, V, Ryden, LE, Cannom, DS, et al. 2011 ACCF/AHA/HRS focused updates incorporated into the ACC/AHA/ESC 2006 guidelines for the management of patients with atrial fibrillation: a report of the American College of Cardiology Foundation/American Heart Association Task Force on Practice Guidelines. *Circulation*, 2011:123;e269–e367.

Jacobson C. Bedside cardiac monitoring. In Burns S, ed. *AACN Protocols for Practice: Noninvasive Monitoring*. 2nd ed. Boston: Jones and Bartlett; 2006.

Wann, LS, Curtis, AB, January, CT, et al. 2011 ACCF/AHA/HRS focused update on the management of patients with atrial fibrillation (updating the 2006 guideline): a report of the American College of Cardiology Foundation/American Heart Association Task Force on Practice Guidelines. Circulation. 2011(a):123; 104-123.

Wann, LS, Curtis, AB, January, CT, et al. 2011 ACCF/AHA/HRS focused update on the management of patients with atrial fibrillation (update on dabigatran): a report of the American College of Cardiology Foundation/American Heart Association Task Force on Practice Guidelines. Circulation. 2011(b):123;1144-1150.

Zipes, D, Camm, A, Borggrefe, M, et al. ACC/AHA/ESC 2006 guidelines for management of patients with ventricular arrhythmias and the prevention of sudden cardiac death: a report of the American College of Cardiology/American Heart Association Task Force and the European Society of Cardiology Committee for Practice Guidelines Circulation, 2006:114;e385-e484.

HEMODYNAMIC MONITORING

4

Leanna R. Miller

KNOWLEDGE COMPETENCIES

1. Identify the characteristics of normal and abnormal waveform pressures for the following hemodynamic monitoring parameters:
   - Central venous pressure
   - Arterial blood pressure
2. Describe the basic elements of arterial and venous pressure-monitoring equipment and methods used to ensure accurate pressure measurements.
3. Discuss the indications, contraindications, and general management principles for the following common hemodynamic monitoring parameters:
   - Central venous pressure
   - Arterial blood pressure
4. Describe the clinical application of $Svo_2/Scvo_2$ monitoring.
5. Discuss the potential use of bioimpedance monitoring in a progressive care population.

The term *hemodynamics* refers to the interrelationship of blood pressure (BP), blood flow, vascular volumes, heart rate, ventricular function, and the physical properties of the blood. While a wide variety of hemodynamic monitoring systems are available in critical care units that are used to monitor these components, hemodynamic monitoring in the progressive care setting is generally limited to central venous pressure (CVP) monitoring and arterial monitoring. These two technologies yield a tremendous amount of useful data and thus it is essential that progressive care nurses have a working knowledge of how to obtain accurate data, analyze associated waveforms, and interpret and integrate the data. The end of this chapter focuses on these specific technologies in addition to providing a brief introductory description of other hemodynamic parameters obtained from a pulmonary artery catheter. The concepts are helpful to understand pathologic conditions discussed later in this book such as heart failure and sepsis. More extensive discussion of other hemodynamic monitoring systems such as the pulmonary artery catheter is found in the *AACN Essentials of Critical Care Nursing*.

Clinical examination can be a poor predictor of hemodynamics. Although noninvasive assessment techniques such as physical examination, history taking, and laboratory analysis are helpful and necessary, they do not provide the specific physiologic data that may be obtained with measurements such as the CVP. These technologies can directly measure the pressures and provide real-time data to clinicians so that appropriate interventions are ensured.

HEMODYNAMIC PARAMETERS

A description of the various parameters derived from the pulmonary artery catheter follows and reference values may be found in Table 4-1.

Cardiac Output

Cardiac output (CO) is the amount of blood pumped by the ventricles each minute. It is the product of the heart rate (HR) and the stroke volume (SV) (the amount of blood ejected by the ventricle with each contraction; Figure 4-1). This is evaluated with a pulmonary artery catheter and some noninvasive monitoring technologies such as bioimpedance systems.

$$CO = HR \times SV$$

The normal value is 4.0 to 8.0 L/min. It is important to note that these values are relative to size. Values within

TABLE 4-1. NORMAL HEMODYNAMIC AND BLOOD FLOW PARAMETERS

Parameter	Abbreviation	Formula	Normal Range
Cardiac output	CO	Stroke volume (SV) × heart rate (HR)	4-8 L/min
Cardiac index	CI	CO/BSA ÷ 1000	2.5-4.3 L/min/m^2
Mean arterial pressure	MAP	2(DBP) + SBP ÷ 3	70-105 mm Hg
Right atrial pressure	RAP	cm H$_2$O = mm Hg × 1.34	2-8 mm Hg
Pulmonary artery wedge pressure	PAOP		8-12 mm Hg
Pulmonary artery diastolic	PAD		10-15 mm Hg
Pulmonary vascular resistance	PVR	PAM–PAOP × 80 ÷ CO	100-250 dynes-sec/cm^{-5}
Pulmonary vascular resistance index	PVRI	PAM–PAOP × 80 ÷ CI	255-285 dynes-sec/cm^{-5}/m^2
Pulmonary artery mean	PAM		15-20 mm Hg
Systemic vascular resistance	SVR	MAP–RAP × 80 ÷ CO	800-1200 dynes-sec/cm^{-5}
Systemic vascular resistance index	SVRI	MAP–RAP × 80 ÷ CI	1970-2390 dynes-sec/cm^{-5}/m^2
Right ventricular stroke work index	RVSWI	(PAM–RAP) SVI × 0.0138	7-12 g-m/M^2
Left ventricular stroke work index	LVSWI	(MAP–PAOP) SVI × 0.0138	35-85 g-m/M^2
Oxygen delivery	DO$_2$	Cao$_2$ × CO × 10	900-1100 mL/min
Oxygen delivery index	DO$_2$I	CaO$_2$ × CI × 10	360-600 mL/min/m^2
Oxygen consumption	VO$_2$	C(a − v)O$_2$ × CO × 10	200-250 mL/min
Oxygen consumption index	VO$_2$I	C(a − v)O$_2$ × CI × 10	108-165 mL/min/m^2
Stroke volume	SV	CO/HR × 1000	50-100 mL/beat
Stroke volume index	SVI	CI/HR × 1000	35-60 mL/beat/m^2
Right ventricular end-diastolic volume	RVEDV	SV/EF	100-160 mol
Right ventricular end-diastolic volume index	RVEDVI	EDV/BSA	60-100 mL/m^2
Right ventricular end-systolic volume	RVESV	EDV − SV	50-100 mol
Right ventricular end-systolic volume index	RVESVI	ESV/BSA	30-60 mL/m^2
Right ventricular ejection fraction	RVEF	SV/EDV	40%-60%
Mixed venous saturation	Svo$_2$		60%-75%
Oxygen extraction ratio	O$_2$ER	(Cao$_2$ − Cvo$_2$)/Cao$_2$ × 100	22%-30%
Oxygen extraction index	O$_2$EI	Sao$_2$ − Svo$_2$/Sao$_2$ × 100	22%-30%

the normal range for a person 5 ft tall weighing 100 lb, may be totally inadequate for a 6-ft, 200-lb individual. Cardiac index (CI) is the CO that has been adjusted to individual body size. It is determined by dividing the CO by the individual's body surface area (BSA), which may be obtained from the DuBois body surface area chart or by pressing the CI button on the cardiac monitor. The normal value is 2.5 to 4.3 L/min/m^2.

$$CI = CO/BSA$$

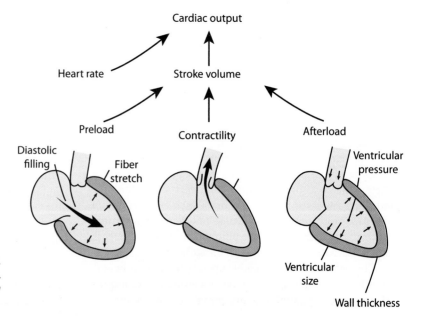

Figure 4-1. Factors affecting CO. (*Reprinted from Price S, Wilson L. Pathophysiology: Clinical Concepts of Disease Processes. Philadelphia, PA: Mosby; 1992: 390, with permission from Elsevier.*)

Cardiac Output measurements are used to assess the patient's perfusion status, response to therapy, and as a rapid means to evaluate the patient's hemodynamic status. As mentioned, CO is composed of HR and SV, or the amount of blood ejected with each contraction of the ventricle. Normal SV range is 60-100 mL/beat. SV depends on preload, afterload, and contractility. Therefore, CO is determined by:

1. HR (and rhythm)
2. Preload
3. Afterload
4. Contractility

Low-Cardiac Output/Cardiac Index

As the SV of the left ventricle is a component used in the determination of CO, any condition or disease process which impairs the pumping (ejection) or filling of the ventricle may contribute to a decreased CO. Alterations that lead to diminished CO can be divided into two general categories: inadequate ventricular filling and inadequate ventricular emptying.

Inadequate Ventricular Filling

Factors that lead to inadequate ventricular filling include arrhythmias, hypovolemia, cardiac tamponade, mitral or tricuspid stenosis, constrictive pericarditis, and restrictive cardiomyopathy. Each of these abnormalities leads to a decrease in preload (the amount of volume in the ventricle at end diastole), which results in a decrease in CO.

Inadequate Ventricular Ejection

Factors that lead to inadequate ventricular emptying include mitral/tricuspid insufficiency, myocardial infarction, increased afterload (hypertension, aortic/pulmonic stenosis), myocardial diseases (myocarditis, cardiomyopathy), metabolic disorders (hypoglycemia, hypoxia, severe acidosis), and use of negative inotropic drugs (beta-blockers, calcium channel blockers).

High-Cardiac Output/Index

In theory, in the normal, healthy individual, any factor that increases HR and contractility and decreases afterload can contribute to an increase in CO. Hyperdynamic states, such as seen in sepsis, anemia, pregnancy, and hyperthyroid crisis, may cause CO values to be increased. Increased HR is a major component in hyperdynamic states; however, in sepsis a profound decrease in afterload also contributes to an increased CO.

Components of Cardiac Output/Cardiac Index

Heart Rate and Rhythm

Rate

Normal HR is 60 to 100 beats/min. In a normal, healthy individual, an increase in HR can lead to an increase in CO. In a person with cardiac dysfunction, increases in HR can lead to a decreased CO and often myocardial ischemia. The increase in HR decreases the ventricular filling time by reducing preload, which decreases SV and leads to decreased CO.

A lower HR does not necessarily result in a decrease in CO. Decreased heart rates with normal COs are often found in athletes. Their training and conditioning strengthens the myocardium such that each cardiac contraction produces an increased SV. In individuals with left ventricular (LV) dysfunction, a slow HR can produce a decrease in CO. This is caused by decreased contractility, as well as fewer cardiac contractions each minute.

Because CO is a product of SV times heart rate, any change in SV normally produces a change in the heart rate. If the SV is elevated, the HR may decrease (eg, as seen in adaptation to exercise). If the SV falls, the HR normally increases. Subsequently, evaluating the cause of the tachycardia becomes an essential component of hemodynamic assessment. Bradycardias and tachycardias are potentially dangerous because they may result in a decrease in CO if adequate SV is not maintained. Bradycardias that develop suddenly are almost always reflective of a falling CO. The cause of tachycardia, on the other hand, must be determined because it may not reflect a low output state but rather a normal physiologic response (eg, tachycardia secondary to fever). Heart rate varies between individuals and is related to many factors. Some are described below.

Decreased Heart Rate

- Parasympathetic stimulation (vagus nerve stimulation) is a common occurrence in the acute care setting. It can occur with Valsalva maneuvers such as excessive bearing down during a bowel movement, vomiting, coughing, and suctioning.
- Conduction abnormalities, especially second- and third-degree blocks, are often seen in patients with cardiovascular diseases. Many drugs used in the progressive care setting may lead to a decreased HR, including digitalis, beta-blockers, calcium channel blockers, and phenylephrine (Neosynephrine).
- Athletes often have resting heart rates below 60 beats/min without compromising CO.
- The actual HR is not as important as the systemic effect of the heart rate. If the patient's HR leads to diminished perfusion (decreased level of consciousness, decreased urinary output, hypotension, prolonged capillary refill, new-onset chest pain, and the like), treatment is initiated to increase the heart rate.

Increased Heart Rate

- Stress, anxiety, pain, and conditions resulting in compensatory release of endogenous catecholamines such as hypovolemia, fever, anemia, and hypotension may all produce tachycardia.
- Drugs with a direct positive chronotropic effect include epinephrine and dopamine.

Tachycardia is very common in acutely ill patients. When evaluating a rapid heart rate, each of the main sources for the tachycardia is evaluated; for example, if a patient has a HR of 120 beats/min, the clinician rules out such factors as fever, pain, and anxiety before assuming that the tachycardia is due to a reduced SV. Once these are ruled out, an investigation of the cause of a low SV is accomplished. The two most common reasons for a low SV are hypovolemia and LV dysfunction. Both causes of low SV can produce an increased HR if no abnormality exists in regulation of the HR (such as autonomic nervous system dysfunction or use of drugs that interfere with the sympathetic or parasympathetic nervous system such as beta-blockers).

An increased HR can compensate for a decrease in SV, although this compensation is limited. The faster the heart rate, the less time exists for ventricular filling. As an increased HR reduces diastolic filling time, the potential exists to eventually reduce the SV. There is no specific HR where diastolic filling is reduced so severely that SV decreases. However, as the HR increases, it is important to remember that SV may be negatively affected.

Increased HR also has the potential to increase myocardial oxygen consumption (MVO_2). The higher the heart rate, the more likely it is that the heart consumes more oxygen. Some patients are more sensitive to elevated MVO_2 than others; for example, a young person may tolerate a sinus tachycardia as high as 160 for several days, whereas a patient with coronary artery disease may decompensate and develop pulmonary edema with a HR in the 130s. Keeping heart rates as low as possible—particularly in patients with altered myocardial blood flow—is one way of protecting myocardial function.

Rhythm

Many of us have observed the deleterious effects produced by a supraventricular tachycardia, or a change from normal sinus rhythm to atrial fibrillation or flutter. Loss of "atrial kick" may contribute to decreased CO. Normally, atrial contraction contributes 20% to 40% of the ventricular filling volume. With tachycardia, that atrial contribution to SV may diminish significantly. Although those with normal cardiac function are unlikely to experience compromise, it is more likely in those with impaired cardiac function.

Stroke Volume and Stroke Volume Index

Stroke volume is the amount of blood ejected from each ventricle with each heartbeat. The right and left ventricle eject nearly the same amount, which normally is from 50 to 100 mL per heartbeat.

$$SV = CO/HR \times 1000$$

Stroke Volume indexed to the patient's BSA is SVI. Indexing helps compare values regardless of the patient's size. Normal SVI is 33-47 mL/beat/m². Common causes of decreased stroke volume/stroke volume index (SV/SVI) is inadequate blood volume (preload), impaired ventricular contractility (strength), increased systemic vascular resistance (SVR; afterload), and cardiac valve dysfunction. High SV/SVI occurs when the vascular resistance is low (sepsis, use of vasodilators, neurogenic shock, and anaphylaxis).

Ejection Fraction

The ejection fraction (EF) is defined as how much blood is pumped with each contraction in relation to the volume of available blood; for example, assume the left ventricular end-diastolic volume (LVEDV is the amount of blood left in the heart just before contraction) is 100 mL. If the SV is 80 mL the EF is 80%; 80 mL of the possible 100 mL in the ventricle were ejected. Right ventricular volumes are roughly equal to those of the left ventricle (RVEF) (Table 4-1). A normal EF is usually over 60%. This is evaluated with a pulmonary artery catheter or with noninvasive methods such as the echocardiogram.

The EF may change before the SV in certain conditions, such as LV failure and sepsis; for example, the left ventricle may dilate in response to LV dysfunction from coronary artery disease, and LVEDV increases. Although the increase in LVEDV may prevent a drop in SV, EF may not be preserved. SV and SVI, then, are the best available measures to assess left and right ventricular dysfunction.

Factors Affecting Stroke Volume/Stroke Volume Index

Preload

Preload is the volume of blood that exerts a force or pressure (stretch) on the ventricles during diastole. It may also be described as the filling pressure of the ventricles at the end of diastole or the amount of blood that fills the ventricles during diastole.

According to the Frank-Starling law of the heart, the force of contraction is related to myocardial fiber stretch prior to contraction. As the fibers are stretched, the contractile force increases up to a certain point. Beyond this point, the contractile force decreases and is referred to as ventricular failure (Figure 4-2). With increased preload there is an increase in the volume of blood delivered to the ventricle,

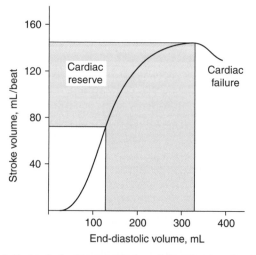

Figure 4-2. Ventricular function curve. As the end-diastolic volume increases, so does the force of ventricular contraction. The SV becomes greater up to a critical point after which SV decreases (cardiac failure). (*From Langley LF.* Review of Physiology. *3rd ed. New York, NY: McGraw-Hill; 1971.*)

the myocardium is stretched, and a more forceful ventricular contraction is produced. This forceful ventricular contraction yields an increase in SV, and therefore, CO. Too much preload causes the ventricular contraction to be less effective. A commonly referred to analogy uses the properties of a rubber band. The more a rubber band is stretched, the greater "snap" is produced when released. The rubber band may be stretched further and further, until it reaches a point where it loses its tautness and fails to recoil. Preload is measured with a CVP catheter and/or a pulmonary artery catheter.

Determinants of Preload

Preload is determined primarily by the amount of venous return to the heart. Venous constriction, venous dilation, and alterations in the total blood volume all affect preload. Preload decreases with volume changes. This can occur in hemorrhage (traumatic, surgical, gastrointestinal [GI], postpartum), diuresis (excessive use of diuretics, diabetic ketoacidosis, diabetes insipidus), vomiting and diarrhea, third spacing (ascites, severe sepsis, heart failure [HF]), redistribution of blood flow (use of vasodilators, neurogenic shock, severe sepsis), and profound diaphoresis. Venous dilatation also results in diminished preload. Etiologies that increase venous pooling and result in decreased venous return to the heart include hyperthermia, septic shock, anaphylactic shock, and drug administration (nitroglycerin, nitroprusside) (Table 4-2).

Factors leading to increased preload include excessive administration of crystalloids or blood products and the presence of renal failure (oliguric phase and/or anuria). Venous constriction results in the shunting of peripheral blood to the central organs (heart and brain). The increased venous return results in an increased preload. This may occur in hypothermia, some forms of shock (hypovolemic, cardiogenic, and obstructive) and with administration of drugs that stimulate the alpha receptors (epinephrine, dopamine at doses greater than 10 mcg/kg/min, norepinephrine) (see Table 4-2).

Clinical Indicators of Preload

The right ventricle pumps blood into the pulmonary circulation and the left ventricle ejects blood into the systemic circulation. Both circulatory systems are affected by preload, afterload, and contractility. These are discussed below and, when appropriate, the clinical indicators are differentiated by right or left heart.

Right Ventricular Preload or Right Atrial Pressure (CVP or RAP)

Normal right ventricular (RV) preload is 2 to 8 mm Hg or 2 to 10 cm H_2O (CVP = central venous pressure; RAP = right atrial pressure). Right atrial pressures are measured to assess right ventricular function, intravascular volume status, and the response to fluid and drug administration. CVP/RAP pressures increase because of intravascular volume overload, cardiac tamponade (effusion, blood, and the like), restrictive cardiomyopathies, and RV failure. There are three etiologies of RV failure: (1) intrinsic disease such as

TABLE 4-2. HEMODYNAMIC EFFECTS OF CARDIOVASCULAR AGENTS

Drug	CO	PAOP	SVR	MAP	HR	CVP	PVR
Norepinephrine (Levophed)	↑(slight)	↑	↑	↑	↔, ↑	↑	↑
Phenylephrine (Neosynephrine)	↔, ↓	↑	↑	↑	↔, ↓	↑	↑
Epinephrine (Asthmahaler)	↑	↑	↑	↑	↑	↑	↑
Dobutamine	↑	↓	↓	↑	↔, ↑	↓	↓
(Dobutrex)				(with ↑CO)	(slight)		
Dopamine (Intropin)	↑	↑	↑	↑	↑	↑	↔
<5 µg/kg/min	↑	↑↑	(slight)	(slight)	↑	↑↑	↑
>5 µg/kg/min			↑↑	↑↑			
Digoxin (Lanoxin)	↑	↔	↔	↔	↓	↔	↔
Isoproterenol (Isuprel)	↑	↓	↓	↓	↑	↓	↓
Levosimendan (Simdox)	↑	↓	↓	↓	↔ (↑in preload-sensitive patient)	↓	↓
Vasopressin	↔, ↓ (related to ↑ SVR)	↑	↑	↑	↔, ↓	↑	↑
Milrinone (Primacor)	↑	↓	↓	↔ (↓in preload-sensitive patient)	↔ (↑in preload-sensitive patient)	↓	↓
Nitroglycerin							
(Tridil)	↔	↓	↔	↔	↔	↓	↔
20-40 µg/min	↑	↓	↓	↓	↑	↓	↓
50-250 µg/min							
Nitroprusside (Nipride)	↑	↓	↓	↓	↑	↓	↓

ESSENTIAL CONTENT CASE

Hypovolemia

A 67-year-old woman is admitted to the progressive care unit with the diagnosis of hypotension secondary to presumed gastrointestinal bleeding. A history of melena for 3 days was provided by her daughter on admission. She is presently unresponsive but is breathing spontaneously. Breath sounds are clear, urine output is 15 mL in 8 hours, and her skin is cool. Laboratory work is pending and 3 U of packed red blood cells have been ordered stat. A CVP catheter is inserted to aid in the provision of fluids, blood, and medications, and to help interpret the situation. The following data are available:

BP	86/54 mm Hg
PR	118/min
RR	30 breaths/min
T	37.3°C
CVP	3 mm Hg

Case Question 1. What findings reinforce that the patient is hypovolemic?

Case Question 2. Which hemodynamic findings are abnormal?

Case Question 3. What treatments are warranted in this patient?

Answers

1. The history of melena for the past 3 days, urinary output 15 mLs in 8 hours, and BP 86/54 mm Hg. Reviewing the patient's BP history would be important—does she usually have a systolic BP less than 90? Lab tests that can be used to trend the volume status would be BUN and Hct. H/H would be especially important in this patient.
2. BP 86/54, PR 118/min, RR 30 breaths/min, CVP 3 mm Hg
3. The exact cause of the hypovolemia cannot be discerned from the CVP by itself but the history and the CVP value are consistent with the need for blood and aggressive fluid resuscitation. The CVP value can be used to target a reasonable preload level, then vasopressors may be added if necessary to further enhance blood pressure should the fluid and blood not do so.

RV infarct or cardiomyopathies; (2) secondary factors that increase pulmonary vascular resistance (PVR) such as pulmonary arterial hypertension, pulmonary embolism, hypoxemia, chronic obstructive pulmonary disease (COPD), acute respiratory distress syndrome (ARDS), sepsis; and (3) severe LV dysfunction as seen in mitral stenosis/insufficiency or LV failure. In contrast, the only clinically significant reason for a decreased CVP/RAP is hypovolemia. CVP/RAP is a late indicator of alterations in LV function therefore limiting its value in clinical decision making.

Left Ventricular Preload (PAOP, PCWP, PAWP, or LAP)

Normal LV preload is 8 to 12 mm Hg and is measured with a pulmonary artery catheter. There are many names that are synonymous with LAP and they include: PCWP = pulmonary capillary wedge pressure; PAOP = pulmonary artery occlusion pressure; and PAWP = pulmonary artery wedge pressure. The most commonly used term is PAOP. The normal PAOP is 8 to 12 mm Hg. The pressure is measured by inserting a small amount of air into the balloon port of the pulmonary artery (PA) catheter: the balloon becomes lodged in a portion of the PA that is smaller than the balloon. This occludes blood flow distal to the catheter tip. The pressure in the left atrium is sensed by the catheter tip. When the mitral valve is open during ventricular diastole, the pressure that is sensed is that of the left ventricle, the left ventricular end-diastolic pressure (LVEDP) or LV preload (Figure 4-3).

Pulmonary artery occlusion pressure increases because of conditions such as intravascular volume overload, cardiac tamponade (blood, effusion, etc), impaired ventricular relaxation (diastolic dysfunction, restrictive cardiomyopathy, and constrictive pericarditis), and LV dysfunction. Common etiologies of LV dysfunction include mitral stenosis/insufficiency, aortic stenosis/insufficiency, and diminished LV compliance (ischemia, fibrosis, hypertrophy). The only clinically significant reason for a decreased PAOP is hypovolemia.

Afterload

Afterload is the resistance to ventricular emptying during systole. It is the pressure or resistance that the ventricles must overcome to open the aortic and pulmonary valves and to pump blood into the systemic and pulmonary vasculature. Vascular resistance is determined by the length of a vessel, its diameter or radius, and the viscosity of the blood. The length of the vessel is considered to be constant. The viscosity of the blood is relatively constant except when gross volume changes occur (eg, hemorrhage) or in polycythemia. Therefore, conditions that alter the diameter of the vessels, or the outflow tract, have a primary effect on the afterload of the ventricles.

As afterload increases (vasoconstriction or obstruction of the outflow tract), the heart must work harder to eject the volume. Afterload affects the isovolumetric contraction phase of the cardiac cycle. During this phase, the ventricular pressure rises so the ventricles are able to overcome the existing vascular resistance, open the semilunar valves, and eject the contents. Once the pressure within the ventricle is higher than the pressure in the aorta/pulmonary system, the valves open and the blood is ejected from the heart. With increased afterload, the heart works harder to eject the contents, leading to increased MVO_2. This is a crucial period of myocardial susceptibility to ischemic injury and is a major reason to consider afterload reduction therapies.

Common causes of increased afterload include aortic/pulmonic stenosis, hypothermia, hypertension, compensatory response to hypotension and decreased CO, classic shock states (hypovolemic, cardiogenic, and obstructive), and response to drugs that stimulate the alpha receptors (epinephrine, norepinephrine, dopamine, phenylephrine) (see Table 4-2). Decreased afterload is seen in hyperthermia, the distributive shocks (septic, anaphylactic, and neurogenic),

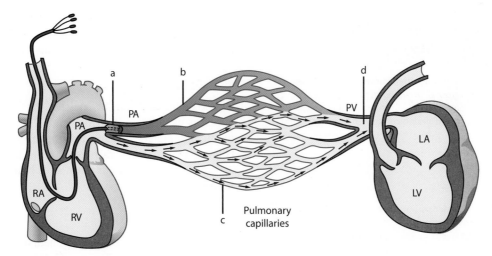

Figure 4-3. Schematic representation of the PA in the wedge position. From its position in small, occluded segment of the pulmonary circulation, the PA catheter in the wedged position allows the electronic monitoring equipment to "look through" a nonactive segment of the pulmonary circulation to the hemodynamically active pulmonary veins and left atrium. (*Reprinted from Darovic GO. Hemodynamic Monitoring: Invasive and Noninvasive Clinical Application. Philadelphia, PA: WB Saunders; 2002:207, with permission from Elsevier.*)

and after administration of vasodilating drugs (nitroprusside, nitroglycerin at higher doses, calcium channel blockers, beta-blockers, and the like) (see Table 4-2).

Clinical Indicators of Afterload

Afterload cannot be directly measured. It is evaluated with a pulmonary artery catheter and is a derived value (ie, is calculated based on other measured variables).

Systemic Vascular Resistance

Systemic vascular resistance (SVR) is normally between 800 and 1200 dynes-sec/cm^{-5}. If the SVR is elevated, the left ventricle faces an increased resistance to the ejection of blood. The SVR commonly elevates as a compensatory response to hypertension or a low CO, such as would occur in shock states. It is important for the clinician to know why the SVR is elevated; for example, if the SVR is elevated because of systemic hypertension, afterload-reducing agents are a critical part of the therapy. However, if the SVR is elevated secondary to a compensation for low CO, therapy should be directed toward the primary goal of improving CO by reducing SVR.

If the SVR is low, the left ventricle faces a lower resistance to the ejection of blood. Generally, the SVR only decreases as a pathologic response to inflammatory conditions (eg, sepsis, fever). The SVR can also be reduced in hepatic disease due to increased collateral circulation or from neurogenic induced central vasodilation. Generally, if the SVR is reduced, administration of fluids and or vasopressor drugs is considered. More important, treating the underlying condition is essential. If the underlying condition is not treated, the use of vasopressors provides only short-term success.

Pulmonary Vascular Resistance

Pulmonary Vascular Resistance is lower in comparison to SVR. Normal PVR is about 100 to 250 dynes/s/cm^{-5}

(see Table 4-1). Generally, only an elevated PVR is considered a problem, because it produces a strain on the right ventricle. If this strain is unrelieved, the right ventricle eventually fails. Failure of the right ventricle results in less blood entering the lungs and the left ventricle. Systemic hypotension follows due to RV dysfunction. The most common causes of an increase in PVR include pulmonary hypertension, hypoxia, end-stage COPD (cor pulmonale), and pulmonary emboli.

Contractility

Contractility is the strength of the myocardial contraction, or the degree of myocardial fiber shortening with contraction. Contractility contributes significantly to CO. If the other determinants of CO were constant, then a heart with a greater contractile force would produce a greater CO. However, contractility depends on many variables including preload (Frank-Starling law of the heart) and afterload.

Electrolyte levels also have a major impact on the contractility of the heart. Monitoring and treating abnormal calcium, sodium, magnesium, potassium, and phosphorus levels is essential to ensure optimal contractility. Other factors that contribute to contractility include myocardial oxygenation (ischemia), amount of functional myocardium (infarction, cardiomyopathy), and administration of positive and negative inotropic drugs.

Clinical Indicators of Contractility

Myocardial contractility is reflected indirectly in the SVI, which is the SV adjusted according to body size, and the right and left stroke work index (RVSWI and LVSWI). The normal value for SVI is 33-47 mL/beat/m^2; RVSWI is 5-10 gm/m/m^2, and LVSWI is 50-62 gm/m/m^2 (see Table 4-1). These are not direct indicators of contractility, but can be used to identify patients at risk for poor contractility and to monitor the effects of therapeutic management.

ESSENTIAL CONTENT CASE

Decreased Afterload

A 65-year-old man is developing hypotension on the acute care floor. He had femoral-popliteal bypass surgery 4 days earlier and was doing well until yesterday. He began to complain of generalized malaise with the following vital signs:

BP: 102/58 mm Hg
RR: 27 breaths/min
PR: 110/min
T: 38.1°C

His wound site is reddened but has no drainage. He does not complain of any discomfort or shortness of breath. His lung sounds are clear and he has a pulse oximeter value of 99%.

Case Question 1. What parameters identify that the patient has a systemic inflammatory response?

Case Question 2. What would be the treatment priorities at this time?

Case Question 3. If the BP drops to 80/50 mm Hg, what is the significance? What would be the priorities of treatment?

Answers

1. The criteria are HR > 90 beats/min, temperature < 36°C or > 38°C; WBC count < 4,000 or > 12,000 or band count > 10%; RR > 20 or $Paco_2$ < 32 mm Hg. This patient has HR (110); RR (27); T (38.1°C).
2. Culture any area suspected of infection. In this patient culture blood, sputum, urine, and wound site. Once cultures are sent, start empiric antimicrobials. CVP monitoring would be helpful to identify hypovolemia (due to vasodilation and third spacing).
3. If the BP drops to 80/50 mm Hg the patient is now in shock (MAP 62 mm Hg). This is a critical drop in BP and requires volume resuscitation with NS until a CVP of 10 mm Hg is reached. If the patient still remains hypotensive, a vasopressor(s) should be added. The recommended drugs are norepinephrine and vasopressin. These drugs require continuous monitoring so transfer to the critical care unit is warranted.

BASIC COMPONENTS OF HEMODYNAMIC MONITORING SYSTEMS

The basic components of hemodynamic monitoring systems include an indwelling catheter connected to a pressure transducer and flush system and a bedside monitor. All components that come in contact with the vascular system must be sterile, with meticulous attention paid to maintaining a closed sterile system during use.

Pulmonary Artery Catheter

The PA catheter is a multilumen catheter inserted into the PA (Figures 4-3, 4-4). Each lumen or "port" has specific functions. The PA catheter typically is inserted through an introducer sheath (large-diameter, short catheter with a diaphragm) placed in a major vein. Veins used for PA catheter insertion include the internal jugular, subclavian, femoral, and less commonly, the brachial vein. More information on the PA catheter is found in *AACN Essentials of Critical Care Nursing.*

Arterial Catheter

The arterial catheter, or "A-line," has only one lumen, which is used for measuring arterial pressures, hemodynamic parameters, and for drawing arterial blood samples (Figure 4-5). Arterial catheters are inserted in any major artery, with the most common sites being the radial and femoral arteries.

Pressure Tubing

The pressure tubing is a key component of any hemodynamic monitoring system (see Figure 4-5). It is designed to be a stiff (noncompliant) tubing to ensure accurate transfer of intravascular pressures to the transducer. The pressure tubing connects the intravascular catheter to the transducer. Many pressure tubings have stopcocks in line to facilitate blood sampling and zeroing the transducer (see below). Normally, the pressure tubing is kept as short as possible (no more than 3-4 ft), with a minimal number of stopcocks, to increase the accuracy of pressure measurements.

Pressure Transducer

The pressure transducer is a small electronic sensor that has the ability to convert a mechanical pressure (vascular pressure) into an electrical signal (see Figure 4-5). This electrical signal can then be displayed on the pressure amplifier.

Pressure Amplifier

The pressure amplifier, or "bedside monitor," augments the signal from the transducer and displays the converted vascular pressure as an electrical signal (see Figure 4-5). This signal is used to display a continuous waveform on the oscilloscope of the monitor and to provide a numerical display of the pressure measurement. Most bedside monitors also have a graphic recorder to print out the pressure waveform.

Pressure Bag and Flush Device

In addition to being attached to the pressure amplifier, the transducer is connected to an intravenous (IV) solution, which is placed in a pressure bag (Figure 4-6). The IV solution is normally 500 to 1000 mL of normal saline (NS), although 5% dextrose in water (D_5W) can be used. The IV solution is placed under 300 mm Hg of pressure to provide a slow, continuous infusion of fluid through the vascular catheter.

The IV solution is placed under pressure for another reason. Included in most pressure systems is a flush device (see Figure 4-6). The flush device regulates fluid flow through the pressure tubing at a slow, continuous rate to prevent occlusion of the vascular catheter. Normally, the flush device restricts fluid flow to approximately 2 to 4 mL/h. If the flush device is activated, normally by squeezing or pulling the flush device,

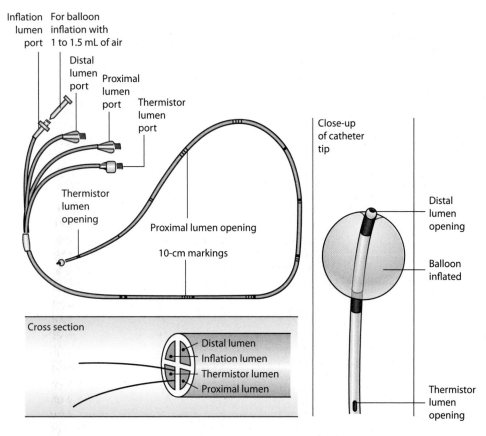

Figure 4-4. Flow-directed PA catheter (Swan-Ganz). (*From Visalli F, Evans P. The Swan-Ganz catheter: a program for teaching safe, effective use. Nursing 1981. 1981;11:1.*)

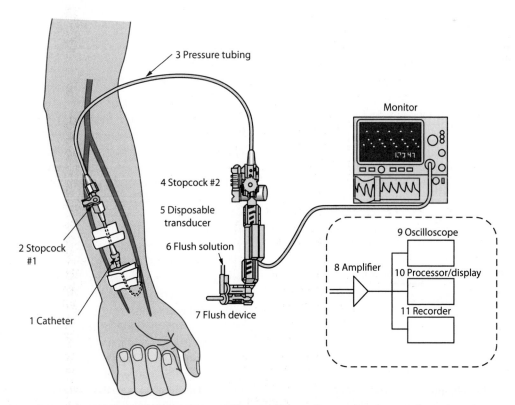

Figure 4-5. Components of a hemodynamic monitoring system. (*Reprinted from Gardner R, Hollingsworth K. Electrocardiography and pressure monitoring: how to obtain optimal results. In: Shoemaker WC, Ayers S, Grenvik A, Holbrook P, eds. Textbook of Critical Care. 3rd ed. Philadelphia, PA: WB Saunders; 1995:272, with permission from Elsevier.*)

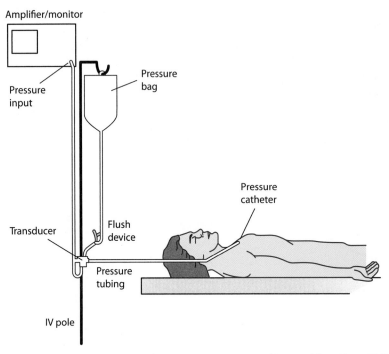

Figure 4-6. Pressure bag and flush device connected to a pressure transducer and monitoring system. (*Reprinted from Ahrens TS, Taylor L. Hemodynamic Waveform Analysis. Philadelphia, PA: WB Saunders; 1992: 210, with permission from Elsevier.*)

a rapid flow of fluid enters the pressure tubing. Flush devices are activated for two reasons: to rapidly clear the tubing of air or blood and to check the accuracy of the tubing/catheter system (square wave test). Measuring the fluid in the IV solution should be done on every shift to determine the amount of fluid infused from the pressure bag. Depending on hospital procedures, unfractionated heparin may be added to the IV solution to aid in keeping the system patent. If this is done, generally about 1 U of 1:1000 unfractionated heparin is added for every cubic centimeter (cc) of the IV solution.

Alarms

Bedside monitors have alarms for each of the hemodynamic pressures being monitored. Normally, every parameter that is being monitored has high and low alarms, which can be set to detect variations from the current value. Alarm limits are generally set to detect significant decreases or increases in pressures or rates, typically ± 10% of the current values.

OBTAINING ACCURATE CVP AND ARTERIAL VALUES

The information obtained from hemodynamic monitoring technology must be verified for accuracy by the bedside clinician.

Zeroing the Transducer

A fundamental step in obtaining accurate hemodynamic values is to zero the transducer amplifier system. Zeroing is the act of electronically compensating for any offset (distortion)

in the transducer. This is normally done by exposing the transducer to air and pushing an automatic zero button on the bedside monitor. This step is performed at least once before obtaining the first hemodynamic reading after catheter insertion. Because it is an electronic function, it normally has to be performed only once when the transducer and amplifier are first attached to the in situ catheter.

Leveling the Transducer to the Catheter Tip

Leveling is the process of aligning the tip of the vascular catheter horizontal to a zero reference position, usually a stopcock in the pressure tubing close to the transducer. The reference point is the phlebostatic axis and is found at the intersection between the fourth intercostal space (ICS) and half the AP diameter of the chest (Figure 4-7).

There are two basic methods for leveling. When the transducer and stopcocks are mounted on a pole close to the bed, the pole height is adjusted to have the stopcock opening horizontal to the external reference location of the catheter tip (Figure 4-8). To ensure horizontal positioning, a carpenter's level is usually necessary. Each time the bed height or patient position is altered, this leveling procedure must be repeated (Figure 4-9).

The other method for leveling places the transducer and stopcock at the correct location on the chest wall or arm (Figure 4-10). Taping or strapping the transducer to the appropriate location on the body eliminates the need for repeating the leveling procedure when bed heights are changed. As long as the transducer/stopcock position remains horizontal to the external reference location, no releveling is required.

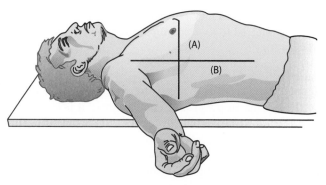

Figure 4-7. Referencing and zeroing the hemodynamic monitoring system in a supine patient. The phlebostatic axis is determined by drawing an imaginary vertical line from the fourth ICS on the sternal border to the right side of the chest. **(A)** A second imaginary line is drawn horizontally at the level of the midpoint between the anterior and posterior surface of the chest. **(B)** The phlebostatic axis is located at the intersection of points A and B. (*Reprinted from Keckeisen M, Chulay M, Gawlinski A, eds. Pulmonary artery pressure monitoring. In: Hemodynamic Monitoring Series. Aliso Viejo, CA: AACN; 1998:11, with permission from Elsevier.*)

Leveling must be performed when obtaining the first set of values and any time the transducer is no longer horizontal to the external reference location. When obtaining the first set of readings, zeroing and leveling are frequently performed simultaneously. After this initial combined effort, zeroing does not need to be performed when leveling is done.

Calibration of the Transducer/Amplifier System

If the transducer/amplifier system is suspected of being inaccurate, calibration can be performed. Calibration is less important today because all disposable transducers are precalibrated by the manufacturer. If calibration needs to

be checked prior to use, or if a reading is in doubt, a simple static pressure check can be done before the transducer is attached to the patient. Detailed descriptions of how to perform static pressure checks are found in most hemodynamic monitoring texts.

Ensuring Accurate Waveform Transmission

For hemodynamic monitoring to provide accurate information, the vascular pressure must be transmitted back to the transducer unaltered and then converted accurately into an electrical signal. For this waveform to be transmitted unaltered, no obstructions or distortions to the signal should be present along the transmission route. Distortion of the waveform leads to inaccurate pressure interpretations. A variety of factors can cause distortions to the waveform, including catheter obstructions (eg, clots, catheter bending, blood or air in tubing), excessive tubing or connectors, and transducer damage. Verification of an accurate transmission of the waveform to the transducer is checked by the bedside nurse by performing a square wave test. This occurs at the beginning of each shift.

Square Wave Test
The square wave test is performed on all hemodynamic pressure systems before assuming that the waveforms and pressures obtained are accurate. The square wave test is performed by recording the pressure waveform while fast flushing the catheter (Table 4-3, Figure 4-11). The fast-flush valve is pulled or squeezed, depending on the model, for at least a second and then rapidly released. The tracing should show a rapid rise in the waveform to the top of the graph paper, with a square pattern. Release of the flush device should show a

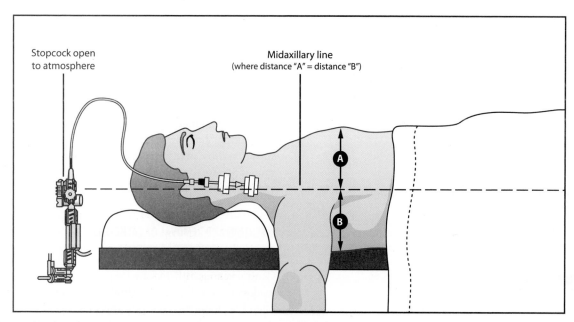

Figure 4-8. Typical leveling of CVP catheter with stopcock attached to the transducer for mounting on a pole. The stopcock close to the transducer is opened to atmospheric pressure (air) horizontal to the fourth ICS at the midaxillary line.

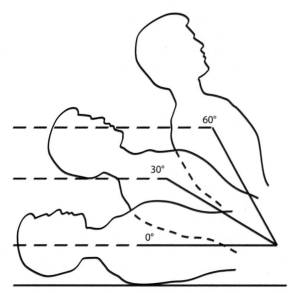

Figure 4-9. The level of the phlebostatic axis as the patient moves flat to a higher level of backrest. The level of the axis for referencing and zeroing the air-fluid interface rotates on the axis and remains horizontal as the patient moves from flat to increasingly higher backrest positions. For accurate hemodynamic pressure readings at different backrest elevations, the air-fluid interface must be at the level of the phlebostatic axis. (*Reprinted from Bridges EJ, Woods SL. Pulmonary artery pressure measurement: state of the art. Heart Lung. 1993;22(2):101, with permission from Elsevier.*)

rapid decrease in pressure below the baseline of the pressure waveform (undershoot), followed immediately by a small increase above the baseline (overshoot) prior to resumption of the normal pressure waveform. Square wave tests with these characteristics are called *optimally damped tests* and represent an accurate waveform transmission. The square wave test is the best method available to the clinician to check the accuracy of hemodynamic monitoring equipment; for example, if an arterial line is to be examined for accuracy, a square wave test should be done. Do not compare the arterial line pressure with an indirect blood pressure reading with a sphygmomanometer, because the indirect method is usually less accurate than the direct method (arterial line pressure). If the square wave test indicates optimal damping, then the arterial line pressure is accurate.

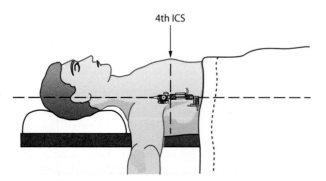

Figure 4-10. Leveling a transducer for mounting on the chest wall at the fourth ICS at the midaxillary line.

Two problems may exist with waveform transmissions, and are referred to as *overdamping* and *underdamping* (see Table 4-3).

Overdamping

If something absorbs the pressure wave (like air or blood in the tubing, stopcocks, or connections), it is said to be *overdamped*. Overdamping decreases systolic pressures and increases diastolic pressures. An overdamped square wave test reflects the obstruction in waveform transmission. Characteristics of overdamping include a loss of the undershoot and overshoot waves after release of the flush valve and a slurring of the downstroke (Figure 4-12).

Underdamping

If something accentuates the pressure wave (like excessive tubing), it is said to be *underdamped*. Underdamping increases systolic pressures and decreases diastolic pressures (Figure 4-13). An underdamped square wave test reflects the amplification of pressure waves and includes large undershoot and overshoot waves after the release of the flush valve. Table 4-4 summarizes the methods of assessing and ensuring the accuracy of hemodynamic monitoring systems.

Care of the Tubing/Catheter System

Nosocomial infections related to the tubing/catheter system are usually caused by the entry of organisms through stopcocks. Stopcocks are opened for blood sampling and zeroing the transducer only when necessary. Closed, needleless systems are used whenever feasible to decrease the risks to the patient and clinician.

Tubing changes, including flush device, transducer, and flush solution, should occur every 72 hours. The frequency of catheter device changes is controversial, but must occur whenever the catheter is suspected as a source of an IV infection or by institutional policy.

Length/duration of indwelling catheter use varies depending upon the need for use, site accessed, patient clinical status, catheter type, and antibiotic coating (if any). There are widespread variations in site care techniques and materials used across hospitals. Current CDC recommendations state central lines should be removed as soon as their exclusive use is no longer required. A multidisciplinary approach to tracking "line days" with removal as soon as possible is supported by many professional organizations. Nurses should adhere to unit policy and work with the care team to remove invasive lines as expediently as reasonable.

INSERTION AND REMOVAL OF CATHETERS

Central Venous Catheters

Central venous catheters are frequently inserted to assess preload in acutely ill patients. However, because these catheters often have more than one port through which to infuse fluids, they may also be used to infuse vasoactive substances, other intravenous medications, and total parenteral nutrition.

TABLE 4-3. **ASSESSING DAMPING CONCEPTS FROM SQUARE WAVE TEST**

Square Wave Test		Clinical Effect	Corrective Action
Optimally damped 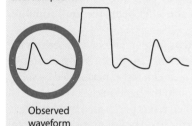 Observed waveform	**Figure 4-11.** Optimally damped system. When the fast flush of the continuous flush system is activated and quickly released, a sharp upstroke terminates in a flat line at the maximal indicator on the monitor and hard copy. This is followed by an immediate and rapid downstroke extending below the baseline with just 1 or 2 oscillations within 0.12 second (minimal ringing) and a quick return to baseline. The patient's pressure waveform is also clearly defined with all components of the waveform, such as the dicrotic notch on an arterial waveform, clearly visible. Intervention: There is no adjustment in the monitoring system required. (*Reprinted from Darovic GO, Vanriper S, Vanriper J. Fluid-filled monitoring systems. In: Darovic GO, ed.* Hemodynamic Monitoring: Invasive and Noninvasive Clinical Application. *3rd ed. Philadelphia, PA: WB Saunders Co; 1995:161-162, with permission from Elsevier.*)	Produces accurate waveform and pressure.	None required.
Overdamped 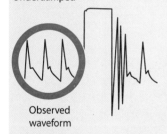 Observed waveform	**Figure 4-12.** Overdamped system. The upstroke of the square wave appears somewhat slurred, the waveform does not extend below the baseline after the fast flush, and there is no ringing after the flush. The patient's waveform displays a falsely decreased systolic pressure and a falsely high diastolic pressure, as well as poorly defined components of the pressure tracing such as a diminished or absent dicrotic notch on arterial waveforms. Interventions: To correct the problem: (1) check for the presence of blood clots, blood left in the catheter following blood sampling, or air bubbles at any point from the catheter tip to the transducer and eliminate them as necessary; (2) use low-compliance (rigid), short (< 3-4 ft) monitoring tubing; (3) ensure there are no loose connections; and (4) check for kinks in the line. (*Reprinted from Darovic GO, Vanriper S, Vanriper J. Fluid-filled monitoring systems. In: Darovic GO, ed.* Hemodynamic Monitoring: Invasive and Noninvasive Clinical Application. *3rd ed. Philadelphia, PA: WB Saunders Co; 1995:161-162, with permission from Elsevier.*)	Produces a falsely low systolic and high diastolic value.	Check the system for air, blood, loose connections, or kinks in the tubing or catheter. Verify extension tubing has not been added.
Underdamped Observed waveform	**Figure 4-13.** Underdamped system. The waveform is characterized by numerous amplified oscillations above and below the baseline following the fast flush. The monitored pressure wave displays falsely high systolic pressure (overshoot), possibly falsely low diastolic pressures, and "ringing" artifacts on the waveform. Intervention: To correct the problem, remove all air bubbles in the fluid system. Use large bore, shorter tubing, or a damping device. (*Reprinted from Darovic GO, Vanriper S, Vanriper J. Fluid-filled monitoring systems. In: Darovic GO, ed.* Hemodynamic Monitoring: Invasive and Noninvasive Clinical Application. *3rd ed. Philadelphia, PA: WB Saunders Co; 1995:161-162, with permission from Elsevier.*)	Produces a falsely high systolic and low diastolic value.	Remove unnecessary tubing and stopcocks. Add a damping device.

Insertion

Central venous catheters can be inserted into most large-diameter veins, with the internal jugular and subclavian veins being the most common insertion sites. Typically, the CVP catheter is advanced into the superior vena cava to a level above the right atrium. Following placement, location is verified with a chest radiograph to rule out the presence of a pneumothorax, kinking of the catheter, or other complications.

The waveform configuration associated with the CVP is readily identifiable (described later) and in combination with the value allows the clinician to monitor the patient's status over time and with interventions.

Removal

Removing the CVP catheter, and/or discontinuing monitoring the CVP value is a clinical decision based on the assessment that the data from the catheter is no longer necessary for care management. This decision may be made anywhere from a few hours to several days after insertion. The removal of the CVP catheter is normally performed by a physician, nurse practitioner, or physician assistant—although in some institutions nurses perform this task. Nurses must be aware of their specific hospital and unit policies regarding removal of the CVP catheter.

Following the discontinuance of IV fluids, all stopcocks to the patient are turned off to avoid air entry into the vascular

TABLE 4-4. SUMMARY OF METHODS FOR ASSESSING AND ENSURING ACCURACY OF HEMODYNAMIC MONITORING SYSTEMS[a]

Method	When Performed
Zero transducer	Should only be performed once. If the transducer zeros properly, a waveform should be visible on the monitor.
Level the transducer	Leveling should be done prior to each pressure reading and with any substantive change in pressures.
Square wave test	Should be performed prior to every reading and after blood has been withdrawn from the catheter.
Calibration	Calibration should be performed once prior to using the transducer.

[a]If a transducer has been zeroed, leveled, and calibrated and has an optimally damped square wave test, the monitor display is accurate.

bed during catheter removal. The patient is placed in a supine position with the head of the bed flat. While the catheter is being gently withdrawn, the patient is instructed to exhale or hold his or her breath to further decrease the chance of air embolus. Resistance during catheter withdrawal may indicate catheter knotting (very rare). A chest x-ray is necessary to confirm the problem and special removal procedures are performed to avoid structural damage to the vessels.

Complications

Complications associated with CVP catheters include those associated with insertion, maintenance, and removal of the device. These include bleeding, pneumothorax or air emboli, and introduction of microorganisms and subsequent infection.

Arterial Catheters

Blood pressure measurement with the indirect method (sphygmomanometer) is not as accurate as direct blood pressure measurement, particularly during conditions of abnormal blood flow (high or low CO states), SVR, or body temperature. The prevalence of these conditions in acutely ill patients may necessitate insertion of an arterial catheter to directly measure blood pressure.

Insertion

Arterial catheters are short (< 4 in) catheters that can be inserted into radial, brachial, axillary, femoral, or pedal arteries. The most common site is the radial artery. Arterial catheters can be placed by cut down or with percutaneous insertion techniques, the latter being the most common insertion method.

General insertion steps for percutaneous insertion are similar to IV catheter insertion. Prior to insertion of a radial artery catheter, however, an Allen test is performed to verify the adequacy of circulation to the hand in the event of radial artery thrombosis. The Allen test is performed by completely obstructing blood flow to the hand by compressing the radial and ulnar arteries for a minute or two. If adequate collateral blood flow exists, there will be rapid return of color to the hand upon release of the ulnar artery (Figure 4-14).

During insertion, care is exercised not to damage the arterial vessel by excessive probing or movement of the needle.

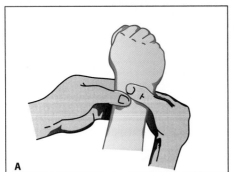
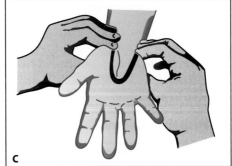
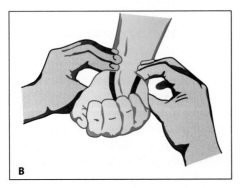
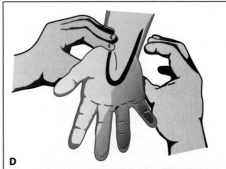

Figure 4-14. The Allen test. (*From DeGroot KD, Damato MB. Monitoring intra-arterial pressure. Crit Care Nurs. 1986;6[1]:74-78.*)

Bleeding into the tissues occurs quite easily if the vessel is damaged, causing obstruction to distal blood flow and nerve pressure. Following artery cannulation, the catheter is connected to the pressure transducer and a high-pressure infusion system to prevent blood from backing up into the tubing and fluid container (see Figure 4-5).

Removal

The removal of the arterial catheter is warranted when an accurate blood pressure can be obtained via noninvasive methods, the blood pressure is no longer labile, or when frequent arterial blood samples are no longer indicated. Removal of arterial catheters is commonly performed by the nurse using procedures similar to IV catheter removal, but because they are in an artery, greater attention to achieving hemostasis is required. Following catheter removal, firm pressure is maintained over the site for at least 5 minutes or until hemostasis occurs. This prevents bleeding and hematoma formation. For patients with coagulation abnormalities, manual pressure may need to be applied for 10 minutes or longer. Pressure dressings, rather than manual pressure, at the site are not recommended as a means to achieve hemostasis. Once hemostasis is achieved, a pressure dressing may be used but is generally not needed.

Frequent assessment of the site after catheter removal is recommended to identify rebleeding and thrombosis of the artery. Checking the extremity for the presence of pulses, circulation, and bleeding is recommended for a few hours after catheter removal.

Complications

A variety of complications are associated with arterial catheters (Table 4-5). The most serious are related to bleeding from the arterial catheter and loss of arterial flow to the extremity from thrombus formation. Loose connections in the arterial system can lead to rapid and massive blood loss. The morbidity and mortality associated with these complications require stringent safeguards (Luer-Lock connections, minimum number of stopcocks, pressure alarm system activated at all times) to prevent bleeding and to rapidly identify disruptions in the arterial system. The catheters are removed as early as possible to prevent the potential for thrombus formation.

OBTAINING AND INTERPRETING HEMODYNAMIC WAVEFORMS

To obtain hemodynamic values, interpretation of waveforms is necessary. A multichannel strip recorder, which provides both an electrocardiographic (ECG) and pressure tracing, is the required element (Figure 4-15). Many institutions also use respiratory pressure waveforms, graphed simultaneously with the ECG, CVP, and arterial waveforms. The larger the scale, the easier is the interpretation of the wave. All waveforms are easily obtained simply by activating the record function of the bedside monitor. When obtaining waveforms for interpretation, make sure the calibration scales on the left side of the paper are properly aligned with the paper grid.

Improperly aligned calibration marks increase the difficulty in reading the waveform and increase potential errors in interpretation.

Patient Positioning

The patient is placed in the supine position, with the backrest elevated anywhere from 0° to 60° (see Figure 4-9). Generally, data should not be obtained if the patient is on his or her side, because it is difficult to identify the location of the catheter tip for purposes of leveling (Figure 4-16). Improper leveling distorts atrial and venous pressure readings.

It is important to remember that patient comfort is a key issue when obtaining waveform readings. Do not position a spontaneously breathing patient with dyspnea flat for the sole reason of obtaining the readings. It is best to obtain values in the position in which the patient is most comfortable.

Interpretation

Correct interpretation of waveforms involves careful assessment of venous and arterial pressure waveforms. Normal values for each of the hemodynamic pressures are listed in Table 4-1.

Central Venous Pressure

The CVP (also known as right atrial pressure) is important because it is used to approximate the right ventricular end-diastolic pressure (RVEDP) and preload. A normal CVP is between 2 and 8 mm Hg. Low CVP values typically reflect hypovolemia or decreased venous return. High CVP values reflect overhydration, increased venous return, or right-sided cardiac failure. The CVP is obtained from the tip of central venous catheter. Measurement of CVP is done simultaneously with the ECG. Using the ECG allows the identification of the point where the CVP best correlates with the RVEDP.

The CVP is read by one of two techniques. The first technique is to take the mean (average) of the A wave of the CVP waveform (Figure 4-17). Although three waves normally exist on atrial waveforms (A, C, and V waves), the mean of the A wave most closely approximates ventricular end-diastolic pressure. The A wave of the CVP waveform starts just after the P wave on the ECG is observed and represents atrial contraction. By taking the reading at the highest point of the A wave, adding it to the reading at the lowest point of that A wave, and dividing by 2, the average or mean CVP reading is obtained (generally a line is drawn though the middle of the A waves to derive a number).

A second method, the Z-point technique, also can be used to estimate ventricular end-diastolic pressures (Figure 4-18). The Z-point is taken just before the closure of the tricuspid valve. This point is located on a CVP tracing in the mid to late QRS complex area. The Z-point technique is especially useful when an A wave does not exist; for example, in atrial fibrillation when atrial contraction is absent.

By isolating the A wave or using the Z-point technique, atrial pressures can reasonably estimate ventricular

TABLE 4-5. PROBLEMS ENCOUNTERED WITH ARTERIAL CATHETERS

Problem	Cause	Prevention	Treatment
Hematoma after withdrawal of needle	Bleeding or oozing at puncture site.	Maintain firm pressure on site during withdrawal of catheter and for 5-15 minutes (as necessary) after withdrawal. Apply elastic tape (Elastoplast) firmly over puncture site. For femoral arterial puncture sites, leave a sandbag on site for 1-2 hours to prevent oozing. If patient is receiving unfractionated heparin, discontinue 2 hours before catheter removal.	Continue to hold pressure to puncture site until oozing stops. Apply sandbag to femoral puncture site for 1-2 hours after removal of catheter.
Decreased or absent pulse distal to puncture site	Spasm of artery. Thrombosis of artery.	Introduce arterial needle cleanly, nontraumatically. Use 1 U unfractionated heparin to 1 mL IV fluid.	Inject lidocaine locally at insertion site and 10 mg into arterial catheter. Arteriotomy and Fogarty catheterization both distally and proximally from the puncture site result in return of pulse in > 90% of cases if brachial or femoral artery is used.
Bleedback into tubing, dome, or transducer	Insufficient pressure on IV bag. Loose connections.	Maintain 300 mm Hg pressure on IV bag. Use Luer-Lock stopcocks; tighten periodically.	Replace transducer. "Fast-flush" through system. Tighten all connections.
Hemorrhage	Loose connections.	Keep all connecting sites visible. Observe connecting sites frequently. Use built-in alarm system. Use Luer-Lock stopcocks.	Tighten all connections.
Emboli	Clot from catheter tip into bloodstream.	Always aspirate and discard before flushing. Use continuous flush device. Use 1 U unfractionated heparin to 1 mL IV fluid. Gently flush < 2-4 mL.	Remove catheter.
Local infection	Forward movement of contaminated catheter. Break in sterile technique. Prolonged catheter use.	Carefully suture catheter at insertion site. Always use aseptic technique. Remove catheter after 72-96 hours. Inspect and care for insertion site daily, including dressing change and antibiotic or iodophor ointment.	Remove catheter. Prescribe antibiotic.
Sepsis	Break in sterile technique. Prolonged catheter use. Bacterial growth in IV fluid.	Use percutaneous insertion. Always use aseptic technique. Remove catheter after 72-96 hours. Change transducer, stopcocks, and tubing every 96 hours. Do not use IV fluid containing glucose. Use sterile dead-end caps on all ports of stopcocks. Carefully flush remaining blood from stopcocks after blood sampling.	Remove catheter. Prescribe antibiotic.

Reprinted from Daily E, Schroeder J. Techniques in Bedside Hemodynamic Monitoring. 5th ed. St. Louis, MO; CV Mosby; 1994:165-166, with permission from Elsevier.

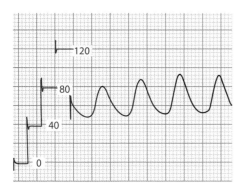

Figure 4-15. Graphic tracing of an arterial waveform preceded by calibration scale markings (0/40/80/120 mm Hg). Note how the scale markers line up with the heavy line of the tracing paper. Each 1-mm line represents 4 mm Hg in this scale.

end-diastolic pressure. It is helpful to read these values off a multichannel strip recorder and not the digital display on the bedside monitor.

Central Venous Pressure: Abnormal Venous Waveforms

Two types of abnormal CVP waveforms are common. Large A waves (also called cannon A waves) occur when the atrium contracts against a closed tricuspid value (Figure 4-19). This occurs most commonly with arrhythmias like PVCs or third-degree heart block. Giant V waves are common in conditions such as tricuspid insufficiency or ventricular failure. Using the Z-point for CVP readings prevents incorrect interpretations associated with the use of large A or V waves.

Arterial Waveforms

An arterial waveform, such as seen in systemic tracings, has three common characteristics: rapid upstroke, dicrotic notch, and progressive diastolic runoff (Figure 4-20). Diastole is read near the end of the QRS complex with systole read before the peak of the T wave. The mean arterial pressure can be calculated (see Table 4-1) or obtained from the digital display on the bedside monitor.

Systemic Arterial Pressures

Direct measurement of systemic arterial pressures is obtained from the tip of an arterial catheter and leveled to the phlebostatic axis (see Figure 4-10), with pressure waveforms interpreted as described. Normal pressures are generally in the region of 100 to 120 mm Hg systolic, 60 to 80 mm Hg diastolic, and 70 to 105 mm Hg mean (see Table 4-1).

Systemic arterial pressures are not interpreted without other clinical information. In general, however, hypotension is assumed if the mean arterial pressure drops below 60 mm Hg. Hypertension is assumed if the systolic blood pressure (SBP) is greater than 140 to 160 mm Hg or the diastolic pressure exceeds 90 mm Hg.

The arterial pressure is one of the most commonly used parameters for assessing the adequacy of blood flow to the tissues. Blood pressure is determined by two factors, CO and SVR. Blood pressure does not reflect early clinical changes in hemodynamics because of the interaction with CO and SVR.

In addition, the CO consists of HR and SV. These two interact to maintain a normal CO. Subsequently, if the SV begins to fall due to loss of volume (hypovolemia) or dysfunction (LV failure), the HR increases to offset the decrease in SV. The net effect is to maintain the CO at near-normal levels. If the CO does not change, then there is no change in the blood pressure.

A key point for the nurse to consider is that because of these compensatory mechanisms, blood pressure may not signal early clinical changes in hemodynamic status. If a patient begins to bleed postoperatively, the blood pressure generally does not reflect this change until compensation is no longer possible. In addition, hypotension is sometimes difficult to evaluate. It is possible that true hypotension exists only when tissue hypoxia is present and end organs are affected. Although tradition dictates that we identify hypotension using predefined levels of blood pressure, other measures such as mixed venous saturation of hemoglobin (Svo_2) and lactate levels may be better indicators. Svo_2 monitoring is described later in the Section Continuous Mixed and Central Venous Oxygen Monitoring (Svo_2/$Scvo_2$).

Although studies identify the role of hypertension in circulatory damage, the specific level of hypertension that results in the damage is unclear. Therefore, any SBP over 140 is considered potentially injurious to the vasculature.

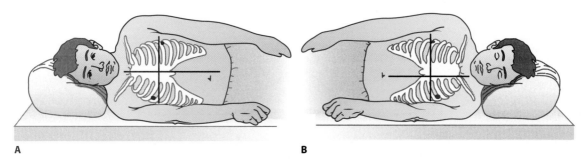

Figure 4-16. Referencing and zeroing the hemodynamic monitoring system in a patient in the lateral position. **(A)** For the right lateral position, the reference point is at the intersection of the fourth ICS and the midsternum. **(B)** For the left lateral position, the reference point is the intersection of the fourth ICS and the left parasternal border. (*Reprinted from Keckeisen M, Chulay M, Gawlinski A, eds. Pulmonary artery pressure monitoring.* In: Hemodynamic Monitoring Series. *Aliso Viejo, CA: AACN; 1998:12, with permission from Elsevier.*)

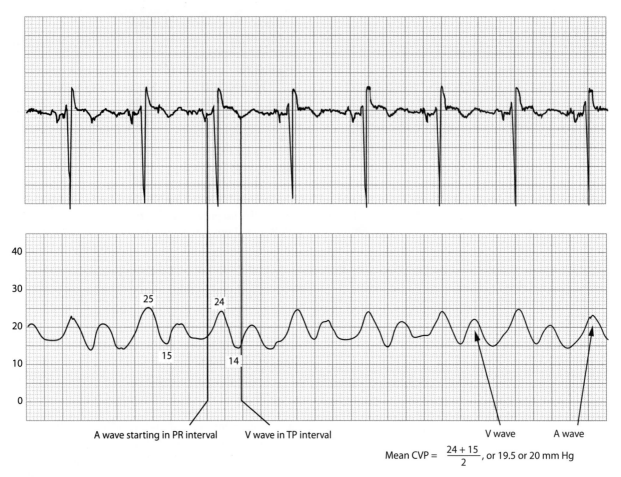

A wave starting in PR interval   V wave in TP interval   V wave   A wave

$$\text{Mean CVP} = \frac{24 + 15}{2}, \text{ or } 19.5 \text{ or } 20 \text{ mm Hg}$$

Figure 4-17. Reading a CVP waveform by averaging the A wave. (*Reprinted from Ahrens TS, Taylor L.* Hemodynamic Waveform Analysis. *Philadelphia, PA: WB Saunders; 1992:31, with permission from Elsevier.*)

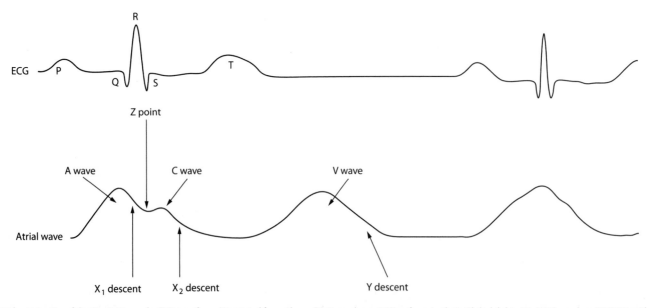

Figure 4-18. Use of the Z-point to read a CVP waveform. (*Reprinted from Ahrens TS.* Hemodynamic Waveform Analysis. *Philadelphia, PA: WB Saunders; 1992:24, with permission from Elsevier.*)

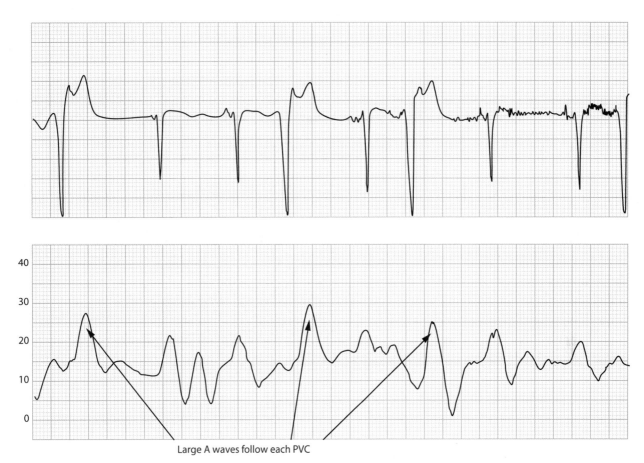

Large A waves follow each PVC

Figure 4-19. Giant A waves with loss of atrioventricular synchrony. (*Reprinted from Ahrens TS.* Hemodynamic Waveform Analysis. *Philadelphia, PA: WB Saunders; 1992:54, with permission from Elsevier.*)

Artifacts in Hemodynamic Waveforms: Respiratory Influence

Respiration can physiologically change hemodynamic pressures. Spontaneous breathing augments venous return and slightly increases resistance to left ventricle filling. Mechanical ventilation does the opposite, potentially reducing venous return and reducing the resistance on the heart. The effect of mechanical ventilation on an arterial pressure is seen in Figure 4-21. The effect of spontaneous breathing on a CVP is noted in Figure 4-22.

A spontaneous breath or a patient-initiated ventilator breath produces a drop in the waveform because of the decrease in pleural pressure. A ventilator breath produces an upward distortion of the baseline due to an increase in pleural and intrathoracic pressure. The key to reading the waveform correctly is to isolate the point where pleural pressure is closest to atmospheric pressure. This point is usually at end expiration, just prior to inspiration (Figure 4-22).

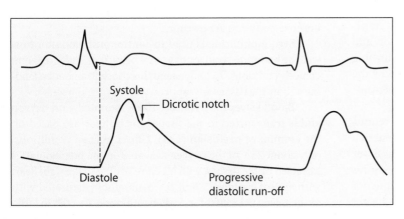

Figure 4-20. Characteristics of an arterial waveform. (*From Ahrens TS, Prentice D.* Critical Care: Certification Preparation and Review, *3rd ed. Stamford, CT: Appleton & Lange; 1993:82.*)

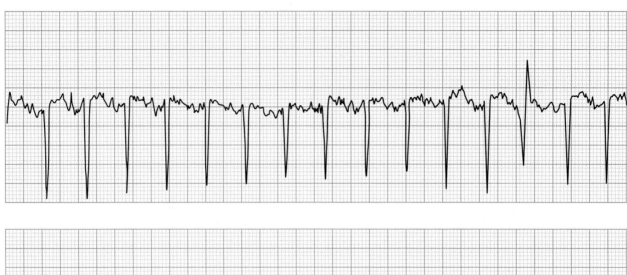

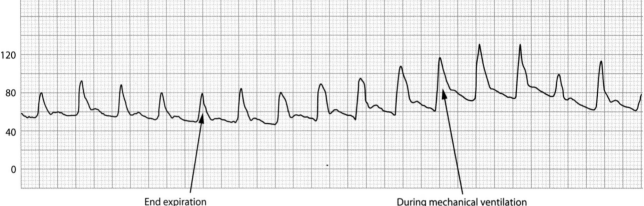

End expiration   During mechanical ventilation

Figure 4-21. Effect of respiration on arterial pressures. (*Reprinted from Ahrens TS.* Hemodynamic Waveform Analysis. *Philadelphia, PA: WB Saunders; 1992:161, with permission from Elsevier.*)

CONTINUOUS MIXED AND CENTRAL VENOUS OXYGEN MONITORING (Svo₂/Scvo₂)

Svo₂/Scvo₂ Monitoring Principles

Mixed venous oxygen saturation (Svo₂) monitoring is generally done in a critical care unit and uses a specialized PA catheter. While a comprehensive discussion of the technology is not within the scope of this book, the associated concepts are important and are briefly discussed below. Svo₂ catheters are different from other PA catheters in that they have two special fiber-optic bundles within the catheter that determine the oxygen saturation of hemoglobin by measuring the wavelength (color) of reflected light. Light is transmitted from the tip of the PA catheter down one bundle and is reflected off the oxygen-saturated hemoglobin, returning up the other bundle. This information is quantified by the bedside computer and numerically displayed as the percentage of saturation of the mixed venous blood.

A newer strategy is measurement of central venous oxygen saturation (Scvo₂). This requires the placement of a central venous catheter, which is easily placed and has fewer complications than a PA catheter. Theoretically, it measures the degree of oxygen extraction from the brain and upper body and trends well with Svo₂. The goal for Scvo₂ is greater than 70%. The Scvo₂ is usually less than the Svo₂ except in shock states. This occurs because of redistribution of blood flow in classic shock states.

Continuous Svo₂ monitoring is used as a diagnostic and therapeutic management tool. It provides early warning of alterations in hemodynamic status and a continuous monitor of the relationship between oxygen delivery and consumption. Many therapeutic strategies are added and adjusted in response to the changes in the Svo₂. If a blood pressure is considered low but the Svo₂ is above 60%, then the blood pressure is not contributing to a decrease in tissue perfusion. However, if the blood pressure and Svo₂ are low, interventions to improve perfusion are essential.

Svo₂ monitoring is used to continuously monitor how well the body's demand for oxygen is being met under different clinical conditions. To understand this concept, an understanding of how the tissues are supplied with oxygen is necessary.

Blood leaves the left heart 100% saturated with oxygen and is transported to the tissues for cellular use based on the amount of perfusion (CO). Under normal conditions, only about 25% of the oxygen available on the hemoglobin is extracted by the tissues, with blood returning to the right heart with approximately 75% of the hemoglobin saturated with oxygen. Normal values for oxygen saturation are 60% to 80%.

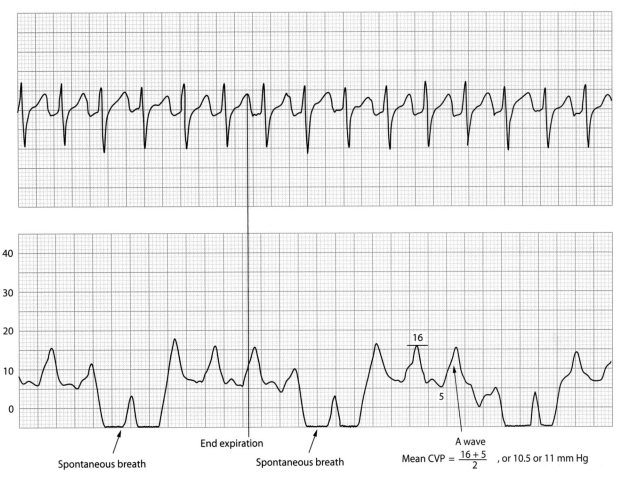

Figure 4-22. Effect of a spontaneous breath on a CVP waveform. (*Reprinted from Ahrens TS. Hemodynamic Waveform Analysis. Philadelphia, PA: WB Saunders; 1992:165, with permission from Elsevier.*)

In situations where tissue demands for oxygen increase, oxygen saturation of blood returning to the right heart will be lower than 70%. Clinical situations of increased tissue demand for oxygen include fever, pain, anxiety, infection, seizures, and some "routine" nursing activities like turning and suctioning. In contrast, hypothermia dramatically decreases oxygen consumption by the tissues. Interventions, then, are directed at decreasing or increasing the oxygen requirements as needed.

The concept of oxygen utilization is often referred to as supply and demand (or more accurately consumption) and is the essential concept inherent in Svo_2 monitoring. Because tissue oxygenation depends on hemoglobin level, saturation of hemoglobin, oxygen consumption, and CO, the saturation of blood returning to the PA tells us much about the interaction of these four variables and can be used to assess the adequacy of interventions.

MINIMALLY INVASIVE HEMODYNAMIC MONITORING

In some acute care units, new noninvasive technology may be used periodically to assess CO and other hemodynamic parameters. While research must still be accomplished to determine the efficacy of the devices, the noninvasive nature of the technologies makes them attractive for use in the progressive care setting. Two, thoracic bioimpedance and pulse contour measurement, are described below.

Thoracic Bioimpedance

The resistance of current flow (impedance) across the chest is inversely related to the thoracic fluid. Using a current that flows from the electrodes on the chest and neck, the SV can be determined. Changes in impedance occur with changes in blood flow and velocity through the ascending aorta. The impedance changes reflect aortic flow, which is directly related to ventricular function (contractility).

Variables that change the bioimpedance and alter the relationship between impedance and SV are changes in hematocrit, lung water, lead contact, shivering, mechanical ventilation, and rhythm changes. Thoracic bioimpedance is a useful method for trend analysis but to date has not found to be accurate enough for diagnostic interpretation. Its major application has been outside the critical care setting (HF clinics, emergency department, pacemaker clinics).

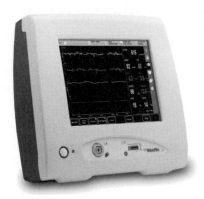

Figure 4-23. Nexfin System for noninvasive continuous hemodynamic monitoring (*Courtesy of: Edwards Lifesciences*).

Pulse Contour Measurement

Pulse contour measurement of hemodynamic parameters can be achieved invasively with an arterial line (PiCCO, LiDCO, Flotrac) and noninvasively with a finger pneumatic cuff (Nexfin). Various formulas are used to compute CCO values from the BP waveform.

The device provides a continuous beat-by-beat finger BP measure through the volume-clamp method (Figure 4-23). It then transforms the finger BP curve into a brachial arterial BP waveform and calculates CCO from the brachial pressure pulse contour.

Hemodynamic parameters that can be measured with the noninvasive system are cardiac output/index, systolic/diastolic blood pressure, mean arterial pressure, HR, SV, stroke volume variation, pulse pressure variation, and systemic vascular resistance. It also includes pulse oximetry and non-invasive hemoglobin. The hemodynamic parameters will allow for the calculation of oxygen delivery.

The technology has been validated for measuring arterial pressure and has been found especially useful in cardiology clinics during tilt-test to detect orthostatic hypotension. It has also been used successfully in the perioperative management of patients. However, studies are needed to test the reliability of the measurement of cardiac index in critically ill patients. The sensor should only be continuously used on a finger for an 8 hour period then moved to another finger.

SELECTED BIBLIOGRAPHY

Hemodynamic Monitoring

Ahrens TS. *Hemodynamic Waveform Recognition.* Philadelphia, PA: WB Saunders; 1993.

Ahrens TS, Taylor L. *Hemodynamic Waveform Analysis.* Philadelphia, PA: WB Saunders; 1992.

Alhashemi JA, Cecconi M, Hofer CK. Cardiac output monitoring: an integrative perspective. *Crit Care.* 2011;15(2):214.

Bigatello LM, George E. Hemodynamic monitoring. *Minerva Anesthesiol.* 2000;68(4):219-225.

Casserly B, Read R, Levy MM. Hemodynamic monitoring in sepsis. *Crit Care Nurs Clin North Am.* 2011;23(1):149-169.

Cocconi M, Johnston E, Rhodes A. What role does the right side of the heart play in circulation? *Crit Care.* 2006;10(suppl 3):1-7.

Cruz K, Franklin C. The pulmonary artery catheter: uses and controversies. *Crit Care Clin.* 2001;17(2):271-291.

Daily EK. Hemodynamic waveform analysis. *J Cardiovasc Nurs.* 2001;15(2):6-22.

Daily EK, Schroeder JS. *Techniques in Bedside Hemodynamic Monitoring.* St. Louis, MO: Mosby; 1994.

Darivuc DO. *Hemodynamic Monitoring: Invasive and Noninvasive Clinical Application.* Philadelphia, PA: Saunders; 2002.

Della Rocca G, Costa MG. Hemodynamic–volumetric monitoring. *Minerva Anesthesiol.* 2004;70(4):229-232.

deWaal EE, Wappler F, Buhre WF. Cardiac output monitoring. *Curr Opin Anaesthesiol.* 2009;22(1):71-77.

Frazier SK, Skinner GJ. Pulmonary artery catheter: state of the controversy. *JCVN.* 2008;32(2):113-121.

Gawlinski A. Cardiac output monitoring. In: Chulay M, Gawlinski A, eds. *Hemodynamic Monitoring Series.* Aliso Viejo, CA: AACN; 1998.

Glickman SW, Cairns CB, Otero RM, et al. Disease progression in hemodynamically stable patients presenting to the emergency department with sepsis. *Acad Emerg Med.* 2010;17(4):383-390.

Hadian M, Pinsky MR. Evidence-based review of the use of the pulmonary artery catheter: impact data and complications. *Crit Care.* 2006;10(suppl 3):1-11.

Imperial-Perez F, McRae M. Arterial pressure monitoring. In: Chulay M, Gawlinski A, eds. *Hemodynamic Monitoring Series.* Aliso Viejo, CA: AACN; 1998.

Keckeisen M. Pulmonary artery pressure monitoring. In: Chulay M, Gawlinski A, eds. *Hemodynamic Monitoring Series.* Aliso Viejo, CA: AACN; 1998.

Kim HK, Pinsky MR. Effect of tidal volume, sampling duration, and cardiac contractility on pulse pressure and stroke volume variation during positive pressure ventilation. *Crit Care Med.* 2008;36(10):2858-2862.

Kohli-Seth R, Oropello JM. The future of bedside monitoring. *Crit Care Clin.* 2000;16(4):557-578.

Latham HE, Rawson ST, Dwyer TT, et al. Peripherally inserted central catheters are equivalent to centrally inserted catheters in intensive care unit patients for central venous pressure monitoring. *J Clin Monit Comput.* 2012;26(2):85-90.

Leeper B. Monitoring right ventricular volumes. *AACN Clin Issues.* 2003;14(2):208-219.

Maar SP. Searching for the holy grail: a review of markers to tissue perfusion in pediatric critical care. *Pediatr Emerg Care.* 2008; 24(12):883-887.

Monnet X, Richard C, Teboul JL. The pulmonary artery catheter in critically ill patients. Does it change outcomes? *Minerva Anesthesiol.* 2004;70(4):219-224.

Muller JC, Kennard JW, Browne JS, et al. Hemodynamic monitoring in the intensive care unit. *Nutr Clin Pract.* 2012;18(3):280-286.

Ott K, Johnson K, Ahrens T. New technologies in the assessment of hemodynamic parameters. *J Cardiovasc Nurs.* 2001;15(2):41-55.

Payen D, Gayat E. Which general intensive care unit patients can benefit from placement of the pulmonary artery catheter? *Crit Care.* 2006;10(suppl 3):1-6.

Pinsky MR. Hemodynamic monitoring in the intensive care unit. *Clin Chest Med.* 2003;24(4):549-560.

Pittman JA, Ping JS, Mark JB. Arterial and central venous pressure monitoring. *Intl Anesthes Clin.* 2004;42(1):13-30.

Plante A, Ro E., Rowbottom JR. Hemodynamic and related challenges: monitoring and regulation in the postoperative period. *Anesthesiol Clin.* 2012;30(3):527-554.

Polanco M, Pinsky M. Practical issues of hemodynamic monitoring at the bedside. *Surg Clin North Am.* 2006;86:1431-1456.

Prentice D, Ahrens T. Controversies in the use of the pulmonary artery catheter. *J Cardiovasc Nurs.* 2001;15(2):1-5.

Quaal SJ. Improving the accuracy of pulmonary artery catheter measurement. *J Cardiovasc Nurs.* 2001;15(2):71-82.

Rajaram SS, Desai NK, Kalra A, et al. Pulmonary artery catheters for adult patients in intensive care. *Cochrane Database Syst Rev.* 2013;28;2:CD003408.

Ranucci M. Which cardiac surgical patients can benefit from placement of a pulmonary artery catheter? *Crit Care.* 2006; 10(suppl 3):1-8.

Reinhart K, Bloos F. The value of venous oximetry. *Curr Opin Crit Care.* 2005;11:259-263.

Richard C, Monnet X, Teboul JL. Pulmonary artery catheter monitoring in 2011. *Curr Opin Crit Care.* 2011;17(3):296-302.

Robin E, Costecalde M, Lebuffe G, Vallet B. Clinical relevance of data from the pulmonary artery catheter. *Crit Care.* 2006; 10(suppl 3):1-10.

Saggar R, Sitbon O. Hemodynamics in pulmonary arterial hypertension: current and future perspectives. *Am J Cardiol.* 2012; 110(6 suppl):9S-15S.

Sandham JD. Pulmonary artery catheter use—refining the question. *Crit Care Med.* 2004;32(4):1070-1071.

Sivarajan VB, Bohn D. Monitoring of standard hemodynamic parameters: heart rate, systemic blood pressure, atrial pressure, pulse oximetry, and end–tidal CO_2. *Pediatr Crit Care Med.* 2011;12(4 suppl):S2-S11.

Tucker D, Hazinski MF. The nursing perspective on monitoring hemodynamics and oxygen transport. *Pediatr Crit Care Med.* 2011;12(4 suppl):S72-S75.

Vender JS, Franklin M. Hemodynamic assessment of the critically ill patient. *Intl Anesthesiol Clin.* 2004;42(1):31-58.

Minimally Invasive Hemodynamic Monitoring

Aherns T, Sona C. Capnography application in acute and critical care. *AACN Clin Issues.* 2003;14(2):123-132.

Akamatsu S, Oda A, Terazawa E. Automated cardiac output measurement by transesophageal color Doppler echocardiography. *Anesth Analg.* 2004;98(5):1232-1238.

Avolio AP, Butlin M, Walsh A. Arterial blood pressure measurement and pulse wave analysis—their role in enhancing cardiovascular assessment. *Physiol Meas.* 2010;31(1):R1-47.

Ayuela Azcarate JM, Clau Terré F, Ochagavia A, Vicho Pereira R. Role of echocardiography in the hemodynamic monitorization of critical patients. *Med Intensiva.* 2012;36(3):220-232.

Bartels SA, Stok WJ, Bezemer R, Boksem RJ, et al. Noninvasive cardiac output monitoring during exercise testing: Nexfin pulse contour analysis compared to an inert gas rebreathing method and respired gas analysis. *J Clin Monit Comput.* 2011 Oct;25(5): 315-321.

Bayram M, Yancy CW. Transthoracic impedance cardiography: a noninvasive method of hemodynamic monitoring. *Heart Fail Clin.* 2009;5(2):161-168.

Bogert LW, van Lieshout JJ. Non-invasive pulsatile arterial pressure and stroke volume changes from the human finger. *Exp Physiol.* 2005;90(4):437-446.

Boswell SA, Scalea TM. Sublingual capnometry. *AACN Clin Issues.* 2003;14(2):176-184.

Boyd JH, Walley KR. The role of echocardiography in hemodynamic monitoring. *Curr Opin Crit Care.* 2009;15(3):239-243.

Camporota L, Beale R. Pitfalls in hemodynamic monitoring based on the arterial pressure waveform. *Crit Care.* 2010;14:124.

Compton F, Schäfer JH. Noninvasive cardiac output determination: broadening the applicability of hemodynamic monitoring. *Semin Cardiothorac Vasc Anesth.* 2009;13(1):44-55.

Compton FD, Zukunft B, Hoffmann C, Zidek W, Schaefer JH. Performance of a minimally invasive uncalibrated cardiac output monitoring system (Flotrac/Vigileo) in haemodynamically unstable patients. *Br J Anaesth.* 2008;100:451-456.

Cottis R, Magee N, Higgins DJ. Haemodynamic monitoring with pulse-induced contour cardiac output (PiCCO) in critical care. *Intensive Crit Care Nurs.* 2003;19:301-307.

Creteur J. Gastric and sublingual capnometry. *Curr Opin Crit Care.* 2006;12:272-277.

de Jong RM, Westerhof BE, Voors AA, van Veldhuisen DJ. Noninvasive haemodynamic monitoring using finger arterial pressure waveforms. *Neth J Med.* 2009;67(11):372-375.

Dueck R, Goedje O, Clopton P. Noninvasive continuous beat-to-beat radial artery pressure via TL-200 applanation tonometry. *J Clin Monit Comput.* 2012;26(2):75-83.

Fellahi JL, Caille V, Charron C, Deschamps-Berger PH, Vieillard-Baron A. Noninvasive assessment of cardiac index in healthy volunteers: a comparison between thoracic impedance cardiography and Doppler echocardiography. *Anesth Analg.* 2009;108(5): 1553-1559.

Garwood S. Measuring renal blood flow with the intraoperative transesophageal echocardiography probe. *Anesth Analg.* 2009; 108(5):1371-1376.

Ghanayem NS, Wernovsky G, Hoffman GM. Near infrared spectroscopy as a hemodynamic monitor in critical illness. *Pediatr Crit Care Med.* 2011:12(4 suppl):S27-S32.

Headley JM. Indirect calorimetry. *AACN Clin Issues.* 2003; 14(2):155-167.

Heard SO. Gastric tonometry: the hemodynamic monitor of choice. *Chest.* 2003;123(5 suppl):469S-474S.

Hett DA, Jonas MM. Non-invasive cardiac output monitoring. *Intensive Crit Care Nurs.* 2004;20(2):103-108.

Horster S, Stemmler HJ, Sparrer J, et al. Mechanical ventilation with positive end-expiratory pressure in critically ill patients: comparison of CW-Doppler ultrasound cardiac output monitoring (USCOM) and thermodilution (PiCCO). *Acta Cardiol.* 2012;67(2):177-185.

Kim SH, Song JG, Park JH, et al. Beat-to-beat tracking of systolic blood pressure using noninvasive pulse transit time during anesthesia induction in hypertensive patients. *Anesth Analg.* 2013;116(1):94-100.

L'E Orme RM, Pigott DW, Mihm FG. Measurement of cardiac output by transpulmonary arterial thermodilution using a long radial artery catheter. A comparison with intermittent pulmonary artery thermodilution. *Anaesthesia.* 2004;59(6):590-594.

Lima A, Bakker J. Noninvasive monitoring of peripheral perfusion. *Intensive Care Med.* 2005;31:1316-1326.

Lima MV, Ochiai ME, Vieira KN, et al. Continuous noninvasive hemodynamic monitoring in decompensated heart failure. *Arq Bras Cardiol.* 2012; 99(3):843-847.

Magder S. Central venous pressure: a useful but not so simple measurement. *Crit Care Med.* 2006;34(8):2224-2227.

Magder S. How to use central venous pressure measurements. *Curr Opin Crit Care*. 2005;11:264-270.

Marik PE. Regional carbon dioxide monitoring to assess the adequacy of tissue perfusion. *Curr Opin Crit Care*. 2005; 11: 245-251.

Marino R, Magrini L, Ferri E, Gagliano G, Di Somma, S. B-Type Natriuretic peptide and non-invasive haemodynamics and hydration status assessments in the management of patients with acute heart failure in the emergency department. *High Blood Press Cardiovasc Prev*. 2010;17 (4):1-7.

Marquél S, Cariou A, Chichel JD, Squara P. Comparison between Flotrac-Vigileo and bioreactance, a totally noninvasive method for cardiac output monitoring. *Crit Care*. 2009; 13(3):1-6.

Martins S, Soares RM, Branco L. Non-invasive monitoring of pulmonary capillary wedge pressure in heart failure. *Eur J Heart Fail*. 2001;3(1):41-46.

Mathews L, Singh K. Cardiac output monitoring. *Ann Card Anaesth*. 2008;11(1):56-68.

Middleton PM, Davies SR. Noninvasive hemodynamic monitoring in the emergency department. *Curr Opin Crit Care*. 2011;17(4):342-350.

Monnet X, Picard F, Lidzborski E, et al. The estimation of cardiac output by the Nexfin device is of poor reliability for tracking the effects of a fluid challenge. *Crit Care*. 2012;16:R212.

Mutoh T, Kazumata K, Ishikawa T, Terasaka S. Performance of bedside transpulmonary thermodilution monitoring for goal-directed hemodynamic management after subarachnoid hemorrhage. *Stroke*. 2009;40:2368.

Napoli AM. Physiologic and clinical principles behind noninvasive resuscitation techniques and cardiac output monitoring. *Cardiol Res Pract*. Volume 2012 (2012), Article ID 531908, 12 pages http://dx.doi.org/10.1155/2012/531908

Napoli AM, Machan JT, Corl K, Forcada A. The use of impedance cardiography in predicting mortality in emergency department patients with severe sepsis and septic shock. *Acad Emer Med*. 2010;17(4):452-455.

Nelson MR, Stepanek J, Cevette M, et al. Noninvasive measurement of central vascular pressures with arterial tonometry: clinical revival of the pulse pressure waveform? *Mayo Clin Proc*. 2010;85(5):460-472.

Nguyen HB, Banta DP, Stewart G, et al. Cardiac index measurements by transcutaneous Doppler ultrasound and transthoracic echocardiography in adult and pediatric emergency patients. *J Clin Monit Comput*. 2010;24(3):237-247.

Noritomi DT, Vieira ML, Mohovic T, Bastos JF, et al. Echocardiography for hemodynamic evaluation in the intensive care unit. *Shock*. 2010;34 (suppl 1):59-62.

Nowak RM, Sen A, Garcia AJ, et al. The inability of emergency physicians to adequately clinically estimate the underlying hemodynamic profiles of acutely ill patients. *Am J Emerg Med*. 2011; 30(6):954-960.

Odenstedt H, Stenqvist O, Lundin S. Clinical evaluation of a partial CO_2 rebreathing technique for cardiac output monitoring in critically ill patients. *Acta Anaesthesiol Scand*. 2002;46(2):152-159.

Ospina-Tascon GA, Cordioli RL, Vincent JL. What type of monitoring has been shown to improve outcomes in acutely ill patients? *Intensive Care Med*. 2008;34:800-820.

Pearse RM, Ikram K, Barry J. Equipment review: an appraisal of the LiDCO trade mark plus method of measuring cardiac output. *Crit Care*. 2004;8(3):190-195.

Peyton PJ, Robinson JB, McCall PR. Noninvasive measurement of intrapulmonary shunting. *J Cardiothorac Vasc Anesth*. 2004;18(1):47-52.

Reinhart K, Kuhn HJ, Hartog C, Bredle D. Continuous central venous and pulmonary artery oxygen saturation monitoring in the critically ill. *Intensive Care Med*. 2004;30:1572-1578.

Silver MA, Cianci P, Brennan S. Evaluation of impedance cardiography as an alternative to pulmonary artery catheterization in critically ill patients. *Congest Heart Fail*. 2004;10 (suppl 2): 17-21.

Summers RL, Parrott CW, Quale C. Use of noninvasive hemodynamics to aid decision making in the initiation and titration of neurohormonal agents. *Congest Heart Fail*. 2004; 10 (suppl 2): 28-31.

Temporelli PL, Scapellato F, Eleuteri E, Imparato A, Giannuzzi P. Doppler echocardiography in advanced systolic heart failure: a noninvasive alternative to Swan-Ganz catheter. *Circ Heart Fail*. (2010);3(3):387-394

Truijen, J, VanLieshout JJ, Wesselink WA, Westerhof BE. Noninvasive continuous hemodynamic monitoring. *J Clin Monit Comput*. 2012;26(4):267-278.

Turner MA. Doppler-based hemodynamic monitoring. *AACN Clin Issues*. 2003;14(2):220-231.

van der Spoel AG, Voogel AJ, Folkers A, Boer C, Bouwman RA. Comparison of noninvasive continuous arterial waveform analysis (Nexfin) with transthoracic Doppler echocardiography for monitoring of cardiac output. *J Clin Anesth*. 2012;24(4): 304-309.

van Genderen ME, van Bommel J, Lima A. Monitoring peripheral perfusion in critically ill patients at the bedside. *Curr Opin Crit Care*. 2012;18(3):273-279.

Wooley JA. Indirect calorimetry: applications in practice. *Respir Care Clin*. 2006;12:619-633.

Young BP, Low LL. Noninvasive monitoring cardiac output using partial CO_2 rebreathing. *Crit Care Clin*. 2010;26(2):383-392.

Yung GL, Fedullo PF, Kinninger K. Comparison of impedance cardiography to direct Fick and thermodilution cardiac output determination in pulmonary arterial hypertension. *Congest Heart Fail*. 2004;10(suppl 2):7-10.

Zhang Z, Xu X, Yao M, et al. Use of PiCCO system in critically ill patients with septic shock and acute respiratory distress syndrome. *Trials*. 2013;1:14-32.

Zimlichman E, Szyper-Kravitz M, Shinar Z, et al. Early recognition of acutely deteriorating patients in non-intensive care units: assessment of an innovative monitoring technology. *J Hosp Med*. 2012 Oct;7(8):628-633.

Therapeutics

Adams KF. Guiding heart failure care by invasive hemodynamic measurements: possible or useful? *J Cardiac Fail*. 2002;8(2): 71-73.

Alvarez J, Bouzada M, Fernandez AL, et al. Hemodynamic effects of levosimendan compared with dobutamine in patients with low cardiac output after cardiac surgery. *Rev Esp Cardiol*. 2006; 59(4):338-345.

Bagshaw SM, Brophy PD, Cruz D, Ronco C. Fluid balance as a biomarker: impact of fluid overload on outcome in critically ill patients with acute kidney injury. *Crit Care*. 2008;12(4):1-7.

Bauer SR, Lam SW. Arginine vasopressin for the treatment of septic shock in adults. *Pharmacotherapy*. 2010;30(10):1057-1071.

Bayer O, Reinhart K, Kohl M, Kabisch B, et al. Effects of fluid resuscitation with synthetic colloids or crystalloids alone on shock reversal, fluid balance, and patient outcomes in patients with severe sepsis. *Crit Care Med.* 2012;40(9):2543-2551.

Brazdzionyte J, Macas A, Sirvinskas E. Application of methods for hemodynamic monitoring in critical cardiac pathology (an experimental model for assessment of hemodynamics). *Medicina.* 2002;38(8):835-842.

Buerke M, Lemm H, Dietz S, Werdan K. Pathophysiology, diagnosis, and treatment of infarction–related cardiogenic shock. *Herz.* 2011;36(2):73-83.

Debacker D, Cretekr J, Dubois M, et al. The effects of dobutamine on microcirculatory alterations in patients with septic shock are independent of its systemic effects. *Crit Care Med.* 2006; 34(2):403-408.

Deedwania PC, Carbajal E. Evidence-based therapy for heart failure. *Med Clin North Am.* 2012;96(5):915-931.

Di Giantomasso D, Morimatsu H, May CN. Increasing renal blood flow: low-dose dopamine or medium-dose norepinephrine. *Chest.* 2004;125(6):2260-2267.

Dünser MW, Mayr AJ, Ulmer H, et al. The effects of vasopressin on systemic hemodynamics in catecholamine-resistant septic and postcardiotomy shock: a retrospective analysis. *Anesth Analg.* 2001;93(1):7-13.

Faybik P, Hetz H, Baker A. Iced versus room temperature injectate for assessment of cardiac output, intrathoracic blood volume, and extravascular lung water by single transpulmonary thermodilution. *J Crit Care.* 2004;19(2):103-107.

Felker GM, Lee KL, Bull DA, et al. Diuretic strategies in patients with acute decompensated heart failure. *N Engl J Med.* 2011;364(9):797-805.

Ferguson-Myrthil N. Vasopressor use in adult patients. *Cardiol Rev.* 2012;20(3):153-158.

Havel C, Arrich J, Losert H, Gamper G, et al. Vasopressors for hypotensive shock. *Cochrane Database Syst Rev.* 2011;11(5): CD003709.

Heart Failure Society of America, Lindenfield J, Albert NM, et al. HFSA 2010 Comprehensive heart failure practice guideline. *J Card Fail.* 2010;16:e1.

Hollenberg SM. Inotrope and vasopressor therapy of septic shock. *Crit Care Clin.* 2009;25(4):781-802.

Jain M, Canham M, Upadhyay D. Variability in interventions with pulmonary artery catheter data. *Intensive Care Med.* 2003; 29(11):2059-2062.

Kampmeier TG, Rehberg S, Westphal M, Lange M. Vasopressin in sepsis and septic shock. *Minerva Anestesiol.* 2010;76(10):844-850.

Kapoor PM, Kakani M, Chowdhury U, et al. Early goal-directed therapy in moderate to high-risk cardiac surgery patients. *Ann Card Anaesth.* 2008;11(1): 27-34.

Khot UN, Novaro GM, Popovic ZB. Nitroprusside in critically ill patients with left ventricular dysfunction and aortic stenosis. *N Engl J Med.* 2003;348(18):1756-1763.

Krejci V, Hiltebrand LB, Higurdsson GH. Effects of epinephrine, norepinephrine and phenylephrine on microcirculatory blood flow in the gastrointestinal tract in sepsis. *Crit Care Med.* 2006;34(1):1456-1463.

Kumar A, Anel R, Bunnell E. Pulmonary artery occlusion pressure and central venous pressure fail to predict ventricular filling volume, cardiac performance, or the response to volume infusion in normal subjects. *Crit Care Med.* 2004;32(3):691-699.

Landoni G, Biondi-Zoccai G, Greco M, Greco T, et al. Effects of levosimendan on mortality and hospitalization. A meta-analysis of randomized controlled studies. *Crit Care Med.* 2012; 40(2):634-646.

Leuchte HH, Schwaiblmair M, Baumgartner RA. Hemodynamic response to sildenafil, nitric oxide, and iloprose in primary pulmonary hypertension. *Chest.* 2004;125(2):580-586.

Liu SS, Monti J, Kargbo HM, Athar MW, et al. Frontiers of therapy for patients with heart failure. *Am J Med.* 2013;126(1):6-12.

Malliotakis P, Xenikakis T, Linardakis M, Hassoulas J. Haemodynamic effects of levosimendan for low cardiac output after cardiac surgery: a case series. *Hellenic J Cardiol.* 2007; 48(2):80-88.

Myburgh J. Norepinephrine: more of a neurohormone than a vasopressor. *Crit Care.* 2010;14(5):196.

O'Connor CM, Starling RC, Hernandez AF, et al. Effect of nesiritide in patients with acute decompensated heart failure. *N Engl J Med.* 2011;365(1):32-43.

Papp A, Uusaro A, Parviainen I. Myocardial function and haemodynamics in extensive burn trauma: evaluation by clinical signs, invasive monitoring, echocardiography and cytokine concentrations. A prospective clinical study. *Acta Anaesthesiol Scand.* 2003;47(10):1257-1263.

Parissis JT, Rafouli-Stergiou P, Stasinos V, et al. Intropes in cardiac patients: update 2011. *Curr Opin Crit Care.* 2010;16(5):432-441.

Pestel GJ, Fukui K, Kimberger O, et al. Hemodynamic parameters change earlier than tissue oxygen tension in hemorrhage. *J Surg Res.* 2010 May 15;160(2):288-293.

Pinto BB, Rehberg S, Etmer C, Westphal M. Role of levosimendan in sepsis and septic shock. *Curr Opin Anaesthesiol.* 2008;21(2):168-177.

Puskarich MA. Emergency management of severe sepsis and septic shock. *Curr Opin Crit Care.* 2012;18(4):295-300.

Richards AM, Troughton RW. Use of natriuretic peptides to guide and monitor heart failure therapy. *Clin Chem.* 2012;58(1):62-71.

Rivers E, Nguyen B, Havestad S, et al. Early goal-directed therapy on the treatment of severe sepsis and septic shock. *NEJM.* 2001; 345(19):1368-1377.

Ruggiero M. Effects of vasopressin in septic shock. *AACN Adv Crit Care.* 2008;19(3):281-287.

Russell JA. Bench-to-bedside review: vasopressin in the management of septic shock. *Crit Care.* 2011;15(4):226.

Sandifer JP, Jones AE. Dopamine versus norepinephrine for the treatment of septic shock EBEM commentators. *Ann Emerg Med.* 2012;60(3):372-373.

Shoemaker WC, Wo CC, Yu S. Invasive and noninvasive hemodynamic monitoring of acutely ill sepsis and septic shock patients in the emergency department. *Eur J Emerg Med.* 2000;7(3):169-175.

Szokol JW, Murphy GS. Transesophageal echocardiographic monitoring of hemodynamics. *Intl Anesthesiol Clin.* 2004;42(1):59-81.

Teerlink JR, Metra M, Zacà V, Sabbah HN, Cotter G, et al. Agents with inotropic properties for the management of acute heart failure syndromes. Traditional agents and beyond. *Heart Fail Rev.* 2009;14(4):243-253.

Vollman KM. Understanding critically ill patients hemodynamic response to mobilization. *Crit Care Nurs Q.* 2013;56(1):17-27.

Zafir B, Amir O. Beta blocker therapy, decompensated heart failure, and inotropic interactions: current perspectives. *Isr Med Assoc J.* 2012;14(3):184-189.

Zanotti Cavazzoni SL, Dellinger RP. Hemodynamic optimization of sepsis-induced tissue hypoperfusion. *Crit Care.* 2006; 10(suppl 3): 1-8.

Evidence-Based Practice Guidelines

AACN Hemodynamic Monitoring Practice Alert. Aliso Viejo, CA: AACN; 2004. http://www.aacn.org. Accessed January 1, 2010.

American Association of Critical-Care Nurses (AACN). Practice Alert: *Pulmonary Artery Pressure Measurement.* Aliso Viejo, CA: AACN; 2009. http://classic.aacn.org/AACN/practiceAlert.nsf/Files/PAP/$file/PAP%20Measurement%2005-2004.pdf. Accessed January 1, 2010.

Gawlinski A. *AACN Protocol for Practice: Cardiac Output Monitoring.* Aliso Viejo, CA: AACN; 1998.

Imperial-Perez F, McRae M. *AACN Protocol for Practice: Arterial Pressure Monitoring.* Aliso Viejo, CA: AACN; 1998.

Jesurum JT. *AACN Protocol for Practice: SvO2 Monitoring.* Aliso Viejo, CA: AACN; 1998.

Keckeisen M. *AACN Protocol for Practice: Pulmonary Artery Pressure Monitoring.* Aliso Viejo, CA: AACN; 1998.

AIRWAY AND VENTILATORY MANAGEMENT

Robert E. St. John and Maureen A. Seckel

KNOWLEDGE COMPETENCIES

1. Interpret normal and abnormal arterial blood gas results and common management strategies for treatment.

2. Identify indications, complications, and management strategies for artificial airways, oxygen delivery, and monitoring devices.

3. Identify pulmonary and nonpulmonary factors important to the promotion of positive weaning outcomes in long-term mechanically ventilated patients.

4. Describe the concepts of respiratory muscle fatigue, rest, and conditioning as they relate to the mechanically ventilated weaning patient.

5. Identify essential components for the successful design and use of weaning predictors, protocols for weaning trials, and multidisciplinary institutional approaches to the care of long-term mechanically ventilated patients.

TESTS, MONITORING SYSTEMS AND RESPIRATORY ASSESSMENT TECHNIQUES

Arterial Blood Gas Monitoring

Arterial blood gas (ABG) monitoring may be used to assess acid-base balance, ventilation, and oxygenation. An arterial blood sample is analyzed for oxygen tension (Pao_2), carbon dioxide tension ($Paco_2$), and pH using a blood gas analyzer. From these measurements, several other parameters are calculated by the blood gas analyzer, including base excess (BE), bicarbonate (HCO_3^-), and oxygen saturation (Sao_2). Fractional arterial Sao_2 can be directly measured if a co-oximeter is available. Normal ABG values analysis are listed in Table 5-1.

Arterial blood gas samples are obtained by direct puncture of an artery, usually the radial artery, or by withdrawing blood through an indwelling arterial catheter system. A heparinized syringe is used to collect the sample to prevent clotting of the blood prior to analysis. Blood gas samples are kept on ice unless there is the ability to immediately analyze to prevent the continued transfer of CO_2 and O_2 in and out of the red blood cells. ABG analysis equipment is often kept in or near progressive care units to maximize accuracy and

decrease the time for reporting of results. Additionally, portable point-of-care devices are available at many hospitals that allow measurement at the bedside. Regardless of the method used to obtain the ABG sample, practitioners should wear gloves and follow universal precautions to prevent exposure to blood during the sampling procedure.

Techniques
Indwelling Arterial Catheters

All the pressure monitoring systems used with indwelling arterial catheters have sites where samples of arterial blood can be withdrawn for ABG analysis or other laboratory testing (Figure 5-1). Using the stopcock closest to the catheter insertion site, or the indwelling syringe or reservoir of the needleless systems, a 3- to 5-mL sample of blood is withdrawn to clear the catheter system of any flush system fluid. A 1-mL sample for ABG analysis is then obtained in a heparinized syringe. Any air remaining in the syringe is then removed, an airtight cap is placed on the end of the syringe, and the sample is placed on ice to ensure accuracy of the measurement. The arterial catheter system is then flushed to clear the line of any residual blood.

TABLE 5-1. LABORATORY AND CALCULATED RESPIRATORY VALUES

Parameter	Value
Arterial Blood Gases	
• pH	7.35-7.45
• $Paco_2$	35-45 mm Hg
• HCO_3^-	22-26 mEq/L
• Base excess	−2 to +2 mEq/L
• Pao_2	80-100 mm Hg (normals vary with age and altitude)
• Sao_2	>95% (normals vary with age and altitude)
Mixed Venous Blood Gases	
• pH	7.32-7.42
• $Pmvco_2$	40-50 mm Hg
• $Pmvo_2$	35-45 mm Hg
• $Smvo_2$	60%-80%
Respiratory Parameters	
• Tidal volume (V_T)	6-8 mL/kg
• Respiratory rate	8-16/min
• Respiratory static compliance	70-100 mL/cm H_2O
• Inspiratory force (IF)	≤ −20 cm H_2O
Respiratory Calculations	
• Alveolar gas equation (Pao_2)	$Pao_2 = Fio_2(P_{ATM} - P_{H_2O}) - \dfrac{Paco_2}{RQ \text{ (Respiratory quotient)}}$
• Static compliance	Vt/(Plateau pressure − PEEP)

Complications associated with this technique for obtaining ABG samples include infection and hemorrhage. Any time an invasive system is used, the potential exists for contamination of the sterile system. The use of needleless systems on indwelling catheter systems decreases patients' risk for infection, as well as the progressive care practitioners' risk for accidental needlestick injuries, and should be used whenever feasible. Hemorrhage is a rare complication, occurring when stopcocks are inadvertently left in the wrong position after blood withdrawal or with tubing disconnections. These complications can be avoided by carefully following the proper technique during blood sampling, limiting sample withdrawal to experienced practitioners, assuring connections are tight, and keeping the pressure alarm system of the bedside monitoring system activated at all times.

Arterial Puncture

When indwelling arterial catheters are not in place, ABG samples are obtained by directly puncturing the artery with a needle and syringe. The most common sites for arterial puncture are the radial, brachial, and femoral arteries. Similar to venipuncture, the technique for obtaining an ABG sample is relatively simple, but success in obtaining the sample requires experience.

An Allen test is performed prior to obtaining an ABG by puncture and prior to the insertion of an arterial line into the radial artery. The Allen test requires that the ulnar and radial pulses be occluded for a brief period of time with the forearm held upward to facilitate blood emptying from the hand.

Once blanching of the hand is observed, the forearm is placed in a downward position, the ulnar artery is released, and the hand is observed for flushing. If the hand flushes, it is clear that the ulnar artery is capable of supplying blood to the fingers should the radial artery be damaged.

Following location of the pulsating artery and antiseptic preparation of the skin, the needle is inserted into the artery at a 45° angle with the bevel facing upward. The needle is slowly advanced until arterial blood appears in the syringe barrel or the insertion depth is below the artery location. If blood is not obtained, the needle is pulled back to just below the skin and relocation of the pulsating artery is verified prior to advancing the needle again.

As soon as the 1-mL sample of arterial blood is obtained, the syringe is withdrawn and firm pressure quickly applied to the insertion site with a sterile gauze pad. Handheld pressure is maintained for at least 5 minutes and the site inspected for bleeding or oozing. If present, pressure should be reapplied until all evidence of oozing has stopped. Pressure dressings are not applied until hemostasis has been achieved.

As described, all air must be removed from the ABG syringe and an airtight cap applied to the end (remove the needle first). Given the importance of maintaining pressure at the puncture site, it is sometimes helpful to have another practitioner assisting during arterial puncture to ensure appropriate handling of the blood sample.

Complications associated with arterial puncture include arterial vessel tears, air embolism, hemorrhage, arterial obstruction, loss of extremity, and infection. Using proper technique during sampling can dramatically decrease the incidence of these complications. Damage to the artery may be decreased by using a small diameter needle (21-23 gauge in adults) and by avoiding multiple attempts at the same site. After one or two failed attempts at entering the artery, a different site should be selected or another experienced practitioner enlisted to attempt the ABG sampling. All facilities have specific policies and procedures providing guidance on sample acquisition and handling of ABGs and the reader is encouraged to follow their institutional guidelines.

Hemorrhage can occur easily into the surrounding tissues if adequate hemostasis is not achieved with direct pressure. Bleeding into the tissue can range from small blood loss with minimal local damage to large blood loss with loss of distal circulation and even exsanguination. Large blood loss is more commonly seen with femoral punctures and is often the result of inadequate pressure on the artery following needle removal. Bleeding from the femoral artery is difficult to visualize, so significant blood loss can occur before practitioners are alerted to the problem. For this reason, the femoral site is the least preferred site for ABG sampling and is used only when other sites are not accessible.

The need for frequent ABG sampling for ventilation and oxygenation assessment and management may require the insertion of an arterial catheter and monitoring system to decrease the risks associated with repetitive arterial punctures.

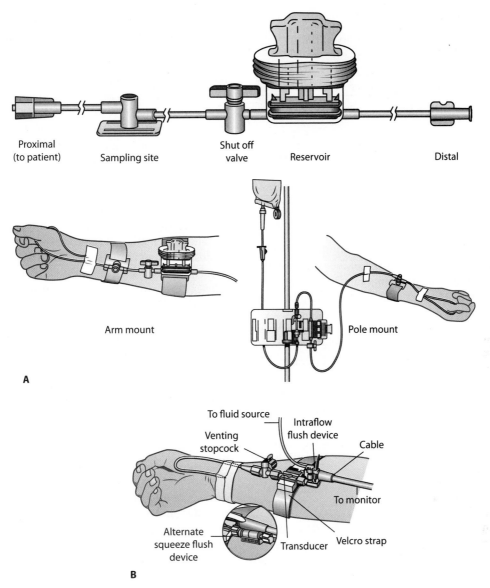

Proximal (to patient)

Sampling site

Shut off valve

Reservoir

Distal

Arm mount

Pole mount

To fluid source

Intraflow flush device

Venting stopcock

Cable

To monitor

Alternate squeeze flush device

Transducer

Velcro strap

A

B

Figure 5-1. Examples of indwelling arterial catheter systems for blood gas analysis. **(A)** Closed blood withdrawal system. **(B)** Open blood withdrawal system. (*Courtesy of: Edwards Lifesciences [A].*)

Analysis

The best approach to analyzing the results of ABGs is a systematic one. Analysis is accomplished by evaluating acid-base and oxygenation status. Upon receipt of ABG results, the practitioner first identifies any abnormal values (see Table 5-1). Then a systematic evaluation of acid-base and oxygenation status is done.

Acid-Base Analysis

Optimal cellular functioning occurs when the pH of the blood is between 7.35 and 7.45. Decreases in pH below 7.35 are termed acidemia, and increases in pH above 7.45 are termed alkalemia. When the amount of acids or bases in the body increases or decreases, the pH changes if the ratio of acids to bases is altered. For example, if acid production increases, and there is no change in the amount of base production, pH decreases. If the base production were to increase as well, as a response to increased acid production, then no change in pH would occur because the ratio of acids to bases would be maintained. Because the body functions best at a pH in the 7.35 to 7.45 range, there are strong systems in place to maintain the balance between acids and bases, even if one of those components is functioning abnormally. Although a variety of regulatory systems are involved in acid-base balance, the bicarbonate (HCO_3^-) and carbon dioxide (CO_2) levels are the primary regulators.

- *Metabolic component:* HCO_3^- levels are controlled primarily by the kidneys and have been termed the metabolic component of the acid-base system.

TABLE 5-2. ACID-BASE ABNORMALITIES

Acid-Base Abnormality	Primary ABG Abnormalities			ABG Changes with Compensation (If Present)	
	pH	Paco₂	HCO₃⁻	Respiratory (Paco₂)	Metabolic (HCO₃⁻)
Alkalemia					
Metabolic	↑		↑	↑	
Respiratory	↑	↓			↓
Acidemia					
Metabolic	↓		↓	↓	
Respiratory	↓	↑			↑

By increasing or decreasing the amount of HCO_3^- excreted in the kidneys, the pH of the blood can be increased or decreased. Changes in HCO_3^- excretion may take up to 24 hours or longer to accomplish, but can be maintained for prolonged periods.

- *Respiratory component:* CO_2 levels are controlled primarily by the lungs and are termed the respiratory component of the acid-base system. By increasing or decreasing the amount of CO_2 excreted by the lungs, the pH of the blood can be increased or decreased. Changes in CO_2 excretion can occur rapidly, within a minute, by increasing or decreasing respiration (minute ventilation). Compensation by the respiratory system is difficult to maintain over long periods of time (24 hours).
- *Acid-base abnormalities:* A variety of conditions may result in acid-base abnormalities (Tables 5-2 and 5-3).

Metabolic alkalemia is present when the pH is above 7.45 and the HCO_3^- is above 26 mEq/L. In metabolic alkalosis there is either a primary increase in hydrogen ion (H_1) loss or HCO_3^- gain. The respiratory system attempts to compensate for the increased pH by decreasing the amount of CO_2 eliminated from the body (alveolar hypoventilation). This compensatory attempt by the respiratory system results in a change in pH, but rarely to a normal value. Clinical situations or conditions that cause metabolic alkalemia include loss of body acids (nasogastric suction of HCl, vomiting, excessive

diuretic therapy, steroids, hypokalemia) and ingestion of exogenous bicarbonate or citrate substances. Management of metabolic alkalosis is directed at treating the underlying cause, decreasing or stopping the acid loss (eg, use of antiemetic therapy for vomiting), and replacing electrolytes.

Metabolic acidemia is present when the pH is below 7.35 and the HCO_3^- is below 22 mEq/L. In metabolic acidosis there is excessive loss of HCO_3^- from the body by the kidneys or the accumulation of acid. The respiratory system attempts to compensate for the decreased pH by increasing the amount of CO_2 eliminated (alveolar hyperventilation). This compensatory attempt by the respiratory system results in a change in pH toward normal. Clinical situations or conditions that cause metabolic acidosis include increased metabolic formation of acids (diabetic ketoacidosis, uremic acidosis, lactic acidosis), loss of bicarbonate (diarrhea, renal tubular acidosis), hyperkalemia, toxins (salicylates overdose, ethylene and propylene glycol, methanol, paraldehyde), and adrenal insufficiency. Management of metabolic acidosis is directed at treating the underlying cause, decreasing acid formation (eg, decreasing lactic acid production by improving cardiac output [CO] in shock), decreasing bicarbonate losses (eg, treatment of diarrhea), removal of toxins through dialysis or cathartics, or administering sodium bicarbonate ($NaHCO_3$) in extreme metabolic acidemia states.

Respiratory alkalemia occurs when the pH is above 7.45 and the $Paco_2$ is below 35 mm Hg. In respiratory alkalosis, there is an excessive amount of ventilation (alveolar hyperventilation) and removal of CO_2 from the body. If these ABG changes persist for 24 hours or more, the kidneys attempt to compensate for the elevated pH by increasing the excretion of HCO_3^- until normal or near-normal pH levels occur. Clinical situations or conditions that cause respiratory alkalosis include neurogenic hyperventilation, interstitial lung diseases, pulmonary embolism, asthma, acute anxiety/stress/ fear, hyperventilation syndromes, excessive mechanical ventilation, and severe hypoxemia. Management of respiratory alkalosis is directed at treating the underlying cause and decreasing excessive ventilation if possible.

Respiratory acidemia occurs when the pH is below 7.35 and the $Paco_2$ is above 45 mm Hg. In respiratory acidosis there is an inadequate amount of ventilation (alveolar

TABLE 5-3. EXAMPLES OF ARTERIAL BLOOD GAS RESULTS

ABG Analysis	pH	Paco₂ (mm Hg)	HCO₃⁻ (mEq/L)	Base Excess	Pao₂ (mm Hg)	Sao₂ (%)
Normal ABG	7.37	38	24	−1	85	96
Respiratory acidosis, no compensation, with hypoxemia	7.28	51	25	−1	63	89
Metabolic acidosis, no compensation, without hypoxemia	7.23	35	14	−12	92	97
Metabolic alkalosis, partial compensation, without hypoxemia	7.49	48	37	+11	84	95
Respiratory acidosis, full compensation, with hypoxemia	7.35	59	33	+6	55	86
Respiratory alkalosis, no compensation, with hypoxemia	7.52	31	24	0	60	88
Metabolic acidosis, partial compensation, with hypoxemia	7.30	29	16	−9	54	85
Laboratory error	7.31	32	28	0	92	96

hypoventilation) and removal of CO_2 from the body. If these ABG changes persist for 24 hours or more, the kidneys attempt to compensate for the decreased pH by increasing the amount of HCO_3^- in the body (decreased excretion of HCO_3^- in the urine) until normal or near-normal pH levels occur. Clinical situations or conditions that cause respiratory acidosis include overall hypoventilation associated with respiratory failure (eg, acute respiratory distress syndrome [ARDS], severe asthma, pneumonia, chronic obstructive pulmonary diseases, and sleep apnea), pulmonary embolism, pulmonary edema, pneumothorax, respiratory center depression, and neuromuscular disturbances in the presence of normal lungs, and inadequate mechanical ventilation. Management of respiratory acidosis is directed at treating the underlying cause and improving ventilation.

Mixed (combined) disturbance is the simultaneous development of a primary respiratory and metabolic acid-base disturbance. For example, metabolic acidosis may occur from diabetic ketoacidosis, with respiratory acidosis occurring from respiratory failure associated with aspiration pneumonia. Mixed acid-base disturbances create a more complex picture when examining ABGs and are beyond the scope of this text.

Oxygenation

After determining the acid-base status from the ABG, the adequacy of oxygenation is assessed. Normal values for PaO_2 depend on age and altitude. Lower levels of PaO_2 are acceptable as normal with increasing age and altitude levels. In general, PaO_2 levels between 80 and 100 mm Hg are considered normal on room air.

SaO_2 levels are also affected by age and altitude, with values above 95% considered normal. Hemoglobin saturation with oxygen is primarily influenced by the amount of available oxygen in the plasma (Figure 5-2). The S shape to the normal oxyhemoglobin curve emphasizes that as long as PaO_2 levels are above 60 mm Hg, 90% or more of the hemoglobin is bound or saturated with O_2. Factors that can shift the oxyhemoglobin curve to the right and left include temperature, pH, $PaCO_2$, and abnormal hemoglobin conditions. In general, shifting the curve to the right decreases the affinity of oxygen for hemoglobin, resulting in an increase in the amount of oxygen released to the tissues. Shifting of the curve to the left increases the affinity of oxygen for hemoglobin, resulting in a decreased amount of oxygen released to the tissues.

A decrease in PaO_2 below normal values is hypoxemia. A variety of conditions cause hypoxemia:

- *Low inspired oxygen:* Usually, the fraction of inspired oxygen concentration (FiO_2) is reduced at high altitudes or when toxic gases are inhaled. Inadequate or inappropriately low FiO_2 administration may contribute to hypoxic respiratory failure in patients with other cardiopulmonary diseases.
- *Overall hypoventilation:* Decreases in tidal volume (V_t), respiratory rate, or both reduce minute ventilation and cause hypoventilation. Alveoli are underventilated, leading to a fall in alveolar oxygen tension (PAO_2) and increased $PaCO_2$ levels. Causes of hypoventilation include respiratory center depression from drug overdose, anesthesia, excessive analgesic administration, neuromuscular disturbances, and fatigue.
- *Ventilation-perfusion mismatch:* When the balance between adequately ventilated and perfused alveoli is altered, hypoxemia develops. Perfusion of blood past underventilated alveoli decreases the availability of oxygen for gas exchange, leading to poorly oxygenated blood in the pulmonary vasculature. Examples of this include bronchospasm, atelectasis, secretion retention, pneumonia, pulmonary embolism, and pulmonary edema.
- *Diffusion defect:* Thickening of the alveolar-capillary membrane decreases oxygen diffusion and leads to hypoxemia. Causes of diffusion defects are chronic disease states such as pulmonary fibrosis and sarcoidosis. Hypoxemia usually responds to supplemental oxygen in conditions of diffusion impairment (eg, interstitial lung disease).
- *Shunt:* When blood bypasses or shunts past the alveoli, gas exchange cannot occur and blood returns to the left side without being oxygenated. Shunts caused anatomically include pulmonary arteriovenous fistulas or congenital cardiac anomalies of the heart and great vessels, such as tetralogy of Fallot. Physiologic shunts are caused by a variety of conditions that result in closed, nonventilated alveoli such as seen in ARDS.
- *Low mixed venous oxygenation:* Under normal conditions, the lungs fully oxygenate the pulmonary arterial blood and mixed venous oxygen tension ($PmvO_2$) does not affect PaO_2 significantly. However, a reduced

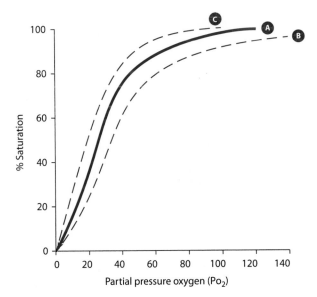

Figure 5-2. Oxyhemoglobin dissociation curve. **(A)** Normal. **(B)** Shift to the right. **(C)** Shift to the left.

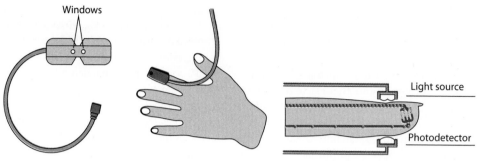

Windows

Light source

Photodetector

Figure 5-3. Pulse oximeter. **(A)** Sensor. **(B)** Schematic of sensor operation on finger.

Pmvo$_2$ can lower the Pao$_2$ significantly when either ventilation-perfusion mismatch or intrapulmonary shunting is present. Conditions that can contribute to low mixed venous oxygenation include low CO, anemia, hypoxemia, and increased oxygen consumption. Improving tissue oxygen delivery by increasing CO or hemoglobin usually improves mixed venous oxygen saturation (Svo$_2$).

Venous Blood Gas Monitoring

Analysis of oxygen and carbon dioxide levels in the venous blood provides additional information about the adequacy of perfusion and oxygen use by the tissues. Venous blood gas analysis, also referred to as a mixed venous blood gas sample, is obtained from the distal tip of a pulmonary artery (PA) catheter or from a central venous pressure (CVP) catheter. Normal values for venous blood gas values are listed in Table 5-1. Central venous oxygen saturation (Scvo$_2$) can be obtained from any central venous catheter with the tip positioned in the superior vena cava. Mixed venous oxygen saturation (Smvo$_2$) can only be obtained from a PA or specialized catheter generally only used in a critical care unit. More information on Smvo$_2$ and Scvo$_2$ monitoring is found in Chapter 4, Hemodynamic Monitoring.

Pulse Oximetry

Pulse oximetry is a common method for the continuous, noninvasive monitoring of Sao$_2$. A sensor is applied to skin over areas with strong arterial pulsatile blood flow, typically one of the peripheral fingers or toes (Figure 5-3). Alternative sites include the bridge of the nose, ear, and the forehead (Figure 5-4). The forehead sensor is a reflectance sensor and provides a central monitoring site location. The Sao$_2$ sensor is connected to a pulse oximeter monitor unit via a cable. Light-emitting diodes on one side of the sensor transmit light of two different wavelengths (infrared and red) through arterial blood flowing under the sensor. Depending on the level of oxygen saturation of hemoglobin in the arterial blood, different amounts of light are detected on the other side of the sensor (transmission) or via scattered light on the same side of the light emitters (reflectance). This photo-detection aspect of the sensor transmits information to the microprocessor within the monitor, which then uses various internal software algorithms for calculation and digital display of the oxygen saturation and pulse rate.

When blood perfusion is adequate and Sao$_2$ levels are greater than 70%, depending on the type of sensor being used and monitoring site, there is generally a close correlation between the saturation reading from the pulse oximeter (Spo$_2$) and Sao$_2$ directly measured from ABGs. In situations where perfusion to the sensor is markedly diminished (eg, peripheral vasoconstriction due to disease, drugs, or hypothermia), the ability of the pulse oximeter to detect a signal may be less than under normal perfusion conditions. Newer generation pulse oximeters have the ability to detect signals during most poor perfusion conditions, as well as certain other sources of signal interference, such as motion or other conditions which create potential for artifact.

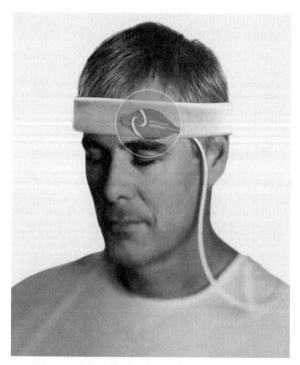

Figure 5-4. Forehead reflectance pulse oximeter sensor. (*With permission, Covidien.*)

ESSENTIAL CONTENT CASE:

Respiratory Failure-Asthma

A 35-year-old woman with a history of asthma was admitted to the emergency department with an asthma exacerbation secondary to a viral pneumonia. Vital signs and laboratory tests on admission were:

Temperature:	38.1°C (oral)
HR:	110/min, slightly labored
BP:	148/90 mm Hg

Lung sounds: pronounced wheezing noted in all lung fields ABGs on room air were:

pH:	7.45
$Paco_2$:	35 mm Hg
HCO_3:	23 mEq/L
BE:	0 mEq/L
Pao_2:	53 mm Hg

She was started on oxygen therapy via a non-rebreather mask at 100% O_2. IV fluids, steroids, and albuterol continuous nebulizers were also initiated along with empiric antibiotics. Within 30 minutes her BP, HR, and RR had decreased to normal values, with improvement in her Pao_2 level (81 mm Hg). She was transferred to the critical care unit 3 hours later. The patient did well until approximately 6 hours following her admission to the hospital. At that time she began experiencing increased shortness of breath, wheezing, and increased HR, BP, and RR. ABGs revealed a respiratory acidosis with partial compensation and hypoxemia despite 4 liters of O_2 by nasal cannula:

pH:	7.31
$Paco_2$:	55 mm Hg
HCO_3:	26.8 mEq/L
BE:	0.9 mEq/L
Pao_2:	48 mm Hg

The patient was intubated with a 7.5-mm oral ET tube without difficulty and placed on a ventilator (mode, SIMV; rate, 15/min; Vt, 600 mL; Fio_2, 0.5; PEEP, 5 cm H_2O). Immediately after intubation and initiation of mechanical ventilation, her BP decreased to 90/64 mm Hg. Following a 500-mL bolus of IV fluids, BP returned to normal values (118/70). ABGs 15 minutes after ventilation were:

pH:	7.36
$Paco_2$:	47 mm Hg
HCO_3:	27.3 mEq/L
BE:	2.1 mEq/L
Pao_2:	65 mm Hg

Case Question 1. Why do you think the patient's BP decreased after intubation?

Case Question 2. What ventilator changes if any would you anticipate?

Answers

1. Hypotension post-intubation is multifactorial. The increased intrathoracic pressure caused by positive end-expiratory pressure (PEEP) and positive pressure ventilation can cause a decreased venous return to the heart along with decrease in cardiac output which may be additionally exaggerated in patient with hypovolemia. This may also be further exacerbated in a patient with severe asthma with hyperinflation and auto-PEEP. Other potential causes may include hemothorax, pneumothorax, or the sequela of medications used to intubate.

2. (A) Increase Fio_2: the patient is on 50% O_2 and her Pao_2 is only 65. She is likely experiencing a late asthmatic response. Once her bronchoconstriction is improved with more bronchodilators and hyperinflation is decreased, the Fio_2 requirements will be less.
(B) Initiate interventions to decrease auto-PEEP and dynamic hyperinflation. A likely cause of hypotension in this patient is hyperinflation and auto-PEEP associated with her history of asthma. There are several strategies to prevent further complications. Auto-PEEP and plateau pressure measurements should be performed. Low tidal volumes, low ventilator rates, short inspiratory times, and long expiratory times may help to prevent hyperinflation. Ensure adequate exhalation time to minimize hyperinflation and auto-PEEP if present.

Pulse oximetry has several advantages for respiratory monitoring. The ability to have continuous information on the Sao_2 level of patients without the need for an invasive arterial puncture decreases infection risks and blood loss from frequent ABG analysis. In addition, these monitors are easy to use, well tolerated by most patients, and portable enough to use during transport.

The major disadvantage of pulse oximeters for assessing oxygen status is that accuracy depends on an adequate arterial pulsatile signal in order for the pulse oximeter to properly function. Clinical situations that decrease the accuracy of the device include:

- Hypotension
- Low CO states
- Vasoconstriction or vasoactive drugs
- Hypothermia
- Movement of the sensor and/or poor skin adherence

Additionally, other sources of potential interference may include direct exposure to ambient light and certain nail polish applications and treatments.

Because these conditions may be found in acutely ill patients, caution is exercised when using pulse oximetry in progressive care units. Proper use (Table 5-4) and periodic validation of the accuracy of the devices with ABG analysis using a co-oximeter instrument is essential to avoid erroneous patient assessment. Routinely used pulse oximeters measure light absorbance at only two wavelengths of light. As such, dyshemoglobinemias such as methemoglobinemia (Met-Hgb) and carboxyhemoglobinemia (CO-Hgb) cannot be measured. Further, the presence of such elevations may cause errors in interpretation of pulse oximetry. Although there are noninvasive devices available for detecting such dyshemoglobinemias, the most widely used and recognized "gold standard" technique for determining the presence of dyshemoglobinemias is co-oximetry via invasive ABG analysis.

TABLE 5-4. TIPS TO MAXIMIZE SAFETY AND ACCURACY OF PULSE OXIMETRY

- Apply sensor to dry finger of nondominant hand according to manufacturer's directions and observe for adequate pulse wave generation or signal on pulse oximeter unit.
- Avoid tension on the sensor cable.
- Rotate application sites and change sensor according to manufacturer's directions whenever adherence is poor.
- In children and elderly patients, assess application sites more often and carefully assess skin integrity when using adhesive sensors.
- Never use pulse oximeter sensors on non-approved monitoring site locations; such as finger or digit sensor use on the ear or forehead.
- If pulse wave generation is inadequate or depending on displayed signal alert message, check for proper adherence to skin and position. Apply a new sensor to another site, if necessary.
- Compare pulse oximeter displayed Sao_2 values with ABGs periodically, when changes in the clinical condition may decrease accuracy and/or when values do not fit the clinical situation.

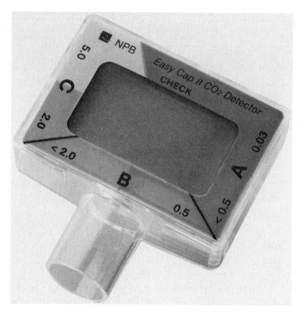

Figure 5-5. Colorimetric carbon dioxide detector. (*With permission, Covidien.*)

Assessing Pulmonary Function

A variety of measurements in addition to ABG analysis can be used to further evaluate the acutely ill patient's respiratory system.

Measurement of selected lung volumes can be easily accomplished at the bedside. V_t, minute ventilation, and negative inspiratory pressure (NIP) are measured with portable, handheld equipment (spirometer and NIP meter, respectively). Lung compliance and alveolar oxygen content can be calculated with standard formulas (see Table 5-1). Frequent trend monitoring of these parameters provides an objective evaluation of the patient's response to interventions.

End-Tidal Carbon Dioxide Monitoring

Carbon dioxide is a byproduct of cellular metabolism and is transported via the venous blood to the lungs where it is eliminated by the lungs during exhalation. End-tidal CO_2 (also referred to as partial pressure of end-tidal CO_2:$PetCO_2$) is the concentration of CO_2 present at the end of exhalation and is expressed either as a percentage ($PetCO_2\%$) or partial pressure ($PetCO_2$ mmHg). The normal range for $PetCO_2$ is typically 1 to 5 mm Hg less than the arterial carbon dioxide tension or $Paco_2$. For this reason, clinicians have sought to use this noninvasive monitoring method for assessing ventilation status over time. Thus, under conditions of normal ventilation and perfusion ($\dot{V}/\dot{Q}$) matching, the relationship between $PetCO_2$ and $Paco_2$ is relatively close. However, when $\dot{V}/\dot{Q}$ relationships are abnormal, this gradient may be as high as 20 mm Hg or more, thus limiting the use of this technology to accurately reflect $Paco_2$. Assessing the arterial to end-tidal CO_2 gradient as a trend may be useful. An increasing gradient reflects a worsening condition and a narrowing gradient may reflect improved ventilation/perfusion matching.

Currently available end-tidal CO_2 monitoring devices fall into one of several categories: colorimetric, capnometric (numeric display only), or capnographic (numeric and graphical display). Colorimetric devices are pH-sensitive, colored paper strips that change color in response to different concentrations of carbon dioxide (Figure 5-5). They are typically used for either initial or intermittent monitoring purposes such as verifying endotracheal tube (ET) placement in the trachea following intubation or in some cases, to rule out inadvertent pulmonary placement of enteral feeding tubes following insertion. A capnometer provides a visual analog or digital display of the concentration of the $PetCO_2$. Capnography includes both capnometry plus the addition of a calibrated graphic recording of the exhaled CO_2 on a breath-by-breath basis and is perhaps the most common instrument used for continuous monitoring. Figure 5-6 demonstrates the various phases of a normal carbon dioxide waveform during exhalation.

Capnography devices measure exhaled carbon dioxide using one of several different techniques: infrared spectrography, Raman spectrography, mass spectrometry, or a laser-based technology called molecular correlation spectroscopy as the infrared emission source. The laser creates an infrared emission precisely matching the absorption rate spectrum of CO_2 and eliminates the need for moving parts. A capnography device using this technology is shown in Figure 5-7. All capnographs sample and measure expired gases either directly at the patient-ventilator interface (mainstream analysis) or collected and transported via small-bore tubing to the sensor in the monitor (sidestream analysis). Each technique has advantages and disadvantages and the user should strictly follow manufacturer recommendations for optimal performance.

Clinical application of capnography includes assessment of endotracheal or tracheostomy tube placement, gastric or small bowel tube placement, pulmonary blood flow, and alveolar ventilation, provided $\dot{V}/\dot{Q}$ relationships are normal. The 2010-2015 AHA Guidelines for ACLS recommend using quantitative waveform capnography during endotracheal tube placement and in intubated patients during CPR.

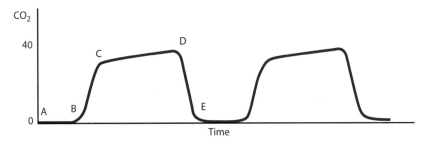

Figure 5-6. Capnogram waveform phases. Phase A to B: Early exhalation. This represents anatomic dead space and contains little carbon dioxide. Phase B to C: Combination of dead space and alveolar gas. Phase C to D: Exhalation of mostly alveolar gas (alveolar plateau). Phase D: End-tidal point, that is, exhalation of carbon dioxide at maximum point. Phase D to E: Inspiration begins and carbon dioxide concentration rapidly falls to baseline or zero. (*With permission, Oridion Systems Ltd., Jerusalem, Israel.*)

Waveform capnography allows nurses and other caregivers to monitor CPR quality, optimize chest compressions, and detect return of spontaneous circulation (ROSC) during chest compressions. Assessment of the capnographic waveform alone can yield useful information in detecting ventilator malfunction, response to changes in ventilator settings and weaning attempts, and depth of neuromuscular blockade. It should be noted that although capnography is commonly used in patients with artificial airways, this monitoring technique can also be used in nonintubated patients via a modified nasal/oral sampling cannula. When using capnography in the clinical setting it is important to always follow manufacturer recommendations regarding set-up, maintenance, and troubleshooting of equipment. Institutional policies and protocols regarding clinical management for patient care should also be followed.

AIRWAY MANAGEMENT

Maintaining an open and patent airway is an important aspect of progressive care management. Patency can be ensured through conservative techniques such as coughing, head and neck positioning, and alignment. If conservative techniques fail, insertion of an oral or nasal airway or ET tube may be required.

Oropharyngeal Airway

The oropharyngeal airway, or oral bite block, is an airway adjunct used to relieve upper airway obstruction caused by tongue relaxation (eg, postanesthesia or during unconsciousness), secretions, seizures, or biting down on oral ETs (Figure 5-8A). Oral airways are made of rigid plastic or rubber material, semicircular in shape, and available in sizes ranging from infants to adults. The airway is inserted with the concave curve of the airway facing up into the roof of the mouth. The oral airway is then rotated down 180° during insertion to fit the curvature of the tongue and ensure the tongue is not obstructing the airway. The tip of the oropharyngeal airway rests near the posterior pharyngeal wall. For this reason, oral airways are not recommended for use in alert patients because they may trigger the gag reflex and cause vomiting. Oropharyngeal airways are temporary devices for achieving airway patency.

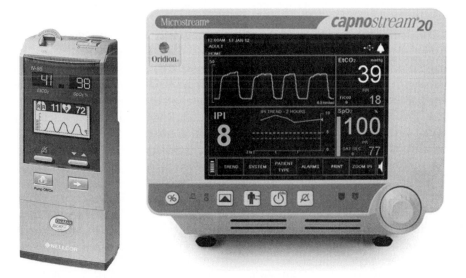

Figure 5-7. Handheld (**A**) and Bedside (**B**) combined capnography (sidestream) and pulse oximetry instruments. (*With permission, Covidien.*)

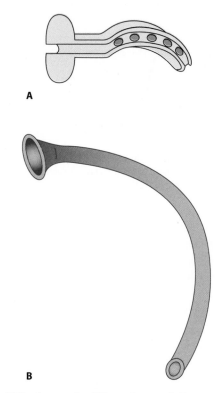

Figure 5-8. (A) Oropharyngeal and (B) nasopharyngeal airways.

Management of oropharyngeal airways includes frequent assessment of the lips and tongue to identify pressure areas. The airway is removed at least every 24 hours to check for pressure areas and to provide oral hygiene.

Nasopharyngeal Airway

The nasopharyngeal airway, or nasal trumpet, is another type of airway adjunct device used to help maintain airway patency, especially in the semiconscious patient (Figure 5-8B). The nasopharyngeal airway is also used to facilitate nasotracheal suctioning. Made of soft malleable rubber or soft plastic, the nasal airway ranges in sizes from 26 to 35 Fr. Prior to insertion, a topical anesthetic (eg, viscous lidocaine), based on hospital policy, may be applied to the nares. The nasopharyngeal airway, lubricated with a water-soluble gel, is gently inserted into one of the nares. The patency of the airway is assessed by listening for, or feeling with your hand, air movement during expiration. The airway should be secured to the nose with a small piece of tape to prevent displacement. Complications of these airways include bleeding, sinusitis, and erosion of the mucous membranes.

Care of the patient with a nasal airway includes frequent assessment for pressure areas and occlusion of the airway with dried secretions. Sinusitis has been documented as a complication. The continued need for the nasal airway is assessed daily and rotation of the airway from nostril to nostril is done on a daily basis. When performing nasotracheal suctioning through the nasal airway, the suction catheter is lubricated with a water-soluble gel to ease passage. Refer to

the following discussion on suctioning for additional standards of care.

Laryngeal Mask Airway

The laryngeal mask airway (LMA) is an ET tube with a small mask on one end that can be passed orally over the larynx to provide ventilatory assistance and prevent aspiration. Placement of the LMA is easier than intubation using a standard ET tube. Commonly used as the primary airway device in the operating room for certain types of surgical procedures, it should, however, only be considered a temporary airway for patients who require prolonged ventilatory support.

Esophageal Tracheal Airway

Esophageal tracheal airways are double-lumen airways that allow for rapid airway establishment through either esophageal or tracheal placement. They are used primarily for difficult or emergency intubation and the design permits blind placement without the need for a laryngoscope. The multifunction design permits positive-pressure ventilation, but an ET tube or tracheostomy is eventually needed. The primary advantages to using the airways include less training required to use than standard intubation, no special equipment required, and the cuff provides some protection against aspiration of gastric contents. The tube is contraindicated in responsive patients with intact gag reflexes, patients with known esophageal pathology, and patients who have ingested caustic substances. The tube is sized to the patient's height.

Artificial Airways

Artificial airways (oral and nasal ET tubes, tracheostomy tubes) are used when a patent airway cannot be maintained with an adjunct airway device for mechanical ventilation or to manage severe airway obstruction. The artificial airway also protects the lower airway from aspiration of oral or gastric secretions and allows for easier secretion removal.

Types of Artificial Airways and Insertion

Endotracheal tubes are made of either polyvinyl chloride or silicone and are available in a variety of sizes and lengths (Figure 5-9A). Standard features include a 15-mm adapter at the end of the tube for connection to various life-support equipments such as mechanical ventilation circuits, closed-suction catheter systems, swivel adapters, or a manual resuscitation bag (MRB). Tubes may be cuffed or uncuffed. For cuffed tubes, air is manually injected into the cuff located near the distal tip of the ET tube through a small one-way pilot valve and inflation lumen. Distance markers are located along the side of the tube for identification of tube position. A radiopaque line is also located on all tubes so as to aid in determining proper position radiographically.

Endotracheal tubes are inserted into the patient's trachea either through the mouth or nose (Figures 5-10 and 5-11). Orally inserted ET tubes are more common than the

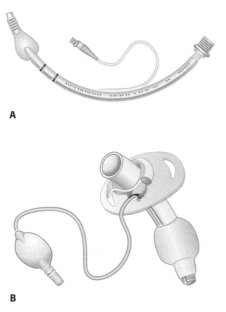

A

B

Figure 5-9. Artificial airways. **(A)** Cuffed endotracheal tube. **(B)** Cuffed tracheostomy tube. (*With permission, Covidien.*)

nasal route because nasal intubation is associated with sinus infections and are considered an independent risk factor for developing ventilator-associated pneumonia (VAP). With use of the laryngoscope, the upper airway is visualized and the tube is inserted through the vocal cords into the trachea, 2 to 4 cm above the carina. The presence of bilateral breath sounds, along with equal chest excursion during inspiration and the absence of breath sounds over the stomach, preliminarily confirms proper tube placement. An end-tidal CO_2 monitor with waveform verification should be used as an immediate assessment for determining tracheal placement. If not available, a colorimetric CO_2 detector may be used. A portable chest x-ray verifies proper tube placement. Once proper placement is confirmed, the tube is anchored to prevent movement with either tape or a special ET tube fixation device (Figure 5-12). The centimeter marking of the ET tube at the lip is documented and checked during each shift to monitor proper tube placement.

Endotracheal tube sizes are typically identified by the tubes' internal diameter in millimeters (mm ID). The size of the tube is printed on the tube and generally also on the outside packaging. Knowledge of the tube ID is critical; the smaller the mm ID, the higher the resistance to breathing through the tube, thus increasing the work of breathing. The most common ET tube sizes used in adults are 7.0 to 9.0 mm ID.

Endotracheal tubes can in some situations be safely left in place for up to 2-3 weeks, but tracheostomy is often considered following 10 to 14 days of intubation or less. If the need for an artificial airway is anticipated for an extended period of time, a tracheostomy tube may be indicated earlier, but the decision is always individualized. Complications of ET intubation are numerous and include laryngeal and tracheal damage, laryngospasm, aspiration, infection, discomfort, sinusitis, and subglottic injury.

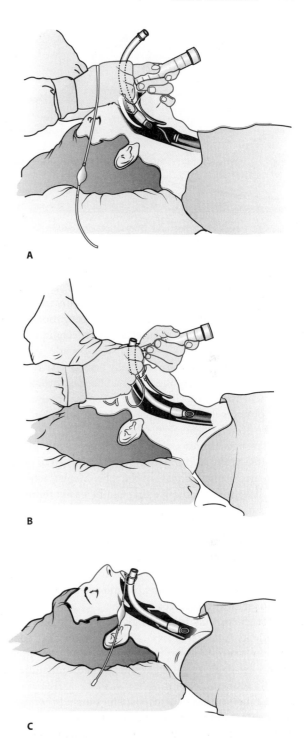

A

B

C

Figure 5-10. Oral intubation with an endotracheal (ET) tube. **(A)** Insertion of ET tube through the mouth with the aid of a laryngoscope. **(B)** ET tube advanced through the vocal cords into the trachea. **(C)** ET tube positioned with the cuff below the vocal cords. (*Reprinted from Boggs Wooldridge-King M.* AACN Procedure Manual for Progressive Care. *3rd ed. Philadelphia, PA: WB Saunders; 1993: 34-36 with permission from Elsevier.*)

The majority of tracheostomy tubes used in acutely ill patients are made of medical-grade plastic or silicone and come in a variety of sizes (Figure 5-9B). Tracheostomy tubes may be cuffed or uncuffed. As with ET tubes, a standard 15-mm adapter at the proximal end ensures universal

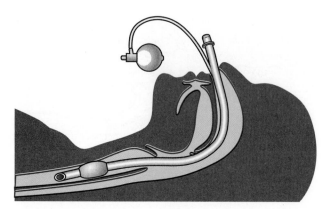

Figure 5-11. Nasal endotracheal tube. (*With permission, Covidien.*)

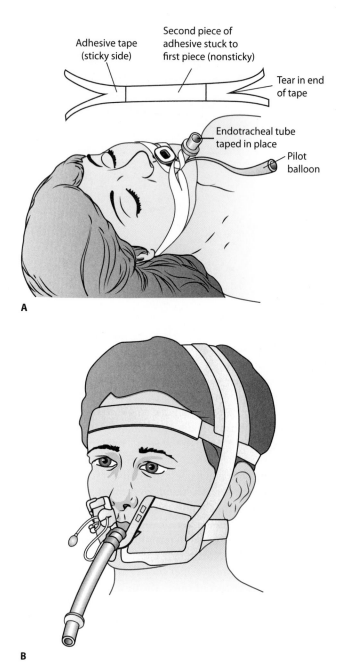

Figure 5-12. Methods for anchoring an endotracheal tube to prevent movement. **(A)** Taping of an oral ET tube. (*Reprinted from Boggs R, Wooldridge-King M. AACN Procedure Manual for Critical Care. 3rd ed. Philadelphia, PA: WB Saunders; 993:108, with permission from Elsevier.*) **(B)** Use of a special fixation device. (*Reprinted from Kaplow R, Bookbinder M. A comparison of four endotracheal tube holders. Heart Lung. 1994;23(1):60, with permission from Elsevier.*)

connection to MRBs and ventilator circuits. Tracheostomy tubes may be inserted as an elective procedure using a standard open surgical technique in the operating room or at the bedside via a percutaneous insertion. This technique involves a procedure in which a small incision is made in the neck and a series of dilators are manually passed into the trachea over a guide wire, creating a stoma opening through which the tracheostomy tube is inserted into place. Bedside placement obviates the need for patient transport out of the unit and the need for general anesthesia.

Tracheostomies are secured with cotton twill tape or latex-free Velcro latching tube holders attached to openings on the neck flange or plate of the tube. Many tracheostomy tubes have inner cannulae that can be easily removed for periodic cleaning (reusable) or replacement (disposable). Some tracheostomy tubes incorporate an additional opening along the outer tube cannula referred to as a fenestration. A fenestrated tracheostomy tube is sometimes used as an aid for facilitating vocalization by allowing airflow upward and through the vocal cords. A fenestration is not necessary to be able to talk with a tracheostomy tube.

Tracheostomy tubes, in general, are better tolerated by patients than oral or nasal ET tubes in terms of comfort. Further, there are more nutrition and communication options available to patients with tracheostomy tubes than with ET tubes.

Complications of tracheostomies include hemorrhage from erosion of the innominate artery; tracheal stenosis, malacia, or perforation; laryngeal nerve injury; aspiration; infection; air leak; and mechanical problems. Most complications rarely occur with proper management.

Cuff Inflation

Following insertion of an endotracheal or tracheostomy tube, the cuff of the tube is inflated with just enough air to create an effective seal. The cuff is typically inflated with the lowest possible pressure that prevents air leak during mechanical ventilation and decreases the risk of pulmonary aspiration. Cuff pressure is maintained at less than 25 mm Hg (30 cm H_2O). Excessive cuff pressure causes

tracheal ischemia, necrosis, and erosion, as well as overinflation-related obstruction of the distal airway from cuff herniation. It is important to recognize that even a properly inflated cuffed artificial airway does not completely protect the patient from aspiration of liquids.

There are two common techniques to ensure proper cuff inflation without overinflation: the minimal leak and minimal occlusive volume techniques (MLT and MOV, respectively). The minimal leak technique involves listening over the larynx during positive pressure breaths with a stethoscope while inflating the tube cuff in 1- to 2-mL increments. Inflation continues until only a small air leak, or rush of air, is heard over the larynx during peak inspiration. The minimal leak technique should result in no more than a 50- to 100-mL air loss per breath during mechanical ventilation. The cuff pressure and amount of air instilled into the cuff are recorded following the maneuver.

The minimal occlusive volume cuff inflation technique is similar to the minimal leak technique. Cuff inflation continues, however, until the air leak completely disappears. The amount of air instilled and the cuff pressure are recorded during cuff inflation and periodically to ensure an intracuff pressure of less than 25 mm Hg (30 cm H_2O). Manual palpation of the tube pilot balloon does not ensure optimal inflation assessment.

Cuff Pressure Measurement

The connection of the ET tube pilot balloon to an intracuff measuring manometer device, such as a manual hand-held cuff inflator, allows for the simultaneous measurement of pressure during inflation or periodic checking (Figure 5-13). The need for excessive pressures to properly seal the trachea may indicate the ET tube diameter is too small for the trachea. In this case, the cuff is inflated to properly seal the trachea until

the appropriately sized ET tube can be electively reinserted. At present, evidence of long-term outcomes is lacking to warrant mandatory cuff pressure monitoring. However, until a more definitive statement may be made, the clinician is encouraged to follow tube manufacturer and hospital policy. Current available evidence from clinical and laboratory testing suggests that intra-cuff pressure may be an important contributing factor to the development of complications related to cuffed endotracheal and tracheostomy tubes so attention to proper inflation is encouraged.

Endotracheal Suctioning

Pulmonary secretion removal is normally accomplished by coughing. An effective cough requires a closed epiglottis so that intrathoracic pressure can be increased prior to sudden opening of the epiglottis and secretion expulsion. The presence of an artificial airway such as an ET tube prevents glottic closure and effective coughing, necessitating the use of periodic endotracheal suctioning to remove secretions.

Currently, two methods are commonly used for ET tube suctioning: the closed and open methods. Closed suctioning means the ventilator circuit remains closed while suctioning is performed, whereas open suctioning means the ventilator circuit is opened, or removed, during suctioning. The open method requires disconnection of the ET tube from the mechanical ventilator or oxygen therapy source and insertion of a suction catheter each time the patient requires suctioning. The closed method refers to a closed suction catheter system device that remains attached to the ventilator circuit, allowing periodic insertion of the suction catheter through a diaphragm to suction without removing the patient from the ventilator. Following suctioning, the catheter is withdrawn into a plastic sleeve of the in-line device until the next suctioning procedure.

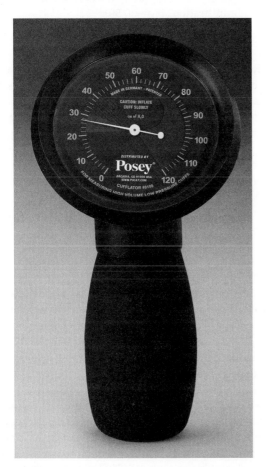

Figure 5-13. Portable endotracheal tube cuff inflator and manometer. (*Courtesy of: Posey Company, Arcadia, CA.*)

Indications

The need for ET suctioning is determined by a variety of clinical signs and symptoms, such as coughing, increased inspiratory pressures on the ventilator, and the presence of adventitious sounds (rhonchi, gurgling) during chest auscultation. Suctioning may also be performed periodically to ensure airway patency. Suctioning is only done when there is a clinical indication and never on a routine schedule.

Procedure

Hyperoxygenation with 100% O_2 for a minimum of 30 seconds is provided prior to each suctioning episode, whether using an open or closed technique (Table 5-5). Hyperoxygenation helps to prevent decreases in arterial oxygen levels after suctioning. Hyperoxygenation can be achieved by increasing the Fio_2 setting on the mechanical ventilator or by using the "suction" button or temporary oxygen-enrichment program available on most microprocessor ventilators. Manual ventilation of the patient using an MRB is not recommended as the best choice and has been

TABLE 5-5. STEPS FOR SUCTIONING THROUGH AN ARTIFICIAL AIRWAY

1. Assess for signs and symptoms of airway obstruction;
   - Secretions in the airway
   - Decreased breath sounds, inspiratory wheezes, or expiratory crackles
   - Restlessness or decreased level of consciousness
   - Ineffective cough
   - Tachypnea, shallow respirations or decreased respirations
   - Tachycardia, or bradycardia
   - Cyanosis
   - Hypertension or hypotension
2. Hyperoxygenate with 100% oxygen for minimum of 30 seconds with one of the following:
   - Press the suction hyperoxygenation button to increase the Fio_2 to 1.0 (100%) on the ventilator, or
   - Manually increase the Fio_2 to 1.0 (100%), or
   - Disconnect from the ventilator and manually ventilate with MRB
3. Insert catheter (closed or open system) gently until resistance is met, then pull back 1 cm.
4. Place the non-dominant thumb over the control vent of the suction catheter to apply continuous or intermittent suction as the catheter is completely withdrawn.
   NOTE: Suction should be applied only as needed and for as short a time as possible.
5. Hyperoxygenate for 30 seconds as described in step 2.
6. Repeat steps 3, 4, and 5 as needed if secretions remain and patient is tolerating the procedure.
7. Monitor cardiopulmonary status before, during, and after suctioning for the following:
   - Decreased arterial or mixed venous oxygen saturation
   - Decreased oxygenation
   - Cardiac dysrhythmias
   - Bronchospasms
   - Respiratory distress
   - Cyanosis
   - Hypertension
   - Increased ICP
   - Anxiety, agitation, pain or change in level of consciousness
   - Increased peak airway pressure
   - Coughing
   - Increased work of breathing

Data from Chulay M, Seckel MA. Suctioning: endotracheal or tracheostomy tube. In Wiegand DL, ed. AACN Procedure Manual for Critical Care. 6th ed. Philadephia, PA: Saunders; 2011.

shown to be ineffective for providing delivered Fio_2 of 1.0. If no other alternative is available to hyperoxygenate, then a MRB can be used. At least 30 seconds of manual breaths with 100% Fio_2 are provided before and after each pass of the suction catheter. In spontaneously breathing patients, encourage several deep breaths of 100% O_2 before and after each suction pass. The number of suction passes are limited to only those necessary to clear the airway of secretions—usually two or three. The mechanical act of inserting the suction catheter into the trachea can stimulate the vagus nerve and result in bradycardia or asystole. Each pass of the suction catheter should be 10 seconds or less.

The instillation of 5 to 10 mL of normal saline is no longer advocated during routine ET tube suctioning. This practice was previously thought to decrease secretion viscosity and increase secretion removal during ET tube suctioning. Bolus saline instillation has not been shown to be beneficial and is associated with Sao_2 decreases and bronchospasm.

Complications

A variety of complications are associated with ET tube suctioning. Decreases in Pao_2 have been well documented when no hyperoxygenation therapy is provided with suctioning. Serious cardiac arrhythmias occur occasionally with suctioning, and include bradycardia, asystole, ventricular tachycardia, and heart block. Less severe arrhythmias frequently occur with suctioning and include premature ventricular contractions, atrial contractions, and supraventricular tachycardia. Other complications associated with suctioning include increases in arterial pressure and intracranial pressure, bronchospasm, tracheal wall damage, and nosocomial pneumonia. Many of these complications can be minimized by using sterile technique, vigilant monitoring during and after suctioning, and hyperoxygenation before and after each suction pass.

Extubation

The reversal or significant improvement of the underlying condition(s) that led to the use of artificial airways usually signals the readiness for removal of the airway. Common indicators of readiness for artificial airway removal include the ability to:

- Maintain spontaneous breathing and adequate ABG values with minimal to moderate amounts of O_2 administration ($Fio_2 < 0.50$).
- Protect the airway.
- Clear pulmonary secretions.

Removal of an artificial airway usually occurs following weaning from mechanical ventilatory support (see the discussion on weaning later). Preparations for extubation include an explanation to the patient and family of what to expect, the need to cough, medication for pain, setting up the appropriate method for delivering O_2 therapy (eg, face mask, nasal cannula), and positioning the patient with the head of the bed elevated at 30° to 45° to improve diaphragmatic function. Suctioning of the artificial airway is performed prior to extubation if clinically indicated. Obtaining a baseline cardiopulmonary assessment also is important for later evaluation of the response to extubation. Extubation should be performed when full ancillary staff is available to assist if reintubation is required.

Hyperoxygenation with 100% O_2 is provided for 30 to 60 seconds prior to extubation in case respiratory distress occurs immediately after extubation and reintubation is necessary. The artificial airway is then removed following complete deflation of the ET or tracheostomy cuff, if present. Immediately apply the oxygen delivery method and encourage the patient to take deep breaths.

Monitor the patient's response to the extubation. Significant changes in heart rate, respiratory rate, and/or blood pressure of more than 10% of baseline values may indicate respiratory compromise, necessitating more extensive assessment and possible reintubation. Pulmonary auscultation is also performed.

Complications associated with extubation include aspiration, bronchospasm, and tracheal damage. Coughing and deep breathing are encouraged while monitoring vital signs and the upper airway for stridor. Inspiratory stridor occurs from glottic and subglottic edema and may develop immediately or take several hours. If the patient's clinical status permits, treatment with 2.5% racemic epinephrine (0.5 mL in 3 mL of normal saline) is administered via an aerosol delivery device. If the upper airway obstruction persists or worsens, reintubation is generally required. A reattempt at extubation is usually delayed for 24 to 72 hours following reintubation for upper airway obstruction.

OXYGEN THERAPY

Oxygen is used for any number of clinical problems (Table 5-6). The overall goals for oxygen use include increasing alveolar O_2 tension (Pao_2) to treat hypoxemia, decreasing the work of breathing, and maximizing myocardial and tissue oxygen supply.

Complications

As with any drug, oxygen should be used cautiously. The hazards of oxygen misuse can be as dangerous as the lack of appropriate use. Alveolar hypoventilation, absorption atelectasis, and oxygen toxicity can be life threatening.

Alveolar Hypoventilation

Alveolar hypoventilation is underventilation of alveoli, and is a side effect of great concern in patients with chronic obstructive pulmonary disease (COPD) with carbon dioxide retention. As the patient with COPD adjusts to chronically high levels of $Paco_2$, the chemoreceptors in the medulla of the brain lose responsiveness to high $Paco_2$ levels. Hypoxemia, then, becomes a primary stimulus for ventilation. However,

TABLE 5-6. COMMON INDICATIONS FOR OXYGEN THERAPY

- Decreased cardiac performance
- Increased metabolic need for O_2 (fever, burns)
- Acute changes in level of consciousness (restlessness, confusion)
- Acute shortness of breath
- Decreased O_2 saturation
- Pao_2 < 60 mm Hg or Sao_2 < 90%
- Normal Pao_2 or Sao_2 with signs and symptoms of significant hypoxia
- Myocardial infarction
- Carbon monoxide (CO) poisoning
- Methemoglobinemia (a form of hemoglobin where ferrous iron is oxidized to ferric form, causing a high affinity for O_2 with decreased O_2 release at tissue level)
- Acute anemia
- Cardiopulmonary arrest
- Reduced cardiac output
- Consider in the presence of hypotension, tachycardia, cyanosis, chest pain, dyspnea, and acute neurologic dysfunction
- During stressful procedures and situations, especially high-risk patients (eg, ET suctioning, bronchoscopy, thoracentesis, PA catheterization, travel at high altitudes)

correction of hypoxemia in the patient with COPD remains important with a target Pao_2 of 55 to 60 mm Hg ($Sao_2 \geq$ 90%), despite the presence of hypercapnia.

Absorption Atelectasis

Absorption atelectasis results when high concentrations of O_2 (> 90%) are given for long periods of time and nitrogen is washed out of the lungs. The nitrogen in inspired gas is approximately 79% of the total atmospheric gases. The large partial pressure of nitrogen in the alveoli helps to maintain open alveoli because it is not absorbed. Removal of nitrogen by inspiring 90% to 100% O_2 results in alveolar closure because oxygen readily diffuses into the pulmonary capillary.

Oxygen Toxicity

The toxic effects of oxygen are targeted primarily to the pulmonary and central nervous systems (CNS). CNS toxicity usually occurs with hyperbaric oxygen treatment. Signs and symptoms include nausea, anxiety, numbness, visual disturbances, muscular twitching, and grand mal seizures. The physiologic mechanism is not understood fully but is felt to be related to subtle neural and biochemical changes that alter the electric activity of the CNS.

Pulmonary oxygen toxicity is due to prolonged exposure to high Fio_2 levels that may lead to ARDS or bronchopulmonary dysplasia. Two phases of lung injury result. The first phase occurs after 1 to 4 days of exposure to higher O_2 levels and is manifested by decreased tracheal mucosal blood flow and tracheobronchitis. Vital capacity decreases because of poor lung expansion and progressive atelectasis persists. The alveolar capillary membrane becomes progressively impaired, decreasing gas exchange. The second phase occurs after 12 days of high exposure. The alveolar septa thickens and an ARDS picture develops, with associated high mortality.

Caring for the patient who requires high levels of oxygen requires astute monitoring by the progressive care nurse. Monitor those patients at risk for absorption atelectasis and oxygen toxicity. Signs and symptoms include nonproductive cough, substernal chest pain, general malaise, fatigue, nausea, and vomiting.

An oxygen concentration of 100% (Fio_2 = 1.0) is regarded as safe for short periods of time (< 24 hours). Oxygen concentrations greater than 50% for more than 24 to 48 hours may damage the lungs and worsen respiratory problems. Oxygen delivery levels are decreased as soon as Pao_2 levels return to clinically acceptable levels (> 60 mm Hg or higher).

Oxygen Delivery

Noninvasive Devices

Face masks and nasal cannulas are standard oxygen delivery devices for the spontaneously breathing patient (Figure 5-14). Oxygen can be delivered with a high- or low-flow device, with the concentration of O_2 delivered ranging from 21% to approximately 100% (Table 5-7). An example of a high-flow

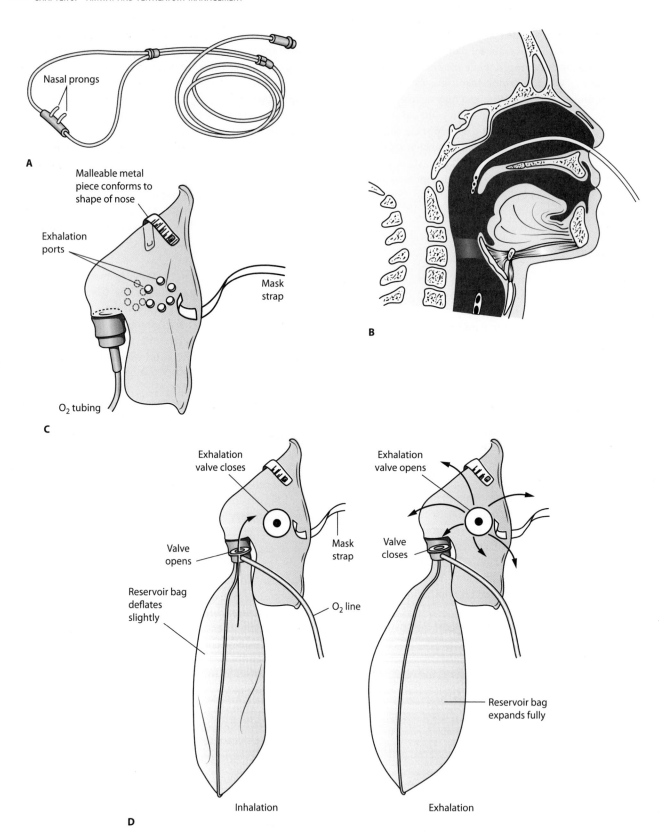

Figure 5-14. Noninvasive and invasive methods of O$_2$ delivery. **(A)** Nasal prongs. **(B)** Nasal catheter. **(C)** Face mask. **(D)** Nonrebreathing mask. (*Reprinted from: Kersten L. Comprehensive Respiratory Nursing. Philadelphia, PA: WB Saunders; 1989:608, 609; with permission from Elsevier.*)

TABLE 5-7. APPROXIMATE OXYGEN DELIVERY WITH COMMON NONINVASIVE AND INVASIVE OXYGEN DEVICES[a]

Device	% O_2
Nasal Prongs/Cannula	
• 2 L/min	28
• 4 L/min	36
• 5 L/min	40
Face Mask	
• 5 L/min	30
• 10 L/min	50
Nonbreathing Mask 10 L/min	60-80
Partial Rebreathing Mask 6-10 L/min	40-70
Venturi Mask	
• 24%	24
• 28%	28
• 35%	35
Manual Resuscitation Bag (MRB)	
• Disposable MRB	Dependent on model

[a]Actual delivery dependent on minute ventilation rates except for Venturi mask.

device is the Venturi mask system that can deliver precise concentrations of oxygen (Figure 5-15). The usual Fio_2 values delivered with this type of mask are 24%, 28%, 31%, 35%, 40%, and 50%. Often, Venturi masks are useful in patients with COPD and hypercapnia because the clinician can titrate the Pao_2 to minimize carbon dioxide retention. An example of a low-flow system is the nasal cannula or prongs. Nasal prongs flow rate ranges are limited to 6 L/min. Flow rates less than 4 L/min need not be humidified. The main advantage of nasal prongs is that the patient can drink, eat, and speak during oxygen administration. The disadvantage is that the exact Fio_2

delivered is unknown, because it is influenced by the patient's peak inspiratory flow demand and breathing pattern. As a general guide, 1 L/min of O_2 flow is an approximate equivalent to an Fio_2 of 24%, and each additional liter of oxygen flow increases the Fio_2 by approximately 4%. Simple oxygen face masks can provide an Fio_2 of 34%-50% depending on fit at flow rates from 5-10 L/min. Flow rates should be maintained at 5 L/min or more in order to avoid rebreathing exhaled CO_2 that can be retained in the mask. Limitations of using a simple face mask include difficulty in delivering accurate delivery of low concentrations of oxygen and long-term use can lead to skin irritation and potential pressure breakdown. Nonrebreathing masks can achieve higher oxygen concentrations (approximately 60%-80%) than partial rebreathing systems. A one-way valve placed between the mask and reservoir bag with a nonrebreathing system prevents exhaled gases from entering the bag, thus maximizing the delivered Fio_2.

A variation of the nonrebreathing mask without the one-way valves is called a partial rebreathing mask. Oxygen should always be supplied to maintain the reservoir bag at least one-third to one-half full on inspiration. At a flow of 6 to 10 L/min, the system can provide 40% to 70% oxygen. High-flow delivery devices such as aerosol masks or face tents, tracheostomy collars, and t-tube adapters can be used with supplemental oxygen systems. A continuous aerosol generator or large-volume reservoir humidifier can humidify the gas flow. Some aerosol generators cannot provide adequate flows at high oxygen concentrations.

Because conventional low-flow nasal cannulae and oxygen masks are constrained by flow, humidity, and accuracy of delivered inspired oxygen, the recent introduction

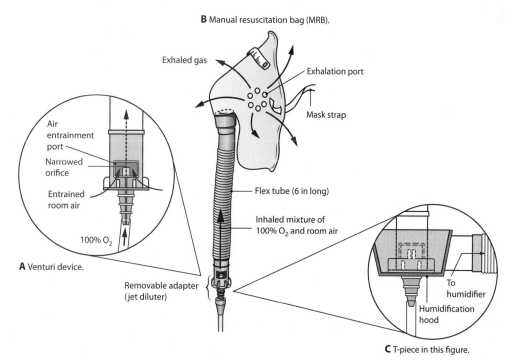

B Manual resuscitation bag (MRB).

Exhaled gas
Exhalation port
Mask strap

Air entrainment port
Narrowed orifice
Entrained room air
100% O_2

A Venturi device.

Flex tube (6 in long)
Inhaled mixture of 100% O_2 and room air

Removable adapter (jet diluter)

To humidifier
Humidification hood

C T-piece in this figure.

Figure 5-15. (A) Venturi device. **(B)** Manual resuscitation bag (MRB). **(C)** T-piece. (*Reprinted from: Kersten L. Comprehensive Respiratory Nursing. Philadelphia, PA: WB Saunders; 1989:611, 629, with permission from Elsevier.*)

of high-flow nasal oxygen devices capable of delivering well-humidified blended oxygen (using vapor) across a wide range of oxygen concentrations has been found to be useful in those patients who require a greater degree of support than what is possible by using traditional low flow oxygen devices. These devices provide oxygen at very high flow rates.

Invasive Devices

Manual Resuscitation Bags

Manual resuscitation bags provide 40% to 100% O_2 at adult V_t and respiratory rates to an ET tube or tracheostomy tube.

Mechanical Ventilators

The most common method for delivering oxygen invasively is with a mechanical ventilator. Oxygen can be accurately delivered from 21% to 100% O_2. Mechanical ventilation is discussed below in more detail.

Transtracheal Oxygen Therapy

Transtracheal oxygen therapy is a method of administering continuous oxygen to patients with chronic hypoxemia. The therapy requires the percutaneous placement of a small plastic catheter into the trachea. The catheter is inserted directly into the trachea above the suprasternal notch under local anesthesia in an outpatient setting. This device allows for low O_2 flow rates (< 1-2 L/min) to treat chronic hypoxemia. Advantages of this method for chronic O_2 delivery include improved mobility and patient aesthetics because the tubing and catheter, unlike the nasal cannula or face mask, can often be hidden from view, avoidance of nasal and ear irritation from nasal cannulas, decreased O_2 requirements, and correction of refractory hypoxemia.

Typically, these patients are managed in the outpatient setting, but occasionally they may be in progressive care units. It is important to maintain the catheter unless specifically ordered to discontinue its use. The stoma formation process takes several weeks and if the catheter is removed, the stoma is likely to close. The catheter is cleaned daily to prevent the formation of mucous plugs. Refer to the manufacturer's guidelines for further recommendations on care of the catheter while the patient is hospitalized.

T-Piece

Oxygen can also be provided directly to an ET or tracheostomy tube with a T-piece, or blow by, in spontaneously breathing patients who do not require ventilatory support. The T-piece is connected directly to the ET tube or tracheostomy tube 15 mm adapter, providing 21% to 80% O_2.

BASIC VENTILATORY MANAGEMENT

Indications

Mechanical ventilation is indicated when noninvasive management modalities fail to adequately support oxygenation and/or ventilation. The decision to initiate mechanical ventilation is based on the ability of the patient to

TABLE 5-8. INDICATIONS FOR MECHANICAL VENTILATION

Oxygenation Indices
1. Calculation of alveolar-arterial gradient of oxygen tension—**A-aDO$_2$** $Pao_2 = Fio_2 (P_{Barr} - PH_2) - (Paco_2/RQ)$ Pao_2 = obtained from ABG $PAo_2 - Pao_2 = A\text{-}aDO_2$ normal value; if Fio_2 (0.21) = 10-20 mm Hg, if Fio_2 (1.0) = 50-70 mm Hg PBARR = barometric pressure (760 mm Hg), PH_2O = pressure of water vapor (47 mm Hg), RQ = repiratory quotient (0.8)
2. Calculation of arterial/alveolar ratio—**a/A ratio** $Pao_2 \div PAo_2$ normal value; 0.8 – 1
3. Calculation of Pao_2/Fio_2 ratio—**P/F ratio** $Pao_2 \div Fio_2$ normal value > 300 Shunt Indices
4. Calculation of Shunt—**Qs/Qt ratio** $Qs/Qt = (CcO_2 - Cao_2)/(CcO_2 - Cvo_2)$ $CcO_2 = (Hgl \times 1.39 \times Sat [1.0]) + (Pao_2 \times 0.003)$ $CaO_2 = (Hgl \times 1.39 \times Sao_2) + (Pao_2 \times 0.003)$ $Cvo_2 = (Hgl \times 1.39 \times Svo_2) + (Pvo_2 \times 0.003)$ Normal value < 0.5% CcO_2 = oxygen content, Cao_2 = arterial oxygen content, Cvo_2 = mixed venous oxygen content, Hgb = hemoglobin, Sat = saturation of hemoglobin, Pvo_2 = partial pressure of mixed venous oxygen

Data from: Burns SM. Indices of oxygenation; Shunt calculation. In: Wiegand DL, ed. AACN Procedure Manual for Critical Care. 6th ed. Philadelphia, PA: Saunders; 2011.

support their oxygenation and/or ventilation needs. The inability of the patient to maintain clinically acceptable CO_2 levels and acid-base status is referred to as respiratory failure and is a common indicator for mechanical ventilation. Refractory hypoxemia—which is the inability to establish and maintain acceptable oxygenation levels despite the administration of oxygen-enriched breathing environments—is also a common reason for mechanical ventilation. Table 5-8 presents a variety of physiologic indicators for initiating mechanical ventilation. By monitoring these indicators, it is possible to differentiate stable or improving values from continuing decompensation. The need for mechanical ventilation may then be anticipated to avoid emergent use of ventilatory support.

Depending on the underlying cause of the respiratory failure, different indicators may be assessed to determine the need for mechanical ventilation. Many of the causes of respiratory failure, however, are due to inadequate alveolar ventilation and/or hypoxemia, with abnormal ABG values and physical assessment as the primary indicators for ventilatory support.

General Principles

Mechanical ventilators are designed to partially or completely support ventilation. Two different categories of ventilators are available to provide ventilatory support. Negative-pressure ventilators decrease intrathoracic pressure by applying negative pressure to the chest wall, typically with a shell placed around the chest (Figure 5-16A). The decrease in intrathoracic pressure causes atmospheric gas to be drawn into the lungs. Positive-pressure ventilators

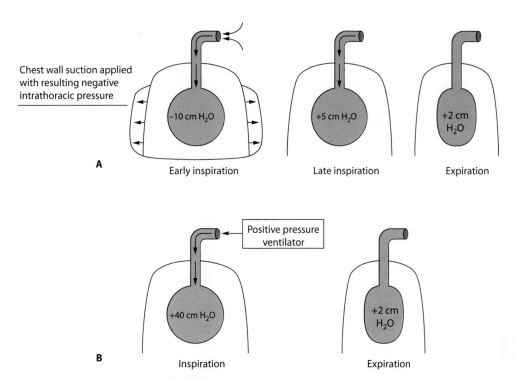

Figure 5-16. Principles of mechanical ventilation as provided by **(A)** negative-pressure and **(B)** positive-pressure ventilators.

deliver pressurized gases into the lung during inspiration (Figure 5-16B). Positive-pressure ventilators can dramatically increase intrathoracic pressures during inspiration, potentially decreasing venous return and CO.

Negative-pressure ventilators are rarely used to manage acute respiratory problems in progressive care. These devices are typically used for long-term noninvasive ventilatory support when respiratory muscle strength is inadequate to support unassisted, spontaneous breathing. Since the emergence of other, noninvasive modes of positive pressure (eg, BiPAP or bilevel), negative pressure ventilators are infrequently selected (described later in this chapter).

Patient-Ventilator System

Positive-pressure ventilatory support can be accomplished invasively or noninvasively. Invasive mechanical ventilation is still widely used in most hospitals for supporting ventilation, although noninvasive technologies, which do not require the use of an artificial airway, are becoming more popular. To provide invasive positive-pressure ventilation, intubation of the trachea is required via an ET tube or tracheostomy tube. The ventilator is then connected to the artificial airway with a tubing circuit to maintain a closed delivery system (Figure 5-17). During the inspiratory cycle, gas from the ventilator is usually directed through a heated humidifier or a heat and moisture exchanger (HME) prior to entering the lungs through the ET tube or tracheostomy tube. Contraindications to HME use are listed in Table 5-9. At the completion of inspiration,

gas is passively exhaled through the expiratory side of the tubing circuit.

Ventilator Tubing Circuit

The humidifier located on the inspiratory side of the circuit is necessary to overcome two primary problems. First, the presence of an artificial airway allows gas entering the lungs to bypass the normal upper airway humidification process. Second, the higher flows and larger volumes typically administered during mechanical ventilation require additional humidification to avoid excessive intrapulmonary membrane drying.

Pressure within the ventilator tubing circuit is continuously monitored to alert clinicians to excessively high or low airway pressures. Airway pressure is dynamically displayed on the front of the ventilator control panel.

Traditionally, ventilator circuits have incorporated special water collection cups in the tubing to prevent the condensation from humidified gas from obstructing the tubing. Recently, however, it has become common to use ventilator

TABLE 5-9. CONTRAINDICATIONS TO USE OF HEATED MOISTURE EXCHANGER (HME)

1. Frank bloody or thick, copious secretions
2. Patients with large bronchopleural fistulas
3. Uncuffed or malfunctioning ET tube cuffs
4. During lung protective strategies such as patients with ARDS
5. Patients with body temperature < 32 degree Celsius

Data from: American Association for Respiratory Care. AARC clinical practice guideline: humidification during invasive and noninvasive mechanical ventilation: 2012. RespCare. 2012;57:782-788.

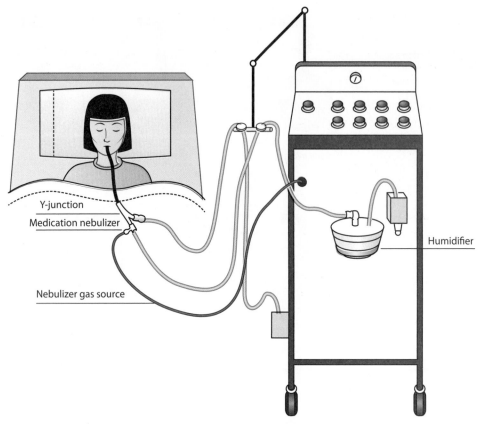

Figure 5-17. Typical setup of a ventilator, closed system tubing circuit, and humidifier connected to an ET tube.

circuits containing heated wires that run through the inspiratory and expiratory limbs of the circuit. These wires maintain the temperature of the gas at or close to body temperature, significantly reducing the condensation and rainout of humidity in the gas, eliminating the need for in-line water traps. Certain medications, such as bronchodilators or steroids, can also be administered via metered dose inhaler (MDI) or nebulized into the lungs through a low volume aerosol-generating device located in the inspiratory side of the circuit.

The ventilator tubing circuit is maintained as a closed circuit as much as possible to avoid interrupting ventilation and oxygenation to the patient, as well as to decrease the potential for VAP. Avoiding frequent or routine changes of the ventilator circuit also decreases the risk of VAP (see Chapter 10, Respiratory System).

Ventilator Control Panel

The user interface or control panel of the ventilator usually incorporates three basic sections or areas: (1) control settings for the type and amount of ventilation and oxygen delivery, (2) alarm settings to specify desired high and low limits for key ventilatory measurements, and (3) visual displays of monitored parameters (Figure 5-18). The number and configuration of these controls and displays vary from ventilator model to model, but their function and principles remain essentially the same.

Control Settings

The control settings area of the user interface allows the clinician to set the mode of ventilation, volume, pressure, respiratory rate, FiO_2, PEEP level, inspiratory trigger sensitivity

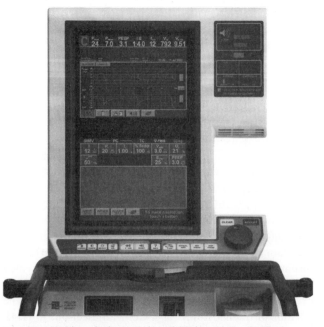

Figure 5-18. Ventilator display control panel. (*With permission, Covidien.*)

TABLE 5-10. TRADITIONAL VENTILATOR ALARMS

Disconnect Alarms (Low-Pressure or Low-Volume Alarms)
- It is essential that when disconnection occurs, the clinician be immediately notified. Generally, this alarm is a continuous one and is triggered when a preselected inspiratory pressure level or minute ventilation is not sensed. With circuit leaks, this same alarm may be activated even though the patient may still be receiving a portion of the preset breath. Physical assessment, digital displays, and manometers are helpful in troubleshooting the cause of the alarms.

Pressure Alarms
- *High-pressure alarms* are set with volume modes of ventilation to ensure notification of pressures exceeding the selected threshold. These alarms are usually set 10-15 cm H_2O above the usual peak inspiratory pressure (PIP). Some causes for alarm activation (generally an intermittent alarm) include secretions, condensate in the tubing, biting on the endotracheal tubing, increased resistance (ie, bronchospasm), decreased compliance (eg, pulmonary edema, pneumothorax), and tubing compression.
- *Low-pressure alarms* are used to sense disconnection, circuit leaks, and changing compliance and resistance. They are generally set 5-10 cm H_2O below the usual PIP or 1-2 cm H_2O below the PEEP level or both.
- *Minute ventilation alarms* may be used to sense disconnection or changes in breathing pattern (rate and volume). Generally, low-minute ventilation and high-minute ventilation alarms are set (usually 5-10 L/min above and below usual minute ventilation). When stand-alone pressure support ventilation (PSV) is in use, this alarm may be the only audible alarm available on some ventilators.
- *Fio_2 alarms*. Most new ventilators provide Fio_2 above and below the selected Fio_2 alarms are generally set 5% above the selected Fio_2.
- *Alarm silence or pause*. Because it is essential that alarms stay activated at all times, ventilator manufacturers have built-in silence or pause options so that clinicians can temporarily silence alarms for short periods (ie, 20 seconds). The ventilators "reset" the alarms automatically. Alarms provide important protection for ventilated patients. However, inappropriate threshold settings decrease usefulness. When threshold gradients are set too narrowly, alarms occur needlessly and frequently. Conversely, alarms that are set too loosely (wide gradients) do not allow for accurate and timely assessments.

Originally written and taken from: Burns SM. Mechanical ventilation and weaning. In: Kinney MR, et al, eds. AACN Clinical Reference for Critical Care Nursing. 4th ed. St Louis, MO: CV Mosby; 1998.

or effort, and a variety of other breath delivery options (eg, inspiratory flow rate, inspiratory waveform pattern).

Alarm Settings

Alarms, which continuously monitor ventilator function, are essential to ensure safe and effective mechanical ventilation. Both high and low alarms are typically set to identify when critical parameters vary from the desired levels. Common alarms include exhaled V_t, exhaled minute volume, Fio_2 delivery, respiratory rate, and airway pressures (Table 5-10).

Visual Displays

Airway pressures, respiratory rate, exhaled volumes, and the inspiratory to expiratory (I:E) ratio are among the most common visually displayed breath-to-breath values on the ventilator. Airway pressures are monitored during inspiration and exhalation and are often displayed as peak pressure, mean pressure, and end-expiratory pressure. A breath delivered by the ventilator produces higher airway pressures than an unassisted, spontaneous breath by the patient (Figure 5-19). The presence of PEEP is identified by a positive value at the end of expiration rather than 0 cm H_2O. Careful observation of the airway pressures provides the clinician with a great deal of information about the patient's respiratory effort, coordination with the ventilator, and changes in lung compliance.

The display of the patient's exhaled V_t reflects the amount of gas that is returned to the ventilator via the expiratory tubing with each respiratory cycle. Exhaled volumes are measured and displayed with each breath. The patient's

total exhaled minute volume is also often displayed. Exhaled V_ts for ventilator-assisted mandatory breaths should be similar (± 10%) to the desired V_t setting selected on the control panel. The V_t of spontaneous breaths, or partially ventilator-supported breaths, however, may be different from the V_t control setting.

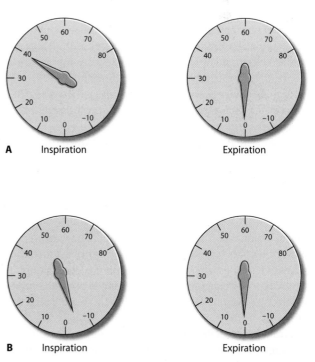

Figure 5-19. Typical airway pressure gauge changes during **(A)** ventilator-assisted breath and **(B)** spontaneous breath (cm H_2O).

Modes

The *mode* of ventilation refers to one of several different methods that a ventilator uses to support ventilation. Modes are often classified as invasive (via an ET tube or tracheostomy tube) or noninvasive (via a face or nasal interface). These modes generate different levels of airway pressures, volumes, and patterns of respiration and, therefore, different levels of support. The greater the level of ventilator support, the less muscle work performed by the patient. This "work of breathing" varies considerably with each of the modes of ventilation and is discussed later in this chapter in the section on respiratory muscle fatigue.

The different modes of ventilation used to support ventilation depend on the underlying respiratory problem and clinical preferences. A brief description of the basic invasive and noninvasive modes of mechanical ventilation follows.

Control Ventilation

The control mode of ventilation ensures that patients receive a predetermined number and volume of breaths each minute. No deviations from the respiratory rate or V_t settings are delivered with this mode of ventilation. Generally the patient is heavily sedated and/or paralyzed with neuromuscular blocking agents in the ICU to achieve the goal; however, in the progressive care setting the use of these agents is unlikely. Instead the "control" mode might be used in the patient who is paralyzed from a spinal cord injury or has a neuromuscular condition that precludes spontaneous breathing, or in the operating room.

Assist-Control Ventilation

The assist-control mode of ventilation ensures that a predetermined number and volume of breaths is delivered by the ventilator each minute should the patient not initiate respirations at that rate or above. If the patient attempts to initiate breaths at a rate greater than the set minimum value, the ventilator delivers the spontaneously initiated breaths at the prescribed V_t; the patient may determine the total rate. Work of breathing with this mode is variable.

Assist-control ventilation is often used when the patient is initially intubated (because minute ventilation requirements can be determined by the patient), for short-term ventilatory support such as postanesthesia, and as a support mode when high levels of ventilatory support are required. Excessive ventilation can occur with this mode in situations where the patient's spontaneous respiratory rate increases for nonrespiratory reasons (eg, pain, CNS dysfunction). The increased minute volume may result in potentially dangerous respiratory alkalosis. Changing to a different mode of ventilation or employing sedation may be necessary in these situations.

Synchronized Intermittent Mandatory Ventilation

The synchronized intermittent mandatory ventilation (SIMV) mode of ventilation ensures (or mandates) that a predetermined number of breaths at a selected V_t are delivered each minute. Any additional breaths initiated by the patient are allowed but, in contrast to the assist-control mode, these breaths are not delivered by the ventilator. The patient is allowed to spontaneously breathe at the depth and rate desired until it is time for the next ventilator-assisted, or mandatory, breath. Mandatory breaths are synchronized with the patient's inspiratory effort, if present, to optimize patient-ventilator synchrony. The spontaneous breaths taken during SIMV are at the same FiO_2 as the mandatory breaths.

Originally designated as a ventilator mode for the gradual weaning of patients from mechanical ventilation, the use of a high-rate setting of SIMV can provide total ventilatory support. Reduction of the number of mandatory breaths allows the patient to slowly resume greater and greater responsibility for spontaneous breathing. SIMV can be used for similar indications as the assist-control mode, as well as for weaning the patient from mechanical ventilatory support. It is common to add pressure support to SIMV as a means of decreasing the work of breathing associated with spontaneous breathing.

The work of breathing with this mode of ventilation depends on the V_t and rate of the spontaneous breaths. When the mandatory, intermittent breaths provide the majority of minute volume, the work of breathing by the patient may be less than when spontaneous breathing constitutes a larger proportion of the patient's total minute volume.

Although strong clinician and institutional biases exist regarding whether to use SIMV or other modes for ventilatory support, little data exist to clarify which mode of ventilation is best. Close observation of the physiologic and psychological response to the ventilatory mode is required, and consideration is given to trials on alternative modes if warranted.

Spontaneous Breathing

Many ventilators have a mode that allows the patient to breathe spontaneously without ventilator. This is similar to placing the patient on a T-piece or blow-by oxygen setup, except it does have the benefit of providing continuous monitoring of exhaled volumes, airway pressures, and other parameters along with a closed circuit. All the work of breathing is performed by the patient during spontaneous breathing. Use of the ventilator rather than the T-piece during spontaneous breathing actually may slightly increase the work of breathing. This occurs because of the additional inspiratory muscle work that is required to trigger flow delivery for each spontaneous breath. The amount of additional work required varies with different ventilator models.

This mode of ventilation is often identified as continuous positive airway pressure (CPAP), flow-by, or spontaneous (SPONT) on the ventilator. Continuous positive airway pressure (CPAP) is a spontaneous breathing setting with the addition of PEEP during the breathing cycle.

Some ventilators have an additional adjunct that compensates for the resistance secondary to ET tube diameter. It is also called automatic tube compensation (ATC). ATC can be used with ventilatory support or alone with spontaneous breathing.

Pressure Support

Pressure support (PS) is a spontaneous breathing mode, available in SIMV and SPONT modes, which maintain a set positive pressure during the spontaneous inspiration. The volume of a gas delivered by the ventilator during each inspiration varies depending on the level of pressure support and the demand of the patient. The higher the pressure support level, the higher the amount of gas delivered with each breath. Higher levels of pressure support can augment the spontaneous V_t and decrease the work of breathing associated with spontaneous breathing. At low levels of support, it is primarily used to overcome the airway resistance caused by breathing through the artificial airway and the breathing circuit. The airway pressure achieved during a pressure support breath is the result of the pressure support setting plus the set PEEP level.

Positive End-Expiratory Pressure/Continuous Positive Airway Pressure

Positive end-expiratory pressure is used in conjunction with any of the ventilator modes to help stabilize alveolar lung volume and improve oxygenation. The application of positive pressure to the airways during expiration may keep alveoli open and prevent early closure during exhalation. Lung compliance and ventilation-perfusion matching are often improved by prevention of early alveolar closure. If alveolar recruitment is not needed and excessive PEEP/CPAP is applied, it may result in adverse hemodynamic (ie, hypotension) or respiratory compromise (ie, auto-PEEP) and lung trauma (ie, barotrauma).

Positive end-expiratory pressure/CPAP is indicated for hypoxemia, which is secondary to diffuse lung injury (eg, ARDS, interstitial pneumonitis). PEEP/CPAP levels of 5 cm Hg or less are often used to provide "physiologic PEEP." The presence of the artificial airway allows intrathoracic pressure to fall to zero, which is below the usual level of intrathoracic pressure at end expiration (2 or 3 cm H_2O).

Use of PEEP may increase the risk of barotrauma due to higher mean and peak airway pressures during ventilation, especially when peak pressures are greater than 40 cm H_2O. Venous return and CO may also be affected by these high pressures. If CO decreases with PEEP/CPAP initiation and oxygenation is improved, a fluid bolus may correct hypovolemia. Other complications from PEEP/CPAP increases in intracranial pressure, decreased renal perfusion, hepatic congestion, and worsening of intracardiac shunts.

Bilevel Positive Airway Pressure

Bilevel positive airway pressure (ie, BiPAP) is a noninvasive mode of ventilation that combines two levels of positive pressure (PSV and PEEP) by means of a full face mask, nasal mask (most common), or nasal pillows. The ventilator is designed to compensate for leaks in the set-up, and a snug fit is needed, often requiring head or chin straps. This form

of therapy can be very labor intensive, requiring frequent assessment of patient tolerance. Full face mask ventilation is cautiously used because the potential for aspiration is high. If full face mask ventilation is chosen, the patient should be able to remove the mask quickly if nausea occurs or vomiting is imminent. Obtunded patients and those with excessive secretions are not good choices for BiPAP ventilation.

A number of options are available with BiPAP and include a spontaneous mode where the patient initiates all the pressure-supported breaths; a spontaneous-timed option, similar to PSV with a backup rate (some vendors call this A/C); and a control mode. The control mode requires the selection of a control rate and inspiratory time.

Bilevel positive airway pressure is used successfully in a wide variety of progressive care patients such as those with sleep apnea, some patients with chronic hypoventilation syndromes, and also to prevent intubation and reintubation following extubation. Use of BiPAP in patients with COPD and heart failure has been associated with decreased mortality and need for intubation. These patients are often difficult to wean from conventional ventilation given their underlying disease processes. Study results also demonstrate that outcomes in immunocompromised patients may also be better with noninvasive ventilation.

Complications of Mechanical Ventilation

Significant complications can arise from the use of any form of mechanical ventilation and can be categorized as those associated with the patient's response to mechanical ventilation or those arising from ventilator malfunctions. Although the approach to minimizing or treating the complications of mechanical ventilation relate to the underlying cause, it is critical that frequent assessment of the patient, ventilator equipment, and the patient's response to ventilatory management be accomplished. Many clinicians participate in activities to assess the patient and ventilator, but the ultimate responsibility for ensuring continuous ventilatory support of the patient falls to the progressive care team including the bedside nurse and the respiratory therapist. Critically evaluating clinical indicators such as pH, $Paco_2$, Pao_2, Spo_2, heart rate, BP, and so on, in conjunction with patient status and ventilatory parameters, is essential to decrease complications associated with this highly complex technology.

Patient Response
Hemodynamic Compromise

Normal intrathoracic pressure changes during spontaneous breathing are negative throughout the ventilatory cycle. Intrapleural pressure varies from about +5 cm H_2O during exhalation to –8 cm H_2O during inhalation. This decrease in intrapleural pressure during inhalation facilitates lung inflation and venous return. Thoracic pressure fluctuation during positive-pressure ventilation is opposite to those that occur during spontaneous breathing. The mean intrathoracic pressure is usually positive and increases during inhalation and decreases during exhalation. The use of positive pressure ventilation increases peak airway pressures during inspiration which in turn, increases mean airway pressures. It is this increase in mean airway pressure which may impede venous return to the right atrium, thus decreasing CO. In some patients, this decrease in CO can be clinically significant, leading to increased heart rate and decreased blood pressure and perfusion to vital organs.

Whenever mechanical ventilation is instituted, or when ventilator changes are made, it is important to assess the patient's cardiovascular response. Approaches to managing hemodynamic compromise include increasing the preload of the heart (eg, fluid administration), decreasing the airway pressures exerted during mechanical ventilation by ensuring appropriate airway management techniques (suctioning, positioning, etc), and by judiciously setting ventilator parameters.

Barotrauma and Volutrauma

Barotrauma describes damage to the pulmonary system due to alveolar rupture from excessive airway pressures or overdistention of alveoli. Alveolar gas enters the interstitial pulmonary structures causing pneumothorax, pneumomediastinum, pneumoperitoneum, or subcutaneous emphysema. The potential for pneumothorax and cardiovascular collapse requires prompt management of pneumothorax and should be considered whenever airway pressure rises acutely, breath sounds are diminished unilaterally, or blood pressure falls abruptly.

Patients with obstructive airway diseases (eg, asthma, bronchospasm), unevenly distributed lung disease (eg, lobar pneumonia), or hyperinflated lungs (eg, emphysema) are at high risk for barotrauma. Techniques to decrease the incidence of barotrauma include the use of small V_ts, cautious use of PEEP, and the avoidance of high airway pressures and development of auto-PEEP in high-risk patients.

Volutrauma describes alveolar damage that results from high pressures resulting from large-volume ventilation in patients with ARDS. A common technique to reduce this risk is the use of smaller V_ts (4-6 ml/kg of ideal body weight) and sometimes this is described as the "low stretch" protocol. Different from barotrauma, this damage results in alveolar fractures and flooding of alveoli (non-ARDS, ARDS). It is linked to the use of V_ts greater than 6 mL/kg in patients with ARDS.

Auto-PEEP occurs when a delivered breath is incompletely exhaled before the onset of the next inspiration. This gas trapping increases overall lung volumes, inadvertently raising the end-expiratory pressure in the alveoli. The presence of auto-PEEP increases the risk for complications from PEEP. Ventilator patients with COPD (eg, asthma, emphysema) or high respiratory rates are at increased risk for the development of auto-PEEP.

Auto-PEEP, also termed intrinsic PEEP, is difficult to diagnose because it cannot be observed on the airway pressure display at end expiration. The technique for assessment for auto-PEEP varies with different ventilatory models and modes, but typically involves measuring the airway pressure close to the artificial airway during occlusion of the expiratory ventilator circuit during end expiration. This method requires that the patient be completely passive and not trigger a breath; it is not possible to measure auto-PEEP in actively breathing patients. Another technique of monitoring auto-PEEP in actively breathing patients is the use of the flow-time curve displayed by the ventilator. If flow does not return to baseline at the end of exhalation before the next breath starts, the patient has auto-PEEP. Auto-PEEP can be minimized by:

- Maximizing the length of time for expiration (eg, increasing inspiratory flow rates)
- Decreasing obstructions to expiratory flow (eg, using larger diameter ET tubes, eliminating bronchospasm and secretions)
- Avoiding overventilation

Ventilator-Associated Pneumonia

Ventilator-associated pneumonia (VAP) is a hospital-acquired complication, and is associated with increased patient morbidity and mortality. Prevention is aimed at avoiding colonization and subsequent aspiration of bacteria into the lower airway. Elevation of the head of the bed (> 30º) and avoiding excessive gastric distention are thought to help minimize the occurrence of aspiration. A specially designed ET tube (Figure 5-20) incorporates a dedicated suction lumen over the ET cuff, which permits continuous or intermittent suctioning of subglottic secretions pooled above the cuff. Removal of the accumulated secretions may be particularly helpful before cuff deflation or manipulation.

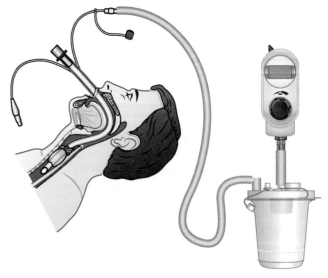

Figure 5-20. Cuffed endotracheal tube with dedicated lumen for continuous aspiration of subglottic secretions accumulated immediately above cuff. The dedicated lumen connector is attached to wall suction. (*With permission, Covidien.*)

Studies have demonstrated that the application of continuous aspiration of subglottic secretions with ET tubes only may prevent or delay the onset of VAP. Although subglottic suctioning is now available in tracheostomy tubes, there are currently no recommendations for the use of subglottic suctioning in these tubes. In addition, recent research suggests that oral care protocols including chlorhexidine gluconate 0.12% mouth rinse and tooth brushing to removal plague may be important adjuncts in VAP prevention.

Positive Fluid Balance and Hyponatremia

Hyponatremia is a common occurrence following the institution of mechanical ventilation and develops from several factors, including applied PEEP, humidification of inspired gases, hypotonic fluid administration and diuretics, and increased levels of circulating antidiuretic hormone.

Upper Gastrointestinal Hemorrhage

Upper gastrointestinal (GI) bleeding may develop secondary to ulceration or gastritis. The prevention of stress ulcer bleeding requires ensuring hemodynamic stability and the administration of proton-pump inhibitors, H_2 receptor antagonists, antacids, or cytoprotective agents as appropriate (see Chapter 7, Pharmacology and Chapter 14, Gastrointestinal System, for discussions of GI prophylaxis).

Ventilator Malfunction

Problems related to the proper functioning of mechanical ventilators, although rare, may have devastating consequences for patients. Many of the alarm systems on ventilators are designed to alert clinicians to improperly functioning ventilatory systems. These alarm systems must be activated at all times if ventilator malfunction problems are to be quickly identified and corrected, and untoward patient events avoided (see Table 5-10).

Many of the "problems" identified with ventilatory equipment are actually related to inappropriate setup or use of the devices. Ventilator circuits that are not properly connected, alarm systems that are set improperly, or inadequate ventilator settings for a particular clinical condition are examples of some of these operator-related occurrences.

There are occasions, however, when ventilator systems do not operate properly. Examples of ventilator malfunctions include valve mechanisms sticking and obstructing gas flow, inadequate or excessive gas delivery, electronic circuit failures in microprocessing-based ventilators, failures with complete shutdown, and power failures or surges in the institution.

The most important approach to ventilator malfunction is to maintain a high level of vigilance to determine if ventilators are performing properly. Ensuring that alarm systems are set appropriately at all times, providing frequent routine assessment of ventilator functioning, and the use of experienced support personnel to maintain the ventilator systems are some of the most crucial activities necessary to avoid patient problems. In addition, whenever ventilator malfunction is suspected, the patient should be immediately removed from the device and temporary ventilation and oxygenation provided with an MRB or another ventilator until the question of proper functioning is resolved. Any sudden change in the patient's respiratory or cardiovascular status alerts the clinician to consider potential ventilator malfunction as a cause.

Weaning From Short-Term Mechanical Ventilation

The process of transitioning the ventilator-dependent patient to unassisted spontaneous breathing is called *weaning from mechanical ventilation*. This is a period of time where the requirement for oxygenation and ventilation is decreased, either gradually or abruptly, while monitoring the patient's response to the resumption of spontaneous breathing. A standardized approach along with weaning readiness criteria has been shown to reduce ventilator days and improve outcomes. Weaning or "liberation" is considered to be complete, or successful, when the patient has been extubated successfully without the need for reintubation within 48 hours. Often, removal of the artificial airway occurs before that time if clinicians are optimistic that the patient's respiratory status will not deteriorate. The majority of patients intubated and ventilated for short periods of time (< 72 hours) are successfully weaned with the first spontaneous breathing trial (SBT) in the ICU. Additionally, there is a subset of patients with long-term tracheostomy tubes who may require short-term ventilation who are able to wean quickly once the clinical issue requiring mechanical ventilation is resolved. Approximately 30% of patients, however, require extended time periods to successfully complete the weaning process, with some being unable to breathe without partial or complete mechanical ventilation.

Weaning proceeds when the underlying pulmonary disorder that led to mechanical ventilation has sufficiently resolved, and the patient is alert and able to protect the airway. Unnecessary delays in weaning from mechanical ventilation increase the likelihood of complications such as ventilator-induced lung injury, pneumonia, discomfort, and increases in hospitalization costs. Thus, aggressive and timely weaning trials such as SBT are encouraged.

Steps in the Weaning Process
Assessment of Readiness

Readiness to wean from short-term mechanical ventilation (STMV) may be assessed with a wide variety of criteria. However, in most institutions, assessment of readiness to wean includes just three or four criteria for most short-term ventilator patients. Along with assessing the patient's clinical stability, some examples are:

- ABGs within normal limits on minimal to moderate amounts of ventilatory support ($Fio_2 \leq 0.50$, minute ventilation # 10 L/min, PEEP ≤ 5 cm H_2O)

ESSENTIAL CONTENT CASE

Long-Term Weaning

A 75-year-old man with COPD and oxygen dependence was admitted to the ED in respiratory distress. He was intubated and placed on the ventilator secondary to profound hypercarbia and acidosis and then transferred to the MICU for management of respiratory failure and right upper lobe pneumonia. He was anticipated to need long-term weaning and received a tracheostomy tube on day 4 to increase his comfort and so that he could be mobilized.

After 7 days of treatment with mechanical ventilation, the patient was transferred to the respiratory stepdown unit for further management and weaning. Major impediments to weaning as assessed by the unit team included factors such as:

- Poor nutritional status (albumin < 1.8 g/dL)
- Anxiety and agitation
- Debilitation and inability to ambulate
- Persistent upper lobe infiltrate
- Copious secretions
- NIP < 15 cm H_2O
- Minute ventilation > 15 L/min with a $Paco_2$ of 50 mm Hg

The team recognized that these factors contributed to his high work of breathing (secretions, respiratory rate, minute ventilation) and his overall weak and debilitated state (nutrition, immobility, NIP). They acknowledged that these factors must be addressed before active weaning could successfully occur. It was likely that prolonged ventilation would be necessary. After 2 days of "complete rest," a ventilatory mode was selected that would allow for gradual respiratory muscle conditioning while overall improvement in physical status occurred. PSV was selected at PSV max (which in this case was 20 cm H_2O). This setting resulted in a respiratory rate of 16 breaths/min, a tidal volume of 8 mL/kg, and an eupneic respiratory pattern. PSV max was used for rest during the day and at night. For gradual conditioning trials, the PSV level was decreased in increments of 5 cm H_2O as defined by the PSV protocol.

Case Question 1. What other weaning modality could have been used in this patient and why?

Case Question 2. What components of the ABCDE protocol were used for this patient?

Answers
1. As the research has not demonstrated any mode or method to be superior for a patient weaning with a tracheostomy, progressively longer spontaneous breathing trials may be used effectively. The modes can vary and include using a t-piece, trach collar, or low levels of PSV with intermittent rest periods on the ventilator (with support settings such as AC or a higher level of PSV). When the patient is able to sustain spontaneous breathing for a full 12 hours during the day, the nighttime ventilator support (at the "rest" level) may then be reduced, or if clinically appropriate, curtailed. The next steps would be to work on removal of the tracheostomy tube following downsizing and or use of a talking trach to determine tolerance. This stepwise approach allows the patient to gradually transition to liberation from the ventilator.
2. The patient received daily spontaneous awakening and assessment for readiness to wean (ABC). His delirium

assessment for readiness to wean (ABC). His delirium was addressed by using a modified sleep protocol and by using the family to reorient the patient as well as encouraging the use of personal items when possible (D). Early exercise was implemented in the ICU and continued after transfer and integrated into his daily routine (E).

Three days later, the patient was sitting in a chair at the bedside and beginning to ambulate with the help of the nurse and physical therapist. Enteral nutrition was provided via a small bore silastic nasal gastric tube. Serial BWAP assessments demonstrated improvement (47%-55%) but it was recognized that his recovery would likely take weeks. It took him 2 more weeks to finally reach a PSV of 5 (the lowest level of the plan), and it was at that time that the team initiated tracheostomy collar trials. Night rest was continued until the patient could tolerate 12 hours without signs of intolerance. He was decannulated and sent home with his family 1 week later.

- Negative inspiratory pressure that is more negative than −20 cm H_2O
- Spontaneous $V_t \geq$ mL/kg
- Vital capacity ≥10 mL/kg
- Respiratory rate < 30 breaths/min
- Spontaneous rapid-shallow breathing index < 105 breaths/min/liter

Following selection of the method for weaning (see the discussion below), the actual weaning trial can begin. It is important to prepare both the patient and the progressive care environment properly to maximize the chances for weaning success. Interventions include appropriate explanations of the process to the patient, positioning and medication to improve ventilatory efforts, and the avoidance of unnecessary activities during the weaning trial. Throughout the weaning time, continuous monitoring for signs and symptoms of respiratory distress or fatigue is essential. They include dyspnea, tachypnea, chest abdominal dyssynchrony, anxiety, tachycardia, changes in blood pressure, and changes in oxygenation or ventilation. Many of these indicators are subtle, but careful monitoring of baseline levels before weaning progresses and throughout the trial provides objective indicators of the need to return the patient to previous levels of ventilator support.

The need to temporarily stop the weaning trial is not viewed as, or termed, a failure. Instead it simply suggests that more time needs to be provided to ensure success. A full evaluation of the multiple reasons for inability to wean is necessary, however.

Weaning Trials

Generally, weaning trials for patients' ventilated short term in the ICU are accomplished with SBT on T-piece or on the ventilator using CPAP or a low level of pressure support. Readiness for weaning is assessed daily using a "safety screen" which includes such factors as hemodynamic stability, oxygenation status, and improvement in the condition that necessitated the use of mechanical ventilation. Once the patient is assessed as "ready" the spontaneous breathing trial is initiated for a duration of at least 30 minutes but no more than 120 minutes. The trial is stopped should the patient show signs of distress and/or deterioration. A decision to extubate is made with the conclusion of a successful trial. The need for reintubation is associated with increased mortality. Thus, premature attempts at extubation are to be avoided. Some suggest that noninvasive positive-pressure ventilation via face or nasal mask may be useful for patients with respiratory failure following extubation. However, research has demonstrated that this therapy does not prevent the need for reintubation or reduce mortality in these cases.

Methods

A variety of methods are available for weaning patients from mechanical ventilation. To date, research on these techniques has not clearly identified any one method as optimal for weaning from short-term mechanical ventilation. Most institutions, however, use one or two approaches routinely. A number of recently published randomized controlled trials demonstrated that the outcomes of patients managed with protocols driven by nonphysician clinicians were better than those managed with standard physician-directed care. Most experts on weaning believe that, with short-term ventilator-dependent patients, the actual method used to wean the patient is less important to weaning success than using a consistently applied protocol strategy.

- *T-piece, blow-by, or trach collar:* The T-piece method of weaning involves removing the patient from the mechanical ventilator and attaching an oxygen source to the artificial airway with a "T" piece for a SBT. A trach collar also provides oxygen but attaches by elastic strap around the neck instead of directly to the artificial airway. No ventilatory support occurs with this device, with the patient completely breathing spontaneously the entire time this device is connected. The advantage of this method of weaning is that the resistance to breathing is low, because no special valves need to be opened to initiate gas flow. Rapid assessment of the patient's ability to spontaneously breathe is another purported advantage. Limitations of this SBT are that it may cause ventilatory muscle overload and fatigue. When this occurs, it usually appears early in the SBT, so the patient must be closely monitored during the initial few minutes. A PEEP valve can be added to the T piece; however, similar to trach collar weaning, there are no alarm or backup systems to support the patient should ventilation be inadequate. It is critical to recognize that this technique relies on the clinician to monitor for signs and symptoms of respiratory difficulty and fatigue. Frequently, the Fio_2 is increased by at least 10% over the Fio_2 setting on the ventilator to prevent hypoxemia resulting from the lower Vt of spontaneous breaths. Patients who fail a SBT should receive a stable, nonfatiguing, comfortable form of ventilatory support for rest following the trial.

- *CPAP:* The use of the ventilator to allow spontaneous breathing periods without mandated breaths, similar to the T-piece, can be done with the CPAP mode. With this approach, ventilator alarm systems can be used to monitor spontaneous breathing rates and volumes, and a small amount of continuous pressure (5 cm H_2O) can be applied if needed. The disadvantage of this approach is that the work of breathing resulting from the need to open the demand valve to receive gas flow for the breath is higher than with the T-piece. For most patients, this slight additional work of breathing is not likely to be a critical factor to their weaning success or failure unless the trial is unduly long. If needed, a low level of pressure support (eg, 5-7 cm H_2O) may also be added to offset this workload (CPAP + PS).

- *Pressure support:* Another method for weaning from ventilation is the use of low level PS ventilation. With this method, patients can spontaneously breathe on the ventilator with a small amount of ventilator *support* to augment their spontaneous breaths. This technique overcomes some of the resistance to breathing associated with ET tubes and demand valves. The main disadvantage with this approach is that clinicians may underestimate the degree of support to spontaneous breathing provided with this method and prematurely stop the weaning process.

- *SIMV:* One of the most popular methods of weaning patients in the past, this modality has recently been shown to prolong the duration of mechanical ventilation in comparison to weaning with SBT or pressure support using the SIMV mode. By progressively decreasing the number of mandated breaths delivered by the ventilator, the patient performs more and more of the work of breathing by increasing spontaneous breathing. Advantages to the SIMV mode are the presence of built-in alarms to alert clinicians when ventilation problems occur and, in some modes, the guarantee of a minimum amount of minute ventilation. The disadvantage of SIMV is that each spontaneous breath requires some additional work of breathing to open a valve, which allows gas flow to the patient for the spontaneous breath. SIMV is used either alone or in conjunction with pressure support (SIMV + PS).

Weaning From Long-Term Mechanical Ventilation

In contrast to patients who require short-term (< 3 days) ventilation, those that require long-term mechanical ventilation (defined as > 3 days), may take weeks or even months to liberate from the ventilator. In these long-term mechanically ventilated (LTMV) patients, the weaning process varies and consists of four stages. The first stage is marked by instability and high ventilatory support requirements. During the second stage, called the prewean stage, many physiologic factors continue to require attention, and the patient's overall status may fluctuate. Ventilatory requirements are less and adjustments are made to maintain oxygenation and acid-base status as well as provide ventilatory muscle conditioning. The third, or weaning stage, is evident when the patient is stable, and rapid progress with weaning trials is possible. Finally, the last stage is called the outcome stage, which consists of extubation, partial or full ventilatory support.

Long-term mechanical ventilation is associated with high morbidity and mortality rates, and institutions lose money on patients ventilated long-term because reimbursement rarely covers the associated costs. As a result, clinicians, scientists, and institutions are interested in testing methods of care delivery that improve the clinical and financial outcomes of the patients. Research in the area of weaning offers guidance to clinicians working with these patients. The following discussions of weaning patients from LTMV address wean assessment, wean planning, and weaning modes and methods, including comprehensive institutional approaches.

Wean Assessment

Traditionally, the decision about when to begin the weaning process is determined once the condition that necessitates mechanical ventilation is improved or resolved. During this prewean stage, other factors that contribute to wean ability are considered prior to attempting weaning trials. In the past, "traditional" weaning predictors were used in an attempt to determine the optimal timing for extubation. More recently, investigators combined pulmonary elements to improve predictive ability in LTMV patients. An example is the index of rapid shallow breathing, also known as the frequency (f_X)/tidal volume (V_t) index, which integrates rate and tidal volume. Unfortunately, predictors have not predicted weanability. This is in part because they focus exclusively on pulmonary specific components to the exclusion of other important nonpulmonary factors (Table 5-11). Although the standard weaning criteria are not predictive, the components are helpful for assessing the patient's overall condition and readiness for weaning.

As noted, assessment of weaning potential starts with an evaluation of the underlying reason for mechanical

ventilation (sepsis, pneumonia, trauma, and the like). Resolution of the underlying cause is necessary before gains in the weaning process can be expected. However, it is important to remember that resolution alone is frequently not sufficient to ensure successful weaning. Patients who require prolonged mechanical ventilation, sometimes referred to as the "chronically, critically ill," often suffer from a myriad of conditions that impede weaning. Even with resolution of the disease or condition that necessitated mechanical ventilation, the patient's overall status is often below baseline (weak, malnourished, etc). Therefore, a systematic, comprehensive approach to weaning assessment is important. One example of a tool that encourages such an approach is the Burns Wean Assessment Program (BWAP) (Table 5-12). The BWAP score is used to track the progress of the patient and keep care planning on target. Factors important to weaning are listed in the BWAP bedside checklist.

Wean Planning

Once impediments to weaning are identified, plans that focus on improving the impediments are made in collaboration with a multidisciplinary team. A collaborative approach to assessment and planning greatly enhances positive outcomes in the LTMV patient. However, for care planning to be successful, it must also be systematic. The wean process is dynamic and regular reassessment and adjustment of plans are necessary. Tools like the BWAP can be used to systematically assess and track weaning progress. Other methods that have demonstrated efficacy in assuring consistency in care management and good outcomes for the patients include care delivery models using clinical pathways, protocols for weaning, and institution-wide approaches to managing and monitoring the patients.

Weaning Trials, Modes, and Methods

A wide variety of weaning modes and methods are available for weaning the patient ventilated short term as described earlier. To date, no data support the superiority of any one mode for weaning those requiring LTMV, however, methods using protocols and other systematic, multidisciplinary approaches do appear to make a difference and are to be encouraged. These methods are described following a discussion of respiratory muscle fatigue, rest, and conditioning because the concepts are integrated into the section on protocols.

Respiratory Fatigue, Rest, and Conditioning

Respiratory muscle fatigue is common in ventilated weaning patients and occurs when the respiratory workload is excessive. When the workload exceeds metabolic stores, fatigue and hypercarbic respiratory failure ensue. Examples of those at risk include patients who are hypermetabolic, weak, or malnourished. Signs of encroaching fatigue include dyspnea, tachypnea, chest-abdominal asynchrony, and elevated $PaCO_2$ (a late sign). These signs and symptoms indicate a need for

TABLE 5-11. PULMONARY SPECIFIC WEAN CRITERIA THRESHOLDS

Traditional Weaning Criteria
- Negative inspiratory pressure (NIP) ≤ -20 cm H_2O
- Positive expiratory pressure (PEP) $\geq +30$ cm H_2O
- Spontaneous tidal volume (SV_t) ≥ 5 mL/kg
- Vital capacity (VC) ≥ 15 mL/kg
- Fraction of inspired oxygen (FiO_2) $\leq 50\%$
- Minute ventilation (MV) ≤ 10 L/min

Integrated Weaning Criteria
- Index of rapid shallow breathing or frequency tidal volume ratio (f_X/V_t) ≤ 105

TABLE 5-12. BURNS' WEAN ASSESSMENT PROGRAM (BWAP)[a]

I. General Assessment

Yes	No	Not Assessed	
___	___	___	1. Hemodynamically stable (pulse rate, cardiac output)?
___	___	___	2. Free from factors that increase or decrease metabolic rate (seizures, temperature, sepsis, bacteremia, hypo/hyperthyroid)?
___	___	___	3. Hematocrit > 25% (or baseline)?
___	___	___	4. Systemically hydrated (weight at or near baseline, balanced intake and output)?
___	___	___	5. Nourished (albumin > 2.5, parenteral/enteral feedings maximized)? *If albumin is low and anasarca or third spacing is present, score for hydration should be "no."
___	___	___	6. Electrolytes within normal limits (including Ca^{++}, Mg^+, PO_4)? *Correct Ca^{++} for albumin level.
___	___	___	7. Pain controlled (subjective determination)?
___	___	___	8. Adequate sleep/rest (subjective determination)?
___	___	___	9. Appropriate level of anxiety and nervousness (subjective determination)?
___	___	___	10. Absence of bowel problems (diarrhea, constipation, ileus)?
___	___	___	11. Improved general body strength/endurance (ie, out of bed in chair, progressive activity program)?
___	___	___	12. Chest x-ray improving?

II. Respiratory Assessment

Yes	No	Not Assessed	

Gas Flow and Work of Breathing

___	___	___	13. Eupneic respiratory rate and pattern (spontaneous RR < 25, without dyspnea, absence of accessory muscle use)? *This is assessed off the ventilator while measuring #20-23.
___	___	___	14. Absence of adventitious breath sounds (rhonchi, rales, wheezing)?
___	___	___	15. Secretions thin and minimal?
___	___	___	16. Absence of neuromuscular disease/deformity?
___	___	___	17. Absence of abdominal distention/obesity/ascites?
___	___	___	18. Oral ETT > #7.5 or trach > #6.5?

Airway Clearance

___	___	___	19. Cough and swallow reflexes adequate?

Strength

___	___	___	20. NIP < 20 (negative inspiratory pressure)?
___	___	___	21. PEP > 30 (positive expiratory pressure)?

Endurance

___	___	___	22. STV > 5 mL/kg (spontaneous tidal volume)?
___	___	___	23. VC > 10-15 mL/kg (vital capacity)?

ABGs

___	___	___	24. pH 7.30-7.45?
___	___	___	25. $Paco_2$ 40 mm Hg (or baseline) with mV < 10 L/min? *This is evaluated while on ventilator.
___	___	___	26. Pao_2 60 on Fio_2 < 40%?

[a]*The BWAP score is obtained by dividing the total number of BWAP factors scored as "yes" by 26. © Burns 1990.*

increased ventilatory support. Once fatigued, the muscles require 12 to 24 hours of rest to recover, and careful application of selected modes of ventilation is required.

For the respiratory muscles to recover from fatigue, the inspiratory workload must be decreased. In the case of volume ventilation (eg, assist-control, intermittent mandatory ventilation), this means complete cessation of spontaneous effort, but in the case of pressure ventilation, a high level of PSV may accomplish the necessary "unloading." Generally, this means increasing the PSV level to attain a spontaneous respiratory rate of 20 breaths per minute or less and the absence of accessory muscle activity. However, in patients with obstructive diseases (eg, asthma and COPD), this higher level of support may result in further hyperinflation and adverse clinical outcomes. If the technique is used in these patients, it should be done cautiously.

Respiratory muscle conditioning employs concepts borrowed from exercise physiology. To condition muscles and attain an optimal training effect from exercise, the concepts of endurance and strength conditioning may be considered. With strength training, a large force is moved a short distance. The muscles are worked to fatigue (short duration intervals) and rested for long periods of time. SBTs on T-piece or CPAP both mimic this type of training because they employ high pressure and low-volume work. Endurance conditioning, which requires that the workload be increased gradually, is easily accomplished with PSV because the level of support can be decreased over time. This kind of endurance training employs low pressure and high-volume work. Central to the application of both conditioning methods is the provision of adequate respiratory muscle rest between trials. Prolonging trials once the patient is fatigued serves no useful purpose and may be extremely detrimental physiologically and psychologically.

Wean Trial Protocols

Study results suggest that no mode of ventilation is superior for weaning, however, the method of weaning, specifically the use of protocols, decreases variations in care and improves outcomes. Protocols direct caregivers by clearly delineating the protocol components. The protocol components consist of weaning readiness criteria (wean screens), weaning trial method and duration (ie, CPAP, T-piece, or PSV), and definitions of intolerance and respiratory muscle rest.

Spontaneous breathing trials (described earlier), primarily using CPAP or T-piece, are commonly used for the trials. As noted, the duration of such trials is generally between 30 minutes and 2 hours, although in those with tracheotomy tubes the duration may be much longer. While CPAP or T-piece is often used for trials, in most cases the choice between PSV (an endurance mode) and T-piece or CPAP (strengthening modes) is somewhat arbitrary if the protocol is appropriately aggressive and easily understood and applied by the caregivers. There are some conditions that require more selective decision making. One example is that

TABLE 5-13. GENERAL WEANING GUIDELINES FOR LTMV PATIENTS

Active Weaning Should Occur
- When patient is stable and reason for mechanical ventilation is resolved or improving.
- When the "wean screen protocol criteria" are attained. A temporary hold and even an increase in support may be necessary when setbacks occur.
- During the daytime, not at night (to allow respiratory muscle rest).

Considerations for Temporary Hold
- With acute changes in condition
- During procedures that require that the patient be flat or in the Trendelenburg position (ie, during line insertion)
- During "road trips" (increased ventilatory support will protect the patient while off the unit)
- If suctioning is excessive (every half hour)
- When febrile, bacteremic, septic, or with *Clostridium difficile* disease.

Rest and Sleep
Rest is important for psychological and physiologic reasons. Complete rest in the mechanically ventilated patient is defined as that level of ventilatory support that offsets the work of breathing and decreases fatigue (refer to detailed description in text). Decisions about when rest is important include the following:
- When an acute event has occurred (ie, hypercarbic respiratory failure, pulmonary embolus, pulmonary edema).
- A reasonable approach for the chronic or nonacute patient is to work on active weaning trials during the day with rest at night until most of the daytime wean is accomplished (≥ 10 hours). Then, nighttime wean trials can be accomplished fairly rapidly. At night, the patient is allowed to sleep—if work of breathing is high, sleep is not possible. Ventilator rate should be high enough to allow for relaxation and optimal resting. If night sleeping aids are used, administer them early in the night to enhance sleep and ventilatory synchronization and so that the drugs can be metabolized before the daytime trials begin.

of patients with heart failure. In these patients, the sudden transition from ventilator support to the use of T-piece or CPAP for a SBT may result in an increased venous return during the wean trial that may overwhelm the heart's ability to compensate. Until appropriate preload and after-load reduction is addressed in these patients, PSV may be a gentler method of weaning. Another example is that of patients with profound myopathies or extremely debilitated states that may benefit from more gradual increases in work such as provided by PSV. Some new pressure modes such as proportional assist ventilation and adaptive support ventilation may potentially decrease the patient's workload during weaning. More on advanced modes of ventilation, including these, may be found in the AACN Essentials of Critical Care Nursing Book, Chapter 20: Advanced Respiratory Concepts: Modes of Ventilation.

A popular and common sense approach to wean trial progression is to attempt weaning trials during the daytime, allowing the patient to rest at night until the protocol threshold for extubation is reached. In the case of the patient with a tracheostomy, progressively longer episodes of spontaneous breathing, usually on tracheostomy collar or T-piece, are accomplished until tolerated for a specified amount of time. Then, decisions about discontinuation of ventilation and tracheostomy downsizing or decannulation may be made. Wean plans need to be

communicated clearly to all members of the healthcare team, and especially the patient, so that the plan is sufficiently aggressive but safe and effective. It is important that the philosophy of weaning is accepted by the healthcare team so that care planning is consistent and effective. Table 5-13 describes some general mechanical ventilator weaning philosophy concepts.

Other Protocols for Use

Patients who require LTMV often are affected by a variety of clinical conditions that prolong ventilator duration and other clinical outcomes such as length of stay and death. Research has demonstrated that outcomes of critically ill patients are improved with protocol-directed management.

Randomized controlled trials (RCT) have demonstrated that decreased sedation infusion use and methods to withdraw sedation daily using a "sedation interruption" improve outcomes such as ventilator duration and LOS. In addition, studies linked sedation use (specifically benzodiazepines) to delirium and subsequent cognitive dysfunction, further stimulating a decrease in sedation use in the ventilated patient population. Further emphasizing the importance of decreasing sedation use in these patients, a multicenter RCT combined sedation interruption with a "wake-up and breathe" trial (ie, SBT). In this study, patients assigned to the intervention (sedation interruption and wake-up) had significantly more days of spontaneous breathing, earlier discharge from ICU and hospital, and better 1-year survival than those in the control group.

The "ABCDE" bundle incorporates sedation awakening trials (Figure 5-21) along with other best evidence-based practice for ICU management (Table 5-14). Bundles are a structured method of improving patient care processes and when collectively performed, have resulted in improved patient outcomes.

The importance of factors such as sedation, delirium, and early mobility to weaning outcomes is essential to understand if the goal of attaining positive outcomes is to be attained. Protocols that assure that these important elements of care are routinely addressed decrease practice variation and improve outcomes.

Critical Pathways

Critical pathways are used to assure that evidence-based care is provided and that variation in care delivery is reduced. The pathways may be very directive in selected categories of patients, such as in patients with hip replacements, progression can be anticipated by hours or days; however, such specificity is not possible in the ventilated patient. Instead, pathways for the LTMV patient combine elements of care by specific time intervals (ie, begin deep vein thrombosis prophylaxis by day 1) with those that are designated by the stage of illness (ie, patient up to the chair during the prewean stage). In addition to providing an evidence-based blueprint

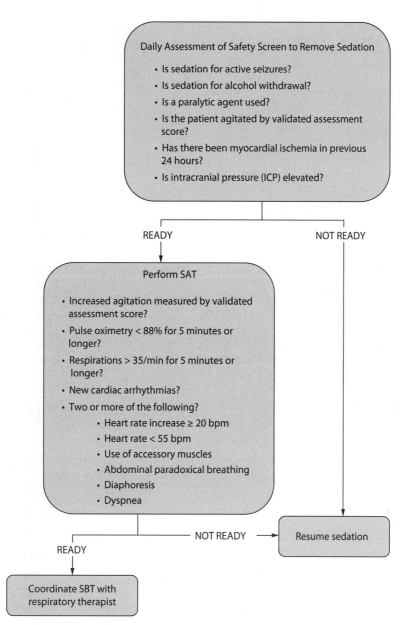

Figure 5-21. Spontaneous Awakening Trial–SAT. (*Data from Balas MC, Vasilevskis EE, Burke WJ, et al. Critical care nurses' role in implementing the "ABCDE Bundle" into practice.* Crit Care Nurse. *2012;32:35-47.*)

for a wide variety of care elements, the pathways encourage multidisciplinary input and collaboration. In general, they are incorporated into systematic institutional approaches to care of the LTMV patient population.

Systematic Institutional Initiatives for the Management of the LTMV Patient Population

Given the importance of systematic assessment and care planning, it is not surprising that many institutions have taken a very comprehensive approach to the care for the LTMV patient. Solutions to reduce variation and promote standardization of care are implemented to ensure that best practices are adhered to and good outcomes result.

In one study, an algorithmic approach to weaning was instituted in three adult ICUs and used nurses to manage the process. In another study, advanced practice nurses called "outcomes managers" managed and monitored long-term ventilated patients using a multidisciplinary clinical pathway and protocols for the management of sedation and weaning trials. The two studies demonstrated that statistically significant positive differences in most variables of interest such as ventilator duration, ICU and hospital lengths of stay (LOS), mortality rate, and cost savings were attainable with the approaches.

The healthcare environment is often chaotic. Short LOS and decreased staffing levels affect the continuity of care and contribute to gaps in practice and care planning. Given the

TABLE 5-14. ABCDE BUNDLE AND COMPONENTS

Requires a coordinated effort between the heathcare team

ABC–Awakening and Breathing Coordination

1. Spontaneous Awakening Trial
   - Daily assessment of safety screen to turn off sedation
   - Daily awakening, sedation vacation, or daily interruption of sedation trial
2. Spontaneous Breathing Trial
   - Daily assessment of safety screen
   - Daily spontaneous breathing trial

D–Delirium Assessment and Management

3. Routine Assessment of Delirium
   - Confusion assessment method for the ICU (CAM-ICU)
   - Intensive care delirium screening checklist (ICDSC)
4. Stop
   - Evaluate risk factors for delirium
5. Think
   - Modify risk factors
     - **T**–Toxic situations
       - CHF, shock, dehydration
       - Medications
       - New organ failure
     - **H**–Hypoxemia
     - **I**–Infection/sepsis
     - **N**–Nonpharmacologic interventions
       - Hearing aids, glasses, reorientation, sleep protocols, music, noise control, ambulation, family
     - **K+** –electrolyte problems
6. Medicate if needed

E–Early Exercise and Progressive Mobility

7. Early Mobility Protocol
   - Daily assessment of mobility readiness
   - Mobility program

Data from American Association for Critical Care. AACN PEARL: Implementing the ABCDE Bundle at the Bedside. http://www.aacn.org/dm/practice/aacnpearl.aspx?menu=practice. Accessed March 10, 2013.

complexity of the care of the ventilated patient, it is clear that approaches to care that decrease variation may improve patient outcomes and are to be encouraged.

Troubleshooting Ventilators

The complexity of ventilators and the dynamic state of the patient's clinical condition, as well as the patient's response to ventilation, create a variety of common problems that may occur during mechanical ventilation. It is crucial that progressive care clinicians be expert in the prevention, identification, and management of ventilator-associated problems in ventilated patients.

During mechanical ventilation, sudden changes in the clinical condition of the patient, particularly respiratory distress, as well as the occurrence of ventilator alarms or abnormal functioning of the ventilator, require immediate assessment and intervention. A systematic approach to each of these situations prevents or minimizes untoward ventilator events (Figure 5-22).

The first step is to determine the presence of respiratory distress or hemodynamic instability. If either is present the patient is removed from the mechanical ventilator and manually ventilated with an MRB and 100% O_2 for a few

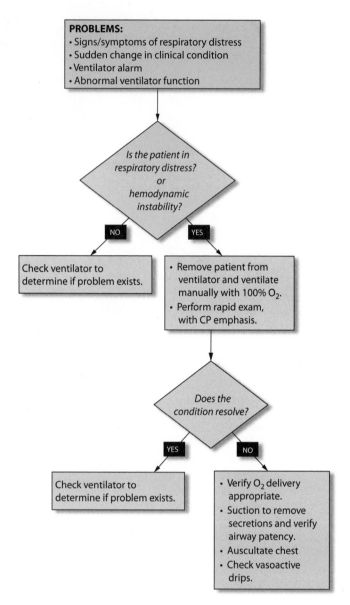

Figure 5-22. Algorithm for management of ventilator alarms and/or development of acute respiratory distress.

minutes. During manual ventilation, a quick assessment of the respiratory and cardiovascular system is made, noting changes from previous status. Clinical improvement rapidly following removal from the ventilator suggests a ventilator problem. Manual ventilation is continued while another clinician corrects the ventilator problem (eg, tubing leaks or disconnections, inaccurate gas delivery) or replaces the ventilator. Continuation of respiratory distress after removal from the ventilator and during manual ventilation suggests a patient-related cause.

Oral Feedings

Being able to eat "regular food" enhances the ventilated patient's sense of well being and optimism. However, it is essential that the patient's ability to swallow is evaluated prior to allowing feeding following extubation (especially in those ventilated long term) and in those who have a tracheostomy tube in place. "Swallow studies" are commonly done in these patients and should be considered for the categories noted above as well as in any patient with a history of aspiration.

Communication

Mechanically ventilated patients are unable to speak and communicate verbally due to the presence of a cuffed ET tube or tracheostomy tube. The inability to speak is frustrating for the patient, nurse, and members of the healthcare team. Impaired communication results in patients experiencing anxiety and fear, symptoms that can have a deleterious effect on their physical and emotional conditions. Patients interviewed after extubation reveal how isolated and alone they felt because of their inability to speak.

Common Communication Problems

Patients' perceptions of communication difficulties related to mechanical ventilation include: (1) inability to communicate, (2) insufficient explanations, (3) inadequate understanding, (4) fears related to potential dangers associated with the inability to speak, and (5) difficulty with communication methods. Except for the problem of inability to vocalize, all of the problems cited by ventilated patients may be resolved easily by progressive care practitioners. For instance, "insufficient explanations" and "inadequate understanding" can be remedied by frequent repetition of all plans and procedures in language that is understandable to a nonmedical person and that takes into account that attention span and cognitive abilities, especially memory, are frequently diminished due to the underlying illness or injury, effects of medications and anesthesia, and the impact of the progressive care environment. Although most messages the ventilated patient needs to communicate lie within a narrow range ("pain," "hunger," "water," and "sleep"), communicating these basic needs is often difficult. Most adults are accustomed to attending to their own basic needs, but in the progressive care unit, not only are they unable to physically perform certain activities, they also may not be able to communicate their needs effectively. Basic needs include such activities as bathing, brushing teeth, combing hair, elimination, eating, drinking, and sleeping. Other examples include simple requests or statements such as "too hot," "too cold," "turn me," "up," "down," "straighten my legs," "my arm hurts," "I can't breathe," and "moisten my lips."

Patients have described difficulties with communication methods while being mechanically ventilated. This also can be avoided by assessing the patient's communication abilities. Is the patient alert and oriented? Can the patient answer simple yes and no questions? Does the patient speak English? Can the patient use at least one hand to gesture? Does the patient have sufficient strength and dexterity to hold a pen and write? Are the patient's hearing and vision adequate? Knowledge of the patient's communication abilities assists the clinician to identify appropriate communication methods.

Once the most successful communication methods have been identified for a particular patient, they should be written into the plan of care. Continuity among healthcare professionals in their approach to communication with nonvocal patients improves the quality of care and increases patient satisfaction.

Methods to Enhance Communication

A variety of methods for augmenting communication are available and can be classified into two categories: nonvocal treatments (gestures, lip reading, mouthing words, paper and pen, alphabet/numeric boards, flashcards, etc) and vocal treatments (talking tracheostomy tubes and speaking valves). The best way to communicate with the patient who has an artificial airway or who is being mechanically ventilated is still unknown.

Nonvocal Treatments

Individual patient needs vary and it is recommended that the nurse use a variety of nonvocal treatments (eg, gestures, alphabet board, and paper and pen). Success with communication interventions varies with the diagnosis, age, type of injury or disease, type of respiratory assist devices, and psychosocial factors. For instance, lip reading can be successful in patients who have tracheostomies because the lips and mouth are visible, but in the ET tube patient, where tape and tube holders limit lip movement and visibility, lip reading may be less successful.

WRITING

Typically the easiest, most common method of communication readily available is the paper and pen. However, the supine position is not especially conducive to writing legibly. The absence of proper eyeglasses, an injured or immobilized dominant writing hand, or lack of strength also can make writing difficult for mechanically ventilated patients. Writing paper should be placed on a firm writing surface (eg, clipboard) with an attached felt-tipped pen that writes in any position. Strength, finger flexibility, and dexterity are required to grasp a pen. Many patients prefer to use a Magic Slate (Western Publishing Co., Racine, WI) or a Magna Doodle (Tyco Industries, Mount Laurel, NJ). These pressure-sensitive, inexpensive toy screens can be purchased at any department store; with them messages can be easily erased, maintaining the privacy of a written message. Although, costly, computer keyboards or touchpads may facilitate writing in patient who are comfortable with "high-tech" solutions.

A phenomenon of decoding exists between patient's written words (which often look like scribbling) and the nurse's ability to read what the patient wrote. The majority of the time, the nurse can read the writing of the patient even when it seems indistinguishable to a casual observer. This is due in part to the fact that over 65% of all communication is nonverbal and many contextual cues exist to assist in understanding and communicating effectively.

GESTURING

Another nonvocal method of communication that can be very effective is the deliberate use of gestures. Gestures are best suited for the short-term ventilated patient who is alert and can move at least one hand, even if only minimally. Generally, well-understood gestures are emblematic, have a low level of symbolism, and are easily interpreted by most people.

For example, ventilated patients often indicate that they need suctioning by curving an index finger (to resemble a suction catheter), raising a hand toward the ET tube, and moving their hand back and forth. This is known as an idiosyncratic gesture, a gesture that is used by a particular community, namely, the nurse and the ventilated patient. Other idiosyncratic gestures include "ice chips," "moisten my mouth," "spray throat," "fan," and "doctor."

One important aspect of communicating by gesture is to "mirror" the gesture(s) back to the patient, at the same time verbalizing the message or idea conveyed by the patient's gesture. This mirroring ensures accuracy in interpretation and assists the clinician and patient to form a repertoire to be used successfully in future gestural conversations. When observing a patient's gestures, stand back from the bed, and watch his or her arms and hands. Most gestures are easily understood, especially those most frequently used by patients (eg, the head nod, indicating "yes" or "no"). Practitioners should ask simple yes-and-no questions, but avoid playing "twenty questions" with ventilated patients because this can be very frustrating. Before trying to guess the needs of ventilated patients, give them the opportunity to use gestures to communicate their needs.

ALPHABET BOARD/PICTURE BOARD

For patients who do not speak English, a picture board is sometimes useful along with well-understood gestures. Picture boards have images of common patient needs (eg, bedpan, glass of water, medications, family, doctor, nurse) that the patient can point to. Picture boards, although commercially available, can be made easily and laminated to more uniquely meet the needs of a specific progressive care population.

Another approach is the use of flash cards that can be purchased or made. Language flash cards contain common words or phrases in English or foreign languages.

Vocalization Techniques

If patients with tracheostomy tubes in place have intact organs of speech, they may benefit from vocal treatment strategies like pneumatic and electrical devices, fenestrated tracheostomy tubes, talking tracheostomy tubes, and tracheostomy speaking valves. Several conditions preclude use of vocalization devices, such as neurologic conditions that impair vocalization (eg, Guillain-Barré syndrome), severe upper airway obstruction (eg, head/neck trauma), or vocal cord adduction (eg, presence of an ET tube).

A number of vocal treatments for tracheostomized patients exist. Generally, they require that the cuff be completely deflated to allow for air to be breathed in and out through the mouth and nose as well as around the sides of the tracheostomy. On exhalation the gases pass through the vocal cords allowing for speech. Some use one-way speaking valves (eg, Passy-Muir valve, shown in Figure 5-23) allow for air to be inhaled through the valve but close during exhalation to direct air up past the vocal cords. A fenestrated tracheostomy tube (Figure 5-24) also allows passage of air through the vocal cords. A cap or speaking valve may be used in conjunction with the fenestrated tube to ensure that all exhaled air moves through the vocal cords for vocalization. There have been reported incidences of granuloma tissue development at the site adjacent to the fenestration, which resolves after removal of the tube. In addition, fenestrated ports often become clogged with secretions, again preventing voicing. It is imperative that if the tracheostomy tube is capped, that the cuff of the tracheostomy be completely deflated.

Another vocal treatment is the talking tracheostomy tube, which is designed to provide a means of verbal communication for the ventilator-dependent patient. Patients who were otherwise considered to be "unweanable" have been reported to take a renewed interest in the weaning process, and some successfully wean upon hearing their own voice. Currently there are two talking tracheostomy tubes available

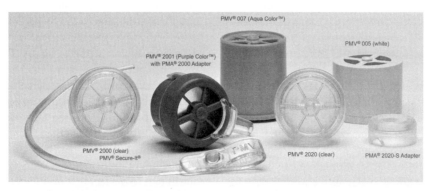

Figure 5-23. Passy-Muir Speaking Valves. (Image courtesy of Passy-Muir, Inc., Irvine, CA.)

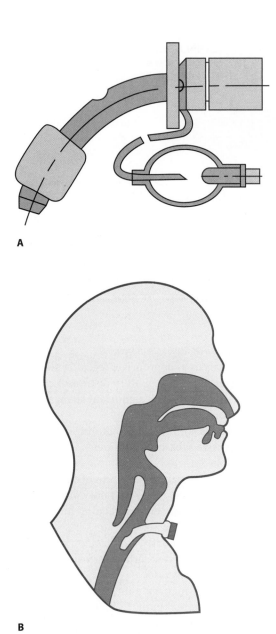

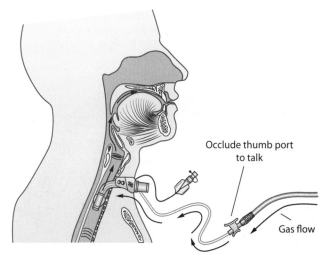

Figure 5-25. Tracheostomy tube with side port to facilitate speech. (*With permission Smith Medical, Keen, NH.*)

Figure 5-24. (A) Fenestrated tracheostomy tube. **(B)** Opening above the cuff site allowing gas, flow past the vocal cords during inspiration and expiration. (*With permission, Covidien.*)

that maintain a closed system with cuff inflation but differ in how they function.

1. *The Portex trachesotomy* operates by gas flowing (4-6 L/min) through an airflow line, which has a fenestration just above the tracheostomy tube cuff (Figure 5-25). The air flows through the glottis, thus supporting vocalization if the patient is able to form words with their mouth. However, an outside air source must be provided, which is usually not humidified and the trachea can become dry and irritated. The line for this air source requires diligent cleaning and flushing of the air port to prevent it from becoming clogged. The patients or staff must be able to manually divert air through the tube via a thumb port control.

2. *The Blom tracheostomy tube* system (Figure 5-26) uses a 2-valve system in a specialized speech inner cannula that redirects air and does not require use of an air source. During inhalation the flap valve opens and the bubble valve seals the fenestration preventing air leak to the upper airway. On exhalation, the flap valve closes and the bubble valve collapses to unblock the fenestration to allow air to the vocal cords. An additional component is the exhaled volume reservoir which attaches to the circuit and returns volume to minimize false low expiratory minute volume alarms.

Teaching Communication Methods

The progressive care environment presents many teaching and learning challenges. Patients and families are under a considerable amount of stress, so the nurse must be a very creative teacher and offer communication techniques that are simple, effective, and easy to learn. The desire to communicate with loved ones, however, often makes the family very willing to learn. Frequently, it is the family who makes up large-lettered communication boards, purchases a Magic Slate, or brings in a laptop computer or touchpad for the patient to use. Suggesting that families do this is usually very well received, because loved ones want so desperately to help in some way.

All patients should be informed prior to intubation that they will be unable to speak during the intubation period. A flipchart illustrating what an endotracheal tube or tracheostomy tube is like, with labeling in simple words, may be shown to patients who will be electively intubated (eg, for planned surgery). Practicing with a few nonverbal communication techniques before intubation (eg, gestures, alphabet

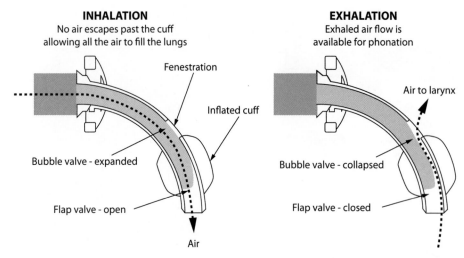

INHALATION
No air escapes past the cuff
allowing all the air to fill the lungs

Fenestration

Inflated cuff

Bubble valve - expanded

Flap valve - open

Air

EXHALATION
Exhaled air flow is
available for phonation

Air to larynx

Bubble valve - collapsed

Flap valve - closed

Figure 5-26. Tracheostomy Tube with inner cannula for speaking (Blom Tracheostomy Tube System). (Courtesy of Pulmodyne, Indianapolis, IN [http://www.dolema.com/uploads/6869E_Blom_Brochure.pdf])

boards, flash cards) is also beneficial. Another important point to emphasize with patients is that being unable to speak is usually temporary, just while the breathing tube is in place. If preintubation explanations are not feasible or possible, provide these explanations to the intubated patient.

Principles of Management

The majority of interventions related to mechanical ventilation focus on maximizing oxygenation and ventilation, and preventing complications associated with artificial airways and the sequelae of assisting the patient's ventilation and oxygenation with an invasive mechanical device.

Maximizing Oxygenation and Ventilation

- Provide frequent explanations of the purpose of the ventilator.
- Monitor the patient's response to ventilator therapy and for signs that the patient is dyssynchronous with the ventilator respiratory pattern. The use of graphic displays, common on many ventilator systems, is often a helpful aid to patient assessment.
- Consider ventilator setting changes to maximize synchrony (eg, changes in flow rates, respiratory rates, sensitivities, and/or modes).
- Administer sedative agents judiciously as required to enhance patient/ventilator synchrony.

Maintain a Patent Airway

- Suction only when clinically indicated according to patient assessment.
- Decrease secretion viscosity by maintaining adequate hydration and humidification of all inhaled gases.
- Monitor for signs and symptoms of bronchospasm and administer bronchodilator therapy as appropriate.
- Prevent obstruction of oral ET tubes by using an oral bite block if necessary.

Monitor Oxygenation and Ventilation Status Frequently

- ABG analysis as appropriate (eg, after some ventilator changes, with respiratory distress or cardiovascular instability, or with significant changes in clinical condition).
- Continuous noninvasive monitoring of Spo_2. Validate noninvasive measures with periodic ABG analysis (see Table 5-4).
- Observe for signs and symptoms of decreases in Pao_2, increases in $Paco_2$, and respiratory distress. Development of respiratory distress requires immediate intervention (see Figure 5-23).
- Reposition frequently and develop a mobilization plan to improve ventilation-perfusion relationships and prevent atelectasis.
- Aggressively manage pain, particularly chest and upper abdominal pain, to increase mobility, deep breathing, and coughing (see Chapter 6, Pain and Sedation Management).

Physiotherapy and Monitoring

- Administer chest physiotherapy for selected clinical conditions (eg, large mucus production, lobar atelectasis).
- Monitor oxygenation status closely during chest physiotherapy for signs and symptoms of arterial desaturation.

Maintain Oxygenation and Ventilatory Support at All Times

- Ensure proper operation of the mechanical ventilator by activation of appropriately set alarms and frequent assessment of device function (commonly checked every 1-2 hours).
- During even brief periods of removal from mechanical ventilation, maintain ventilation and oxygenation with MRB. During intrahospital transport, verify adequacy of ventilatory support equipment, particularly the

maintenance of PEEP (when > 10 cm H$_2$O is required) as well as ensuring adequate portable oxygen supply tank pressure. When possible, a portable mechanical ventilator should be used versus MRB.
- Emergency sources of portable oxygen should be readily available in the event of loss of wall oxygen capabilities.

Weaning from Mechanical Ventilation
- Systematically assess wean potential and address factors impeding weaning.
- Use a weaning protocol with a "wean screen." Assure that the patient, family, and key caregivers are aware of weaning trials.
- Stop weaning trial if signs of intolerance emerge.
- Use a systematic evidence-based multidisciplinary approach to weaning.

Preventing Complications
- Maintain ET or tracheostomy cuff pressures less than 25 mm Hg (30 cm H$_2$O).
- Maintain artificial airway position by securing with a properly fitting holder device or selected tapes. Frequently verify proper ET position by noting ET marking at lip or nares placed after intubation.
- Ensure tape or devices used to secure the artificial airway are properly applied and are not causing pressure areas or skin breakdown. Periodic repositioning of ET tubes may be required to prevent skin integrity problems.
- Use a bite block with oral ET tubes if necessary to prevent accidental biting of the tube.
- Provide frequent mouth care and assess for development of pressure areas from ET tubes. Move the ET from one side of the mouth to the other daily or more frequently if necessary.
- Assess for signs and symptoms of sinusitis with nasal ET tube use (eg, pain in sinus area with pressure, purulent drainage from nares, fever, increased white blood cell count).

Maximizing Communication
- Assess communication abilities and establish at least a method for nonverbal communication (see the discussion of communication previously). Assist family members in using that approach with the patient.
- Anticipate patient needs and concerns in the planning of care.
- Ensure that call lights, bells, or other methods for notifying unit personnel of patient needs are in place at all times.
- Frequently repeat information about communication limitations and how to use different nonverbal communication methods.

Reducing Anxiety and Providing Psychosocial Support
- Maintain a calm, supportive environment to avoid unnecessary escalation of anxiety. Provide brief explanations of activities and procedures. The vigilance and presence of healthcare providers during anxiety periods is crucial to avoid panic by patients and visiting family members.
- Teach the patient relaxation techniques to control anxiety.
- Administer mild doses of anxiolytics if needed (eg, lorazepam or diazepam) that do not depress respiration (see Chapter 6, Pain and Sedation Management and Chapter 9, Cardiovascular System).
- Encourage the family to stay with the patient as much as desired and to participate in caregiver activities as appropriate. Presence of a family member provides comfort to the patient and assists the family member to better cope with the illness.
- Promote sleep at night by decreasing light, noise, and unnecessary patient interruptions.

SELECTED BIBLIOGRAPHY

General Critical Care

Ahrens T, Sona C. Capnography application in acute and progressive care. *AACN Clin Issues*. 2003;14:123-132.

Balas MC, Rice M, Chaperon C, et al. Management of delirium in critically ill adults. *Crit Care Nurs*. 2012;32:15-25.

Balas MC, Vasilevskis EE, Burke WJ, et al. Critical care nurses' role in implementing the "ABCDE Bundle" into practice. *Crit Care Nurs*. 2012;32:35-47.

Berry E, Zecca H. Daily interruptions of sedation: a clinical approach to improve outcomes in clinically ill patients. *Crit Care Nurs*. 2012;32:43-51.

Branson RD, Mannheimer PD. Forehead oximetry in critically ill patients: the case of a new monitoring site. *Respir Care Clin N Am*. 2004;10(3):359-367.

Chang L, Wang KK, Chao F. Influence of physical restraint on unplanned extubation of adult intensive care patients: a case-control study. *Am J Crit Care*. 2008;17:408-415.

Cuccio L, Cerullo E, Paradis H, et al. An evidence-based oral care protocol to decrease ventilator-associated pneumonia. *Dimens Crit Care Nurs*. 2012;31:301-308.

Dolovich MB, Ahrens RC, Hess DR, et al. Device selection and outcomes of aerosol therapy: evidence-based guidelines. *Chest*. 2006;127:335-371.

Ely EW, Shintani A, Truman B. Delirium as a predictor of mortality in mechanically ventilated patients in the intensive care unit. *JAMA*. 2004;291:1753-1762.

Girard TD, Jackson JC, Pandharipande PP, et al. Delirium as a predictor of long-term cognitive impairment in survivors of crtical illness. *Crit Care Med*. 2010;38:1513-1520.

Halm M, Amrola R. Effect of oral care on bacterial colonization and ventilator-associated pneumonia. *Am J Crit Care*. 2009;18:275-278.

Hellstom A, Fagerstom C, Willman A. Promoting sleep by nursing interventions in health care settings: a systematic review. *Worldviews Evid Based Nurs*. 2011;8:128-142.

Jarachovic M, Mason M, Kerber K, McNett M. The role of standardized protocols in unplanned extubations in a medical intensive care unit. *Am J Crit Care*. 2011;20:304-311.

Jongerden IP, Rovers MM, Grypdonck MH, Bonten MJ. Open and closed endotracheal suction systems in mechanically ventilated intensive care patients: a meta-analysis. *Crit Care Med.* 2007;35:260-270.

Kazmarek RM, Stoller JK, Heur AJ, eds. *Egan's Fundamentals of Respiratory Care.* 10th ed. St. Louis, MO: Elsevier Mosby; 2013.

Kjonegaard R, Fields W, King ML. Current practice in airway management: a descriptive evaluation. *Am J Crit Care.* 2009;doi: 10.4037/ajcc2009803.

MacLeod DB, Cortinez LI, Keifer JC, et al. The desaturation response time of finger pulse oximeters during mild hypothermia. *Anaesthesia.* Jan 2005;60(1):65-71.

Matthews EE. Sleep disturbances and fatigue in critically ill patients. *AACN Adv Crit Care.* 2011;22:204-224.

Munro CL, Grap MJ, Jones DJ, et al. Chlorhexidine, tooth brushing, and preventing ventilator-associated pneumonia in critically ill adults. *Am J Crit Care.* 2009;18:428-437.

Neumar RW, Otto CW, Link MS, et al. Part 8: adult advanced cardiovascular life support: 2010 American Heart Association Guidelines for Cardiopulmonary Resuscitation and Emergency Cardiovascular Care. *Circulation.* 2010;122(18 suppl 3): S729-767.

Seckel MA. Ask the experts: does the use of a closed suction system help to prevent ventilator-associated pneumonia? *Crit Care Nurs.* 2008;28(1):65-66.

Seckel MA. Ask the experts: normal saline and mucous plugging. *Crit Care Nurs.* 2012;32:66-68.

Seckel MA, Schulenburg K. Ask the experts: eating while receiving mechanical ventilation. *Crit Care Nurs.* 2011;31:95-97.

Stauffer JL. Complications of endotracheal intubation and tracheotomy. *Respir Care.* 1999;44(7):828-844.

St John RE, Malen JF. Airway management. *Crit Care Nurs Clin N Am.* 2004;16:413-430.

Stonecypher K. Ventilator-associated pneumonia: the importance of oral care in intubated adults. *Crit Care Nurs Q.* 2010;33(4):339-347.

Unoki T, Serita A, Grap MJ. Automatic tube compensation during weaning from mechanical ventilation: evidence and clinical implications. *Crit Care Nurs.* 2008;28:34-42.

Valdez-Lowe C, Ghareeb SA, Artinian NT. Pulse oximetry in adults. *AJN.* 2009;109(6):52-59.

Ventilator Management

Aloe K, Ryan M. Creation of an intermediate respiratory care unit to decrease intensive care utilization. *JONA.* 2009;39:494-498.

Burns SM. Mechanical ventilation and weaning. In: Carlson KK, ed. *AACN Advanced Critical Care Nursing.* St Louis, MO: Saunders-Elsevier; 2009.

Burns SM. Pressure modes of mechanical ventilation: the good, the bad, and the ugly. *AACN Advance Crit Care.* 2008;19:399-411.

Esteban A, Frutos-Vivar F, Ferguson ND, et al. Noninvasive positive-pressure ventilation for respiratory failure after extubation. *N Engl J Med.* 2004;350:2452-2460.

Kane C, York NL. Understanding the alphabet soup of mechanical ventilation. *Dimens Crit Care Nurs.* 2012;31:217-222.

MacIntyre NR, Branson RD. *Mechanical Ventilation.* Philadelphia, PA: Saunders; 2009.

Pierce LN. *Management of the Mechanically Ventilated Patient.* Philadelphia, PA: Saunders-Elsevier; 2007.

Restrepo RD, Walsh BK. Humidification during invasive and noninvasive mechanical ventilation: 2012. *Resp Care.* 2012;57: 782-788.

St. John R. End-tidal CO_2 monitoring. In Burns SM. ed. *AACN's Protocols for Practice: Non-Invasive Monitoring Series.* Sudbury, MA: Jones and Bartlett; 2006.

Tobin MJ. *Principles and Practice of Mechanical Ventilation.* New York, NY: McGraw-Hill Medical Publishing Division; 2006.

Unroe M, Kahn JM, Carson SS, et al. One-year trajectories of care and resource utilization for recipients of prolonged mechanical ventilation: a cohort study. *Ann Intern Med.* 2010;153:167-175.

Walkey AJ, Wiener RS. Use of noninvasive ventilation in patient with acute respiratory failure, 2000-2009. *Annals ATS.* 2013;10: 10-17.

White AC. Long-term mechanical ventilation: management strategies. *Resp Care.* 2012;57:889-897.

Weaning From Mechanical Ventilation

Blackwood B, Alderdice F, Burns K, et al. Use of weaning protocols for reducing duration of mechanical ventilation in critically ill adult patients: Cochrane systematic review and meta-analysis. *BMJ.* 2011;342c7237doi:1-.1136/bmj.b7237.

Boles JM, Blon J, Connors A, et al. Task force: weaning from mechanical ventilation. *Eur Respir J.* 2007;29:1033-1056.

Bou Aki I, Bou-Khalil P, Kanazi G. Weaning from mechanical ventilation. *Curr Opin Anesthesiol.* 2012;25:42-47.

Brochard L, Thille AW. What is the proper approach to liberating the weak from mechanical ventilation? *Crit Care Med.* 2009;37:S410-S415.

Burns SM. Adherence to sedation withdrawal protocols and guidelines in ventilated patients. *Clin Nurs Spec.* 2012;26:22-8. doi: 10.1097/NUR.0b013e31823bfae8.

Burns SM. Weaning from mechanical ventilation: where were we then, and where are we now? *Crit Care Nurs Clin N Am.* 2012;24:457-458.

Burns SM, Fisher C, Tribble SS, et al. The relationship of 26 clinical factors to weaning outcome. *Am J Crit Care.* 2012;21:52-58.

Epstein SK. Weaning from ventilatory support. *Curr Opin Crit Care.* 2009;15:36-43.

Eskandar N, Apostolakos MJ. Weaning from mechanical ventilation. *Crit Care Clin.* 2007;23:263-274.

Girard TD, Kress JP, Fuchs BD, et al. Efficacy and safety of a paired sedation and ventilator weaning protocol for mechanically ventilated patients in intensive care (Awakening and Breathing Controlled trial): a randomised controlled trial. *Lancet.* 2008;371:126-134.

Haas CF, Loik PS. Ventilator discontinuation protocols. *Resp Care.* 2012;57:1649-1662.

MacIntyre N. Discontinuing mechanical ventilator support. *Chest.* 2007;132:1049-1056.

MacIntyre NR. Evidence-based assessments in the ventilator discontinuation process. *Resp Care.* 2012;57:1611-1618.

McConville JF, Kress JP. Current concepts: weaning patients from the ventilator. *NEJM.* 2012;367:2233-2239.

Mendes-Tellez PA, Needham DM. Early physical rehabilitation in the ICU and ventilator liberation. *Resp Care.* 2012;57:1663-1669.

Olff C, Clark-Wadkins C. Tele-ICU partners enhanced evidence-based practice: ventilator weaning intiative. *AACN Adv Crit Care.* 2012;23:312-322.

Penuelas O, Frutos-Vivar F, Fernandez C, et al. Characteristics and outcomes of ventilated patients according to time to liberation from mechanical ventilation. *Am J Respir Crit Care Med.* 2011;184:430-437.

Tobin MJ, Guenther SM, Perez W, et al. Konno-Mead analysis of ribcage-abdominal motion during successful and unsuccessful trials of weaning from mechanical ventilation. *Am Rev Respir Dis.* 1987;135:1320-1328.

White V, Currey J, Botti M. Multidisciplinary team developed and implemented protocols to assist mechanical ventilation weaning: a systematic review of literature. *Worldviews Evid Based Nurs.* 2011;8:51-59.

Communication

Batty S. Communication, swallowing and feeding in the intensive care unit patient. *Nurs Crit Care.* 2009;14:175-179.

Baumgartner CA, Bewyer E, Bruner D. Management of communication and swallowing in intensive care. *AACN Adv Crit Care.* 2008;19:433-443.

Happ MB. Communicating with mechanically ventilated patients: state of the science. *AACN Clin Issues.* 2001;12:247-258.

Windhorst C, Harth R, Wagoner C. Patients requiring tracheostomy and mechanical ventilation: a model for interdisciplinary decision-making. *AHSA Leader.* 2009;14:10-13.

Evidence-Based Resources

A Collective Task Force Facilitated by the American College of Chest Physicians, the American Association for Respiratory Care, and the American College of Medicine. Evidence-based guidelines for weaning and discontinuing ventilator support. *Resp Care.* 2002;47:69-90.

American Association of Respiratory Care. AARC clinical practice guideline: capnography/capnometry during mechanical ventilation: 2011. *Resp Care.* 2011;56:503-509.

American Association for Respiratory Care. AARC clinical practice guideline: care of the ventilator circuit and its relation to ventilator-associated pneumonia. *Resp Care.* 2003;48:869-879.

American Association of Respiratory Care. AARC clinical practice guideline: endotracheal suctioning of mechanically ventilated patients with artificial airway. *Resp Care.* 2010;55:758-764.

American Association for Respiratory Care. AARC clinical practice guideline: oxygen therapy for adults in the acute care facility 2002 revision and update. *Resp Care.* 2002;47;717-720.

American Association for Respiratory Care. AARC clinical practice guideline: removal of the endotracheal tube-2007 revision and update. *Resp Care.* 2007;52;81-93.

American Association of Critical Care Nurses (AACN). Practice alert: delirium assessment and management. Alisio Viejo, CA: AACN: 2011. www.aacn.org. Accessed March 1, 2013.

American Association of Critical Care Nurses (AACN). Practice alert: oral care in the critically Ill. Alisio Veijo, CA: AACN: 2010. www.aacn.org. Accessed March 1, 2013.

American Association of Critical Care Nurses (AACN). Practice alert: prevention of aspiration. Alisio Viejo, CA: AACN: 2011. www.aacn.org. Assessed March 1, 2013.

American Association of Critical Care Nurses (AACN). Practice alert: ventilator associated pneumonia. Alisio Veijo, CA: AACN: 2008. www.aacn.org. Accessed January 10, 2010.

American Thoracic Society and the Infectious Diseases Society of America. Guidelines for the management of adults with hospital acquired, ventilator-associated, and healthcare-associated pneumonia. *Am J Respir Crit Care Med.* 2005;171:388-416.

Barden, C, Davis T, Seckel M, et al. C. AACN Tele-ICU Nursing Practice Guidelines. 2013. Available at http://www.aacn.org/wd/practice/docs/tele-icu-guidelines.pdf.

Barr J, Fraser Gl, Puntillo K, et al. Clinical practice guidelines for the management of pain, agitation, and delirium in adult patients in the intensive care unit. *Crit Care Med.* 2013;41:263-306.

Burns SM. Practice protocol: weaning from mechanical ventilation. In: *Care of the Mechanically Ventilated Patient.* 2nd ed. Sudbury, MA: Jones and Bartlett; 2007.

Centers for Disease Control and Prevention. Guidelines for preventing health-care-associated pneumonia, 2003: recommendations of CDC and the Health Care Infection Control Practices Advisory Committee. *MMWR.* 2004;53(No. RR-3):1-35.

Grap MJ. Pulse oximetry. In: Burns SM, ed. *AACN's Protocols for Practice: Noninvasive Monitoring Series.* Sudbury, MA: Jones and Bartlett; 2006.

MacIntyre, NR, Cook DJ, Ely EW, Jr., et al. Evidence-based guidelines for weaning and discontinuing ventilatory support: a collective task force facilitated by the American College of Chest Physicians; the American Association for Respiratory Care; and the American College of Critical Care Medicine. *Chest.* 2001;120(6 suppl):375S-395S.

Muscedere J, Dodek P, Keenan S, et al. Comprehensive evidence-based clinical practice guidelines for ventilator-associated pneumonia: prevention. *J Crit Care.* 2008;23:126-137.

Pierce LN. Invasive and noninvasive modes and methods of mechanical ventilation. In: Burns SM, ed. *AACN's Protocols for Practice: Care of the Mechanically Ventilated Patient Series.* Sudbury, MA: Jones and Bartlett; 2006.

St John RE. End-tidal carbon dioxide monitoring. In: Burns SM, ed. *AACN's Protocols for Practice: Noninvasive Monitoring Series.* Sudbury, MA: Jones and Bartlett; 2006.

St John RE, Seckel MA. Airway management. In: Burns SM, ed. *AACN's Protocols for Practice: Care of the Mechanically Ventilated Patient Series.* Sudbury, MA: Jones and Bartlett; 2006.

Wiegand DL, ed. AACN Procedure Manual for Critical Care. 6th ed. Philadelphia, PA: Saunders; 2011.

PAIN AND SEDATION MANAGEMENT

6

Yvonne D'Arcy and Suzanne M. Burns

KNOWLEDGE COMPETENCIES

1. Describe the elements of pain assessment in progressive care patients.

2. Compare and contrast pain-relieving modalities for the critically ill:
   - Nonsteroidal anti-inflammatory drugs
   - Opioids, including patient-controlled analgesia
   - Epidural analgesia with opioids and/or local anesthetics
   - Elastomeric pumps with local anesthetic (LA)
   - Nonpharmacologic modalities: distraction, cutaneous stimulation, imagery, and relaxation techniques

3. Identify the important elements of pain control for a patient who is an addict.

4. Describe special considerations for pain management in vulnerable populations such as the elderly.

5. Identify the need for sedation, common sedative drugs, and how to monitor and manage the patient requiring sedation.

Pain management is central to the care of the acutely ill or injured patient. Unfortunately acutely ill patients may not be able to self-report their pain management needs to their healthcare team. Patients identify physical care that promotes pain relief and comfort as an important element of their hospitalization and recovery, especially while in the hospital environment. Providing optimum pain relief for acutely ill patients not only enhances their psychoemotional well-being, but can also help avert additional physiologic injury. This chapter explores a multimodal approach to pain management in acutely ill patients based on the physiologic mechanisms of pain transmission and human responses to pain. Using a multimodal approach, specific pharmacologic and nonpharmacologic pain management techniques are described, including the integral relationships among relaxation, sedation, and pain relief. Strategies also are presented that promote comfort and are easy to incorporate into a plan of care for progressive care patients. Finally, special considerations are delineated for vulnerable populations within the acute care setting.

PHYSIOLOGIC MECHANISMS OF PAIN

Peripheral Mechanisms

The pain response is elicited with tissue injuries, whether actual or potential. Undifferentiated free nerve endings, or nociceptors, are the major receptors signaling tissue injury (Figure 6-1). Nociceptors are polymodal and can be stimulated by thermal, mechanical, and chemical stimuli. Nociception refers to the transmission of impulses by sensory nerves, which signal tissue injury.

At the site of injury, the release of a variety of neurochemical substances potentiates the activation of peripheral nociceptors. Many of these substances are also mediators of the inflammatory response and they can facilitate or inhibit the pain impulse. These substances include histamine, kinins, prostaglandins, serotonin, and leukotrienes (Figure 6-2).

The nociceptive impulse travels to the spinal cord via specialized, afferent sensory fibers. Small, myelinated A-delta (Aδ) fibers conduct nociceptive signals rapidly to

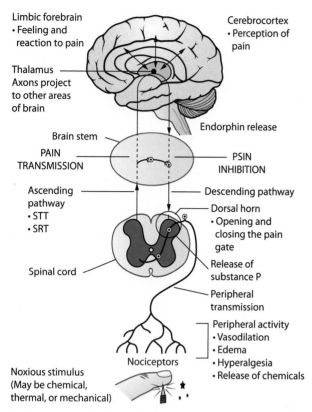

Figure 6-1. Physiologic pathway of pain transmission. (*Reprinted from Wild LR, Evans L. Pain. In: Copstead L, ed.* Perspectives on Pathophysiology. *Philadelphia, PA: WB Saunders;1995:934, with permission from Elsevier.*)

the spinal cord. The A-delta fibers transmit sensations that are generally localized and sharp in quality. In addition to A-delta fibers, smaller, unmyelinated C fibers also transmit nociceptive signals to the spinal cord. Because C fibers are unmyelinated, their conduction speed is much slower than their A-delta counterparts. The sensory quality of signals carried by C fibers tends to be dull and unlocalized (Figure 6-3).

Spinal Cord Integration

Sensory afferent fibers enter the spinal cord via the dorsal nerve, synapsing with cell bodies of spinal cord interneurons in the dorsal horn (see Figure 6-1). Most of the A-delta and C fibers synapse in laminae I through V, in an area referred to as the substantia gelatinosa. Numerous neuro-transmitters (eg, substance P, glutamate, and calcitonin gene-related peptide) and other receptor systems (eg, opiate, alpha-adrenergic, and serotonergic receptors) modulate the processing of nociceptive inputs in the spinal cord.

Central Processing

Following spinal cord integration, nociceptive impulses travel to the brain via specialized, ascending somatosensory pathways (see Figure 6-1). The spinothalamic tract conducts nociceptive signals directly from the spinal cord to the thalamus. The spinoreticulothalamic tract projects signals to the reticular formation and the mesencephalon in the midbrain,

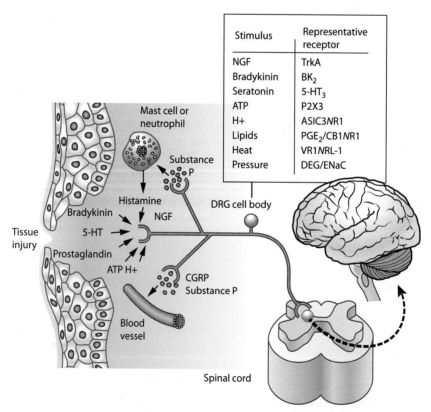

Stimulus	Representative receptor
NGF	TrkA
Bradykinin	BK_2
Seratonin	$5\text{-}HT_3$
ATP	P2X3
H+	ASIC3/VR1
Lipids	PGE_2/CB1/VR1
Heat	VR1/VRL-1
Pressure	DEG/ENaC

Figure 6-2. Peripheral nociceptors and the inflammatory response at the site of injury. (*From Julius D, Basbaum AI. Molecular mechanisms of nociception. Nature. 2001;413:203-210.*)

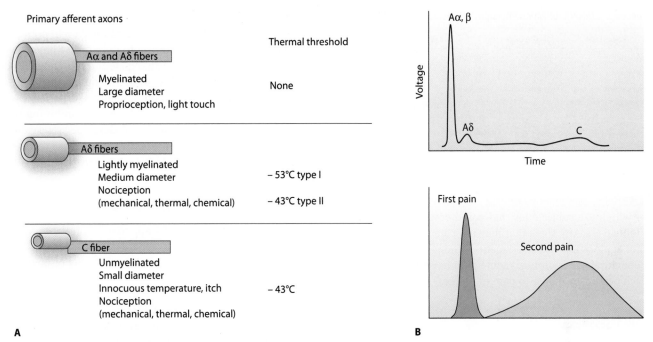

Figure 6-3. Different nociceptors detect different types of pain. **(A)** Peripheral nerves include small-diameter (Aδ) and medium- to large-diameter (Aα- β) myelinated afferent fibers, as well as small-diameter unmyelinated afferent fibers (C). **(B)** The fact that conduction velocity is directly related to fiber diameter is highlighted in the compound action potential recording from a peripheral nerve. Most nociceptors are either Aδ or C fibers, and their different conduction velocities (6-25 and ~1.0 m/s, respectively) account for the first (fast) and second (slow) pain responses to injury.

as well as to the thalamus. From the thalamus, axons project to somatosensory areas of the cerebrocortex and limbic forebrain. The unique physiologic, cognitive, and emotional responses to pain are determined and modulated by the specific areas to which the somatosensory pathways project. The stimulus to the cerebrocortex can also activate the patient's previous memories of the experience of pain; for example, the thalamus regulates the neurochemical response to pain, and the cortical and limbic projections are responsible for the perception of pain and aversive response to pain, respectively. Similarly, the reticular activating system regulates the heightened state of awareness that accompanies pain. The modulation of pain by activities in these specific areas of the brain is the basis of many of the analgesic therapies available to treat pain.

RESPONSES TO PAIN

Human responses to pain can be both physical and emotional. The physiologic responses to pain are the result of hypothalamic activation of the sympathetic nervous system associated with the stress response. Sympathetic activation leads to:

- Blood shifts from superficial vessels to striated muscle, the heart, the lungs, and the nervous system.
- Dilation of the bronchioles to increase oxygenation.
- Increased cardiac contractility.
- Inhibition of gastric secretions and contraction.
- Increase in circulating blood glucose for energy.

Signs and symptoms of sympathetic activation which frequently accompany nociception and pain:

- Increased heart rate
- Increased blood pressure
- Increased respiratory rate
- Pupil dilation
- Pallor and perspiration
- Nausea and vomiting

Although patients experiencing acute pain often exhibit signs and symptoms as noted above, it is critical to note that the absence or presence of any or all of these signs and symptoms does not negate or confirm the presence of pain. In fact some patients, especially those who are seriously ill and with little or no compensatory reserves, may exhibit a shock-like clinical picture in the presence of pain. Patients who are accustomed to underlying chronic pain may have a decreased physiologic response to pain while the actual intensity of the pain remains high (Table 6-1).

Acutely ill patients also express pain both verbally and nonverbally. The expressions can take many forms, some

TABLE 6-1. TYPES OF PAIN

Pain is defined as an unpleasant sensory and emotional experience associated with actual or potential tissue damage (APS, 2008). There are three main types of pain that can occur alone or in combination:
- Acute pain from which the patient expects to recover
- Chronic pain that lasts beyond the normal healing period
- Neuropathic pain is a special type of chronic pain that is the result of nerve damage

TABLE 6-2. EXAMPLES OF PAIN EXPRESSION IN CRITICALLY ILL PATIENTS

Verbal Cues	Facial Cues	Body Movements
Moaning	Grimacing	Splinting
Crying	Wincing	Rubbing
Screaming	Eye signals	Rocking
Silence		Rhythmic movement of extremity
		Shaking or tapping bed rails
		Grabbing the nurse's arm

From: Herr K, Coyne P, Kry T, et al. Pain assessment in the nonverbal patient: position statement with clinical practice recommendations. Pain Manage Nurs. 2006 7(2):44-52.

of which are subtle cues that could easily be overlooked (Table 6-2). Any signs that may indicate pain warrant further exploration and assessment. Although physiologic and behavioral expressions of acute pain have been described, each person's response to pain is unique.

PAIN ASSESSMENT

Pain assessment is a core element of ongoing surveillance of the acutely ill patient. Self-report of pain intensity and distress should be used whenever possible, especially for patients who can talk or communicate effectively. Regular documentation of pain assessment not only helps monitor the efficacy of analgesic modalities, but also helps ensure communication among caregivers regarding patient's pain. A variety of tools to assess pain intensity are available. There are three commonly used scales. The numeric rating scale (NRS) uses numbers between 0 and 10 to describe pain intensity; the anchors are "no pain to worst pain imaginable." Some patients find it easier to use adjectives to describe their pain. The verbal descriptive scale offers patients a standardized list of adjectives to describe their pain intensity. The descriptors are "none," "mild," "moderate," and "severe." With the visual analogue scale (VAS), a tool developed primarily for research, patients indicate their pain intensity by drawing a vertical line, bisecting a horizontal baseline. The baseline is anchored at either end by the terms "no pain" or "worst pain imaginable." A numeric conversion is done by measuring the line from the left anchor to the patient's mark, in millimeters.

Any of these scales can be used with patients who are intubated or unable to speak for other medical reasons; for example, patients can be asked to use their fingers to indicate a number between 0 and 10; similarly, patients can be asked to indicate by nodding their head or pointing to the appropriate adjective or number as they either hear or read the list of choices. With the VAS, the line can be printed on a sheet of paper or marker board and the patients asked to mark the line to indicate their level of pain. While the VAS has been used in acute care patients it may be difficult to use in many as it requires dexterity that may be inhibited by invasive lines, bandages, etc.

Unfortunately, some acutely ill patients are unable to indicate their pain intensity either verbally or nonverbally. In these situations, nurses must often use other clues to assess their patient's pain. Using a behavioral pain scale provides a guide for identifying and assessing pain in nonverbal patients (Table 6-3). In addition to monitoring physiologic parameters, nurses may also anticipate and recognize clinical situations where pain is likely to occur and use their knowledge of physiology and pathophysiology and experience with other patients with similar problems. By combining their knowledge and experience with well-developed interviewing and observational skills, progressive care nurses can assess patient's pain effectively and intervene appropriately.

A MULTIMODAL APPROACH TO PAIN MANAGEMENT

Today there are numerous approaches and modalities available to treat acute pain. Whereas, pharmacologic techniques traditionally have been the mainstay of analgesia, other complementary or nonpharmacologic methods are growing in their acceptance and use in clinical practice. Most modalities used in the treatment of acute pain can be used effectively in patients in progressive care units. Evidence-based practice guidelines to maximize analgesia in acutely ill patients are summarized in Table 6-4.

One of the central goals of pain management is to combine therapies or modalities that target as many of the processes involved in nociception and pain transmission as possible. Analgesic modalities, both pharmacologic and nonpharmacologic, exert their effects by altering nociception at specific structures within the peripheral or central nervous system (CNS), ie, the peripheral nociceptors, the spinal cord, or the brain or by altering the transmission of nociceptive impulses between these structures (Figure 6-4). By understanding where analgesic modalities work, nurses can more effectively select a combination of modalities working at different sites to best treat the source or type of pain patients experience and, subsequently, help patients achieve optimal analgesia.

To assist nurses to select and maximize analgesic modalities, for each of the analgesic modalities presented here, there is a brief description of where and how the selected modality works, clinical situations where it can be used most effectively, and strategies for titrating the modality. Finally, because few modalities exert a singular effect, a summary of secondary or side effects commonly associated with them, and strategies to minimize their occurrence, are also addressed.

NONSTEROIDAL ANTI-INFLAMMATORY DRUGS

Nonsteroidal anti-inflammatory drugs (NSAIDs) target the peripheral nociceptors. The NSAIDs exert their effect by modifying or reducing the amount of prostaglandin produced at the site of injury by inhibiting the formation of the enzyme cyclooxygenase, which is also responsible for the breakdown of arachidonic acid and formation of the neurotransmitter prostaglandin. As prostaglandin inhibitors, the NSAIDs have been shown to have opioid-sparing effects and are very effective in managing pain associated with inflammation, trauma

TABLE 6-3. DMC PAIN ASSESSMENT BEHAVIOR SCALE (NONVERBAL) FOR PATIENTS UNABLE TO PROVIDE A SELF-REPORT OF PAIN

	0	1	2	
FACE	Face muscles relaxed.	Facial muscle tension, frown, grimace.	Frequent to constant frown, clenched jaw.	**Face Score**
RESTLESSNESS	Quite, relaxed appearance, normal movement.	Occasional restless movement shifting position.	Frequent restless movement may include extremities or head.	**Restlessness Score**
MUSCLE TONE*	Normal muscle tone, relaxed.	Increased tone, flexion of fingers and toes.	Rigid tone.	**Muscle Tone Score**
VOCALIZATION**	No abnormal sounds.	Occasional moans, cries, whimpers or grunts.	Frequent or continuous moans, cries, whimpers or grunts.	**Vocalization Score**
CONSOLABILITY	Content, relaxed.	Reassured by touch or talk. Distractible.	Difficult to comfort by touch or talk.	**Consolability Score**
Behavioral Pain Assessment Scale Total (0 -10)				

*Assess muscle tone in patients with spinal cord lesion or injury at a level above the lesion or injury. Assess patients with hemiplegia on the unaffected side.

**This item cannot be measured in patients with artificial airways.

How to use the pain assessment behavioral scale:

1. Observe behaviors and mark appropriate number for each category.

2. Total the numbers in the pain assessment behavioral score column.

3. **Zero = No evidence of pain. Mild pain = 1-3. Moderate pain = 4-6. Severe uncontrolled pain is ≥ 6.**

Considerations:

4. Use the standard pain scale whenever possible to obtain the patient's self-report of pain. Self-report is the best indicator of the presence and intensity of pain.

5. Use this scale for patients who are unable to provide a self-report of pain.

6. In addition, a "proxy pain evaluation" from family, friends or clinicians close to the patient may be helpful to evaluate pain based on previous knowledge of patient response.

7. When in doubt, provide an analgesic. "If there is reason to suspect pain, an analgesic trial can be diagnostic as well as therapeutic."

Used with permission by the Detroit Medical Center via Margaret L. Campbell, PhD, RN.

TABLE 6-4. EVIDENCE-BASED GUIDELINES: PAIN MANAGEMENT

- Pain should be routinely monitored
- Use the behavioral pain scale BPS or critical-care pain observation tool (CPOT) for patients who cannot self-report pain
- Do not use vital signs alone for pain assessment in ICU patients
- Use preemptive analgesia prior to procedures
- Consider IV opioids as the first line to treat non-neuropathic pain
- Non-opioids and co-analgesics such as gabapentin or carbamazepine be considered for use with opioids
- Epidural analgesia is recommended for rib fractures and postoperative analgesia for abdominal aortic aneurysm

Data from Barr J, Fraser G. Puntillo K, et al. Clinical practice guidelines for the management of pain, agitation, and delirium in adult patients in the intensive care unit. Crit Care Med. 2013;41(1):263-306.

to peripheral tissues (eg, soft tissue injuries), bone pain (eg, fractures, metastatic disease), and pain associated with indwelling tubes and drains (eg, chest tubes).

One of the NSAIDs commonly used in the acute care setting is ketorolac tromethamine (Toradol). Ketorolac is currently the only parenteral NSAID preparation available in the United States and can be administered safely via the intravenous (IV) route. Intramuscular administration is not recommended due to the potential for irregular and unpredictable absorption. Recommended dosing for ketorolac is a 30-mg loading dose followed by 15 mg every 6 hours. Like all NSAIDs, ketorolac has a ceiling effect where administration of higher doses offers no additional therapeutic benefit yet

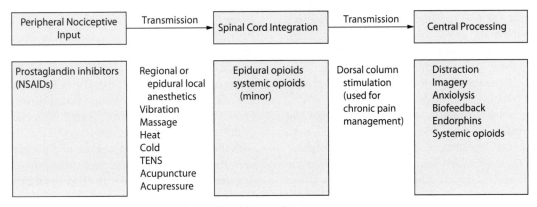

Figure 6-4. A multimodal approach to pain management.

significantly increases the risk of toxicity. Another non-opioid alternative to ketorolac is acetaminophen IV for patients who can tolerate the drug and do not have liver disease or other potential contraindications. The Society of Critical Care Medicine (SCCM) recommends the use of adjuvant analgesics such as NSAIDs to reduce opioid analgesic use and reduce opioid-related side effects.

Side Effects

The side effects associated with the use of NSAIDs relate to the function of prostaglandins in physiologic processes in addition to nociception; for example, gastrointestinal (GI) irritation and bleeding may result from NSAID use because prostaglandins are necessary for maintaining the mucous lining of the stomach. Similarly, the enzyme cyclooxygenase is needed for the eventual production of thromboxane, a key substance involved in platelet function. As a result, when NSAIDs are used chronically or in high doses, platelet aggregation may be altered, leading to bleeding problems. NSAID use can also lead to renal toxicity. Cross-sensitivities with other NSAIDs have also been documented (eg, ibuprofen, naproxen, indomethacin, piroxicam, aspirin). For these reasons, ketorolac and other NSAIDs should be avoided for patients who have a history of gastric ulceration, renal insufficiency, and coagulopathies or a documented sensitivity to aspirin or other NSAIDs. In addition, NSAID use is not recommended in patients with heart disease, recent heart bypass surgery, or patients with a history of ischemic attacks or strokes. An alternative to ketorolac for patients who are not good candidates for NSAIDs is intravenous acetaminophen, as noted above. The severity of all NSAID-related side effects increases with high doses or prolonged use. For this reason, ketorolac and other such drugs are designed for short-term modality only and should not be used for more than 5 days.

OPIOIDS

The principal modality of pain management in the acute care setting continues to be opioids. The SCCM recommends that opioids be considered as first line treatment for non-neuropathic pain. Traditionally referred to as narcotics, opioids produce their analgesic effects primarily by binding with specialized opiate receptors throughout the CNS and thereby altering the perception of pain. Opiate receptors are located in the brain, spinal cord, and GI tract. Although opioids work primarily within the CNS, they also have been shown to have some local or peripheral effects as well. There are at least 45 variations of opiate receptors, which account for the varied response in individual patients.

Opioids are well tolerated by most acutely ill patients and can be administered by many routes including IV, IM, oral, buccal, nasal, rectal, transdermal, and intraspinal. Morphine sulfate is still the most widely used opioid and serves as the gold standard against which others are compared. Other opioids commonly used in the care of the acutely ill include hydromorphone (Dilaudid) and fentanyl (Sublimaze).

Opioid polymorphisms may cause opioids to affect patients differently, thus careful use and assessment of the drugs are necessary to determine optimal dosing.

Side Effects

Patient's responses to opioids, both analgesic responses and side effects, are highly individualized. Just as all the opioid agents have similar pain-relieving potential, all opioids currently available share similar side effect profiles. When side effects do occur, it is important to remember that they are primarily the result of opioid pharmacology, as opposed to the route of administration.

Nausea and Vomiting

Nausea and vomiting are distressing side effects often related to opioids that, unfortunately, many patients experience. Generally, nausea and vomiting result from stimulation of the chemoreceptor trigger zone (CTZ) in the brain and/or from slowed GI peristalsis. Nausea and vomiting often can be managed effectively with antiemetic modality. Metoclopramide (Reglan), a procainamide derivative, works both centrally at the CTZ and at the GI level to increase gastric motility. However, there are significant risks with metoclopramide use such as the potential for seizures and tardive dyskinesia. These conditions occur more commonly in the elderly and with prolonged use of the drug.

The vestibular system also sends input to the CTZ. For this reason, opioid-related nausea frequently is exacerbated by movement. If patients complain of movement-related nausea, the application of a transdermal scopolamine patch can help prevent and treat opioid-induced nausea. The use of transdermal scopolamine is best avoided in patients older than 60 years because the drug has been reported to increase the incidence and severity of confusion in older patients.

The phenothiazines (ie, prochlorperazine [Compazine], 2.5-10 mg IV) and the butyrophenones (droperidol [Inapsine], 0.625 mg IV) treat nausea through their effects at the CTZ. The serotonin antagonist ondansetron (Zofran) is also effective for treatment of opioid-related nausea. The doses required for postoperative or opioid-related nausea are significantly smaller doses (4 mg IV) than those used with emetogenic chemotherapy.

Pruritus

Pruritus is another opioid-related side effect commonly reported by patients. The actual mechanisms producing opioid-related pruritus are unknown. Although antihistamines can provide symptomatic relief for some patients, the role of histamine in opioid-related pruritus is unclear. One of the drawbacks of using antihistamine agents, such as diphenhydramine (Benadryl), is the sedation associated with their use. In addition, the use of diphenhydramine has been shown to have a 70% increase in cognitive deterioration in geriatric patients. Similar to other opioid side effects, the incidence and severity of pruritus is dose-related and tends to diminish with ongoing use. Another option to treat pruritis is nalbuphine (Nubain), dosed at small doses of 2.5 to 5.0 milligrams IV every 6 hours as needed.

Constipation

Constipation, another common side effect, results from opioid binding at opiate receptors in the GI tract and decreased peristalsis. The incidence of constipation may be low in acutely ill patients, but it is important to remember that it is likely to be a problem for many patients following the acute initial phase of their illness or injury. The best treatment for constipation is prevention by ensuring adequate hydration, as well as by administering stimulant laxatives and stool softeners, as needed. For patients with opioid induced constipation, the use of methylnaltrexone (Relistor) can be given as a subcutaneous injection for palliative care patients with advanced illness.

Urinary Retention

Urinary retention can result from increased smooth muscle tone caused by opioids, especially in the detrusor muscle of the bladder. Opioids have no effect on urine production and neither cause nor worsen oliguria.

Respiratory Depression

Opioid modality can result in respiratory depression through its effects on the respiratory centers in the brain stem. Both respiratory rate and the depth of breathing can decrease as a result of opioids, usually in a dose-dependent fashion. Patients at increased risk for respiratory depression include the elderly, those with preexisting cardiopulmonary diseases, patients receiving other respiratory depressive medications such as benzodiazipines, and those who receive large doses. Frequently, the earliest sign of respiratory depression is an increased level of sedation, making this an important component of patient assessment. Other signs and symptoms of respiratory depression include decreased depth of breathing, often combined with slowed respiratory rate, constriction of pupils, hypoxemia, and hypercarbia.

Clinically significant respiratory depression resulting from opiate use is usually treated with IV naloxone (Narcan). Naloxone is an opioid antagonist; it binds with opiate receptors, temporarily displacing the opioid and suspending its pharmacologic effects. As with other medications, naloxone should be administered in very small doses and titrated to the desired level of alertness (Table 6-5). It should be emphasized that the half-life of naloxone is short—approximately

TABLE 6-5. ADMINISTRATION OF NALOXONE

1. Support ventilation.
2. Dilute 0.4 mg (400 mcg) ampule of naloxone with normal saline to constitute a 10-mL solution.
3. Administer in 1-mL increments, every 2-5 minutes, titrating to desired effect. Onset of action: approximately 2 minutes.
4. Continue to monitor patient; readminister naloxone as needed. Duration of action: approximately 45 minutes.
5. For patients requiring ongoing doses, consider naloxone infusion: administer at 50-250 mcg/h, titrating to desired response.

30 to 45 minutes. Careful assessment of the patient should continue and because of its short half-life, additional doses of naloxone may be needed.

Naloxone should be used with caution in patients with underlying cardiovascular disease. The acute onset of hypertension, pulmonary hypertension, and pulmonary edema with naloxone administration has been reported. Also, naloxone should be avoided in patients who have developed a tolerance to opioids since opioid antagonists can't precipitate withdrawal or acute abstinence syndrome.

Intravenous Opioids

Many acutely ill patients are unable to use the oral route, thus the IV route is used most often. One of the advantages of IV opioids is their rapid onset of action, allowing for easy titration. Loading doses of IV opioids should be administered to achieve an adequate blood level of the drug. Additional doses can then be administered intermittently to maintain analgesic levels.

Many progressive care patients may benefit from the addition of a continuous IV opioid infusion; for example, patients who may not be able to communicate their pain needs effectively, such as those that are mechanically ventilated, are good candidates for continuous opioid infusions. The continuous infusion not only helps achieve the appropriate blood levels, but also can be easily titrated to maintain consistent blood levels. Patients who experience significant fluctuations in analgesia or side effects related to opioid administration may also benefit from the constant blood levels provided by continuous infusions. Whenever possible, the maintenance dose for the infusion should be based on patient's previous opioid requirements.

Patient-Controlled Analgesia

Patient-controlled analgesia (PCA) pumps can also be used effectively in the progressive care setting with patients who are alert and able to activate the PCA button. With PCA, patients self-administer small doses of an opioid infusion using a programmable pump. PCA prescriptions typically include a bolus dose of the selected drug, a lockout or delay interval, and either a 1- to 4-hour limit; many of the PCA devices also can be programmed to deliver a basal or background infusion. The bolus dose refers to the amount of the drug the patient receives following pump activation. The initial dose usually ranges between 0.5 and 2.0 mg of morphine or its equivalent. The lockout or delay interval typically ranges between 5 and 10 minutes, which is enough time for the prescribed drug to circulate and take effect, yet allows the patient to easily titrate the medication over time. The 1- to 4-hour limit serves as an additional safety feature by regulating the amount of medication the patient can receive over this period of time.

Assessing whether an acutely ill patient is capable of using a PCA is significant to the success of this analgesic modality. PCA should not be prescribed for the patient who is unable to reliably self-administer pain medication (eg, a patient with a decreased level of consciousness). A patient, however, who is cognitively intact but unable to activate the PCA button due to lack of manual dexterity or strength may utilize a PCA device that has been ergonomically adapted to suit the patient with impaired motor abilities (eg, a pressure switch pad). Lastly, if PCA is prescribed, patients, family members, and visitors should be educated that the patient is the only person to activate the PCA device. Family members and friends may think they are helping by activating the PCA device for the patient and not realize this can produce life-threatening sedation and respiratory depression.

Titrating Patient-Controlled Analgesia

Patients using PCAs usually find a dose and frequency that balances pain relief with other medication-related side effects such as sedation. It is best to start PCA modality after the patient has received loading doses to achieve adequate blood levels of the prescribed opioid. For patients who continue to experience pain while using the PCA pump, the first step in titration is to give an additional loading dose and increase the bolus dose, usually by 25%-50% depending on the pain intensity. If patients continue to have pain in spite of the increased dose, the lockout interval or delay should then be reduced, if possible.

Continuous PCA infusions are no longer recommended for the majority of patients as they increase sedation and do not provide additional pain relief. However, in patients who have preexisting opioid tolerance, a continuous infusion may maintain their baseline opioid requirements while the patient-controlled bolus doses are available to help manage any new pain they experience. The hourly dose of the continuous infusion should be equianalgesic to, and calculated from, patients' preexisting opioid requirements.

Regional Analgesia

One additional method of reducing pain for acutely ill patients is to combine standard options such as opioids with a regional analgesia. Commonly, this is done with a block during surgery lasting 6 to 8 hours using local anesthetics or a continuous infusion using a small self-continued elastomeric pump. These pumps include the drug reservoir for the local anesthetic (LA) that resembles a filled softball, and there is a preset flow control that allows the LA to infuse at the preset rate. The pump is attached to a catheter that can be placed as a soaker hose configuration along the surgical incision or along a nerve, such as the femoral nerve, for patients undergoing such procedures as a total knee replacement where a continuous flow can be provided for a period of several days. The concentrations of regional analgesics do not cause motor blockade. This technique is especially helpful for thoracotomy patients where pain with respiratory effort may be significantly reduced.

Switching From IV to Oral Opioid Analgesia

Most often switching from IV to oral opioids is accomplished when acute pain subsides and the patient is able to tolerate oral or enteral nutrition. Patients who receive analgesics by mouth or via the enteral route can experience comparable pain relief to parenteral analgesia with less risk of infection and at lowered cost. Calculating the equianalgesic dose increases the likelihood that the transition to the oral route will be made without loss of pain control. A creative way to wean PCA is to substitute oral or enteral opioid (like morphine or oxycodone) for the amount of drug given by continuous infusion plus one-half of the total dosage of PCA demand doses. Over the next 24 hours, reducing PCA consumption by increasing the lockout period or reducing the bolus size may help transition the patient and narrow the "analgesic gap" between different routes. To prevent opioid overdosage, controlled-release preparations of morphine and oxycodone, designed to be taken less frequently than their immediate-release counterparts, should not be crushed, halved, or administered into enteral feeding tubes to prevent opioid overdosage.

ESSENTIAL CONTENT CASE

Pain Management Using an Epidural Catheter

A 59-year-old man was admitted to the surgical step-down unit following a thoracotomy with wedge resection of the left lung for small-cell lung cancer. On his second postoperative day, his two left pleural chest tubes had a moderate amount of drainage and continuing air leaks. He was alert, responsive, and able to communicate his pain to the nurse. He had a thoracic epidural catheter in place (T7-T8) with a bupivacaine (0.625 mg/mL) and fentanyl (4 mcg/mL) combination infusing at 6 mL/h. He also had an elastomeric infusion device that was providing a localized block at the incision site using a LA only. When asked about his pain level, he said it was 5 on a scale of 0 (no pain) to 10 (worst pain imaginable).

His nurse noticed he was reluctant to cough and seemed to have some difficulty taking a deep breath. She also noticed his oxygen saturation was slowly drifting downward from 97% to 95%. His respiratory rate was increasing, as was his heart rate. When she listened to his breath sounds, they were bilateral and equal, but diminished throughout with scattered rhonchi. When she asked him about his pain, he said his pain was still a 5 as long as he did not move or cough. He also indicated that he tried to avoid taking a deep breath because it would make him cough and that made the pain go to an 8 or 10.

The nurse knew it would be important for this patient to breathe deeply and cough to clear his lungs, but his pain and discomfort were limiting his ability to perform those maneuvers. He also refused to move from the bed to a chair. The nurse discussed strategies to help minimize the pain associated with activity. First, she found an extra pillow for him not only to use as a splint to support his incision and chest wall, but also to stabilize his chest tubes.

Then she called the anesthesiologist to confer about increasing the rate of the bupivacaine/fentanyl infusion to increase the pain relief. She also inquired about adding ketorolac or IV acetaminophen to his analgesic regimen to help with pain associated with the chest tubes. Because the patient also had an elastomeric infusion pump with LA along the surgical incision the nurse checked to make sure the clamp was open and the medication was infusing.

The anesthesiologist prescribed a bolus of 3 mLs of the epidural solution via the pump and increased the continuous rate to 8 mL/h and added ketorolac, 15 mg, IV every 6 hours and a dose of IV acetaminophen. Over the course of the next 2 hours, the patient was able to cough more effectively, with less pain. His oxygen saturation returned to 97% and he was also able to sit in his chair for lunch.

Case Question 1. What are the advantages of using epidural analgesia?

(A) Local anesthetic blocks the entire surgical area.
(B) Combining an opioid with LA improves pain relief, decreases opioid needs, and can increase respiratory efforts.
(C) An epidural provides the patient with a method of continuous pain relief.
(D) Patients like epidurals because they provide superior pain relief.

Case Question 2. What is the value of adding toradol or acetaminophen to the pain regimen?

(A) IV medications work very quickly.
(B) The two medications do not make the patient sedated.
(C) Adding non-opioid medications can reduce opioid needs and decrease opioid-related side effects.
(D) Patients have fewer allergies to non-opioid medications.

Answers
1. B
2. C

ESSENTIAL CONTENT CASE

The Addicted Patient

A 22-year-old woman was admitted to the cardio-vascular ICU (CVICU) following a tricuspid valve replacement related to recurrent subacute bacterial endocarditis. She has a self-reported history of heroin use (approximately 2 g/day).

She was extubated within the first 24 hours after surgery and was transferred to the cardiovascular step-down unit for further management. During the unit transfer report the CVICU nurse commented that "... she is a constant whine. She refuses to do anything. All she wants is to go out for a smoke and more drugs. She had 10 mg of IV morphine from the PCA pump."

When the step-down unit nurse came into this patient's room to make her initial assessment, the patient said, "I can't take much more of this pain." The nurse probed further and asked her to use some numbers to describe her pain. She replied, "It's at 10!"

The nurse noticed that the patient was reluctant to move and refused to cough. Her vital signs were:

Heart rate	130 beats/min
BP	150/85 mm Hg
Temperature	38.5°C (orally)
Respiration rate	26 breaths/min, shallow

The nurse was concerned that because of this patient's preoperative use of heroin, she might not be receiving adequate doses of morphine. She consulted the clinical nurse specialist for assistance in calculating an equivalent dose of morphine based on the usual heroin use. Using an estimated equivalence of heroin of 1 g = 10 to 15 mg morphine, the nurse calculated that the patient would need approximately 20 to 30 mg of morphine per day to account for her pre-existing opioid tolerance. Consequently, analgesic dosing related to her surgery would need to be relative to this baseline requirement. The patient's nurse approached the surgical team to discuss the potential benefits of using a PCA pump in addition to a continuous infusion of morphine. "By doing this," the nurse explained, "she will receive her baseline opioid requirements related to her tolerance by the continuous infusion, while using the patient-controlled boluses to treat her new surgical pain. The PCA may also offer her some control during a time in her recovery when there are few options to do so. In addition to starting the PCA with a continuous infusion, the surgical team and the primary nurse also discussed using other nonopioid agents such as NSAIDs to augment her analgesia. The team also discussed adding morphine sulfate controlled-release (MS-Contin) to the patient's regimen once she was more comfortable on the PCA and titrating the oral medication doses up while decreasing the PCA. Once the MS-Contin was titrated to an effective dose, the PCA could be discontinued and short-acting oral breakthrough medication used for additional pain relief. The nurse noted she would also need to monitor the patient for any signs or symptoms of withdrawal.

In addition to the changes in the medications, the primary nurse worked with the patient to use relaxation techniques. The nurse explained that relaxation techniques could be thought of as "boosters" to her pain medications and were something that she could do to control the pain. They also agreed to try massage in the evening to try to promote sleep and relaxation.

Case Question 1. In order to maintain adequate pain control after surgery in a patient who is addicted to heroin or takes regular opioids the nurse will need to:

(A) Provide a continuous rate on the PCA.
(B) Provide a continuous rate on the PCA to account for her pre-surgical heroin usage and add additional pain medications for the surgical pain.
(C) Try to limit the patient's opioid use because she is an addict.
(D) Substitute a non-opioid medication such as acetaminophen or ketorolac because the patient is an addict.

Case Question 2. The best way to control postoperative pain is to:

(A) Use opioids exclusively.
(B) Use only medications.
(C) Encourage the patient to cough and deep breathe.
(D) Use a multimodal approach with medications and complementary techniques such as relaxation.

Answers
1. B
2. D

EPIDURAL ANALGESIA

Over the past decade the use of epidural analgesia has grown rapidly. The advantages of epidural analgesia include improved pain control with less sedation, lower overall opioid doses, and generally longer duration of pain management. Epidural analgesia has been associated with a lower morbidity and mortality in acutely ill patients. Both opioids and local anesthetics (LAs), either alone or in combination, commonly are administered via the epidural route. Epidural analgesia may be administered by several methods, including intermittent bolus dosing, continuous infusion, or PCA technology. The mechanisms of action and the resultant clinical effects produced by epidurally administered opioids and LAs are distinct. For this reason, these agents not only are discussed separately, but also should be distinguished when used in clinical practice.

Epidural Opioids

When opioids are administered epidurally, they diffuse into the cerebrospinal fluid and into the spinal cord (Figure 6-5). There, the opioids bind with opiate receptors in the substantia gelatinosa, preventing the release of the neurotransmitter, substance P, and subsequently alter the transmission of nociceptive impulses from the spinal cord to the brain. Because the opioid is concentrated in the areas of high opiate receptor density and where nociceptive impulses are entering the spinal cord, lower doses offer enhanced analgesia, with few, if any, supraspinal effects such as drowsiness.

A variety of opioids are commonly used for epidural analgesia including morphine, fentanyl, and hydromorphone. Preservative-free (PF) preparations are usually preferred because some preservative agents can have neurotoxic effects. The opioids can be administered either by intermittent bolus or continuous infusion depending on the pharmacokinetic activity of the selected agent; for example, fentanyl is generally administered via continuous infusion due to its high lipid solubility, resulting in a short duration of action. In contrast, the low lipid solubility of PF morphine results in a delayed onset of action (30-60 minutes) and a prolonged duration of action (6-12 hours). Because of the delayed onset of action taking as long as 60 minutes, PF morphine is recommended for use as a continuous infusion but not as a patient-controlled bolus dose.

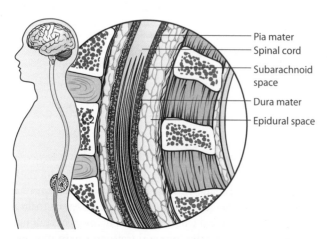

Figure 6-5. Epidural space for catheter placement.

- Pia mater
- Spinal cord
- Subarachnoid space
- Dura mater
- Epidural space

Side Effects

The side effects associated with epidural opioids are the same as those described for oral opioids. It is important to remember that side effects are related more closely to the drug administered than by the route of administration; for example, the incidence of nausea and vomiting with epidural morphine is similar to that associated with IV morphine. Although epidural opioids were once feared to be associated with a higher risk of respiratory depression, clinical studies and experience have not confirmed this risk. The incidence of respiratory depression has been reported as being no higher than 0.2%. Risk factors for respiratory depression are similar to those seen with IV opioids: increasing age, high doses, underlying cardiopulmonary dysfunction, obstructive sleep apnea, obesity, and the use of perioperative or supplemental parenteral opioids or other agents causing sedation such as benzodiazipines in addition to epidural opioids.

Epidural Local Anesthetics

Epidural opioids can also be combined with dilute concentrations of LAs. When administered in combination, these agents work synergistically, reducing the amount of each agent that is needed to produce analgesia. Whereas epidurally administered opioids work in the dorsal horn of the spinal cord, epidural LAs exert work primarily at the dorsal nerve root by blocking the conduction of afferent sensory fibers. The extent of the blockade is dose related. Higher LA concentrations block more afferent fibers within a given region, resulting in an increased density of the blockade. Higher infusion rates of LA-containing solutions increase the extent or spread of the blockade because more afferent fibers are blocked over a broader region.

Bupivacaine is the LA most commonly used for epidural analgesia and is usually administered in combination with either fentanyl or PF morphine as a continuous infusion. The concentration of bupivacaine used for epidural analgesia usually ranges between 1/16% (0.065 mg/mL) and 1/8% (1.25 mg/mL). These concentrations are significantly lower than those used for surgical anesthesia, which usually range between 1/4% and 1/2% bupivacaine. The type and concentration of opioid used in combination with bupivacaine vary by practitioner and organizational preferences, but usually range between 2 and 5 mcg/mL fentanyl or between 0.02 and 0.04 mg/mL PF morphine. Ropivacaine, a LA alternative to bupivacaine, has a lower profile for causing motor block. For older patients with rib fractures or flail chest, an epidural catheter with LA only may provide positive results with less respiratory compromise and reduced pain.

Side Effects

The side effects accompanying LAs are a direct result of the conduction blockade produced by the agents. Unfortunately, the LA agents are relatively nonspecific in their capacity to block nerve conduction. That is, LAs not only block sensory afferent fibers, but also can block the conduction of motor efferent and autonomic nerve fibers within the same dermatomal regions. Side effects associated with epidural LAs include hypotension—especially postural hypotension from sympathetic blockade—and functional motor deficits from varying degrees of efferent motor fiber blockade. Sensory deficits, including changes in proprioception in the joints of the lower extremities, can accompany epidural LA administration due to the blockade of non-nociceptive sensory afferents.

The extent and type of side effects that can be anticipated with epidural LAs depend on three primary factors: the location of the epidural catheter, the concentration of the LA administered, and the volume or rate of infusion; for example, if a patient has an epidural catheter placed within the midthoracic region, one can anticipate signs of sympathetic nervous blockade, such as postural hypotension, because the sympathetic nerve fibers are concentrated in the thoracic region. In contrast, a patient with a lumbar catheter may experience a mild degree of motor weakness in the lower extremities because the motor efferent and nerves exit the spine in the lumbar region. This usually presents clinically as either heaviness in a lower extremity or an inability to "lock" the knee in place when standing.

Also, as noted, both the concentration and infusion rate of the LA influence the severity and extent of side effects. The density of the blockade and intensity of observed side effects may be increased with high LA concentrations. With higher infusion volumes, greater spread of the LA can be anticipated which can, in turn, lead to a greater number or extent of side effects. If side effects occur, the dose of the LA often is reduced either by decreasing the concentration of the solution or by decreasing the rate.

Titrating Epidural Analgesia

To maximize epidural analgesia, doses may need to be adjusted. With opioids alone, the dose needed to produce effective analgesia is best predicted by the patient's age as opposed to body size. Older patients typically require lower doses to achieve pain relief than those who are younger. Small bolus doses of fentanyl (50 mcg) can help safely titrate the epidural dose or infusion to treat pain. Similarly, a small bolus dose of fentanyl can also help treat breakthrough pain that may occur with increased patient activity or procedures. For patients receiving combinations of LAs and opioids, a small bolus dose of the prescribed infusate in conjunction with an increased rate can help titrate pain relief. Recall, however, that increasing the rate of the LA infusion increases the spread of the drug to additional dermatomes, whereas increasing the LA concentration increases the depth or intensity of the blockade and subsequent analgesia.

CUTANEOUS STIMULATION

One of the primary nonpharmacologic techniques for pain management used in the acute care setting is cutaneous stimulation. Cutaneous stimulation produces its analgesic effect by the altering conduction of sensory impulses as they move from the periphery to the spinal cord through the stimulation of the largest sensory afferent fibers, known as the A-alpha (α) and A-beta (β) fibers. The sensory information transmitted by these large fibers is conducted more rapidly than that carried by their smaller counterparts (A-delta (δ) and C fibers) (see Figure 6-3). As a result, nociceptive input from the A-delta and C fibers is believed to be *preempted* by the sensory input from the non-noxious cutaneous stimuli. Examples of cutaneous stimulation include the application of heat, cold, vibration, or massage. Transcutaneous electrical nerve stimulation units produce similar effects by electrically stimulating large sensory fibers.

Cutaneous stimulation can produce analgesic effects whether used as a complementary modality with other pharmacologic treatments or as an independent treatment modality. Nurses can integrate these modalities easily and safely into analgesic treatment plans for the acutely ill, especially for patients who may be unable to tolerate higher opioid doses. To apply or administer cutaneous stimulation, one simply needs to stimulate sensory fibers anywhere between the site of injury and the spinal cord, but within the sensory dermatome (Figure 6-6). Massage, especially back massage, has additional analgesic benefits; it has been shown to promote relaxation and sleep, both of which can influence patient's responses to pain.

DISTRACTION

Distraction techniques such as music, conversation, television viewing, laughter, and deep breathing for relaxation can be valuable adjuncts to pharmacologic modalities. These techniques produce their analgesic effects by sending intense stimuli through the thalamus, midbrain, and brain stem which can increase the production of modulating substances such as endorphins. Also, because the brain can process only a limited amount of incoming signals at any given time, the input provided by distraction techniques *competes* with nociceptive inputs. This is particularly true for the reticular activating system.

When planning for and using distraction techniques, keep in mind that they are most effective when activities are interesting to the patient (eg, their favorite type of music, television program, or video) and when they involve multiple senses such as hearing, vision, touch, and movement. Activities should be consistent with patient's energy levels and, most of all, be flexible to meet changing demands.

IMAGERY

Imagery is another technique that can be used effectively with acutely ill patients, particularly during planned procedures. Imagery alters the perception of pain stimuli within the brain, promotes relaxation, and increases the production of endorphins in the brain. Patients can use imagery independently or use guided imagery where either a care provider,

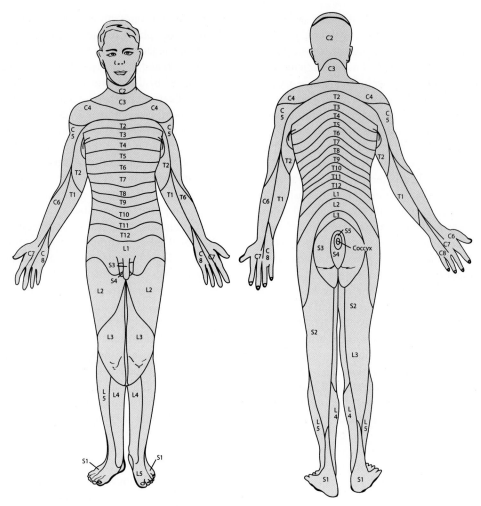

Figure 6-6. Sensory dermatomes.

family member, or friend helps *guide* the patient in painting an imaginary picture. The more details that can be pictured with the image, the more effective it can be. As with distraction techniques, tapping into multiple sensations is beneficial. Some patients prefer to involve the pain in their picture and imagine it melting or fading away. Other patients may prefer to paint a picture in their mind of a favorite place or activity. Strategies to help guide patients include the use of details to describe the imaginary scene (eg, "smell the fresh scent of the ocean air" or "see the intense red hue of the sun setting beyond the snow-capped mountains") and the use of relaxing sensory terms such as floating, smooth, dissolving, lighter, or melting. If the patients are able to talk, it can be helpful to have them describe the image they see using appropriate detail, although some patients will prefer not to talk and instead focus on their evolving image. Again, it is important to be flexible in the approach to imagery to maximize its benefits.

RELAXATION TECHNIQUES

Because acutely ill patients experience numerous stressors, most patients benefit from the inclusion of relaxation or anxiolytic therapies. The use of relaxation techniques can help interrupt the vicious cycle involving pain, anxiety, and muscle tension that often develops when pain goes unrelieved. The physiologic response associated with relaxation includes decreased oxygen consumption, respiratory rate, heart rate, and muscle tension; blood pressure may either normalize or decrease.

A wide variety of pharmacologic and nonpharmacologic techniques can be used safely and effectively with progressive care patients to achieve relaxation and/or sedation. Relaxation techniques are simple to use and can be particularly useful in situations involving brief procedures such as turning or minor dressing changes, and following coughing or endotracheal suctioning or other stressful events.

Deep Breathing and Progressive Relaxation

Guided deep breathing and progressive relaxation can be incorporated easily into a plan of care for the progressive care patient. Nurses can coach patients with deep breathing exercises by helping them to focus on and guide their breathing patterns. As patients begin to control their breathing, nurses can work with them to begin progressive relaxation of their muscles. To do this, the nurse can say to the patient as he or she just begins to exhale, "Now begin to relax, from the top of your head to the tips of your toes." Change the pitch of the voice to be higher for "top of your head," lower for "tips of your toes," and be timed such that the final phrase ends as the patient completes exhalation. This procedure capitalizes on the positive aspects of normal body functions, as the body tends to relax naturally during exhalation. This process can and should be *practiced* during nonstressful periods to augment its efficacy. In fact, teaching and coaching patients to use deep breathing exercises helps equip them with a lifelong skill that can be used any time stressful or painful situations arise.

Presence

Probably the single most important aspect of promoting comfort in the ill or injured is the underlying relationship between the patient, the family, and his or her care providers. Family presence at the patient's bedside has been shown to decrease anxiety and promote healing. Including the people identified by the patient as his or her family support (with a broad definition of family) can provide enormous comfort for the patient resulting in relaxation. Presence not only refers to physically "being there," but also refers to psychologically "being with" a patient. Although presence has not been well-defined as an intervention protocol, patients regularly describe the importance of the support that their nurses render simply by "being there" and "being with" them.

SPECIAL CONSIDERATIONS FOR PAIN MANAGEMENT IN THE ELDERLY

The pain experience of elderly patients has often been shadowed by myths and misperceptions. Some believe that older patients have less pain because their extensive life experiences have equipped them to cope with discomfort more effectively. This may be true for some individuals—to accept this generalization as truth for all elderly patients is short sighted. In fact, the incidence of and morbidity associated with pain is higher in the elderly than in the general population. Many elderly patients continue to experience chronic pain in addition to any acute pain associated with their illness or injury. Major sources of underlying pain in the elderly include low back pain, arthritis, headache, chest pain, and neuropathies.

Assessment

Elderly patients often report pain very differently from younger patients due to physiologic, psychological, and cultural changes accompanying age. Some patients may fear loss of control, loss of independence, or being labeled as a "bad patient" if they report pain-related concerns. Also, for some patients the presence of pain may be symbolic of impending death, especially in the acute care setting. In such cases, a patient may be reticent to report his or her pain to a care provider or family member as if to deny pain is to deny death. For reasons such as these, it is important for nurses not only to assure patients about the nature of their pain and the

importance of reporting any discomfort. Nurses may also use a variety of pain assessment strategies to incorporate behavioral or physiologic indicators of pain.

Similar strategies are often needed to assess pain in persons who are cognitively impaired. Preliminary reports from ongoing work among nursing home patients suggest that many patients with moderate to severe cognitive impairment are able to report acute pain reliably at the time they are asked. For these patients, pain recall and integration of pain experience over time may be less reliable.

Interventions

Acutely ill elderly patients can benefit from any of the analgesic therapies discussed. Older patients can tolerate opioids well if the doses are individualized and the patient is monitored for effect. However, it is important to recognize that medication requirements may be reduced in some elderly patients due to age-related renal insufficiency and the potential for decreased renal clearance of the drugs. In addition, they have a reduced muscle to body fat ratio which affects the way that opioids bind and activate in the body. Analgesic requirements are highly individualized and doses should be carefully titrated to achieve pain relief.

SEDATION

The progressive care environment can be uncomfortable and anxiety provoking for patients. Once pain is addressed, anxiolysis may be appropriate to enhance comfort, decrease anxiety, reduce awareness of noxious stimuli, and induce sleep. In some cases, the use of sedatives may be necessary to ensure tolerance of medical modalities, clinical stability, and to protect patients from inadvertent self-harm. While the treatment of anxiety is an important aspect of the care of patients who are acutely ill, frequent dosing methods (infusions or IV boluses) intended to induce a more depressed sensorium (ie, amnesia) in these patients is discouraged. The use of sedation infusions in mechanically-ventilated patients has been associated with negative outcomes such as prolonged mechanical ventilation, increased lengths of stay, and even death. To that end, in critical care and progressive care units where mechanically-ventilated patients are cared for, nurses must focus on how best to minimize infusion use. Daily interruptions of sedation infusions have been associated with improved outcomes and do not appear to incur additional psychological stress. This finding is in direct opposition to the commonly held philosophy that amnesia protects the patient from the psychological stress induced by critical or acute care environments. Further, there is a strong association between sedation infusion use and delirium. Compounding the issue is the fact that those who develop delirium are then at risk for the development of long-term cognitive dysfunction. Because of this finding and other studies demonstrating the positive effect of less sedation use in ventilated patients, recent Society of Critical Care Medicine (SCCM) evidence-based guidelines recommend treating pain first, light sedation if necessary, and the use of nonpharmacologic means of promoting sleep. To ensure that appropriate and adequate anxiolysis is achieved in the acutely ill patient, the nurse must be able to identify the reason for sedation, the drugs most commonly used, the level of sedation required, and how to monitor and manage the sedated patient. Clear identification of the reason for sedation is the first step in the process.

Reasons for Sedation

Amnesia

One of the most common reasons for sedative use is to ensure amnesia. Many of the procedures and interventions performed in acute care units may potentially cause pain and anxiety. In anticipation of this, sedatives are proactively administered, often concomitantly with analgesics. Moderate sedation (also called conscious sedation) is commonly employed in these situations; it is discussed later in this chapter.

Ventilator Tolerance

Ineffective, dyssynchronous, and excessive respiratory effort results in increased work of breathing and oxygen consumption. The reason for the dyssynchronous breathing should be quickly assessed and managed. Efforts should be made to improve tolerance by first treating potential pain and adjusting the ventilator to optimize patient-ventilator interaction. But sedative use in severe cases of patient/ventilator dyssynchrony may also be necessary, and in some cases, lifesaving. These patients are generally transferred to a critical care unit for care management. For more in-depth information on advanced modes of ventilation see Chapter 20 in the *AACN Essentials of Critical Care Nursing, 3rd edition.*

Anxiety and Fear

Anxiety and fear are symptoms that can be experienced by acutely ill patients. However, these symptoms may be difficult to assess in acutely ill patients, especially if they are unable to adequately communicate their feelings secondary to the underlying condition, the presence of an artificial airway, or a reduced sensorium.

When the patient can identify anxiety or fear, the treatment goals are clear. However, in the patient who cannot, the presence of behaviors and signs that are associated with anxiety and/or fear are used as evidence and are the reason sedatives are provided. Manifestations of severe anxiety and/or fear include nonspecific signs of distress such as agitation, thrashing, diaphoresis, facial grimacing, blood pressure elevation, and increased heart rate. These nonspecific signs may also be indicative of pain or may be due to delirium. Pain management requirements must be addressed prior to the administration of sedation in such cases as well as assessing the patient for potential delirium.

Patient Safety and Agitation

Agitation includes any activity that appears unhelpful or potentially harmful to the patient. The patient may be aware of the activity and be able to communicate the reason for the activity; more commonly they are not aware, making it difficult to identify the reason for the agitation. The patient appears distressed and the associated activity includes episodic or continuous nonpurposeful movements in the bed, severe thrashing, attempts to remove tubes, efforts to get out of bed, or other behaviors which may threaten patient or staff safety. Reasons for agitation include pain and anxiety, delirium, preexisting conditions that require pharmacologic interventions (ie, preexisting psychiatric history), withdrawal from certain medications such as benzodiazepines (especially if they have been on them for a long time), and delirium tremens secondary to alcohol withdrawal (see Chapter 11 Multisystem Problems, section on alcohol withdrawal). Patients who experience inadequately controlled agitation face a high risk of morbidity and mortality. Thus potential reasons for the agitation are explored so that appropriate therapy may be initiated.

Sleep Deprivation

Sleep deprivation is common among hospitalized patients. Although patients may appear restful, physiologically they may never experience stages of sleep that ensure a "rested" state (ie, rapid eye movement sleep, and stages 2, 3, and 4). These restorative stages of sleep are adversely affected by many factors, including a wide variety of medications. Sleep deprivation is also common among those with pain, discomfort, and anxiety. Additionally, sleep deprivation may be a result of the increased auditory, tactile, and visual stimuli ubiquitous to the hospital environment. The SCCM guidelines recommend the use of nonpharmacologic interventions when possible.

Delirium

Delirium is more prevalent in acutely ill patients than previously assumed. Patients are especially at risk if they have been on sedatives, especially by infusion for longer than 24 hours, are elderly, have preexisting dementia, a history of hypertension, and high severity of illness at admission. Coma is an independent risk factor for the development of delirium. As noted earlier, the risk of long-term cognitive dysfunction is increased in patients who experience delirium. In the past delirium was commonly associated with agitation. In fact, the agitated presentation of delirium accounts for less than 5% of those who experience the condition. The remainder presents with the hypoactive (calm, quiet) or mixed presentation of the condition. This hypoactive category is underdiagnosed and the associated outcomes are worse than for those with the agitated/active form of delirium. The hallmarks of the condition are disorientation and disorganized thinking. Awareness of the potential for delirium and early recognition are essential for effective management and prevention of undesirable outcomes. Routine assessment of delirium should be done with the use of a valid and reliable delirium-monitoring tool such as the confusion assessment method for the ICU (CAM-ICU) that many acute care units are increasingly adopting for use in selected patients. The drugs of choice for delirium in the acute care setting are described later in this chapter under "Drugs for Delirium" and further discussed in Chapter 7 Pharmacology.

Drugs for Sedation

After ensuring that the presence of pain is either ruled out or addressed with the appropriate administration of analgesics, sedatives may be selected based on patient-specific factors such as the level and duration of sedation required. Sedative category summaries follow and comprehensive descriptions of the drugs are discussed in Chapter 7 Pharmacology.

Short-Term Sedatives

These sedatives have a rapid onset of action and a short duration of effect.

- *Midazolam* is a popular benzodiazepine that fits in this category. It can be administered intermittently in a bolus IV form or as a continuous infusion. Generally continuous infusions of midazolam are reserved for the critical care unit.
- *Ketamine* is an IV *general* anesthetic that produces analgesia, anesthesia, and amnesia without loss of consciousness. It may be given in an IV bolus form, intranasally, or orally. Although contraindicated in those with elevated intracranial pressure, its bronchodilatory properties make it a good choice in those with asthma. A well-known side effect of ketamine is hallucinations; however, these may be prevented with concurrent use of benzodiazepines. It is rarely a first-line sedative of choice, but is commonly used in patients requiring painful, frequent skin debridement procedures (eg, burn patients). The nurse needs to be aware of the hospital policy for use of this medication as some hospitals limit it to physician use only and/or use in ICUs.

Intermediate-Term Sedatives

These drugs have an intermediate onset of action and duration of effect. However, when given as infusions they may last much longer as they are lipophilic. Generally, continuous infusions of the drug are reserved for the critical care unit.

- *Lorazepam* is the most common benzodiazepine in acute care and can be administered orally and IV as an intermittent bolus or continuous infusion. When given orally or in a bolus intermittent form, the drug effect is intermediate; however, when used as a continuous infusion (24 hours), its effect is more long term (and it should be considered as such) because awakening may take hours to days to accomplish. Lorazepam, if given frequently or by infusion, may accumulate in those with decreased metabolic function such as the elderly or those with hepatic dysfunction.

Long-Acting Sedatives

- *Diazepam,* a long acting benzodiazepine, and *chlordiazepoxide* are infrequently used in acute care; however, they may be selected for treatment of severe alcohol withdrawal. They may be given orally or as an IV bolus.

Drugs for Delirium

In the past, the drug of choice for treatment of delirium was haloperidol. However, no evidence supports the use of haloperidol as a pharmacologic agent to reduce the duration of delirium. The drug has been popular in the past because it sedates without significant respiratory depression and is not associated with potential development of tolerance or dependence. It does, however, have potential adverse side effects that must be closely monitored. Extrapyramidal reactions such as dystonia and the potential for neuroleptic malignant syndrome are possible. Another is the effect of haloperidol on QTc intervals; QTc interval monitoring is essential and required when using the drug. Atypical antipsychotics such as risperidone and olanzapine have been used, but little data exist to support widespread use of the drugs for the treatment of delirium. Critical care units are now encouraged to decrease benzodiazepine use due to the association of the drugs with delirium. It is hoped that this will result in less delirium in those transferred to progressive care units as well. In addition, the use of nonpharmacologic interventions may be helpful in decreasing the incidence of delirium in acute care (see Chapter 7 Pharmacology for more on these classes of drugs).

Goals of Sedation, Monitoring, and Management

The goal of sedation administration is important to identify (anxiety, sleep, ventilator tolerance, amnesia, etc) and once accomplished an appropriate level of sedation may be determined. When the sedation goal is to produce deep sedation, as in the case of an agitated, ventilated patient with oxygenation problems, intubation and ventilation may be necessary and the patient may need to be transferred to a critical care unit for vigilant monitoring. Monitoring of the patient's sedation level is often accomplished using sedation scales. Sedation scales have been developed in an effort to assist with the management of sedation in these cases, especially if the sedation requirements are anticipated to last for longer than a few hours. The SCCM evidence-based guidelines recommend the use of two tested and reliable sedation scales that may be used for these patients (see Table 6-6).

Moderate or Conscious Sedation

A technique referred to as "moderate sedation" (also known as conscious sedation) is common in progressive, acute care, and special procedure units (interventional radiology, endoscopy, etc). It refers to the use of a combination of analgesics and sedatives to minimize discomfort during a procedure while assuring that the patient is able to communicate throughout

TABLE 6-6. SEDATION ASSESSMENT SCALES WITH VALIDITY AND RELIABILITY IN ADULT PATIENTS

Sedation-Agitation Scale[a]	Richmond Agitation-Sedation Scale[b]
1 Unarousable (minimal or no response to noxious stimuli, does not communicate or follow commands)	– 5 Unresponsive (no response to voice or physical stimulation)
2 Very sedated (arouses to physical stimuli but does not communicate or follow commands; may move spontaneously)	– 4 Deep sedation (no response to voice, but any movement to physical stimulation)
3 Sedated (difficult to arouse, awakens to verbal stimuli or gentle shaking but drifts off again, follows simple commands)	– 3 Moderate sedation (any movement, but no eye contact to voice)
4 Calm and cooperative (calm, awakens easily, follows commands)	– 2 Light sedation (briefly, < 10 seconds, awakening with eye contact to voice)
5 Agitated (anxious or mildly agitated, attempting to sit up, calms down to verbal instructions)	– 1 Drowsy (not fully alert, but has sustained, > 10 seconds, awakening with eye contact to voice)
6 Very agitated (does not calm, despite frequent verbal reminding of limits; requires physical restraints, biting ET tube)	0 Alert and calm
7 Dangerous agitation (pulling at ET tube, trying to remove catheter, climbing over bed rail, striking at staff, thrashing side to side)	1 Restless (anxious or apprehensive but movements not aggressive or vigorous)
	2 Agitated (frequent nonpurposeful movement or patient-ventilator dysynchrony)
	3 Very agitated (pulls on or removes tubes or catheters or has aggressive behavior toward staff)
	4 Combative (overly combative or violent; immediate danger to staff)

Data compiled from: [a]Riker R, Picard J, Fraser G, et al (1994); and [b]Sessler C, Gosnet M, Grap MJ, et al (2002).

the procedure. Amnesia is anticipated and often desired. The patient's ability to maintain a patent airway is central to the decision related to the use of moderate sedation. Patients considered "lowest risk" are generally those who are recommended for the technique, although higher risk individuals may also be recommended based on consultation with the healthcare team. The American Society of Anesthesiology Patient Classification Status is used to determine level of risk (Table 6-7). Institutional guidelines for the use of moderate sedation vary somewhat however, they generally include the use of continuous real-time monitoring such as respiratory rate and pattern, pulse oximetry and heart rhythm in addition to very frequent (ie, every 5 minutes during the procedure) assessment of vitals signs and evaluation of level of consciousness.

In contrast, there are times when the sedation goal is to produce deeper sedation as in the case of an agitated ventilated patient with oxygenation problems. Sedation scales have

TABLE 6-7. ASA CONTINUUM OF DEPTH OF SEDATION: DEFINITION OF GENERAL ANESTHESIA AND LEVELS OF SEDATION/ANALGESIA

	Minimal Sedation (Anxiolysis)	Moderate Sedation/Analgesia (Conscious Sedation)	Deep Sedation/Analgesia	General Anesthesia
Responsiveness	Normal response to verbal stimulation	Purposeful* response to verbal or tactile stimulation	Purposeful* response after repeated or painful stimulation	Unarousable, even with painful stimulus
Airway	Unaffected	No intervention required	Intervention may be required	Intervention often required
Spontaneous ventilation	Unaffected	Adequate	May be inadequate	Frequently inadequate
Cardiovascular function	Unaffected	Usually maintained	Usually maintained	May be impaired

Minimal Sedation (Anxiolysis) = a drug-induced state during which patients respond normally to verbal commands. Although cognitive function and coordination may be impaired, ventilatory and cardiovascular functions are unaffected.

Moderate Sedation/Analgesia (Conscious Sedation) = a drug-induced depression of consciousness during which patients respond purposefully* to verbal commands, either alone or accompanied by light tactile stimulation. No interventions are required to maintain a patent airway, and spontaneous ventilation is adequate. Cardiovascular function is usually maintained.

Deep Sedation/Analgesia = a drug-induced depression of consciousness during which patients cannot be easily aroused but respond purposefully* following repeated or painful stimulation. The ability to independently maintain ventilatory function may be impaired. Patients may require assistance in maintaining a patent airway, and spontaneous ventilation may be inadequate. Cardiovascular function is usually maintained.

General Anesthesia = a drug-induced loss of consciousness during which patients are not arousable, even by painful stimulation. The ability to independently maintain ventilatory function is often impaired. Patients often require assistance in maintaining a patent airway, and positive pressure ventilation may be required because of depressed spontaneous ventilation or drug-induced depression of neuromuscular function. Cardiovascular function may be impaired.

Because sedation is a continuum, it is not always possible to predict how an individual patient will respond. Hence, practitioners intending to produce a given level of sedation should be able to rescue patients whose level of sedation becomes deeper than initially intended. Individuals administering Moderate Sedation/Analgesia (Conscious Sedation) should be able to rescue patients who enter a state of Deep Sedation/Analgesia, while those administering Deep Sedation/Analgesia should be able to rescue patients who enter a state of general anesthesia.

* Reflex withdrawal from a painful stimulus is not considered a purposeful response.

Reproduced with permission from American Society of Anesthesiologists Task Force on Sedation and Analgesia by Non-Anesthesiologists: Practice guidelines for sedation and analgesia by non-anesthesiologists. Anesthesiology. 2002 Apr;96(4):1004-1017.

been developed in an effort to assist with the management of sedation in these cases, especially if the sedation requirements are anticipated to last for longer than a few hours.

Sedation Scales: Goals and Monitoring

Sedation scales allow the nurse to select a level of sedation for the patient in collaboration with the healthcare team. Descriptors of each level of sedation are provided so that the sedative may be adjusted appropriately. When patients in the progressive care areas require aggressive sedation management (eg, for ventilator intolerance), the scales noted above may be helpful. Sedation monitoring in these cases is done at least hourly and the level of sedation achieved is recorded.

Sedation Management

Management of sedation is an essential step in attaining positive outcomes for acutely ill patients. Patients may require sedatives for the treatment of mild to moderate anxiety while in the progressive care unit. Treatment of such anxiety is appropriate and rarely results in adverse effects. Generally the sedatives are provided orally and occasionally as an IV bolus. The doses are adjusted to prevent excessive drowsiness or respiratory depression. Appropriately dosed, use of the sedatives does not interfere with clinical progress such as weaning or rehabilitation. In contrast, it is especially important to consider the effects associated with sedation infusions on outcomes. Generally if a sedation infusion is used in a progressive care unit, its use is short lived and the patient is converted to PO or IV bolus sedation as soon as possible.

In patients who require high levels of sedation to prevent self-harm, sedation infusions and/or frequent IV bolus sedation may be essential. These patients may need to be transferred to a critical care unit if the condition persists.

SELECTED BIBLIOGRAPHY

Pain Management

American Pain Society. *Principles of Analgesic Use in the Treatment of Acute Pain and Cancer Pain*. 6th ed. Glenview, IL: American Pain Society; 2008.

American Society of Pain Management Nursing. *Core Curriculum for Pain Management Nursing*. Dubuque IA: Hunt Publishing; 2009.

Barr J, Fraser G, Puntillo K, et al. Clinical practice guidelines for the management of pain, agitation, and delirium in adult patients in the intensive care unit. *Crit Care Med*. 2013;41(1):263-306.

Barthelmey O, Limbourg T, Collet J, et al. Impact of non-steroidal anti-inflammatory drugs (NSAIDs) on cardiovascular outcomes in patients with stable atherothrombosis or multiple risk factors. *Int J Cardiol*. June 28, 2011.

Bavry A, Khaliq A, Gong Y, Handberg E, Cooper-DeHoff R, Pepine C. Harmful effects of NSAIDs among patients with hypertension and coronary artery disease. *Am J Med*. 2011;124:614-620.

Bennett JS, Daugherty A, Herrington D, Greeneland P, Roberts H, Taubert K. The use of non-steroidal anti-inflammatory drugs (NSAIDs): a science advisory from the American Heart Association. *Circulation*. 2005;111(13):1713-1716.

Berry P, Covington E, Dahl J, Katz J, Miaskowski C. Pain: current understanding of assessment, management, and treatments. Reston VA: National Pharmaceutical Council, Inc., and the Joint Commission on Accreditation of Healthcare Organizations. 2006.

D'Arcy Y. *A Compact Clinical Guide to Acute Pain Management*. New York, NY: Springer Publishing, 2011.

Faucett J. Care of the critically ill patient in pain: the importance of nursing. In: Puntillo KA, ed. *Pain in the Critically Ill*. Gaithersburg, MD: Aspen;1991.

Fine P, Portenoy R. *A Clinical Guide to Opioid Analgesia* New York, NY: Vendome Group LLC, 2007.

Gardner DL. Presence. In: Bulechek GM, McCloskey JC, eds. *Nursing Interventions: Essential Nursing Treatments*. Philadelphia, PA: WB Saunders; 1992:316-324.

Gordon DB, Dahl J, Phillips P, et al. The use of "as-needed" range orders for opioid analgesics in the management of acute pain: a consensus statement of the American Society for Pain Management Nursing and the American Pain Society. *Pain Manag Nurs*. 2004;5:53-58.

Julius D, Basbaum AI. Molecular mechanisms of nociception. *Nature*. 2001;413:203-210.

Khatta M. A complementary approach to pain management. *Adv Pract Nurs*. 2007. Available at www.medscape.com.

Marmo L, D'Arcy Y. *A Compact Clinical Guide to Critical Care, ER, and Trauma Pain Management*. New York, NY: Springer Publishing, 2013.

Maxam-Moore VA, Wilkie DJ, Woods SL. Analgesics for cardiac surgery patients in critical care: describing current practice. *Am J Crit Care*. 1994;3:31-39.

Melton S, Liu S. Regional anesthesia techniques. In: S Fishman, J Ballantyne, J Rathmell (eds). *Bonica's Management of Pain*, 5th ed, Philadelphia PA: Lippincott Williams and Wilkins, 2010, 92-106.

Morrison RS, Ahronheim JC, Morrison GR, et al. Pain and discomfort associated with common hospital procedures and experiences. *J Pain Symptom Manage*. 1998,15:91-101.

Pasternak GW. Molecular biology of opioid analgesia. *J Pain Symptom Manag*. 2005;29(5S):S2-S9.

Pettigrew J. Intensive nursing care: the ministry of presence. *Crit Care Nurs Clin North Am*. 1990;2(3):503-508.

Puntillo K. Advances in management of acute pain: great strides or tiny footsteps? Capsules comments. *Crit Care Nurs*. 1995; 3:97-100.

Puntillo K. Pain experience in intensive care patients. *Heart Lung*. 1990;19:526-533.

Puntillo K, Weiss SJ. Pain: its mediators and associated morbidity in critically ill cardiovascular surgical patients. *Nurs Res*. 1994;43:31-36.

Puntillo KA, Morris AB, Thompson CL, et al. Pain behaviors observed during six common procedures: results from Thunder Project II. *Crit Care Med*. 2004;32(2):421-427.

Puntillo KA, White C, Morris AB, et al. Patients' perceptions and responses to procedural pain: results from Thunder Project II. *Am J Crit Care*. 2001;10(4):238-251.

Puntillo KA, Wild LR, Morris AB, et al. Practices and predictors of analgesic interventions for adults undergoing painful procedures. *Am J Crit Care*. 2002;11(5):415-429.

Puntillo KA, Wilke DJ. Assessment of pain in the critically ill. In: Puntillo KA, ed. *Pain in the Critically Ill*. Gaithersburg, MD: Aspen; 1991:45-64.

Richman J, Liu S, Courpas C, Wong R, Rowlinson A. McGready J Wu C. Does peripheral nerve block provide superior pain control to opioids? A metanalysis. *Anesth and Analg.* 2006;102(1):248-257.

Rose L, Smith O, Gelinas C, et al. Critical care nurses' pain assessment and management practices: a survey in Canada. *Am J Crit Care.* 2012;21(4):151-259.

Schulz-Stübner S, Boezaart A, Hata JS. Regional analgesia in the critically ill. *Crit Care Med.* 2005;33:1400-1407.

Stanik-Hutt JA, Soeken KL, Belcher AE, Fontaine DK, Gift AG. Pain experiences of traumatically injured patients in a critical care setting. *Am J Crit Care.* 2001;10:252-259.

Summer G, Puntillo K. Management of surgical and procedural pain in the critical care setting. *Crit Care Clin North Am.* 2001;13:233-242.

Sun X, Weissman C. The use of analgesics and sedatives in critically ill patients: physicians' orders versus medications administered. *Heart Lung.* 1994;23:169-176.

Thompson C, White C, Wild L, et al. Translating research into practice. *Crit Care Nurs Clin North Am.* 2001;13:541-546.

Tittle M, McMillan SC. Pain and pain-related side effects in an ICU and on a surgical unit: nurses' management. *Am J Crit Care.* 1994;3:25-39.

Wong DL, Baker CM. Pain in children: comparison of assessment scales. *Pediatr Nurs.* 1988;14(1):9-17.

Wu CL, Cohen SR, Richman JM, et al. Efficacy of postoperative patient-controlled and continuous infusion epidural analgesia versus intravenous patient-controlled analgesia with opioids: a meta-analysis. *Anesthesiology.* 2005;103:1079-1088.

Sedation

Brook AD, Ahrens TS, Schaff R, et al. Effect of a nursing-implemented sedation protocol on the duration of mechanical ventilation. *Crit Care Med.* 1999;27:2609-2615.

Ely W, Truman B, Shintani A, et al. Monitoring sedation status over time in ICU patients: reliability and validity of the Richmond Agitation-Sedation Scale (RASS). *JAMA.* 2003;22 (289):2983-2991.

Girard TD, Pandharipande PP, Ely EW. Review: delirium in the intensive care unit. *Crit Care.* 2008;12(suppl 3):1-9.

Kress JP, Gehlbach B, Lacy M, et al. The long-term psychological effects of daily sedative interruption on critically ill patients. *Am J Respir Crit Care Med.* 2003;168:1457-1461.

Kress JP, Pohlman A, O'Connor MF, Hall JB. Daily interruption of sedative infusions in critically ill patients undergoing mechanical ventilation. *N Engl J Med.* 2000;342:1471-1477.

Kress JP, Pohlman AS, Hall JB. Sedation and analgesia in the intensive care unit. *Am J Respir Crit Care Med.* 2002;166:1024-1028.

Riker R, Picard J, Fraser G. Prospective evaluation of the sedation-agitation scale for adult critically ill patients. *Crit Care Med.* 1999;27:1325-1329.

Sessler C, Gosnet M, Grap MJ. The Richmond agitation-sedation scale: validity and reliability in adult intensive care unit patients. *Am J Respir Crit Care Med.* 2002;166:1338-1344.

Evidence-Based Practice Guidelines

American Geriatric Society (AGS). The pharmacological management of persistent pain in older persons. *J Am Geriatr Soc.* 2009;57:1331-1346.

American Society of Anesthesiologists. Practice guidelines for sedation and analgesia by non-anesthesiologists: an updated report by the American Society of Anesthesiologists Task Force on Sedation and Analgesia by non-Anesthesiologists. *Anesthesiology.* 2002; 96:1004-1017.

American Psychiatric Association. Practice guideline for the treatment of patients with delirium. *Am J Psychiatry.* 1999;156:1-20.

American Society of Anesthesiologists Taskforce on Acute Pain Management. Practice guidelines for acute pain management in the perioperative setting. *Anesthesiology,* 2004;100(6):1573-1581.

Barr J, Fraser G, Puntillo K, et al. Clinical practice guidelines for the management of pain, agitation, and delirium in adult patients in the intensive care unit. *Crit Care Med.* 2013;41(1):263-306.

Herr K, Coyne P, Kry T, et al. Pain assessment in the nonverbal patient: position statement with clinical practice recommendations. *Pain Manage Nurs.* 2006; 7(2):44-52.

Woods S. Spiritual and complementary therapies to promote healing and reduce stress. In: Molter NC, ed. *AACN's Protocols for Practice: Creating Healing Environments.* 2nd ed. Sudbury, MA: Jones and Bartlett Publishers; 2007.

PHARMACOLOGY 7

Earnest Alexander

KNOWLEDGE COMPETENCIES

1. Discuss advantages and disadvantages of various routes for medication delivery in acutely ill patients.

2. Identify indications for use, mechanism of action, administration guidelines, side effects, and contraindications for drugs commonly administered in acute illness.

Acutely ill adult patients often receive multiple medications during their admissions to an acute care ward or stepdown unit. These patients may be at risk for increased adverse effects from their medications because of altered metabolism and elimination that is commonly seen in the acutely ill patient. Organ dysfunction or drug interactions may produce increased serum drug or active metabolite concentrations, resulting in enhanced or adverse pharmacologic effects. Therefore, it is important to be familiar with each patient's medications, including the drug's metabolic profile, drug interactions, and adverse effect profile. This chapter reviews medications commonly used in progressive care units and discusses mechanisms of action, indications for use, common adverse effects, contraindications, and usual doses. A summary of intravenous (IV) medication information is provided in Chapter 22: Pharmacology Tables.

MEDICATION SAFETY

In the care of the acutely ill, the medication use process is particularly complex. Each step in the process is fraught with the potential for breakdowns in medication safety (ie, adverse drug events [ADEs], medication errors). Improvement in medication safety requires interdisciplinary focus and attention. The Institute for Safe Medication Practices (ISMP) has highlighted the following key elements which must be optimized in order to maintain patient safety in the medication-use process:

- *Patient information:* Having essential patient information at the time of medication prescribing, dispensing, and administration will result in a significant decrease in preventable ADEs.
- *Drug information:* Providing accurate and usable drug information to all healthcare practitioners involved in the medication-use process reduces the amount of preventable ADEs.
- *Communication of drug information:* Miscommunication between physicians, pharmacists, and nurses is a common cause of medication errors. To minimize medication errors caused by miscommunication, it is important to always verify drug information and eliminate communication barriers.
- *Drug labeling, packaging, and nomenclature:* Drug names that look alike or sound alike, as well as products that have confusing drug labeling and nondistinct drug packaging significantly contribute to medication errors. The incidence of medication errors is reduced with the use of proper labeling and the use of unit dose systems within hospitals.
- *Drug storage, stock, standardization, and distribution:* Standardizing drug administration times, drug concentrations, and limiting the dose concentration of drugs available in patient-care areas will reduce the risk of medication errors or minimize their consequences, should an error occur.

- *Drug device acquisition, use, and monitoring:* Appropriate safety assessment of drug delivery devices should be made both prior to their purchase and during their use. Also, a system of independent double checks should be used within the institution to prevent device-related errors such as, selecting the wrong drug or drug concentration, setting the rate improperly, or mixing the infusion line up with another.
- *Environmental factors:* Having a well-designed system offers the best chance of preventing errors; however, sometimes the acute care environment in which we work may contribute to medication errors. Environmental factors that can often contribute to medications errors include poor lighting, noise, interruptions, and a significant workload.
- *Staff competency and education:* Staff education should focus on priority topics, such as new medications being used in the hospital, high-alert medications, medication errors that have occurred both internally and externally, protocols, policies, and procedures related to medication use. Staff education can be an important error-prevention strategy when combined with the other key elements for medication safety.
- *Patient education:* Patients must receive ongoing education from physicians, pharmacists, and the nursing staff about the brand and generic names of medications they are receiving, their indications, usual and actual doses, expected and possible adverse effects, drug or food interactions, and how to protect themselves from errors. Patients can play a vital role in preventing medication errors when they are encouraged to ask questions and seek answers about their medications before drugs are dispensed at a pharmacy or administered in a hospital.
- *Quality processes and risk management:* The way to prevent errors is to redesign the systems and processes that lead to errors rather than focus on correcting the individuals who make errors. Effective strategies for reducing errors include making it difficult for staff to make an error and promoting the detection and correction of errors before they reach a patient and cause harm.

MEDICATION ADMINISTRATION METHODS

Intravenous

Intravenous administration is the preferred route for medications in acutely ill patients because it permits complete and reliable delivery. Depending on the indication and the therapy, medications may be administered by IV push, intermittent infusion, or continuous infusion. Typically, IV push refers to administration of a drug over 3 to 5 minutes; intermittent infusion refers to 15-minute to 2-hour drug administration

several times per day, and continuous infusion administration occurs over a prolonged period of time.

Intramuscular or Subcutaneous

Intramuscular (IM) or subcutaneous (SC) administration of medications should rarely be used in acutely ill patients. This is due to a number of factors, including delayed onset of action, unreliable absorption because of decreased peripheral perfusion, particularly in patients who are hypotensive or hypovolemic, or inadequate muscle or decreased SC fat tissue. Furthermore, SC/IM administration may result in incomplete, unpredictable, or erratic drug absorption. If the medication is not absorbed from the injection site, a depot of medication can develop. If this occurs, once perfusion is restored, absorption can potentially lead to supratherapeutic or toxic effects. Additionally, patients with thrombocytopenia or who are receiving thrombolytic agents or anticoagulants may develop hematomas and bleeding complications due to SC or IM administration. Finally, administering frequent IM injections may also be inconvenient and painful for patients.

Oral

Oral (PO) administration of medication in the acutely ill patient can also result in incomplete, unpredictable, or erratic absorption. This may be caused by a number of factors including the presence of an ileus impairing drug absorption, or to diarrhea decreasing gastrointestinal (GI) tract transit time and time for drug absorption. Diarrhea may have a pronounced effect on the absorption of sustained-release preparations such as theophylline, procainamide, or calcium channel–blocking agents, resulting in a suboptimal serum drug concentration or clinical response. Several medications such as fluconazole and the fluoroquinolones have been shown to exhibit excellent bioavailability when orally administered to acutely ill patients. The availability of an oral suspension for some of these agents makes oral administration a reliable and cost-effective alternative for patients with limited IV access.

In patients unable to swallow, tablets are often crushed and capsules opened for administration through nasogastric or orogastric tubes. This practice is time-consuming and can result in blockage of the tube, necessitating removal of the clogged tube and insertion of a new tube. If enteral nutrition is being administered through the tube, it often has to be stopped for medication administration, resulting in inadequate nutrition for patients. Also, several medications (eg, phenytoin, carbamazepine, and warfarin) have been shown to compete, or interact, with enteral nutrition solutions. This interaction results in decreased absorption of these agents, or complex formation with the nutrition solution leading to precipitation and clogging of the feeding tube.

Liquid medications may circumvent the need to crush tablets or open capsules, but have their own limitations. An example is ciprofloxacin (Cipro) oral solution which is an oil-based preparation that should not be given via feeding tube because of the high probability of clogs. Many liquid dosage forms contain sorbitol as a flavoring agent or as the primary delivery vehicle. Sorbitol's hyperosmolarity is a frequent cause of diarrhea in acutely ill patients, especially in patients receiving enteral nutrition. Potassium chloride elixir is extremely hyperosmolar and requires dilution with 120 to 160 mL of water before administration. Administering undiluted potassium chloride elixir can result in osmotic diarrhea.

Lastly, sustained-release or enteric-coated preparations are difficult to administer to acutely ill patients. When sustained-release products are crushed, the patient absorbs the entire dose immediately as opposed to gradually over a period of 6, 8, 12, or 24 hours. This results in supratherapeutic or potentially toxic effects soon after the administration of the medication, with subtherapeutic effects at the end of the dosing interval. Sustained-release preparations must be converted to equivalent daily doses of immediate-release dosing forms and administered at more frequent dosing intervals. Enteric-coated dosage forms that are crushed may be inactivated by gastric juices or may cause stomach irritation. Enteric-coated tablets are specifically formulated to pass through the stomach intact so that they can enter the small intestine before they begin to dissolve.

Sublingual

Because of the high degree of vascularity of the sublingual mucosa, sublingual administration of medication often produces serum concentrations of medication that parallel IV administration, and an onset of action that is often faster than orally administered medications.

Traditionally, nitroglycerin has been one of the few medications administered sublingually (SL) to acutely ill patients. Several oral and IV medications, however, have been shown to produce therapeutic effects after sublingual administration. Captopril has been shown to reliably and predictably lower blood pressure in patients with hypertensive urgency. Oral lorazepam tablets have been administered SL to treat patients in status epilepticus; preparations of oral triazolam and IV midazolam have been shown to produce sedation after sublingual administration.

Intranasal

Intranasal administration is a way to effectively administer sedative and analgesic agents. The high degree of vascularity of the nasal mucosa results in rapid and complete absorption of medication. Agents that have been administered successfully intranasally include meperidine, fentanyl, sufentanil, butorphanol, ketamine, and midazolam.

Transdermal

Transdermal administration of medication is of limited value in acutely ill patients. Although nitroglycerin ointment is extremely effective as a temporizing measure before IV access is established in the acute management of patients with angina, heart failure (HF), pulmonary edema, or hypertension, nitroglycerin transdermal patches are of limited benefit. Transdermal patches are limited by their slow onset of activity and their inability for dose titration. Also, patients with decreased peripheral perfusion may not sufficiently absorb transdermally administered medications to produce the desired therapeutic effect. Transdermal preparations of clonidine, nitroglycerin, or fentanyl may be beneficial in patients who have been stabilized on IV or oral doses, but require chronic administration of these agents. Chronic use of nitroglycerin transdermal patches is further complicated by the development of tolerance. However, the development of tolerance can be avoided by removing the patch at bedtime, allowing for an 8- to 10-hour "nitrate-free" period.

A eutectic mixture of local anesthetic (EMLA) is a combination of lidocaine and prilocaine. This local anesthetic mixture can be used to anesthetize the skin before insertion of IV catheters or the injection of local anesthetics that may be required to produce deeper levels of topical anesthesia.

Although transdermal administration of medications is an infrequent method of drug administration in acutely ill patients, its use should not be overlooked as a potential cause of adverse effects in this patient population. Extensive application to burned, abraded, or denuded skin can result in significant systemic absorption of topically applied medications. Excessive use of viscous lidocaine products or mouthwashes containing lidocaine to provide local anesthesia for mucositis or esophagitis also can result in significant systemic absorption of lidocaine. Lidocaine administered topically to the oral mucosa has resulted in serum concentrations capable of producing seizures. The diffuse application of topical glucocorticosteroid preparations also can lead to absorption capable of producing adrenal suppression. This is especially true with the high-potency fluorinated steroid preparations such as betamethasone dipropionate, clobetasol propionate, desoximetasone, or fluocinonide.

CENTRAL NERVOUS SYSTEM PHARMACOLOGY

Sedatives

Sedatives can be divided into four main categories: benzodiazepines, barbiturates, neuroleptics, and miscellaneous agents. Benzodiazepines are the most commonly used sedatives in acutely ill patients. Neuroleptics typically are used in patients who manifest a psychological or behavioral component to their sedative needs, and barbiturates are reserved for patients with head injuries and increased intracranial pressure. Propofol is a short-acting IV general anesthetic that is approved for use as a sedative for mechanically ventilated, acutely ill patients. Dosing of sedatives should be guided by frequent assessment of the level of sedation with a valid and reliable sedation assessment scale (see Chapter 6 Pain and Sedation Management).

Benzodiazepines

Benzodiazepines are the most frequently used agents for sedation in acutely ill patients. These agents provide sedation, decrease anxiety, have anticonvulsant properties, possess indirect muscle-relaxant properties, and induce antegrade amnesia. Benzodiazepines bind to gamma-aminobutyric acid (GABA) receptors located in the central nervous system, modulating this inhibitory neurotransmitter. These agents have a wide margin of safety as well as flexibility in their routes of administration.

Benzodiazepines are frequently used to provide short-term sedation and amnesia during imaging procedures, other diagnostic procedures, and invasive procedures such as central venous catheter placement or bronchoscopy. A common long-term indication for using benzodiazepines is sedation and amnesia during mechanical ventilation.

Excessive sedation and confusion can occur with initial doses, but these effects diminish as tolerance develops during therapy. Elderly and pediatric patients may exhibit a paradoxical effect manifested as irritability, agitation, hostility, hallucinations, and anxiety. Respiratory depression may be seen in patients receiving concurrent narcotics, as well as in elderly patients and patients with chronic obstructive pulmonary disease (COPD) or obstructive sleep apnea (OSA). Benzodiazepines have also been associated with the development of ICU delirium, which has been linked with worse clinical outcomes.

Monitoring Parameters

- Mental status, level of consciousness, respiratory rate, and level of comfort should be monitored in any patient receiving a benzodiazepine. Signs and symptoms of withdrawal reactions should be monitored for patients receiving short-acting agents (ie, midazolam).

Midazolam

Midazolam is a short-acting, water-soluble benzodiazepine that may be administered IV, IM, SL, PO, intranasally or rectally. Clearance of midazolam has been shown to be extremely variable in acutely ill patients. The elimination half-life can be increased by as much as 6 to 12 hours in patients with liver disease, shock, or concurrently receiving enzyme-inhibiting drugs such as erythromycin or fluconazole; and hypoalbuminemia. Midazolam's two primary metabolites, 1-hydroxymidazolam and 1-hydroxymidazolam glucuronide, have been shown to accumulate in acutely ill patients, especially those with renal dysfunction, contributing additional pharmacologic effects. Geriatric patients demonstrate prolonged half-lives secondary to age-related reduction in liver function.

Dose

- *IV bolus:* 0.025 to 0.05 mg/kg
- *Continuous infusion:* 0.5 to 5 mcg/kg/min

Lorazepam

Lorazepam is an intermediate-acting benzodiazepine that offers the advantage of not having its metabolism affected by impaired hepatic function, age, or interacting drugs. Glucuronidation in the liver is the route of elimination of lorazepam. Because lorazepam is relatively water insoluble, it must be diluted in propylene glycol, and it is propylene glycol that is responsible for the hypotension that may be seen after bolus IV administration. Large volumes of fluid are required to maintain the drug in solution, so that only 20 to 40 mg can be safely dissolved in 250 mL of dextrose-5%-water (D_5W). In-line filters are recommended when administering lorazepam by continuous infusion because of the potential for the drug to precipitate. Finally, lorazepam's long elimination half-life of 10 to 20 hours limits its dosing flexibility by continuous infusion. Patients requiring high-dose infusions may be at risk for developing propylene glycol toxicity, which is manifested as a hyperosmolar state with a metabolic acidosis.

Dose

- *IV bolus:* 0.5 to 2 mg q1-4h
- *Continuous infusion:* 0.06 to 0.1 mg/kg/h
- *Oral:* 1 to 10 mg daily divided 2 to 3 times/day

Diazepam

Diazepam is a long-acting benzodiazepine with a faster onset of action than lorazepam or midazolam. Although its duration of action is 1 to 2 hours after a single dose, it displays cumulative effects because its active metabolites contribute to its pharmacologic effect. Desmethyldiazepam has a half-life of approximately 150 to 200 hours, so it accumulates slowly and then is slowly eliminated from the body after diazepam is discontinued. Diazepam metabolism is reduced in patients with hepatic failure and in patients receiving drugs that inhibit hepatic microsomal enzymes. Diazepam may be used for one or two doses as a periprocedure anxiolytic and amnestic, but should not be used for routine sedation of mechanically ventilated patients.

Dose

- *IV bolus:* 2.5 to 10 mg q2-4h
- *Continuous infusion:* Not recommended
- *Oral:* 2 to 10 mg bid-qid

Benzodiazepine Antagonist

Flumazenil

Flumazenil is a specific benzodiazepine antagonist indicated for the reversal of benzodiazepine-induced moderate sedation, recurrent sedation, and benzodiazepine overdose. It should be used with caution in patients who have received benzodiazepines for an extended period of time to prevent the precipitation of withdrawal reactions.

Dose

- *Reversal of conscious sedation:* 0.2 mg IV over 2 minutes, followed in 45 seconds by 0.2 mg repeated every minute as needed to a maximum dose of 1 mg. Reversal of recurrent sedation is the same as for conscious sedation, except doses may be repeated every 20 minutes as needed.

- *Benzodiazepine overdose:* 0.2 mg over 30 seconds followed by 0.3 mg over 30 seconds; repeated doses of 0.5 mg can be administered over 30 seconds at 1-minute intervals up to a cumulative dose of 3 mg. With a partial response after 3 mg, additional doses up to a total dose of 5 mg may be administered. In all of the above-mentioned scenarios, no more than 1 mg should be administered at any one time, and no more than 3 mg in any 1 hour. Continuous infusion: 0.1 to 0.5 mg/h (for the reversal of long-acting benzodiazepines or massive overdoses).

Monitoring Parameters

- Level of consciousness and signs and symptoms of withdrawal reactions

Neuroleptics

Haloperidol

Haloperidol is a major tranquilizer that has commonly been used for the management of agitated or delirious patients who fail to respond adequately to nonpharmacologic interventions or other sedatives. This agent has the advantage of limited respiratory depression and little potential for the development of tolerance or dependence. Although its exact mechanism of action is unknown, it probably involves dopaminergic receptor blockade in the central nervous system, resulting in central nervous system depression at the subcortical level of the brain.

Intravenous haloperidol is the most frequently used neuroleptic for controlling agitation in acutely ill patients. Initial doses of 2 to 5 mg may be doubled every 15 to 20 minutes until the patient is adequately sedated. Single IV doses as large as 150 mg as well as total daily doses of approximately 1000 mg have been safely administered to patients. As soon as the patient's symptoms are controlled, the total dose required to calm the patient should be divided into four equal doses and administered every 6 hours on a regularly scheduled basis. When the patient's symptoms are stable, the daily dose should be rapidly tapered to the smallest dose that controls the patient's symptoms. Continuous IV infusions have also been advocated to allow flexible dosing to control the patient's symptoms. Higher doses and IV administration of haloperidol may prolong the QTc interval in patients, especially those patients receiving haloperidol by IV injection or continuous infusions. Monitoring the QTc interval is mandatory for all patients receiving haloperidol by continuous infusion.

The major side effect of haloperidol is its extrapyramidal reactions, such as akathisia and dystonia. These reactions usually occur early in therapy and may resolve with dose reduction or discontinuation of the drug. However, in more severe cases, diphenhydramine, 25 to 50 mg IV, or benztropine, 1 to 2 mg IV, may be required to relieve the symptoms. Extrapyramidal reactions appear to be more common after oral haloperidol than after IV haloperidol administration. Neuroleptic malignant syndrome may also be seen with this agent, manifested by hyperthermia, severe extrapyramidal reactions, severe muscle rigidity, altered mental status, and autonomic instability. Treatment involves supportive care and the administration of dantrolene. Cardiovascular side effects include hypotension. It is important to note that despite the common usage of this agent to treat delirium, there is no published evidence that haloperidol reduces the duration of delirium. The lack of this supporting evidence is leading to the reconsideration of the role of haloperidol in this setting compared with other potentially more well-tolerated agents (ie, atypical antipsychotics).

Dose

- *IV bolus:* 1 to 10 mg (titrated up as clinically indicated)
- *Continuous infusion:* 10 mg/h (not generally recommended)
- *Oral:* 0.5 to 10 mg bid-tid

Monitoring Parameters

- Mental status, blood pressure, electrocardiogram (ECG), bedside delirium monitoring, and electrolytes (especially with continuous infusions)

Atypical Antipsychotics

Atypical antipsychotic agents such as quetiapine, olanzapine, risperidone, and ziprasidone have been suggested as possible alternatives to haloperidol, due to their similar mechanism of action and more favorable side effect profile, including reduced incidence of extrapyramidal reactions and QT prolongation. The use of atypical antipsychotics to manage ICU delirium has increased during recent years with reported usage as high as 40% in some studies. Despite these increases, additional well-controlled studies are warranted.

Monitoring Parameters

- Mental status, level of consciousness, electrocardiogram (ECG), bedside delirium monitoring

Quetiapine

Quetiapine is the most well studied of these agents to this point, with a randomized, placebo-controlled trial demonstrating a reduction in duration of delirium. Quetiapine can be administered as a scheduled dosing, with additional doses of haloperidol as needed. Dose escalation of the scheduled quetiapine may be required in 50 mg increments in patients still requiring breakthrough management with haloperidol. Sedation is the most commonly-associated adverse effect.

Dose

- *PO or per tube:* 50-200 mg q12h

Monitoring Parameters

- Mental status, level of consciousness, electrocardiogram (ECG), bedside delirium monitoring

Miscellaneous Agents

Propofol

Propofol is an IV general anesthetic that has become popular for sedation of mechanically ventilated patients. Propofol use is typically limited to fewer than 3 days because of the rapid development of tolerance or is used as the primary sedative in daily awakening protocols. The advantages of propofol are its rapid onset and short duration of action compared to the benzodiazepines. Propofol is associated with pain on injection, respiratory depression, and hypotension in acutely ill patients, especially those who are hypotensive or hypovolemic. Hypotension can be avoided by limiting bolus doses to 0.25 to 0.5 mg/kg and the initial infusion rate to 5 mcg/kg/min. The fat emulsion vehicle of propofol has been shown to support the growth of microorganisms. The manufacturer recommends changing the IV tubing of extemporaneously prepared infusions every 6 hours, or every 12 hours if the infusion bottles are used. Propofol is formulated in a fat-emulsion vehicle that provides 1.1 calories/mL and its infusion rate must be accounted for when determining a patient's nutrition support regimen because the fat-emulsion base can be considered as a calorie source. High infusion rates can be a cause of hyper-triglyceridemia. The agent also causes a rare but serious adverse effect known as propofol infusion syndrome (PRIS). PRIS is associated with the use of propofol for more than 48 hours and at doses greater than 75 mcg/kg/min. Hyperkalemia, tachyarrhythmia, and bradycardia combined with hypertriglyceridemia as previously described are common signs of PRIS. The bedside nurse should monitor closely for these signs as discontinuance of therapy may avoid the serious outcomes of PRIS: myocardial failure, metabolic acidosis, rhabdomyolysis, dysrhythmias, and renal failure. Propofol is available in 50- and 100-mL infusion vials. To decrease waste, 50-mL vials may be used when changing vials in patients who are scheduled for IV line changes, extubation from mechanical ventilation, and low infusion rates.

Dose

- *IV bolus:* 0.25 to 0.50 mg/kg
- *Continuous infusion:* 5 to 50 mcg/kg/min

Monitoring Parameters

- Level of consciousness, blood pressure, lactic acid, creatinine kinase, and serum triglyceride level, especially at high infusion rates

Ketamine

Ketamine is an analog of phencyclidine that is commonly used as an IV general anesthetic. It is an agent that produces analgesia, anesthesia, and amnesia without the loss of consciousness. The onset of anesthesia after a single 0.5- to 1.0-mg/kg bolus dose is within 1 to 2 minutes and lasts approximately 5 to 10 minutes. Ketamine causes sympathetic stimulation that normally increases blood pressure and heart rate while maintaining cardiac output. This may be important in patients with hypovolemia. Ketamine is useful in patients who require repeated painful procedures such as wound debridement. The bronchodilatory effects of ketamine may be beneficial in patients experiencing status asthmaticus. However, ketamine may increase intracranial pressure and should be avoided or used with caution in patients with head injuries, space-occupying lesions, or any other conditions that may cause an increase in intracranial pressure. Emergence reactions or hallucinations, commonly seen after ketamine anesthesia, may be prevented with the concurrent use of benzodiazepines.

Dose

- *IV bolus:* 0.1 to 1 mg/kg
- *Continuous infusion:* 0.1 to 3 mcg/kg/min
- *Oral:* 10 mg/kg diluted in 1 to 2 oz of juice
- *Intranasal:* 5 mg/kg

Monitoring Parameters

- Levels of sedation and analgesia, heart rate, blood pressure, and mental status

Dexmedetomidine

Dexmedetomidine is a relatively selective alpha-2-adrenergic agonist with sedative properties indicated for the short-term (up to 24 hour) sedation of intubated and mechanically ventilated patients. Dexmedetomidine is not associated with respiratory depression but has been associated with reductions in heart rate and blood pressure. Some patients may complain of increased awareness while receiving the drug in the intensive care unit. Dexmedetomidine has minimal amnestic properties and most patients require breakthrough doses of sedatives and analgesics while receiving the drug. The agent has been evaluated for longer term sedation, up to 28 days in a limited number of patients. In this setting, a reduction of the loading infusion is advised to minimize cardiovascular depression. However, a higher maintenance infusion (up to 1.5 mcg/kg/h) may be required compared to short-term sedation.

Dose

- *IV bolus:* 1 mcg/kg over 10 minutes
- *Continuous infusions:* 0.2 to 1.5 mcg/kg/h

Monitoring Parameters

- Levels of sedation and analgesia, heart rate, and blood pressure

Analgesics

Opioids

Opioids, also known as narcotics produce their effects by reversibly binding to the mu, delta, kappa, and sigma opiate receptors located in the central nervous system. Mu-1 receptors are associated with analgesia, and mu-2 receptors are associated with respiratory depression, bradycardia, euphoria, and dependence. Delta receptors have no selective agonist and modulate mu receptor activity. Kappa receptors function at the spinal and supraspinal levels and are associated with sedation. Sigma receptors are associated with dysphoria and psychotomimetic effects.

Monitoring Parameters

- Level of pain or comfort, blood pressure, renal function, and respiratory rate

Morphine

Morphine is a commonly used narcotic analgesic. Morphine is hepatically metabolized to several metabolites, including morphine-6-glucuronide (M6G), which is approximately 5 to 10 times more potent than morphine. M6G is renally eliminated and after repeated doses can accumulate in patients with renal dysfunction, producing enhanced pharmacologic effects. Morphine's clearance is reduced in acutely ill patients due to increased protein binding, decreased hepatic blood flow, or reduced hepatocellular function. Morphine possesses vasodilatory properties and can produce hypotension because of either direct effects on the vasculature or histamine release.

Dose

- *IV bolus:* 2 to 5 mg
- *Continuous infusion:* 2 to 30 mg/h
- *Oral*: 10 to 30 mg q3-4h prn

Patient-Controlled Analgesia (PCA)

- *IV bolus:* 0.5 to 3.0 mg
- *Lockout interval:* 5 to 20 minutes

Meperidine

Meperidine is a short-acting opioid that has one-seventh the potency of morphine. It is hepatically metabolized to normeperidine, which is renally eliminated and is also a neurotoxin. Normeperidine can accumulate in patients with renal dysfunction, resulting in seizures. Meperidine should be avoided in patients taking monoamine oxidase inhibitors because of the potential for development of a hypertensive crisis when these agents are administered concurrently.

Dose

- *IV bolus:* 25 to 100 mg
- *Oral*: 50 to 150 mg q2-4h prn

Fentanyl

Fentanyl is an analog of meperidine that is 100 times more potent than morphine. After single doses, its duration of action is limited by its rapid distribution into fat tissue. However, after repeated dosing or continuous infusion administration, fat stores become saturated, thereby prolonging its terminal elimination half-life to more than 24 hours. Fentanyl does not have active metabolites, although accumulation can occur in hepatic dysfunction. Unlike morphine, fentanyl does not cause histamine release.

Dose

- *IV bolus:* 25 to 100 mcg q1-2h
- *Continuous infusion:* 50 to 300 mcg/h
- *Transdermal:* Patients not previously on opioids: 25 mcg/h
- *Opioid-tolerant patients*: 25 to 100 mcg/h

Patient-Controlled Analgesia

- *IV bolus:* 25 to 100 mcg
- *Lockout interval:* 5 to 10 minutes

Opioid Antagonist

Naloxone

Naloxone is a pure opiate antagonist that displaces opioid agonists from the mu, delta, and kappa receptor-binding sites. Naloxone reverses narcotic-induced respiratory depression, producing an increase in respiratory rate and minute ventilation, a decrease in arterial Pco_2, and normalization of blood pressure if reduced. Narcotic-induced sedation or sleep is also reversed by naloxone. Naloxone reverses analgesia, increases sympathetic nervous system activity, and may result in tachycardia, hypertension, pulmonary edema, and cardiac arrhythmias. Naloxone administration produces withdrawal symptoms in patients who have been taking narcotic analgesics chronically. Diluting and slowly administering naloxone in incremental doses can prevent the precipitation of acute withdrawal reactions as well as prevent the increase in sympathetic stimulation that may accompany the reversal of analgesia. One 0.4-mg ampule should be diluted with 0.9% NaCl (saline) to 10 mL to produce a concentration of 0.04 mg/mL. Sequential doses of 0.04 to 0.08 mg should be administered slowly until the desired response is obtained. Because its duration of action is generally shorter than that of opiates, the effect of opiates may return after the effects of naloxone dissipate, approximately 30 to 120 minutes.

Dose

- *Opiate depression:* Initial dose: 0.1 to 0.2 mg given at 2- to 3-minute intervals until the desired response is obtained. Additional doses may be necessary depending on the response of the patient and the dose and duration of the opiate administered.
- *Continuous infusion:* 3 to 5 mcg/kg/h.
- *Known or suspected opiate overdose:* Initial dose: 0.4 to 2.0 mg administered at 2- to 3-minute intervals if necessary. If no response is observed after a total of 10 mg has been administered, other causes of the depressive state should be determined.
- *Continuous infusion:* Loading dose: 0.4 mg, followed by 2.5 to 5 mcg/kg/h and titrated to the patient's response.

Monitoring Parameters

- Signs and symptoms of withdrawal reactions, respiratory rate, blood pressure, mental status, level of consciousness, and pupil size

Nonsteroidal Anti-Inflammatory Drugs

Ketorolac

Ketorolac is a nonsteroidal anti-inflammatory drug (NSAID) that is indicated for the short-term treatment of moderately severe acute pain that requires analgesia at the opioid level. The drug exhibits anti-inflammatory, analgesic, and antipyretic properties. Its mechanism of action is thought to be due to inhibition of prostaglandin synthesis by inhibiting cyclooxygenase, an enzyme that catalyzes the formation of endoperoxidases from arachidonic acid. NSAIDs are more efficacious in the treatment of prostaglandin-mediated pain. Ketorolac is the only currently available NSAID approved for IM, IV, and oral administration, and it is often used in combination with other analgesics because pain often involves multiple mechanisms. Combination therapy may be more efficacious than single-drug regimens, and combinations with narcotics can decrease narcotic requirements, minimizing narcotic side effects.

Ketorolac is associated with the same adverse effects as orally administered NSAIDs, such as reversible platelet effects, GI bleeding, and reduced renal function. Ketorolac is contraindicated in patients with advanced renal failure and in patients at risk for renal failure due to volume depletion. Therefore, volume depletion should be corrected before administering ketorolac. Because of the potential for significant adverse effects, the maximum combined duration of parenteral and oral use is limited to 5 days.

Dose

- *Loading dose:* <65 years: 60 mg; >65 years or <50 kg: 30 mg
- *Maintenance dose:* <65 years: 30 mg q6h; >65 years or <50 kg: <15 mg q6h

Monitoring Parameters

- Renal function and volume status

Acetaminophen

Acetaminophen is an analgesic and antipyretic that is now available in the United States in an IV formulation. This agent has been used extensively in European countries. In the United States, IV acetaminophen is indicated for the management of mild to moderate pain, and management of moderate to severe pain with adjunctive opioid analgesics. The preferred route of administration for acetaminophen continues to be oral, but the IV route has proven beneficial in the perioperative setting when oral is not feasible. The IV form of this agent is not cost-effective for antipyretic usage as better options exist (eg, acetaminophen rectal suppositories). Use of IV acetaminophen should be restricted to post-surgical patients who are unable to take oral or rectal acetaminophen.

Dose

- *IV bolus:* 1-gm IV every 6 hours for 24-48 hours post-operative (maximum of 4 gm in 24 hours)

Monitoring Parameters

- Liver function test, pain control

Anticonvulsants

Hydantoins

Phenytoin

Phenytoin is an anticonvulsant used for the acute control of generalized tonic clonic seizures, following the administration of benzodiazepines, and for maintenance therapy once the seizure has been controlled. Phenytoin stabilizes neuronal cell membranes and decreases the spread of seizure activity. Phenytoin may inhibit neuronal depolarizations by blocking sodium channels in excitatory pathways and prevent increases in intracellular potassium concentrations and decreases in intracellular calcium concentrations.

The bioavailability of oral phenytoin is approximately 90% to 100%. Dissolution is the rate-limiting step in phenytoin absorption with peak serum concentrations occurring 3 to 12 hours after a dose. The rate of absorption is dose dependent, with increasing times to peak concentration with increasing doses. In addition, the dissolution and absorption rate depend on the phenytoin formulation administered. The Dilantin Kapseal brand of phenytoin capsules has the dissolution characteristics of an extended-release preparation, whereas generic phenytoin products possess rapid-release characteristics and are absorbed more quickly. Extended-release and rapid-release products are not interchangeable, and only extended-release products may be administered in a single daily dose.

Phenytoin is 90% to 95% bound to albumin. In acutely ill patients the pharmacologically free fraction is highly variable and ranges between 10% and 27% of the total serum concentration. The free fraction has been shown to increase by more than 100% from baseline during the first week of illness and is generally associated with a significant reduction in serum albumin concentration. Alterations in albumin binding also may be seen in hypoalbuminemia (<2.5 g/dL), major trauma, sepsis, burns, malnutrition, and surgery, as well as liver or renal disease, and may result in an increase in a free concentration with potentially toxic effects. Significant alterations in phenytoin metabolism usually do not occur until the serum albumin falls below 2.5 g/dL. Equations used to normalize the phenytoin concentration in patients with hypoalbuminemia are usually unreliable, and direct measurement of the free phenytoin concentration should be used to adjust therapy.

Phenytoin is metabolized by the cytochrome P-450 enzyme system to its inactive primary metabolite 5-(p-hydroxyphenyl)-5-phenylhydantoin, which is glucuronidated and renally eliminated. Phenytoin undergoes dose-dependent metabolism such that proportional increases in the dose may result in greater than proportional increases in the serum concentration. It is difficult to predict the concentration at which a patient's metabolism will become saturated, so that any changes in dose above 400 to 500 mg/day need to be carefully monitored. Because phenytoin displays nonlinear metabolism, half-life is an inappropriate term to describe phenytoin elimination. Phenytoin metabolism is usually referred to as the time it takes to eliminate 50% (t50) of a given daily dose.

In normal patients taking 300 mg/day, the t50 is about 22 hours. As the dose is increased, the t50 increases, with the time to reach steady-state becoming progressively longer. The time to steady-state may vary from several days to several weeks depending on the dose and the patient's ability to metabolize the drug. Phenytoin metabolism can be affected by drugs that induce or inhibit its metabolic pathway. The effects of enzyme induction can occur within 2 days to 2 weeks after starting an agent. Inhibition usually occurs within 1 to 2 days after a drug is started and its effects usually last until the inhibiting drug is eliminated from the body. Phenytoin clearance is increased in acutely ill patients, resulting in serum concentrations less than 10 mg/L. The mechanism for the increase in clearance is unclear, but may be caused by changes in protein binding, induction in phenytoin metabolism, or a stress-related transient increase in hepatic metabolic function.

The recommended phenytoin loading dose of 15 to 20 mg/kg produces serum concentrations between 20 and 30 mg/L. Loading doses of 18 to 20 mg/kg are recommended for treating status epilepticus, and loading doses of 15 to 18 mg/kg are recommended for seizure prophylaxis after head injury or neurosurgery. The serum concentration increases approximately 1.4 mg/L for each 1 mg/kg of phenytoin administered.

The maintenance dose should be started 8 to 12 hours after the loading dose. The usual adult maintenance dose is 5 to 6 mg/kg/day, although acutely ill patients or patients with neurotrauma may require doses of 6.0 to 7.5 mg/kg/day. Intravenous maintenance doses should be administered every 6 to 8 hours to maintain therapeutic serum concentrations.

Phenytoin precipitates in dextrose-containing solutions and should only be mixed in 0.9% sodium chloride solutions. To prevent phlebitis, the maximum concentration for peripheral administration is 10 mg/mL; a final concentration of 20 mg/mL may be used if the dose is being administered through a central venous catheter. Phenytoin solution must be administered through an in-line 1.2- or 5.0-µ filter to prevent the administration of phenytoin crystals into the systemic circulation. Phenytoin doses should not be administered at a rate faster than 50 mg/min because hypotension and arrhythmias may occur because of its propylene glycol diluent. The infusion rate should be decreased by 50% if hypotension or arrhythmias develop.

Oral administration is not usually recommended in acutely ill patients because of the risk of erratic or incomplete absorption. Phenytoin oral suspension may adhere to the inside walls of oro- or nasogastric tubes, reducing the dose delivered to the patient. If phenytoin is administered through a feeding tube, the tube should be flushed with 30 to 60 mL of 0.9% sodium chloride before and after administering the dose. After the dose is administered, the feeding tube should be clamped for an hour before restarting the feeding solution. Oral absorption may be impaired by concomitant administration with enteral nutrition solutions, reducing its bioavailability and resulting in erratic serum concentrations with seizures occurring as a result of subtherapeutic serum concentrations. Phenytoin oral solution must be shaken prior to use to ensure uniformity in the distribution of the phenytoin particles throughout the suspension. If the suspension is not shaken before obtaining a dose, the phenytoin powder settles to the bottom of the bottle producing subtherapeutic doses when the bottle is first opened and toxic doses as the bottle is used.

Hemodialysis and hemofiltration have no effect on phenytoin clearance. Agents known to inhibit or enhance this enzymatic pathway may affect phenytoin's clearance. Early adverse effects that may be associated with increasing serum concentrations are nystagmus (>20 mg/L), ataxia (>30 mg/L), and lethargy, confusion, and impaired cognitive function (>40 mg/L).

The normal therapeutic range for the total phenytoin serum concentration is 10 to 20 mg/L with the free fraction therapeutic range of 1 to 2 mg/L. Serum concentration of 20 to 30 mg/L may be required in patients who are having seizures. Phenytoin serum concentrations can be obtained 30 to 60 minutes after the loading dose is infused to assess the adequacy of the dose. Trough concentrations should be monitored 2 to 3 times a week, particularly after the first week of therapy. Measurement of free phenytoin concentrations may be indicated in acutely ill patients, patients with serum albumin concentrations less than 2.5 g/dL, renal failure, or receiving drugs known to displace phenytoin from albumin-binding sites. Other monitoring parameters include the patient's seizure activity and medication profile for agents known to alter phenytoin's metabolism.

Dose

- *Loading dose:* 15 to 20 mg/kg IV
- *Maintenance dose:* 5 mg/kg/day IV or PO

Monitoring Parameters

- Seizure activity, electroencephalogram (EEG), serum phenytoin concentration (free phenytoin concentration if applicable), albumin, liver function, infusion rate, blood pressure, ECG with IV administration, and IV injection site

Fosphenytoin

Fosphenytoin is a phenytoin prodrug with good aqueous solubility that was developed to be a water-soluble alternative to phenytoin. In patients unable to tolerate oral phenytoin, equimolar doses of fosphenytoin have been shown to produce equal or greater plasma phenytoin concentrations. Although phenytoin sodium 50 mg is equal to fosphenytoin sodium 75 mg, phenytoin should be converted to fosphenytoin on a milligram-per-milligram basis (eg, phenytoin 300 mg should be converted to fosphenytoin 300 mg).

Fosphenytoin, administered IM or IV, is rapidly and completely converted to phenytoin in vivo, resulting in essentially 100% bioavailability. The conversion half-life to phenytoin is about 33 minutes following IM administration and about 15 minutes after IV infusion. After IM administration, peak plasma fosphenytoin concentrations occur approximately 30 minutes postdose, with peak phenytoin concentrations occurring in about 3 hours. Fosphenytoin's peak concentration following IV administration occurs at the end of the infusion, with peak phenytoin concentrations occurring in approximately 40 to 75 minutes. In patients with renal or hepatic dysfunction or hypoalbuminemia, there is enhanced conversion to phenytoin without an increase in clearance. Fosphenytoin is 90% to 95% bound to plasma proteins and is saturable with the percent of bound fosphenytoin decreasing as the fosphenytoin dose increases.

The maximum total phenytoin concentration increases with increasing fosphenytoin doses, but the total phenytoin concentration is less affected by increasing fosphenytoin infusion rates. Maximum free phenytoin concentrations are nearly constant at infusion rates up to 50 mg phenytoin equivalents (PE)/min, whereas they increase with faster infusion rates secondary to phenytoin displacement from albumin-binding sites in the presence of high fosphenytoin concentrations.

For the treatment of status epilepticus, the recommended loading dose of IV fosphenytoin is 15 to 20 PE/kg, and it should not be administered faster than 150 mg PE/min because of the risk of hypotension. Fosphenytoin 15 to 20 mg PE/kg infused at 100 to 150 mg PE/min yields plasma-free phenytoin concentrations over time that approximate those achieved when an equimolar dose of IV phenytoin is administered at 50 mg/min. In the treatment of status epilepticus, total phenytoin concentrations greater than 10 mg/L and free phenytoin concentrations greater than 1 mg/mL are achieved within 10 to 20 minutes after starting the infusion.

In nonemergent situations, loading doses of 10 to 20 PE/kg administered IV or IM is recommended. In nonemergent situations, IV administration of infusion rates of 50 to 100 mg PE/min may be acceptable, but results in slightly lower and delayed maximum free phenytoin concentrations as compared with administration at higher infusion rates. The initial daily maintenance dose is 4 to 6 mg PE/kg/day. Dosing adjustments are not required when IM fosphenytoin is substituted temporarily for oral phenytoin. However, patients switched from once-daily extended-release phenytoin capsules may require twice-daily or more frequent administration of fosphenytoin to maintain similar peak and trough phenytoin concentrations.

The incidence of adverse effects tends to increase as both dose and infusion rate are increased. At doses above 15 mg PE/kg and infusion rates higher than 150 mg PE/min, transient pruritus, tinnitus, nystagmus, somnolence, and ataxia occur more frequently than at lower doses or infusion rates. Severe burning, itching, and paresthesias of the groin are commonly associated with infusion rates greater than 150 mg PE/min. Slowing or temporarily stopping the infusion can

minimize the frequency and severity of these reactions. Continuous cardiac rate and rhythm, blood pressure, and respiratory function should be monitored throughout the fosphenytoin infusion and for 10 to 20 minutes after the end of the infusion.

Following fosphenytoin administration, phenytoin concentrations should not be monitored until the conversion to phenytoin is complete. This occurs within 2 hours after the end of an IV infusion and 5 hours after an IM injection. Prior to complete conversion, commonly used immunoanalytic techniques such as fluorescence polarization and enzyme-mediated assays may significantly overestimate plasma phenytoin concentrations because of cross-reactivity with fosphenytoin. Blood samples collected before complete conversion to phenytoin should be collected in tubes containing ethylenediamine tetraacetic acid (EDTA) as an anticoagulant to minimize the ex vivo conversion of fosphenytoin to phenytoin. Monitoring is similar to phenytoin. In acutely ill patients with renal failure receiving fosphenytoin, one or more metabolites of adducts of fosphenytoin accumulate and display significant cross-reactivity with several phenytoin immunoassay methods.

Levetiracetam

Levetiracetam is a second-generation antiepileptic drug with increasing usage in acute care settings. The agent leads to selective prevention of burst firing and seizure activity. Levetiracetam is commonly prescribed for adjunctive treatment of partial onset seizures with or without secondary generalization. Other approved indications include monotherapy treatment of partial onset seizures with or without secondary generalization, and adjunctive treatment of myoclonic seizures associated with juvenile myoclonic epilepsy and primary generalized tonic-clonic (GTC) seizures associated with idiopathic generalized epilepsy. Seizure prophylaxis in post-traumatic brain injury patients is also an established role for levetiracetam.

Levetiracetam lacks cytochrome P450 isoenzyme-inducing potential and is not associated with clinically significant interactions with other drugs, including other antiepileptic drugs. Sedation is the most common adverse effect noted.

Dose

- *Maintenance dose:* 250 mg to 1000 mg q12 IV or PO

Monitoring Parameters

- Seizure activity, electroencephalogram (EEG), sedation

Benzodiazepines

Benzodiazepines are the primary agents in the management of status epilepticus. These agents suppress the spread of seizure activity but do not abolish the abnormal discharge from a seizure focus. Although IV diazepam has the fastest onset of action, lorazepam or midazolam are equally efficacious in controlling seizure activity. They are the agents of choice to temporarily control seizures and to gain time for the loading of phenytoin or phenobarbital. Phenytoin may also be used prophylactically in patients who are at risk for seizures after neurosurgery or following head injuries.

Monitoring Parameters

- Seizure activity, EEG, and respiratory rate and quality

CARDIOVASCULAR SYSTEM PHARMACOLOGY

Miscellaneous Agents

Nesiritide

Nesiritide is a recombinant human b-type natriuretic peptide, which is a cardiac hormone that regulates cardiovascular homeostasis and fluid volume during states of volume and pressure overload. The agent is effective in reducing pulmonary capillary wedge pressure and improving dyspnea symptoms in patients with acutely decompensated HF who have dyspnea at rest or with minimal activity. The most common adverse effects include hypotension, tachycardia, and/or bradycardia.

Dose

- *IV bolus:* 2 mcg/kg
- *Continuous infusion:* 0.01 mcg/kg/min

Monitoring Parameters

- Blood pressure, heart rate, urine output, and hemodynamic parameters

Parenteral Vasodilators (see Chapter 22)

Nitrates
Sodium Nitroprusside

Sodium nitroprusside is a balanced vasodilator affecting the arterial and venous systems. Blood pressure reduction occurs within seconds after an infusion is started, with a duration of action of less than 10 minutes once the infusion is discontinued. Sodium nitroprusside is considered the agent of choice in acute hypertensive conditions such as hypertensive encephalopathy, intracerebral infarction, subarachnoid hemorrhage, carotid endarterectomy, malignant hypertension, microangiopathic anemia, and aortic dissection, and after general surgical procedures, major vascular procedures, or renal transplantation.

If sodium nitroprusside is used for longer than 48 hours, there is the risk of thiocyanate toxicity. However, this may only be a concern in patients with renal dysfunction. In this setting, thiocyanate serum concentrations should be monitored to ensure that they remain below 10 mg/dL. Other potential side effects include methemoglobinemia and cyanide toxicity. Nitroprusside should be used with caution in the setting of increased intracranial pressure, such as head trauma or postcraniotomy, where it may cause an increase in cerebral blood flow. Nitroprusside's effects on intracranial pressure may be attenuated by a lowered $PaCO_2$ and raised PaO_2. In pregnant women, nitroprusside should be reserved only for refractory hypertension associated with eclampsia, because of the potential risk to the fetus.

Dose

- *Continuous infusion:* 0.5 to 10.0 mcg/kg/min

Monitoring Parameters

- Blood pressure, renal function, thiocyanate concentration (prolonged infusions), acid-base status, and hemodynamic parameters

Nitroglycerin

Nitroglycerin is a preferential venous dilator affecting the venous system at low doses, but relaxes arterial smooth muscle at higher doses. The onset of blood pressure reduction after starting a nitroglycerin infusion is similar to sodium nitroprusside, approximately 1 to 3 minutes, with duration of action of less than 10 minutes. Headaches are a common adverse effect that may occur with nitroglycerin therapy and can be treated with acetaminophen. Tachyphylaxis can be seen with the IV infusion, similar to what is seen after the chronic use of topical nitroglycerin preparations. In patients receiving unfractionated heparin in addition to nitroglycerin, increased doses of unfractionated heparin may be required to maintain a therapeutic partial thromboplastin time (PTT). The mechanism by which nitroglycerin causes unfractionated heparin resistance is unknown. However, the PTT should be closely monitored in patients receiving nitroglycerin and unfractionated heparin concurrently.

Nitroglycerin is the preferred agent in the setting of hypertension associated with myocardial ischemia or infarction because its net effect is a reduction in oxygen consumption.

Dose

- *Continuous infusion:* 10 to 300 mcg/min
- *Oral:* 2.5 to 9 mg bid-qid

Monitoring Parameters

- Blood pressure, heart rate, signs and symptoms of ischemia, hemodynamic parameters (if applicable), and PTT (in patients receiving unfractionated heparin concurrently)

Arterial Vasodilating Agents
Hydralazine

Hydralazine reduces peripheral vascular resistance by directly relaxing arterial smooth muscle. Blood pressure reduction occurs within 5 to 20 minutes after an IV dose and lasts approximately 2 to 6 hours. Common adverse effects include headache, nausea, vomiting, palpitations, and tachycardia. Reflex tachycardia may precipitate anginal attacks. Co-administration of a beta-receptor antagonist can decrease the incidence of tachycardia.

Dose

- 10 to 25 mg IV q2-4h
- Oral: 10 to 125 mg bid-qid

Monitoring Parameters

- Blood pressure and heart rate

Diazoxide

Diazoxide is a nondiuretic that reduces peripheral vascular resistance by directly relaxing arterial smooth muscle. Side effects such as hypotension, nausea and vomiting, dizziness, weakness, hyperglycemia, and reflex tachycardia have been associated with the use of the higher than 300-mg dosing regimen. Using lower dose regimens produces similar but less severe side effects. Caution should be used when diazoxide is administered with other antihypertensive agents because excessive hypotension may result.

Blood pressure reduction occurs within 1 to 2 minutes and lasts 3 to 12 hours after a dose. Blood pressure should be monitored frequently until stable, and then monitored hourly.

Dose

- *IV bolus:* 50 to 150 mg q5min
- *Continuous infusion:* 7.5 to 30.0 mg/min
- *Oral:* 3 to 8 mg/kg/day divided 2 to 3 times/day

Monitoring Parameters

- Blood pressure, heart rate, and serum glucose

Alpha- and Beta-Adrenergic Blocking Agents

Labetalol

Labetalol is a combined alpha- and beta-adrenergic blocking agent with a specificity of beta receptors to alpha receptors of approximately 7:1. Labetalol may be administered parenterally by escalating bolus doses or by continuous infusion. The onset of action after the administration of labetalol is within 5 minutes with duration of effect from 2 to 12 hours. Because labetalol possesses beta-blocking properties, it may produce bronchospasm in individuals with asthma or reactive airway disease. It also may produce conduction system disturbances or bradycardia in susceptible individuals, and its negative inotropic properties may exacerbate symptoms of HF.

Labetalol may be considered as an alternative to sodium nitroprusside in the setting of hypertension associated with head trauma or postcraniotomy, spinal cord syndromes, transverse lesions of the spinal cord, Guillain-Barré syndrome, or autonomic hyperreflexia, as well as hypertension associated with sympathomimetics (eg, cocaine, amphetamines, phencyclidine, nasal decongestants, or certain diet pills) or withdrawal of centrally acting antihypertensive agents (eg, beta-blockers, clonidine, or methyldopa). It also may be used as an alternative to phentolamine in the setting of pheochromocytoma because of its alpha- and beta-blocking properties.

Dose

- *IV bolus:* 20 mg over 2 minutes, then 40 to 80 mg IV q10min to a total of 300 mg
- *Continuous infusion:* 1 to 4 mg/min and titrate to effect
- *Oral:* 100 to 400 mg bid

Monitoring Parameters

- Blood pressure, heart rate, ECG, and signs and symptoms of HF or bronchospasm (if applicable)

Alpha-Adrenergic Blocking Agents

Phentolamine

Phentolamine is an alpha-adrenergic blocking agent that may be administered parenterally by bolus injection or continuous infusion. Onset of action is within 1 to 2 minutes, with duration of action of 3 to 10 minutes. Potential adverse effects that may occur with phentolamine include tachycardia, GI stimulation, and hypoglycemia.

Phentolamine is considered the drug of choice for the treatment of hypertension associated with pheochromocytoma because of its ability to block alpha-adrenergic receptors. Also, it is the primary agent used to treat acute hypertensive episodes in patients receiving monoamine oxidase inhibitors.

Dose

- *IV bolus:* 5 to 10 mg q5-15min
- *Continuous infusion:* 1 to 10 mg/min

Monitoring Parameters

- Blood pressure and heart rate

Beta-Adrenergic Blocking Agents

Beta-adrenergic blocking agents available for IV delivery include propranolol, esmolol, and metoprolol. Propranolol and metoprolol may be administered by bolus injection or continuous infusion. Atenolol typically is administered by bolus injection, and esmolol is administered by continuous infusion. A continuous infusion of esmolol may or may not be preceded by an initial bolus injection.

Esmolol has the fastest onset and shortest duration of action, approximately 1 to 3 minutes and 20 to 30 minutes, respectively. Propranolol and metoprolol have similar onset times, but durations of action vary between 1 and 6 hours. The duration of action after a bolus dose of atenolol is approximately 12 hours.

All agents may produce bronchospasm in individuals with asthma or reactive airway disease and may produce conduction system disturbances or bradycardia in susceptible individuals. Also, because of their negative inotropic properties, they may exacerbate symptoms of HF.

Beta-blocking agents typically are used as adjuncts with other agents in the treatment of acute hypertension. They may be used with sodium nitroprusside in the treatment of acute aortic dissections. They should be administered to patients with hypertension associated with pheochromocytoma only after phentolamine has been given. Also, they are the agents of choice in patients who have been maintained on beta-blocking agents for the chronic management of hypertension but who have abruptly stopped therapy.

Beta-blocking agents should be avoided in patients with hypertensive encephalopathy, intracranial infarctions, or subarachnoid hemorrhages because of their central nervous system depressant effects. They also should be avoided in patients with acute pulmonary edema because of their negative inotropic properties. Finally, beta-blocking agents should be avoided in hypertension associated with eclampsia and renal vasculature disorders.

Dose

- *Esmolol:* IV bolus 500 mcg/kg; continuous infusion: 50 to 400 mcg/kg/min
- *Metoprolol:* IV bolus: 5 mg IV q2min × 3 doses or maintenance 1.25 to 5 mg IV q6-12h. Oral: 25 to 450 mg daily divided 2 to 3 times/day
- *Propranolol:* IV bolus: 0.5 to 1.0 mg q5-15min; *continuous infusion:* 1 to 4 mg/h. Oral: 30 to 320 mg daily divided 2 to 4 times/day

Monitoring Parameters

- Blood pressure, heart rate, ECG, and signs and symptoms of HF or bronchospasm (if applicable)

Angiotensin-Converting Enzyme Inhibitors

Angiotensin-converting enzyme (ACE) inhibitors competitively inhibit angiotensin-converting enzyme, which is responsible for the conversion of angiotensin I to angiotensin II (a potent vasoconstrictor). In addition, these agents inactivate bradykinin and other vasodilatory prostaglandins, resulting in an increase in plasma renin concentrations and a reduction in plasma aldosterone concentrations. The net effect is a reduction in blood pressure in hypertensive patients and a reduction in afterload in patients with HF.

Angiotensin-converting enzyme inhibitors are indicated in the management of hypertension and HF. Adverse effects associated with ACE inhibitors include rash, taste disturbances, and cough. Initial-dose hypotension may occur in patients who are hypovolemic, hyponatremic, or who have been aggressively diuresed. Hypotension may be avoided or minimized by starting with low doses or withholding diuretics for 24 to 48 hours. Worsening of renal function may occur in patients with bilateral renal artery stenosis.

Enalapril

Enalapril is a prodrug that is converted in the liver to its active moiety, enalaprilat, a long-acting ACE inhibitor. Enalapril is available in an oral dosage form, and enalaprilat is available in the IV form. Following an IV dose of enalaprilat, blood pressure lowering occurs within 15 minutes and lasts 4 to 6 hours.

Dose

- *Enalaprilat:* IV bolus: 0.625 to 1.250 mg over 5 minutes q6h; continuous infusion: not recommended
- *Enalapril:* Oral: 2.5 to 40.0 mg qd

Monitoring Parameters

- Blood pressure, heart rate, renal function, and electrolytes

Angiotensin Receptor Blockers

Angiontensin receptor blockers (ARBs) selectively block the binding of angiotensin II (a powerful vasoconstrictor in vascular smooth muscle) to the receptors in tissues such as vascular smooth muscle and the adrenal gland. This receptor blockade results in vasodilation and decreased secretion of aldosterone, which leads to increased sodium excretion and potassium sparing effects. ARBs are indicated for both hypertension and HF. ARBs currently available in oral formulations include valsartan, candesartan, irbesartan, azilsartan, eprosartan, losartan, and olmesartan. The most common adverse effects of ARBs are hypotension, dizziness, and headache. Although rare, cough can also be associated with ARBs. This cough can be reversed by discontinuance of therapy. Overall, these agents are relatively well tolerated and thus used quite commonly for the chronic management of stages 1 and 2 hypertension. The role in acute blood pressure lowering is limited due to the lack of a parenteral formulation.

Monitoring Parameters

- Blood pressure and heart rate, and electrolytes

Calcium Channel–Blocking Agents

Calcium channel–blocking agents may be used as alternative therapy in the treatment of hypertension resulting from hypertensive encephalopathy, myocardial ischemia, malignant hypertension, or eclampsia, or after renal transplantation.

Nicardipine

Nicardipine is an IV calcium channel–blocking agent that is primarily indicated for the treatment of hypertension. Onset is within 5 minutes with duration of approximately 30 minutes. Nicardipine also is available in an oral dosage form so that patients started on IV therapy can convert to oral therapy when indicated.

Dose

- *Continuous infusion:* 5 mg/h, increase every 15 minutes to a maximum of 15 mg/h
- *Oral:* 20 to 40 mg q8h

Monitoring Parameters

- Blood pressure and heart rate

Clevidipine

Clevidipine is an IV calcium channel blocking agent that is also indicated for the treatment of hypertension. An onset of 2 minutes is faster than nicardipine with a shorter duration of 10 minutes. Clevidipine is delivered as an injectable lipid emulsion (20%), similar to intralipids, and is not available in an oral dosage form. Similar to propofol, vials of clevidipine and IV tubing must be changed every 12 hours during therapy because the phospholipids support microbial growth.

Dose

- *Continuous infusion:* 1 to 2 mg/h, increase by doubling dose every 90-second intervals initially to achieve blood pressure reduction. As the blood pressure approaches goal, increase dose less aggressively every 5 to 10 minutes. Maximum recommended dose is 16 mg/h.

Monitoring Parameters

- Blood pressure and heart rate

Central Sympatholytic Agents

Clonidine

Clonidine is an oral agent that stimulates alpha-2-adrenergic receptors in the medulla oblongata, causing inhibition of sympathetic vasomotor centers. Although clonidine typically is used as maintenance antihypertensive therapy, it can be used in the setting of hypertensive urgencies or emergencies. Its antihypertensive effects may be seen within 30 minutes and last 8 to 12 hours. Once blood pressure is controlled, oral maintenance clonidine therapy may be started.

Centrally acting sympatholytics rarely are indicated as first-line agents except when hypertension may be due to the abrupt withdrawal of one of these agents.

Dose

- *Hypertensive urgency:* 0.2 mg PO initially, then 0.1 mg/h PO (to a maximum of 0.8 mg)
- *Transdermal:* TTS-1 (0.1 mg/day) to TTS-3 (0.3 mg/day) topically q1wk

Monitoring Parameters

- Blood pressure, heart rate, and mental status

Antiarrhythmics

Antiarrhythmic agents are divided into five classes. Dosage information for individual antiarrhythmic agents is listed in Chapter 22 (see Table 22-4).

Class I Agents

Class I agents are further divided into three subclasses: Ia (procainamide, quinidine, disopyramide), Ib (lidocaine, mexiletine), and Ic (flecainide, propafenone). All class I agents block sodium channels in the myocardium and inhibit potassium-repolarizing currents to prolong repolarization.

Class Ia Agents

Class Ia agents inhibit the fast sodium channel (phase 0 of the action potential), slow conduction at elevated serum drug concentrations, and prolong action potential duration and repolarization. Class Ia agents can cause proarrhythmic complications by prolonging the QT interval or by depressing conduction and promoting reentry.

Monitoring Parameters

- ECG (QRS complex, QT interval, arrhythmia frequency)

Class Ib Agents

Class Ib agents have little effect on phase 0 depolarization and conduction velocity, but shorten the action potential duration and repolarization. QT prolongation typically does not occur with class Ib agents. Class Ib agents act selectively on diseased or ischemic tissue where they block conduction and interrupt reentry circuits.

Monitoring Parameters

- ECG (QT interval, arrhythmia frequency)

Class Ic Agents

Class Ic agents inhibit the fast sodium channel and cause a marked depression of phase 0 of the action potential and slow conduction profoundly, but have minimal effects on repolarization. The dramatic effects of these agents on conduction may account for their significant proarrhythmic effects, which limit their use in patients with supraventricular arrhythmias and structural heart disease.

Monitoring Parameters

- ECG (PR interval and QRS complex, arrhythmia frequency)

Class II Agents

Beta-blocking agents inactivate sodium channels and depress phase 4 depolarization and increase the refractory period of the atrioventricular node. These agents have no effect on repolarization. Beta-blockers competitively antagonize catecholamine binding at beta-adrenergic receptors.

Beta-blocking agents can be classified as selective or nonselective agents. Nonselective agents bind to beta-1 receptors located on myocardial cells and beta-2 receptors located on bronchial and skeletal smooth muscle. Stimulation of beta-1 receptors causes an increase in heart rate and contractility, whereas stimulation of beta-2 receptors results in bronchodilation and vasodilation. Selective beta-blocking agents block beta-1 receptors in the heart at low or moderate doses, but they become less selective with increasing doses.

Class II agents are used for the prophylaxis and treatment of both supraventricular arrhythmias and arrhythmias associated with catecholamine excess or stimulation, slowing the ventricular response in atrial fibrillation, lowering blood pressure, decreasing heart rate, and decreasing ischemia. Esmolol is useful especially for the rapid, short-term control of ventricular response in atrial fibrillation or flutter.

Nonselective beta-blocking agents should be avoided or used with caution in patients with HF, atrioventricular nodal blockade, asthma, COPD, peripheral vascular disease, Raynaud phenomenon, and diabetes. Beta-1 selective beta-blocking agents should be used with caution in these populations.

Monitoring Parameters

- ECG (heart rate, PR interval, arrhythmia frequency)

Class III Agents

Class III agents (amiodarone, dofetilide, and sotalol) lengthen the action potential duration and effective refractory period and prolong repolarization. Additionally, amiodarone possesses alpha- and beta-blocking effects and calcium channel–blocking properties and inhibits the fast sodium channel. Sotalol possesses nonselective beta-blocking properties. Although torsades de pointes is relatively rare with amiodarone, precautions should be taken to prevent hypokalemia- or digitalis-toxicity–induced arrhythmias. Sotalol may be associated with proarrhythmic effects in the setting of hypokalemia, bradycardia, high sotalol dose, and QT-interval prolongation, and in patients with preexisting HF. Sotalol is also contraindicated in patients with severe renal impairment.

Amiodarone

The antiarrhythmic effect of amiodarone is due to the prolongation of the action potential duration and refractory period, and secondarily through alpha-adrenergic and beta-adrenergic blockade. In patients with recent-onset (<48 hours) atrial fibrillation or atrial flutter, IV amiodarone has been shown to restore normal sinus rhythm within 8 hours in approximately 60% to 70% of treated patients. Although IV amiodarone has been associated with negative inotropic effects, minimal side effects are associated with its short-term administration. Amiodarone is recommended as an option for the treatment of wide-complex tachycardia; stable, narrow-complex supraventricular tachycardia; stable, monomorphic or polymorphic ventricular tachycardia; atrial fibrillation and flutter; ventricular fibrillation; and pulseless ventricular tachycardia.

Monitoring Parameters

- ECG (PR and QT intervals, QRS complex, arrhythmia frequency)

Dofetilide

Dofetilide is a class III antiarrhythmic (potassium channel blocker) agent used for rhythm conversion in patients with atrial fibrillation. The agent has been FDA approved with substantial restrictions, as prescribers must undergo drug specific training before being permitted to prescribe. Initiation of drug therapy is also limited to hospitalized patients with continuous ECG monitoring and dosing based on a prespecified dosing algorithm. Proarrhythmic events and sudden cardiac death are the most substantial adverse events associated with dofetilide administration leading to these restrictions. The dose should be adjusted according to QT prolongation and creatinine clearance. If the QTc is greater than 400 millisecond, dofetilide is contraindicated. Dofetilide is also contraindicated in patients with severe renal impairment.

Dose

- Modified based on creatinine clearance and QT or QTc interval. The usual recommended oral dose is 250 mcg bid.

Ibutilide

Ibutilide is a class III antiarrhythmic agent indicated for the conversion of recent-onset atrial fibrillation and atrial flutter to normal sinus rhythm. Ibutilide causes the prolongation of the refractory period and action potential duration, with little or no effect on conduction velocity or automaticity. Its electrophysiologic effects are predominantly derived from activation of a slow sodium inward current. Ibutilide can cause slowing of the sinus rate and atrioventricular node conduction, but has no effect on heart rate, PR interval, or QRS interval. The drug is associated with minimal hemodynamic effects with no significant effect on cardiac output, mean pulmonary arterial pressure, or pulmonary capillary wedge pressure. Ibutilide has not been shown to lower blood pressure or worsen HF.

Ibutilide has been shown to be more effective than procainamide and sotalol in terminating atrial fibrillation and atrial flutter. In addition, ibutilide has been shown to decrease the amount of joules required to treat resistant atrial fibrillation and atrial flutter during cardioversion. Depending on the duration of atrial fibrillation or flutter, ibutilide has an efficacy rate of 22% to 43% and 37% to 76%, respectively, for terminating these arrhythmias. Ibutilide is only available as an IV dosage form and cannot be used for the long-term maintenance of normal sinus rhythm.

Sustained and nonsustained polymorphic ventricular tachycardia is the most significant adverse effect associated with ibutilide. The overall incidence of polymorphic ventricular tachycardia diagnosed as torsades de pointes was 4.3%, including 1.7% of patients in whom the arrhythmia was sustained and required cardioversion. Ibutilide administration should be avoided in patients receiving other agents that prolong the QTc interval, including class Ia or III antiarrhythmic agents, phenothiazines, antidepressants, and some antihistamines. Before ibutilide administration, patients should be screened carefully to exclude high-risk individuals, such as those with a QTc interval greater than 440 millisecond or bradycardia. Serum potassium and magnesium levels should be measured and corrected before the drug is administered. The ibutilide infusion should be stopped in the event of nonsustained or sustained ventricular tachycardia or marked prolongation in the QTc interval. Patients should be monitored for at least 4 hours after the infusion or until the QTc returns to baseline, with longer monitoring if nonsustained ventricular tachycardia develops.

Monitoring Parameters

- ECG (heart rate, PR interval, ST segment, T wave, arrhythmia frequency)

Class IV Agents

Calcium channel–blocking agents inhibit calcium channels within the atrioventricular node and sinoatrial node, prolong conduction through the atrioventricular and sinoatrial nodes, and prolong the functional refractory period of the nodes, as well as depress phase 4 depolarization. Class IV agents are used for the prophylaxis and treatment of supraventricular arrhythmias and to slow the ventricular response in atrial fibrillation, flutter, and multifocal atrial tachycardia.

Monitoring Parameters

- ECG (PR interval, arrhythmia frequency)

Class V Agents

Adenosine, digoxin, and atropine possess different pharmacologic properties but ultimately affect the sinoatrial node or atrioventricular node.

Monitoring Parameters

- ECG (heart rate, PR interval, ST segment, T wave, arrhythmia frequency)

Adenosine

Adenosine depresses sinus node automaticity and atrioventricular nodal conduction. Adenosine is indicated for the acute termination of atrioventricular nodal and reentrant tachycardia, and for supraventricular tachycardias, including Wolff-Parkinson-White syndrome.

Atropine

Atropine increases the sinus rate and decreases atrioventricular nodal conduction time and effective refractory period by decreasing vagal tone. The major indications for the use of atropine include symptomatic sinus bradycardia and type I second-degree atrioventricular block.

Digoxin

Digoxin is indicated for the treatment of supraventricular tachycardia and for controlling ventricular response associated with supraventricular tachycardia.

Vasodilators and Remodeling Agents

Idiopathic pulmonary arterial hypertension (IPAH), formerly called primary pulmonary hypertension, is characterized by elevations in pulmonary arterial pressure in the absence of a demonstrable cause. Vasoconstriction in the pulmonary vasculature is thought to play an important role in the pathogenesis of IPAH. This vasoconstriction occurs secondary to either impaired production of endogenous vasodilators (prostacyclin and nitric oxide), or from increased production of endothelin, an endogenous vasoconstrictor.

Nitric Oxide
Prostacyclin analogues

Epoprostenol (Flolan), treprostinil (Remodulin), and iloprost (Ventavis) are potent vasodilators, which also inhibit platelet aggregation and smooth muscle proliferation and are the mainstay of IPAH therapy. Epoprostenol is delivered intravenously via continuous infusion. For long-term therapy, a permanently implanted central venous catheter and portable infusion pump are useful for drug administration. Side effects include jaw pain, diarrhea, and arthralgias. The doses are typically titrated based on impact on systemic

blood pressure, therefore monitoring is recommended whenever therapy is initiated. Treprostinil has an advantage of continuous SC delivery, a longer half-life (possibly less immediately life-threatening if interrupted), and the lack of a need for refrigeration. A major disadvantage of treprostinil is the high rate of significant infusion site discomfort if the SC rate is used. Iloprost is an aerosolized preparation which is delivered via a specialized nebulizer device. This agent was recently FDA approved with its role yet to be clearly defined compared to other prostacyclin analogues.

Endothelin receptor antagonist

Bosentan (Tracleer) works by blocking the vasoconstrictive properties of endothelin and is only available orally. The main adverse event associated with therapy is elevations in liver enzymes, therefore close monitoring of liver function tests is required. Bosentan is often combined with prostacyclin analogues to treat refractory cases of IPAH.

Phosphodiesterase inhibitors

Numerous studies of patients with IPAH have demonstrated improvements in pulmonary hemodynamics after treatment with sildenafil (Viagra, Revatio). Tadalafil (Cialis) and vardenafil (Levitra) have similar mechanisms of action; however, there appear to be some differences in the degree of phosphodiesterase inhibition, leading to questions of whether these agents are interchangeable. Sildenafil is the most widely studied and therefore the most commonly prescribed phosphodiesterase inhibitor. Similar to bosentan, sildenafil's most prominent role appears to be in combination with prostacyclin analogues.

Calcium channel blockers

Nifedipine (Procardia, Adalat), amlodipine (Norvasc), and diltiazem (Cardizem) all have proven beneficial in IPAH therapy due to vasodilatory properties. Relatively high doses are required to see responses, with systemic hypotension and edema being the most significant adverse effects in these patients. The historical role for these agents has been first-line management; however many clinicians currently opt for prostacyclin therapy or phosphodiesterase therapy initially.

Vasopressor Agents

The 2012 Surviving Sepsis Campaign international guidelines for management of severe sepsis and septic shock recommend norepinephrine as the first-choice vasopressor in this setting. It is recommended that vasopressor therapy initially target a mean arterial pressure (MAP) of 65 mm Hg. Norepinephrine is a direct-acting vasoactive agent. It possesses alpha- and beta-adrenergic agonist properties producing mixed vasopressor and inotropic effects. Dopamine is recommended as an alternative vasopressor agent to norepinephrine only in highly selected patients (eg, patients with low risk of tachyarrhythmias and absolute or relative bradycardia). Dopamine is both an indirect-acting and a direct-acting agent. Dopamine works indirectly by causing the release of norepinephrine from nerve terminal storage vesicles as well as directly by stimulating alpha and beta receptors. Dopamine is unique in that it produces different pharmacologic responses based on the dose infused. At doses less than 5 mcg/kg/min, dopamine stimulates dopaminergic receptors in the kidneys. Doses between 5 and 10 mcg/kg/min are typically associated with an increase in inotropy resulting from stimulation of beta receptors in the heart, and doses above 10 mcg/kg/min stimulate peripheral alpha-adrenergic receptors, producing vasoconstriction and an increase in blood pressure. Dopamine and norepinephrine are both effective for increasing blood pressure. Dopamine raises cardiac output more than norepinephrine, but its use is limited by tachyarrhythmias. Norepinephrine may be a more effective vasopressor in some patients, thus the first line designation. Epinephrine is an option for addition to norepinephrine as needed to maintain adequate blood pressure in refractory patients. Epinephrine possesses alpha- and beta-adrenergic effects, increasing heart rate, contractility, and vasoconstriction with higher doses. Epinephrine's use is reserved for when other, vasoconstrictors are inadequate. Adverse effects include tachyarrhythmias; myocardial, mesenteric, renal, and extremity ischemia; and hyperglycemia. Phenylephrine is not recommended in the treatment of septic shock except in the following circumstances: (a) norepinephrine is associated with serious arrhythmias, (b) cardiac output is known to be high and blood pressure persistently low, or (c) as salvage therapy when combined inotrope/vasopressor drugs and low-dose vasopressin have failed to achieve the MAP target. Phenylephrine is a pure alpha-adrenergic agonist. It produces vasoconstriction without a direct effect on the heart, although it may cause a reflex bradycardia. Phenylephrine may be useful when dopamine, dobutamine, norepinephrine, or epinephrine cause tachyarrhythmias and when a vasoconstrictor is required.

Vasopressin is an emerging therapeutic agent for the hemodynamic support of septic and vasodilatory shock. Vasopressin is a hormone that mediates vasoconstriction via V1 receptor activation on vascular smooth muscle. During septic shock, vasopressin levels are particularly low. Exogenous vasopressin administration is based on the theory of hormone replacement. Vasopressin (up to 0.03 unit/min) can be added to norepinephrine with the intent of raising MAP to target or decreasing norepinephrine dosage. Low-dose vasopressin is not recommended as the single initial vasopressor for treatment of sepsis-induced hypotension, and vasopressin doses higher than 0.03-0.04 units/min should be reserved for salvage therapy (failure to achieve an adequate MAP with other vasopressor agents). It is important to note that harmful vasoconstriction of the gut vasculature will occur with dose escalation greater than 0.04 units/min.

Dose

- See Table 22-3.

Monitoring Parameters

- Blood pressure, heart rate, ECG, urine output, and hemodynamic parameters

Inotropic Agents (see Table 22-3)

Catecholamines

Dobutamine

Dobutamine produces pronounced beta-adrenergic effects such as increases in inotropy and chronotropy along with vasodilation. Dobutamine is useful especially for the acute management of low cardiac output states. Adverse effects associated with the use of dobutamine include tachyarrhythmias and ischemia.

A trial of dobutamine infusion up to 20 mcg/kg/min may be administered or added to vasopressors (if in use) in the presence of: (a) myocardial dysfunction as suggested by elevated cardiac filling pressures and low cardiac output, or (b) ongoing signs of hypoperfusion, despite achieving adequate intravascular volume and adequate MAP. Norepinephrine and dobutamine can be titrated separately to maintain both blood pressure and cardiac output.

Dopamine

Dopamine in the range of 5 to 10 mcg/kg/min typically produces an increase in inotropy and chronotropy. Doses above 10 mcg/kg/min typically produce alpha-adrenergic effects.

Isoproterenol

Isoproterenol is a potent pure beta-receptor agonist. It has potent inotropic, chronotropic, and vasodilatory properties. Its use typically is reserved for temporizing life-threatening bradycardia. Adverse effects associated with isoproterenol include tachyarrhythmias, myocardial ischemia, and hypotension.

Epinephrine

Epinephrine produces pronounced effects on heart rate and contractility and is used when other inotropic agents have not resulted in the desired pharmacologic response. Epinephrine is associated with tachyarrhythmias; myocardial, mesenteric, renal, and extremity ischemia; and hyperglycemia.

Dose

- See Table 22-3.

Monitoring Parameters

- Blood pressure, heart rate, ECG, urine output, and hemodynamic parameters

ANTIBIOTIC PHARMACOLOGY

There are a wide variety of antibiotic agents used in hospitalized patients. Commonly used antibiotic classes include beta lactams or penicillins (eg, penicillin G potassium, ampicillin ± sulbactam, oxacillin, nafcillin, ticarcillin ± clavulanic acid, and piperacillin ± tazobactam), carbapenems (eg, meropenem, doripenem, and imipenem/cilastatin), monobactams (eg, aztreonam), cephalosporins (eg, cefazolin, cefotetan, cefoxitin, cefotaxime, ceftazidime, ceftriaxone, and cefepime), fluoroquinolones (eg, levofloxacin, moxifloxacin, and ciprofloxacin), macrolides (eg, azithromycin, erythromycin), lincosamides (eg, clindamycin), nitroimidazoles (eg, metronidazole), lipopetides (eg, daptomycin), oxazolidinones (eg, linezolid), glycopeptides (eg, vancomycin, telavancin), and aminoglycosides (eg, amikacin, tobramycin, and gentamicin). Since the development of the first antibiotic (penicillin) in 1944, microorganisms have consistently evolved by developing resistance to these agents. This has led to the need for newer and more innovative classes of antibiotics with different targets and ways to avoid resistance. Selection of the correct agent(s) is a key consideration, along with correct identification of the site of infection, and knowledge of resistance patterns within your institution. In some instances, combinations of different antibiotic classes (eg, aminoglycoside + beta lactam, or fluoroquinolone + beta lactam) may be used as a strategy to address resistance patterns. This is used particularly with gram negative organisms, and may be advocated vs monotherapy for certain indications. Additionally, the antibiotic dose, frequency, and/or length of infusion can also be modified as well.

As noted, there are a number of factors related to optimal antibiotic therapy. A complete review of all antibiotic classes is beyond the scope of this text, and the focus of this section is on aminoglycosides and vancomycin due to the commonality of their usage and the link to therapeutic drug monitoring.

Aminoglycosides

Gentamicin, tobramycin, and amikacin are the most commonly used aminoglycoside antibiotics in acutely ill patients. These agents are typically used with antipseudomonal penicillins or third- or fourth-generation cephalosporins for additional gram-negative bacteria coverage. Occasionally they are added to vancomycin or penicillin for synergy against staphylococcal, streptococcal, or enterococcal organisms.

Aminoglycosides are not metabolized but are cleared from the body through the kidney by glomerular filtration with some proximal tubular reabsorption occurring. The clearance of aminoglycosides parallels glomerular filtration, and a reduction in glomerular filtration results in a reduction in clearance with elevation in serum concentrations. Additional factors accounting for the reduced aminoglycoside clearance in acutely ill patients include the level of positive end-expiratory pressure and the use of vasoactive agents to maintain blood pressure and perfusion. Aminoglycosides are removed from the body by hemodialysis, peritoneal dialysis, continuous renal replacement therapy (CRRT), extracorporeal membrane oxygenation, exchange transfusion, and cardiopulmonary bypass.

The major limiting factors in the use of aminoglycosides are drug-induced ototoxicity and nephrotoxicity. Ototoxicity results from the loss of sensory hair cells in the cochlea and vestibular labyrinth. Gentamicin is primarily vestibulotoxic, amikacin causes primarily cochlear damage, and tobramycin affects vestibular and cochlear function equally. Symptoms of ototoxicity typically appear within the first 1 to 2 weeks of therapy but may be delayed as long as 10 to 14 days after stopping therapy.

Early damage may be reversible, but it may become permanent if the agent is continued. Vestibular toxicity may be manifested by vertigo, ataxia, nystagmus, nausea, and vomiting, but these symptoms may not be apparent in a sedated or paralyzed, acutely ill patient. Cochlear damage occurs as subclinical high-frequency hearing loss that is usually irreversible and may progress to deafness even if the drug is discontinued. It is difficult to diagnose hearing loss in the absence of pretherapy audiograms. Risk factors for ototoxicity include advanced age, duration of therapy for more than 10 days, total dose, previous aminoglycoside therapy, and renal impairment.

Nephrotoxicity has been estimated to occur in up to 30% of acutely ill patients and typically develops 2 to 5 days after starting therapy. An increase in serum creatinine of 0.5 mg/dL above baseline has been arbitrarily defined as significant and as possible evidence of nephrotoxicity. Nephrotoxicity is associated with a reduction in glomerular filtration rate, impaired concentrating ability, increased serum creatinine, and increased urea nitrogen. In most cases, the renal insufficiency is nonoliguric and reversible. The mechanism of nephrotoxicity is possibly related to the inhibition of intracellular phospholipases in lysosomes of tubular cells in the proximal tubule, resulting in rupture or dysfunction of the lysosome, leading to proximal tubular necrosis. Risk factors for the development of aminoglycoside nephrotoxicity include advanced age, prolonged therapy, preexisting renal disease, preexisting liver disease, volume depletion, shock, and concurrent use of other nephrotoxins such as amphotericin B, cyclosporine, or cisplatin.

Aminoglycosides are effectively removed during hemodialysis. However, there is a rebound in the serum concentration within the first 2 hours after the completion of hemodialysis as the serum and tissues reach a new equilibrium. Therefore, a serum concentration should be drawn at least 2 hours after a dialysis treatment. Typically a dose of 1 to 2 mg/kg of gentamicin or tobramycin (amikacin 4-8 mg/kg) is sufficient to increase the serum level into the therapeutic range after dialysis. Continuous hemofiltration is also effective at removing aminoglycosides. Up to 35% of a dose can be removed during a 24-hour period of CRRT. Initially, several blood samples may be required to determine the drug's pharmacokinetic profile for dosing regimen adjustments. If the hemofiltration rate remains constant, aminoglycoside clearance should remain stable, permitting the administration of a stable dosing regimen. In this setting, drug concentration monitoring may only be required 2 to 3 times a week.

Vancomycin

Vancomycin is a glycopeptide antibiotic active against gram-positive and certain anaerobic organisms. It exerts its antimicrobial effects by binding with peptidoglycan and inhibiting bacterial cell wall synthesis. In addition, the antibacterial effects of vancomycin also include alteration of bacterial cell wall permeability and selective inhibition of RNA synthesis.

Vancomycin is minimally absorbed after oral administration. After single or multiple doses, therapeutic vancomycin concentrations can be found in ascitic, pericardial, peritoneal, pleural, and synovial fluids. Vancomycin penetrates poorly into cerebrospinal fluid (CSF), with CSF penetration being directly proportional to vancomycin dose and degree of meningeal inflammation. Vancomycin is eliminated through the kidneys primarily via glomerular filtration with a limited degree of tubular secretion. Nonrenal elimination occurs through the liver and accounts for about 30% of total clearance. The elimination half-life of vancomycin is 3 to 13 hours in patients with normal renal function and increases in proportion to decreasing creatinine clearance. In acute renal failure, nonrenal clearance is maintained but eventually declines approaching the nonrenal clearance in chronic renal failure. In acutely ill patients with reduced renal function, the increase in half-life may be due to a reduction in clearance as well as an increase in the volume of distribution.

Vancomycin is removed minimally during hemodialysis with cuprophane filter membranes, so that dosage supplementation after hemodialysis is not necessary. Vancomycin's half-life averages 150 hours in patients with chronic renal failure. With the newer high-flux polysulfone hemodialysis filters, vancomycin is removed to a greater degree, resulting in significant reductions in vancomycin serum concentrations. However, there is a significant redistribution period that takes place over the 12-hour period after the high-flux hemodialysis procedure with postdialysis concentrations similar to predialysis concentrations. Therefore, dose supplementation should be based on concentrations obtained at least 12 hours after dialysis.

Vancomycin is removed very effectively by CRRT, resulting in a reduction in half-life to 24 to 48 hours. Up to 33% of a dose can be eliminated during a 24-hour hemofiltration period. Supplemental doses of vancomycin may need to be administered every 2 to 5 days in patients undergoing CRRT.

The most common adverse effect of vancomycin is the "red-man syndrome," which is a histamine-like reaction associated with rapid vancomycin infusion and characterized by flushing, tingling, pruritus, erythema, and a macular papular rash. It typically begins 15 to 45 minutes after starting the infusion and abates 10 to 60 minutes after stopping the infusion. It may be avoided or minimized by infusing the dose over 2 hours or by pretreating the patient with diphenhydramine, 25 to 50 mg, 15 to 30 minutes before the vancomycin infusion. Other rare, but reported, adverse effects include rash, thrombophlebitis, chills, fever, and neutropenia.

PULMONARY PHARMACOLOGY

Theophylline

Theophylline is a phosphodiesterase inhibitor, which produces bronchodilatation possibly by inhibiting cyclic AMP phosphodiesterase, inhibition of cellular calcium translocation, inhibition of leukotriene production, reduction in the reuptake or metabolism of catecholamines, and blockade of adenosine receptors. The use of theophylline for bronchospastic or lung disease has declined over the past decade. Most clinicians no longer use it as standard therapy for patients admitted to the hospital with bronchospasm; however, occasional patients may benefit from theophylline therapy. Theophylline should be used with caution in acutely ill patients for several reasons. First, theophylline is metabolized in the liver and illnesses such as low cardiac output, HF, or hepatic failure may impair the ability of the liver to metabolize theophylline, resulting in increased serum concentrations. Second, antibiotics and anticonvulsants routinely administered to acutely ill patients are known to alter theophylline's metabolism.

In patients without a recent history of theophylline ingestion, the parenteral administration of 6 mg/kg of IV aminophylline (aminophylline = 85% theophylline) produces a serum theophylline concentration of approximately 10 mg/L. In patients with a recent history of theophylline ingestion, a serum theophylline concentration should be obtained before administering a loading dose. Once the serum concentration is known, a partial loading dose may be administered to increase the concentration to the desired level. Each 1.2 mg/kg aminophylline (theophylline 1.0 mg/kg) increases the theophylline serum concentration approximately 2 mg/L. The loading dose should be administered over 30 to 60 minutes to avoid the development of tachycardia or arrhythmias.

The maintenance infusion should be started following the completion of the loading dose and should be adjusted according to the patient's underlying clinical status (smokers: 0.9 mg/kg/h; nonsmokers: 0.6 mg/kg/h; liver failure or HF: 0.3 mg/kg/h). These infusion rates are designed to achieve a serum concentration of approximately 10 mg/L. In most patients, concentrations above 10 mg/L are rarely indicated and may be associated with adverse effects.

When an IV regimen is converted to an oral regimen, the total daily theophylline dose should be calculated and divided into two to four equal doses depending on the theophylline product selected for chronic administration. When switching to a sustained-release product, the IV infusion should be discontinued with administration of the first sustained-release dose to maintain constant serum theophylline concentrations. Overlapping of the oral dose and IV infusion is not recommended because of the increase in serum theophylline concentrations and the potential development of toxicity resulting from the absorption of the sustained-release product.

Adverse effects occur more frequently at serum concentration above 20 mg/L and include anorexia, nausea, vomiting, epigastric pain, diarrhea, restlessness, irritability, insomnia, and headache. Serious arrhythmias and convulsions usually occur at serum concentrations above 35 mg/L, but have occurred at lower concentrations and may not be preceded by less serious toxicity.

Theophylline concentrations should be determined daily until they are stable. In addition, theophylline concentrations should be obtained daily in unstable patients and in whom interacting drugs are started or stopped. Levels may be measured once or twice weekly if the patient, theophylline level, and drug regimen are stable.

Dose

- *Loading dose:* 6 mg/kg IV or PO (each 1.2 mg/kg aminophylline increases the theophylline serum concentration by 2 mg/L)
- *Continuous infusion:* Smokers: 0.9 mg/kg/h; nonsmokers: 0.6 mg/kg/h; liver failure, HF: 0.3 mg/kg/h

Monitoring Parameters

- Serum theophylline concentration, signs and symptoms of toxicity such as tachycardia, arrhythmias, nausea, vomiting, and seizures

Albuterol

Albuterol is a selective beta-2 agonist, used to treat or prevent reversible bronchospasm. Adverse effects tend to be associated with inadvertent beta-1 stimulation leading to cardiovascular events including tachycardia, premature ventricular contractions, and palpitations.

Monitoring Parameters

- Heart rate and pulmonary function tests

Levalbuterol

Levalbuterol is the active enantiomer of racemic albuterol. Dose ranging studies in stable ambulatory asthmatics and patients with COPD have documented that levalbuterol 0.63 mg and albuterol 2.5 mg produced equivalent increases in the magnitude and duration of FEV_1. There are no studies evaluating the efficacy of levalbuterol in hospitalized or acutely ill patients. One study assessing the tachycardic effects of these agents in acutely ill patients showed a clinically insignificant increase in heart rate following the administration of either agent.

Monitoring Parameters

- Heart rate and pulmonary function tests

GASTROINTESTINAL PHARMACOLOGY

Stress Ulcer Prophylaxis

Stress ulcers are superficial lesions commonly involving the mucosal layer of the stomach that appear after stressful events such as trauma, surgery, burns, sepsis, or organ failure. Risk factors for the development of stress ulcers include coagulopathy, patients requiring mechanical ventilation for more than 48 hours, patients with a history of GI ulceration or bleeding within the past year, sepsis, an ICU stay longer than 1 week, occult bleeding lasting more than 6 days, and the use of high-dose steroids (>250 mg of hydrocortisone or the equivalent). Numerous studies support the use of antacids, H2-receptor antagonists, and sucralfate. There are

limited prospective comparative studies supporting the use of proton pump inhibitors (PPI) for preventing stress ulcer formation in acutely ill patients. More studies are warranted to highlight the role of PPIs in this setting.

Antacids

Antacids once were considered the primary agents for the prevention of stress gastritis. Their main attributes were their effectiveness and low cost. However, this was offset by the need to administer 30- to 120-mL doses every 1 to 2 hours. Large doses of antacids had the potential to produce large gastric residual volumes, resulting in gastric distention and bloating, as well as increasing the risk for aspiration. Magnesium-containing antacids are associated with diarrhea and can produce hypermagnesemia in patients with renal failure. Aluminum-containing antacids are associated with constipation and hypophosphatemia. Large, frequent doses of antacids prevent the effective delivery of enteral nutrition. Finally, antacids are known to impair the absorption of digoxin, fluoroquinolones, and captopril. Also, alkalinization of the GI tract may predispose patients to nosocomial pneumonias with gram-negative organisms that originate in the GI tract.

Dose

- 30 to 120 mL PO, NG q1-4h

Monitoring Parameters

- Nasogastric aspirate pH, serum electrolytes, bowel function (diarrhea, constipation, bloating), hemoglobin, hematocrit, and nasogastric aspirate and stool guaiac

H2 Antagonists

Ranitidine and famotidine essentially have replaced antacids as therapy for the prevention of stress gastritis. These agents have the benefit of requiring administration only every 6 to 12 hours or may be delivered by continuous infusion. When they are administered by continuous infusion, they may be added to parenteral nutrition solutions, decreasing the need for multiple daily doses. Each agent has been associated with thrombocytopenia and mental status changes. Mental status changes typically occur in elderly patients or in patients with reduced renal function in whom the doses have not been adjusted to account for the reduction in renal function. Also, similar to antacids, alkalinization of the GI tract with H2 antagonists may predispose patients to nosocomial pneumonias with gram-negative organisms that originate in the GI tract.

Dose

- *Ranitidine:* Intermittent IV: 50 mg q8h; continuous infusion: 6.25 mg/h. Oral: 300 to 600 mg daily divided 1 to 2 times/day
- *Cimetidine:* Oral: 300 mg qid or 800 mg qhs, or 400 mg bid
- *Famotidine:* Intermittent IV: 20 mg q12h; continuous infusion: not recommended. Oral: 20 to 40 mg daily divided 1 to 2 times/day

Monitoring Parameters

- Nasogastric aspirate pH, platelet count, hemoglobin, hematocrit, and nasogastric aspirate and stool guaiac

Other Agents
Sucralfate

Sucralfate is an aluminum disaccharide compound that has been shown to be safe and effective for the prophylaxis of stress gastritis. Sucralfate may work by increasing bicarbonate secretion, mucus secretion, or prostaglandin synthesis to prevent the formation of stress ulcers. Sucralfate has no effect on gastric pH. It can be administered either as a suspension or as a tablet that can be partially dissolved in 10 to 30 mL of water and administered orally or through a nasogastric tube. Although sucralfate is free from systemic side effects, it has been reported to cause hypophosphatemia, constipation, and the formation of bezoars. Because sucralfate does not increase gastric pH, it lacks the ability to alkalinize the gastric environment and may decrease the development of gram-negative nosocomial pneumonias. Sucralfate has a limited role as an alternative to H2 antagonists in patients with thrombocytopenia or mental status changes.

Dose

- 1 g PO, NG q6h

Monitoring Parameters

- Hemoglobin, hematocrit, nasogastric aspirate, and stool guaiac

Acute Peptic Ulcer Bleeding

Proton Pump Inhibitors

Proton pump inhibitors have demonstrated efficacy in preventing rebleeding and reducing transfusion requirements in several randomized-controlled trials. The rationale for adjunctive acid-suppressant therapy is based on in vitro data demonstrating clot stability and platelet aggregation enhancement at high gastric pHs (> 6). High-dose IV PPI therapy in conjunction with therapeutic endoscopy is the most cost-effective approach for the management of hospitalized patients with acute peptic ulcer bleeding.

Pantoprazole and esomeprazole are available in oral and injectable forms, while lansoprazole and omeprazole are available in oral forms only. It is advisable to transition to oral/enteral PPI therapy, if possible, after 72 hours of IV therapy. The 72-hour time period for continuous infusions is the longest duration that has been studied.

Dose

- *Pantoprazole and esomeprazole:* IV bolus dosing: 40 to 80 mg IV q12h for 72 hours; continuous infusion: 80 mg IV bolus; then 8 mg/h for 72 hours

Monitoring Parameters

- Hemoglobin, hematocrit, and stool guaiac

Variceal Hemorrhage

Upper GI bleeding is a common problem encountered in the intensive care unit. Its mortality remains around 10%. Vasoactive drugs to control bleeding play an important role in the immediate treatment of acute upper GI bleeding associated with variceal hemorrhage.

Vasopressin

Vasopressin remains a commonly used agent for acute variceal bleeding. Vasopressin is a nonspecific vasoconstrictor that reduces portal pressure by constricting the splanchnic bed and reducing blood flow into the portal system. Vasopressin is successful in stopping bleeding in about 50% of patients. Many of the adverse effects of vasopressin are caused by its relative nonselective vasoconstrictor effect. Myocardial, mesenteric, and cutaneous ischemia have been reported in association with its use. Drug-related adverse effects have been reported in up to 25% of patients receiving vasopressin. The use of transdermal or IV nitrates with vasopressin reduces the incidence of these adverse effects.

Dose

- 0.3 to 0.9 units/min

Monitoring Parameters

- Hemoglobin, hematocrit, nasogastric aspirate, stool guaiac, ECG, signs and symptoms of ischemia, blood pressure, and heart rate

Octreotide

Octreotide, the longer acting synthetic analog of somatostatin, reduces splanchnic blood flow and has a modest effect on hepatic blood flow and wedged hepatic venous pressure with little systemic circulation effects. Although octreotide produces the same results as vasopressin in the control of bleeding and transfusion requirements, it produces significantly fewer adverse effects. Continuous infusion of octreotide has been shown to be as effective as injection sclerotherapy in control of variceal hemorrhage.

Dose

- Initial bolus dose: 100 mcg, followed by 50-mcg/h continuous infusion

Monitoring Parameters

- Hemoglobin, hematocrit, nasogastric aspirate, and stool guaiac

Propranolol

Propranolol has been shown to reduce portal pressure both acutely and chronically in patients with portal hypertension by reducing splanchnic blood flow. The primary use of propranolol has been in the prevention of variceal bleeding. Propranolol or other beta-blockers should be avoided in patients experiencing acute GI bleeding, because beta-blocking agents may prevent the compensatory tachycardia needed to maintain cardiac output and blood pressure in the setting of hemorrhage.

Monitoring Parameters

- Hemoglobin, hematocrit, heart rate, and blood pressure

RENAL PHARMACOLOGY

Diuretics

Diuretics may be categorized in a number of ways, including site of action, chemical structure, and potency. Although many diuretics are available for oral and IV administration, intravenously administered agents typically are given to acutely ill patients because of their guaranteed absorption and more predictable responses. Therefore, the primary agents used in intensive care units are the intravenously administered loop diuretics, thiazide diuretics, and osmotic agents. However, the oral thiazide-like agent, metolazone, is used commonly in combination with loop diuretics to maintain urine output for patients with diuretic resistance.

Monitoring Parameters

- Urine output, blood pressure, renal function, electrolytes, weight, fluid balance, and hemodynamic parameters (if applicable)

Loop Diuretics

Loop diuretics (furosemide, bumetanide, torsemide) act by inhibiting active transport of chloride and possibly sodium in the thick ascending loop of Henle. Administration of loop diuretics results in enhanced excretion of sodium, chloride potassium, hydrogen, magnesium, ammonium, and bicarbonate. Maximum electrolyte loss is greater with loop diuretics than with thiazide diuretics. Furosemide, bumetanide, and torsemide have some renal vasodilator properties that reduce renal vascular resistance and increase renal blood flow. Additionally, these three agents decrease peripheral vascular resistance and increase venous capacitance. These effects may account for the decrease in left ventricular filling pressure that occurs before the onset of diuresis in patients with HF.

Loop diuretics typically are used for the treatment of edema associated with HF or oliguric renal failure, the management of hypertension complicated by HF or renal failure, in combination with hypotensive agents in the treatment of hypertensive crisis, especially when associated with acute pulmonary edema or renal failure, and in combination with 0.9% sodium chloride to increase calcium excretion in patients with hypercalcemia.

Common adverse effects associated with loop diuretic administration include hypotension from excessive reduction in plasma volume, hypokalemia and hypochloremia resulting in metabolic alkalosis, and hypomagnesemia. Reduction in these electrolytes may predispose patients to the development of supraventricular and ventricular ectopy. Tinnitus, with reversible or permanent hearing impairment, may occur

with the rapid administration of large IV doses. Typically, IV bolus doses of furosemide should not be administered faster than 40 mg/min.

Dose

- *Furosemide:* IV bolus: 10 to 100 mg q1-6h; continuous infusion: 1 to 15 mg/h. Oral: 20 to 600 mg daily divided 1 to 4 times/day
- *Bumetanide:* IV bolus: 0.5 to 2.5 mg q1-2h; continuous infusion: 0.08 to 0.30 mg/h. Oral: 0.5 to 5 mg qd-bid (maximum of 10 mg)
- *Torsemide:* IV bolus: 5 to 20 mg qd. Oral: 2.5 to 20 mg qd

Thiazide Diuretics

Thiazide (IV chlorothiazide) and thiazide-like (PO metolazone) diuretics enhance excretion of sodium, chloride, and water by inhibiting the transport of sodium across the renal tubular epithelium in the cortical diluting segment of the nephron. Thiazides also increase the excretion of potassium and bicarbonate.

Thiazide diuretics are used in the management of edema and hypertension as monotherapy or in combination with other agents. They have less potent diuretic and antihypertensive effects than loop diuretics. Intravenously administered chlorothiazide or oral metolazone is often used in combination with loop diuretics in patients with diuretic resistance. By acting at a different site in the nephron, this combination of agents may restore diuretic responsiveness. Thiazide diuretics decrease glomerular filtration rate, and this effect may contribute to their decreased efficacy in patients with reduced renal function (glomerular filtration rate, < 20 mL/min). Metolazone, unlike thiazide diuretics, does not substantially decrease glomerular filtration rate or renal plasma flow and often produces a diuretic effect even in patients with glomerular filtration rates less than 20 mL/min.

Adverse effects that may occur with the administration of thiazide diuretics include hypovolemia and hypotension, hypochloremia and hypokalemia resulting in a metabolic alkalosis, hypercalcemia, hyperuricemia, and the precipitation of acute gouty attacks.

Dose

- Chlorothiazide: 500 to 1000 mg IV q12h
- Metolazone: 2.5 to 20.0 mg PO qd

Osmotic Diuretics

Mannitol

Mannitol is an osmotic diuretic commonly used in patients with increased intracranial pressure. Mannitol produces a diuretic effect by increasing the osmotic pressure of the glomerular filtrate and preventing the tubular reabsorption of water and solutes. Mannitol increases the excretion of sodium, water, potassium, and chloride, as well as other electrolytes.

Mannitol is used to treat acute oliguric renal failure, and reduce intracranial and intraocular pressures. The renal protective effects of mannitol may be due to its ability to prevent nephrotoxins from becoming concentrated in the tubular fluid. However, its ability to prevent or reverse acute renal failure may be owing to restoring renal blood flow, glomerular filtration rate, urine flow, and sodium excretion. To be effective in preventing or reversing renal failure, mannitol must be administered before reductions in glomerular filtration rate or renal blood flow have resulted in acute tubular damage. Mannitol is useful in the treatment of cerebral edema, especially when there is evidence of herniation or the development of cord compression.

The most severe adverse effect of mannitol is overexpansion of extracellular fluid and circulatory overload, producing acute HF and pulmonary edema. This effect typically occurs in patients with severely impaired renal function. Therefore, mannitol should not be administered to individuals in whom adequate renal function and urine flow have not been established.

Dose

- 0.25 to 0.50 g/kg, then 0.25 to 0.50 g/kg q4h

Monitoring Parameters

- Urine output, blood pressure, renal function, electrolytes, weight, fluid balance, hemodynamic parameters (if applicable), serum osmolarity, and intracranial pressure (if applicable)

HEMATOLOGIC PHARMACOLOGY

Anticoagulants

Unfractionated Heparin

Unfractionated heparin consists of a group of mucopolysaccharides derived from the mast cells of porcine intestinal tissues. It binds with antithrombin III, accelerating the rate at which antithrombin III neutralizes coagulation factors II, VII, IX, X, XI, and XII. Unfractionated heparin is used for prophylaxis and treatment of venous thrombosis and pulmonary embolism, atrial fibrillation with embolization, and treatment of acute disseminated intravascular coagulation.

Subcutaneously administered unfractionated heparin is absorbed slowly and completely over the dosing interval. The total amount of unfractionated heparin required to achieve the same degree of anticoagulation over the same time period does not appear to differ whether the unfractionated heparin is administered subcutaneously or intravenously. The apparent volume of distribution of unfractionated heparin is directly proportional to body weight, and it has been suggested that the dose should be based on ideal body weight in obese patients. Others suggest that in obese patients the dose should be normalized to total body weight.

The metabolism and elimination of unfractionated heparin involves the process of depolymerization and desulfation. Enzymes reported to be involved in unfractionated heparin metabolism include unfractionated heparinase and desulfatase, which cleave unfractionated heparin into oligosaccharides. The half-life of unfractionated heparin ranges from 0.4 to 2.5 hours. Patients with underlying thromboembolic disease have been shown to have shorter elimination half-lives, faster clearance, and require larger doses to maintain adequate thrombotic activity.

A weight-based nomogram is utilized with a loading dose followed by a continuous infusion. The infusion is titrated based on activated PTT monitoring. The main adverse effects may be attributed to excessive anticoagulation. Bleeding occurs in 3% to 20% of patients receiving short-term, high-dose therapy. Bleeding is increased threefold when the PTT is 2.0 to 2.9 times above control and eightfold when the PTT is more than 3 times the control value. Unfractionated heparin-induced thrombocytopenia may occur in 1% to 5% of patients receiving the drug.

The PTT is the test used to monitor and adjust unfractionated heparin doses. Although unfractionated heparin is typically administered as a continuous infusion, it is important that samples are collected as close to steady state as possible. After starting unfractionated heparin therapy or adjusting the dose, PTT values should be drawn at least 6 to 8 hours after the change. Samples drawn too early are misleading and may result in inappropriate dose adjustments. Once the unfractionated heparin dose has been determined, daily monitoring of the PTT for minor adjustments in the unfractionated heparin dose is indicated. Large variations in subsequent coagulation tests should be investigated to ensure that the patient's condition has not changed or the patient is not developing thrombocytopenia.

Platelet counts should be monitored every 2 to 3 days while a patient is receiving unfractionated heparin to assess for unfractionated heparin–induced thrombocytopenia, thrombosis, or hemorrhage. Hemoglobin and hematocrit should be monitored every 2 to 3 days to assess for the presence of bleeding. Additionally sputum, urine, and stool should be examined for the presence of blood. Patients should be examined for signs of bleeding at IV access sites and for the development of hematomas and ecchymosis. In addition, IM injections should be avoided in patients receiving unfractionated heparin and elective invasive procedures should be avoided or rescheduled.

Dose

- *Individualized dosing:* Bolus: 80 units/kg followed by a continuous infusion of 18 units/kg/h; infusion rates should be adjusted to maintain a PTT between 1.5 and 2.0 times the control value

Monitoring Parameters

- PTT, hemoglobin, hematocrit, and signs of active bleeding

Low-Molecular-Weight Heparins

Low-molecular-weight heparins have a role in the treatment of deep venous thrombosis, pulmonary embolism, and acute MI.

Low-molecular-weight heparins are less time consuming for nurses and laboratories and more comfortable for patients by allowing them to be discharged earlier from the hospital. The use of a fixed-dose regimen avoids the need for serial monitoring of the PTT and follow-up dose adjustments. Enoxaparin is the most studied low-molecular-weight unfractionated heparin. Its dose for the treatment of deep venous thrombosis, pulmonary embolism, and acute MI is 1 mg/kg q12h. Dalteparin is another agent that has been shown to be as effective as unfractionated heparin in the treatment of thromboembolic disease and acute MI. Dalteparin 200 units/kg once daily is the typical dose used for the treatment of thromboembolic disease; 120 units/kg followed by 120 units/kg 12 hours later has been used in patients with acute MI receiving streptokinase. Warfarin can be started with the first dose of enoxaparin or dalteparin. Enoxaparin or dalteparin should be continued until two consecutive therapeutic international normalized ratio (INR) values are achieved, typically in about 5 to 7 days.

Both dalteparin and enoxaparin are primarily renally eliminated with the potential for drug accumulation in patients with renal impairment. The approach for managing these patients differs between the two drugs. Because these agents work by inhibiting factor Xa activity, it is possible to monitor their anticoagulation by measuring antifactor Xa levels. This is a useful monitoring tool, particularly when compared with serum drug levels. Doses of either agent may be adjusted based on antifactor Xa levels in patients with significant renal impairment (ie, creatinine clearance, <30 mL/min). The dosing adjustment for enoxaparin in patients with creatinine clearances less than 30 mL/min is to extend the dosing interval from 12 hours to 24 hours in both prophylaxis and treatment of thrombosis. No such dosage adjustment guideline has been approved for dalteparin; thus antifactor Xa levels may be required.

Several studies have documented that acutely ill patients have significantly lower anti-Xa levels in response to single daily doses when compared to patients on general medical wards. Factor Xa activity may need to be monitored in acutely ill patients to adjust doses to ensure adequate anticoagulation to prevent deep venous clots from developing.

Dose

- *Enoxaparin:* 1 mg/kg SC q12h.

Monitoring Parameters

- Hemoglobin, hematocrit, signs of active bleeding, and antifactor Xa levels

Warfarin

Warfarin prevents the conversion of vitamin K back to its active form from the vitamin K epoxide, impairing the formation of vitamin K–dependent clotting factors II, VII, IX, X, protein C, and protein S. Warfarin is indicated in the treatment of venous thrombosis or pulmonary embolism following full-dose parenteral anticoagulant (eg, unfractionated or low-molecular weight heparin) therapy. Warfarin is also used for chronic therapy to reduce the risk of thromboembolic episodes in patients with chronic atrial fibrillation.

Warfarin is rapidly and extensively absorbed from the GI tract. Peak plasma concentrations occur between 60 and 90 minutes after an oral dose with bioavailability ranging between 75% and 100%. Albumin is the principal binding protein with 97.5% to 99.9% of warfarin being bound.

Warfarin's metabolism is stereospecific. The R-isomer is oxidized to 6-hydroxywarfarin and further reduced to 9S, 11R-warfarin alcohols. The S-isomer is oxidized to 7-hydroxywarfarin and further reduced to 9S, 11R-warfarin alcohols. The stereospecific isomer alcohol metabolites have anticoagulant activity in humans. The warfarin alcohols are renally eliminated. The elimination half-lives of the two warfarin isomers differ substantially. The S-isomer half-life is approximately 33 hours and the R-isomer half-life is 45 hours.

Warfarin therapy may be started on the first day of unfractionated or low-molecular weight heparin therapy. Traditionally, warfarin 5 mg daily is started for the first 2 to 3 days then adjusted to maintain the desired prothrombin time (PT) or INR. The timing of INR measurements relative to changes in daily dose is important. After the administration of a warfarin dose, the peak depression of coagulation occurs in about 36 hours. It is important to select an appropriate time during a given dosing interval and perform coagulation tests consistently at that time. After the first four to five doses, the fluctuation in the INR over a 24-hour dosing interval is minimal. The time course of stabilization of warfarin plasma concentrations and coagulation response during continued administration of maintenance doses is less clear. A minimum of 10 days appears to be necessary before the dose-response curve shows interval-to-interval stability. During the first week of therapy, two INR measurements should be determined to assess the impact of warfarin accumulation on INR. Several factors should be assessed when evaluating an unexpected response to warfarin. Laboratory results should be verified to exclude inaccurate or spurious results. The medication profile should be reviewed to exclude drug-drug interactions including changes in warfarin product, and the patient should be evaluated for disease-drug interactions, nutritional-drug interactions, and noncompliance.

Bleeding is the major complication associated with the use of warfarin, occurring in 6% to 29% of patients receiving the drug. Bleeding complications include ecchymoses, hemoptysis, and epistaxis, as well as fatal or life-threatening hemorrhage.

Dose

- 5 mg PO qd × 3 days, then adjusted to maintain the INR between 2 and 3.
- To prevent thromboembolism associated with prosthetic heart valves, the dose should be adjusted to maintain an INR between 2.5 and 3.5.

Monitoring Parameters

- INR, hemoglobin, hematocrit, and signs of active bleeding

Factor Xa Inhibitors

Rivaroxaban

Rivaroxaban is an oral factor Xa inhibitor, indicated for venous thromboembolism (VTE) prophylaxis post hip or knee replacement, or prophylaxis of embolism, or cerebrovascular accident (CVA) in patients with nonvalvular atrial fibrillation. Additionally, the agent is also indicated for PE and deep venous thrombosis (DVT) treatment.

Dose

- *VTE prophylaxis post-surgery:* 10 mg PO qd
- Atrial fibrillation, nonvalvular-CVA prophylaxis: 20 mg PO qd
- DVT or PE treatment, and secondary prophylaxis: 15 mg PO bid × 21 days followed by 20 mg PO qd

Monitoring Parameters

- Hemoglobin, hematocrit, renal function, and signs of active bleeding

Direct Thrombin Inhibitors

Dabigatran

Dabigatran is an oral direct thrombin inhibitor indicated for use for stroke prevention in patients with non-valvular atrial fibrillation. In clinical trials, dabigatran was superior to warfarin in reducing the risk for stroke and systemic embolism with lower minor bleed risk comparatively. Dabigatran also has a developing role as a VTE prophylaxis after total knee or hip arthroplasty, as well as the treatment of DVT and PE. It is important to note that dabigatran capsules cannot be opened for feeding tube or oral administration.

Dose

- 150 mg PO bid

Monitoring Parameters

- Hemoglobin, hematocrit, aPTT, ecarin clotting time (ECT), and signs of active bleeding

Bivalirudin

Bivalirudin is an anticoagulant with direct thrombin inhibitor properties. Bivalirudin, when given with aspirin, is indicated for use as an anticoagulant in patients with unstable angina undergoing coronary angioplasty. It has been used as a substitute for unfractionated heparin; potential advantages over unfractionated heparin include activity against clot-bound thrombin, more predictable anticoagulation, and no inhibition by components of the platelet release reaction. A study has suggested the efficacy of SC bivalirudin in preventing deep vein thrombosis in orthopedic surgery patients. The place in therapy of bivalirudin will

be determined by further comparisons with unfractionated heparin, low-molecular-weight unfractionated heparins, and recombinant hirudin.

Dose

- Bolus: 1 mg/kg
- *Continuous infusion:* 2.5 mg/kg/h × 4 hours, if necessary 0.2 mg/kg/h for up to 20 hours

Monitoring Parameters

- Activated PTT, activated clotting time (ACT), hemoglobin, hematocrit, and signs of active bleeding

Argatroban

Argatroban is a selective thrombin inhibitor indicated for the prevention or treatment of thrombosis in unfractionated heparin–induced thrombocytopenia and for use in percutaneous coronary interventions (PCIs). It has also shown effectiveness in ischemic stroke and as an adjunct to thrombolysis in patients with acute MI. Further studies are needed to establish effectiveness for other indications. Argatroban is dosed as a continuous infusion that is titrated based on activated PTT, similar to unfractionated heparin. During PCI, the ACT may be used. A notable drug-laboratory value interaction is the increase in PT and INR values that occurs with argatroban therapy, which may complicate the monitoring of warfarin therapy once oral anticoagulation is initiated.

Dose

- *Percutaneous coronary intervention:* Bolus: 350 mcg/kg; continuous infusion: 25 mcg/kg/min
- *Heparin-induced thrombocytopenia with thrombosis:* Continuous infusion: 2 mcg/kg/min

Monitoring Parameters

- Activated PTT, ACT, PT, INR, hemoglobin, hematocrit, and signs of active bleeding

Glycoprotein IIb/IIIa Inhibitor

Glycoprotein IIb/IIIa inhibitors are recommended, in addition to aspirin and unfractionated heparin, in patients with acute coronary syndrome awaiting PCI. If the glycoprotein IIb/IIIa inhibitor is started in the catheterization laboratory just before PCI, abciximab is the agent of choice.

Dose

- *Abciximab:* Bolus: 0.25 mg/kg over 10 to 60 minutes; continuous infusion: 0.125 mcg/kg/min for 12 hours (maximum infusion of 10 mcg/kg/min)
- *Tirofiban:* Bolus infusion: 0.4 mcg/kg/min over 30 minutes; continuous infusion: 0.1 mcg/kg/min for 12 to 24 hours after angioplasty or atherectomy
- *Eptifibatide:* Bolus: 180 mcg/kg; continuous infusion: 2 mcg/kg/min until discharge or coronary artery bypass grafting (maximum of 72 hours)

Monitoring Parameters

- Platelet count, hemoglobin, hematocrit, and signs of active bleeding

Thrombolytic Agents

Thrombolytic agents may be beneficial as reperfusion therapy in ST-elevation myocardial infarction (STEMI). The 2013 American College of Cardiology Foundation/American Heart Association guidelines for the management of STEMI include the following recommendations in order from most supported by published literature (class I) to least supported (class III):

Class I Recommendations

- In the absence of contraindications, fibrinolytic therapy should be given to patients with STEMI and onset of ischemic symptoms within the previous 12 hours when it is anticipated that primary percutaneous coronary intervention (PCI) cannot be performed within 120 minutes of first medical contact.

Class IIa Recommendations

- In the absence of contraindications and when PCI is not available, fibrinolytic therapy is reasonable for patients with STEMI if there is clinical and/or electrocardiographic evidence of ongoing ischemia within 12 to 24 hours of symptom onset and a large area of myocardium at risk or hemodynamic instability.

Class III Recommendations

- Fibrinolytic therapy should not be administered to patients with ST depression except when a true posterior (inferobasal) MI is suspected or when associated with ST elevation in lead aVR.

Absolute contraindications to the use of thrombolytic agents include any active or recent bleeding, suspected aortic dissection, intracranial or intraspinal neoplasm, arteriovenous malformation or aneurysms, neurosurgery or significant closed head injury within the previous 3 months, ischemic stroke within the previous 3 months (except acute ischemic stroke within 3 hours), or facial trauma in the preceding 3 months. Relative contraindications include acute or chronic severe uncontrolled hypertension, ischemic stroke more than 3 months prior, traumatic or prolonged cardiopulmonary resuscitation greater than 10 minutes in duration, major surgery within the previous 3 weeks, internal bleeding within 2 to 4 weeks, noncompressible vascular punctures, prior allergic reaction to thrombolytics, pregnancy, active peptic ulcer, and current anticoagulation (risk increasing with increasing INR).

Adverse effects include bleeding from the GI or genitourinary tracts, as well as gingival bleeding and epistaxis. Superficial bleeding may occur from trauma sites such as those for IV access or invasive procedures. Intramuscular injections, with noncompressible arterial punctures, should be avoided during thrombolytic therapy.

Monitoring Parameters

- For short-term thrombolytic therapy of MI: ECG, signs and symptoms of ischemia, and signs and symptoms of bleeding at IV injection sites (laboratory monitoring is of little value)
- *Continuous infusion therapy:* Thrombin time, activated PTT, and fibrinogen, in addition to above-mentioned monitoring parameters

Alteplase

Alteplase (recombinant tissue-type plasminogen activator) has a high affinity for fibrin-bound plasminogen, allowing activation on the fibrin surface. Most plasmin formed remains bound to the fibrin clot, minimizing systemic effects. Alteplase is nonantigenic and should be considered in patients who have received streptokinase or anistreplase in the previous 6 to 9 months. The risk of an intracerebral bleed is approximately 0.5%.

Dose

- *Acute MI-accelerated infusion:* Patients over 67 kg, total dose 100 mg IV (15 mg IV bolus, then 50 mg over 30 minutes, then 35 mg over 60 minutes)
- *Acute MI-accelerated infusion:* Patients 67 kg or less, (15 mg IV bolus, then 0.75 mg/kg over 30 minutes, then 0.5 mg/kg over 60 minutes); total dose not to exceed 100 mg
- *Acute MI-3-hour infusion:* Weight 65 kg or more, 60 mg IV in the first hour (6 to 10 mg of which to be given as bolus), then 20 mg over the second hour, and 20 mg over the third hour
- *Acute MI-3-hour infusion:* Weight less than 65 kg, 1.25 mg/kg IV administered over 3 hours, give 60% in the first hour (10% of which to be given as bolus), give remaining 40% over the next 2 hours
- *Pulmonary embolism:* 100 mg IV over 2 hours

Tenecteplase

Tenecteplase (recombinant TNK-tissue type plasminogen activator) has a longer elimination half-life (20 to 24 minutes) and is more resistant to inactivation by plasminogen activator inhibitor-1 than alteplase. Tenecteplase appears more fibrin specific than alteplase, which may account for a lower rate of noncerebral bleeding comparatively. However, there have been reports of antibody development to tenecteplase. Tenecteplase and alteplase have similar clinical efficacy for thrombolysis after MI.

Dose

- *Acute MI:* 30 to 50 mg (based on weight) IV over 5 seconds

Reteplase

Reteplase is a recombinant plasminogen activator for use in acute MI and pulmonary embolism as a thrombolytic agent. Reteplase has a longer half-life (13 to 16 minutes) than that of alteplase, allowing for bolus administration. The dosing regimen requires double bolus doses.

Dose

- *Acute MI and pulmonary embolism:* Two 10-U IV bolus doses, infused over 2 minutes via a dedicated line. The second dose is administered 30 minutes after the initiation of the first injection.

IMMUNOSUPPRESSIVE AGENTS

Cyclosporine

Cyclosporine is used to prevent allograft rejection after solid organ transplantation and graft-vs-host disease in bone marrow transplant patients. Unlike other immunosuppressive agents, cyclosporine does not suppress bone marrow function. Cyclosporine inhibits cytokine synthesis and receptor expression needed for T-lymphocyte activation by interrupting signal transduction. A lack of cytokine disrupts the activation and proliferation of the helper and cytotoxic T-cells that are essential for rejection.

Cyclosporine is poorly absorbed from the GI tract with bioavailability averaging 30%. Its absorption is influenced by the type of organ transplant, time from transplantation, presence of biliary drainage, liver function, intestinal dysfunction, and the use of drugs that alter intestinal function. Cyclosporine is metabolized by cytochrome P-450 isoenzyme 3A to numerous metabolites with more than 90% of the dose excreted into the bile and eliminated in the feces. The kidneys eliminate less than 1% of the dose. There is no evidence that the metabolites have significant immunosuppressive activity compared with cyclosporine and none of the metabolites are known to cause nephrotoxicity.

Because of poor oral absorption, the oral dose is 3 times the IV dose. When converting from IV to oral administration, it is important to increase the oral dose by a factor of three to maintain stable cyclosporine concentrations. The oral solution can be administered diluted with chocolate milk or juice and administered through a nasogastric tube. The tube should be flushed before and after cyclosporine is administered to ensure complete drug delivery and optimal absorption.

The microemulsion formulation of cyclosporine capsules and solution has increased bioavailability compared to the original formulation of cyclosporine capsules and solution. These formulations are not bioequivalent and cannot be used interchangeably. Converting from cyclosporine capsules and solution for microemulsion to cyclosporine capsules and oral solution using as 1:1 mg/kg/day ratio may result in lower cyclosporine blood concentrations. Conversion between formulations should be made utilizing increased monitoring to avoid toxicity due to high concentrations or possible organ rejection due to low concentrations.

Nephrotoxicity is cyclosporine's major adverse effect. Three types of nephrotoxicity have been shown to occur. The first is an acute reversible reduction in glomerular filtration; second, tubular toxicity with possible enzymuria and aminoaciduria; and third, irreversible interstitial fibrosis and arteriopathy. The exact mechanism of cyclosporine nephrotoxicity is unclear, but may involve alterations in the various vasoactive substances in the kidney. Other side effects include a dose-dependent increase in bilirubin that occurs within the first 3 months after transplantation. Hyperkalemia can develop secondary to cyclosporine nephrotoxicity. Cyclosporine-induced hypomagnesemia can cause seizures. Neurotoxic effects such as tremors and paresthesias may occur in up to 15% of treated patients. Hypertension occurs frequently and may be due to the nephrotoxic effects or renal vasoconstrictive effects of the drug.

Tacrolimus (FK506)

Tacrolimus is a macrolide antibiotic produced by the fermentation broth of *Streptomyces tsukubaensis*. Although it bears no structural similarity to cyclosporine, its mode of action parallels cyclosporine. Tacrolimus exhibits similar in vitro effects to cyclosporine, but at concentrations 100 times lower than those of cyclosporine.

Tacrolimus is primarily metabolized in the liver by the cytochrome P-450 isoenzyme 3A4 to at least 15 metabolites. There is also some evidence to suggest that tacrolimus may be metabolized in the gut. The 13-*O*-demethyl-tacrolimus appears to be the major metabolite in patient blood. Less than 1% of a dose is excreted unchanged in the urine of liver transplant patients. Renal clearance accounts for less than 1% of total body clearance. The mean terminal elimination half-life is 12 hours but ranges from 8 to 40 hours. Patients with liver impairment have a longer tacrolimus half-life, reduced clearance, and elevated tacrolimus concentrations. The elevated tacrolimus concentrations are associated with increased nephrotoxicity in these patients. Because tacrolimus is primarily metabolized by the cytochrome P-450 enzyme system, it is anticipated that drugs known to interact with this enzyme system may affect tacrolimus disposition.

In most cases, IV therapy can be switched to oral therapy within 2 to 4 days after starting therapy. The oral dose should start 8 to 12 hours after the IV infusion has been stopped. The usual initial oral dose is 150 to 300 mcg/kg/day, administered in two divided doses every 12 hours.

Nephrotoxicity is the most common adverse effect associated with the use of tacrolimus. Nephrotoxicity occurs in up to 40% of transplant patients receiving tacrolimus. Other side effects observed during tacrolimus therapy include headache, tremor, insomnia, diarrhea, hypertension, hyperglycemia, and hyperkalemia.

Sirolimus (Rapamycin)

Sirolimus is an immunosuppressive agent used to the prophylaxis of organ rejection in patients receiving renal transplants.

It typically is used in regimens containing cyclosporine and corticosteroids. Sirolimus inhibits T-lymphocyte activation and proliferation that occurs in response to antigenic and cytokine stimulation. Sirolimus also inhibits antibody production.

Sirolimus is administered orally once daily. The initial dose of sirolimus should be administered as soon as possible after transplantation. It is recommended that sirolimus be taken 4 hours after cyclosporine modified oral solution or capsules.

Routine therapeutic drug level monitoring is not required in most patients. Sirolimus levels should be monitored in patients with hepatic impairment, during concurrent administration of cytochrome P-450 cyp3a4 inducers and inhibitors, or when cyclosporine dosing is reduced or discontinued. Mean sirolimus whole blood trough concentrations, as measured by immunoassay, are approximately 9 ng/mL for the 2-mg/day dose and 17 ng/mL for the 5-mg/day dose. Results from other assays may differ from those with an immunoassay. On average, chromatographic methods such as HPLC or mass spectroscopy yield results that are 20% lower than immunoassay whole blood determinations.

SPECIAL DOSING CONSIDERATIONS

Drug Disposition in the Elderly

The elderly population is the fastest growing segment of the population in the United States. Older patients consume nearly 3 times as many prescription drugs as younger patients and therefore are at risk for experiencing significantly more drug-drug interactions and ADEs. The most common risk factors that contribute to adverse events include polypharmacy, low body mass, preexisting chronic disease, excessive length of therapy, organ dysfunction, and prior history of drug reaction. Special attention must be paid on the part of healthcare professionals when dosing medications in these patients with low body mass and potentially impaired metabolism and clearance of drug secondary to age-related organ dysfunction (eg, renal or hepatic impairment). Agents that are of particular interest in this population include sedatives, antihypertensives, narrow therapeutic index drugs, and anti-infectives. These agents often require a decrease in dose or the extension of the dosing interval to facilitate drug clearance and minimize the likelihood of toxicity.

Therapeutic Drug Monitoring

Therapeutic drug monitoring (TDM) is the process of using drug concentrations, pharmacokinetic principles, and pharmacodynamics to optimize drug therapy (see Table 22-5). The goal of TDM is to maximize the therapeutic effect while avoiding toxicity. Drugs that are toxic at serum concentrations close to those required for therapeutic effect are the drugs most commonly monitored. The indications for therapeutic drug monitoring include narrow therapeutic range, limited objective monitoring parameters, potential for poor patient response, the need for therapeutic confirmation, unpredictable dose-response relationship, serious consequences of toxicity or lack of efficacy, correlation between serum concentration and efficacy or toxicity, suspected toxicity, identification of drug interactions, determination of individual pharmacokinetic parameters, and changes in patient pathophysiology or disease state. The specific indication for TDM is important, because it affects the timing of the sample. Timing of sample collection depends on the question being asked.

The timing of serum drug concentrations is critical for the interpretation of the results. The timing of peak serum drug concentrations depends on the route of administration and the drug product. Peak serum drug concentrations occur soon after an IV bolus dose, whereas they are delayed after IM, SC, or oral doses. Oral medications can be administered as either liquid or rapid- or slow-release dosage forms (eg, theophylline). The absorption and distribution phases must be considered when obtaining a peak serum drug concentration. The peak serum concentration may be much higher and occur earlier after a liquid or rapid-release dosage form compared to a sustained-release dosage form. Trough concentrations usually are obtained just prior to the next dose. Drugs with long half-lives (eg, phenobarbital) or sustained-release dosage forms (eg, theophylline) have minimal variation between their peak and trough concentrations. The timing of the determination of serum concentrations may be less critical in patients taking these dosage forms. Serum drug concentrations may be drawn at any time after achieving a steady state in a patient who is receiving a drug by continuous IV infusion. However, in patients receiving a drug by continuous infusion, the serum specimen should be drawn from a site away from where the drug is infusing. If toxicity is suspected, serum drug concentrations can be obtained at any time during the dosing interval.

Appropriate interpretation of serum concentrations is the step that requires an understanding of relevant patient factors, pharmacokinetics of the drug, and dosing regimen. Misinterpretation of serum drug concentrations can result in ineffective and, at worst, harmful dosage adjustments. Interpreting serum concentrations includes an assessment of whether the patient's dose is appropriate, if the patient is at a steady state, the timing of the blood samples, an assessment of whether the time of blood sampling is appropriate for the indication, and an evaluation of the method of delivery to assess the completeness of drug delivery. Serum drug concentrations should be interpreted within the context of the individual patient's condition. Therapeutic ranges serve as guidelines for each patient. Doses should not be adjusted on the basis of laboratory results alone. Individual dosage ranges should be developed for each patient as various patients may experience therapeutic efficacy, failure, or toxicity within a given therapeutic range.

ESSENTIAL CONTENT CASE

Tips for Calculating IV Medication Infusion Rates

Information Required to Calculate IV Infusion Rates to Deliver Specific Medication Doses

- Dose to be infused (eg, mg/kg/min, mg/min, mg/h)
- Concentration of IV solution (eg, dopamine 400 mg in D_5W 250 mL = 1.6 mg/mL; nitroglycerin 50 mg in D_5W 250 mL = 200 mcg/mL)
- Patient's weight

1. Calculate the IV infusion rate in milliliters per hour for a 70-kg patient requiring dobutamine 5 mcg/kg/min using a dobutamine admixture of 500 mg in D_5W 250 mL.

   - Dose to be infused: 5 mcg/kg/min
   - Dobutamine concentration: 500 mg/250 mL = 2 mg/mL or 2000 mcg/mL
   - Patient weight: 70 kg

Calculation:

5 mcg/kg/min × 70 kg = 350 mcg/min
350 mcg/min × 60 min/h = 21,000 mcg/h
21,000 mcg/h ÷ 2000 mcg/mL = 10.5 mL/h

Answer: Setting the infusion pump at 10.5 mL/h will deliver dobutamine at a dose of 5 mcg/kg/min.

2. Calculate the IV infusion rate in milliliters per hour for a 70-kg patient requiring nitroglycerin 50 mcg/min using a nitroglycerin admixture of 50 mg in D_5W 250 mL.

   - Dose to be infused: 50 mcg/min
   - Nitroglycerin concentration: 50 mg/250 mL = 0.2 mg/mL or 200 mcg/mL
   - Patient weight: 70 kg

Calculation:

50 mcg/min × 60 min/h = 3000 mcg/h
3000 mcg/h ÷ 200 mcg/mL = 15 mL/h

Answer: Setting the infusion pump at 15 mL/h will deliver nitroglycerin at a dose of 50 mcg/min.

3. Calculate the IV loading dose and infusion rate in milliliters per hour for a 70-kg patient requiring aminophylline 0.6 mg/kg/h using an aminophylline admixture of 1 g in D_5W 500 mL. The loading dose should be diluted in D_5W 100 mL and infused over 30 minutes.

   - Desired dose: Loading dose: 6 mg/kg
     Maintenance infusion: 0.6 mg/kg/h
   - Aminophylline concentration:
     Aminophylline vial: 500 mg/20 mL = 25 mg/mL
     Aminophylline infusion: 1 g/500 mL = 2 mg/mL
   - Patient weight: 70 kg

Calculation:

Loading dose: 6 mg/kg × 70 kg = 420 mg
420 mg ÷ 25 mg/mL = 16.8 mL
Infusion rate: Aminophylline 16.8 mL + D_5W 100 mL = 116.8 mL
116.8 mL ÷ 0.5/h = 233.6 mL/h

Answer: Setting the infusion pump at 234 mL/h will infuse the aminophylline loading dose over 1/2 hour.

Maintenance dose: 0.6 mg/kg/h × 70 kg = 42 mg/h
42 mg/h ÷ 2 mg/mL = 21 mL/h

Answer: Setting the infusion pump at 21 mL/h will deliver the aminophylline maintenance dose at 42 mg/h, or 0.6 mg/kg/h.

SELECTED BIBLIOGRAPHY

General

Institute of Safe Medication Practices. nwww.ismp.org. Accessed February 8, 2013.

Martin SJ, Olsen KM, Susla GM. *The Injectable Drug Reference.* 2nd ed. Des Plaines, IL: Society of Critical Care Medicine; 2006.

Sulsa GM, Suffredini AF, McAreavey D, et al. *The Handbook of Critical Care Drug Therapy.* 3rd ed. Philadelphia, PA: Lippincott William and Wilkins; 2006.

Vincent J, Abraham E, Kochanek P, et al. *Textbook of Critical Care.* 6th ed. Philadelphia, PA: Elsevier; 2011.

Evidence-Based Practice Guidelines

Barr J, Fraser GL, Puntillo K, et al. Clinical practice guidelines for the management of pain, agitation, and delirium in adult patients in the intensive care unit. *Crit Care Med.* 2013;41:263-306.

Dellinger RP, Levy MM, Rhodes A, et al. Surviving sepsis campaign: international guidelines for management of severe sepsis and septic shock: 2012. *Crit Care Med.* DOI: 10.1097/CCM.0b013e31827e83af.

O'Gara PT, Kushner FG, Ascheim DD, et al. American College of Cardiology Foundation/American Heart Association Guidelines for Management of ST-Elevation Myocardial Infarction. Executive summary. *Circulation.* 2013;127:529-555.

Task Force of the American College of Critical Care Medicine (ACCM) of the Society of Critical Care Medicine (SCCM), American Society of Health-System Pharmacist, American College of Chest Physicians. Clinical practice guidelines for sustained neuromuscular blockage in the adult critically ill patient. *Crit Care Med.* 2002;30:142-156.

ETHICAL AND LEGAL CONSIDERATIONS 8

Sarah Delgado

KNOWLEDGE COMPETENCIES

1. Characterize the nurse's role in recognizing and addressing ethical concerns.

2. Identify ethical principles and describe their application in the healthcare setting.

3. Describe the steps involved in analyzing an ethical problem.

As new ethical issues in progressive care continue to emerge, practitioners must develop skills in ethical decision making. An ethical dilemma occurs when two (or more) ethically acceptable but mutually exclusive courses of action are present. The dilemma is further complicated as either choice can be supported by an ethical principle, yet there are consequences for either choice. Moral distress, another common ethical problem, occurs when a provider believes he knows the ethically acceptable action to take but feels unable to do so. Competence in moral decision making evolves throughout one's professional career. However, there are general moral principles and guidelines that direct ethical reasoning and provide a standard to which professional nurses are held. Beginning clinicians, as well as more experienced nurses, should be familiar with the moral expectations and ethical accountability embedded in the nursing profession. This chapter introduces the elements that serve as a foundation for addressing ethical problems, including professional codes and standards, institutional policies, and ethical principles. Advance directives, end-of-life issues, and ethical environment are also discussed.

THE FOUNDATION FOR ETHICAL DECISION MAKING

Professional Codes and Standards

The purpose of professional codes is to identify the moral requirements of a profession and the relationships in which they engage. The Code for Nurses developed by the American Nurses Association (ANA) articulates the essential values, principles, and obligations that guide nursing actions. The nine provisions of the ANA *Code of Ethics for Nurses* identify the ethical obligations of nurses and are applicable across all nursing roles (American Nurses Association, Code of Ethics for Nurses with Interpretive Statements, 2001. http://www.nursingworld.org/MainMenuCategories/EthicsStandards/CodeofEthicsforNurses). While these provisions do not address specific ethical problems, they do provide a framework for examining issues and understanding the nurse's role in resolving them.

In addition to the ANA Code, nurses function in accordance with particular standards of practice. Standards of nursing practice are delineated by professional organizations and statutory bodies that govern the practice of nursing in various jurisdictions. Derived from nursing's contract with society, professional nursing standards define the criteria for the assessment and evaluation of nursing practice. External bodies, such as state boards of nursing, impose certain regulations for licensure, regulate the practice of nursing, and evaluate and monitor the actions of professional nurses. Many organizations also delineate standards of practice for registered nurses practicing in a defined area of specialty; for example, the American Association of Critical-Care Nurses (AACN) has established standards and expectations of performance for nurses practicing in critical care.

Standards of practice outlined by statutory bodies and specialty organizations are not confined to clinical skills and knowledge. Nurses are expected to function within the profession's code of ethics and are held morally and legally accountable for unethical practice. When allegations of unsafe, illegal, or unethical practice arise, the regulatory body serves to protect the public by investigating and disciplining the culpable professional. Although specialty organizations do not have authority to retract professional licensure, issues of professional misconduct are reviewed and may result in revocation of certification and notification of external parties.

Position Statements and Guidelines

In an effort to address specific issues in clinical practice, many professional organizations develop position statements or guidelines. The purpose of position statements is to apply the values, principles, and rules described in the ANA *Code of Ethics for Nurses* to particular contemporary ethical issues. Familiarity with the AACN and ANA position statements helps the progressive care nurse to clarify and articulate a position consistent with the professional values of nursing.

To illustrate the application of position statements, consider a situation in which a progressive care nurse is asked to intentionally hasten a patient's death. The Code for Nurses and ANA position statement on assisted suicide and active euthanasia clarify the nurse's role when such requests are made. In addition, the ANA position statement on pain management and control of distressing symptoms in dying patients provides guidance for addressing the physical and emotional needs of patients at the end of life. In this case, the nurse and physician should explore the patient's request for an accelerated death and explain the legal and moral boundaries of his request. The option to withdraw treatment and provide aggressive palliative care should be offered and examined with the patient. The Essential Content Case "Working Together" provides a further example of the application of professional organization's position statements to clinical practice.

Institutional Policies

Because nurses practice within organizations, institutional policies and procedures also guide their practice. Institutional guidelines for assessing decision-making capacity, caring for un-represented patients who lack capacity, or policies for the determination of brain death are intended to guide employees of an organization when they are faced with ethical uncertainty. These policies usually reflect ethical expectations congruent with the professional codes of ethics. However, in some circumstances, organizations may assume a particular position or value and therefore expect the employees to uphold this position; for example, some hospitals endorse particular religious positions and may prohibit professional practices that violate these positions. Ideally, the nurse and institution have complementary values and beliefs about professional responsibilities and obligations. Institutions often provide internal resources to help clinicians resolve difficult ethical issues. Institutional ethics committees provide consultation on ethical situations and institutional policies outline the procedures of case review, which

---

ESSENTIAL CONTENT CASE

Working Together

Julia is 28-year-old registered nurse who recently married and moved to a new city. She was pleased to land a job in a telemetry unit in a large academic medical center. While still on orientation, she was caring for a patient who had undergone CABG and subsequently developed sternal wound infection. The family had many questions about this complication and, after answering them to the best of her ability, Julia called the patient's CT surgeon. As she began describing her conversation with the family, the CT surgeon, stated "you are a nurse and it's not your place to talk to the patient's family. Stop trying to practice medicine without a license" and then hung up on her. When she spoke with her preceptor about the phone call, he advised "Oh don't worry, he's made every nurse here cry at one time or another. He's just like that. But he's a great surgeon and the hospital is really lucky to have him." As Julia leaves at the end of her shift, she starts to question her "luck" in getting a position on this unit.

Case Question: How does Julia's position as a new nurse on the floor affect her response to this situation?

Answer: As a new nurse, Julia has not had the time to demonstrate the leadership and strong clinical skills that would make her an opinion leader among the nurses on the unit. However, being new also has an advantage. While other nurses may have reached a state of accepting the unprofessional, verbally abusive conduct of this surgeon because "it's always been that way," Julia's fresh perspective lends conviction to her belief that the behavior should not be tolerated. In addition, she can observe the interactions of other nurses and begin to identify opinion leaders to support her effort as a change agent.

The AACN position statement *Zero Tolerance for Abuse* addresses Julia's surprise and disgust that the neurosurgeon's disrespectful behavior is tolerated and accepted by the nurses on her unit. In addition, the AACN position statement on moral distress describes how nurses and managers are obligated to recognize and address sources of moral distress, including verbal abuse from colleagues. Moral distress occurs when one knows the right action but feels unable to take it. Julie's colleagues have experienced verbal abuse and felt the surgeon should be reported to a higher authority but they felt unable to do so because the surgeon is highly regarded for his skill and reputation. Applying these position statements to her current situation, Julia knows that the neurosurgeon's behavior is abusive and therefore not acceptable and furthermore, that accepting such abuse can generate moral distress and therefore she is compelled to take action. The fifth provision of the ANA *Code of Ethics for Nurses* similarly advises nurses of the ethical obligation to care for themselves and supports Julia's decision to report the neurosurgeon's behavior to her manager.

ESSENTIAL CONTENT CASE

Who Decides?

A 82-year-old grandmother has been on the general medical floor for 4 weeks following a large anterolateral myocardial infarction. She has suffered from CHF, pulmonary edema, and hypotension, and now has developed pneumonia. Her family is very supportive and visits her often. The physicians have communicated with the family, and because the patient does not have an advance directive, the family has entrusted the physicians with making the "right decisions."

Despite treatment for her pneumonia, the patient becomes progressively more confused while on the unit and at times tries to pull on her Foley catheter, her IV line, and oxygen mask. As a result she is sometimes placed in soft wrist restraints. The nurses believe that it is inappropriate to continue treating her aggressively, particularly when her actions suggest she is trying to refuse care and her prolonged illness makes her unlikely to regain her prior functional status.

After multiple complaints from staff involved in the care of this patient, the unit's clinical nurse specialist, Rhonda, asks the physician to discuss the goals of care with the patient's family. The physician states that "the family has already told me to make the right decisions" and that gives him the authority to decide what is best for this patient without further discussion. Rhonda is uncomfortable asking her staff to continue to restrain the patient and provide aggressive care based on the physician's perspective rather than a clear understanding of the patient's values and goals regarding continued treatment.

Case Question: What steps can be taken to address the discomfort that Rhonda and her colleagues are experiencing?

Answer: As described in *AACN's 4 A's to Address Moral Distress*, a stepwise approach is appropriate to addressing the distress these nurses are experiencing. The first step, to "Ask," has already been completed in this case; the staff recognizes there is a significant problem. The next step is to "Affirm" their feelings, which may require a meeting with all the nurses involved in the care of this patient, giving each the chance to voice his or her feelings and to be validated by other members of the group. The third step, "Assess," requires the nurses to evaluate the severity of their distress and determine their motivation to take action. The final step is to "Act," which may involve working with the medical team to identify an appropriate course of action, calling an ethics committee consult, asking the family to take a more active role in making decisions about the patient's care, or seeking support from the nurse manager or supervisor. Rhonda and her colleagues may feel hesitant to advocate for this patient but also need to remember that inaction will worsen the distress, and may ultimately affect the care of all patients on the unit. Furthermore, health care teams in which all members share their perspectives deliver high quality nursing care. Addressing morally distressing situations such as this empowers nurses to remain involved in difficult patient situations and to recognize that information gained through nursing care is critical to effective and appropriate care.

should be available to all employees. In the case example "Who Decides?" the nurse should consider what resources, such as the ethics committee, another physician, or the nurse manager, might assist her in advocating for this patient, and clarifying the goals of care. While the ANA Code states that nurses are obligated to advocate for patients, finding support is an essential step in that process.

Legal Standards

Public policies and state and federal laws also influence the practice of healthcare professionals. Policies from agencies such as the Centers for Disease Control and Prevention (CDC) or the Department of Health and Human Services (DHHS) generate changes in practice and in the actions of health professionals. In addition, the Centers for Medicare and Medicaid Services (CMS), a major payor for healthcare, sets standards for hospitals and providers that must be abided to ensure reimbursement for services. State legislation can also influence nursing practice; for instance, some states have laws that support hospitals and providers in refusing to provide futile medical care.

The Affordable Care Act (ACA) passed in 2010 includes tracking quality indicators such as the rate of hospital readmission (CMS) and tying these indicators to Medicare reimbursement for services. The ACA thus creates financial incentives for hospitals to ensure that patients are adequately supported at the time of discharge to decrease the likelihood that the patient returns to the hospital in the first 30 days. In this way, the ACA offers a legal manifestation of the ethical principle of non-maleficence, discussed below. The Health Information Portability and Accountability Act (HIPAA) Privacy Rule similarly creates a legal mandate to honor the ethical obligation of confidentiality (DHHS).

When faced with an ethical problem, professional guidelines, institutional policies, or legal standards can assist, and sometimes resolve, the issue. Thus, it is imperative that nurses be familiar with these resources and how to access them. However, nurses also need to recognize that guidelines and policies and even the law do not always answer the question of what action should be taken. In such situations, the nurse must be prepared to identify the ethical principles involved and follow a step wise approach to addressing the problem.

Principles of Ethics

One of the most influential perspectives in biomedical ethics is that of principle-based ethics. This framework arose in the 1970s through the work of Beauchamp and Childress and continues to be a dominant method of thinking today. Inherent in this viewpoint is the belief that some basic moral principles define the essence of ethical obligations in human society. Four basic principles, and derivative imperatives or rules, are considered prima facie or binding. In other words, to breach a principle is wrong unless there are prevailing and compelling reasons that outweigh the necessary infringement. The principles and rules are binding, but not absolute.

Because many approaches to ethics integrate the rules and principles outlined by the principle-oriented approach, understanding the fundamental concepts of principle-based ethics is helpful to the progressive care nurse. The primary principles used are nonmaleficence, beneficence, justice, and respect for persons (or autonomy). The derivative principles or rules include privacy, confidentiality, veracity, and fidelity. The principles are not ordered in a particular hierarchy, but their application and interpretation are based on the specific features of the dilemma and the values of the team members involved. Articulating the principles involved and recognizing the personal values of the providers and family members are essential steps to resolving an ethical problem.

Nonmaleficence

The principle of nonmaleficence imposes the duty to do no harm. This injunction suggests that the nurse should not knowingly inflict harm and is responsible if negligent actions result in detrimental consequences. In general, progressive care nurses preserve the principle of nonmaleficence by maintaining competence and practicing within accepted standards of care.

When the patient's safety or well-being is threatened by the actions of others, the nurse is obligated to remove and prevent harm. Knowledge of unsafe, illegal, or unethical practice by any healthcare provider obligates the nurse both morally and legally to intervene. The nurse must remove the immediate danger and communicate the infringement to the appropriate sources to prevent further harm. The nurse should turn to institutional policies and state nurse practice acts for guidance on the appropriate process of reporting.

Beneficence

The ethical principle of beneficence affirms an obligation to prevent harm, remove harm, and promote good by actively helping others to advance and realize their interests. Intrinsic to this principle is action. The nurse moves beyond the concept of not inflicting harm (nonmaleficence) by actively promoting the best interests of the patient and family.

To optimize the patient's well-being and prevent harm, nurses must practice with the essential knowledge and skills required of the clinical setting. Nurses are expected to practice according to established standards of practice, to continue professional learning to improve clinical practice, and to refrain from providing care measures in which they are not proficient.

Beyond the provision of safe nursing care, the promotion of the patient's well-being requires that the patient's perspective be known and valued. Therefore, the nurse must gain an understanding of the patient's underlying value structure to ensure that the care provided is consistent with the patient's wishes. The duty to do good requires that the healthcare team understand the patient's interpretation of what is "good."

The obligations to do no harm (nonmaleficence) and to promote good or remove harm (beneficence) extend beyond provider incompetence and safe care. In ethically challenging situations, the potential harms associated with each of the available treatment options should be considered before deciding the best action. This can be difficult because sometimes an identified harm is death and in some of these cases death is not the worst harm. Careful and thorough thinking with regard to harms and benefits to a patient can often clarify not only which actions might be "right" for a patient, but also which actions might be "wrong."

Respect for Persons (Autonomy)

The principle of respect for persons or autonomy affirms the freedom and right of an individual to make decisions and choose actions based on that individual's personal values and beliefs. In other words, an autonomous choice is an informed decision made without coercion that reflects the individual's underlying interests and values.

To respect a person's autonomy is to recognize that patients may hold certain views and take particular actions that are incongruent with the values of the healthcare providers. Often this concept is difficult for healthcare providers to accept and endorse, particularly when the patient's choice conflicts with the caregivers' view of what is best in this situation. As an advocate, the nurse appreciates this diversity and continues to provide care as long as the patient's choice is an informed decision and does not infringe on the autonomous actions of others.

Patients in the progressive care setting frequently have varying degrees of autonomy. The capacity of ill patients to participate in the decision-making process often is compromised and constrained by internal factors such as the effects of pharmacologic agents, the emotional elements associated with a sudden acute illness, and the physiologic factors related to the underlying illness. External factors, such as the hospital environment, also influence the patient's potential to make autonomous choices. As demonstrated in the case example "Who Decides," providers may differ in their assessment of patient capacity. Often, institutions have policies outlining a process for determining a patient's capacity. In the case of "Who Decides," the nurses involved in the patient's care may find these policies helpful in guiding their thinking as well as their action. The progressive care nurse advocates for the patient by limiting, as much as possible, the factors that constrain the patient's freedom to make autonomous choices. In this way the nurse supports the principle of respect for personal autonomy and upholds the ethical duty of beneficence.

Justice

The principle of justice is defined as fairness and in healthcare, is often applied to the manner in which goods, burdens, and services are distributed among a population. When resources are limited, justice demands that they be fairly allocated. There are three interpretations of the justice principle that will be described here by the following example. Imagine a population of people who have a set of goods that must be shared fairly among them. Egalitarian justice would demand that the goods be divided into equal portions and every member of the population given the same share. Humanitarian justice would demand that the goods be divided according to the needs of each member, with the neediest members getting larger portions. Libertarian justice would demand the goods be distributed according to the contributions made by each member of the population; those making the greatest contributions get the greater share.

Organ transplant offers a clear example of the justice principle in healthcare. Organs are a scarce resource and some of those listed for transplant will not survive the wait. Priority for transplant can be based strictly on time spent waiting (an egalitarian approach), or on illness severity (a humanitarian approach) or based on an assessment of an individual's contributions and potential contributions to society (libertarian approach).

On a day-to-day basis, nurses make decisions involving the allocation of nursing care—which patient to assess first or how to assign patients on the unit to the staff on the next shift. The complex and competing demands for nursing resources can lead to chaotic and random decisions. The principle of justice argues for a comprehensive, thoughtful approach to address competing claims to resources.

Privacy and Confidentiality

Privacy and confidentiality are associated, but distinct, concepts that are derived from the principles of respect for autonomy, beneficence, and nonmaleficence. Privacy refers to the right of an individual to be free from unjustified or unnecessary access by others.

In the progressive care setting the patient's privacy often is disregarded. The design of many units includes easy visualization of patients from the nurses' station, and open access to the patient is presumed by most caregivers. This suggests a breach of individual privacy. Practitioners should be particularly attentive to requesting permission from the patient for any bodily intrusion or physical exposure. The casual infringement of an individual's privacy erodes the foundation for establishing a trusting and caring practitioner-patient relationship.

Confidentiality refers to the protection of information. When the patient shares information with the nurse or a member of the healthcare team, the information should be treated as confidential and discussed only with those directly involved in the patient's care. Exceptions to confidentiality include quality improvement activities, mandatory disclosures to public health agencies, reporting abuse, or required disclosure in a judicial setting. Most other disclosures of information obtained in a confidential manner should be shared with appropriate persons only when strong

and compelling reasons to do so exist. The patient should be informed of the impending disclosure, and ideally the patient should authorize the disclosure.

Violations of patient confidentiality occur in many subtle ways. The use of electronic medical records and the transmission of patient information via facsimile are common practices in many institutions. Persons unrelated to the patient's medical care who have access to the computers or facsimile may view confidential information without the individual's permission. Other ways in which confidentiality is unprotected include casual conversations in hallways or elevators in which patient information is shared within earshot of strangers, the unauthorized release of patient information to friends or the media, and healthcare professionals within the institution taking the liberty to view a coworker's medical record.

Nurses may feel conflicted when a patient discloses confidential information. The profession of nursing strongly values the principle of respect for persons and highly regards the concept of protecting confidential information. Therefore, decisions to break a patient's confidentiality must be well considered and require balancing competing obligations and claims; for example, a nurse may consider breaking a patient's confidentiality if there is a clear indication that, without doing so, harm may come to another individual. Clearly, this decision should not be made in isolation, and the nurse should seek advice when confronted with this difficult situation.

Fidelity

Fidelity is the obligation to be faithful to commitments and promises, and uphold the implicit and explicit commitments to patients, colleagues, and employers. The nurse portrays this concept by maintaining a faithful relationship with the patient, communicating honestly, and meeting the obligations to oneself, the profession of nursing, other healthcare professionals, and the employer.

The concept of fidelity is particularly important when caring for very sick patients. The vulnerability of these patients increases their dependency on the relationship with the nurse, thus making the nurse's faithfulness to that relationship essential. Nurses demonstrate this faithfulness by fulfilling the commitments of the relationship, which include the provision of competent care and advocacy on the patient's behalf. In addition, the nurse is obligated to demonstrate fidelity in relationships with colleagues and employers. In this way, the principle of fidelity can be difficult to uphold as institutions may have policies, such as those related to resource utilization, that the nurse finds are in conflict with the patient's best interests. When confronted with such situations, the nurse is wise to carefully weigh the ethical principles involved, to seek guidance if necessary, and to consider a role as a moral agent of change if appropriate.

Veracity

The rule of veracity simply means that one should tell the truth and not lie or deceive others. Derived from the principle of respect for persons and the concept of fidelity, veracity is fundamental to relationships and society. The nurse-patient relationship is based on truthful communication and the expectation that each party will adhere to the rules of veracity. Deception, misrepresentation, or inadequate disclosure of information undermines and erodes the patient's trust in healthcare providers.

Patients expect that information about their condition will be relayed in an open, honest, and sensitive manner. Without truthful communication, patients are unable to assess the options available and make fully informed decisions. However, the complex nature of acute illness does not always manifest as a single truth with clear boundaries. Uncertainty about the course of the illness, the appropriate treatment, or the plan of care is common in progressive care and a single "truth" may not exist. As emphasized in a model of patient-centered care, patients or surrogate decision makers must be kept informed of the plan of care and areas of uncertainty should be openly acknowledged. Disclosure of uncertainty enables the patient or surrogate to realistically examine the proposed plan of care and reduces the likelihood that the healthcare team will proceed in a paternalistic manner.

The Ethics of Care

The ethic of care is viewed as an alternative to the principled approach in bioethics. Rather than distinguish the ethical dilemma as a conflict of principles, the ethic of care involves the analysis of important relationships in a case, and emphasizes that the correct ethical action is one that preserves the key relationships (patient-spouse or patient-child). Carol Gilligan (1984) first described the ethic of care after observing how children make ethical decisions. Some adhere to rules ("do not steal" or "do not lie"), others consider how an action will affect others involved (hurt feelings, loss of trust). These ways of thinking carry through to adulthood. Most adults can view a situation through both the rules lens and the relationship lens.

The ethic of care begins from an attached, involved, and interdependent position. From this standpoint, morality is viewed as caring about others, developing relationships, and maintaining connections. Moral problems result from disturbances in interpersonal relationships and disruptions in the perceived responsibilities within relationships. The resolution of moral issues emerges as the involved parties examine the contextual features and embrace the relevance of the relationship and the related responsibilities.

In contrast, a principle-oriented or justice approach typically originates from a position of detachment and individuality. This approach recognizes the concepts of fairness, rights, and equality as the core of morality. Therefore, dilemmas arise when these elements are compromised. From this perspective, the approach to moral resolution is a reliance on formal logic, deductive reasoning, and a hierarchy of principles.

For nursing, the ethic of care provides a useful approach to moral analysis. Traditionally, nursing is a profession that necessitates attachment, caring, attention to context, and the development of relationships. To maintain this position, nurses develop proficiency in nurturing and sustaining relationships with patients and within families. The importance of relationships is also suggested in the first provision of the ANA *Code of Ethics for Nurses*. The ethic of care legitimizes and values the emotional, intuitive, and informal interpretation of moral issues. This perspective expands the sphere of inquiry and promotes the understanding and resolution of moral issues.

In addition to the care-based and principle-based approaches, there are other frameworks for examining ethical problems. Examples include the casuistry approach, which applies outcomes of past cases to the current situation, the narrative approach which examines the contextual features of the ethical problem, and the feminist approach which emphasizes addressing power imbalances. A full description of these approaches is beyond the scope of this chapter; however, an awareness of the variety of approaches to ethical problems is essential to collaborative decision making. The nurse, as member of the healthcare team, recognizes that other team members and patients and families may adopt different approaches when faced with the same ethical problem. Active listening and open-ended questions enable the nurse to recognize the approach adopted by another provider or family member, and this recognition improves communication and resolution of the ethical problem.

Paternalism

In ethics, paternalism refers to instances in which the principle of beneficence overrides that of autonomy. In such cases healthcare providers select and implement interventions that they believe will lead to the best outcomes without (or even against) consent from the patient. Sometimes, these actions are appropriate. An example of paternalism in progressive care is requiring mentally-competent patients to call for assistance before getting out of bed to use the bathroom. Fall prevention overrides the patient's autonomy but is justified by the benefit of ensuring patient safety. Most times, however, paternalism is not justified. It is generally not acceptable to override an autonomous patient's decisions without their consent. The case manager in the Essential Content case above was exercising paternalism in suggesting that the patient's daughter be contacted despite the patient's clear statement that she did not desire this course of action.

Progressive care nurses may find the balance between the patient's beliefs and the duty to promote good difficult and confusing. In the acute care setting it is often unclear what actions or course of treatment will most benefit the patient physiologically and which plan best reflects the patient's values. This uncertainty may result in fragmented discussions with the patient or surrogate and a treatment plan that reflects the values of the healthcare team rather than the patient. The nurse's moral obligation is to continue

ESSENTIAL CONTENT CASE

Examples of Different Ethical Frameworks and How They Affect Conclusions

An 85-year-old female with chronic obstructive pulmonary disease and atrial fibrillation is on the surgical unit following hip repair after a fall at home. The patient is evaluated by physical therapy who advises that the patient go to a skilled nursing facility for further care. The patient declines this advice, preferring to go back to her assisted living facility with home health physical therapy because she would "rather die than go to place with a lot of depressing sick people." Two weeks after discharge, the patient returns to the emergency room with a COPD flare and is admitted to the medical unit. Her INR is supratherapeutic at 8.6, she's lost 6 pounds, and she reports her albuterol inhaler is empty and she was unable to refill it. During the admission, physical therapy evaluates the patient and again recommends SNF placement for rehabilitation. The case manager places a call to the patient's daughter, who lives in a neighboring city, spends her days caring for her grandchildren and states she is not able to assist in her mother's care. The staff nurse caring for the patient is in her room when the hospitalist rounds, and tells the patient that she can probably be discharged the following day, assuming her INR is down, and her breathing continues to improve. The case manager then enters the room to begin discharge planning and the patient tells all three providers that she plans to go back to her assisted living facility. "Don't bother" she says, when the case manager offers to contact her daughter again, "she doesn't have time for me." Outside the patient's room, the case manager questions the safety of the patient's plan to return to the assisted living facility.

The three providers all witness the same situation but they interpret it through different ethical frameworks and arrive at different conclusions as to how to proceed:

The hospitalist believes the patient is competent to make her own decisions and should be discharged back to the assisted living facility as she requested. In adopting a principle-based approach, the hospitalist preferences the ethical principle of autonomy and feels that the patient's wishes, even if they are not consistent with what providers feel is in her best interest, ought to be honored.

The case manager similarly adopts a principle-based approach but she prefers the principle of beneficence and objects to discharging the patient to the assisted living facility. She points out that the patient's fall that lead to her prior hospital admission occurred at the assisted living facility indicating that this level of care is inadequate. In addition, the patient receives no medication assistance at the facility, and medication error contributed to her readmission. The case manager's desire to do good and ensure the patient's safety and well-being leads her to suggest further efforts to persuade the patient to go SNF, including possibly calling the daughter and enlisting her support, and consulting social work to consider an APS report if the patient continues to refuse.

The nurse adopts a care-based approach and focuses on the relationships in the situation. She notes that the daughter and the patient appear to be similarly distant from each other so she asks the patient about this relationship. The patient states that they grew apart over religious differences, specifically after the patient became a Jehovah's Witness. The patient goes on to tell the nurse "that's why I need to go back home. My church friends can come and see me since it's so close by and I know they are counting on me." Recognizing that the essential relationship for this patient is not with her daughter but with her church, she asks if her friends would be able to assist her with her medications, or to assume a regular schedule of visits to check on her after discharge. The patient reluctantly admits that she probably needs more assistance than she is currently receiving and then identifies the pastor's wife as the person who could be enlisted to coordinate more formal support from the church. The nurse therefore supports the patient's preference for discharge back to the assisted living with home health, including a home health social worker to ensure that the patient follows through in getting increased support from her fellow church members.

This case illustrates how professionals adopting different frameworks can arrive at different conclusions about the correct course of action. It also offers an example of ethical creativity, which is required in difficult situations, particularly in ethical dilemmas where two opposing courses of action can both be justified. What is needed in such situations is often a third option.

to promote the patient's interests by pursuing an accurate representation of the patient's beliefs and values, and to raise concerns of conflicting interpretations to appropriate members of the healthcare team.

Patient Advocacy

Patient advocacy is an essential role of the nurse, as emphasized in the ANA *Code of Ethics*. Although there are many models for defining and interpreting the relationship between the nurse and patient and no model can thoroughly describe its complexity and uniqueness, the patient advocacy role offers an essential description of the moral nature of this relationship. In addition, the third provision of the ANA *Code of Ethics*, "The nurse promotes, advocates for, and strives to protect the health, safety, and rights of the patient," specifically identifies the nurse's role as a patient advocate.

The term advocacy refers to the use of one's own skills and knowledge to promote the interests of another. Nurses, through their education and experience, are able to interpret healthcare information and understand the impact of disease and medical interventions in a unique way. A nurse acts as a patient advocate by applying this unique understanding to ensure that the patient's beliefs and values guide the plan of care. The nurse does not impose personal values or preferences when acting as an advocate, but instead guides the patient or surrogate decision maker through values clarification, identification of the patient's best interests, and the process of communicating decisions. Thus, the patient or surrogate is empowered by the nurse to direct the healthcare plan.

Assuming the role of patient advocate is not without risk. Nurses may find that obligations to oneself, the patient, the patient's family, other members of the healthcare team, or the institution are in conflict and have competing claims on nursing resources. These situations are intensely troubling to nurses and the support of colleagues is essential to resolving these dilemmas. In circumstances of conflict, nurses should clarify the nature and significance of the moral problem, engage in a systematic process of moral decision making, communicate concerns openly, and seek mutually acceptable resolutions. A framework within which to identify and compare options provides the necessary structure to begin the process of moral resolution.

THE PROCESS OF ETHICAL ANALYSIS

When faced with an ethical problem, the nurse is expected to implement a formal process that promotes resolution. A structured approach to ethical dilemmas provides consistency, eliminates the risks of overlooking relevant contextual features, and invites thoughtful reflection on moral problems. Even so, analysis of ethical dilemmas is not easy. It often requires the assistance of an ethics consult service, the members of which have specific training in handling ethical dilemmas. While there are a variety of ethical decision-making processes, the one described here mirrors the nursing process. The following steps are involved in case analysis:

Assessment

- Identify the problem. Is it an ethical dilemma? Is it moral distress? Clarify the competing ethical claims, the conflicting obligations, and the personal and professional values in contention. Acknowledge the emotional components and communication issues.
- Gather the data. Distinguish the morally relevant facts. Identify the medical, nursing, legal, social, and psychological facts. Clarify the patient's and family's religious and philosophical beliefs and values.
- Identify the individuals involved in the problem. Clarify who is involved in the problem's development and who should be involved in the decision-making process. Identify who should make the final decision, and discern what factors may impede that individual's ability to make the decision.

Plan

- Consider all possible courses of action and avoid restricting choices to the most obvious.
- Identify the risks and benefits likely to arise from each option.
- Analyze each course of action. In a principle-based approach, identify which principles support the alternative courses of action. In a care-based approach, consider the impact of each course of action on the existing relationships.
- Search for professional organizations' position statements and institutional guidelines that address this issue.

- Seek input from the resources available to help with ethical problems. In many cases, this is an ethics consult service or an ethics committee. Any hospital that is accredited by the Joint Commission must have in place a mechanism for dealing with ethical issues.

Implementation

- Choose a plan and act.
- Anticipate objections.

Evaluation

- Outline the results of the plan. Identify what harm or good occurred as a result of the action.
- Identify the necessary changes in institutional policy, professional organizations' position statements or other strategies to avoid similar conflicts in the future.

This stepwise process of ethical analysis incorporates ethical principles and rules, relevant medical and nursing facts, and specific contextual features, and reflects a model of shared decision making. This ideology is essential if current and future moral issues are to be addressed and negotiated.

CONTEMPORARY ETHICAL ISSUES

Informed Consent

As a patient advocate, the progressive care nurse recognizes the patient's or surrogate's central role in decision making. Patients must make informed decisions based on accurate and appropriate information. By uncovering the patients' primary values and beliefs, the nurse empowers patients and surrogates to articulate their preferences. Therefore, the nurse does not speak for the patient, but instead maintains an environment in which the patient's autonomy and right to self-determination are respected and preserved.

The doctrine of informed consent encompasses four elements: disclosure, comprehension, voluntariness, and competence. The first two of these elements are related because the patient's comprehension often depends on how the information is disclosed. Information must be provided in a manner that promotes the patient's understanding of the current medical status, the proposed interventions (including the nature of the therapy and its purpose, risks, and benefits), and the reasonable alternatives to the proposed treatment. Full disclosure in clear language is supported by the principle of veracity.

The overall goal of the treatment, rather than just the procedure, should be discussed with the patient and family and the goals should reflect the desirable and likely outcomes for this individual. The nurse can contribute significantly to the comprehension portion of the consent process by clarifying the patient's or surrogate's perception of the situation. Questions such as "What additional information do you need to help you make this decision?" or "What do you understand are the goals of this treatment?" help highlight the patient's interests and comprehension of the situation.

Decisions must be reached voluntarily, and any threat of coercion, manipulation, duress, or deceit is unethical. Voluntary decisions uphold the principle of respect for persons and support the concept of self-determination. In addition, the patient must be capable of making decisions about medical care. Competence is a legal term and reflects judicial involvement in the determination of a patient's decision-making capacity. Capacity reflects the ability of an individual to participate in the medical decision-making process. Determining capacity is discussed in the next section.

The intent of the informed consent process is based on the principle of autonomy. In theory, the consent process provides an individual with the necessary information to compare options and make a reasoned choice. Unfortunately, the consent process is handled more as an event than a process. The focus is to "get consent" rather than to help the patient gain an understanding of the proposed treatment. The progressive care nurse must be sensitive to the timing of such discussions and should attempt to optimize the environment and enhance the patient's and family's ability to participate in the decision-making process. Interactions should be uninterrupted, free from distractions, during intervals when the patient is fully awake, and, if desired by the patient, in the presence of loved ones.

Nurses have both a moral and a legal duty in the consent process. Incorrect information given with the intent to deceive or mislead the patient or family must be reported according to institutional guidelines and in some states may qualify as professional misconduct to be reported to the profession's state board. The ANA *Code of Ethics for Nurses* portrays the nurse's role during the consent process as a patient advocate upholding the patient's right to self-determination. Therefore, the nurse must respect the competent patient's choice and support the patient's decisions even if the decision is contrary to the judgments of the healthcare team.

Determining Capacity

Patients are presumed to possess decision-making capacity unless there are clear indications that the individual's choices are harmful or inconsistent with previously stated wishes. Questioning another's ability to engage in the decision-making process should be executed with caution. Value laden judgments of an individual's capacity, such as restricting involvement based on mental illness or advanced age, should be avoided. Cultural, religious, or ethical differences should not be misinterpreted as evidence of incapacity. In addition, evaluations of capacity based on the presumed outcome of the decision are equally unjust. Capacity to make decisions is based on the patient's physical and mental health and the ability to be consistent in addressing issues. Capacity is not based on the ability to concur with healthcare providers or family members. Instead, a functional standard to evaluate capacity is recommended. At many institutions, this functional standard is used to create a policy for establishing decisional capacity.

The functional standard of determining capacity focuses on the patient's abilities as a decision maker rather than on the condition of the patient or the projected outcome of the decision. The three elements necessary for a patient to meet the functional standard are the abilities to comprehend, to communicate, and to form and express a preference.

The ability to comprehend implies that the patient understands the information relevant to the decision. A patient must exhibit abilities sufficient to understand only the facts pertinent to the prevailing issue. Therefore, orientation to person, place, and time does not guarantee or preclude the patient's ability to understand and comprehend the relevant information.

Decision-making capacity requires a communication of the decision between the patient and healthcare team. Communication with very ill patients often is compromised by pharmacologic or technological interventions. The progressive care nurse should attempt to remove barriers to communication and advance the patient's opportunity to engage in the decision-making process.

The final component essential for evaluating functional capacity is evidence of the patient's ability to reason about his or her choices. An individual's choices should reflect the person's own goals, values, and preferences. To evaluate this aspect, comments such as "Tell me about some of the most difficult healthcare decisions that you had to make in the past," or "Describe how you reached the decision you did," are useful. The patient should recount a pattern of reasoning that is consistent with personal goals and that reflects an accurate understanding of the consequences of the decision.

When the patient lacks decision-making capacity, and attempts to control factors and return the patient to an autonomous state are unsuccessful, the healthcare team must rely on other sources for direction in approximating the patient's preferences. Advance directives and surrogate decision makers are two ways in which the patient's choices can be understood.

Advance Directives

The Patient Self Determination Act (PSDA), effective December 1, 1991, is a federal law that requires healthcare institutions receiving Medicare or Medicaid funds to inform patients of their legal rights to make healthcare decisions and execute advance directives. The purpose of the PSDA is to preserve and protect the rights of adult patients to make choices regarding their medical care. The PSDA also requires institutions to inform individuals of relevant state laws surrounding the preparation and execution of advance directives.

Advance directives are statements made by an individual with decision-making capacity that describe the care or treatment he or she wishes to receive when no longer competent. Most states recognize two forms of advance directives, the treatment directive, or "living will," and the proxy directive. The treatment directive enables the individual to specify in advance his or her treatment choices and which interventions are desired. Usually treatment directives focus on cardiopulmonary resuscitation (CPR), mechanical ventilation, nutrition and hydration, and other life-sustaining technologies.

Proxy directives, also called the durable power of attorney for health care, expand the sphere of decision making by identifying an individual to make treatment decisions when the patient is unable to do so. The appointed individual, a relative or close friend, assumes responsibility for healthcare decisions as soon as the patient loses the capacity to participate in the decision-making process. Treatment decisions by the healthcare proxy are based on a knowledge and understanding of the patient's values and wishes regarding medical care. Most states have statutory provisions that recognize the legal authority of the healthcare proxy, and this individual is given complete authority to accept or refuse any procedure or treatment on behalf of a patient who lacks capacity.

Although most adults should complete both, a treatment and proxy directive, the proxy directive has some important advantages over a treatment directive. Many treatment directives are valid only under certain conditions. Terminal illness and/or an imminent death are common limitations required before the patient's treatment directive is enacted. Such restrictions are not relevant in proxy directives, and the sole requirement before the proxy assumes responsibility on the individual's behalf is that the patient lacks decisional capacity. Furthermore, the proxy directive enables the authorized decision maker to consider the contextual and unique features of the specific situation before arriving at a decision. A treatment directive may indicate refusal of mechanical ventilation but a durable power of attorney speaking for the patient with a reversible acute respiratory process may consent to a trial of noninvasive ventilation. In this way, the benefits and burdens of proposed interventions are considered in partnership with the knowledge and understanding of the patient's preferences and values.

If a patient lacks decision-making capacity and has not previously designated a proxy decision maker in an advance directive, the healthcare team must identify an appropriate surrogate to make decisions on the patient's behalf. Guidelines for identifying surrogate decision makers vary from state to state. Generally, family members have the patient's best interests in mind, and many state statutes identify a hierarchy of relatives as appropriate surrogate decision makers.

Regardless of whether the decision maker is a designated proxy or family member, the process of making decisions on behalf of the incapacitated patient is difficult and arduous. If the patient left no written treatment directive, the surrogate decision maker and the designated proxy follow the same guidelines for making decisions. The decisions are made based on either the substituted judgment standard or the best interest standard.

Substituted Judgment

When a patient previously has expressed his or her wishes regarding medical care, the surrogate decision maker invokes the standard of substituted judgment. The patient's goals, beliefs, and values serve to guide the surrogate in constructing and shaping a decision that is congruous with the patient's expressed wishes. An ideal interpretation of substituted judgment is that the patient, if competent, would arrive at the same decision as the surrogate. This standard originates in the belief that when we know someone well enough, we often are able to determine how he or she would have reacted to a particular situation, and therefore can make decisions on that person's behalf.

Best Interests

The best interest standard is used when the patient's values, ideals, attitudes, or philosophy are not known; for example, a patient who never gained decision-making capacity and lacked competence throughout his or her life would not have the opportunity to articulate wishes and beliefs about health care. Using the best interest standard, the surrogate decision maker determines the course of treatment based on what would be in the patient's best interests, considering the needs, risks, and benefits to the affected person. This burden/benefit analysis includes considering the relief of suffering, restoration of function, likelihood of regaining capacity, and quality of an extended life.

Although neither the best interest standard nor the substituted judgment standard is problem free, when possible the decision maker for an incapacitated patient should follow the principles of substituted judgment. Knowledge of the patient's underlying values should guide the surrogate and will most likely result in a decision reflective of the patient's interests and well-being. Nurses support surrogate decision makers in the same way that they serve as patient advocates by providing consistent, accurate information and asking questions to clarify the patient's values.

End-of-Life Issues

Decisions to Forego Life-Sustaining Treatments

Decisions to forego life-sustaining treatments are made almost daily in the hospital setting. The prevalence of these decisions does not diminish the difficulty that patients, families, nurses, and physicians face when considering this treatment decision. The model for this decision-making process is a collaborative approach that promotes the patient's interests and well-being.

The patient's interests are best served when information is shared among the caregivers, patient, and family in an open and honest manner. Through this process, a plan of care that reflects the patient's goals, values, and interests is developed. Continued collaboration is essential to ensure that the plan promotes the patient's well-being and reflects the patient's preferences. However, the patient may determine that the current treatment plan imposes more burdens than benefits, and may choose to forego new or continued therapies.

Grounded in the principle of patient autonomy, patients with capacity have the moral and legal right to forego life-sustaining treatments. The right of a capable patient to refuse treatment, even beneficial treatment, must be upheld if the elements of informed consent are met and innocent or third parties are not injured by the refusal. Ongoing dialogue among the healthcare team, family, and patient is appropriate so that mutually satisfactory realistic goals are adopted. Patients must understand that refusal of treatment will not lead to inadequate care or abandonment by members of the healthcare team.

In patients without decisional capacity, the determination to withdraw or withhold treatments is made by the identified surrogate. If the wishes and values of the patient are known, the surrogate makes treatment decisions based on this framework. If, however, the patient's values or wishes are unknown, or the patient never had capacity to express underlying beliefs, the decision maker must consider and weigh the benefits and burdens imposed by the particular treatments. Any treatment that inflicts undue burdens on the patient without overriding benefits or that provides no benefit may be justifiably withdrawn or withheld. If the benefits outweigh the burdens, the obligation is to provide the treatment to the patient.

In cases where the identified surrogate is not acting in the patient's best interests, healthcare professionals have a moral obligation to negotiate an acceptable resolution to the problem. Progressive care nurses should intervene when the best interest of the patient is in question. If extensive attempts to resolve the differences through the use of internal and external resources are unsuccessful in facilitating an acceptable solution, the healthcare professional should seek the appointment of an alternative surrogate. Often, the burden of proof is on the healthcare professional to justify the need for an alternative decision maker. In situations in which the patient's life is threatened and the refusal of treatment by the surrogate would jeopardize the patient's safety, the healthcare team must seek an alternative surrogate without prolonged discussion with the identified surrogate. This situation arises when parents who are Jehovah's Witnesses refuse a life-saving blood transfusion for their child. The healthcare team can rapidly acquire court approval to transfuse the minor. In less emergent situations, attempts to convince the surrogate of the need for treatment and to reach a satisfactory settlement may take more time.

In the case "The Patient's Wishes," members of the healthcare team interpreted the patient's actions as a decision made by a competent individual. They realized that even after aggressive treatment the patient would most likely be dependent on hemodialysis, and therefore his independence and living environment would change. On the other hand, his daughter saw her father's act as a reflection of his depression from Parkinson disease and the loss of his wife. His daughter believed that additional antidepressant medications and more frequent psychiatric evaluations would renew her father's desire to live. In this case, both parties believe they are advancing the patient's best interests. Reflection on the patient's life, work, actions, religion, and beliefs helps all parties to clarify the patient's values, and may help in the development of an acceptable resolution.

Conflicts regarding the withdrawal of life-sustaining treatments often reflect differences in values and beliefs.

ESSENTIAL CONTENT CASE

The Patient's Wishes

An 86-year-old widower, Mr. Johnson, resides in an assisted living facility. He has an adult daughter who lives out of town and regularly visits him twice a month. One morning, the care providers at the facility find him unresponsive with shallow respirations and bradycardia. A note, written by Mr. Johnson, is attached to his body and states that he intentionally took a lethal overdose and that he does not wish to be resuscitated. Empty bottles of levodopa and amitriptyline are found in his room next to a glass partially filled with alcohol. Residents of the facility said that Mr. Johnson had continued to express sadness over the loss of his wife 2 years ago and that progression of Parkinson disease was also troubling to him. The providers at the assisted living facility call 911, and he is rapidly transported to the hospital. The patient is hypotensive and unresponsive on admission to the emergency room. Laboratory tests reflecting his renal and hepatic function are grossly abnormal. Gastric lavage and activated charcoal are initiated to remove the drugs. The patient's daughter requests that everything be done to save her father. The healthcare team respects the daughter's wishes as surrogate, but is concerned that this is not what the patient wanted. They believe that the likelihood of a full recovery is remote and he should be allowed a peaceful death.

Case Question 1: What factors need to be considered to evaluate Mr. Johnson's capacity when he wrote the statement indicating he did not desire resuscitation?

Case Question 2: What guidance can Mr. Johnson's nurse offer to his daughter to help her in her role as surrogate decision maker?

Answers

1. If Mr. Johnson had untreated or undertreated depression or dementia then his capacity when he wrote his wish not to be resuscitated is called into question. Contacting his outpatient providers or seeking to review records from outpatient appointments may assist in determining if the patient had capacity and if his statement in his note should dictate a do not resuscitate (DNR) order, and influence the care provided.

2. The patient's daughter should be encouraged to consider what kind of care her father, in the absence of mental illness or dementia, would desire. While she is grieving, and probably feeling guilty about the drastic action her father has taken, her ethical obligation is to speak on her father's behalf and not to speak for herself. The nurse can encourage the daughter to recall conversations the two had during her visits in which he may have indicated his preferences regarding resuscitation, life support, and the use of medical hydration and nutrition.

Typically, healthcare professionals value life and health. When patients or surrogates choose to forego treatments that have minimal benefit, relinquishing the original goal of restoring health is difficult. This dilemma is particularly apparent in the acute care setting, where actions and interventions are aggressive, dramatic, and often life saving. Shifting from this model to a paradigm that advocates for a calm and peaceful death requires the progressive care nurse and healthcare team to relinquish control and to change the treatment goals to promote comfort and support the grieving process. The intensity required to support the patient and family during the process of withdrawal of treatment must also be valued and appreciated by healthcare professionals in all settings.

In some circumstances, surrogate decision makers insist on treatment that members of the healthcare team believe is burdensome and nonbeneficial for the patient. Frequently, the request for futile treatment reflects the surrogate or patient's desire to be assured that "everything" is being done to eradicate the disease or restore health. Emotional, financial, and social concerns can all motivate individuals to pursue nonbeneficial, and even harmful, treatments. If patients and surrogates are kept fully informed of the goals and the successes and failures throughout the course of treatment, the request for futile therapies is less likely. If, after numerous discussions, the patient or surrogate continues to request futile treatment, eliciting help from an uninvolved party, such as an ethics committee, can facilitate discussions. Healthcare institutions often have policies that delineate the responsibilities of the caregiver and the resources within the institution to resolve these unusual situations. In rare circumstances, judicial involvement is necessary to determine the outcome of the case.

Nutrition and Hydration

To many nurses and healthcare consumers, the provision of nutrition and hydration is fundamental to patient care. Therefore, nurses may be distressed when the withdrawal of nutrition and hydration are considered. However, the provision of nutrition and hydration is a medical intervention and thus has both risks and benefits. Medical nutrition and hydration are administered through intravenous access, nasogastric and duodenal feeding tubes, or via gastrostomy. The image of gently spoon feeding a dying patient is replaced with the reality of meeting the nutritional requirements through invasive and uncomfortable technologies.

Provision of medical nutrition and hydration should occur following a careful burden-benefit analysis. If medical nutrition and hydration support can expedite the patient's return to an acceptable level of functioning (as defined by the patient or surrogate), then provision of the therapy is beneficial. When uncertainty exists, the presumption should be to provide nutrition and hydration. On the other hand, when continued provision of nutrition and hydration will not effectively restore the patient to a functional status consistent with the patient's values, the treatment may be discontinued.

Pain Management

When faced with a potentially life-limiting disease process, issues regarding the aggressive management of pain and comfort develop. Although palliation or relief of troubling symptoms is a priority in the care of all patients, once the decision to forego life-sustaining measures is made, palliation becomes the main focus of all care. In some circumstances, patients experience distressing symptoms despite the availability of pharmacologic agents to manage the uncomfortable effects of chronic and terminal illness. Whether due to a lack of knowledge, time, or a deliberate unwillingness to prescribe the necessary medication, inadequate symptom management is unethical. Nurses are obligated to ensure that patients receive care and treatments that are consistent with their choices. There are few patients in whom adequate pain management cannot be achieved. The ANA Position Statement on pain management and control of distressing symptoms in dying patients delineates the role of the nurse in the assessment and management of pain.

When patients require large doses of medications, such as narcotics, to effectively alleviate their symptoms, providers may be concerned that the side effects of such doses may hasten the patient's death. The ANA *Code for Nurses* helps clarify this concern for nurses by affirming that nurses "should provide interventions to relieve pain and other symptoms in the dying patient even when those interventions entail risks of hastening death." The essential element in this situation is the nurse's intent in providing the medication. Because the intent is to relieve pain and suffering, and not to deliberately hasten death, the action is morally justified.

The concept that supports this reasoning is called the principle of double effect.

This principle states that if an action has both a good and bad effect, a person is justified in taking that action if the intent was the good effect, the bad effect was a possible but not certain outcome of the action, and there was no additional course of action which could produce the good effect and avoid the bad one. The Supreme Court cited the principle of double effect in a decision that distinguished palliative care from assisted suicide. A provider who assists in a patient's death intends to cause that persons death, which is ethically and legally distinct from a provider who seeks to control symptoms and gives medications that may, inadvertently, hasten death.

Resuscitation Decisions

Acutely ill patients are susceptible to sudden and unpredictable changes in cardiopulmonary status. Most hospitalized patients presume that, unless discussed otherwise, resuscitation efforts will be instituted immediately upon cardiopulmonary arrest. In-hospital resuscitation is moderately successful, and delay in efforts significantly reduces the chance of the victim's survival. The emergent nature, the questionable effectiveness, and the presumed provision of CPR contribute to the ethical dilemmas that surround this intervention.

Do Not Resuscitate Orders

"Do not resuscitate" (DNR) or "no code" are orders to withhold CPR in the event of cardiac or respiratory arrest. Other medical or nursing interventions are not influenced directly by a DNR order. In other words, the decision to forego CPR is not a decision to forego any other medical interventions. The communication surrounding this decision is one of the most important elements in designing a mutually acceptable treatment plan for a particular patient. Appropriate discussions with the patient or surrogate must occur before a resuscitation decision is made. Conversations about resuscitation status and the overall treatment goals should occur with the patient or surrogate, physician, nurse, and other appropriate members of the healthcare team. Open communication and a shared understanding of the treatment plan are essential to understanding and responding to the patient's interests and preferences. Once a decision is made regarding resuscitation status, the physician must document the discussion and decision in the medical record according to the institution's policy. When the issue of resuscitation status is not addressed with the patient or surrogate or the decision is not documented or communicated with caregivers, then a code is initiated, risking the provision of unwanted care.

Slow Codes or Partial Codes

The failure to define the DNR status and other treatment or nontreatment decisions often reflects the absence of an overall treatment goal. Patients or their surrogates must be involved in decisions surrounding resuscitation. Although some providers believe that decisions to withhold CPR can be made without involving patients or surrogates, such decisions violate the principle of patient autonomy. Just as patient's consent to other interventions in the plan of care, including decisions to omit particular treatments, the provision or withholding of CPR is based on discussions with the patient and family. In some instances healthcare providers rely on "slow" or "partial" codes, in which interventions are administered with less effort and speed than the emergent situation demands, increasing the likelihood that the resuscitative effort will be unsuccessful. Slow or partial codes are always unethical and often indicate failed communication between the patient and family and the healthcare team. It is the responsibility of healthcare providers to explain CPR, ensure that the family and patient understand both the risks and benefits and likely outcomes of the procedure, and either provide or withhold the intervention in accordance with the patient and family's wishes.

Most institutions have policies that address the process of writing and implementing a DNR order. In addition, many states have an approved process and format to indicate a desire to forgo life support so that this wish can be conveyed across all healthcare settings. Examples of such forms include the Durable DNR form in Virginia and the Physician Order for Life Sustaining Treatment or POLST form in California. Nurses should be familiar with the forms available in the states where they practice, understand institutional policies for recognizing such forms, and encourage patients and families to use these means to convey their wishes. These forms are tools for preventing the provision of undesired care.

Family Presence During Resuscitation

The practice of allowing family members to be present during resuscitative efforts and other invasive procedures is a key consideration in the ethical care of critically and acutely ill patients. Protocols or procedures for allowing family presence may be available on an individual nursing unit or for all nursing units in a given institution and can guide nurses in providing this care. Some considerations include having a staff member available to narrate the experience for the family members, and documenting family presence in the patient's chart. AACN's 2010 Practice Alert lists the strong evidence in favor of allowing family members to be present during resuscitation and invasive procedures, noting primarily the benefit of this practice for family and patients. Thus, the principle of beneficence supports family presence during resuscitation and other invasive procedures. The ethic of care similarly supports this practice as it acknowledges the priority of family relationships.

BUILDING AN ETHICAL ENVIRONMENT

Values Clarification

One of the most useful and essential skills offered by nurses is that of assisting the patient and family in values clarification. This process helps families to weigh the burdens and benefits of medical interventions and develop a framework of the patient's preferences and interests. Additionally, families are less encumbered during the bereavement process, when reflecting on the patient's hospitalization, if they feel the decisions they made for the patient reflect the patient's values.

Provide Information and Clarify Issues

Patients and families rely on nurses to clarify medical information and support their exploration of the meaning of different treatment decisions. The trusting relationship that develops is based on the nurse's ability to communicate and understand the patient's needs. Questions that help unveil patients' families' perceptions of the situation include: "What information do you need to make this decision?" "What do you understand of your (or your loved one's) condition?" and "What are your fears about being sick?"

The information provided to patients and surrogates must be more than simply disclosing facts. The dialogue must be ongoing, open, honest, and expressed with concern. Because the understanding of new knowledge is often rooted in past learning, the nurse begins by assessing the patient's or surrogate's prior experiences with the healthcare system. Patients and families often draw conclusions or create relationships based on incomplete or inaccurate interpretations of information. Nurses play a key role in facilitating communication and translating discrepancies in perceptions.

Recognize Moral Distress

Moral distress refers to the suffering that occurs when individuals feel compelled to act in ways they think are unethical. Nurses can feel trapped between institutional constraints, medical directives, patient and family wishes, and personal beliefs, duties, and values. Although all ethical problems are challenging, situations that result in moral distress are particularly troubling because they may have lasting effects on the individual's professional and personal life. Recognizing situations that contribute to moral distress and developing strategies to preserve moral integrity are essential tools for the progressive care nurse. The AACN booklet *4 A's to Rise above Moral Distress* provides an approach to address the situations that create moral distress and to prevent the harmful consequences that it causes. Increasingly, institutions are recognizing the importance of addressing moral distress in the workplace. Many other strategies are being designed and implemented, such as unit-based conversations in ethics and moral distress consult services.

Engage in Collaborative Decision Making

Nursing offers a distinct perspective that is grounded in humanistic and caring values. Nurses recognize, interpret, and react to the patient's and family's response to health problems. Factors such as the patient's ability to adapt to changes in health, cope with a diagnosis, or adjust to a treatment are valuable contributions to a model of shared decision making. Because nursing embraces this viewpoint, nurses must have a consistent presence on the healthcare team. Patients and families expect and need nurses to be actively involved in planning and implementing the plan of care.

In a collaborative model, the nurse's contributions and perspectives are valued, heard, and acknowledged. The nurse, in exchange, is open to the contributions of other team members, actively listening and encouraging their participation. When nurses are absent from the circle of decision making, moral problems occur and communication falters. Every progressive care nurse must remain involved, attached, and committed to the process of shared decision making and collaborative interaction.

SELECTED BIBLIOGRAPHY

Ahronheim J, Moreno JC, Zuckerman C. *Ethics in Clinical Practice.* 2nd ed. Gaithersburg, MD: Aspen; 2000.

Beauchamp TL, Childress JF. *Principles of Biomedical Ethics.* 6th ed. Oxford, England: Oxford University Press; 2009.

Burkhardt MA, Nathaniel AK. *Ethics and Issues in Contemporary Nursing.* 2nd ed. Independence, KY: Delmar Thomson Learning; 2001.

Campbell GM, Delgado S, Heath JE, et al. *The 4A's to Rise Above Moral Distress.* Wavra T. ed. Aliso Viejo, CA: AACN; 2004.

Campbell ML. *Foregoing Life-Sustaining Therapy.* Aliso Viejo, CA: AACN; 1998.

CMS regulations. http://www.cms.gov/apps/docs/aca-update-implementing-medicare-costs-savings.pdf. Accessed February 27, 2013.

Coughennower M. Physician assisted suicide. *Gastroenterol Nurs.* 2003;26(2):55-59.

Davis AJ, Aroskar MA, Liaschenko J, Drought TS. *Ethical Dilemmas and Nursing Practice.* 4th ed. Stamford, CT: Appleton & Lange; 1997.

Fry ST, Killen AR, Robinson EM. Care-based reasoning, caring, and the ethic of care: a need for clarity. *J Clin Ethics.* 1996;7(1):41-47.

Fry ST, Veatch RM. *Case Studies in Nursing Ethics.* 2nd ed. Boston, MA: Jones & Bartlett Publishers; 2000.

Georges J-J, Grypdonck M. Moral problems experienced by nurses when caring for terminally ill people: a literature review. *Nurs Ethics.* 2002;9:155-178.

Gilligan C. Moral orientation and moral development. In: Kittay EF, Meyers DT, eds. *Women and Moral Theory.* New York, NY: Rowman & Littlefield Publishers, Inc; 1987:19-33.

Gordon EJ, Hamric AB. The courage to stand up: the cultural politics of nurses' access to ethics consultation. *J Clin Ethics.* 2006;17(3):231-254.

Grisso T, Applebaum PS. *Assessing Competence to Consent to Treatment: A Guide for Physicians and Other Health Professionals.* New York, NY: Oxford University Press; 1998.

Hamric AB, Davis WS, Childress MD. Moral distress in health care providers: what is it and what can we do about it? *The Pharos.* 2006; Winter:17-23.

Hamric, AB, Wocial, LD, Epstein, EG. Transforming moral distress into moral agency. Panel presentation, ASBH annual conference, Minneapolis, MN; October 2011.

Ivy SS. Ethical considerations in resuscitation decisions: a nursing ethics perspective. *J Cardiovasc Nurs.* 1996;10(4):47-58.

Kuczewski MG. Ethics committees at work: the illegal alien who needs surgery. *Camb Q Healthc Ethics.* 2000;9:128-135.

La Puma J, Orentlicher D, and Moss RJ. Advance directives on admission. Clinical implications and analysis of the Patient Self Determination Act of 1990. *J Am Med Assoc.* 1991;266(3):402-405.

Lo B. *Resolving Ethical Dilemmas: A Guide for Clinicians.* 2nd ed. Philadelphia, PA: Lippincott Williams & Wilkins; 2000.

Manojlovich M. Power and empowerment in nursing: looking backward to inform the future. *Online J Issues Nurs.* January 31, 2007:12(1). Manuscript 1. www.nursingworld.org/MainMenu Categories/ANAMarketplace/ANAPeriodicals/OJIN/Tableof Contents/Volume122007/No1Jan07/LookingBackwardto InformtheFuture.aspx.

Matzo M, Sherman D, Penn B, Ferrell B. The End of Life Nursing Education Consortium (ELNEC) experience. *Nurse Educ.* 2003;28(6):266-270.

Meisel A, Snyder L, Quill T. Seven legal barriers to end of life care: myths, realities and grains of truth. *J Am Med Assoc.* 2000;284(19):2495-2501.

Naden D, Eriksson K. Understanding the importance of values and moral attitudes in nursing care in preserving human dignity. *Nurs Sci Q.* 2004;17(1):86-91.

National Consensus Project for Quality Palliative Care. *Clinical Practice Guidelines for Quality Palliative Care.* Brooklyn, NY: National Consensus Project for Quality Palliative Care; 2004.

Oberle K, Hughes D. Doctors' and nurses' perceptions of ethical problems in end-of-life decisions. *J Advanced Nurs.* 2001;33(6):707-715.

Rushton CH, Penticuff JH. A framework for analysis of ethical dilemmas in critical care nursing. *AACN Advanced Critical Care.* 2007;19(3):323-329.

Westphal C, Wavra T. Acute and Critical Choices: Guide to Advance Directives. American Association of Critical Care Nurses, 2005, online at http://www.aacn.or/wd/Practice/Docs/Acute_and_Critical_Care_Choices_to Advance_Directives.pdf.

Wocial LD, Hancock M, Bledsoe PD, Chamness AR, Helft PR. An evaluation of unit-based ethics conversations. *JONA's Healthcare Law, Ethics, and Regulation.* 2010;12(2): 48-54.

Professional Codes, Standards, and Position Statements

AACN Position Paper: Zero Tolerance for Violence: http://www.aacn.org/wd/practice/docs/publicpolicy/zero_tolerance_for_abuse.pdf. Accessed February 7, 2013.

AACN Position Paper: moral distress: http://www.aacn.org/wd/practice/docs/moral_distress.pdf. Accessed February 7, 2013.

ACCN Practice Alert: family presence during resuscitation and invasive procedures. http://www.aacn.org/wd/practice/docs/practicealerts/family%20presence%2004-2010%20final.pdf. Accessed February 27, 2013.

American Nurses' Association. *Code for Nurses With Interpretive Statements.* Washington, DC: ANA; 2001.

American Nurses' Association. *Position Statement on Nursing Care and Do-Not-Resuscitate (DNR) Decisions.* Washington, DC: ANA; 2003.

American Nurses' Association. *Position Statement on Pain Management and Control of Distressing Symptoms in Dying Patients.* Washington, DC: ANA; 2003.

Evidence-Based Guidelines

Puntillo K, Medina J, Rushton C, et al. End-of-life and palliative care issues in critical care. In: Medina J, Puntillo K, eds. *Protocols for Practice: End of Life and Palliative Care Issues in Critical Care.* Aliso Viejo, CA: AACN; 2007.

On-line References of Interest: Related to Legal and Ethical Considerations

The ANA Center for Ethics and Human Rights. http://www.nursingworld.org/MainMenuCategories/ThePracticeofProfessionalNursing/EthicsStandards.aspx. Accessed January 10, 2010.

American Association of Critical-Care Nurses: AACN Ethics website: http://www.aacn.org/WD/AACNNews/Content/2008/oct-practice.pcms?menu=Practice. Accessed January 10, 2010.

NIH site for ethics resources: http://bioethics.od.nih.gov/. Accessed January 10, 2010. The American Journal of Bioethics: http://www.bioethics.net/. Accessed January 10, 2010.

The Hastings Center: http://www.thehastingscenter.org/. Accessed January 10, 2010.

The Office for Human Research Protections http://www.hhs.gov/ohrp/. Accessed January 10, 2010.

Pathologic Conditions

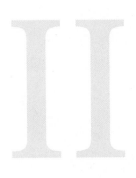

CARDIOVASCULAR SYSTEM

Barbara Leeper

KNOWLEDGE COMPETENCIES

1. Identify indications for, complications of, and nursing management of patients undergoing coronary angiography and percutaneous coronary interventions.

2. Describe the etiology, pathophysiology, clinical presentation, patient needs, and principles of management of patients with ischemic heart disease.

3. Discuss the indications for, complications of, and management of patients undergoing electrophysiology studies.

4. Discuss the etiology, pathophysiology, clinical presentation, patient needs, and principles of management of patients in shock, heart failure, and hypertensive crisis.

SPECIAL ASSESSMENT TECHNIQUES, DIAGNOSTIC TESTS, AND MONITORING SYSTEMS

Assessment of Chest Pain

Obtaining an accurate assessment of chest pain history is an important aspect of differentiating cardiac chest pain from other sources of pain (eg, musculoskeletal, respiratory, anxiety). Ischemic chest pain, caused by lack of oxygen to the myocardium, must be quickly identified for therapeutic interventions to be effective. The most important descriptors of ischemic pain include precursors of pain onset, quality of the pain, pain radiation, severity of the pain, what relieves the pain, and timing of onset of the current episode of pain that brought the patient to the hospital. Each of these descriptors can be assessed using the "PQRST" nomogram (Table 9-1). This nomogram prompts the clinician to ask a series of questions which help clarify the characteristics of the cardiac pain.

Coronary Angiography

Coronary angiography is a common and effective method for visualizing the anatomy and patency of the coronary arteries. This procedure, also known as cardiac catheterization, is used to diagnose atherosclerotic lesions or thrombus in the coronary vessels. Cardiac catheterization is also used for evaluation of valvular heart disease, including stenosis or insufficiency, atrial or ventricular septal defects, congenital anomalies, and cardiac wall motion abnormalities (Table 9-2).

Procedure

Prior to cardiac catheterization, the patient should be NPO for at least 6 to 12 hours, in the event that emergency intubation is required during the procedure. NPO may indicate everything except medications which should be taken with small sips of water the day of the procedure. Typically, if the patient is on insulin or taking oral hypoglycemics the doses may need to be adjusted or held the day of the procedure. There are other medications that may need to be held. Benadryl may be administered prior to beginning the procedure as a precautionary measure against allergic reaction to the dye. Unfractionated heparin and platelet inhibitor agents (including aspirin, glycoprotein IIb/IIIa receptor inhibitors, and/or clopidogrel) may be administered to prevent catheter-induced platelet aggregation during the procedure. Typically, patients remain awake during the procedure, allowing them to facilitate the catheterization process by controlling

TABLE 9-1. CHEST PAIN ASSESSMENT

	Ask the Question	Examples
P (Provoke)	What *provokes* the pain or what precipitates the pain?	Climbing the stairs, walking; or may be unpredictable—comes on at rest
Q (Quality)	What is the *quality* of the pain?	Pressure, tightness; may have associated symptoms such as nausea, vomiting, diaphoresis
R (Radiation)	Does the pain *radiate* to locations other than the chest?	Jaw, neck, scapular area, or left arm
S (Severity)	What is the *severity* of the pain (on a scale of 1-10)?	On a scale of 1-10, with 10 being the worst, how bad is your pain?
T (Timing)	What is the *time* of onset of this episode of pain that caused you to come to the hospital?	When did this episode of pain that brought you to the hospital start? Did this episode wax and wane or was it constant? For how many days, months, or years have you had similar pain?

respiratory patterns (eg, breath holding during injection of radiopaque dye to improve the quality of the image). An anxiolytic agent, such as diazepam, is frequently administered during the procedure to decrease anxiety or restlessness.

An intracoronary catheter is inserted through a "sheath" or vascular introducer placed in a large artery, most commonly the femoral artery (Figure 9-1A). In recent years there has been an increase in the use of the radial artery as catheters have been made smaller, allowing easier access to the vessel. If inserted via the femoral artery the catheter is then advanced into the ascending abdominal aorta, across the aortic arch, and into the coronary artery orifice located at the base of the aorta (Figure 9-1B). Ionic dye, visible to the observer or operator under fluoroscopy (x-ray), is then injected into the coronary arterial tree by the catheter. If the cardiac valves, septa, or ventricular wall motion is being evaluated, the catheter is advanced directly into the left ventricle,

TABLE 9-2. INDICATIONS FOR CARDIAC CATHETERIZATION

Right Heart
- Measurement of right-sided heart pressures:
  Suspected cardiac tamponade
  Suspected pulmonary hypertension
- Evaluation of valvular disease (tricuspid or pulmonic)
- Evaluation of atrial or ventricular septal defects
- Measurement of AVO$_2$ difference

Left Heart
- Diagnosis of obstructive coronary artery disease
- Identification of lesion location prior to CABG surgery
- Measurement of left-sided heart pressures:
  Suspected left heart failure or cardiomyopathy
- Evaluation of valvular disease (mitral or aortic)
- Evaluation of atrial or ventricular septal defects

followed by injection of dye (Figure 9-1C). During a right heart catheterization, the catheter is inserted into the venous system through the inferior vena cava, passed through the right ventricle, and advanced into the pulmonary artery.

Interpretation of Results

The coronary vascular tree consists of a left and a right system (Figure 9-2). The left system consists of two main branches, the left anterior descending (LAD) artery and the left circumflex (LCx) artery. The right system has one main branch, the right coronary artery (RCA). Both systems have a number of smaller vessels that branch off these three primary arterial vessels. A clinically significant stenosis is considered to be an obstruction of 75% or greater in a major coronary artery or one of its major branches. If there is significant disease in only one of the major arteries, the patient is said to have single-vessel disease. If two major vessels are affected, the patient has two vessel disease. If significant disease exists in all three major coronary arteries then the patient has three-vessel disease. Frequently, the microvasculature, or smaller vessels branching off the major coronary artery, may also have blockages. It is common to refer to these multiple lesions as diffuse disease.

A cineventriculogram is obtained by radiographic imaging during the injection of dye after advancing the catheter from the aorta, through the aortic valve, and into the left ventricle (see Figure 9-1C). The cineventriculogram provides information on ventricular wall motion, ejection fraction, and the presence and severity of mitral regurgitation and aortic regurgitation. Ejection fraction, or the percentage of blood volume ejected from the left ventricle with each contraction, is the gold standard for determining left ventricular function and is helpful in selecting treatment strategies. A left ventricular ejection fractions (LVEF) normal value is 55% to 60%. The LVEF is one of the most important predictors of long-term outcome following acute myocardial infarction (AMI). Patients with ejection fractions less than 20% have nearly 50% 1-year mortality. Another important measurement is the pressure in the left ventricle at the end of diastole. This is called "left ventricular end-diastolic pressure (LVEDP)." It, too, is an important determinant of ventricular function and is considered to be a predictor of morbidity and mortality in patients with heart failure (HF) and those undergoing cardiac surgery. The normal LVEDP is 6-12 mm Hg.

Complications

During cardiac catheterization, a number of complications may occur, including arrhythmia; coronary vasospasm; coronary dissection; allergic reaction to the dye; atrial or ventricular perforation resulting in pericardial tamponade; embolus to an extremity, a lung, or, rarely, the brain; acute closure of the left main coronary; myocardial infarction (MI); or death. Common management and prevention strategies for catheterization complications are summarized in Table 9-3.

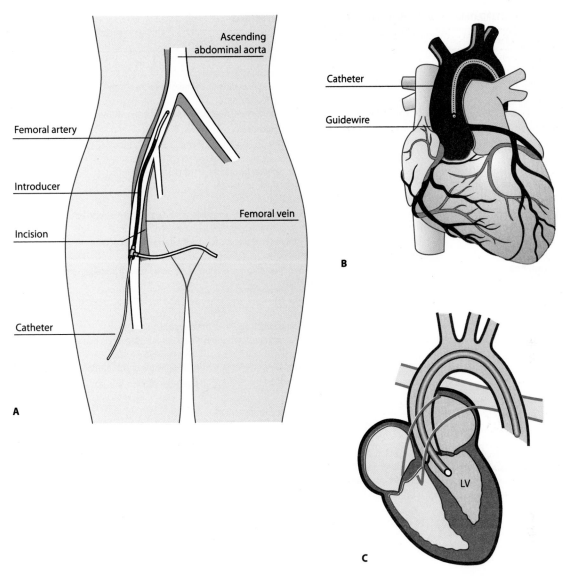

Figure 9-1. Coronary angiography. **(A)** Insertion of the coronary catheter into the femoral artery through a percutaneously inserted introducer sheath. **(B)** Coronary catheter advancement into the aorta and the left coronary artery. **(C)** Catheter advancement into the left ventricle.

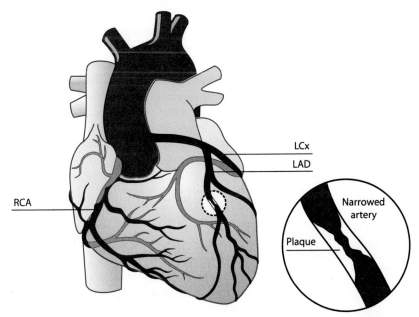

Figure 9-2. Coronary artery circulation with a coronary vessel narrowed with plaque formation.

TABLE 9-3. CARDIAC CATHETERIZATION: COMMON COMPLICATIONS AND NURSING INTERVENTIONS

Complication	Intervention
Local bleeding due to catheter site artery damage (hematoma, hemorrhage, pseudoaneurysm)	Keep patient flat; head of bed (HOB) < 30°. Discontinue unfractionated heparin infusion if present. Compress the artery just above the incision (pedal pulse should be faint). Monitor for hypotension, tachycardia, or arrhythmia. Embolectomy or vascular repair may be deemed necessary following groin ultrasound.
Coronary artery dissection	Stent will typically be placed during procedure. Monitor for arrhythmia or tamponade. Administer heparin.
Tamponade due to perforation of the heart or bleeding due to antiplatelet medications	Typically this will be evident in the catheter laboratory at the time of perforation. Monitor patient for equalization of cardiac pressures. Emergency surgery may be required for repair.
Peripheral thromboembolism	Extremity will exhibit pain, pallor, pulselessness, paresthesias, and paralysis; may also be cool to touch. Unfractionated heparin or other anticoagulant should be continued. Thrombolytic therapy may be administered directly to the clot using a tracking catheter. Surgical intervention may be necessary.
Thromboembolism: CVA due to embolus	Monitor for signs and symptoms of neurologic compromise including speech patterns, orientation, vision, equal grips and pedal pushes, and sensation.
Pulmonary embolism	Provide supplemental O_2. Monitor for adequate arterial oxygen saturation and respiratory rate. Continue administration of unfractionated heparin or other anticoagulant IV. Direct thrombolytic therapy may be administered using a tracking catheter; direct extraction of the clot may also be attempted. Ventilation-perfusion scan or pulmonary arteriograms may be done to verify thrombus location.
Arrhythmia	Direct irritation of the ventricular wall by the catheter tip poses the greatest risk; postprocedure risk is extremely low. Monitor the patient in lead V_1.
Infection	Use aseptic technique for all dressing changes. Monitor catheter insertion sites for erythema, inflammation, heat, or exudate. Monitor patient temperature trends.
Pulmonary edema due to recumbent position, stress of angiographic contrast, or poor left ventricular function	Elevate HOB 30°. Administer diuretics as necessary. Consider use of flexible sheath or brachial access.
Acute tubular neurosis and renal failure	Hydrate patient well prior to and following procedure with continuous infusion of normal saline (typically 8 hours before and 8 hours after at 100 mL/h). Monitor for elevations in serum creatinine.
Vasovagal reaction	Administer pain medications prior to sheath removal. Monitor BP and heart rate before and after sheath removal, then every 15 minutes for 4 times after removal.

Percutaneous Coronary Interventions

Percutaneous coronary interventions (PCIs) include percutaneous transluminal coronary angioplasty (PTCA), insertion of one or more stents, and coronary atherectomy. PTCA, also termed angioplasty or balloon angioplasty, is a cardiac catheterization with the addition of a balloon apparatus on the tip of the catheter for revascularizing the myocardium (Figure 9-3). The catheter tip is advanced, generally over a guidewire, into the coronary artery until the balloon is positioned across the atherosclerotic lesion in the vessel. Once properly positioned, the balloon is inflated to stretch the vessel wall, resulting in fracture and compression of the atherosclerotic plaque improving blood flow through the vessel. As a result, the degree of stenosis is reduced. This allows a higher rate and volume of blood flow through the vessel, which translates clinically into fewer symptoms of angina and better exercise tolerance.

Complications

Angioplasty is associated with the same complications found during cardiac catheterization. In addition, complications related to manipulation of the coronary artery itself may also occur. The most common serious complications include a 2% to 10% incidence of complete occlusion of the vessel (abrupt closure), AMI (1%-5% incidence), and the need for emergency coronary artery bypass surgery (1%-2% incidence). The most important predictor of complications of MI and abrupt vessel closure is reduced coronary flow through the lesion prior to the procedure. A universal scale, the TIMI Scale, is used to quantify this rate of coronary flow. The scale rates coronary blood flow as follows: no perfusion, penetration without perfusion, partial perfusion, and complete perfusion.

Other Percutaneous Coronary Interventions

In addition to routine balloon angioplasty, a number of other devices are now commonly used for percutaneous coronary

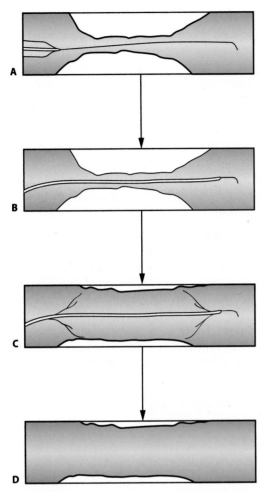

Figure 9-3. Percutaneous transluminal coronary angioplasty (PTCA). **(A)** PTCA catheter being advanced into the narrowed coronary artery over a guidewire. **(B)** Catheter position prior to balloon inflation. **(C)** Balloon inflation. **(D)** Coronary vessel following catheter removal.

revascularization. Intracoronary stents are small metallic mesh tubes placed across the stenotic area and expanded with an angioplasty balloon (Figure 9-4). Once expanded, the tube is permanently anchored in the vessel wall. Stents are effective in decreasing the rate of abrupt vessel closure seen with traditional PTCA. Some stents are coated with a drug that is bonded to a material on the stent causing the drug to be released directly onto the arterial wall over several months to years. These drug-coated stents have been shown to significantly reduce the restenosis rate associated with metal stents. Atherectomy catheters and lasers are used infrequently; however, patient outcomes are not significantly better than those achieved with traditional balloon catheters and stent deployment and may result in higher rates of complication, including AMI. Each of these devices may offer advantages over traditional balloon angioplasty catheters in situations involving specific vascular anatomy (eg, ostial lesions) or lesion morphology (eg, high degree of calcified plaque).

PATHOLOGIC CONDITIONS

Acute Ischemic Heart Disease

Myocardial ischemia is the lack of adequate blood supply to the heart, resulting in an insufficient supply of oxygen to meet the demands of the heart muscle. This supply-demand mismatch, known as ischemia, is most often caused by thrombus formation at a site of atherosclerotic plaque rupture within a coronary artery. Decreased oxygen supply to myocardial tissue may cause a variety of symptoms such as chest discomfort (angina), shortness of breath, diaphoresis, and nausea. Unstable angina, defined as angina that is of new onset, increasing in frequency, or occurring at rest, and

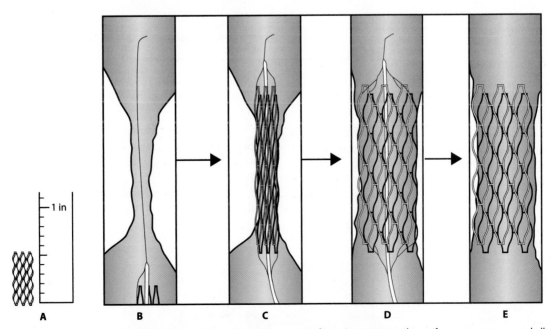

Figure 9-4. Intracoronary stent. **(A)** Size of stent device when fully deployed. **(B)** Insertion of stent into a narrowed area of a coronary artery on a balloon-inflatable catheter. **(C)** Inflation of the balloon catheter to expand the stent. **(D)** Inflation complete with stent fully expanded. **(E)** Stent following removal of balloon catheter.

AMI are referred to as the acute coronary syndromes (ACS), which form the spectrum of acute ischemic heart disease.

Etiology and Pathophysiology

Intracoronary thrombus formation, and the resulting obstruction of coronary blood flow, is the pathophysiologic mechanism of acute ischemic heart disease. Preexisting atherosclerosis and spasm of the smooth muscle wall of the coronary arteries, termed fixed obstructions, may also contribute to reduced flow. In some situations, coronary artery spasm may play a major role, unrelated to underlying atherosclerosis, causing MI. These occurrences are sometimes associated with cocaine abuse seen in MI in young patients.

The formation of a thrombus in coronary arteries is initiated by the fissuring and rupture of atherosclerotic plaque in the vessel wall of the coronary artery (Figure 9-5). A continuous, dynamic process occurs whereby plaque may become unstable during periods of active accumulation of more lipid into the core of the plaque. The plaque then ruptures, dispelling its contents into the lumen of the coronary artery and causing activation of clotting factors at the site of plaque rupture. The rupture of plaque and resultant thrombus formation may eventually occlude the coronary artery.

Although most people have some degree of atherosclerotic plaque formation by age 30, the vast majority of these plaques are considered "stable." They are covered by smooth fibrous caps allowing adequate blood flow through the coronary arteries, and are not prone to development of unstable angina or MI. In young, growing plaques, the fibrous cap may become thin and rupture, resulting in unstable angina, ischemia, or MI.

A variety of factors predispose a plaque to fissure and rupture. Characteristics of plaque at increased risk for rupture include:

- *Location of the lesion in the vascular tree:* Areas of greater turbulence of flow and dynamic activity during the cardiac cycle are at higher risk.
- *Size of the lipid pool within the plaque:* A large amount of lipid inside the plaque core is more likely to be associated with plaque disruption.
- *Infiltration of the plaque with macrophages:* Macrophages are thought to weaken the integrity of the fibrous cap of the plaque, making it more susceptible to rupture.

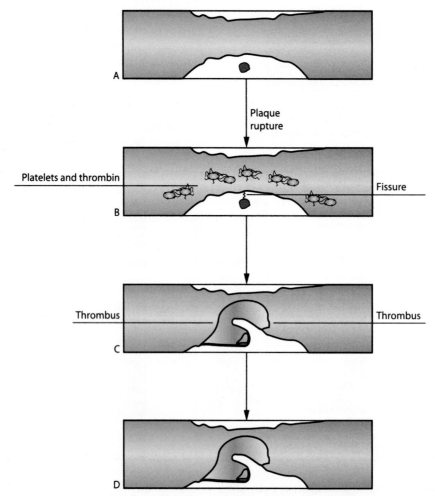

Figure 9-5. Atherosclerotic plaque formation. **(A)** Stable plaque. **(B)** Plaque with cap disruption. **(C)** Moderate amount of layered thrombus. **(D)** Occlusive thrombus.

ESSENTIAL CONTENT CASE

Unstable Angina

A 62-year-old man presents to the emergency department (ED) with complaints of pain in his chest and jaw. The pain, originally occurring only with exertion and resolving with rest, became increasingly persistent over the past 2 to 3 days. On the evening of his arrival, the patient experienced a 15-minute episode of severe pain while watching television. This episode he characterized as a "tight, burning feeling in my chest, and an aching in my jaw" that did not vary with respiratory effort and was accompanied by diaphoresis, nausea, and shortness of breath.

On arrival to the ED, his pain and nausea had resolved, pulse oximetry showed oxygen saturation of 98% on room air, and his vital signs were:

BP	148/86 mm Hg
HR	90 beats/min
RR	18 breaths/min
T	37.6 °C orally

On physical examination, heart sounds were normal, without S_3, S_4, or murmurs. Initial diagnostic tests revealed:

- ECG: Normal sinus rhythm with nonspecific ST-T wave changes
- Chest x-ray: Normal cardiac silhouette, clear lungs

A more detailed assessment of his history revealed increasing dyspnea on exertion and fatigue for the previous 6 months. Despite these symptoms, he had continued his daily 2.5-mile walking routine, sometimes experiencing shortness of breath several times during the walk. The patient reported smoking cigarettes in the past, one pack per day for 20 years, but quit 25 years ago. No ankle swelling, nocturnal dyspnea, or orthopnea were reported, nor was he aware of any family history of cardiac problems, coronary artery disease, diabetes, or hypertension.

He was started on aspirin based on his history and the likelihood of underlying coronary artery disease. He was then admitted for observation and evaluation of cardiac enzymes. (See section on cardiac enzymes I section on MI below.)

	CK Total	CK-MB	Troponin I
ED	169 mcg/L	5 ng/mL	0.4
4 hours later	163 mcg/L	5 ng/mL	0.4

Six hours after presenting to the ED, the patient had recurrent tightness in his chest. An ECG showed T-wave inversion in the anterior leads. Sublingual nitroglycerin 0.4 mg was administered every 5 minutes with complete relief of the pressure following the second tablet. An unfractionated heparin drip was started. Subsequent cardiac enzymes showed:

	CK Total	1 CK-MB	Troponin I
8 hours	159 mcg/L	4 ng/mL	0.4
12 hours	152 mcg/L	4 ng/mL	0.4

Other laboratory results were normal with the exception of elevated cholesterol and triglycerides on the lipid panel. Following receipt of these results, he was scheduled for an exercise tolerance test.

The ECG recorded a heart rate of 118 beats/min after 6 minutes of exercise. Onset of chest tightness during the last minute of exercise was described as similar to that which brought him to the hospital and correlated with 1.5-mm ST depression in leads V_4 to V_6. A cardiac catheterization was scheduled.

Coronary angiography showed a 75% obstruction of the LAD artery and 90% obstruction of the diagonal branch of the same artery. LVEF was 55%. A coronary angioplasty (PTCA) was performed on both lesions.

Case Question 1. While in the ED, an important aspect of his care would be to:

(A) Obtain repeat ECGs intermittently every 4 hours
(B) Monitor the patient's ECG continuously with continuous ST-segment monitoring
(C) Monitor platelet levels every 6 hours
(D) Assess breath sounds every 2 hours

Case Question 2. The ST-segment depression and T-wave inversion would be indicative of a:

(A) Non–ST-segment elevation MI
(B) ST-segment elevation MI
(C) Coronary spasm
(D) Pericarditis

Case Question 3. Following the PTCA, which of the following would be a clear sign of acute closure of one or both target vessels?

(A) Increased heart rate of 115 beats/min
(B) Hypotension
(C) 4 mm ST-segment elevation in leads V3-V4
(D) All of the above

Answers: 1: B; 2: A; 3: C

Although these characteristics determine the likelihood of plaque rupture, they are not easily identified by clinical assessment, stress testing, or cardiac catheterization. Plaque rupture may be caused by a number of environmental or hormonal factors, known as triggers (Table 9-4). These triggers may disrupt the plaque and precipitate an acute coronary event. Some of the triggers for atherosclerotic plaque rupture can be manipulated or controlled, such as blood

TABLE 9-4. HORMONAL AND ENVIRONMENTAL TRIGGERS OF PLAQUE RUPTURE

Acute	Chronic
Hemodynamic Reactivity	**Basal Hemodynamic Forces**
• Morning increase in BP	• Increased resting BP
• Morning increase in heart rate	• Increased resting heart rate
• Physical exertion	**Basal Hemostatic Variables**
• Emotional stress	• Location of the plaque
• Exposure to cold	• Size of the lipid pool within the core plaque
Hemostatic Reactivity	• Degree of macrophage infiltration of the plaque
• Increased coronary blood flow velocity	**Chronic Risk Factors**
• Increased viscosity of blood	• Gender (male > female)
• Decreased tPA activity	• Increasing age
• Increased platelet aggregation	• Diabetes mellitus
Vasoreactivity	• Hypercholesterolemia
• Increased plasma epinephrine	• Cigarette smoking
• Increased plasma cortisol	

pressure (BP), blood glucose level, and stress. In the clinical setting, management of these variables may decrease the risk for AMI, reinfarction, and reocclusion. They should be closely monitored.

When these triggers combine to cause plaque rupture, the lipid pool is exposed and a rough surface on the intima of the vessel wall occurs, stimulating the local effects of hormonal and immune factors and initiating thrombus formation. At the same time, the fibrinolytic system is stimulated, creating a dynamic process of simultaneous attempts to form and dissolve the clot. Because of the dynamic nature of the clotting process, the thrombus may be completely or only partially obstructive, or may fluctuate intermittently between the two stages. Regardless of the maturity of the clot, the process of thrombus formation may lead to obstruction of blood flow, diminishing oxygen delivery to distal myocardium and creating a mismatch between the supply of and demand for oxygen.

Because the underlying pathology of the ischemia-related diagnoses is the same (plaque rupture and thrombus formation), ischemic heart disease encompasses the entire spectrum of ischemic coronary events that are referred to as the ACS. ACS represents a continuum of clinical events that may result from the supply-demand mismatch including unstable angina, non–ST-segment elevation MI (NSTEMI), or ST-segment elevation MI (STEMI) (Figure 9-6).

Following a decrease in oxygen supply to the myocardium, the cell membranes lose their integrity and fluid moves into the cell. The cell is no longer able to regulate its internal and external environment. The cell dies, releasing cytotoxic substances into the bloodstream. When they die, cardiac myocytes release significant amounts of myoglobin, troponin I and T, as well as cardiac-specific creatine kinase (CK-MB), causing elevation in these laboratory values and confirming the MI diagnosis.

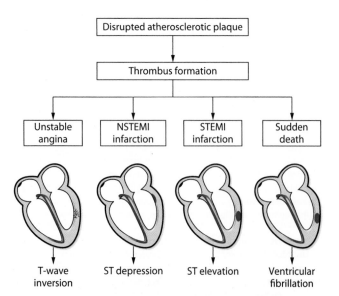

Figure 9-6. Pathophysiologic steps leading to acute coronary events.

Clinical Presentation

Clinical presentation across the spectrum of ACS is similar, with slight differences depending on the involved vessels (Table 9-5).

1. Pain or discomfort, usually in the chest (see Table 9-1)
   - Pressure or tightness in the chest
   - Jaw or neck pain
   - Left arm ache or pain
   - Epigastric discomfort
   - Scapular back pain
2. Nausea/vomiting
3. Hemodynamic instability
   - Hypotension (systolic BP < 90 mm Hg or 20 mm Hg below baseline)
   - Cardiac index (CI) (< 2.0 L/min/m^2)
   - Elevated pulmonary artery diastolic (PAD) and/or pulmonary artery occlusion pressure (PAOP)
   - Skin cool, clammy, diaphoretic
4. Dyspnea
5. Dysrhythmia/Conduction Defects
   - Left bundle branch block (LBBB)
   - Tachycardia/bradycardia
   - Frequent premature ventricular contractions
   - Ventricular fibrillation
6. Anxiety, sense of impending catastrophe
7. Denial

Some patient populations are predictably different in their description of chest discomfort, such as women and diabetics. Women frequently present with symptoms that are more vague such as feeling tired, short of breath, and lack of energy. Women may be prone to deny their symptoms for longer periods of time than men, delaying their arrival to the ED and often rendering them ineligible for thrombolytic therapy. In addition, women are typically postmenopausal when signs and symptoms of atherosclerotic disease become apparent. This predominantly older patient population may pose problems of its own such as anxiety, fear of the inability to care for oneself following MI, and other concerns to geriatric patient populations, which must be considered.

Diabetics are another patient population with atypical differences in symptoms when experiencing an MI. Diabetics have atypical pain secondary to neuropathies, and early development of atherosclerotic disease. Coronary artery disease (CAD) in this patient population is diffuse, and poor distal vascular anatomy is common. Lesion morphology in diabetic patients is also more difficult to revascularize, either using percutaneous or surgical methods.

Diagnostic Tests
Unstable Angina

1. *12-lead electrocardiogram (ECG):* Transient changes may occur and resolve; most commonly T-wave inversion or ST-segment depression.

2. *Cardiac enzymes (Troponin [I or T], myoglobin, and CK-MB):* Normal (Figure 9-7).
3. *Cardiac catheterization:* Not recommended in the acute setting, except in the case of continued pain/discomfort without relief from nitroglycerin. Catheterization results may be normal, or with visible atherosclerotic disease, but without a complete occlusion or thrombus.

Myocardial Infarction

1. *12-lead ECG:* Thirty-five percent of patients with AMI have ST-segment elevation (see Chapter 18, Advanced ECG Concepts). Approximately 65% of those with AMI have no ECG or other diagnostic changes.
2. *Creatine kinase (CK and CK-MB):* (see Figure 9-7).
   - Total CK > 150 to 180 mcg/L
   - MB band > 10 ng/mL or 0.3% of total.
   - Peaks at 12 hours after symptom onset.
   - CK-MB isoforms have better sensitivity and specificity for detecting MI within the first 6 hours.
3. *Troponin T:* > 0.1 to 0.2 ng/mL.
   - Begins to increase 3 to 5 hours after symptom onset
   - Remains elevated for 14 to 21 days
4. *Troponin I:* > 0.4 ng/mL.
   - Begins to increase 3 hours after onset of myocardial ischemia
   - Peaks at 14 to 18 hours
   - Remains elevated for 5 to 7 days
5. *Myoglobin:* Present in serum, 17.4 to 105.7 ng/mL
   - Released from myocardium within 2 hours of coronary occlusion
   - Peaks in 6 to 7 hours
   - Better marker for early detection of MI; better negative indicator if negative
6. Cardiac catheterization: Ventricular wall motion abnormalities (also may be seen by echocardiography); total occlusion of one or more coronary arteries.

Principles of Management of Acute Ischemic Heart Disease

Because most complications of acute ischemic heart disease directly result from reduced coronary flow, a primary objective in patient management is to optimize blood flow to the myocardium. Additional goals are to prevent complications of ischemia and infarction, alleviate chest discomfort/pain, and reduce anxiety.

Optimize Blood Flow to the Myocardium

Regardless of whether a patient presents with unstable angina or AMI, restoration and maintenance of coronary blood flow is important to improve patient outcomes. Interventions to optimize blood flow to the myocardium include pharmacologic measures, such as antiplatelet or antithrombin agents, and mechanical measures, such as percutaneous coronary revascularization (eg, angioplasty, stent, or

other) or coronary artery bypass grafting (CABG). Refer to Table 9-6 for evidence-based guidelines for AMI. The intervention selected and the optimal timing of the intervention depends on whether the occlusion of the artery is total or partial. This determination must be made as accurately and as quickly as possible, as a totally occluded artery will soon result in tissue necrosis or MI (Figure 9-8 for algorithm on acute chest pain management). All unstable arteries benefit from the following interventions which stabilize the artery and optimize coronary arterial flow.

MEDICAL MANAGEMENT

1. Decrease activity of coagulation system with pharmacologic therapy (Figure 9-9).
   - Antiplatelet agents: Aspirin, GP IIb/IIIa receptor blocking agents (eg, abciximab [Reopro®], eptifibatide [Integrilin®], and tirofiban [Aggrastat®]), thienopyridine agents (eg, clopidogrel [Plavix®])
   - Antithrombin agents: Indirect (eg, unfractionated heparin, low-molecular-weight heparin), direct (eg, bivalirudin [Angiomax®])
2. Increase ventricular filling time (decrease heart rate).
   - Beta-blockers
   - Bed rest for 24 hours
3. Decrease preload.
   - Nitrates
   - Diuretics
   - Morphine sulfate
4. Decrease afterload.
   - Angiotensin-converting enzyme (ACE) inhibitors or angiotensin receptor blockers (ARBs)
   - Hydralazine
5. Decrease myocardial oxygen consumption (MVO_2).
   - Beta-blockers
   - Bed rest for 24 hours
6. Reduce risk for sudden cardiac death due to ventricular tachycardia/ventricular fibrillation.
   - Beta blockers

Totally occluded arteries require, in addition to the above pharmacologic interventions, further reperfusion therapy, such as fibrinolysis, angioplasty, or CABG, to effectively restore blood flow to the coronary artery. In the event of left main coronary artery stenosis or three-vessel disease, urgent or emergent CABG is usually considered. In the acute setting, for ST-segment elevated MI (STEMI) fibrinolytic therapy is often the fastest, most universally available method for reperfusion if a catheterization laboratory is not available or operational 24 hours a day. The indications, contraindications, and common complications of fibrinolytic therapy are listed in Tables 9-7 and 9-8. In those settings where the catheterization laboratory is operational 24 h/day, primary PCI is indicated. Studies have indicated that primary PCI may be associated with better outcomes and fewer complications than with the use of fibrinolytic agents.

TABLE 9-5. CLINICAL PRESENTATION OF MYOCARDIAL ISCHEMIA AND INFARCTION

Type MI	Arterial Involvement	Muscle Area Supplied	Assessment
Anteroseptal wall	LAD	Anterior LV wall, Anterior LV septum, Apex LV, Bundle of His, Bundle branches	↓ LV function → ↓ CO, ↓ BP, ↑ PAD, ↑ PAOP, S_3 and S_4, with HF, Rales with pulmonary edema
Posterior septal lateral	RCA circumflex branches (right and left)	Posterior surface of LV, SA node 45%, AV node 10%, Left atrium, Lateral wall of LV	Murmurs indicating VSD (septal), PA catheter to assess, R to L shunt in VSD, Signals/symptoms of LV aneurysm with lateral displaced PMI leading to signs and symptoms of mitral regurgitation
Inferior or "diaphragmatic"	RCA	RV, RA, SA node 50%, AV node 90%, RA, RV, Inferior LV, Posterior, IV septum, Posterior LBBB, Posterior LV	Symptomatic bradycardia: ↓ BP LOC changes diaphoresis, ↓ CO ↑ PAD ↑ PAOP, Murmurs: associated with papillary muscle dysfunction mid/holosystolic rates, pulmonary edema, nausea
Right ventricular infarction	RCA	RA, RV, inferior LV, SA node, AV node, Posterior, IV septum	Kussmaul sign, JVD, Hypotension, ↑ SVR, ↓ PAOP, ↑ CVP, S_3 with noncompliant RV, Clear breath sounds initially, Hepatomegaly; peripheral edema; cool, clammy, pale skin

ECG Changes	Likely Arrhythmias	Possible Complications
Indicative ST elevation with or without abnormal Q waves in V$_{1-4}$ Loss of R waves in precordial leads **Reciprocal** ST depression in II, III, aVF.	RBBB, LBBB AV blocks Atrial fibrillation or flutter Ventricular tachycardia (VT) Tachycardia (septal)	Cardiogenic shock VSD Myocardial rupture Heart blocks may be permanent (LBBB) High mortality associated with this location of MI
Lateral Indicative ST elevation with or without abnormal Q waves in I, aVL, V$_{5,6}$ Loss of R wave and ↑ ST in I, aVL, V5-6 **Posterior Indicative** Tall, broad R waves (> 0.04 seconds) in V$_{1-3}$ ↑ ST V$_4$R (right-sided 12 lead, V$_4$ position) **Posterior Reciprocal** ST depression in V$_{1,2}$, upright T wave in V$_{1,2}$	Bradycardia Mobitz I (posterior)	RV involvement Aneurysm development Papillary muscle dysfunction Heart blocks frequently resolve
Indicative ↑ ST segments in II, III, aVF Q waves in II, III, aVF **Reciprocal** ST depression in I, aVL, V$_{1-4}$	AV blocks; often progress to CHB which may be transient or permanent; Wenckebach; bradyarrhythmias	Hiccups Nausea/vomiting Papillary muscle dysfunction MR Septal rupture (0.5%-1.0%) RV involvement associated with atrial infarcts especially with atrial arrhythmias
Indicative 1- to 2-mm ST-segment elevation in V$_4$R ST- and T-wave elevation in II, III, aVF Q waves in II, III, aVF ST-elevation decreases in amplitude over V$_{1-6}$	First-degree AV block Second-degree AV block, type I Incomplete RBBB Transient CHB Atrial fibrillation VT/VF	Hypotension requiring large fluid volumes initially to maintain systemic pressure. Once RV contractility improves, fluids will mobilize, possibly requiring diuresis

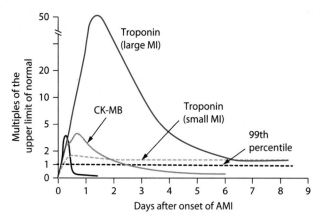

Figure 9-7. Timing and levels of biomarkers associated with heart injury. (*Modified from Antman EM: Decision making with cardiac troponin tests. N Engl J Med 346:2079, 2002; and Jaffe AS, Babiun L, Apple FS: Biomarkers in acute cardiac disease: The present and the future. J Am Coll Cardiol 48:1, 2006.*)

SURGICAL MANAGEMENT

Coronary artery bypass grafting is one method of revascularization generally used in patients with atherosclerosis of three or more coronary vessels or in the case of significant left main CAD. CABG is performed both electively, as well as emergently, and may be performed either prior to or following an MI. The CABG procedure requires *induction* with general anesthesia, and possible initiation of cardiopulmonary bypass (blood is diverted outside of the body to a pump that mechanically oxygenates the blood before returning it to the arterial circulation) and placement of a graft into the

TABLE 9-6. EVIDENCE-BASED PRACTICE: ACS—ST ELEVATION MI AND NON–ST-ELEVATION MI

Diagnosis
- Diagnosis of AMI is based on two of three findings:[a,b]
  1. History of ischemic-like symptoms
  2. Changes on serial ECGs
  3. Elevation and fall in level of serum cardiac biomarkers
- Of AMI patients, 50% do not present with ST-segment elevation. Other indicators:[a,b]
  1. ST-segment depression may indicate non–ST-elevation MI (NSTEMI).
  2. New LBBB.
  3. ST-segment depression that resolves with relief of chest pain.
  4. T-wave inversion in all chest leads may indicate NSTEMI with a critical stenosis in the proximal LAD.

Acute Management
- Optimal time for initiation of therapy is within 1 hour of symptom onset. Rarely feasible due to delay in treatment-seeking behavior.[a,b]
- Initial ECG should be obtained within 10 minutes of emergency department arrival.[a,b]
- Oxygen, nitroglycerine, and aspirin should be administered if not contraindicated.[a,b]
- Reperfusion strategy for STEMI only[a,b]
  1. Fibrinolytic agent should be initiated within 30 minutes of arrival if no contraindication.
  2. If primary PCI to be done, culprit vessel should be opened within 90 minutes of arrival.
- Reperfusion strategy for NSTEMI.[a,b]
  1. Fibrinolytics not recommended.
  2. PCI to be done within 24 hours of arrival.
- Weight-based heparin or low-molecular-weight heparin.[a,b]
- IV beta-blocker should be given within 12 hours of arrival.[a,b]
- Lipid-lowering agent should be initiated.[a,b]

Data compiled from [a]O'Gara et al. (2013) [b]Adams et al. (2012).

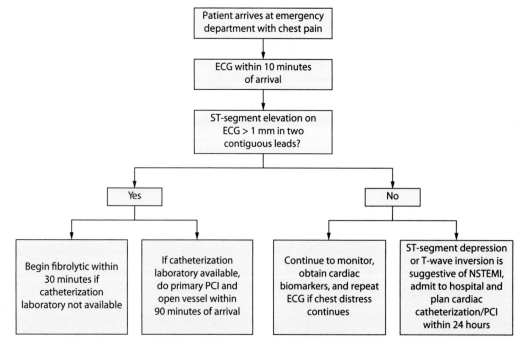

Figure 9-8. Algorithm for management of acute chest pain.

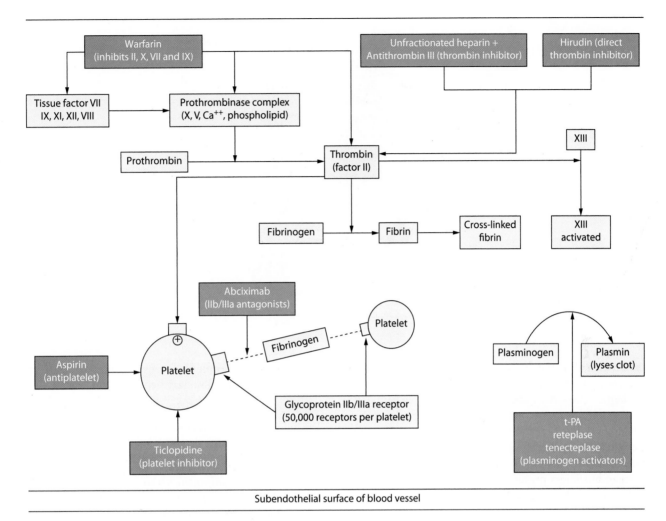

Figure 9-9. Coagulation sequence and site of antithrombotic/antiplatelet drug activity.

TABLE 9-7. INDICATIONS AND CONTRAINDICATIONS FOR THROMBOLYTIC THERAPY

Indications
- Chest pain > 20 minutes, but typically < 12 hours
- ST elevation ≥ 1 mm in two contiguous leads
- LBBB
- High-risk patients with chest pain > 12 hours in duration may still be candidates if pain persists

Absolute Contraindications
- Active internal bleeding
- History of intracranial bleeding, cerebral neoplasm, or other intracranial pathology
- Stroke or head trauma within 6 months
- Known allergy to the drug chosen

Relative Contraindications
- Major surgery or GI bleeding within 2 months
- Traumatic puncture of noncompressible vessel
- Pregnancy or 1 month postpartum
- Uncontrolled hypertension (systolic > 200 or diastolic > 110)
- Trauma within 2 weeks, including CPR with rib fracture

TABLE 9-8. COMPLICATIONS OF FIBROLYTIC THERAPY

Complication	Percentage Occurrence
Groin bleeding, local (compressible external)	25-45
Intracerebral bleeding	1.45
Retroperitoneal bleeding (noncompressible internal)	1
Gastrointestinal bleeding	4-10
Genitourinary bleeding	1-5
Other bleeding	1-5

coronary arterial tree (Figure 9-10). Technological advances have resulted in the development of stabilizer devices permitting CABG to be performed without placing the patient on cardiopulmonary bypass. The heart continues to beat while the surgeon places a device over the coronary artery site where the bypass graft is to be anastomosed, which stabilizes

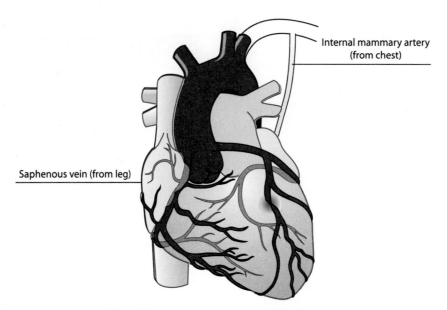

Figure 9-10. Coronary artery bypass grafting (CABG).

the small area allowing for suturing to occur. This is often referred to as "beating heart surgery" or "off pump" coronary artery bypass (OPCAB). The graft, generally a leg vein, left internal mammary artery, or radial artery, is inserted past the distal end of the blockage in the coronary artery and, in the case of a leg vein graft and radial artery graft, anastomosed to the aorta. Multiple grafts may be inserted based on the number of blockages present and the availability of viable insertion sites in the patient's native coronary tree.

INDICATIONS

The indications for CABG and long-term patient outcome following this procedure have been intensively reviewed over the past decade. In general, patients with three-vessel disease, poor LVEF (< 35%), or significant disease in the left main coronary artery have lower long-term morbidity and mortality with surgical revascularization (CABG) compared to medical therapy or percutaneous interventions such as angioplasty or stent. Diabetics with multivessel disease have also been found to fare better following CABG than following percutaneous interventions including drug-eluting stents. CABG may also be indicated as an emergent "rescue" procedure in patients whose coronary artery severely dissects or fractures during an attempted percutaneous procedure.

CONTRAINDICATIONS

Several populations of patients may be considered poor candidates for coronary bypass, including the very elderly, debilitated patients, patients with severely diseased distal coronary vasculature (eg, some diabetics), and patients with extremely low LVEF (eg, < 5%-15%). Patients with low ejection fractions often have difficulty being weaned from cardiopulmonary bypass following the procedure. Other contraindications are those related to general anesthesia risk,

including severe chronic obstructive pulmonary disease, pulmonary edema, or pulmonary hypertension.

POSTOPERATIVE MANAGEMENT

The following is a general overview of the early postoperative management of CABG patients:

1. *Maintain hemodynamic stability:* A variety of cardiac drugs are administered to maintain hemodynamic stability in the first 24 hours postoperatively. The following hemodynamic values may serve as guides for inotropic and vasopressor administration along with intravascular fluid therapy. In general, values greater or lower than the following require intervention:
   - Mean arterial pressure: 70 to 80 mm Hg
   - CI: 2.0 to 3.5 L/min/m^2
   - PAD/PAOP: 10 to 12 mm Hg (used primarily to evaluate need for volume replacement)
   - Central venous pressure (CVP): 5 to 10 mm Hg (used primarily to evaluate need for volume replacement)
   - HR: Intrinsic or paced rhythm in range of 80 to 100 beats/min to keep CI ≥ 2.0
   - If radial artery graft used, monitor for arterial spasm. Prophylactic nitroglycerin drip and nitro paste.
2. *Maintain ventilation and oxygenation:* Ventilation and oxygenation are maximized in the early postoperative period with mechanical ventilation. Within 2 to 12 hours, most patients have recovered from the anesthesia effects and are sufficiently stable to allow weaning from mechanical ventilation and extubation. Individuals with preexisting pulmonary problems may require longer periods of intubation until weaning can be successfully accomplished.

Following weaning and extubation, supplemental O_2 therapy usually is required for 1 to 2 days to maintain PaO_2 or SaO_2 in normal ranges. Postoperative atelectasis and pleural effusions are a common occurrence after cardiopulmonary bypass, requiring frequent pulmonary interventions (eg, coughing and deep breathing, incentive spirometry, ambulation) to maintain ventilation and oxygenation.

3. Prevention of postoperative complications:
   - *Bleeding from vascular graft anastomosis sites:* Frequent monitoring of mediastinal tube drainage, hematocrit, and coagulation status; avoidance of even brief periods of hypertension.
   - *Cardiac tamponade:* Frequent assessment for signs and symptoms of tamponade which include tachycardia, SOB, anxiety/decreased LOC, paradoxus, sinus tachycardia, decreased mediastinal tube drainage, increased CVP, PAD, and PAOP (note: these are often within 2 to 3 mm Hg of each other, which is called equalization of pressures or diastolic plateau), muffled heart sounds, decreased BP, and cardiac output.
   - *Infection:* Antibiotics may be used prophylactically for 48 hours; temperature spike within 24 hours postoperatively is not abnormal (may be related to pulmonary atelectasis).
   - *Cardiac arrhythmias:* ECG and continuous ST-segment monitoring, treat unstable rhythms, maintain K^+ and Mg^+ within normal limits with IV replacement.
   - *Relief of postoperative pain and anxiety:* Analgesic administration is typically required to ensure pain relief, especially to facilitate ambulation, coughing, and deep breathing.
   - If median sternotomy performed ensure sternal precautions are implemented, eg, avoid hyperextension of chest (arms and shoulders pulled posteriorly).

Preventing Complications Associated with Coronary Obstruction

Complications associated with acute ischemic syndromes include recurrent ischemia, infarction or reinfarction, onset of HF, and arrhythmias.

1. Prevent recurrent ischemia, infarction, or reinfarction: Continue pharmacologic interventions to inhibit prothrombotic events, including ischemia and infarction (eg, antiplatelet and antithrombin agents). Assess for recurrent angina with frequent chest pain assessment and serial 12-lead ECG and continuous ST-segment ischemia monitoring. (See *AACN Practice Alert: ST-Segment Monitoring.*)
2. Continuously monitor for arrhythmias: Monitor, if possible, for 24 to 72 hours following an ischemic episode.
3. Minimize potential for HF: Minimize myocardial oxygen consumption with the administration of beta-blockers, limit physical activity (bed rest), and avoid increases in metabolic rate (eg, fever). Reduce left ventricular afterload with the administration of ACE inhibitors or ARBs and hydralazine.

Alleviating Pain

Pain relief improves coronary flow by decreasing the level of circulating catecholamines, thereby decreasing BP (afterload) and heart rate (myocardial oxygen consumption). Nitrates typically relieve anginal pain by dilating coronary arteries and increasing blood flow, thereby improving myocardial oxygenation and directly treating the source of the pain. Another pharmacologic intervention commonly used to relieve pain in ischemia is morphine sulfate. Although morphine is a potent narcotic that has been criticized for masking cardiac pain, it is also a potent vasodilator and effectively vasodilates coronary as well as peripheral arteries, resulting in mild afterload reduction. Severe pain, unable to be relieved with nitrates or a combination of nitrates and morphine, is typically an indication for immediate PCI if available or transfers to a referring institution for emergency PCI.

Reducing Anxiety

The reduction of anxiety in ischemic heart disease is important for a number of reasons. The most important physiologically is the reduction of catecholamine secretion and decrease in sympathetic tone following relaxation in the anxious patient. This effect has been shown to decrease the incidence of dysrhythmia and promote vasodilation and afterload reduction. Decreasing anxiety may also increase the patient's ability to process new information regarding his or her diagnosis, and to better understand instructions for tests or procedures that will be done.

Relief of pain typically is most effective in reducing patient anxiety. In the event that pain is not relieved with nitroglycerin, or fibrinolytics in the initial treatment of ischemia, pain relievers such as morphine sulfate or anxiolytics such as midazolam or lorazepam (short- or intermediate-acting benzodiazepines respectively) are usually effective.

A number of interventions may be done at the bedside to promote relaxation, including specific relaxation and imagery techniques, meditation, music therapy, and the use of relaxation tapes. Providing the patient and family with adequate information regarding unfamiliar surroundings, when the physician may be available to speak with them, possible "unknowns" such as tests or procedures, and important expectations such as visitation guidelines helps provide a sense of security and facilitates relaxation by increasing the patient's level of comfort with the situation. Anxiety can also be decreased by offering the patient opportunities for control in the acute setting. Examples include the timing of simple activities such as visitor presence, bathing, and eating.

Electrophysiology Studies

In the past 25 years, the cardiology subspecialty of electro-physiology (EP) has grown significantly and continues to expand. An electro-physiology study involves the insertion of several catheters with multiple electrodes on each into the right atrium and ventricle, the coronary sinus and, in some cases across the intra-atrial septum (trans-septal) into the left atrium. The multiple electrode locations (Figure 9-11) are used to record the impulse initiative and/or the conduction of the electrical waveform (depolarization process) through the myocardial tissue. The purpose of the EP may be for a variety of reasons such as: (1) to identify the site of origin for a dysrhythmia like atrial fibrillation or ventricular tachycardia; (2) to map the conduction pathway to identify the location of a conduction disturbance; (3) to identify the presence of an anomalous pathway which may be seen with Wolf-Parkinson-White Syndrome; (4) to determine the need for an implantable device for instance a pacemaker, or cardiovertor defibrillator (ICD or PCD). If the study identifies the site of origin for a dysrhythmia or abnormal pathway, the EP physician is able to use radiofrequency (electricity) ablation or cryoablation (extreme cold) to destroy the site or the abnormal pathway. Following the procedure, the patient needs to be monitored for similar groin complications as seen with cardiac catheterization. Additional monitoring includes observing for the onset of AV blocks as the AV node and/or Bundle of His tissue might have been injured during ablation of the anomalous pathway. If there is evidence of the AV block during the EP study, a pacemaker will be implanted at that time.

Heart Failure

Heart failure is a broad term referring to the inability of the heart to eject an adequate cardiac output to meet the oxygen

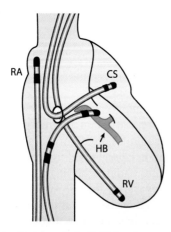

Figure 9-11. Electrophysiology study: Multiple catheters with electrodes are threaded into the right side of the heart. This allows for local monitoring and recording of the electrical activity as the heart depolarizes and repolarizes. The recordings help to locate the origin of the arrhythmia or conduction abnormality across the anomalpous pathway. (Source: *Medtronic, Inc. Minneapolis, MN.*) Abbreviations: RA, right atrium; RV, right ventricle; HB, his bundle; CS, coronary sinus.

and metabolic requirements of the body. A number of underlying disease processes may contribute to this "weak pump" syndrome, with coronary atherosclerosis, valvular heart disease, hypertension, and cardiomyopathy as the most common causes. Although the underlying causes are diverse, the progressive process which occurs in response to one of these initiating events is the same.

Etiology, Risk Factors, and Pathophysiology

Although HF may result from a number of underlying etiologies, those causing left ventricular systolic dysfunction are the most common contributors. The pathophysiology of HF is a three-stage process, beginning with an initial insult to the myocardium (phase I), followed by a response phase (phase II), and resulting in the clinical syndrome known as HF, characterized by exhaustion of compensatory mechanisms (phase III) (Figure 9-12). Regardless of the precipitating event, the physiologic progression of the syndrome, once initiated, is the same.

Phase I

Phase I of HF is characterized by an initiating event (eg, MI, viral infection, chemotherapeutic agents, valvular heart disease, hypertension, idiopathic cardiomyopathy), which causes loss of myocytes. This cell loss or permanent damage to the myocytes can be either localized or diffuse, resulting in compromised ventricular function. To date, over 700 initiating factors, such as acute ischemic damage, viruses, and toxins, have been isolated as contributors to myocardial insult and HF.

- *Result of phase I:* Decreased stroke volume secondary to an initial insult to the myocardium.

Phase II

A number of adaptive mechanisms occur in response to the initial insult in an effort to maintain adequate cardiac output to meet the body's needs. This phase is sometimes referred to as the compensatory phase (Figures 9-12 and 9-13). These compensatory mechanisms or responses include the Frank-Starling response, myocardial remodeling, and the neurohormonal response.

Frank-Starling Response

As cardiac output decreases and the sympathetic nervous system is activated, alpha-1 receptors are stimulated, resulting in arteriolar and venous vasoconstriction. This adaptive response initially results in increased venous return to the ventricle, increased ventricular end-diastolic volume, stretching of the ventricular myocytes, and improved stroke volume. Later, as overstretching of the ventricle occurs, this compensatory mechanism is lost, resulting in left ventricular decompensation and myocardial hypertrophy (Figure 9-14). Additionally, there is increased expression of granules in the left ventricle causing an increased release of brain natriuretic peptide (BNP).

Increased BNP levels in the serum are used as markers of severity of ventricular failure.

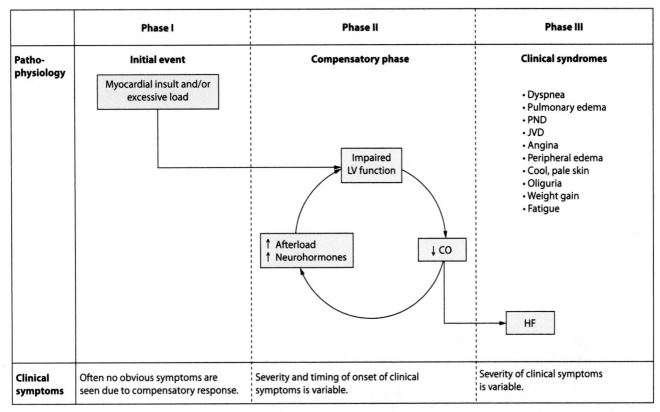

Figure 9-12. Pathophysiology of heart failure during phases I, II, and III.

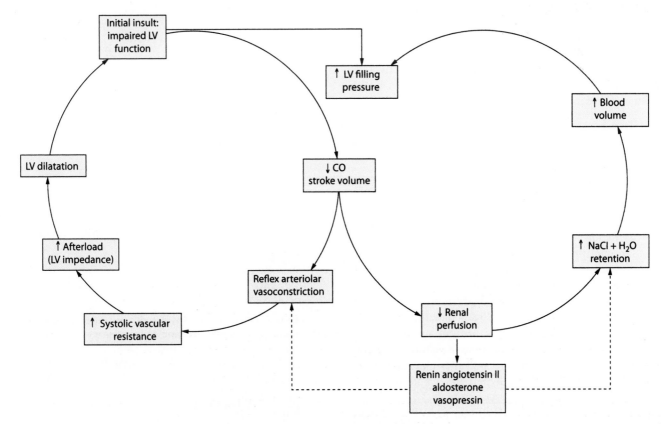

Figure 9-13. Compensatory mechanisms of heart failure.

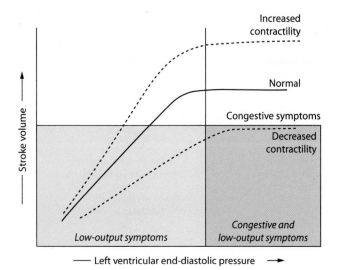

Figure 9-14. Frank-Starling curve.

MYOCARDIAL HYPERTROPHY (REMODELING)

In response to increased vascular volume and decreased myocardial function (loss of the Frank-Starling response), the left ventricle dilates and hypertrophies. This distortion of the normal left ventricular anatomy causes mitral regurgitation and further left ventricular dilatation. Angiotensin II, a by-product of the renin-angiotensin system activation, directly induces myocyte hypertrophy as well. The result of these factors is decreased left ventricular reserve (stretch), increased preload (high residual volume in the ventricle following systole), and further mitral regurgitation.

NEUROHORMONAL RESPONSE

In response to decreased stroke volume and decreased renal perfusion, several neurohormonal systems are activated, each of which acts to compensate for the decrease in stroke volume. These include:

1. *Adrenergic nervous system:* Adrenergic nervous system activity is heightened in the setting of impaired ventricular function as a direct result of baroreceptor stimulation. These baroreceptors mediate the sympathetic nervous system, which in turn stimulates the beta-1 receptors. This results in an increase in heart rate and contractility.

2. *Renin-angiotensin-aldosterone system:* Decreased renal perfusion stimulates the release of renin, increasing the production of angiotensin I and II and the release of aldosterone. This causes arteriolar vasoconstriction, decreased cardiac output, increased arterial BP and peripheral resistance, increased ventricular filling pressures, sodium and potassium retention (imbalance), increased volume overload, increased left ventricular wall stress, increased ventricular dilation and hypertrophy, and increased sympathetic nervous system arousal.

3. *Arginine vasopressin (AVP) system:* AVP is a potent vasoconstrictor that is normally inhibited by stretch

ESSENTIAL CONTENT CASE

Heart Failure

A 75-year-old man presents to the ED with diaphoresis and severe dyspnea. Initial assessment revealed the following:

RR	32 breaths/min
BP	110/90 mm Hg
HR	110 beats/min, irregular
JVD	Bilateral 7-mm elevation
Lungs	Bibasilar crackles throughout the lower lobes
Cardiovascular	S_1, S_2 with an S_3

A pulse oximeter revealed 83% oxygen saturation.

Laboratory work, including an arterial blood gas sample, was done with the following results:

Pao_2	60 mm Hg
$Paco_2$	28 mm Hg
pH	7.51
Sao_2	93%

Oxygen was initiated at 4 L/min via nasal cannula. An ECG was done and showed left ventricular hypertrophy, and left bundle branch block. His chest x-ray showed an enlarged cardiac silhouette and bilateral infiltrates. A pulmonary artery catheter was placed and the following parameters were found (refer Chapter 3 for hemodynamic parameters):

RA	10 mm Hg
PA	41/35 mm Hg
PAOP	32 mm Hg
CO	3.8 L/min
CI	1.9 L/min/m^2

A dobutamine drip was started at 2.5 mcg/kg/min, and furosemide 40 mg IV was given. Cardiac catheterization was performed the next morning with the following findings:

LAD	95% occlusion
RCA	50% occlusion
LCx	75% occlusion
EF	28%

Severe asyneresis

Case Question 1. The purpose of starting the dobutamine infusion and administering the furosemide is to:

(A) Increase myocardial contractility and reduce ventricular preload

(B) Increase myocardial contractility and reduce ventricular afterload

(C) Reduce myocardial contractility and increase ventricular preload

(D) Increase myocardial contractility and increase ventricular afterload

Case Question 2. Following the initiation of dobutamine and administration of furosemide, you would expect which of the following to occur?

(A) HR 120 beats/min; PA 40/38, PAOP unchanged

(B) HR 110 beats/min; PA 32/25 mm Hg; PAOP 24 mm Hg

(C) HR 95 beats/min; PA unchanged; RA 14 mm Hg

(D) BP 105/80 mm Hg, PA 49/38 mm Hg; RA 14 mm Hg

Case Question 3. After reviewing the cardiac catheterization results, you would anticipate the patient having one of the following procedures:

(A) Implantation of a HeartMate II LVAD as destination therapy
(B) Ventricular aneurysmectomy/reconstruction surgery
(C) Mitral valve repair
(D) Insertion of a dual chamber biventricular pacemaker

Answers: 1: A; 2: B; 3: D

receptors in the atria during atrial distension. In HF, these receptors are less sensitive, causing a decrease in AVP inhibition. This results in systemic vasoconstriction, further increasing afterload (the pressure the ventricle must work against to eject blood out to the system). Increases in AVP availability also lead to an inability to excrete free water, hypoosmolarity, and, in general, inability to autoregulate further AVP production.

4. *Atrial natriuretic peptide (ANP):* ANP is a counterregulatory hormone that opposes all three of the above systems, resulting in vasodilation and sodium excretion. ANP is produced in response to atrial distension and results in decreased formation of renin, decreased effects of angiotensin II, decreased release of aldosterone and vasopressin, and enhanced renal excretion of sodium and water. In chronic HF, the

levels of ANP remain elevated, but are less so than in the acute decompensation phase (phase III).

The effects of the compensatory mechanisms in phase II lead to an increase in circulating volume and perfusion to vital organs. Eventually, these mechanisms are self-limiting and a vicious cycle of increased afterload and volume overload results. The neurohormonal response is no longer beneficial in the chronic state but, as seen in phase III, becomes detrimental leading to changes in the myocyte DNA, resulting in programmed cell death (apoptosis) and further loss of myocytes.

- *Result of phase II:* Ventricular hypertrophy, weakened myocytes, increased arteriolar resistance, increased vascular volume, and increased ventricular wall stress occur in an effort to maintain adequate cardiac output.

Phase III

When the adaptive mechanisms of phase II fail, the clinical syndrome of HF follows. This third phase of HF is extremely variable in onset and presentation. The clinical expression and course of the disease is determined by the extent of the initial insult and myocyte damage, the severity of hemodynamic burden (volume overload), and the patient's individual neurohormonal response to these changes. Phase III is characterized by a progressive deterioration of cardiovascular functioning due to the relationship between compromised left ventricular function and excessive cardiac afterload (Figure 9-15). As ventricular dilation occurs, brain natriuretic peptide (BNP) levels in the serum increase.

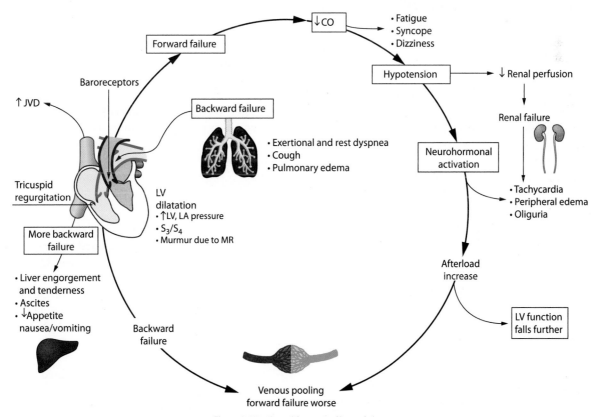

Figure 9-15. Clinical features of heart failure.

- *Result of phase III:* Clinical signs and symptoms of HF are evident, resulting in decreased functional status and activity intolerance for the patient.

Clinical Presentation

Regardless of the underlying cause of the weak pump, patients with HF present with clinical signs and symptoms of intravascular and interstitial volume overload, as well as manifestations of inadequate tissue perfusion. Common findings in HF include:

- Dyspnea (especially with exertion, commonly severe in the acute setting)
- Paroxysmal nocturnal dyspnea
- Pulmonary edema (pronounced crackles)
- Jugular venous distention (JVD)
- Chest discomfort or tightness
- Peripheral edema
- Cool, pale, cyanotic skin
- Oliguria
- Reported weight gain
- Fatigue

More specific physical signs and symptoms may vary in individuals depending on the ventricle which is primarily involved. A summary of clinical findings specific to left and right ventricular failure is presented in Table 9-9.

Because subjective assessment of symptoms and their severity may vary from clinician to clinician, classification systems have been developed to standardize symptom severity as well as the evolution and progression of HF. The American College of Cardiology and the American Heart Association developed a staging system that addresses the evolution and progression of HF. A second system, known as the New York Heart Association (NYHA) Functional Classification System, is used to provide systematic assessment of patient status and to benchmark improvement or deterioration from initial evaluation (Table 9-10).

A number of conditions, both cardiac and noncardiac, are similar to HF in their clinical presentation and should be ruled out as possible diagnoses in the initial assessment. These conditions include MI, pulmonary disease, dysrhythmias, anemia, renal failure, nephrotic syndrome, and thyroid disease.

Diagnostic Tests

- *12-lead ECG:* Acute ST-T wave changes, low voltage, left ventricular hypertrophy, atrial fibrillation or other tachyarrhythmias, bradyarrhythmias, Q waves from previous MI, LBBB
- *Chest x-ray:* Cardiomegaly, cardiothoracic ratio 0.5
- *Complete blood count:* Low red cell count (anemia)
- *Urinalysis:* Proteinuria, red blood cells, or casts
- *Creatinine:* Elevated
- *Albumin:* Decreased
- *Serum sodium and potassium:* Decreased
- *PAP:* Elevated
- *CI:* < 2.0 L/min/m^2

TABLE 9-10. CLASSIFICATION OF CARDIOVASCULAR DISABILITY

AHA/ACC Stages of Heart Failure	
Stage A:	Patients at high risk for HF due to the presence of conditions strongly associated with the development of HF. Asymptomatic.
Stage B:	Patients with structural disease, such as previous MI, but have never shown signs or symptoms of HF.
Stage C:	Patients with structural heart disease who have current or prior symptoms of HF.
Stage D:	Patients with advanced structural heart disease and marked symptoms at rest in spite of optimal medical therapy and who require specialized interventions.
New York Heart Association Functional Classification	
Class	
I	Patients with cardiac disease but without resulting limitations of physical activity. Ordinary physical activity does not cause undue fatigue, palpitation, dyspnea, or anginal pain.
II	Patients with cardiac disease resulting in slight limitation of physical activity. They are comfortable at rest. Ordinary physical activity results in fatigue, palpitation, dyspnea, or anginal pain.
III	Patients with cardiac disease resulting in marked limitation of physical activity. They are comfortable at rest. Less than ordinary physical activity causes fatigue, palpitation, dyspnea, or anginal pain.
IV	Patient with cardiac disease resulting in inability to carry on any physical activity without discomfort. Symptoms of cardiac insufficiency or of the anginal syndrome may be present even at rest. If any physical activity is undertaken, discomfort is increased.

TABLE 9-9. CLINICAL SIGNS AND SYMPTOMS SPECIFIC TO RIGHT- AND LEFT-SIDED HEART FAILURE

Right Heart Failure	Left Heart Failure
Signs and Symptoms of Hepatic Congestion	**Signs and Symptoms of Pulmonary Congestion**
JVD	Pulmonary edema
Liver enlargement and tenderness	Rales
Positive hepatojugular reflex (pressure on liver increases JVD)	Atrial fibrillation or other atrial arrhythmias secondary to atrial distension
Dependent edema	Pulsus alternans (every other beat diminished)
Ascites	Dyspnea
Decreased appetite, nausea, vomiting	Cough
Cardiac Pressures	Hyperventilation
Increased RV pressure	Dizziness, syncope, fatigue
Increased RA pressure	**Cardiac Pressures**
Heart Sounds	Increased LV and LA pressure
S$_3$ (early sign)	Increased pulmonary artery pressures
S$_4$ (may also present)	**Heart Sounds**
Wide split S$_2$	S$_3$ and (occasionally) S$_4$
Pansystolic murmur at lower left sternal border secondary to stretching of tricuspid ring	Pansystolic murmur at apex secondary to mitral regurgitation

- *Brain natriuretic peptide:* Elevated
- *Echocardiography:* Dilated left ventricle, right ventricle, or right atria; hypertrophied left ventricle; AV valve incompetence; diffuse or segmental hypocontractility; atrial thrombus; pericardial effusion; LVEF < 40%
- *Radionuclide ventriculography:* More precise measure of right ventricular dysfunction and LVEF

Principles of Management for Heart Failure

Acute management of HF has changed dramatically over the past decade, from an emphasis on the micromanagement of hemodynamic parameters, primarily using positive inotropes, to an emphasis on functional capacity and long-term survival with the use of neurohormonal blocking agents. This shift is due to a better understanding of the neurohormonal response and the dependence of the body on these mechanisms for compensation in low-output states. Goals of patient management in HF revolve around four general principles: (1) treatment of the underlying cause (eg, ischemia, valvular dysfunction), (2) management of fluid volume overload, (3) improvement of ventricular function, and (4) patient and family education.

Limiting the Initial Insult and Treating the Underlying Cause

The most effective, but often the most difficult, management strategy for HF is to limit the damage done by the initial insult. This limitation of myocardial damage and cell loss maximizes the amount of viable ventricular muscle, myocardial contractility, and overall ventricular function.

- Administer fibrinolytic therapy as soon as possible for eligible patients in the setting of AMI or facilitate immediate transfer to the cardiac catheterization laboratory for primary PCI (see the previous section on acute ischemic heart disease).
- Revascularization may be warranted in patients with persistent ischemia as a preventive measure against eventual tissue necrosis.
- Valve replacement or repair or other surgical corrections (ventricular reconstruction surgery) should be undertaken as soon as possible to prevent prolonged overstretching of the ventricular myocardium.

Management of Fluid Volume Overload

Decrease preload by the use of diuretic therapy, limitation of dietary sodium, and restriction of free water.

- Diuretics should be initiated according to the severity of the patient's signs and symptoms. More severe symptoms require intravenous therapy and loop diuretics, and less severe symptoms may be managed adequately on loop diuretics. Thiazide diuretics may be added later if the patient does not respond to the loop diuretics. Caution must be taken not to diurese the patient too fast as rapid loss of fluid can lead to activation of the renin-angiotensin system.

- Sodium and fluid restriction should be monitored carefully, with sodium intake not exceeding 2 g/day and free water not exceeding 1500 mL in a 24-hour period. Obtain nutrition consult to reinforce sodium and water restrictions.
- Serum sodium and potassium should be monitored on a regular basis to prevent inadvertent electrolyte imbalances (each day or two in the acute setting, depending on the aggressiveness of therapy).

Improvement of Left Ventricular Function

Improvement in left ventricular function is accomplished by decreasing the workload on the heart with preload and after-load reduction and by augmenting ventricular contractility. Ventricular function may be measured directly in the acute setting by monitoring CI using a noninvasive cardiac output monitor. As has been demonstrated by a number of large clinical trials, traditional micromanagement of hemodynamic variables, such as CI with inotropic drugs, may be detrimental to long-term patient outcome. Current recommendations do not advocate this as an initial management strategy.

- Decrease preload (see above).
- Decrease afterload by administration of pharmacologic therapy, including ACE inhibitors and vasodilators. ACE inhibitors are recommended in all HF patients with a LVEF < 40% unless otherwise contraindicated or not tolerated. Contraindications to ACE inhibitor therapy include previous intolerance, potassium > 5.5 mEq/L, hypotension with systolic blood pressure less than 90 mm Hg, and serum creatinine greater than 3.0 mg/dL. Cautious initiation of low-dose therapy in patients with contraindications may still be considered. If the patient is ACE inhibitor intolerant (eg, experiences a cough), an ARB may be administered. Vasodilators may also be used in conjunction with diuretics and ACE inhibitors if further afterload reduction is necessary. Nitrates are often used concomitantly with ACE inhibitors and diuretics to augment afterload reduction, especially in the case of underlying atherosclerotic disease, still the largest single contributor to HF. Angiotensin receptor blockers may be used if the patient does not tolerate the side effects of an ACE inhibitor (eg, cough).
- ACE inhibitors and beta-blockers are considered cornerstone therapy for HF in an effort to reverse the remodeling of the left ventricle. Aldosterone antagonists may be used as add on therapy. Lastly isosorbide, dinitrate, and hydralazine are used for special populations. Digoxin has been shown to improve symptoms but is no longer considered to be first-line therapy unless paroxysmal atrial fibrillation or atrial flutter is present. Digoxin may be used to control the ventricular rate in this situation.

- Beta-blockers are also used to reduce the incidence of ventricular tachycardia and ventricular fibrillation, the most common cause of death in HF patients. Recommended beta-blockers for the management of HF include carvedilol, metoprolol, and bisoprolol. Caution should be taken when initiating a beta-blocker in a patient with reactive airway disease.

- BNP (nesiritide [Natrecor®]) has been another recent addition to the management of decompensated HF. Nesiritide's effects include promoting diuresis and vasodilation, thereby decreasing ventricular preload and afterload. The agent may also inhibit angiotensin II as well as some of the other neuroendocrine compensatory mechanisms associated with HF. Nesiritide is recommended for acutely decompensated ventricular failure.

- *Dual-chamber biventricular pacemaker/implantable cardioverter defibrillator (ICD):* Approximately 60% of patients with dilated cardiomyopathy develop LBBB. In the presence of LBBB, the right and left ventricles no longer contract simultaneously but in a series causing the intraventricular septum to shift inappropriately, interfering with the aortic and mitral valve functioning. There have been several studies demonstrating significantly improved outcomes (quality of life, survival rates, etc) with the use of a dual chamber biventricular pacemaker. This technology stimulates both ventricles simultaneously, causing both to contract at the same time resulting in a narrowing of the QRS complex and improved myocardial contractility and cardiac output. Often the pacing technology is combined with an ICD because sudden cardiac death related to ventricular tachycardia/fibrillation is the most common cause of death in these patients.

- Cardiac assist devices (left ventricular, right ventricular, or both) can provide temporary maintenance or preservation of ventricular function, especially as a bridge to recovery, bridge to cardiac transplantation, or as destination therapy (discharge to home). These devices may be inserted percutaneously via the femoral artery or femoral vein or surgically using the medial sternotomy or thoracotomy approach (see Chapter 19, Advanced Cardiovascular Concepts). Left ventricular apical cannulation allows ambulation and physical rehabilitation. Technological developments have contributed to the development of small axial flow pumps allowing many to be implanted with the drive line (power source) exiting the skin. Risks related to insertion of these devices include infection, peripheral embolization including stroke, and, for some, long-term weaning difficulties in the event that an organ donor is not available. Presently, the Heart Mate II* is approved for destination therapy (a replacement for heart transplant).

1. *Intra-aortic balloon pump (IABP):* Femoral artery cannulation with the IABP allows for ventricular support, but restricts the patient to bed rest and compromises arterial flow to the cannulated limb. These patients will be in the intensive care unit (ICU).

2. *Minimally invasive catheter-based micro-axial flow ventricular assist devices:* These are frequently used to reduce ventricular afterload and myocardial work. They may be inserted through the femoral artery across the aortic valve into the left ventricle or introduced via the femoral vein into the right atrium and through an atrial septostomy, and positioned in the left atrium. As with the IABP, the patient is restricted to bedrest.

3. *Ventricular reconstruction:* Many patients with end-stage HF have a previous history of CAD and MI resulting in the development of a ventricular aneurysm on the anterior wall of the left ventricle. A surgical procedure can be performed removing the aneurysm, reducing the size of the ventricle resulting in increased contractility and cardiac output. Studies have shown that some patients experience improvement in physical functioning and NYHA Functional Class following this procedure.

4. *Extracoporeal membrane oxygenation (ECMO):* In recent years the use of ECMO has become more common for severely decompensated HF patients who are in cardiogenic shock. This is used as a bridge to recovery, a link to a ventricular assist device (VAD), or a bridge to transplant. The use of this technology is limited to the ICU.

Patient Education

Patients who present with HF to the progressive care unit have high acuity levels, require more pharmacological interventions, and have an increased need for emotional support surrounding the serious nature of the hospital admission. Previous admissions for HF make patients more aware of the serious nature of acute episodes. Patient education, which is appropriately addressed in the acute-care setting, includes the following:

1. Both patient and family may require crisis interventions. The nurse may help by encouraging the verbalization of fears related to role adaptations or changes in family responsibility, lifestyle alterations and limitations, and death and dying. The completion of advanced directives and living wills should be initiated if not previously addressed.

2. Family involvement in the acute-care phase should be strongly encouraged, including assistance with activities of daily living such as bathing, and "patterning" of daily activities to allow for frequent periods of rest and spacing of exertional activity. In addition, family involvement in reading or other leisure activity with the patient is often restful and relaxing, and may be useful as a diversional activity. If possible, the family

should also be present for reinforcement of patient teaching regarding the medical regimen, the importance of fluid and sodium restriction, and the need for daily weights.

Shock

Shock is the inability of the circulatory system to deliver enough blood to meet the oxygen and metabolic requirements of body tissues. This clinical syndrome may result from ineffective pumping of the heart (cardiogenic shock), insufficient volume of circulating blood (hypovolemic shock), or massive vasodilation of the vascular bed causing maldistribution of blood (distributive shock). Although the specific definition of shock and strategies for patient management vary according to the underlying pathophysiology, the principle of ineffective or insufficient oxygen delivery to meet the needs of body tissues remains consistent.

Etiology, Risk Factors, and Pathophysiology

The ineffective delivery of oxygen to the tissues leads to cellular dysfunction, rapidly progressing to organ failure and finally to total body system failure. The cause of the initial onset of the shock syndrome may be from any number of underlying problems, including heart problems, fluid loss, and trauma. Because the body responds in the same way, differences between cardiogenic, hypovolemic, and distributive shock are obvious to the clinician only after the initial assessment has provided key information about the patient's acute illness. Given the history, the clinician can classify shock into one of three major pathologic groups and proceed to further determine the patient's needs with the help of diagnostic testing. Because interventions for patient management are directed at the cause, it is essential for the underlying pathophysiology to be clearly understood.

Cardiogenic Shock

In cardiogenic shock, the heart is unable to pump enough blood to meet the oxygen and metabolic needs of the body. Pump failure is caused by a variety of factors, the most common being CAD. A number of other factors may cause pump failure, however, and are typically categorized as coronary or noncoronary causes (Table 9-11).

TABLE 9-11. CAUSES OF CARDIOGENIC SHOCK

Coronary Causes
- MI with resultant cell death in a significant portion of the ventricle
- Rupture of ventricle or papillary muscle secondary to MI
- Dysfunctional ischemic—"shock ventricle"—which occurs as a result of myocardial ischemia, not involving cell death, and is therefore transient

Noncoronary Causes
- Myocardial contusion
- Pericardial tamponade
- Ventricular rupture
- Arrhythmia (PEA—pulseless electrical activity—new name)
- Valvular dysfunction resulting in ventricular congestion
- Cardiomyopathies
- End-stage HF

ESSENTIAL CONTENT CASE

Shock Following AMI

A 49-year-old man was found slumped in his living room chair, cool and clammy but still breathing. His wife phoned emergency medical services, which arranged air transportation to the local emergency room. On arrival, his vital signs were as follows:

BP	68/44 mm Hg
HR	122 beats/min
RR	33 breaths/min
T	36.1°C, orally
Sao_2	91%

Oxygen at 60% by face mask had been initiated in flight, as well as intravenous normal saline running wide open, 450 mL having already infused. Dopamine was started at a rate of 5 mcg/kg/min. A stat ECG showed "tombstone" ST elevation in anterior leads (V_2, V_3, V_4), with reciprocal changes in leads II, III, and aVF. The patient was taken for immediate PTCA. In the laboratory, cardiac catheterization findings were as follows:

LAD	99% proximal lesion
RCA	70% mid lesion
LCx	Normal
LVEF	13%
Wall motion	Left ventricular akinesis

On return to the progressive care unit, the nurse obtained hemodynamic parameters as follows:

PA	45/25 mm Hg
RA	15 mm Hg
PAOP	22 mm Hg
CO	4.0 L/min
CI	1.5 L/min/m^2

Case Question 1. Given the patient's history, ECG changes, and hemodynamic profile, you know the type of shock this patient is experiencing is:

(A) Hypovolemic
(B) Distributive
(C) Cardiogenic
(D) Neurogenic

Case Question 2. Following the interventional procedure the primary goal for this patient is to:

(A) Reduce myocardial workload
(B) Dilate the pulmonary vascular bed
(C) Administer a diuretic
(D) Intubate the patient to improve oxygen delivery

Case Question 3. You anticipate the next intervention for this patient will be:

(A) Initiate a vasodilator to reduce afterload
(B) Give volume to improve preload
(C) Titrate the dopamine infusion up to 7.5 mcg/kg/min
(D) Insertion of an intra-aortic balloon

Answers: 1: C; 2: A; 3: D

In all cardiogenic shock cases, the heart ceases to function effectively as a pump, resulting in decreases in stroke volume and cardiac output. This leads to a decrease in blood pressure and tissue perfusion. The inadequate emptying of the ventricle increases left atrial pressure, which then increases pulmonary venous pressure. As a result, pulmonary capillary pressure increases, resulting in pulmonary edema.

Hypovolemic Shock

Hypovolemic shock occurs when there is inadequate volume in the vascular space. This volume depletion may be caused by blood loss, either internal or external, or by the vascular fluid volume shifting out of the vascular space into other body fluid spaces (Table 9-12). The loss of vascular volume results in insufficient circulating blood to maintain tissue perfusion.

The pathophysiology of hypovolemic shock is related directly to a decreased circulating blood volume. When an insufficient amount of blood is circulating, the venous blood returning to the heart is insufficient. As a result, right and left ventricular filling pressures are insufficient, decreasing stroke volume and cardiac output. As in cardiogenic shock, when cardiac output is decreased, BP is low and tissue perfusion is poor.

Distributive Shock

Distributive shock is characterized by an abnormal placement or distribution of vascular volume, occurring in three situations: (1) sepsis, (2) neurologic damage, and (3) anaphylaxis. In each of these situations, the pumping function of the heart and the total blood volume are normal, but the blood is not appropriately distributed throughout the vascular bed. Massive vasodilation occurs in each of these situations for various reasons, causing the vascular bed to be much larger than normal. In this enlarged vascular bed, the usual volume of circulating blood (approximately 5 L) is no longer sufficient to fill the vascular space, causing a decrease in blood pressure and inadequate tissue perfusion. For this reason distributive shock is also referred to as relative hypovolemic shock.

Of the distributive shock syndromes, septic shock is most commonly seen in the critical care setting. In the field or emergency department setting, anaphylaxis and neurogenic shock are also common and typically result from allergic reactions and trauma-related spinal cord injury.

Stages of Shock

Regardless of underlying etiology, all three types of shock (cardiogenic, hypovolemic, distributive) activate the sympathetic nervous system, which in turn initiates neural, hormonal, and chemical compensatory mechanisms in an attempt to improve tissue perfusion (Figure 9-16). Cellular changes that occur as a result of these compensatory mechanisms are similar in all types of shock. Progression of these cellular changes follows a predictable, four-stage course.

Initial Stage

The initial stage of shock represents the first cellular changes resulting from the decrease in oxygen delivery to the tissue. These changes include decreased aerobic and increased anaerobic metabolism, leading to increases in serum lactic acid. No obvious clinical signs and symptoms are apparent during this stage of shock.

Compensatory Stage

The compensatory stage is composed of a number of physiologic events that represent an attempt to compensate for decreases in cardiac output and restore adequate oxygen and nutrient delivery to the tissues (Figure 9-17). These events can be organized into neural, hormonal, and chemical responses. Neural responses involve the baroreceptors in the aortic arch and carotid arteries, detecting changes in the arterial BP, and responding by activating the vasomotor center of the medulla. Hypovolemia and resultant hypotension lead to activation of the sympathetic nervous system. The sympathetic nervous system initiates neural, hormonal, and chemical compensatory mechanisms causing peripheral vasoconstriction and elevation of the BP. The sympathetic nervous system activation produces vasoconstriction of the peripheral circulation, shunting blood to vital organs (autoregulation). Vasoconstriction of the peripheral circulation shunts blood to the vital organs, reducing renal blood flow, which activates the hormonal response.

Hormonal responses include increased production of catecholamines and adrenocorticotropic hormone (ACTH) and activation of the renin-angiotensin-aldosterone system. As a direct result of decreased renal blood flow, renin is released from the juxtaglomerular cells in the kidney, combining with angiotensinogen from the liver resulting in the production of angiotensin I. Angiotensin I, circulating in the blood, is converted to angiotensin II in the lungs. As was discussed in more detail in the HF section, this hormonal response results in direct peripheral vasoconstriction, as well as release of aldosterone from the adrenal cortex and antidiuretic hormone (ADH) from the pituitary gland. Sodium and potassium retention, in conjunction with increased ADH, ACTH, and circulating catecholamines, effectively

TABLE 9-12. CAUSES OF HYPOVOLEMIC SHOCK

Sources of External Loss of Body Fluid
- Hemorrhage (loss of whole blood)
- Gastrointestinal tract (vomiting, diarrhea, ostomies, fistulas, nasogastric suctioning)
- Renal (diuretic administration, diabetes insipidus, Addison disease, hyperglycemic osmotic diuresis)

Sources of Internal Loss of Body Fluid
- Internal hemorrhage
- Movement of body fluid into interstitial spaces ("third spacing," often the result of bacterial toxin, thermal injury, or allergic reaction)

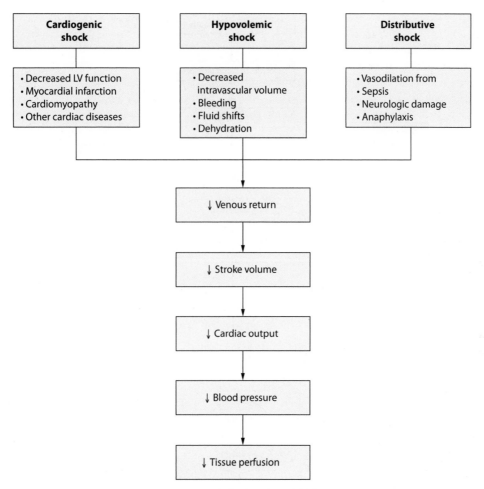

Figure 9-16. Pathophysiology of shock.

increases intravascular volume, heart rate, and blood pressure, and decreases urine output.

Chemical responses during the compensatory stage are related to the respiratory ventilation-perfusion imbalance, which occurs as a result of sympathetic stimulation, redistribution of blood flow, and decreased pulmonary perfusion. A respiratory alkalosis ensues, adversely affecting the patient's level of consciousness, and causing restlessness, and agitation.

These compensatory mechanisms are effective for finite periods of time, which may vary depending on the individual and presence of comorbidities. The younger and healthier the patients prior to the shock episode, the more likely they are to survive a prolonged episode of shock. In the absence of vascular volume replacement, these intrinsic vasopressors eventually fail as a compensatory mechanism, and the patient enters the progressive, and finally refractory, stages of shock, usually resulting in death.

Progressive Stage
The progressive stage is characterized by end-organ failure due to cellular damage from prolonged compensatory changes. The compensatory changes, which were effective in supporting blood pressure and therefore tissue perfusion, are no longer effective and severe hypoperfusion ensues. Impaired oxygen delivery to the tissues results in multiple organ system dysfunction (MODS)—typically beginning with gastrointestinal and renal failure—followed by respiratory and/or cardiac failure and loss of liver and cerebral function. See Chapter 11 for more on sepsis and MODS.

Refractory Stage
The refractory stage, as its name implies, is the irreversible stage of shock. At this stage, cell death has progressed to such a point as to be irreparable, and death is imminent.

Clinical Presentation
Clinical signs and symptoms vary depending on the underlying cause of shock and the stage of shock in which the patient presents.

- *Initial stage:* No visible signs and symptoms evident from ongoing cellular changes
- *Compensatory stage*
  - Consciousness: Restless, agitated, confused
  - Blood pressure: Normal or slightly low

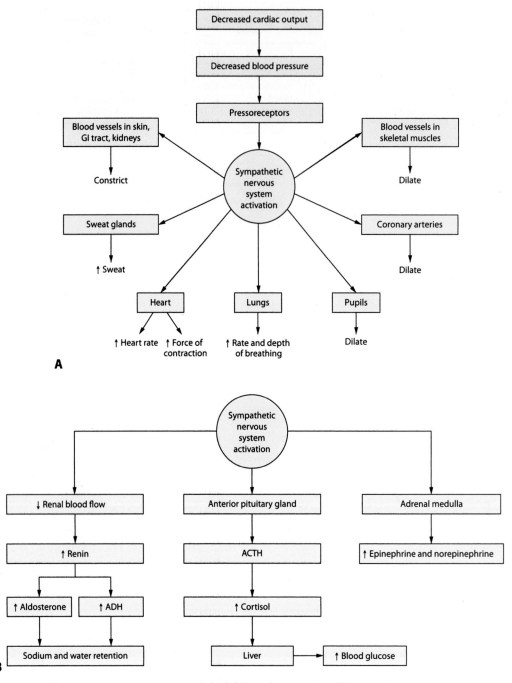

Figure 9-17. Compensatory response to shock. **(A)** Neural compensation. **(B)** Hormonal compensation.

- Heart rate: Increased
- Respiratory rate: Increased (> 20 breaths/min)
- Skin: Cool, clammy, may be cyanotic
- Peripheral pulses: Weak and thready
- Urine output: Concentrated and scant (< 30 mL/h)
- Bowel sounds: Hypoactive, possible abdominal distension
- Laboratory results
  - Glucose: Increased
  - Sodium: Increased

- Pao_2: Decreased
- $Paco_2$: Decreased
- pH: Increased
- *Progressive stage*
  - Consciousness: Unresponsive to verbal stimuli
  - Blood pressure: Inadequate (< 90 mm Hg systolic)
  - Heart rate: Increased > 90/min
  - Respiratory rate: Increased, shallow
  - Skin: Cold, cyanotic, mottled
  - Peripheral pulses: Weak and thready, may be absent

- Urine output: Scant (< 20 mL/h) and concentrated
- Bowel sounds: Absent
- Laboratory results
  - Amylase: Increased
  - Lipase: Increased
  - SGPT/SGOT: Increased
  - Lactate: Increased
  - CPK: Increased
  - Creatinine: Increased
  - Blood urea nitrogen: Increased
  - Pao_2: Decreased
  - $Paco_2$: Increased
  - pH: Decreased
  - HCO_3: Decreased

Diagnostic Tests

- ECG: Tachycardia
- Pulmonary arterial pressure: PAD/PAOP high (> 12 mm Hg), RAP high (> 8 mm Hg)
- Echocardiogram: Ventricular wall motion abnormalities, cardiac tamponade, ventricular rupture
- *Hypovolemic*
  - Pulmonary arterial pressure: PAD/PAOP low (< 8 mm Hg), RAP low (< 5 mm Hg), RVEDVI low
  - Ultrasound: Groin or retroperitoneal hemorrhage
- *Distributive*
  - Septic: WBC ≥ 12,000 or ≤ 4,000 > 10% neutrophils, serum lactate > 4 mmol/L, positive blood cultures (in 50% of patients).
  - Anaphylactic: Arterial blood gas shows inadequate oxygenation.
  - Neurogenic: Computed tomography (CT) scan and magnetic resonance imaging (MRI) shows spinal cord damage.

Principles of Management for Shock

Differences in the underlying cause of shock lead to some variation in the principles of management. The basic goals of therapy for all forms of shock, however, include the need to correct the underlying cause of shock, improvement of oxygenation, and restoration of adequate tissue perfusion. Generally a patient in shock will be transferred to the critical care unit for management of their shock state.

Correction of the Underlying Cause of Shock

- *Cardiogenic:* Remove coronary obstruction or correct tamponade, if present, and support ventricular contractility to increase cardiac output.
- *Hypovolemic:* Identify source and stop bleeding if possible; correct fluid shunting or third spacing with electrolyte management.
- *Distributive*
- Anaphylactic: Intubate for oxygenation and treat the underlying allergic reaction using antidote or steroid therapy.

- Septic: Implement 3 hour "bundle" including obtaining blood cultures and serum lactate; administer broad spectrum antibiotics and 30 mL/kg crystalloid for hypotension; implement early goal-directed therapy protocol, removal of infected tissue or device, refer to *AACN Practice Alert: Severe Sepsis* for evidence-based practices for the management of severe sepsis and septic shock. (See Chapter 11 for more on sepsis.)
- Neurogenic: Severing of the cord may be irreversible; however, intubation provides respiratory support while the underlying cause is identified.

Improve Oxygenation

- Assess for patent airway and intubate if necessary.
- Administer oxygen at 100% or as necessary until Pao_2 is adequate (> 60 to 70 mm Hg).

Restore Adequate Tissue Perfusion

- Administer fluid volume expanders (normal saline, lactated Ringer solution, or plasmanate) in large rapid boluses. Type and cross-match for blood type and administer blood as necessary for hypovolemic shock.
- Initiate vasoactive drug therapy.

Hypertension

Hypertension is typically a chronic disease of BP elevation that is often masked, especially in the early years of onset, by lack of warning signs or symptoms. Hypertensive crisis is an acute episode or exacerbation, occurring infrequently in a small percentage of hypertensive patients and characterized by the pivotal effect the particular episode and its treatment may have on the patient's long-term outcome. In most cases, the numerical or absolute value of the arterial BP is less important than its impact on the individual's underlying risk of target organ damage, specifically cerebrovascular, coronary, and renal diseases.

Etiology, Risk Factors, and Pathophysiology

Although a number of clinical syndromes commonly are associated with hypertension and many underlying etiologies may contribute to the progression of hypertensive disease, the pathophysiology of hypertension is similar regardless of the underlying cause.

An acute hypertensive crisis begins with elevation of the systolic or diastolic BP causing a threat, direct or indirect, to an organ or body system. Acute, severe increases in pressure may cause serious, life-threatening cerebrovascular and cardiovascular compromise. Prolonged hypoperfusion of an organ system leads to ischemia, necrosis, and organ system failure.

Classification

Because of the increased risk of such events in all hypertensive patients, morbidity and mortality directly related to hypertension is high, and long-term, consistent therapy in

TABLE 9-13. CLASSIFICATION OF BLOOD PRESSURE FOR ADULTS

Blood Pressure Classification	SBP (mm Hg)	DBP (mm Hg)
Normal	< 120	And < 80
Prehypertension	120-139	or 80-89
Stage 1 hypertension	140-159	or 90-99
Stage 2 hypertension	≥160	or ≥100

SBP, systolic blood pressure; DBP, diastolic blood pressure; mm Hg, millimeters of mercury.

all stages of hypertension is necessary. Hypertension can be described in stages as described below or classified according to the value of the blood pressure. Refer Table 9-13 for the classification of blood pressure for adults.

- *Stage 1 hypertension:* Benign hypertension is characterized by slightly elevated blood pressure (140-160 mm Hg systolic/90 mm Hg diastolic, in adults) for long periods of time, with little if any end-organ damage. Stage 1 hypertension does not tend to cause acute problems or complications, unless other comorbid conditions, such as atherosclerotic disease, are present. The pressure does not typically exacerbate or precipitate an acute emergent event (generally not > 140-160 mm Hg systolic/90 mm Hg diastolic, in adults).
- *Accelerated hypertension:* Often used interchangeably with malignant hypertension, the stage known as accelerated hypertension is generally considered a precursor to malignant hypertension, and is characterized by an increase in the patient's baseline BP.
- *Malignant hypertension:* Hypertension typically is a chronic disease in which elevation in BP occurs slowly, over a period of several years. Because of its gradual onset, the body adapts to increased pressures in the vascular bed and the patient frequently is asymptomatic for years, eventually able to tolerate pressures of up to 200/120 mm Hg without experiencing significant symptoms or clinical events. This type of presentation often is identified "accidentally," secondary to hospitalization for another problem. Generally patients with malignant hypertension are at risk for significant end-organ damage because of the severity of high pressure in the vascular bed and inability of the circulatory system to further adapt or compensate in the event of additional stressors.
- *Hypertensive crisis:* Hypertensive crisis is characterized by a severe elevation in BP, relative to the individual's baseline BP, which causes risk of end-organ damage and poor long-term outcome due to permanent organ system damage if the immediate episode is not treated quickly and aggressively.
- Special populations: In pregnant women and in children a less severe elevation in blood pressure may result in significant end-organ damage and is therefore considered to be a "hypertensive crisis" at values much lower than would be expected to be problematic in the average adult. The absolute value of the

blood pressure varies significantly depending on the situation and the individual involved; for example, pre-eclampsia, considered to be a hypertensive crisis in pregnancy, may occur at pressures as low as 130/100 to 160/100 mm Hg.

Clinical Presentation

Diagnosis of hypertensive crisis is not based on the absolute value of the blood pressure, but rather on the following combined criteria:

- Rapidity of the rise of the BP
- Duration of prior hypertension
- Clinical determination of the immediate threat to vital organ function
- Headache
- Blurred vision
- Nosebleed
- Dizziness or vertigo
- Transient ischemic attack
- Diminished peripheral pulses or bruits
- Carotid or abdominal bruit
- Heart sounds with S_3 and/or S_4
- Systolic and/or diastolic murmurs
- Gastrointestinal bleeding
- Pulmonary edema
- Shortness of breath
- Fatigue
- Malaise
- Weakness
- Nausea and vomiting
- Hematuria
- Dysuria
- *Funduscopic findings:* Arteriovenous thickening, arteriolar narrowing, hemorrhage, papilledema, or exudates

Diagnostic Tests

- *Chest x-ray:* Myocardial hypertrophy, pulmonary infiltrates
- *Computed tomography:* Arteriolar narrowing and arteriovenous thickening
- Specific tests to target organ damage
- Renal angiography
- Coronary angiography
- Carotid/cerebral angiography
- *Magnetic resonance imaging:* Cerebral vascular malperfusion

Principles of Management for Hypertension

Management of the patient with acute exacerbation of hypertension, or hypertensive crisis, revolves around three primary objectives: reduction of arterial pressure, evaluation and treatment of target organ damage, and preparation and planning for continuous and consistent outpatient follow-up.

Reduction of Arterial Pressure

Ascertain correct arterial blood pressure. Verify arterial blood pressure, being sure to assess bilateral measurements with the correct cuff size if using sphygmomanometry, as well as orthostatic pressures if possible (lying and sitting up, if standing is not possible). Each measurement should be 2 minutes apart and both right and left measurements should be documented. If differences between the right and left measurements are greater than 10 mm Hg, the higher reading should be used to gauge therapy. In most acute situations, priority should be given to establishing a stable arterial access site for direct, invasive monitoring of BP.

Initiate pharmacologic intervention. For acute high arterial pressure, intravenous pharmacologic intervention is the fastest, most effective means of reducing arterial blood pressure. A number of agents are used in the acute setting for management of hypertensive crisis (Table 9-14). Aggressiveness of pharmacologic intervention should be based on the severity of blood pressure elevation (immediate risk of stroke), the immediate risk of irreversible target organ damage (renal and hepatic function related to drug metabolism and clearance also should be considered), and any confounding conditions or risk factors which are present (for example, the fetus in pre-eclampsia). In general, acute, severe (accelerated malignant/stages 3 and 4) hypertension should be treated as quickly and aggressively as can be tolerated by the patient in order to prevent the immediate risk of hypertensive encephalopathy, dissecting aortic aneurysm, MI, or intracranial hemorrhage. Maintenance of cerebral perfusion pressure is imperative during treatment, and overly aggressive pharmacologic management poses the threat of cerebrovascular compromise due to a sudden drop in arterial pressure and inability of the autoregulatory mechanism to adjust. Other organ systems dependent on higher pressure for perfusion include the renal and coronary systems. A sudden, severe drop in systemic arterial pressure may result in ischemic episodes or acute renal failure.

For non-acute hypertension, dietary alteration and relaxation, or biofeedback techniques may be used in addition to pharmacologic measures to reduce the morbidity and mortality of hypertension. Although these measures are most effective when employed long term as part of a cohesive outpatient follow-up program, initiating these strategies in the acute setting may help emphasize their importance.

Evaluation and Treatment of Target Organ Disease

Concomitant to initiation of pharmacologic intervention, the assessment and prevention of target organ disease is important to avoid irreversible damage. Target organs typically at risk include the brain, heart, kidneys, and eyes. Strategies to prevent damage to these organ systems during hypertensive crisis include the following:

- *Brain:* Reduce diastolic pressure by one-third (not to go < 95 mm Hg) using aggressive pharmacologic measures (see Table 9-14).
- *Heart:* Reduce diastolic and systolic pressure by one-third; administer combination therapy if possible (vasodilator and beta-blocker) or ACE inhibitor for afterload reduction; monitor for ischemic changes on ECG.
- *Kidneys:* Reduce systolic and diastolic BP using pharmacologic measures; monitor serum creatinine and urine specific gravity as well as proteinuria and hematuria; for patients with severe existing renal impairment, use of ACE inhibitors may exacerbate their renal compromise and is therefore contraindicated in patients with bilateral renal artery stenosis; administer diuretics to maintain serum sodium and adequate diuresis.
- *Eyes:* Reduce systolic and diastolic BP; observe retina for evidence of hemorrhage, exudate, or papilledema; instruct the patient with blurring of vision regarding his or her environment, especially location of the call bell.

Patient Education on Lifestyle Modification and Follow-Up

Following control of hypertension in the acute phase, patient education should be initiated regarding the serious and chronic nature of the disease. Often, the clinician may have an opportunity in the acute stage to make an impact regarding

TABLE 9-14. COMMON DRUGS USED TO MANAGE ACUTE HYPERTENSIVE EPISODES

Enalapril	• An ACE inhibitor. • Administer IV at a rate of 5 mg/min.
Esmolol	• Beta1 selective blocker and at higher doses inhibits $\beta2$ receptors in the blood vessels • Useful for treating hypertension • Administer 0.5 mg/Kg over 1 min loading dose followed by 50 mcg/Kg/min infusion • Titrate to achieve desired lower BP • Onset of action within minutes • Peak effect in less than 5 minutes
Labetalol	• Beta-receptor agonist (beta-blocker) • Particularly indicated in patients with suspected MI or angina. • Administer 5 mg bolus over 5 minutes and repeat 3 times. IV drip may then be started.
Nicardipine	• Calcium channel blocker • Administer 5 mg/h initially, titrate 2.5 mcg/h at 5- to 15-minute intervals to a maximum dose of 15 mg/h.
Nitroglycerin	• Dilates veins more than arterioles. • Administer IV at a rate of 5 to 100 mcg/min. Mix 100 mg in 100 mL NS or D_5 IV.
Nitroprusside	• Dilates arterioles and veins. • Administer IV at 0.5 to 10.0 mcg/kg/min (mix in normal saline only; 100 mg in 500 mL). Cover bottle with foil to avoid light exposure. • Titrate up to desired blood pressure, recognizing that the effect will be evident within 1 minute of change in dose.

ESSENTIAL CONTENT CASE

Thinking Critically

You are taking care of a patient, 4 days post anterior MI, who is just transferred to the progressive care unit from a medicine floor with severe shortness of breath. Your initial assessment reveals the following:

HR	128 beats/min
BP	110/82 mm Hg
RR	36 breaths/min
T	37.6 °C, orally
Pulse oximetry	88%
Lung sounds	Coarse, bilateral crackles in lower lobes, poor respiratory effort
Heart sounds	S_1, S_2, S_3
Skin	Flushed, diaphoretic, 2+-pedal edema
ECG	Sinus tachycardia, with tall R-waves in V5-V6 indicating left ventricular hypertrophy

Case Question 1. What is your initial intervention?

(A) Obtain an arterial blood gas measurement
(B) Initiate a nesiritide infusion
(C) Prepare to intubate the patient
(D) Call a Code Blue

Case Question 2. What is the most likely underlying cause for this patient's respiratory compromise?

(A) Acute decompensated HF with pulmonary edema
(B) Abrupt onset of septic shock with ARDS
(C) Acute anxiety attack
(D) Hypovolemic shock

Case Question 3. Management of this condition would most likely include what interventions?

1. Administration of a diuretic to reduce preload
2. Initiation of a dobutamine infusion at 5 mcg/kg/min
3. Consideration for mechanical support
4. Consideration for intubation and ventilator support

(A) 4
(B) 1 and 2
(C) 3 and 4
(D) All of the above

Answers: 1: C; 2: B; 3: D

the seriousness of uncontrolled hypertension and its potentially debilitating effects. Prior to beginning the educational process, assessment should include:

1. Family history of hypertension, cardiovascular disease, coronary artery disease, stroke, diabetes mellitus, and hyperlipidemia
2. Lifestyle history including weight gain, exercise, and smoking habits
3. Dietary patterns including high sodium, alcohol, and dietary fat intake or low potassium intake
4. Knowledge of hypertension and impact of previous medical therapy for hypertension (compliance, side effects, results, or efficacy)

SELECTED BIBLIOGRAPHY

General Cardiovascular

Bonow RO, Mann DL, Zipes DP, Libby P, eds. *Braunwald's Heart Disease: A Textbook of Cardiovascular Medicine.* 9th ed. Philadelphia, PA: WB Saunders; 2012.

Moser DK, Riegel B. *Cardiac Nursing: A Companion to Braunwald's Heart Disease.* Canada: Saunders; 2008.

Woods SL, Froelicher ESS, Motzer SA, Bridges EJ. *Cardiac Nursing.* 6th ed. Philadelphia, PA: Lippincott, Williams & Wilkins; 2010.

Coronary Revascularization

Hardin S, Kaplow R. *Cardiac Surgery Essentials for Critical Care Nursing.* Dudbury, MA: Jones & Bartlett Publishing; in press; 2010.

South T. Coronary artery bypass surgery. *Crit Care Nurs Clin NA.* 2011;23(4):573-586.

Todd BA. *Cardiothoracic Surgical Nursing Secrets.* St Louis, MO: Mosby-Year Book, Inc; 2005.

Acute Ischemic Heart Disease

Cahoon W, Flattery MP. ACC/AHA non-ST elevation myocardial infarction guidelines revision: 2007: implications for nursing practice. *Prog Cardiovasc Nurs.* 2008;23(1):53-56.

Naples RM, Harris JW, Ghaemmaghami CA. Critical care aspects in the management of patients with acute coronary syndromes. *Emerg Med Clin N Am.* 2008;26:685-702.

Thygesen K, Alpert JS, Jaffe AS, et al. Third universal definition of myocardial infarction. *Circulation.* 2012;126:2020-2035.

Heart Failure

Albert NM. Fluid management strategies in heart failure. *Crit Care Nurs.* 2012;32(2):20-33.

Albert NM. Heart failure with preserved systolic function: giving well-deserved attention to the "other" heart failure. *Crit Care Nurs Q.* 2007;30(4):287-296.

Daleiden-Burns A, ed. Heart failure. *Crit Care Nurs Q.* 2007;30(4):285-286.

English MA. Advanced concepts in heart failure. *Crit Care Nurs Q.* 1995;18(1):56-64.

Fara-Erny A. Heart failure: challenges and outcomes. *J Cardiovasc Nurs.* 2000;14(4):v-vii.

Litton KA. Demystifying ventricular assist devices. *Crit Care Nurs Q.* 2011;34(2):200-207.

Shock

Bridges EJ, Dukes S. Cardiovascular aspects of septic shock. *Crit Care Nurs.* 2005;25(2):14-42.

Cheng JM, den Ull CA, Hoeks SE, et al. Percutaneous left ventricular assist devices vs intra-aortic balloon pump counterpulsation for treatment of cardiogenic shock: a meta-analysis on controlled trials. *Eur Heart J.* 2009;30(17):2101-2108.

Kelley DM. Hypovolemic shock: an overview. *Crit Care Nurs Q.* 2005;28(1):2-19.

McAtee ME. Cardiogenic shock. *Crit Care Nurs Clin of NA.* 2011;23(4):607-616.

Reynolds HR, Hochman JS. Cardiogenic shock: current concepts and improving outcomes. *Circulation.* 2008;117(5):686-697.

Rivers E, Nguyen B, Havstad S, et al. Early goal-directed therapy in the treatment of severe sepsis and septic shock. *N Eng J Med.* 2001;345(19):1368-1377.

Topalian S, Ginsberg F, Parillo JE. Cardiogenic shock. *Crit Care Med.* 2008;36(suppl 1):S66-S74.

Hypertension

Schulenburg M. Management of hypertensive emergencies: implications for the critical care nurse. *Crit Care Nurs Q.* 2007;30(2):80-93.

Smithburger PL, Kane-Gill SL, Seybert AL. Recent advances in the treatment of hypertensive emergencies. *Crit Care Nurs.* 2010;30(5).

Whelton PK, Appel LJ, Sacco RL, et al. Sodium, blood pressure, and cardiovascular disease: further evidence supporting the American Heart Association sodium reduction recommendations. *Circulation.* 2012;126:2880-2889.

Evidence-Based Practice Guidelines

Adams D, Bridges CR, Casey DE, et al. 2012 ACCF/AHA focused update of the guideline for the management of patients with unstable angina/non-ST-elevation myocardial infarcton: a report of the American College of Cardiology Foundation/American Heart Association Task Force on Practice Guidelines. *Circulation.* 2012;126:875-910.

American Association of Critical-Care Nurses. *AACN Practice Alert: Noninvasive Blood Pressure Monitoring.* Aliso Viejo, CA: American Association of Critical-Care Nurses; 2010, June.

American Association of Critical-Care Nurses. *AACN Practice Alert: Severe Sepsis.* Aliso Viejo, CA: American Association of Critical-Care Nurses; 2006, April.

American Association of Critical-Care Nurses. *AACN Practice Alert: ST-Segment Monitoring.* Aliso Viejo, CA: American Association of Critical-Care Nurses; 2008, April.

Dellinger RP, Carlet JM, Masur H, Gerlach H. The surviving sepsis guidelines for the management of severe sepsis and septic shock: background, recommendations, and discussion from an evidence-based review. *Crit Care Med.* 2004;32(suppl 11).

Dellinger RP, Levy MM, Rhodes A, et al. Surviving sepsis campaign: international guidelines for management of severe sepsis and septic shock: 2012. *Crit Care Med.* 2013;41(2):580-637.

Drew BJ, Calif RM, Funk M, et al. Practice standards for electrocardiographic monitoring in hospital settings. *Circulation.* 2004;110:2721-2746.

Hillis LD, Smith PK, Anderson JL, et al. 2011 ACCF/AHA guideline for coronary artery bypass surgery: a report of the American College of Cardiology Foundation/American Heart Association Task Force on Practice Guidelines. *Circulation.* 2011;124:e652-e735.

Levine GN, Bates ER, Blankenship JC, et al. 20100 ACCF/AHA/SCAI Guidelines for percutaneous coronary intervention: a report of the American College of Cardiology Foundation/American Heart Association Task Force on Practice Guidelines and the Society for Cardiovascular Angiography and Interventions. *Circulation.* 2011;124:e574-e651.

Lindenfeld J, Albert NM, Boehmer JP, et al. Executive summary: HSFA 2010 comprehensive heart failure practice guideline. *J Card Fail.* 2010;16(6):475-539.

Masoudi FA, Bonow RO, Brindis RG, et al. ACC/AHA 2008 statement on performance measurement and reperfusion therapy: a report of the ACC/AHA Task Force on Performance Measures. *Circulation.* 2008;118:2649-2661.

National Institute of Health. The seventh report of the Joint National Committee on Prevention, Detection, Evaluation and Treatment of High Blood Pressure. U.S. Department of Health and Human Services. [NIH Publication No. 04-5230]. Bethesda, MD: NIH: August 2004.

O'Gara PT, Kushner FG, Ascheim DD, et al. 2013 ACCF/AHA Guideline for the management of ST-elevation myocardial infarction: a report of the American College of Cardiology Foundation/American Heart Association Task Force on Practice Guidelines. *Circulation.* 2013;127:529-555.

Peura JL, Colvin-Adams M, Francis GS, et al. Recommendations for the use of mechanical circulatory support: device strategies and patient selection: a scientific statement from the American Heart Association. *Circulation.* 2012;126:2648-2667.

RESPIRATORY SYSTEM

10

Maureen A. Seckel

KNOWLEDGE COMPETENCIES

1. Identify various radiologic and pulmonary anatomic features relevant to interpretation of chest x-rays.

2. Describe different systems and principles of management for chest tubes.

3. Describe the etiology, pathophysiology, clinical presentation, patient needs, and principles of management of acute respiratory failure (ARF).

4. Compare and contrast the pathophysiology, clinical presentation, patient needs, and

management approaches for common diseases leading to ARF:
- Acute respiratory distress syndrome (ARDS)
- ARF in the chronic obstructive pulmonary disease patient (asthma, emphysema, bronchitis)
- COPD exacerbation
- Acute asthma
- Pulmonary hypertension
- Pneumonia
- Interstitial lung disease
- Pulmonary embolism (PE)
- Venous thromboembolism (VTE)

SPECIAL ASSESSMENT TECHNIQUES, DIAGNOSTIC TESTS, AND MONITORING SYSTEMS

Chest X-Rays

Chest radiography is an important tool in respiratory assessment, providing visualization of the heart and lungs. Chest x-rays are a complement to bedside assessment. Progressive care nurses need to know basic radiographic concepts and how to optimize portable chest x-ray technique, as well as how to systematically view a chest x-ray image.

Chest x-rays are obtained as part of routine screening procedures, when respiratory disease or an acute change is suspected, to evaluate the status of respiratory abnormalities (eg, pneumothorax, pleural effusion, tumors), to confirm proper invasive tube placement (ie, endotracheal, tracheostomy, or chest tubes, and central line catheters), or following traumatic chest injury.

Basic Concepts

An x-ray is a form of radiant energy, and a radiographic image is made by x-ray machines. Only a few rays are absorbed by air as beams pass through the atmosphere, whereas all rays are absorbed by metal as the beams attempt to pass through a sheet of metal. When nothing but air lies between the film cassette and the x-ray source, the radiographic image is blackness or radiolucency. If density increases, more beams are absorbed between the film cassette or detector and the x-ray source, and the radiographic image is whiteness or radiopacity. Many institutions are replacing traditional x-ray film with detectors that convert the x-ray energy to a digital radiograph. These can then be stored and distributed in a digital format. As the x-ray beam passes through the patient, the denser tissues absorb more of the beam, and the less dense tissues absorb less of the beam.

The lungs are primarily sacs of air or gas, so normal lungs look black on chest films. Conversely, the skeletal thorax appears white, because bone is very dense and absorbs the most x-rays (Table 10-1). The heart and mediastinum appear gray because those structures are made up of mostly water. Breast tissue is made up of mostly fat and it appears whitish-gray.

TABLE 10-1. BASIC X-RAY DENSITIES

Radiolucent (black)
Gas, air (dark or black)
• Lungs, trachea, bronchi, alveoli
Water (dark or gray)
• Heart, muscle, blood, blood vessels, diaphragm, spleen, liver
Fat (lighter or whitish-gray)
• Breasts, marrow, hilar streaking
Radiopaque (white)
Metal, bone (lightest or white)
• Ribs, scapulae, vertebrae
• Bullets, coins, teeth, ECG electrodes

Basic Views of the Chest

The most common method of obtaining a chest x-ray is the posterior-anterior (PA) view. PA chest x-rays are typically done in the radiology department with the machine about 6 ft away from the x-ray film cassette and the patient standing with the anterior chest wall against the x-ray plate and the posterior chest wall toward the x-ray machine. The patient is told to take a deep breath and hold it as the x-ray beam is delivered through the posterior chest wall to the x-ray film cassette. The PA view results in a very accurate, sharp picture of the chest.

Acutely ill patients are rarely able to tolerate the positioning requirements of a PA chest x-ray. Many chest x-rays in progressive care are obtained with an anterior-posterior (AP) view with the patient supine in bed, with or without back rest elevation. With portable AP chest films, the film cassette is placed behind the patient and the x-ray beam is delivered through the anterior chest to the x-ray film. The x-ray machine is only 3 ft away from the patient, which results in greater distortion of chest images, making the AP chest x-ray less accurate than the PA method. Of particular concern is that the heart size is enlarged on an AP film. When viewing chest x-rays, it is important to know whether a PA or an AP view was used to avoid misinterpretation of heart size as cardiomegaly.

Distortions can be minimized by placing the patient in a high Fowler position, or as erect as possible, with the thorax symmetrically placed on the x-ray film cassette. Explain the procedure to the patient and the need to avoid movement. All unnecessary objects lying on the anterior chest (such as ventilator tubing, safety pins, jewelry, ECG wires, nasogastric tubes, etc) are removed or repositioned as possible. If the patient is unconscious, taping the forehead in a neutral position may be necessary, especially in the high Fowler position to avoid mispositioning of the head. All caregivers assisting with the chest x-ray need to protect themselves from radiation exposure by positioning themselves behind the x-ray machine or by using lead aprons covering the neck, chest, and abdomen.

Other chest x-ray views include: (1) lateral views to identify normal and abnormal structures behind the heart, along the spine, and at the base of the lung; (2) oblique views to localize lesions without interference from the bony thorax or to get a better picture of the trachea, carina, heart, and great vessels; (3) lordotic views to better visualize the apical and middle regions of the lungs and to differentiate anterior from posterior lesions; and (4) lateral decubitus (cross-table) views, done with the patient supine or side-lying, to assess for air-fluid levels or free-flowing pleural fluid.

Systematic Approach to Chest X-Ray Interpretation

A systematic approach should be used when analyzing a chest x-ray image including reviewing the results. It is important to first make sure that the report and image have been properly labeled (correct name and medical record number), and to identify the right and left sides before viewing the images. If previous images are available, place them next to the new images for comparison. View the chest x-ray from the lateral borders, moving to the medial aspects of the thorax and asking the series of questions found in Table 10-2. Begin the chest x-ray analysis by comparing the right side to the left side using the following sequence (Figures 10-1 and 10-2): (1) soft tissues—neck, shoulders, breasts, and subcutaneous fat; (2) trachea—the column of radiolucency readily visible above the clavicles; (3) bony thorax—note size, shape, and symmetry; (4) intercostal spaces (ICS)—note width and angle; (5) diaphragm—dome-shaped with distinct margins, right dome 1 to 3 cm higher than left dome; (6) pleural surfaces—visceral and parietal pleura appear like a thin, hairlike line along the apices and lateral chest; (7) mediastinum—size varies with age, gender, and size; (8) hila—large pulmonary arteries and veins; (9) lung fields—largest area of the chest and most radiolucent; and (10) catheters, tubes, wires, and line.

Normal Variants and Common Abnormalities

When the soft tissues are examined, the two sides of the lateral chest should be symmetric. A mastectomy makes one lung look more radiolucent than the other due to the

TABLE 10-2. STEPS FOR INTERPRETATION OF A CHEST X-RAY FILM

Step 1
Look at the different densities (black, gray, and white), and answer the question, "What is air, fluid, tissue, and bone?"
Step 2
Look at the shape or form of each density, and answer the question, "What normal anatomic structure is this?"
Step 3
Look at both right and left sides, and answer the question, "Are the findings the same on both sides or are there differences (both physiologic and pathophysiologic)?"
Step 4
Look at all the structures (bones, mediastinum, diaphragm, pleural space, and lung tissue), and answer the question, "Are there any abnormalities present?"
Step 5
Look for all tubes, wires, and lines, and answer the question, "Are the tubes, wires, and lines in the proper place?"

Reprinted from: Urden L, Stacy KM, Lough M. Thelan's Critical Care Nursing: Diagnosis and Management. 5th ed. St Louis, MO: Mosby; 2006:612, with permission from Elsevier.

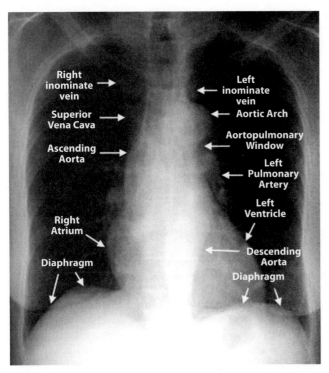

Figure 10-1. Normal chest x-ray with anatomical references. Courtesy of University of Virginia Health Sciences Center, Department of Radiology (From Spencer B. Gay, MD, Juan Olazagasti, MD, Jack W. Higginbotham, MD, et al. Introduction to Chest Radiology. University of Virginia Health Sciences Center–http://www.med-ed.virginia.edu/courses/rad/cxr/anatomy4chest.html)

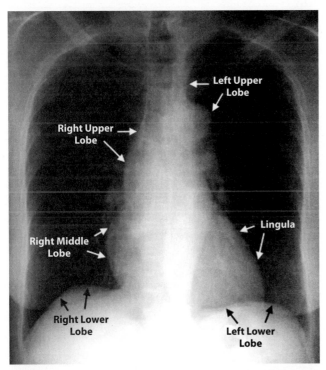

Figure 10-2. Normal chest x-ray with anatomical references. Courtesy of University of Virginia Health Sciences Center, Department of Radiology (From Spencer B. Gay, MD, Juan Olazagasti, MD, Jack W. Higginbotham, MD, et al. Introduction to Chest Radiology. University of Virginia Health Sciences Center–http://www.med-ed.virginia.edu/courses/rad/cxr/anatomy4chest.html)

absence of fatty tissue. The trachea should be midline, with the carina visible at the level of the aortic knob or second ICS. The most common cause of tracheal deviation is a pneumothorax, which causes a tracheal and mediastinal shift to the area away from the pneumothorax (Table 10-3, Figures 10-3 and 10-4).

Bony thorax inspection reveals general body build. Clavicles should be symmetric and may have an irregular notch or indentation in the inferior medial aspect of the clavicle called a rhomboid fossa, a normal variant. Deformities of the thorax can be detected, such as scoliosis, pectus excavatum (also called funnel chest), or pectus carinatum (also known as pigeon chest). Decreases in the density (less white) of the spine, ribs, and other bones may indicate loss of calcium from the bones due to osteoporosis or long-term steroid dependency. Careful examination of the ICSs and rib angles may indicate pathology. Patients with chronic obstructive pulmonary disease (COPD) have widened ICS and the angle of the ribs to the spine increases to 90° instead of the normal 45° angle because of severe hyperinflation (see Figure 10-3). Conversely, narrowed ICS may be visible in cystic fibrosis patients with severe interstitial fibrosis. Rib fractures, if present, are commonly visible along the lateral borders of the rib cage.

Elevation of the diaphragm can be a result of abdominal distention, phrenic nerve paralysis, or lung collapse. Depression or flattening of the diaphragm can occur when 11 or 12 ribs show on a chest x-ray as a result of COPD or severe hyperinflation due to asthma. Normal costophrenic angles can be seen where the tapered edges of the diaphragm and the chest wall meet. Because breast tissue can obscure the angles in women, these angles are more distinct in men. Obliteration or "blunting" of the costophrenic angle may occur with pleural effusion or atelectasis.

Identification of a pleural space on a chest x-ray is an abnormal finding (see Figure 10-4). The pleural space is not visible unless air (pneumothorax) or fluid (pleural effusion) enters it. These findings commonly are seen in the *progressive care unit* population.

Two terms often heard regarding the mediastinum are shifting and widening. Mediastinal structures, usually the trachea, bronchi, and heart, can shift with atelectasis, with the shift directed toward the alveolar collapse. Pneumothorax shifts the mediastinum away from the area of involvement. A widening of the mediastinum can indicate several pathologic conditions, such as cardiomegaly, aneurysms, or aortic disruption. Bleeding into the mediastinum, following chest trauma or cardiac surgery, also may cause widening of the mediastinum.

Heart size can be estimated easily by measuring the cardiothoracic ratio on a PA film. It is measured with a PA chest x-ray and is measured by comparing the ratio of the maximal horizontal cardiac diameter to the maximal horizontal thoracic diameter. A normal measurement is less than 50%. Greater percentages are indicative of cardiac enlargement.

TABLE 10-3. CHEST X-RAY FINDINGS

Assessed Area	Usual Adult Findings	Remarks
Trachea	Midline, translucent, tubelike structure found in the anterior mediastinal cavity	Deviation from the midline suggests tension, pneumothorax, atelectasis, pleural effusion, mass, or collapsed lung
Clavicles	Present in upper thorax and are equally distant from sternum	Malalignment or break indicates fracture
Ribs	Thoracic cavity encasement	Widening of intercostal spaces indicates emphysema; malalignment or break indicates fractured sternum or ribs
Mediastinum	Shadowy-appearing space between the lungs that widens at the hilum	Deviation to either side may indicate pleural effusion, fibrosis, or collapsed lung
Heart	Solid-appearing structure with clear edges visible in the left anterior mediastinal cavity; heart should be less than one-half the width of the chest wall on a PA film	Shift may indicate atelectasis or tension pneumothorax; if heart is greater than one-half the chest wall width, heart failure or pericardial fluid may be present
Carina	The lowest tracheal cartilage at which the bronchi bifurcate	If the end of the endotracheal tube is seen 3 cm above the carina, it is in the correct position
Main-stem bronchus	The translucent, tubelike structure visible to approximately 2.5 cm from hilum	Densities may indicate bronchogenic cyst
Hilum	Small, white, bilateral densities present where the bronchi join the lungs; left hilum should be 2 to 3 cm higher than the right hilum	A shift to either side indicates atelectasis; accentuated shadows may indicate emphysema or pulmonary abscess
Bronchi (other than main stem)	Not usually visible	If visible, may indicate bronchial pneumonia
Lung fields	Usually not completely visible except as fine white areas from hilum; fields should be clear as normal lung tissue is radiolucent; normal "lung markings" should be present to the periphery	If visible, may indicate atelectasis; patchy densities may be signs of resolving pneumonia, silicosis, or fibrosis; nasogastric tubes, pulmonary artery catheters, and chest tubes will appear as shadows and their positions should be noted
Diaphragm	Rounded structures visible at the bottom of the lung fields; right side is 1 to 2 cm higher than the left; the costophrenic angles should be clear and sharp	An elevated diaphragm may indicate pneumonia, pleurisy, acute bronchitis, or atelectasis; a unilateral flattened diaphragm suggests COPD; elevation indicates a pneumothorax or pulmonary infection; the presence of scarring or fluid causes blunting of costophrenic angles; 300 to 500 mL of pleural fluid must be present before blunting is seen

Reprinted from: Talbot I, Meyers-Marquardt M. Pocket Guide to Critical Assessment. *St Louis, MO: CV Mosby; 1990, with permission from Elsevier.*

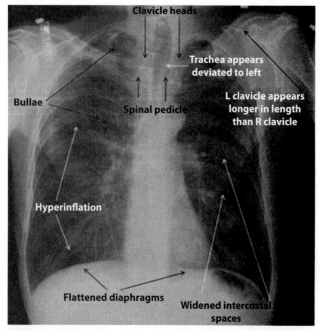

Figure 10-3. COPD, flattened diaphragms, hyperinflation, widened intercostals spaces, apical bullae, and chest rotation. (*Reprinted from: Siela D. Chest radiograph evaluation and interpretation.* AACN Adv Crit Care. *2008;19:444-473.*)

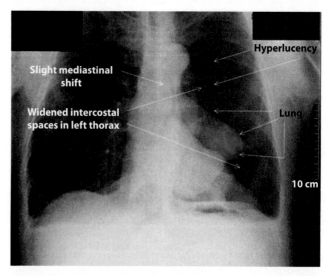

Figure 10-4. Left pneumothorax, hyperlucency, and widened intercostals spaces. (*Reprinted from: Siela D. Chest radiograph evaluation and interpretation.* AACN Adv Crit Care. *2008;19:444-473.*)

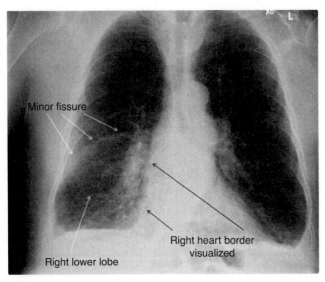

Figure 10-5. Right lower lobe pneumonia with minor fissure visualized. (*Reprinted from: Siela D. Chest radiograph evaluation and interpretation. AACN Adv Crit Care. 2008;19:444-473.*)

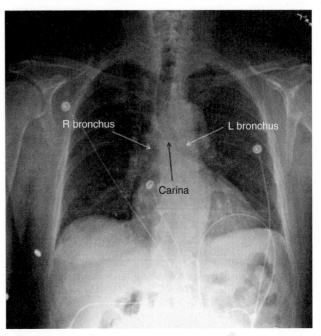

Figure 10-6. Carina and right bronchus. (*Reprinted from: Siela D. Chest radiograph evaluation and interpretation. AACN Adv Crit Care. 2008;19:444-473.*)

This method for determining normal heart size is not accurate using AP chest x-rays, the most common type taken of the acutely ill.

The lung fields should be assessed for any areas of increased density (whiteness) or increased radiolucency (blackness), which can indicate an abnormality. Density increases when water, pus, or blood accumulates in the lungs, as in pneumonia (Figure 10-5). Increased radiolucency is caused by increased air in the lungs, as may occur with COPD. A fine line present on the right side of the lung at the sixth rib level (midlung) is a normal finding, representing the horizontal fissure separating the right upper and middle lobes.

Invasive Lines

Chest x-rays are frequently obtained in progressive care to confirm proper emergent and nonemergent placement of invasive equipment (endotracheal tubes, central venous catheters including peripherally inserted central catheter [PICC] nasogastric or orogastric tubes, and chest tubes). All invasive tubes have radiopaque lines running the length of the tube that are visible on the x-ray (Figures 10-6 and 10-7).

All lines should be identified and followed through their paths. The nasogastric or orogastric tube should run the length of the esophagus with the tip of the tube beyond the gastroesophageal junction in the stomach. The stomach can be identified by the radiolucency just under the diaphragm on the left side, which is called the gastric air bubble. Small bore nasoenteric tubes may be positioned with the tip in the stomach or small bowel depending on whether gastric or small bowel feedings are intended. Central line catheters should be viewed with the tip in the superior vena cava.

All items in the chest should be identified, such as temporary or permanent pacing wires, pacing generators,

automatic implantable defibrillators, airway stents, tracheostomy tubes, chest tubes, and surgical wires, drains, or clips (see Figure 10-7).

Helpful Hints

Chest x-rays should be taken after every attempt to insert central venous catheters to detect the presence of an accidental pneumothorax. A common error is to mistake the area above the clavicles as a pneumothorax, especially on AP views.

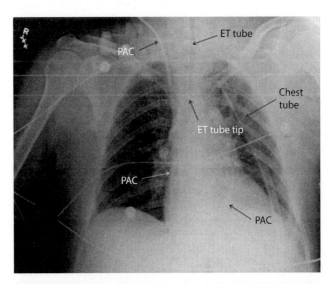

Figure 10-7. Pulmonary artery catheter, endotracheal tube, and left chest tube. (*Reprinted from: Siela D. Chest radiograph evaluation and interpretation. AACN Adv Crit Care. 2008;19:444-473.*)

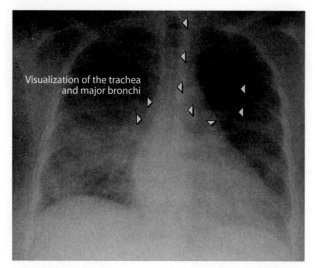

Visualization of the trachea
and major bronchi

Figure 10-8. Air Bronchogram. (*Courtesy of: Yale School of Medicine–http://www.yale.edu/imaging/findings/air_bronchogram/index.html. Accessed September 1, 2013.*)

Two common abnormal x-ray signs frequently discussed are the silhouette sign and the air bronchogram. For any structure to be visible, the density of its edge must contrast with the surrounding density. The loss of contrast is called the *silhouette sign*. It means that two structures of the same density have come in contact with each other and the borders are lost; for example, the heart is a water density, so if the alveoli near the left heart border fill with fluid, the two densities are the same and there is a loss of contrast and no left heart border. An air bronchogram is air showing through a greater density, such as water (Figure 10-8). The bronchi are not seen on a normal chest x-ray, except for the main-stem bronchi, because they have thin walls, contain air, and are surrounded by air in the alveoli (two structures of the same density). If water surrounds the bronchi, as in pneumonia and pulmonary edema, then the bronchi filled with air are in contrast to the water density and are visible.

Computed Tomography and Magnetic Resonance Imaging

Computed tomography (CT) and magnetic resonance imaging (MRI) allow for the three-dimensional examination of the chest in situations where two-dimensional chest x-rays are insufficient. CT and MRI are particularly advantageous over chest x-rays to evaluate mediastinal and pleural abnormalities, particularly those with fluid collections. Pleural effusions or empyemas, malpositioned or occluded chest tubes, mediastinal hematomas, and mediastinitis are problems for which CT and MRI are more sensitive than chest x-rays.

The need for transportation to the radiology department and positioning restrictions within the scanning devices pose certain risks to acutely ill patients. Of particular concern is the automatic movement of patients during the procedure into and out of the scanning device. Accidental disconnection of invasive devices can easily occur if additional tubing lengths and potential obstructions are not considered.

Decreased visualization of patients during the procedures requires vigilant monitoring of cardiovascular and respiratory parameters and devices, as well as establishing a method for conscious patients to alert nearby clinicians in case of difficulties. The strong magnetic field of MRI units may interfere with ventilator performance and a non-magnetic ventilator is required.

Magnetic resonance imaging testing can be a frightening experience for the patient. Anxiety-related reactions, occurring in up to almost one-third of patients, range from mild apprehension to severe anxiety. These reactions can result in cancellation of the test or interference with its results. It is suggested that all patients receive basic information regarding the MRI procedure, including details of the small chamber they will be placed in, the noise and temperature they will experience, and the duration of the procedure. If possible, use of some form of relaxation or music tapes, ear plugs or headsets, and the presence of a family member or friend should be considered. In addition, short-acting anxiolytics should be used for patients who need them.

Pulmonary Angiograms/CTPA and V/Q Scans

Pulmonary angiograms are one of the most sensitive tools for diagnosis of pulmonary emboli. A catheter is advanced into the pulmonary artery and contrast material is injected during rapid filming. Emboli appear as filling defects, or dark circumscribed areas, within the white vascular images of the artery.

The invasive nature of this diagnostic test, coupled with potential reactions to the contrast material, restricts its use. As a result the use of computed tomography of the pulmonary arteries (CTPA) is quickly replacing pulmonary angiograms as the gold standard for detecting PE.

Computed tomography of the pulmonary arteries is a less invasive but very specific method of diagnosing a PE. The CTPA only requires a peripheral line through which to inject the contrast material. Similar to the pulmonary angiogram, defects may be readily seen in the pulmonary artery and the study can be done very quickly. This technology is not available in all institutions; however, it is quickly emerging as the diagnostic choice and gold standard for PE detection.

Some still use ventilation-perfusion (V/Q) scans to diagnose a PE although they are also being outdated by the CTPA. A V/Q scan is a nuclear medicine diagnostic tool that requires that medical isotopes are inhaled or injected in order to view the lungs and pulmonary arteries respectively. Generally the perfusion (or blood circulation) part of the test is done first. If there is no defect detected, the scan is read as "low probability." If the scan detects a defect, then the inhaled (ventilation) portion of the test is done. If no matching defect is seen in the lung, the test is interpreted as "high probability." But if a "matched defect" is noted (ie, there is a defect in the lung scan that corresponds with that of the perfusion scan), then the interpretation is "indeterminate" or "matched defect." This may be the result of an atelectasis, pneumonia, or other infiltrate where circulation to that inactive area of

TABLE 10-4. INDICATIONS FOR CHEST TUBE INSERTION

Pneumothorax
- Open: Both chest wall and pleural spaces are penetrated.
- Closed: Pleural space is penetrated with an intact chest wall, allowing air to enter the pleural space from the lungs.
- Tension: Air leaks into the pleural space through a tear in the lungs, with no means to escape the space, leading to lung collapse.

Hemothorax
Hemopneumothorax
Thoracostomy
Pyothorax or empyema
Chylothorax
Cholothorax
Hydrothorax
Pleural effusion
Special application
- Instillation of anesthetic or sclerosing agent

Adapted from: Lusardi PA, Scott SS, Scott F. Chest Tube Placement (Perform). In Wiegand DI, ed. AACN Procedure Manual for Critical Care. 6th ed. Philadelphia, PA: Saunders 2011.

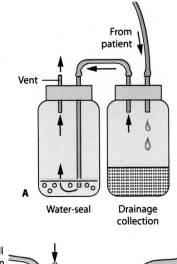
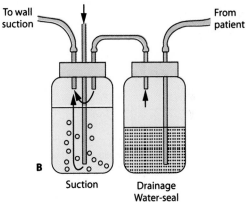

Figure 10-9. Two-bottle chest drainage system. **(A)** Drainage collection bottle and a water-seal bottle. **(B)** Water-seal/drainage collection bottle and suction control bottle. (*Reprinted from: Luce JM, Tyler ML, Peirson DJ. Intensive Respiratory Care. Philadelphia, PA: WB Saunders; 1984:164, with permission from Elsevier.*)

the lung is redistributed to other active areas thus resulting in a "matched defect." In addition to the cumbersome nature of the V/Q scan, the progressive care patient may require both tests (perfusion and ventilation) rather than just one, and the diagnostic yield is often poor.

Chest Tubes

Chest tubes are commonly used in acutely ill patients to drain air, blood, or fluid from the pleural spaces (pleural chest tubes) or from the mediastinum (mediastinal tubes). Indications for chest tube insertion are varied (Table 10-4), with no contraindications to chest tube insertion because the need to restore lung function supersedes any potential complications associated with insertion. Pleural tube insertion sites vary based on the type of drainage to be removed (air: second ICS, midclavicular line; fluid: fifth or sixth ICS, midaxillary line). Mediastinal tubes are placed during surgery, exiting from the mediastinum below the xiphoid process. Type of chest tube insertions include tube thoracostomy (traditional rigid tubes) or smaller percutaneously inserted catheters (pigtails).

Following insertion, chest tubes are connected to a closed drainage collection system which uses gravity or suction to restore negative pressure in the pleural space and facilitate drainage of fluids or air (Figure 10-9). A Heimlich flutter valve is an alternative to the closed drainage system and consists of a one-way valve that allows air or drainage to collect in a vented drain bag (Figure 10-10). The PleurX® catheter also has a one-way valve and connects as needed to a drainage system (Figure 10-11). Patients may be discharged home with either a Heimlich flutter valve or PleurX catheter for long-term use. Connections to the drainage system must be airtight and secure for proper functioning and to prevent inadvertent entry of air into the pleural space (Figure 10-12). Patency of the system is ensured by avoiding kinking of the drainage tubing, periodic inspection of the tubing for visible

clot formation, and gentle squeezing of the tubing between the thumb and index finger.

Removal of the chest tube occurs when restoration of lung expansion and fluid or air removal has been accomplished and the underlying lung abnormality has been resolved or corrected. An occlusive dressing at the chest tube removal site is typically used to prevent introduction of air into the pleural space until the skin has formed a protective seal. Analgesic administration is appropriate prior to removal; discomfort associated with removal is often as much or even greater than during insertion.

Thoracic Surgery and Procedures

Thoracic surgery and procedures are terms inclusive of a number of procedures involving the thoracic cavity and the lungs. See Table 10-5 for definitions and indications.

Principles of Management for Thoracic Surgery and Procedures

Management of the patient after lung surgery or post procedure is similar to the patient with trauma to the chest. Refer to the section on thoracic trauma in Chapter 17, Trauma, with the following additions:

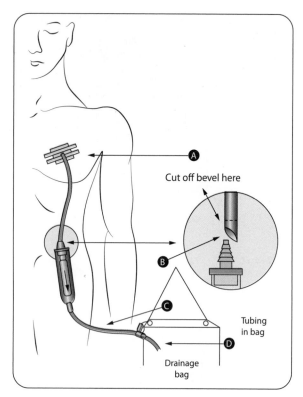

Cut off bevel here

Tubing in bag

Drainage bag

Figure 10-10. Heimlich chest drain valve with connection to drain bag. (*From: BD Medical Systems, Franklin Lakes, NJ.*)

Pain Control

The thoracotomy incision is one of the most painful surgical incisions and pain control is an important factor in recovery and prevention of respiratory complications. The routine use of epidural catheters, intercostal blocks, intrapleural local anesthetic administration, or PCA narcotics has improved pain management significantly. Relaxation therapy, deep breathing exercises, and guided imagery may also be effective in helping to reduce pain and anxiety.

Positioning

- It was once thought that optimal patient ventilation and perfusion matching would be improved and should be prioritized with "good lung" positioned in the dependent position. While blood flow is improved to the dependent lung, patients require frequent repositioning side to side to prevent atelectasis and other complications.
- Early ambulation and sitting at the bedside or in a chair improves diaphragmatic excursion, enhancing ventilation and maximum inflation.
- Deep breathing and use of incentive spirometry is encouraged regularly. These activities both help promote lung reexpansion of collapsed lung tissue and prevent atelectasis.

Maintenance of Chest Tube System

See section "Chest Tubes" explained earlier.

PATHOLOGIC CONDITIONS

Acute Respiratory Failure

Each of the case studies below represents a common situation in a progressive care unit—respiratory dysfunction. This rapid onset of respiratory impairment, which is severe enough to cause potential or actual morbidity or mortality if untreated, is termed acute respiratory failure (ARF). Although, the origin of the respiratory failure may be a medical or surgical problem, the management approaches share similar features.

Acute respiratory failure is a change in respiratory gas exchange (CO_2 and O_2) such that normal cellular function is jeopardized. ARF is defined as a Pao_2 less than 60 mm Hg and $Paco_2$ greater than 50 mm Hg with a pH less than or equal to 7.30. Actual Pao_2 and $Paco_2$ values that define ARF vary, depending on a variety of factors that influence the patient's normal (or baseline) arterial blood gas values. Factors such as age, altitude, chronic cardiopulmonary disease, or metabolic disturbances may alter the normal blood gas values for an individual, requiring an adjustment to the classic definition of ARF; for example, if $Paco_2$ levels in a 75-year-old man with COPD are normally 56 mm Hg, ARF would not be diagnosed until pH is less than or equal to 7.30.

Etiology, Risk Factors, and Pathophysiology

Many abnormalities can lead to ARF (Table 10-6). Regardless of the specific underlying cause, the pathophysiology of ARF can be organized into four main components: impaired ventilation, impaired gas exchange, airway obstruction, and ventilation-perfusion abnormalities.

Impaired Ventilation

Conditions that disrupt the muscles of respiration or their neurologic control can impair ventilation and lead to ARF (see Table 10-6). Decreased or absent respiratory muscle movement may be due to fatigue from excessive use, atrophy from disuse, inflammation of nerves, nerve damage (eg, surgical damage to the vagus nerve during cardiac surgery), neurologic depression, or progressive disease states such as Guillian Barre or amyotrophic lateral sclerosis (ALS). Impaired respiratory muscle movement decreases movement of gas into the lungs, resulting in alveolar hypoventilation. Inadequate alveolar ventilation causes retention of CO_2 and hypoxemia.

Impaired Gas Exchange

Conditions that damage the alveolar-capillary membrane impair gas exchange. Direct damage to the cells lining the alveoli may be caused by inhalation of toxic substances (gases or gastric contents), pneumonia and/or other pulmonary conditions leading to two detrimental alveolar changes. The first is an increase in alveolar permeability, increasing the potential for interstitial fluid to leak into the alveoli and causing noncardiac pulmonary edema (Figure 10-13A). The second alveolar change is a decrease in surfactant production

Procedure Pack

Vacuum Bottle with Drainage Line

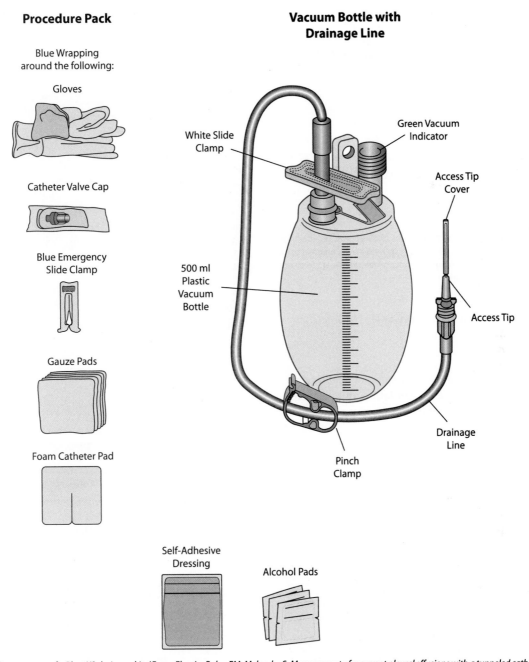

Blue Wrapping around the following:

Gloves

Catheter Valve Cap

Blue Emergency Slide Clamp

Gauze Pads

Foam Catheter Pad

Self-Adhesive Dressing

Alcohol Pads

White Slide Clamp

500 ml Plastic Vacuum Bottle

Pinch Clamp

Green Vacuum Indicator

Access Tip Cover

Access Tip

Drainage Line

Figure 10-11. Components of a PleurX® drainage kit. (*From: Elsevier Baker EM, Melander S. Management of recurrent pleural effusions with a tunneled catheter. Heart Lung. 2010;39:314-318.*)

by alveolar type II cells, increasing alveolar surface tension, which leads to alveolar collapse (Figure 10-13B).

Another cause of impaired gas exchange occurs when fluid leaks from the intravascular space into the pulmonary interstitial space (Figure 10-13C). The excess fluid increases the distance between the alveolus and the capillary, decreasing the efficiency of the gas exchange process. Interstitial edema also compresses the bronchial airways, which are surrounded by interstitial tissue, causing bronchoconstriction. Capillary leakage may occur when pressures within the cardiovascular system are excessively high (eg, in heart failure) or when pathologic conditions elsewhere in the body

release biochemical substances (eg, serotonin, endotoxin) that increase capillary permeability.

Airway Obstruction

Conditions that obstruct airways increase resistance to airflow into the lungs, causing alveolar hypoventilation and decreased gas exchange (Figure 10-14). Airway obstructions can result from conditions that: (1) block the inner airway lumen (eg, excessive secretions or fluid in the airways, inhaled foreign bodies), (2) increase airway wall thickness (eg, edema or fibrosis) or decrease airway circumference (eg, bronchoconstriction) as occurs in asthma, or (3) increase

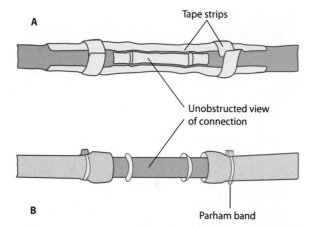

Figure 10-12. Methods for securing connections of chest tube and drainage system. **(A)** Tape. **(B)** Parham bands. (*Reprinted from: Kersten LD. Comprehensive Respiratory Nursing: A Decision-Making Approach. Philadelphia, PA: WB Saunders; 1989:783, with permission from Elsevier.*)

peribronchial compression of the airway (eg, enlarged lymph nodes, interstitial edema, tumors).

Ventilation-Perfusion Abnormalities

Conditions disrupting alveolar ventilation or capillary perfusion lead to an imbalance in ventilation and perfusion. This decreases the efficiency of the respiratory gas exchange process (Figure 10-15A). In an effort to keep the ventilation and perfusion ratios balanced, two compensatory changes occur: (1) to avoid wasted alveolar ventilation when capillary perfusion is decreased (eg, with pulmonary embolism [PE]),

TABLE 10-6. CAUSES OF ACUTE RESPIRATORY FAILURE IN ADULT

Impaired Ventilation
- Spinal cord injury (C4 or higher)
- Phrenic nerve damage
- Neuromuscular blockade
- Guillain-Barré syndrome
- CNS depression
  Drug overdoses (narcotics, sedatives, illicit drugs)
  Increased intracranial pressure
  Anesthetic agents
- Respiratory muscle fatigue

Impaired Gas Exchange
- Pulmonary edema
- ARDS
- Aspiration pneumonia

Airway Obstruction
- Aspiration of foreign body
- Thoracic tumors
- Asthma
- Bronchitis
- Pneumonia

Ventilation-Perfusion Abnormalities
- Pulmonary embolism
- Emphysema

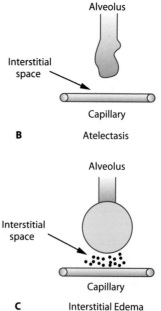
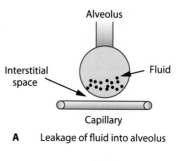

Figure 10-13. Pathophysiologic processes in ARF that impair gas exchange. **(A)** Increased alveolar membrane permeability. **(B)** Alveolar collapse from decreased surfactant production. **(C)** Increased capillary membrane permeability and interstitial edema.

TABLE 10-5. THORACIC SURGERY AND PROCEDURES

	Definitions
Thoracic Surgery	
Pneumonectomy	Removal of entire lung
Lobectomy	Resection of one or more lobes of the lung
Wedge resection	Removal of small wedge-shaped section of lung tissue
Segmental resection	Removal of bronchovascular segment of the lung lobe
Bullectomy	Resection of emphysematous bullae
Lung volume reduction surgery (LVRS)	Resection of diseased and functionless lung tissue
Open lung biopsy	Resection of portion of lung for biopsy through a thoracotomy incision
Decortication	
Video-assisted thoracic surgery (VATS)	Endoscopic procedure through small incision
Procedure	
Pulmonary stent	Device(s) placed by flexible or rigid bronchoscopes to keep airways open in the central tracheobronchial tree
Bronchoscopy (rigid or flexible)	Invasive procedure used to visualize the oropharynx, larynx, vocal cords, and tracheal bronchial tree for diagnosis and treatment

ESSENTIAL CONTENT CASE

Motor Vehicle Accident

A 22-year-old man was admitted to the progressive care unit following a motor vehicle accident in which he suffered blunt chest trauma. During his second day in the unit, his Spo$_2$ began deteriorating and he required increasing amounts of supplemental oxygen to maintain Pao$_2$ levels greater than 60 mm Hg. He was dyspneic, restless, and somewhat agitated. He verbalized a fear of impending death.

The rapid response team was called and the patient was transferred to the ICU.

	Admission	Day 2
Respiration rate	24 breaths/min	34 breaths/min
Chest x-ray	clear	bilateral diffuse infiltrates
ABGs	40% FM	100% non-rebreather mask
Pao$_2$	120 mm Hg	58 mm Hg
Paco$_2$	33 mm Hg	50 mm Hg
pH	7.42	7.35
HCO$_3$	24 mEq/L	27 mEq/L

Case Question 1: What signs and symptoms of ARF is this patient exhibiting?

Case Question 2: What intervention do you next anticipate based on his arterial blood gases and transfer to the ICU?

Answers

1. Signs and symptoms include dyspnea, restless, agitated, fear of impending death, and hypoxemia despite increasing Fio$_2$ to 100% non-rebreather mask.
2. Intubation and initiation of mechanical ventilation to improve hypoxemia along with analgesia and sedation. Patient has known bilateral diffuse infiltrates by chest x-ray. See next section on Acute Respiratory Distress Syndrome.

ESSENTIAL CONTENT CASE

Postanesthesia

A woman was admitted to the progressive care unit following an open lung biopsy. She was receiving oxygen by humidified face mask at 40%. A right pleural chest tube was draining minimal amounts of blood, with no evidence of air leak or obstruction.

The patient was minimally responsive to verbal and pain stimulation on admission. Respiratory rate was 8-10 breaths/min with an Spo$_2$ of 92%. She was receiving hydromorphone by continuous patient-controlled analgesia (PCA). Ten minutes after naloxone (Narcan) was given, assessment was:

	Admission	Post-Narcan
Pao$_2$	70 mm Hg	140 mm Hg
Paco$_2$	52 mm Hg	38 mm Hg
pH	7.31	7.40
HCO$_3$	24 mEq/L	23 mEq/L
Respiratory rate	8-10 breaths/min	22 breaths/min

Case Question 1. What was the etiology of her impaired ventilation?

Case Question 2. What is the next intervention that you anticipate?

Answers

1. Excessive use of narcotics can cause CNS depression leading to decreased ventilator muscle movement resulting in alveolar hypoventilation. Narcan was used as a reversal agent with resulting improvement in respiratory rate and ABGs.
2. Anticipate an adjustment in the patient's narcotic dose and delivery. Due to the short half-life of narcan as a reversal agent, careful assessment and reassessment of the patient's respiratory rate along with level of pain needs to be done. See Chapter 6 Pain, Sedation, and Neuromuscular Blockade Management for additional information.

alveolar collapse occurs to limit ventilation to alveoli with poor or absent capillary perfusion (Figure 10-15B); (2) to avoid capillary perfusion of alveoli that are not adequately ventilated (eg, with atelectasis), arteriole constriction (ie, hypoxic vasoconstriction) occurs and shunts blood away from hypoventilated alveoli to normally ventilated alveoli (Figure 10-15C). As the number of alveolar-capillary units affected by these compensatory changes increases, gas exchange eventually is affected negatively.

Each of these pathophysiologic changes results in inadequate CO_2 removal, O_2 absorption, or both. The severity of ARF can be further increased when anxiety and fear of impending death develop, a common consequence of severe dyspnea and hypoxemia. These symptoms increase oxygen demands and the work of breathing, further compromising O_2 availability for crucial organ function and depleting respiratory muscle strength.

Clinical Presentation

Signs and Symptoms

- Hypoxemia (Pao$_2$ < 60 mm Hg)
- Restlessness
- Tachypnea
- Dyspnea
- Tachycardia
- Confusion

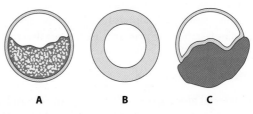

Figure 10-14. Mechanism of airway obstruction. **(A)** Fluid secretions present within airway. **(B)** Intraluminal edema narrowing airway diameter. **(C)** Peribronchial compression of airway.

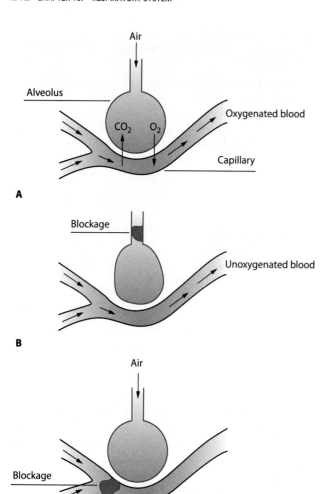

Figure 10-15. Pathophysiologic processes in ARF from ventilation-perfusion abnormalities. **(A)** Normal ventilation and perfusion relationship. **(B)** Decreased ventilation and normal perfusion. **(C)** Normal ventilation and decreased perfusion.

- Diaphoresis
- Anxiety
- Hypercarbia ($Paco_2 > 50$ mm Hg)
- Hypertension
- Irritability
- Somnolence (late)
- Cyanosis (late)
- Loss of consciousness (late)
- Pallor or cyanosis of skin
- Use of accessory muscles of respiration
- Abnormal breath sounds (crackles, wheezes)
- Manifestations of primary disease (see description of individual diseases later on)

Diagnostic Tests

- Arterial blood gases—Pao_2 less than 60 mm Hg and $Paco_2$ more than 50 mm Hg; with pH less than or equal to 7.30; or Pao_2 and $Paco_2$ in abnormal range for that individual

- Tests specific to underlying cause (see description of individual diseases later on)

Principles of Management for Acute Respiratory Failure

The management of the patient in ARF revolves around four primary areas: improving oxygenation and ventilation, treating the underlying disease state, reducing anxiety, and preventing and managing complications.

Improving Oxygenation and Ventilation

Most causes of ARF are treatable, with a return of normal respiratory function following resolution of the pathophysiologic condition. Aggressive support of respiratory function is required, though, until there is resolution of the underlying condition.

1. Provide supplemental O_2 to maintain Pao_2 greater than 60 mm Hg. The use of noninvasive methods for O_2 administration (nasal cannula or face masks) is preferable if acceptable Pao_2 levels can be achieved. Continued hypoxemia despite noninvasive O_2 delivery methods necessitates intubation and mechanical ventilation and transfer to a critical care unit.

2. Improve ventilation with the administration of bronchodilators, mucolytic agents, and other airway management modalities (suctioning, positioning, mobilization) as indicated. The routine use of chest physiotherapy has not been shown to be supported by the literature and is not recommended.

3. Intubate and initiate mechanical ventilation if noninvasive methods fail to correct hypoxemia and hypercarbia, or if cardiovascular instability develops. The mode of mechanical ventilation, rate, and tidal volume vary, depending on the underlying cause of respiratory failure and a variety of clinical factors.

4. Depending on the cause of ARF, the patient's response to treatment along with the institution's resources (specialized respiratory care units), the patient may need to be moved into intensive care for noninvasive ventilation or intubation and mechanical ventilation.

5. If suctioning is required, closely observe for signs and symptoms of complications: oxygenation (Spo_2), cardiac arrhythmias, respiratory distress, bronchospasm, increased respiratory rate, increased blood pressure or intracranial pressure, anxiety, pain, or change in mental status. Hyperoxygenate with 100% oxygen using a manual resuscitation bag (MRB) that delivers 100% O_2 as well as a PEEP valve when ventilator PEEP levels are more than 5 cm H_2O. Suctioning should only be performed when clinically indicated, and never on a routine schedule. The use of in-line suction catheters is encouraged as the catheters do not affect oxygenation as

dramatically as complete disconnection, and they decrease the potential contamination of the clinician doing the suctioning.

6. Prior to intrahospital transport, verify adequacy of ventilatory support equipment to maintain cardiopulmonary stability. Verify that PEEP on the transport equipment is maintained.

Treating the Underlying Disease State

Correction of the underlying cause of the ARF should be done as soon as possible. See specific management approaches later in the chapter for selected disease states.

Reducing Anxiety

Maintain a calm, supportive environment to avoid unnecessary escalation of anxiety. Give brief explanations of activities and approaches being done to relieve ARF. Vigilance and presence of healthcare providers during anxious periods is crucial to avoid panic by patients and visiting family members.

Teach diaphragmatic breathing to slow the rate and increase the depth of respirations. Place one hand on the patient's abdomen. Instruct the patient to inhale deeply, causing the hand on the abdomen to rise. During exhalation, have the patient feel the hand on the belly sink down toward the spine. Explain that the chest should move minimally. After a minute or two, ask the patient to place his or her hands on the belly to continue the exercise.

If necessary, administer mild doses of anxiolytics (ie, lorazepam or diazepam) that do not depress respiration.

Preventing and Managing Complications

See Chapter 5, Airway and Ventilatory Management, for additional strategies, Chapter 11, Multisystem Problems for preventing selected hospital acquired conditions, and Chapter 14, Gastrointestinal System for GI prophylaxis.

Acute Respiratory Distress Syndrome (ARDS)

The case study of the patient in a motor vehicle accident is typical of a patient who develops acute respiratory distress syndrome (ARDS). ARDS has a very high morbidity and mortality. It is characterized by non-cardiac pulmonary edema caused by increased alveolar capillary membrane permeability. ARDS affects both lungs and hypoxemia refractory to oxygenation is a hallmark of the condition. ARDS was previously described as the most severe presentation of acute lung injury (ALI) but recently the term ALI has been eliminated in favor of the labels "mild," "moderate," and "severe" ARDS. The definition is called the "Berlin Definition of ARDS" and consists of categories that identify the timing of the condition, chest imaging criteria, origin of lung edema, and oxygenation status. The severity stratification of mild, moderate, and severe is based on the Pao_2/Fio_2 score and PEEP level. The Pao_2/Fio_2 (also called P/F ratio) ratio is calculated by dividing the Pao_2 by the Fio_2 (with a decimal; 50% = 0.5).

TABLE 10-7. PRIMARY AND SECONDARY CAUSES OF ARDS

Primary Causes (Direct Damage to the Alveolar Membrane)
- Aspiration of gastric contents
- Pulmonary contusion
- Near drowning
- Inhalation of smoke or toxic substances
- Diffuse pneumonias (viral and bacterial)

Secondary Causes (Mediated by Cellular or Humoral Injury to the Capillary Endothelium)
- Systemic sepsis
- Hypovolemic shock associated with chest trauma or sepsis
- Acute pancreatitis
- Fat emboli
- Trauma
- DIC
- Massive blood transfusions

Etiology, Risk Factors, and Pathophysiology

Risk factors for the development of ARDS can be categorized into conditions that lead to direct damage to the alveolar-capillary membrane (primary causes) and those that are thought to be mediated by cellular or humoral injury to the capillary endothelial wall (secondary causes) (Table 10-7). Whether primary or secondary causes, the pathologic processes involved in ARDS are characterized by excessive alveolar–capillary membrane permeability, interstitial edema, and diffuse alveolar injury (see Figure 10-13). Direct damage to the alveolar membrane can easily occur when toxic substances are inhaled, such as during fires or chemical spills.

Alveolar and interstitial edema, microatelectasis, and ventilation-perfusion mismatching in ARDS lead to severe hypoxemia and poor lung compliance ("stiff lungs"). In the setting of trauma and sepsis, this abnormality in microvascular permeability occurs in capillary beds throughout the body. Typically, this multisystem organ dysfunction is not clinically apparent, with clinical manifestations isolated to the respiratory system. When multiple organ dysfunction syndrome does occur, it is seen in ARDS patients who develop bacterial infections and sepsis (see Chapter 11, Multisystem Problems).

The ARDS process disrupts normal macrophage function and increases the risk of infection. Mortality and long-term disability from ARDS is high.

Clinical Presentation

Signs and Symptoms

- Dyspnea
- Tachypnea (rates often > 40 breaths/min)
- Intercostal retractions
- Copious secretions
- Panic, fear of impending death
- Crackles and/or wheezes

Diagnostic Tests

- Chest x-ray shows diffuse, bilateral pulmonary infiltrates without increased cardiac size
- Pao_2/Fio_2 less than or equal to 300 mm Hg

Principles of Management for ARDS

Much of the management of ARDS relies on supportive care and the prevention of complications. To date, interventions to limit the disease progression or reverse the underlying structural defects are not known.

Improving Oxygenation and Ventilation

Interventions specific to ARDS to improve oxygenation and ventilation include the following:

1. Administer high Fio_2 levels with high-flow system or rebreathing mask. A constant positive airway pressure (CPAP) mask may be tolerated in alert, cooperative patients. Continuous, vigilant monitoring for contraindications of noninvasive CPAP (decreased loss of consciousness, nausea/vomiting, increased dyspnea, or panic) is imperative.
2. Intubation, mechanical ventilation, and transfer to intensive care if cardiovascular instability is present, severe hypoxemia persists, or if fatigue develops. The majority of these patients will need transfer to the ICU for additional management.

Reducing Anxiety

Same as previously described for ARF management.

Achieving Effective Communications

Refer Chapter 5, Airway and Ventilatory Management, for detailed discussion of communication techniques for intubated patients.

Maintaining Hemodynamic Stability and Adequate Perfusion

1. Minimize cardiovascular instability by careful monitoring; administer fluids to correct hypovolemia.
2. Vasoactive drugs may be required to maintain adequate perfusion.

Acute Respiratory Failure in the Patient with Chronic Obstructive Pulmonary Disease

Individuals with COPD are at high risk for exacerbations and the development of ARF due to progressive airflow limitation with chronic inflammatory airway and lung response. Acute asthma will be discussed in the next section. Altered host defenses, increased secretion volume and viscosity, impaired secretion clearance and airway changes, and common pathophysiologic changes predispose the patient with COPD to acute exacerbations or episodes of ARF requiring hospitalizations.

Etiology, Risk Factors, and Pathophysiology

Any systemic or pulmonary illness can precipitate exacerbations and the development of ARF in patients with COPD. In addition to the etiologies of ARF listed in Table 10-6, diseases or situations that decrease ventilatory drive, muscle strength, chest wall elasticity, or gas exchange capacity, or increase airway resistance or metabolic oxygen requirements can easily

TABLE 10-8. PRECIPITATING EVENTS OF ACUTE RESPIRATORY FAILURE IN COPD

Decreased Ventilatory Drive
- Oversedation
- Hypothyroidism
- Brain stem lesions

Decreased Muscle Strength
- Malnutrition
- Shock
- Myopathies
- Hypophosphatemia
- Hypomagnesemia
- Hypocalcemia

Decreased Chest Wall Elasticity
- Rib fractures
- Pleural effusions
- Ileus
- Ascites

Decreased Lung Capacity for Gas Exchange
- Atelectasis
- Pulmonary edema
- Pneumonia
- Pulmonary embolus
- Heart failure

Increased Airway Resistance
- Bronchospasm
- Increased secretions
- Upper airway obstructions
- Airway edema

Increased Metabolic Oxygen Requirements
- Systemic infection
- Hyperthyroidism
- Fever

lead to ARF in patients with COPD (Table 10-8). The most common precipitating events include:

- *Airway infection (pneumonia, bronchitis):* Frequent antibiotic administration, hospitalization, and impaired cough and host defenses in COPD increase acute airway infections. Infections are commonly caused by gram-negative enteric bacteria or Legionella, with *Haemophilus influenzae* and *Streptococcus pneumoniae* causing acute bronchitis. Moraxella catarrhalis is also a common respiratory organism causing infection in these patients.
- *Pulmonary embolus:* The high incidence of right ventricular failure in COPD increases the risk of pulmonary embolus from right ventricular mural thrombi.
- *Heart failure:* In the presence of pulmonary hypertension and right-sided heart failure, treatment of left-sided heart failure is often delayed due to difficulties in early diagnosis.
- *Nonadherance to medication regime:* The complicated treatment regime for management of COPD, which includes frequent administration of both oral and inhaled agents, frequently leads to underuse of medications.

The development of ARF in COPD patients places a tremendous burden on the pulmonary system. The chronic disease process leads to impairment of ventilation, poor gas exchange, and airway obstruction. The additional burden of an acute disease process, even a relatively minor one, further impairs ventilation and gas exchange and increases airway obstruction. Compensatory mechanisms can easily be overwhelmed, with lethal consequences.

Clinical Presentation

Signs and symptoms are similar to ARF, but usually more pronounced.

Diagnostic Tests

- *Chest x-ray:* Evidence of COPD (flat diaphragms, hyperinflation of air fields), in addition to x-ray findings specific to the cause of the ARF (see Figure 10-3).
- *Arterial blood gases:* $Paco_2$ greater than 50 mm Hg and higher than baseline levels during stable, chronic disease periods.

Principles of Management for ARF in Patients with COPD

The presence of chronic respiratory dysfunction and an acute respiratory problem leads to some changes in the typical management of ARF.

Treating the Underlying Disease State

Treatment is directed at both the acute precipitating event and the chronic airflow obstruction problems associated with COPD.

1. Increase airway diameter with bronchodilators and reduce airway edema with corticosteroids. Beta-adrenergic and anticholinergic agents are often used concurrently (Table 10-9). Higher than usual doses may be necessary until the precipitating event is resolved. Systemic corticosteroids are used to decrease airway inflammation and thus bronchospasm, and may enhance secretion clearance as well.
2. Treat pulmonary infections with appropriate antibiotics.
3. Improve secretion removal. Strategies to improve secretion removal include adequate hydration, patient mobilization, coughing, and heated moist aerosolization. The routine use of chest physiotherapy has not been shown to be supported by the literature and is not recommended. Secretions may

TABLE 10-9. BRONCHODILATOR CATEGORIES

Category	Examples
Beta-agonists (short-acting) (goal is beta$_2$ specificity)	Albuterol, beta$_2$-specific (often given as a continuous aerosol treatment) Epinephrine (beta$_1$ and beta$_2$)
Beta-agonists (long acting)	Salmeterol
Anticholinergics	Ipratropium bromide Glycopyrrolate
Combination Beta-agonist (short-acting) and anticholinergic	Ipratropium bromide and albuterol
Methylxanthines	Aminophylline

be thick and tenacious in asthma patients. Monitor response to these therapies and discontinue them if no additional benefits are observed.

Improving Oxygenation and Ventilation

Correction of hypoxemia (saturation < 90%) is done by small increases in Fio_2 levels, preferably with a controlled O_2 delivery device such as a Venturi mask, biphasic intermittent positive airway pressure (BiPAP), or CPAP. Frequent monitoring of arterial blood gases is essential to ensure adequate arterial oxygenation (Pao_2 of 55-60 mm Hg or baseline values during nonacute situations) without significantly increasing $Paco_2$ levels. The administration of oxygen to COPD patients was once felt to eliminate the "hypoxic drive," putting the patient at risk for hypercarbia, acidosis, and death. This drive is responsible for only approximately 10% of the total drive to breathe. Oxygen should never be withheld and is essential to prevent further deleterious effects of hypoxia and potential organ failure. While it is correct that higher than necessary Fio_2 levels may increase $Paco_2$, this effect occurs by three physiologic mechanisms:

1. *The Haldane effect*: As hemoglobin becomes desaturated with oxygen, the affinity for carbon dioxide increases. The administration of oxygen then displaces carbon dioxide on hemoglobin and increases carbon dioxide levels in the plasma. Patients with COPD are unable to increase minute ventilation or "blow off" carbon dioxide. This leads to an increase in carbon dioxide, lowering the pH and resulting in a respiratory acidosis.
2. *Hypoxic vasoconstriction*: This physiologic adaptive mechanism is a response to a decrease in alveolar oxygen and moves capillary blood flow from a closed or atelectatic alveolus to an open alveolus. In patients with COPD, this adaptive mechanism no longer occurs. As a result, dead space ventilation or decreased perfusion (see Figure 10-15C) occurs with resulting increased carbon dioxide levels.
3. *Decreased minute ventilation*: As a result of increased dead space ventilation with resulting increased carbon dioxide, some COPD patients will decrease their minute ventilation. This decrease will further limit the patient's inspiratory reserve capacity.

Oxygen administration in COPD patients is necessary to prevent hypoxia and organ failure and should never be withheld. Titration and considerations for mechanical ventilation in the COPD patient with CO_2 retention ($Paco_2$ > 50 mm Hg) should be guided by the pH and Pao_2. These include (Figure 10-16):

- pH less than 7.35 with Pao_2 greater than 60 mm Hg: consider noninvasive mechanical ventilation or intubation.
- pH greater than 7.35 with Pao_2 less than 60 mm Hg: increase oxygen to increase Pao_2 to greater than 60 mm Hg. Reassess ABG.

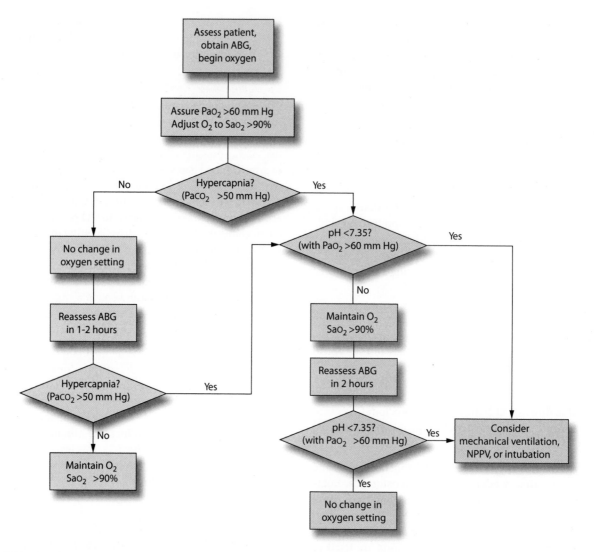

Figure 10-16. Algorithm to correct hypoxemia in an acutely ill COPD patient. ABG: arterial blood gas; NPPV: noninvasive positive pressure ventilation; O_2: oxygen; $PaCO_2$: arterial carbon dioxide tension; PaO_2: arterial oxygen tension; SaO_2: arterial oxygen saturation. (*From: American Thoracic Society and European Respiratory Society. Standards for the diagnosis and management of patients with COPD. 2004;183. Available: http://www.thoracic.org/sections/copd/resources. Accessed January 23, 2014.*)

Position the patient to maximize ventilatory efforts and relaxation/rest during spontaneous breathing. A high Fowler position and leaning on an overbed table may be a position of comfort.

Relaxation techniques and diaphragmatic, pursed lip breathing may be helpful to decrease anxiety and improve ventilatory patterns. Anxiolytics and other sedatives should be used cautiously to avoid decreasing minute ventilation. COPD patients with ARF may benefit from early use of noninvasive mechanical ventilation.

The decision to intubate and mechanically ventilate the patient is based primarily on the deterioration of mental status, coupled with knowledge of the patient's baseline pulmonary function and functional status, and the reversibility of the underlying cause. Weaning from mechanical ventilation is frequently more difficult, and in some cases not possible, in the presence of COPD. Informed discussions with the patient and family regarding intubation options should be undertaken. The presence of an advanced directive and power of attorney designee for healthcare decisions can help in guiding clinician's actions when patients are unable to make treatment decisions themselves (see Chapter 8, Ethical and Legal Considerations).

Nutritional Support

Typically, patients with COPD have protein-calorie malnutrition, as well as low levels of phosphate, magnesium, and calcium. These chronic nutritional deficits lead to muscle weakness and may interfere with the weaning process if mechanical ventilation becomes necessary. Early enteral feeding (oral or by feeding tube) of these patients is essential to avoid further deterioration in their nutritional status during acute illness and should be initiated as soon as hemodynamically stable. Enteral feeding is preferred over parenteral nutrition due to decreased risk of infectious complications. COPD patients who are malnourished have greater air trapping, lower diffusing capacity, and are less able to mobilize (see Chapter 14, Gastrointestinal System). If used, non-invasive positive pressure ventilation makes oral feeding difficult and the insertion of a small bore nasoenteric tube may be necessary.

Preventing and Managing Complications

In addition to the complications associated with ARF, the following complications are commonly observed in COPD exacerbation patients with ARF:

- *Arrhythmia:* High incidence of both atrial and ventricular arrhythmia in patients with COPD due to hypoxemia, acidosis, heart disease, medications, and electrolyte abnormalities. Cardiac monitoring and correction of the underlying cause is the goal, with pharmacologic treatment of arrhythmia only for life-threatening situations.
- *Pulmonary embolus:* High incidence. Observe for signs and symptoms and follow the usual treatment and prevention guidelines.
- *GI distention and ileus:* Aerophagia is common in dyspneic patients, increasing the incidence of this complication.
- *If ventilated* (auto-PEEP and barotrauma): High incidence, especially in the elderly and in individuals with high ventilation needs.

Patient Teaching

- Smoking cessation continues to be the single most-effective way to stop the progression of COPD (Table 10-10).
- Immunizations to prevent pneumococcal pneumonia (year round) and influenza (during flu season) remain important preventive measures (Table 10-11).

Acute Respiratory Failure in the Patient with Asthma

Individuals with asthma are at risk for exacerbations that are characterized by a progressive increase in shortness of breath, cough, wheezing, or decrease in expiratory airflow. Acute/severe asthma, status asthmaticus, and asthma attack are also terms that have been used to describe this condition. Asthma differs from COPD in both pathophysiology and therapeutic response and the airway restriction is usually reversible with aggressive treatment (Figure 10-17).

Etiology, Risk Factors, and Pathophysiology

Asthma exacerbations are first and foremost due to uncontrolled airway inflammation. The pathology results in the severe bronchospasm and increased mucus production present during asthma "attacks," both of which contribute to the overall airway obstruction. Triggers vary and include infection, inhaled seasonal antigens, foods, exercise, or

TABLE 10-10. HELPING SMOKERS QUIT: A GUIDE FOR NURSES

Ask

Ask about tobacco use at every admission.
- Implement a system in your clinical setting that ensures that tobacco-use status is obtained and recorded at every contact.

Advise

Advise tobacco users to quit.
- Tell your patient, "quitting smoking is the most important thing you can do to protect your health."

Assess

Assess readiness to quit.
- Ask every tobacco user if he or she is willing to quit at this time.
  - If willing to quit, provide resources and assistance.
  - If unwilling to quit, provide resources and help patient identify barriers to quitting.

Assist

Assist tobacco users with a plan to quit.
Advise the smoker to:
- Set a quit date, ideally within 2 weeks.
- Get support from family, friends, and coworkers.
- Review past quit attempts, what helped, what led to relapse.
- Anticipate challenges.
- Identify reasons for quitting and benefits of quitting.

Arrange

Arrange follow-up visits.
- Provide information for follow-up visits with his or her healthcare provider.

Adapted from: Helping Smokers Quit: A Guide for Nurses. March 2005. Agency for Healthcare Research and Quality, Rockville, MD. Available at: http://www.ahrq.gov/about/nursing/hlpssmksqt.htm.

medications to name just a few. While triggers may stimulate an exacerbation of asthma, they are not causal.

Bronchoconstriction results from mediator release from mast cells and include histamine, prostaglandins, and leukotrienes that contract the smooth muscle. Mucus plugging is thought to be because of eosinophil and shed bronchial epithelial cells as well as impaired mucus transport. Additionally, over time some patients may exhibit airway remodeling (thickening that contributes to airflow narrowing and airflow obstruction) especially if their airway inflammation is not controlled. All of these contribute to the severe and often unrelenting nature of the asthma "attack."

Some risk factors for the development of an acute severe asthma episode include frequent need for use of their "rescue" inhalers, recent illness, frequent past emergency room visits or hospitalizations, prior intubations and ICU admissions, noncompliance with medical therapy, and inadequate access to healthcare.

Clinical Presentation

Clinical findings are related to severe airflow obstruction and may include the inability to say a whole sentence, shortness of breath, wheezing, pulsus paradoxus, use of accessory muscles of inspiration, diaphoresis, and need to maintain upright position. However, peak flow measurement is one of the best assessment tools for determining the severity of the exacerbation. An absolute peak flow measurement of < 100L/min in an adult generally indicates

TABLE 10-11. INFLUENZA AND PNEUMOCOCCAL VACCINE RECOMMENDATIONS

Influenza Vaccine Recommendations

- Persons aged ≥ 50 years
- Women who will be pregnant during the influenza season
- Persons who have chronic pulmonary (including asthma), cardiovascular (except hypertension), renal, hepatic, hematologic, or metabolic disorders (including diabetes mellitus)
- Persons who have immunosuppression (including immunosuppression caused by medications or by HIV)
- Persons who have any condition (eg, congnitive dysfunction, spinal cord injuries, seizure disorders, or other neuromuscular disorders) that can compromise respiratory function or the handling of respiratory secretions or that can increase the risk of aspiration
- Residents of nursing homes and other chronic-care facilities
- Healthcare personnel
- Household contacts and caregivers of children aged > 5 years and adults aged ≥ 50 years, with particular emphasis on vassination contacts of children aged > 6 months
- Household contacts and caregivers of persons with medical conditions that put them at high risk for severe complications from influenza
- Children aged 6 months to 18 years

Pneumococcal Vaccine Recommendations

- All adults 65 years of age and older
- Anyone over 2 through 64 years of age who has a long-term health problem such as heart disease, lung disease, sickle cell disease, diabetes, alcoholism, cirrhosis, leaks of cerebrospinal fluid, or cochlear implant
- Anyone over 2 through 64 years of age who has a disease or condition that lowers the body's resistance to infection, such as Hodgkin disease; lymphoma or leukemia; kidney failure; multiple myeloma; syndrome; HIV infection or AIDS; damaged spleen no spleen; organ transplant
- Anyone over 2 through 65 years of age who is taking a drug or treatment that lowers the body's resistance to infection, such as: long-term steroids, certain cancer drugs, radiation therapy
- Any adult 19 through 64 years of age who is a smoker or has asthma

Adapted from: Fiore AE, Shay DK, Broder K, et al. Prevention and control of influeza: recommendations of the advisory committee on immunization practices (ACIP), 2008. MMWR. 2008;57(RR-7):1-60. Department of Health and Human Services: Centers for Disease Control and Prevention: Pneumococcal polysaccharide vaccine: what you need to know (4-16-009). 2009. Available at: http://www.cdc.gov/vaccines/pubs/vis/download/vis-ppv.pdf. Accessed January 23, 2014.

severe bronchoconstriction, especially in combination with failure to respond to aggressive bronchodilator treatments. These patients are generally admitted to a critical care unit or progressive care unit for close monitoring and aggressive therapy (see Figure 10-17).

Diagnostic Tests

- *Arterial blood gases:* Initial findings may show pH greater than 7.45, $Paco_2$ less than 35 mm Hg, and mild to moderate hypoxia (respiratory alkalosis). In severe airflow obstruction, findings may progress to pH less than 7.35 and $Paco_2$ greater than 50 mm Hg (metabolic acidosis).
- *Pulsus paradoxus:* A decrease of greater than 10 mm Hg in systolic blood pressure during inspiration.
- *Pulmonary function tests:* FEV_1 of less than 20% or peak expiratory flow rate (PEFR) of less than 40% of predicted despite aggressive bronchodilator therapy.
- *Spo_2:* Observe for hypoxia. The Spo_2 should be greater than 92%.

Principles of Management for Asthma Patients
Treat the Underlying Disease State

Treatment is directed at decreasing airway inflammation, reversal of airflow obstruction, and correction of hypercapnia or hypoxemia if present.

1. Reduce airway inflammation with systemic corticosteroids and provide aggressive bronchodilation. Beta-2 specific bronchodilators (eg, albuterol) are the drug of choice and may be provided continuously by nebulizer through a mouthpiece, mask or if ventilated, through the ventilator circuit. Concomitant use of anticholinergic bronchodilators is generally provided to enhance rapid reversal of bronchospasm. If bronchospasm is refractory to aggressive pharmacologic management (beta-2 specific drugs and anticholinergics), then subcutaneous epinephrine may be used. However, epinephrine should be avoided in adults except in extreme cases as it may precipitate heart attacks, especially in those with pre-existing cardiac disease. The use of magnesium sulfate is not supported in the literature although it is still sometimes used in patients with acute severe asthma.

2. Treat pulmonary infections with appropriate antibiotics.

3. Improve secretion removal. Generally secretions will be easier to mobilize as bronchodilation is enhanced. Until then, strategies are limited. Adequate hydration (generally provided parenterally) is important as the asthma patient is often dehydrated.

4. Once improved, treatment is directed at long-term "control" of the disease.

Education during recovery is crucial to prevent future exacerbations and should focus on self-management techniques such as regular use of their "controller" medications to decrease inflammation, "rescue' inhalers for bronchodilation, identification and avoidance of "triggers," and smoking cessation (see Table 10-10). Additionally, provision of pneumococcal and influenza (seasonal) vaccines (see Table 10-11) should be done prior to discharge if they have not already received the vaccines.

Improving Oxygenation and Ventilation

Severe hypoxemia should be corrected by providing high Fio_2 levels until an adequate oxygen saturation is obtained (90% or greater). Oxygen masks and high flow O_2 systems may be used to deliver oxygen. Mechanical ventilation may be necessary if the patient does not respond to more conservative methods. The use of non-invasive ventilation in an asthmatic is discouraged as it may lead to increased hyperinflation and respiratory failure.

Frequent monitoring of arterial blood gases is essential to monitor pH and $Paco_2$. Helium-oxygen (heliox) mixtures may be used to decrease work of breathing and improve ventilation. Heliox can be administered via mask, or invasive ventilation. Due to the high levels of helium in the heliox

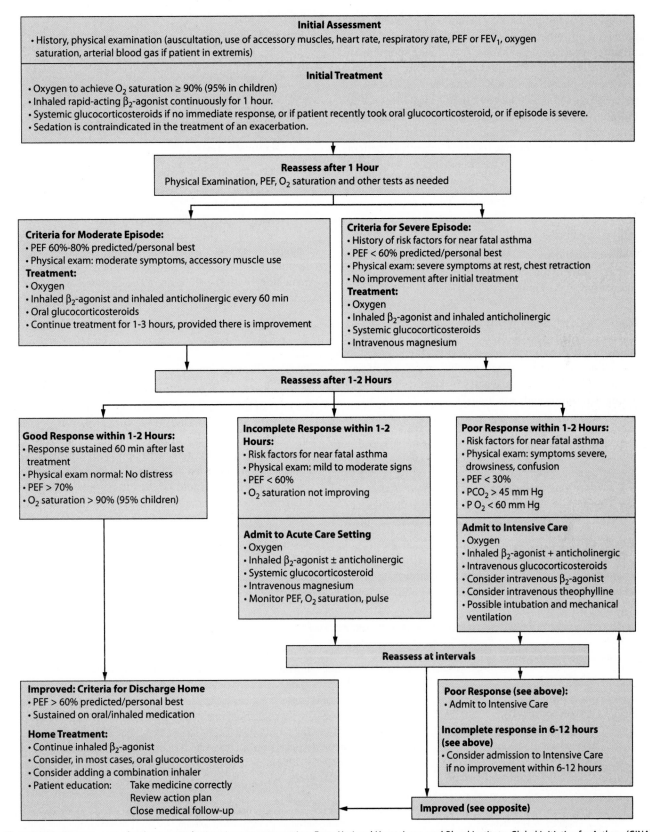

Figure 10-17. Management of asthma exacerbations in acute care setting. From National Heart, Lung, and Blood Institute. Global Initiative for Asthma (GINA) Global Strategy for Asthma Management and Prevention. 2013. Available at: http://www.ginasthma.org/uploads/users/files/GINA_Report_2012Feb13.pdf. Accessed September 1, 2013.

mixtures, the use of heliox may be limited in patients with high Fio_2 requirements. Position the patient to maximize ventilatory efforts and relaxation/rest during spontaneous breathing. Relaxation techniques may be helpful to decrease anxiety and improve ventilatory patterns. Anxiolytics and other sedatives should not be given unless the patient is intubated. Studies have demonstrated that doing so increases the potential for death. The decision to intubate and mechanically ventilate the patient may be made urgently in patients who are failing to respond to treatment and are fatiguing. If intubation is done the patient should be transferred to a critical care unit for management.

Interstitial Lung Disease

Interstitial lung disease (ILD) is a broad category of over 130 lung disorders that are characterized by fibrosis and/or inflammation of the lungs.

Etiology, Risk Factors, and Pathophysiology

The lung tissue or interstitium is damaged by a known or unknown causes leading to inflammation. The interstitium may include the alveolar space, small airways, blood vessels, and/or the pleura. Fibrosis and scarring then occur with resulting hypoxemia and "stiff lungs."

Some known causes include:

- Occupational and environmental exposure to irritants, asbestos, silica.
- Infections, tuberculosis.
- Medications, amiodarone, chemotherapy agents.
- Connective tissue or collagen disorders, rheumatoid arthritis, systemic sclerosis, systemic lupus erythematosis.
- Genetic/familial.

Unknown causes are classified as idiopathic pulmonary fibrosis.

Clinical Presentation

Signs and symptoms

- Dyspnea
- Nonproductive cough
- Clubbing
- Lung auscultation fine crackles
- Signs of right-sided heart failure

Diagnostic Tests

- *Chest x-ray:* May be normal or show lung volume loss
- *CT chest:* Classic description of honeycombing or "ground glass"
- *Lung biopsy:* To determine pathogenesis

Principles of Management

Treatment is same as previously described for ARF management along with the addition of therapy directed toward the cause of the ILD and may include the following:

- Corticosteroids
- Cytoxic agents

Pulmonary Hypertension

Pulmonary hypertension is a progressive, life-threatening disorder of the pulmonary circulation characterized by high pulmonary artery pressures (> 25 mm Hg). This persistent high pulmonary artery pressure ultimately leads to right ventricular failure. Patients with pulmonary arterial hypertension (PAH) are often on a chronic regimen of therapy to decrease PAH that should not be interrupted during hospitalization. Abrupt cessation of therapy can lead to rebound pulmonary hypertension that can be fatal.

Etiology, Risk Factors, and Pathophysiology

Pulmonary hypertension may result from a number of etiologies (Table 10-12). The pathophysiology is multifactoral with evidence that endothelial dysfunction leads to remodeling of

TABLE 10-12. WORLD HEALTH ORGANIZATION CLASSIFICATION OF PULMONARY HYPERTENSION[a]

Group	Main classification	Diseases included
1.	Pulmonary arterial hypertension (PAH)	PAH: Idiopathic, familial, associated with corrective tissue disease, associated with congenital heart disease, associated with HIV infection, associated with drugs or toxins
2.	Pulmonary hypertension due to left-sided heart disease	Systolic dysfunction, diastolic dysfunction, valvular disease
3.	Pulmonary hypertension due to lung disease and/or hypoxia	Chronic obstructive pulmonary disease, interstitial lung disease, mixed restrictive and obstructive pattern, sleep disordered breathing, alveolar hypoventilation disorders, chronic exposure to high altitude, developmental abnormalities
4.	Chronic thromboembolic pulmonary hypertension	Chronic thromboembolic disease
5.	Pulmonary hypertension with unclear multifactorial mechanisms	Hematologic disorders: myeloproliferative disorders, splenectomy; systemic disorders: sarcoidosis, pulmonary Langerhans cell histiocytosis: lymphangioleiomyomatosis, neurofibromatosis, vasculitis; metabolic disorders: glycogen storage disease, Gaucher disease, thyroid disorders; others: tumoral obstruction, fibrosing mediastinitis, chronic renal failure on dialysis

[a]Revisions made at the 4th World Symposium on Pulmonary Hypertension held at Dana Point, California, in 2008.

Source: *Reproduced with permission from Poms AI, Kingman M. Inhaled treprostinil for the treatment of pulmonary arterial hypertension. Crit Care Nurse. 2011 Dec;31(6):e1-10.*

the pulmonary artery vessel wall causing exaggerated vasoconstriction and impaired vasodilatation. This results in decreased blood flow and return of deoxygenated blood to the lungs.

Clinical Presentation

Signs and symptoms include pallor, dyspnea, fatigue, chest pain, and syncope. Cor pulmonale or enlargement of the right ventricle can be a result of pulmonary hypertension and may lead to right ventricular failure (see Table 9-10). The diagnostic strategy is related to both establishing the diagnosis of pulmonary hypertension and if possible the underlying cause.

Diagnostic Tests

- *Echocardiogram*: Valvular heart disease, left ventricular dysfunction, and intracardiac shunts.
- *Chest x-ray:* Enlarged hilar and pulmonary arterial shadows and enlargement of the right ventricle.
- *12-lead ECG:* Right ventricular strain, right ventricular hypertrophy, and right axis deviation.
- *CTPA, Ventilation-perfusion scan, or pulmonary angiogram:* These are done to rule out thromboembolism.
- *CT chest:* Assess for presence or absence of parenchymal lung disease.
- *6-minute-walk test:* Measurement of distance used to monitor exercise tolerance, response to therapy, and progression of disease.
- *Right-heart cardiac catheterization:* Gold standard for diagnosis with vasodilator (adensosine, nitric oxide, epoprostentol) testing for benefit from long-term therapy with calcium channel blockers. Positive response is a decrease in mean PAP of 10 to 40 mm Hg with an increased or unchanged CO from baseline values.
- *Serology testing:* Antinuclear antibodies.
- *Pulmonary function testing:* Used to rule out any other diseases contributing to shortness of breath.
- *Sleep study:* Done as a screen for sleep apnea, which may also contribute to the pulmonary hypertension.

Principles of Management

Current treatment options can slow the progression of the disease.

- Long-term anticoagulation therapy to prevent thrombosis.
- Avoidance of beta blockers, decongestants, or other medications that worsen pulmonary hypertension or decrease right heart function.
- Symptom limited physical activity.
- Oxygen to prevent additional pulmonary vasoconstriction due to low oxygen levels. Maintain Sao_2 greater than 90% if possible.
- Diuretics to control edema and ascites if right-sided heart failure present.
- Calcium channel blockers only if positive response to vasodilator during cardiac catheterization.

Newer Medical Treatment Options

Prostacylin therapy is a potent vasodilator of both the systemic and pulmonary arterial vascular beds and is an inhibitor of platelet aggregation. Patients must be preapproved through their insurance prior to starting these costly medications and be able to self-administer.

- Remodulin (treprostinil sodium) is a continuous subcutaneous or intravenous infusion.
- Veletri (epoprostenol sodium, room temperature stable) is a continuous intravenous infusion.
- Ventavis (iloprost sodium) and Tyvaso (treprostinil) are intermittent inhalation treatments using medication specific nebulizers.

Endothelin receptor antagonists block the neurohormone endothelin from binding in the endothelium and vascular smooth muscle.

- Tracleer (bosentan) and Letairis (ambrisentan) are oral agents.

Phosphodiesterase inhibitors block phosphodiesterase type 5 which is responsible for the degradation of cyclic guanosine monophosphate (cGMP). Increased cGMP concentration results in pulmonary vasculature relaxation; vasodilation in the pulmonary bed and the systemic circulation (to a lesser degree) may occur.

- Revatio (sildenafil) and Adcirca (tadalafil) are oral agents specific for the use in patients with pulmonary hypertension.

Surgical options include the following:

- Atrial septostomy to create a right-to-left shunt to help decompress a failing right ventricle in select patients who are unresponsive to medical therapies. This also leads to significant hypoxemia in an already compromised patient.
- Pulmonary thromboendarterectomy for those with suspected chronic thromboembolic pulmonary hypertension to improve hemodynamics and functional status.
- Lung transplantation is indicated when the pulmonary hypertension has progressed despite optimal medical and surgical therapy.

Pneumonia

Respiratory infection is a common cause of ARF. Infections developed before hospitalization (community-acquired), during medical treatment (healthcare acquired), and those acquired during hospitalization (hospital-acquired and ventilator-associated) can lead to significant morbidity and mortality, and require progressive care management. A variety of respiratory infections occur in acutely ill patients, including bronchitis, and pneumonia. This section focuses on pneumonia, the most common respiratory infection and the most common cause of respiratory failure in acutely ill patients.

Etiology, Risk Factors, and Pathophysiology

At high risk for the development of pneumonia are the young, the elderly, those with chronic cardiopulmonary disease, and immunocompromised individuals. In addition, immobility, decreased level of consciousness, and mechanical ventilation place hospitalized patients at high risk for development of hospital-acquired pneumonias. These latter pneumonias are most commonly referred to as ventilator-associated pneumonias or VAPs.

The major routes of entry of causative organisms for pneumonia are aspiration of oropharyngeal or gastric contents into the lungs, inhalation of aerosols or particles containing the organisms, and hematogenous spread of the organism into the lung from another site in the body (Figure 10-18). Most hospital-acquired pneumonias are due to aspiration of bacteria colonizing the oropharynx or upper GI tract. Pneumonia develops when the normal bronchomucociliary clearance mechanism or phagocytic cells are overwhelmed by the number or virulence of organisms aspirated or inhaled into the airways. The proliferation of organisms in the pulmonary parenchyma elicits an inflammatory response, with large influxes of phagocytic cells into the alveoli and airways and production of protein-rich exudates. This inflammatory response impairs the distribution

of ventilation and decreases lung compliance, resulting in increased work of breathing and the sensation of dyspnea. Hypoxemia results from the shunting of blood through poorly ventilated areas of pulmonary consolidation. The inflammatory response leads to fever and leukocytosis.

Pneumonia also can develop through hematogenous spread, when organisms remote from the lungs gain access to the blood, become lodged in the pulmonary vasculature, and proliferate. Pneumonias with a hematogenous origin usually are distributed diffusely in both lung fields, rather than localized to a single lung or lobe.

Several factors present in acutely ill patients increase the risk for the development of hospital-acquired pneumonias including VAP. Aspiration of oropharyngeal and gastric secretions is increased in the presence of tracheostomy tubes, nasogastric tubes, poor GI motility, gastric distention, and immobility, all of which are common situations in acutely ill patients. Treatments that neutralize the normally acidic gastric contents, such as antacids, H_2 blockers, or tube feeding, allow increased growth of gram-negative bacteria in gastric contents. This increases the potential for aspiration of gram-negative bacteria and/or hematogenous spread.

Acutely ill patients at high risk for hospital-acquired pneumonias are those immunocompromised from malignancy, AIDS, and chronic cardiac or respiratory disease; the elderly; or those with depressed alveolar macrophage function (oxygen, corticosteroids). Although a variety of

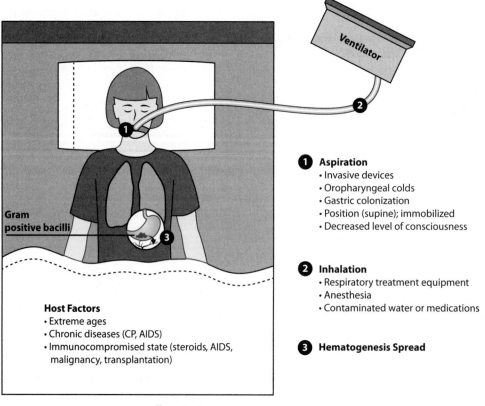

Figure 10-18. Pathogenesis of pneumonia.

TABLE 10-13.   INFECTIOUS ETIOLOGIC AGENTS IN SEVERE COMMUNITY-ACQUIRED PNEUMONIA REQUIRING INTENSIVE CARE SUPPORT AND HOSPITAL-ACQUIRED PNEUMONIA IN CRITICALLY ILL PATIENTS

	Etiologic Agent (Decreasing Rank)
Community-acquired pneumonias	Streptococcus pneumonia
	Staphylococcus aureus
	Legionella species
	Gram-negative bacilli
	Haemophilus influenzae
Ventilator-acquired pneumonias	Staphyloccous aureus
	Pseudomonas aeruginosa
	Klebseilla oxytoca
	Enterobacter species
	Acinetobactor baumannii
	Escherichia coli
	Serratia spp

Data from: Mandell LA, Wunderink RG, Anzueto A, et al. Infections Diseases Society of America/American Thoracic Society consensus guidelines on the management of community-acquired pneumonia in adults. Clin Infect Dis. 2007;44:(suppl 2):S27-S72. Sievert DM, Ricks P, Edwards JR, et al. Antimicrobial-resistant pathogens associated with healthcare-associated infections: summary of data reported to the National Healthcare Safety Network at the Centers for Disease Control and Prevention. 2009-2010. Infect Control Hosp Epidemiol. 2013;34:1-14.

similar organisms cause community-acquired and hospital-acquired pneumonias, their frequency distribution is different (Table 10-13). Of particular concern in hospital-acquired infections is the polymicrobial origin of the pneumonia and the potential for causative organisms to be resistant to antimicrobial therapy.

Development of a hospital-acquired pneumonia is a serious complication in acutely ill patients. Increased morbidity and mortality, in addition to increases in progressive care and hospital lengths of stay and costs, make hospital-acquired pneumonias one of the most important sources of negative outcomes for acutely ill patients.

Clinical Presentation
Signs and Symptoms

- Fever
- Cough, typically productive
- Purulent sputum or hemoptysis
- Dyspnea
- Pleuritic chest pain
- Tachypnea
- Abnormal breath sounds (crackles, bronchial breath sounds)

Diagnostic Tests

- Gram stain and culture of sputum for causative organisms. May require fiberoptic bronchoscopy with brush specimen or bronchoalveolar lavage specimen retrieval in situations where pneumonia responds poorly to treatment. This may also be necessary early in admission in those patients who are immunocompromised, such as those with HIV/AIDS. The pneumonias in these immune deficient patients are often

due to opportunistic organisms that may require very specific antibiotic coverage.
- New or progressive infiltrates on chest x-ray. Infiltrates may be either localized or diffuse in nature (see Figure 10-5).
- Elevated WBC.
- Abnormal arterial blood gases (hypoxemia, hypocapnia).

Principles of Management for Pneumonia
Treating the Underlying Disease

Appropriate empirical broad spectrum antimicrobial therapy should be initiated based on likely causative organisms until definitive culture results are obtained. Fluids should be administered to correct hypovolemia and hypotension, if present. Hypotension unresponsive to fluid therapy should alert the clinician to the potential for septic shock.

Improving Oxygenation and Ventilation

Similar to ARF management, with the following additions:

- PEEP and CPAP are unlikely to improve oxygenation in the presence of a unilateral pneumonia, and may exacerbate the associated ventilation-perfusion abnormalities. These techniques should be used with caution in pneumonia.
- Voluminous, tenacious respiratory secretions may require endotracheal intubation to assist with clearance. Fiberoptic bronchoscopy may also be required to assist with secretion management.

Assessment and Surveillance of Ventilator-Associated Pneumonia in Progressive Care Units who Care for Chronic and Weaning Ventilator Patients

Although the signs and symptoms of VAP are known, clinical diagnosis is complicated by lack of specific and sensitive criteria. In 2013, the National Healthcare Safety Network lead by the Centers for Disease Control began collecting new surveillance criteria for ventilator-associated events, which include ventilator-associated conditions (VAC), infection-related ventilator-associated conditions (IVAC), possible VAP, and probable VAP (Figure 10-19).

Preventing Hospital-Acquired Pneumonias

In addition to the high morbidity and mortality associated with pneumonia in acutely ill patients, high priority must be given to strategies to prevent the development of hospital-acquired pneumonias. The development of a hospital-acquired pneumonia in an acutely ill patient increases requirements for ventilatory support (mechanical ventilation, oxygen, duration of treatment). It is estimated that a hospital-acquired pneumonia increases hospitalization 4 to 10 days, and increases costs by $20,000 to $40,000 per episode. Prevention strategies (Table 10-14) include the following:

- Decrease the risk of cross-contamination or colonization via the hands of hospitalized personnel. Hand washing is the most effective strategy.

Patient has a baseline period of stability or improvement on the ventilator, defined by ≥ 2 calendar days of stable or decreasing daily minimum FiO_2 or PEEP values. The baseline period is defined as the 2 calendar days immediately preceding the first day of increased daily minimum PEEP or FiO_2.

After a period of stability or improvement on the ventilator, the patient has at least one of the following indicators of worsening oxygenation:
1. Minimum daily FiO_2 values increase ≥ 0.20 (20 points) over the daily minimum FiO_2 in the preceding 2 calendar days (the baseline period), for ≥ 2 calendar days.
2. Minimum daily PEEP values increase ≥ 3 cmH_2O over the daily minimum PEEP in the preceding 2 calendar days (the baseline period), for ≥ 2 calendar days.

Ventilator-Associated Condition (VAC)

On or after calendar day 3 of mechanical ventilation and within 2 calendar days before or after the onset of worsening oxygenation, the patient meets both of the following criteria:
1. Temperature > 38°C or < 36°C, **OR** white blood cell count ≥ 12,000 cells/mm³ or ≤ 4,000 cells/mm³
AND
2. A new antimicrobial agent(s)* is started, and is continued for ≥ 4 calendar days.

Infection-related Ventilator-Associated Complication (IVAC)

On or after calendar day 3 of mechanical ventilation and within 2 calendar days before or after the onset of worsening oxygenation; ONE of the following criteria is met:

1. Purulent respiratory secretions (from one or more specimen collections)
   - Defined as secretions from the lungs, bronchi, or trachea that contain > 25 neutrophils and ≤ 10 squamous epithelial cells per low power field [lpf, x 100].
   - If the laboratory reports semi-quantitative results, those results must be equivalent to the above quantitative thresholds.

2. Positive culture (qualitative, semi-quantitative or quantitative) of sputum*, endotracheal aspirate*, bronchoalveolar lavage*, lung tissue, or protected specimen brushing*

Excludes the following:

   - Normal respiratory/oral flora, mixed respiratory/oral flora or equivalent
   - *Candida* species or yeast not otherwise specified
   - Coagulase-negative *Staphylococcus* species
   - *Enterococcus* species

On or after calendar day 3 of mechanical ventilation and within 2 calendar days before or after the onset of worsening oxygenation; ONE of the following criteria is met:

1. Purulent respiratory secretions (from one or more specimen collections– and defined as for possible VAP) AND one of the following:
   - Positive culture of endotracheal aspirate*, ≥ 10⁵ CFU/ml or equivalent semi-quantitative result
   - Positive culture of bronchoalveolar lavage*, ≥ 10⁴ CFU/ml or equivalent semi-quantitative result
   - Positive culture of lung tissue, ≥ 10⁴ CFU/g or equivalent semi-quantitative result
   - Positive culture of protected specimen brush*, ≥ 10³ CFU/ml or equivalent semi-quantitative result
     Same organism exclusions as noted for Possible VAP.

2. One of the following (without requirement for purulent respiratory secretions):
   - Positive pleural fluid culture (where specimen was obtained during thoracentesis or initial placement of chest tube and NOT from an indwelling chest tube)
   - Positive lung histopathology
   - Positive diagnostic test for *Legionella* spp.
   - Positive diagnostic test on respiratory secretions for influenza virus, respiratory syncytial virus, adenovirus, parainfluenza virus, rhinovirus, human metapneumovirus, coronavirus

Possible Ventilator-Associated Pneumonia

Probable Ventilator-Associated Pneumonia

Figure 10-19. Ventilator-Associated Events (VAE) Surveillance Definition Algorithm. (From: the Centers for Disease and Control and Prevention [CDC]). NHSN e-News ventilator-associated event (VAE) surveillance for adults special edition. 2012. Available at: www.cdc.gov/nhsn/psc_da-vae.html.)

- Decrease the risk of aspiration during enteral nutrition. Avoid supine positioning and keep the head of the bed elevated at all times, unless medically contraindicated. Assess for, and correct, gastric reflux problems. Ambulate as soon as possible.
- Eliminate invasive devices and equipment as soon as possible.

For Ventilator Patients

- Avoid supine positioning and keep the head of the bed elevated to 30 to 45 degrees at all times.
- Implement a comprehensive oral hygiene program that includes oral suctioning, teeth brushing, and use of oral 0.12% chlorhexidine gluconate for ventilator patients.

TABLE 10-14. EVIDENCE-BASED PRACTICE GUIDELINES FOR THE PREVENTION OF VENTILATOR-ASSOCIATED PNEUMONIA

Preventing Gastric Reflux

1. All mechanically ventilated patients, as well as those at high risk for aspiration (eg, decreased level of consciousness; enteral tube in place), should have the head of the bed elevated at an angle of 30°-45° unless medically contraindicated.[a,b,c]
2. Routinely verify appropriate placement of the feeding tube.[a]

Airway Management

1. If feasible, use an endotracheal tube with a dorsal lumen above the endotracheal cuff to allow drainage (by continuous or intermittent suctioning) of tracheal secretions that accumulate in the patient's subglottic area.[a,b]
2. Unless contraindicated by the patient's condition, perform orotracheal rather than nasotracheal intubation.[a]
3. ET cuff management: Before deflating the cuff of an endotracheal tube in preparation for tube removal, or before moving the tube, ensure that secretions are cleared from above the tube cuff.[a]
4. Use only sterile fluid to remove secretions from the suction catheter if the catheter is to be used for reentry into the patient's lower respiratory tract.[a]
5. Perform tracheostomy under aseptic conditions.[a]
6. Sedation interruption and daily assessment for readiness to wean.[c]

Oral Care

1. Develop and implement a comprehensive oral hygiene program.[a,c]
2. Use an oral chlorhexidine gluconate (0.12%) rinse.[c]

Cross-Contamination

1. Hand washing: Decontaminate hands with soap and water or a waterless antiseptic agent after contact with mucous membranes, respiratory secretions, or objects contaminated with respiratory secretions, whether or not gloves are worn.[a]
2. Decontaminate hands with soap and water or a waterless antiseptic agent before and after contact with a patient who has an endotracheal or tracheostomy tube, and before and after contact with any respiratory device that is used on the patient, whether or not gloves are worn.[a]
3. Wear gloves for handling respiratory secretions or objects contaminated with respiratory secretions of any patient.[a]
4. When soiling with respiratory secretions is anticipated, wear a gown and change it after soiling and before providing care to another patient.[a]
5. Room-air humidifiers: Do not use large-volume room-air humidifiers that create aerosols (nebulizers) unless they can be sterilized or subjected to high-level disinfection at least daily and filled only with sterile water.[a]

Mobilization

1. Ambulate as soon as medically indicated in the postoperative period.[a]

Equipment Changes

1. Do not change routinely, on the basis of duration of use, the patient's ventilator circuit. Change the circuit when it is visibly soiled or mechanically malfunctioning. Periodically drain or discard any condensate that collects in the tubing. Do not allow condensate to drain toward the patient.[a,b]
2. Between use on different patients, sterilize or subject to high-level disinfection all MRBs.[a]

Data from: [a]Centers for Disease Control and Prevention (2004), [b]AACN VAP Practice Alert (2008), and [c]Institute for Healthcare Improvement (2012).

- Use sterile technique for tracheal suctioning and suction only when necessary to clear secretions from large airways.
- Maintain a closed system on ventilator/humidifier circuits and avoid pooling of condensation or secretions in the tubing. Do not routinely change the ventilator circuit, except when visibly soiled or malfunctioning. Use sterile water or saline for use with any respiratory equipment.

- Provide nutritional support to improve host defenses.
- Eliminate invasive devices and equipment as soon as possible. Assess weaning readiness daily and limit the use of sedatives (see Chapter 6, Pain and Sedation Management).

Pulmonary Embolism

Etiology, Risk Factors, and Pathophysiology

Pulmonary embolism is a complication of deep venous thrombosis (DVT), long bone fracture, or air entering the circulatory system. There are many risk factors for PE (Table 10-15), with acutely ill patients being especially prone due to the presence of central venous catheters, immobility, use of muscle relaxants, and heart failure.

Venous Thromboembolism (VTE)

Venous thrombi form at the site of vascular injuries or where venous stasis occurs, primarily in the leg or pelvic veins. Thrombi that dislodge travel through the venous circulation until they become wedged in a branch of the pulmonary circulation. Depending on the size of the thrombi, and the

TABLE 10-15. RISK FACTORS FOR THE DEVELOPMENT OF PULMONARY EMBOLISM

Thromboemboli

- Obesity
- Prior history of thromboembolism
- Advanced age
- Malignancy
- Estrogen
- Immobility
- Paralysis
- Heart failure
- Postpartum
- Postsurgical
- Posttrauma
- Hypercoagulability states
- Central venous and PA catheters

Air Emboli

- Neurosurgery
- Liver transplant
- Harrington rod insertion
- Open heart surgery
- Arthroscopy
- Pacemaker insertion
- Cardiopulmonary resuscitation
- Gastroscopy
- Positive pressure ventilation
- Scuba diving
- Intravenous infusion
- Central venous catheter insertion or removal

Fat Emboli

- Long bone fracture
- Blunt trauma to liver
- Pancreatitis
- Lipid infusions
- Sickle cell crisis
- Burns
- Cardiopulmonary bypass
- Cyclosporine administration

location of the occlusion, mild to severe obstruction of blood flow occurs beyond the thrombi.

The primary sequela, and major contributor to mortality, of the pulmonary obstruction is circulatory impairment. The physical obstruction of the pulmonary capillary bed increases right ventricular afterload, dilates the right ventricle, and impedes coronary perfusion. This predisposes the right ventricle to ischemia and right ventricular failure (cor pulmonale).

A secondary consequence of thromboemboli is a mismatching of ventilation to perfusion in gas exchange units beyond the obstruction (see Figure 10-15C), resulting in arterial hypoxemia. This hypoxemia further compromises oxygen delivery to the ischemic right ventricle.

Air Emboli

Air or other nonabsorbable gases entering the venous system also travel to the right heart, pulmonary circulation, arterioles, and capillaries. A variety of surgical and non-surgical situations predispose patients to the development of air embolization (see Table 10-15). Damage to the pulmonary endothelium occurs from the abnormal air-blood interface, leading to increased capillary permeability and alveolar flooding. Bronchoconstriction also occurs with air embolization. In addition to hypoxemia, Pco_2 removal is also impaired.

Arterial embolization may occur if air passes to the left heart through a patent foramen ovale, present in approximately 30% of the population. Peripheral embolization to the brain, extremities, and coronary perfusion leads to ischemic manifestations in these organs.

Fat Emboli

Fat enters the pulmonary circulation most commonly when released from the bone marrow following long bone fractures (see Table 10-15). Nontraumatic origins of fat embolization also occur and are thought to be due to the agglutination of low-density lipoproteins or liposomes from nutritional fat emulsions. The presence of fat in the pulmonary circulation injures the endothelial lining of the capillary, increasing permeability and alveolar flooding.

Clinical Presentation

The diagnosis of PE is based primarily on clinical signs and symptoms. Because many of the signs and symptoms are nonspecific, PE frequently is difficult to diagnosis. In acutely ill patients, diagnosis is especially difficult owing to alterations in communication and level of consciousness, and the nonspecific nature of other cardiopulmonary alterations.

Signs and Symptoms

- Dyspnea
- Pleuritic chest pain
- Cough
- Rales
- Apprehension
- Diaphoresis
- Evidence of DVT
- Hemoptysis
- Tachypnea
- Fever
- Tachycardia
- Syncope
- Hypoxia
- Hypotension

Diagnostic Tests

- *Chest x-ray:* Evaluate for basilar atelectasis, elevation of the diaphragm, and pleural effusion, although most patients have nonspecific findings on chest x-ray; diffuse alveolar filling in air embolism.
- *Arterial blood gas analysis:* Hypoxemia with or without hypercarbia.
- *ECG:* Signs of right ventricular strain (right axis deviation, right bundle branch block) or precordial strain; sinus tachycardia.

See earlier discussion of diagnostics for PE.

Principles of Management for Pulmonary Emboli

The key to preventing morbidity and mortality from PE is primarily prevention and secondarily early diagnosis and treatment to prevent reembolization. Objectives include the improvement of oxygenation and ventilation, improvement of cardiovascular function, prevention of reembolization, and prevention of pulmonary embolus.

Improving Oxygenation and Ventilation

Oxygen therapy is usually very effective in relieving hypoxemia associated with PE. When cardiopulmonary compromise is severe, the patient may need to be moved into the ICU for intubation and mechanical ventilation to achieve optimal oxygenation.

Improving Cardiovascular Function

Controversy exists as to the benefit of vasoactive drug administration (such as norepinephrine and/or inotropic agents) to improve myocardial perfusion of the right ventricle. In severe embolic events, where cardiac failure is profound, additional therapy to hasten clot resolution, such as use of thrombolytic agents and/or interventional removal of massive emboli may be warranted.

Preventing Reembolization

Several strategies are employed to prevent the likelihood of future embolization and cardiopulmonary compromise:

- Limiting activity to prevent dislodgement of additional clots.
- Use of anticoagulation therapy with unfractionated heparin to maintain a PTT 1.5 to 2.5 times the control when no contraindication exists.
- Insertion of vena cava filters to prevent emboli from legs, pelvis, and inferior vena cava from migrating to pulmonary circulation if anticoagulation therapy is

TABLE 10-16. RISK FACTORS, ASSESSMENT AND THROMBOPROPHYLAXIS FOR VTE

Risk Factor for VTE	Risk Assessment	Suggested Thromboprophylaxis
• Surgery • Trauma • Immobility • Cancer	**Low Risk** Minor surgery in mobile patients Medical patient who are fully mobile	Early and aggressive ambulation

• Venous compression
• Previous VTE
• Age
• Pregnancy and postpartum
	Moderate Risk
	Most general, open gynecologic or urologic
	  surgery patients
	Medical patients who are immobile
		Low-molecular-weight heparin, unfractionated heparin,
		  or fondaparinux

• Oral contraceptives and hormone
  replacement therapy
• Erythropoiesis-stimulating agents
• Acute medical illness
	Moderate Risk plus Bleeding Risk	Mechanical thromboprophylaxis, consider switch to
		  pharmacologic prophylaxis when bleeding risk
		  decreases

• Inflammatory bowel disease • Nephritic syndrome • Myeloproliferative disorders • Paroxysmal nocturnal hemoglobinuria • Obesity • Central venous catheter	**High Risk** Hip or knee arthroplasty Hip fracture surgery Major trauma Spinal cord injury **High Risk plus bleeding Risk**	Low-molecular-weight heparin, fondaparinux, oral vitamin K antagonist
• Thrombophilia		Low-molecular-weight heparin, unfractionated heparin, or fondaparinux

contraindicated. Filters are placed percutaneously in the inferior vena cava.

Preventing Venous Thromboembolism (VTE)

- An important recommendation for the prevention of VTE is awareness and access to a hospital prevention policy including risk assessment (Table 10-16).
- A risk assessment should be done on admission to the unit and discussion daily on rounds should take place. Discussion should also include current VTE prevention intervention, risk for bleeding, and response to treatment.
- If ordered, graduated compression stocking or IPCs (Figure 10-20; Table 10-17) should be in use at all times except when being removed for correct fitting or skin assessment.
- Placement of prophylactic vena cava filters in high-risk patients.

- Early fixation of long bone fractures to prevent fat emboli.
- Early mobilization. As soon as hemodynamic stability is achieved, and there are no other contraindications to mobilization, activity level should begin increasing to include sitting in a chair several times per day and short periods of ambulation.

ESSENTIAL CONTENT CASE

COPD Exacerbation

You are caring for a patient with COPD who was admitted with the following ABGs:

- -pH   7.31
- -Pao$_2$ 63 mm Hg
- -Paco$_2$ 86 mm Hg

He was awake but somewhat confused and was placed on BiPAP support (IPAP 16 cm H$_2$O, EPAP 5 cm H$_2$O, Fio$_2$ 0.40).

After 2 hours he is becoming increasingly difficult to arouse. His RR is 22 breaths/min and labored, and his heart rate is 122 beats/min.

Case Question: What assessment criteria lead you to suspect this patient is not tolerating noninvasive mechanical ventilation and may need to be intubated?

Answer

The patient's level of consciousness is decreased, and he has labored respirations, and an elevated heart rate. An ABG should be obtained, as it is likely his Paco$_2$ is high and his pH is very low. His decrease in consciousness requires that he be intubated and ventilated while further assessment is accomplished or he will likely code.

**BiBAP is contraindicated in patients with decreased mental status and inability to protect the airway (see Chapter 5, Airway and Ventilatory Management).

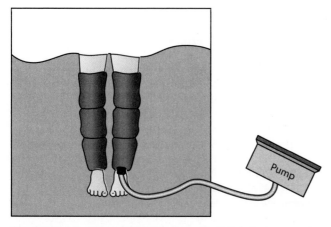

Figure 10-20. Intermittent pneumatic compression (IPC) device for prevention of DVT and PE.

TABLE 10-17. TIPS FOR SAFE AND EFFECTIVE USE OF INTERMITTENT PNEUMATIC COMPRESSION DEVICES

- Follow manufacturer recommendations for the correct fit, including patient measurement.
- Include ongoing assessment for fit as changes in weight and fluid shifts occur.
- Monitor that the devices are on the patient and in correct placement.
- Implement patient and family teaching regarding VTE and the role of mechanical prophylaxis COPD.
- Ensure that devices do not impede ambulation.

SELECTED BIBLIOGRAPHY

Critical Care Management of Respiratory Problems

Burns S, ed. *Protocols for Practice: Care of the Mechanically Ventilated Patient*. Sudbury, MA: Jones and Bartlett Publishers; 2006.

Burns SM. Ventilating patient with acute severe asthma: what do we really know? AACN *Adv Crit Care*. 2006;17:186-193.

Carlson KK. ed. *Advanced Critical Care Nursing*. St Louis, MO: Saunders Elsevier; 2008.

Collins PF, Stratton RJ, Elia M. Nutritional support in chronic obstructive pulmonary disease: a systematic review and meta-analysis. *Am J Clin Nutr*. 2012;95:1385-1395.

Epstein SK. Noninvasive ventilation to shorten the duration of mechanical ventilation. *Resp Care*. 2009;54:198-211.

Geiger-Bronsky M, Wilson DJ, eds. *Respiratory Nursing: A Core Curriculum*. New York, NY: Springer Publishing Company; 2008.

Ginn MB, Cox G, Health J. Evidence-based approach to an inpatient tobacco cessation protocol. *AACN Adv Crit Care*. 2008;19: 268-278.

Halm MA. Relaxation: a self-care healing modality reduces harmful effects of anxiety. *Am J Crit Care*. 2009;18:169-172.

Louie S, Morrissey BM, Kenyon NJ, Albertson TE, Avdalovic M. The critically ill asthmatic; from ICU to discharge. *Clin Rev Allerg Immunol*. 2012;43:30-44.

Maki MB, Martin SA, Burns S, Philbrick D, Rauen C. Putting evidence into nursing practice: four traditional practices not supported by evidence. *Crit Care Nurse*. 2013;33:28-42.

Matthay MA, Ware LB, Zimmerman GA. The acute respiratory distress syndrome. *J Clin Invest*. 2012;122:2731-2740.

McLean B. Acute respiratory failure and intensive measures, *Crit Care Nurs Clin N Am*. 2012;24:361-375.

Raghavendran K, Napolitano LM. Definition of ALI/ARDS. *Crit Care Clin*. 2011;27:429-437.

Raoff S, Goulet K, Esan A, Hess DR, Sessler C. Severe hypoxemic respiratory failure, part 2; nonventilatory strategies. *Chest*. 2010;137:1437-1448.

Rauen CA, Flynn Makic MB, Bridges E. Evidence-based practice habits: transforming research into bedside practice. *Crit Care Nurs*. 2009;29:46-59.

The ARDS Definition Task Force. Acute respiratory distress syndrome; the Berlin definition. 2012;307:2526-2533.

Urden LD, Stacy KM, Lough ME. *Thelan's Critical Care Nursing: Diagnosis and Management*. 6th ed. St Louis, MO:Mosby; 2010.

Chest X-Ray Interpretation

Connolly MA. Black, white, and shades of gray: common abnormalities in chest radiographs. *AACN Clin Issues*. 2001;12(2):259-269.

Eisenhuber E, Schaefer-Prokop CM, Prosch H, Schima W. Bedside chest radiography. *Resp Care*. 2012;57:427-443.

Godoy MC, Leitman BS, deGroot PM, Viahos J, Naidich DP. Chest radiography in the ICU: part 1; evaluation of airway, enteric, and pleural tubes. *Am J Roentgenol*. 2012;198:563-571.

Sanchez F. Fundamentals of chest x-ray interpretation. *Crit Care Nurse*. 1986;6:41-52.

Siela D. Chest radiography evaluation and interpretation. *Adv Crit Care*. 2008;19:444-473.

Miscellaneous

Lynn-McHale DJ. *AACN Procedure Manual for Critical Care*, 5th ed. Philadelphia, PA: Elsevier-Saunders; 2011.

Evidence-Based Practice Guidelines

AACN Deep Vein Thrombosis Prevention Practice Alert. Aliso Viejo, CA: AACN; 2010. http://www/aacn.org. Accessed February 18, 2013.

AACN VAP Practice Alert. Aliso Viejo, CA: AACN; 2008. http://www.aacn.org. Accessed February 18, 2013.

American College of Chest Physician. Antithrombotic and thrombolytic therapy: American College of Chest Physicians evidence based clinical practice guidelines. 2012 (9th ed). http://journal.publications.chestnet.org/issue.aspx?journalid=99&issueid=23443. Accessed February 21, 2013.

American Thoracic Society and the European Respiratory Society. International multidisciplinary consensus classification of the idiopathic interstitial pneumonias. *Am J Respir Crit Care Med*. 2002;165:277-304.

American Thoracic Society and the Infectious Diseases Society of America. Guidelines for the management of adults with hospital-acquired, ventilator-associated, and healthcare-associated pneumonia. *Am J Respir Crit Care Med*. 2005;171:388-416.

Centers for Disease Control and Prevention. Guidelines for prevention of health-care-associated pneumonia, 2003: Recommendations of CDC and the Healthcare Infection Control Practices Advisory Committee. *MMWR*. 2004;53(No. RR-3):1-35.

Ernst A, Silvestri GA, Johnstone D. Interventional pulmonary procedures: Guidelines from the American College of Chest Physicians. *Chest*. 2003;123:1693-1717.

Filore MC, Jaen CR, Baker TB. Treating tobacco use and dependence: 2008 Update. Quick Reference Guide for Clinicians. Rockville, MD: U.S. Department of Health and Human Services. Public Health Services: April 2009.

Gold Executive Committee. Global strategy for the diagnosis, management, and prevention of chronic obstructive pulmonary disease (Updated 2013). http://www.goldcopd.org/. Accessed February 20, 2013.

Mandell LA, Wunderink RG, Anzueto A, et al. Infectious Diseases Society of America/American Thoracic Society consensus guidelines on the management of community-acquired pneumonia in adults. *Clin Infect Dis*. 2007;44(suppl 2):S27-S72.

McClave SA, Martindale RG, Vanek VW. Guidelines for the provision and assessment of nutrition support therapy in the adult critically ill patient: Society of Critical Care Medicine (SCCCM) and the American Society for Parenteral and Enteral Nutrition (ASPEN). *J Parenter Enteral Nutr.* 2009;33:277-316.

McLaughlin VV, Archer SL, Badesch DB, et al. ACCF/AHA 2009 expert concensus document on pulmonary hypertension: a report of the American College of Cardiology foundation task force on expert consensus documents and the American Heart Association. *Circulation.* 2009;119:2250-2294.

National Heart, Lung, and Blood Institute. Expert Panel Report 3: Guidelines for the Diagnosis and Management of Asthma, Full Report 2007. http://www.nhlbi.nih.gov/guidelines/asthma/asth-gdln.pdf. Accessed February 21, 2013.

National Heart, Lung, and Blood Institute. Global Initiative for Asthma (GINA) Global Strategy for Asthma Management and Prevention. http://www.ginasthma.org/uploads/users/files/GINA_Report_2012Feb13.pdf. Accessed February 21, 2013.

National Heart, Lung, and Blood Institute. Global Initiative for Chronic Obstructive Lung Disease (GOLD) Global Strategy for the Diagnosis, Management, and Prevention of Chronic Obstructive Pulmonary Disease. http://www.goldcopd.org/uploads/users/files/GOLD_Report_2013_Feb20.pdf. Accessed February 21, 2013.

Parshall MB, Schwartzstein RM, Adams L, et al. An official America Thoracic Society statement: update on the mechanisms, assessment, and management of dyspnea. *Am J Respir Crit Care Med.* 2012;185:435-452.

Qaseem A, Wilt TJ, Weingberger SE, et al. Diagnosis and management of stable chronic obstructive pulmonary disease: a clinical practice guideline update from the American College of Physicians, American College of Chest Physicians, American Thoracic Society, and European Respiratory Society. *Annals Intern Med.* 2011;155:179-192.

Raghu G, Collard HR, Egan JJ. An official ATS/ERS/JRS/ALAT statement: idiopathic pulmonary fibrosis: evidence-based guidelines for diagnosis and management. *Am J Respir Crit Care Med.* 2011;183:788-824.

Task Force for Diagnosis and Treatment of Pulmonary Hypertension of European Society of Cardiology (ESC), European Respiratory Society (ERS), International Society of Heart and Lung Transplantation (ISHLT). Guidelines for the diagnosis and treatment of pulmonary hypertension. *Eur Respir J.* 2009:34: 1219-1263.

The ARDS Definition Task Force. Acute Respiratory Distress Syndrome: the Berlin Definition. *JAMA.* 2012;307:2526-2533.

MULTISYSTEM PROBLEMS

11

Ruth M. Kleinpell

KNOWLEDGE COMPETENCIES

1. Identify the relationship between the cellular mediators and clinical manifestations of systemic inflammatory response syndrome (SIRS).

2. Describe the etiology, pathophysiology, clinical manifestations, patient needs, and principles of management of SIRS, sepsis, and associated conditions leading to multisystem problems.

3. Compare and contrast the pathophysiology, clinical manifestations, patient needs, and

management approaches for multisystem problems resulting from SIRS, sepsis, multiple organ dysfunction, and overdoses.

4. Describe the symptoms and pharmacologic management of the patient suffering from alcohol withdrawal syndrome.

5. Describe treatment considerations for complex wounds and pressure ulcers.

PATHOLOGIC CONDITIONS

Sepsis and Multiple Organ Dysfunction Syndrome

Any acute illness can predispose patients to several complex conditions including sepsis and multiple organ dysfunction syndrome (MODS) (Table 11-1). Sepsis results from an infectious process and represents a systemic response to infection. Sepsis with acute organ dysfunction (severe sepsis) commonly occurs in patients cared for in progressive or critical care units. Sepsis is a serious worldwide healthcare condition that is associated with high mortality rates, despite improvements in the ability to manage infection. Severe sepsis incidence increases annually by 13% with associated mortality rates of 15% to 29%. It is the third most common cause of death in the United States. Patients in any progressive care unit are vulnerable to the condition. Thus, understanding the syndrome and initiating early therapy may prevent deterioration, transfer to a critical care unit, and ultimately death. Systemic inflammatory response syndrome (SIRS) is a systemic response to a clinical insult, such as an infection or burn (Figure 11-1). In some cases, the syndrome may progress to sepsis and

MODS. The stimulus for SIRS can be singular or multifactorial. Examples of situations that can precipitate SIRS are burns, trauma, transfusions, pancreatitis, or infection. Following the insult, an inflammatory response is initiated as a normal physiologic response. The inflammatory response consists of vasodilatation, increased microvascular permeability, cellular activation and release of mediators, and coagulation (see Figure 11-1). In SIRS, there is an excessive release of these mediators, which may lead to severe tissue damage, with hypoperfusion of organ systems.

Systemic inflammatory response syndrome is manifested in a variety of ways: fever, tachycardia, tachypnea, altered level of consciousness, and decreased urine output. These findings may or may not be the result of an infection. If the response progresses unchecked, the result may be the development of sepsis or dysfunction of one or more organ systems, or MODS. The SIRS, sepsis, and MODS may be thought of as progressively severe conditions along a continuum. The key is early identification of the signs and symptoms of SIRS, and prompt development of a treatment plan to avoid further progression. Early intervention is important to ensure good outcomes in these patients.

TABLE 11-1. INFLAMMATORY RESPONSES: DEFINITIONS

Term	Definition
Bacteremia	The presence of viable bacteria in the blood.
Hypotension	A systolic BP of < 90 mm Hg or a reduction of > 40 mm Hg from baseline in the absence of other causes for hypotension.
Infection	Microbial phenomenon characterized by an inflammatory response to the presence of microorganisms or the invasion of normally sterile host tissue by those organisms.
MODS	Presence of altered organ function in an acutely ill patient such that homeostasis cannot be maintained without intervention.
Sepsis	The systemic response to infection. This systemic response is manifested by two or more of the following conditions as a result of infection: • Temperature > 38.0°C (100.4°F) • Heart rate > 90 beats/min • Respiratory rate > 20 breaths/min or $Paco_2$ < 32 mm Hg • WBC > 12,000 cells/mm³, < 4000 cells/mm³, or > 10% immature (band) forms
Septic shock	Sepsis with hypotension, despite adequate fluid resuscitation, along with the presence of perfusion abnormalities that may include, but are not limited to, lactic acidosis, oliguria, or an acute alteration in mental status. Patients who are on inotropic or vasopressor agents may not be hypotensive at the time that perfusion abnormalities are measured.
Severe sepsis	Sepsis associated with organ dysfunction, hypoperfusion, or hypotension. Hypoperfusion and perfusion abnormalities may include, but are not limited to, lactic acidosis, oliguria, or an acute alteration in mental status.
SIRS	The systemic inflammatory response to a variety of severe clinical insults. The response is manifested by two or more of the following conditions: • Temperature > 38.0°C (100.4°F) • Heart rate > 90 beats/min • Respiratory rate > 20 breaths/min or $Paco_2$ < 32 mm Hg • WBC > 12,000 cells/mm³, < 4000 cells/mm³, or > 10% immature (band) forms

Data from: ACCP/SCCM Consensus Committee: definitions for sepsis and organ failure and guidelines for the use of innovative therapies in sepsis. Crit Care Med. 1992;20:866.

Etiology, Risk Factors, and Pathophysiology
Systemic Inflammatory Response Syndrome

Systemic inflammatory response syndrome consists of a series of systemic events that occur in response to an insult to the body. This response is a cellular reaction that initiates a number of mediator-induced responses, and is both inflammatory and immune in nature (Figure 11-2).

There are essentially four different types of cells that are activated as part of the response to an insult or stimulus: polymorphonuclear cells (neutrophils), macrophages, platelets, and endothelial cells. These cells are activated to become either directly involved in the reaction (ie, platelet aggregation) or are stimulated to produce and release chemical mediators into the circulation, such as cytokines or plasma enzymes. Once activated, "a checks and balances system" is normally in place to control the inflammatory response. In some situations, however, when the response is large or the injury diffuse, local control of the response is lost, leading

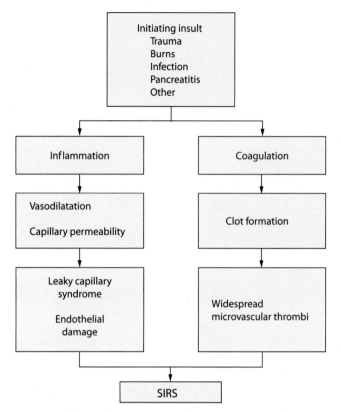

Figure 11-1. SIRS results from activation of interactive cascades of inflammation and coagulation.

to excessive mediator release with consequent organ damage. The cellular activation response is highly individualized, and subsequent organ compromise is also variable.

A general understanding of the various mediators responsible for the SIRS is important. Mediators can be divided into five groups: cytokines, plasma enzyme cascades, lipid mediators, toxic oxygen-derived metabolites, and unclassified mediators such as nitric oxide and proteases. These mediators are stimulated after cellular activation in response to a certain stimulus (eg, infection, trauma, pancreatitis). Cytokines are active chemical substances secreted by cells in response to a stimulus. If secreted by lymphocytes, they are called lymphokines, and if secreted by monocytes or macrophages, they are called monokines. Examples of cytokines include tumor necrosis factor, interleukin, interferon, and colony-stimulating factors such as granulocyte colony-stimulating factor.

In addition to cytokines, there is also activation of different enzymatic plasma cascades. Examples of these include the complement cascade and the various coagulation cascades. In addition, there are various lipid mediators that are either stimulated or produced as part of a cellular destructive process. These lipid mediators include arachidonic acid metabolites, leukotrienes, prostaglandins, and platelet-activating factor. Oxygen-derived free radicals are another group of mediators that exert a negative effect as part of the SIRS. Examples of these include hydrogen peroxide and hydroxyl radical. Nitric oxide and proteases are other mediators that

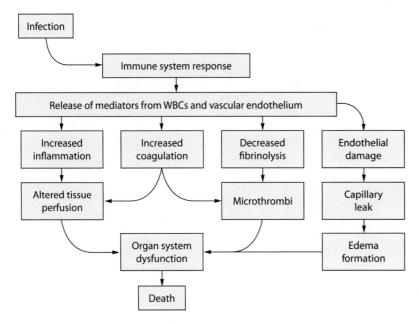

Figure 11-2. Interactive cascade of inflammation and coagulation, leading to endothelium damage, diffuse thrombi, and organ system dysfunction. (*Reprinted with permission: Kleinpell R. New initiatives focus on prevention and early recognition of sepsis. Nurs Spectrum. 2004;17[12]:24-26.*)

are not grouped into any of the previous categories, but are mediators that enhance the SIRS.

In addition to the mediators stimulated as part of the inflammatory and immune responses, mediators related to hormonal stimulation and regulation are also produced. The hormonal response component of the SIRS is characterized by the release of stress hormones (catecholamines, glucagon, cortisol, and growth hormone), suppression of thyroid hormone, and hormonal regulation of fluid and electrolyte balance. Toll-like receptors, or transmembrane proteins that are expressed on various immune cells such as neutrophils and macrophages, have been implicated in ischemia-reperfusion injury that can further alter perfusion and contribute to inflammation.

Sepsis

Sepsis is the manifestation of the SIRS in response to an infectious process (see Table 11-1). The source of infection may be bacterial, viral, fungal, or on rare occasions, rickettsial or protozoal.

The risk factors for development of sepsis are many and include malnutrition, immunosuppression, prolonged antibiotic use, and the presence of invasive devices (Table 11-2). It is important to remember that a large number of infections in acutely ill patients are hospital acquired and can lead to sepsis. Many of these hospital-acquired infections can be prevented with simple measures. The role of the progressive care nurse is instrumental in preventing hospital acquired infections. Hand washing remains the single most effective method for preventing nosocomial infections. Recent research suggests that relatively simple measures such as ensuring head-of-bed elevation and meticulous mouth care may prevent ventilator-associated pneumonia, a common source of sepsis in acutely ill patients. Therefore, nursing measures to target sepsis prevention as well as early recognition and treatment are important in reducing the high mortality rates associated with severe sepsis (Table 11-3).

TABLE 11-2. RISK FACTORS FOR THE DEVELOPMENT OF SEPSIS

Host-Related Factors	Treatment-Related Factors
Malnutrition	
Immune deficiency disorders	Invasive diagnostic devices
Immunosuppression	Invasive therapeutic devices
Skin breakdown	Surgical procedures
Fragile skin/mucous membranes	Prolonged hospitalization
Traumatic injuries	Therapeutic immunosuppression
Burns	Chemotherapy
Pressure sores	Radiation therapy
IV drug abuse	Splenectomy
EtOH abuse	Urinary catheters
Chronic illness	Use of H_2 receptor antagonists (leading
Diabetes mellitus	to gastric bacterial overgrowth and
Neoplastic disease	aspiration pneumonia)
Cirrhosis	Aggressive resuscitation
Renal failure	Prolonged TPN
Cardiac disease	Extensive antibiotic therapy
Pulmonary disease	Pain/stress
Pregnancy associated with prolonged rupture of membranes	
Immune senescence (elderly)	
Poor mobility	
Bedridden status	
BPH	
Decreased mucociliary transport mechanisms	
Decreased cough and clearance function	
Increased response to influenza vaccine	
UTI	
Vaginal colonization with GBS	
Perineal colonization with *Escherichia coli*	
Premature rupture of membranes	

Adapted with permission from: Klein DM, Witek-Janusek L. Advances in immunotherapy of sepsis. Dimensions Crit Care Nurs. 1992;11(2):75-81.

TABLE 11-3. NURSING CARE OF PATIENTS WITH SEVERE SEPSIS

Recognition	Early identification of patients at risk for developing sepsis
	• Elderly
	• Immunocompromised
	• Patients with surgical/invasive procedures
	• Patients with indwelling catheters
	• Mechanically ventilated patients
Monitoring physical assessment parameters	Vital signs
	• Fever/hypothermia
	• Tachycardia
	• Tachypnea
	• Hypotension
	Hemodynamic parameters
	• Heart rate/rhythm and presence of ectopy
	• Hemodynamic monitoring parameter changes (elevated CO and low systemic vascular resistance)
	Ventilatory parameters
	• Respiratory rate
	• Lung sounds
	• Oxygenation status (pulse oximetry, arterial blood gases, mixed venous oxygen saturation levels)
	Renal parameters
	• Hourly urine output monitoring
	• Note sudden/gradual decreases in urine output
	• Monitor laboratory parameters of renal function (creatinine, BUN levels, fractional excretion of sodium levels)
	Coagulation parameters
	• Monitor coagulation indices (thrombocytopenia, prothrombin time, activated partial thromboplastin time, INR)
	• Monitor for bruising, bleeding
	Metabolic parameters
	• Provide nutritional support
	• Recognize role of intact gut barrier in preventing translocation of gram-negative bacteria
	• Maintain nitrogen balance in hypermetabolic state
	• Provide normalization of hyperglycemia
	Mental status parameters
	• Mental status changes (restlessness, confusion)
	• Changes in GCS
Provide comprehensive sepsis treatment	• Circulatory support with fluids, inotropes, and vasopressors
	• Implement the sepsis bundles
	• Supportive treatment with oxygenation and ventilation
	• Antibiotic administration
	• Monitoring and reporting patient response to treatment
Promote patient and family comfort care	Promote patient comfort/pain relief/sedation
	• Turning/skin care
	• Patient and family teaching
	• Address needs of families of critically ill patients
Sepsis prevention	Prevention remains the best treatment
	• Hand washing
	• Universal precautions
	• Measures to prevent hospital-acquired infections and iatrogenic complications:
	• Ventilator-associated pneumonia (see practice guidelines in Chapter 10, Respiratory System)
	• DVT and GI prophylaxis
	• Invasive catheter care
	• Wound care
	• Urinary catheter care
	• Astute clinical assessment
	• Maintain mucosal integrity
	• Prevent translocation
	• Formulate a sepsis prevention plan
	• Educate members of the healthcare team on identification and treatment of sepsis
	• Screen patients daily for signs of sepsis
	• Monitor sepsis cases and outcomes
	• Track changes in sepsis incidence rates and outcomes

Data from: Kleinpell R, Aitken L, and Schorr CA. Implications of the new international sepsis guidelines for nursing care. Am J Crit Care. 2013;22:212-220.

TABLE 11-4. SIGNS OF ACUTE ORGAN SYSTEM DYSFUNCTION

Cardiovascular	• Tachycardia • Arrhythmias • Hypotension • Elevated central venous and pulmonary artery pressures
Respiratory	• Tachypnea • Hypoxemia
Renal	• Oliguria • Anuria • Elevated creatinine
Hematologic	• Jaundice • Elevated liver enzymes • Decreased albumin • Coagulopathy
Gastrointestinal	• Ileus (absent bowel sounds)
Hepatic	• Thrombocytopenia • Coagulopathy • Decreased protein C levels • Increased D-dimer levels
Neurologic	• Altered consciousness • Confusion • Psychosis

Data from: Balk R: Pathogenesis and management of multiple organ dysfunction or failure in severe sepsis and septic shock. Crit Care Clin. 2000;16(2):337-352, with permission from Elsevier.

Severe Sepsis

Sepsis can progress to severe sepsis, with organ dysfunction, hypoperfusion, or severe hypotension. Severe sepsis (sepsis that has progressed to cellular dysfunction and organ damage or evidence of hypoperfusion) and septic shock (sepsis with persistent hypotension despite adequate fluid resuscitation) are associated with high mortality rates, despite improvements in the ability to manage infection. Hypoperfusion and perfusion abnormalities that occur in severe sepsis may include oliguria, lactic acidosis, hypoxemia, and alteration in mental status (Table 11-4). Severe sepsis is associated with three integrated responses: activation of inflammation, activation of coagulation, and impairment of fibrinolysis. The result is systemic inflammation, widespread coagulopathy, and microvascular thrombosis, conditions that often lead to multiple organ dysfunction.

Multiple Organ Dysfunction Syndrome

Multiple organ dysfunction syndrome (MODS) is the worsening progression of the SIR. If SIRS is allowed to persist unchecked, or becomes overwhelming, the patient develops clinical manifestations of organ dysfunction. The mortality rates for MODS vary depending on the underlying cause, with mortality rates ranging from 50% to 100% as the number of involved organs increases.

Multiple organ dysfunction syndrome can be classified as either primary or secondary. In primary MODS, organ dysfunction is a direct effect of an insult to an organ that has been compromised; for example, aspiration causes lung dysfunction, or acetaminophen overdose causes liver dysfunction. With primary MODS, the onset occurs relatively soon after the insult. In secondary MODS, the organ dysfunction occurs as the result of persistent and prolonged mediator release following an insult such as a thermal burn or pancreatitis. Generally, the time frame for secondary MODS is 7 to 10 days; however, this onset is variable.

ESSENTIAL CONTENT CASE

Sepsis

A 67-year-old man with a 6-year history of hypertension and a 30-pack per year cigarette history was admitted to the progressive care unit with a diagnosis of cirrhosis secondary to biliary obstruction. He underwent an exploratory laparotomy and cholecystectomy 3 days ago. Postoperatively, he was relatively stable, experiencing an episode of hypotension 12 hours postoperatively, which was corrected by fluid administration. He remains intubated and attempts at weaning have been delayed due to periodic hypoxemia.

He currently has an arterial line and a central venous pressure (CVP) monitoring, T-tube drain, and an indwelling urinary catheter. He is alert and oriented, moving in bed with little assistance. Physical examination reveals that his skin is pale pink and warm to touch, lungs have a few bibasilar crackles, and pedal edema is present bilaterally. His abdomen is nondistended, no active bowel sounds. His 5 inch midline abdominal wound requires dressing changes 3 times daily and is approximated with retention sutures. Current vital signs are:

T	38.6°C (101.0°F) core
HR	122 beats/min

Sinus tachycardia
RR	34 breaths/min
BP	82/60 mm Hg

Current laboratory results are:
ABG: pH 7.30, Pao_2 62, $Paco_2$ 46, HCO_3 18, Sao_2 94%
WBC: 22,000, 65 neutrophils, 50 segs, 12 bands, 40,000 platelets
RBC: 4.5, Hct 39, Hgb 13, bili 2.2 mg, LDH 220, Na^1 140, K^1 3.5, Cl 100, CO_2 20, BUN 22, Creat 1.1

Case Question 1. Why might this patient be at risk for developing sepsis?

Case Question 2. What clinical signs and symptoms may be evidence of early sepsis?

Case Question 3. Is he exhibiting SIRS criteria?

Answers
1. Postoperative status, intubated, invasive lines and catheters, abdominal wound requiring dressing changes are risk factors for sepsis in this patient.
2. Elevated temperature, elevated white blood cell count with bandemia, sinus tachycardia, elevated respiratory rate are clinical symptoms of early sepsis.
3. Yes.

Clinical Presentation

Systemic Inflammatory Response Syndrome

Systemic inflammatory response syndrome is the clinical manifestation of two or more of the following conditions:

- Temperature > 38°C (100.4°F) or < 36°C (96.8°F)
- Heart rate > 90 beats/min
- Respiratory rate > 20 breaths/min or $Paco_2$ < 32 mm Hg
- WBC > 12,000 cells/mm^3, < 4000 cells/mm^3 or > 10% immature neutrophils (band) forms

Close monitoring and assessment are essential for the detection of early signs of SIRS.

Severe Sepsis

The clinical manifestation of severe sepsis is the result of altered perfusion to vital organ systems. Organ system dysfunction develops due to hypoperfusion and microvascular thrombosis. Table 11-4 summarizes the common manifestations of severe sepsis. Signs of organ system dysfunction include cardiovascular alterations (hypotension, tachycardia, dysrhythmias), respiratory system alterations (tachypnea, hypoxemia), renal system alterations (oliguria, elevated creatinine), hematologic system alterations (thrombocytopenia), gastrointestinal alteration (change in bowel sounds, ileus), hepatic alterations (elevated liver enzymes, jaundice, coagulopathies), and neurologic system alterations (confusion, agitation). Early recognition and treatment are extremely important as the prognosis of patients with severe sepsis is related to the number or organs involved and the severity of dysfunction.

Multiple Organ Dysfunction Syndrome

The clinical manifestations of primary and secondary MODS depend on which organs are affected. In patients with severe sepsis, MODS appears to result from a cascade of inflammatory mediators, endothelial injury, altered perfusion, and microcirculatory failure. Mortality in severe sepsis is directly related to the number of failing organ systems and the severity of dysfunction. MODS is regarded as one of the most common causes of death among patients in the ICU.

Diagnostic Tests

- *Complete blood cell count:* White blood cell count > 12,000 cells/mm^3, or < 4000 cells/mm^3, or > 10% immature bands
- *Arterial blood gas:* $Paco_2$ < 32 mm Hg
- *Serum lactate:* More than 4 mmol/L (36 mg/dL)
- *Chest x-ray:* May be normal or show signs of infiltrates
- *Culture and sensitivity:* Generally is positive from a normally sterile source
- *Axial computed tomography scan:* May be negative or show abscess collection

Principles of Management of Severe Sepsis

The treatment of a patient with severe sepsis (SIRS + infection + new organ dysfunction) consists of several objectives: treating or eliminating the underlying cause, maximizing oxygen delivery, and use of evidence-based practice guidelines to include early antibiotic administration and ensure that initial resuscitation, organ system support, and targeted interventions are provided. Additional components of the management plan include providing nutrition and psychological support for the patient and family.

Treating the Underlying Cause

The management plan begins with recognition and treatment of the source or stimulus of the response. Until this is done, no other therapy may be successfully applied. Examples include the drainage of an abscess or the removal of an infected invasive line, vascular graft, or orthopedic device. Once the source (or presumed source) has been identified, empiric antibiotic therapy is initiated and adjusted when definitive culture results are available.

Maximizing Oxygen Delivery

Parallel to the administration of antibiotics are measures to maximize oxygen delivery. The components of oxygen delivery include cardiac output (CO), oxygen saturation (Sao_2), hemoglobin (Hgb), and to a lesser extent, partial pressure of oxygen (Pao_2). Oxygen demands can be significantly increased in sepsis, especially when patients have fever and/or tachycardia. Administration of supplemental oxygen may help maintain the balance between oxygen supply and oxygen demand.

Maximize Cardiac Output

A significant number of patients with sepsis increase their CO as a compensatory response to meet increased cellular oxygen demands. However, a major pathological problem of sepsis is the increase in the permeability of the capillary bed and vasodilation. As a result, intravascular volume is difficult to maintain and generally transfer to the critical care unit is necessary for aggressive monitoring and management. Protocolized, quantitative resuscitation of patients with severe sepsis with tissue hypoperfusion (defined as hypotension persisting after initial fluid challenge or blood lactate concentration greater than or equal to 4 mmol/L) is recommended. The goals of resuscitation should include all of the following:

1. CVP 8-12 mm Hg
2. MAP > 65 mm Hg
3. Urine output > 0.5 ml/kg/h
4. Superior vena cava oxygenation saturation ($Scvo_2$) or mixed venous oxygen saturation (Svo_2) 70% or 65% respectively.
5. Normalization of lactate in patients with elevated lactate levels.

This often necessitates the liberal administration of fluids. A patient may require a combination of both crystalloid and colloid fluid replacement. Pharmacologic support also may be required to maximize CO.

Maximize Oxygenation

Maintaining Sao$_2$ more than 90% and Pao$_2$ more than 60 mm Hg are acceptable goals.

Hemoglobin

Sufficient hemoglobin is necessary to ensure adequate oxygen-carrying capacity. Disagreement exists as to the appropriate hemoglobin and hematocrit levels for this type of patient; however, as a general rule, 7 to 9 g of hemoglobin and 21%-27% hematocrit are acceptable depending on the patient's tolerance.

Decrease Oxygen Demand

Decreasing oxygen demand is an important aspect of maximizing oxygen delivery. Methods to reduce oxygen demand include:

1. Reducing tachycardia and tachypnea
2. Reducing hyperthermia
3. Alleviating pain
4. Preventing shivering
5. Providing comfort measures
6. Consolidating activities
7. Placing the patient on mechanical ventilation

By addressing these aspects of supply and demand, unnecessary oxygen consumption may be minimized, thus improving the supply to other tissues in greater need of oxygen.

Notice that there has been no mention of maintaining an optimal blood pressure. The reason for this is that although maintenance of blood pressure is critical, adequate blood pressure does not imply adequate perfusion. For this reason, measurements of oxygen delivery and consumption are used to assess adequacy of perfusion, and not blood pressure alone. There is great variability in perfusion among patients with similar mean arterial pressures (MAPs). A patient with a MAP of 100 mm Hg may not have adequate tissue perfusion. In contrast, a patient with a MAP of 50 may have sufficient tissue perfusion. The point is that an evaluation of perfusion should not be based on pressure assessment alone (this concept is also reviewed in Chapter 4, Hemodynamic Monitoring).

Supporting Dysfunctional Systems

An important objective in the management of sepsis and MODS is to support dysfunctional organ systems. Renal dysfunction, a common sequela of sepsis, is aggressively managed to prevent fluid and electrolyte imbalances, which contribute to the risk of death. Refer the chapter in this book specific to each organ system for approaches used to support failing organs.

Evidence-Based Practice Strategies

Evidence-based practice guidelines for managing patients with severe sepsis highlight the use of the sepsis bundles (Table 11-5). Key recommendations include initial resuscitation to restore perfusion, organ system support, appropriate

TABLE 11-5. SURVIVING SEPSIS CAMPAIGN CARE BUNDLES

Within 3 Hours of Severe Sepsis
1. Measure lactate level
2. Obtain blood cultures prior to administration of antibiotics
3. Administer broad spectrum antibiotics
4. Administer 30 ml/kg crystalloid for hypotension or lactate ≥ 4mmol/L

Within 6 Hours of Initial Symptoms for Septic Shock
5. Apply vasopressors for hypotension that does not respond to initial fluid resuscitation to maintain a mean arterial pressure (MAP) ≥ 65 mmHg
6. In the event of persistent arterial hypotension despite volume resuscitation (septic shock) or initial lactate ≥ 4 mmol/L (36 mg/dl)
   - Measure central venous pressure (CVP)*
   - Measure central venous oxygen saturation (Scvo$_2$) *
7. Remeasure lactate if initial lactate was elevated*

*Targets for quantitative resuscitation included in the guidelines are CVP of ≥8 mm Hg, Scvo$_2$ of ≥70% and lactate normalization.
Reproduced with permission from Dellinger RP, Levy ML, Opal S, et al. Surviving sepsis campaign: international guidelines for management of severe sepsis and septic shock: 2012. Crit Care Med. 2013;41:580-637.

diagnostic studies, early administration of broad-spectrum antibiotic therapy, vasopressor and inotropic support, lung protective ventilation strategies, limiting the use of sedation, glucose control, and goal-directed therapy to improve outcomes for patients with severe sepsis (Table 11-6). Several of the evidence-based practice recommendations have direct implications for nursing care because they require monitoring and oversight. Control of glucose (blood glucose, 180 mg/dL) in critically ill patients has been shown to decrease mortality rates and improve outcomes. The use of intravenous insulin to maintain glycemic control requires frequent monitoring of glucose (every 1 hour) and is a nurse-driven intervention.

Providing Nutritional Support

Enteral nutritional support is the gold standard and preferred route of specialized nutrition support (SNS) delivery unless contraindicated (ASPEN guidelines). If unable to eat, most acutely ill patients can tolerate a standard type of tube feeding or parenteral formula, with rare situations that require feeding modifications (eg, volume overload, organ dysfunction, or gastrointestinal abnormalities). General guidelines for nutritional support include 25 to 35 kcal/kg/day for total caloric intake and 1.5 to 2.0 g protein/kg/day. It is helpful to have a nutrition specialist assist with nutritional planning. Refer Chapter 14, Gastrointestinal System, for more on nutrition.

Providing Psychological Support

Chapter 1, Assessment of Progressive Care Patients and Their Families, and Chapter 2, Planning Care for Progressive Care Patients and Their Families, discuss many aspects of psychosocial support of progressive care patients and their families. The updated international sepsis care guidelines identify that setting goals of care, including the discussion of prognosis, should be incorporated into care of the patient with sepsis. Palliative care and end-of-life care planning should also

TABLE 11-6. EVIDENCE-BASED PRACTICE GUIDELINES: SURVIVING SEPSIS CAMPAIGN GUIDELINES FOR THE MANAGEMENT OF SEVERE SEPSIS

Initial resuscitation for sepsis-induced hypoperfusion	Goals: CVP of 8-12 mm Hg • Mean arterial pressure ≥ 65 mm Hg • Urine output ≥ 0.5 mL/kg/h • Central venous (superior vena cava or mixed venous oxygen saturation ≥ 70%) Initial fluid challenge goal in patients with sepsis-induced tissue hypoperfusion with suspicion of hypovolemia is to achieve a minimum of 30 mL/kg of crystalloids (a portion of this may be albumin equivalent). More rapid administration and greater amounts of fluid may be needed in some patients. Administration of vasopressors when appropriate fluid challenge fails to restore adequate blood pressure and organ perfusion (eg, norepinephrine) Transfusion of packed red blood cells to achieve a hemoglobin concentration of 7.0 to 9.0 g/dL in adults. Administration of inotropic infusion (eg, dobutamine) to increase CO
Diagnosis	Obtain cultures: At least two blood cultures with one drawn percutaneously and one drawn through each vascular access device; obtain cultures of other sites such as urine, wounds, and respiratory secretions before initiating antibiotic therapy. Diagnostic studies (eg, ultrasound, imaging studies)
Antibiotic therapy	Empirical antibiotics
Source control	Removal of potentially infected device, drainage of abscess, debridement of infected necrotic tissue
Enhance perfusion	Fluid therapy Vasopressors Inotropic therapy
Steroids	For patients with septic shock that have not responded to fluid resuscitation or vasopressor
Blood product administration	To target hemoglobin of 7.0-9.0 g/dL
Mechanical ventilation	Lung protective ventilation for acute lung injury/acute respiratory distress syndrome (eg, low tidal volume 6 mL/kg of predicted body weight with the goal of maintaining end inspiratory plateau pressure < 30 cm H_2O)
Sedation, analgesia, and neuromuscular blockade	To provide comfort yet avoid prolonged sedation
Glucose control	To maintain blood glucose < 180 mg/dL
Renal replacement	For acute renal failure
Prophylaxis measures	Deep vein thrombosis Stress ulcer
Setting goals of care	Discuss goals of care, prognosis for achieving those goals and level of certainty for the prognosis with patients and families, incorporating palliative care principles and as appropriate, end-of-life care planning Address goals of care as early as feasible but no later than within 72 hours of ICU admission

Adapted from: Dellinger RP, Levy ML, Opal S,. et al. Surviving Sepsis Campaign: International guidelines for management of severe sepsis and septic shock: 2012. Crit Care Med. 2013;41:580-637.

be addressed. The new guidelines identify that a family care conference to discuss goals of care should be addressed as early as feasible, but no later than within 72 hours of ICU admission. Table 11-3 outlines important considerations for nursing care of patients with sepsis or MODS.

OVERDOSES

Drug or alcohol overdoses, as well as poisonings, can result in multiple organ dysfunction. Overdoses can be deliberate or accidental. Accidental overdose may involve one or multiple substances, and can be acute (eg, inaccurate dosing of pediatric medications) or chronic (eg, inadvertent, unnecessary dosing of asthma medication or over-the-counter medications). The Center for Disease Control and Prevention reports that prescription abuse is the fastest growing drug problem in the United States, with drug overdoses from opioid analgesia misuse among the highest.

The level of intoxication or overdose varies with the element and amount ingested, the time until the patient is treated, and the underlying physical and emotional condition of the patient. The priority of care, as in all emergency situations, is maintenance of the patient's airway, breathing, and circulation. These patients are often cared for in critical care units, however, some, following the delivery of emergency department care, may be triaged to a progressive care unit for continued therapy and monitoring.

Etiology, Risk Factors, and Pathophysiology

Alcohol Overdose

Alcohol overdose is most often seen in alcoholics, in young persons who have not yet reached legal drinking age, or in combination with other drugs as a suicidal gesture. There are four types of alcohol intoxication:

- Ethanol (ethyl or grain alcohol)
- Methanol (wood alcohol)
- Ethylene glycol (antifreeze)
- Isopropyl alcohol (rubbing alcohol)

Alcohol dissolves readily in the lipid components of the plasma membranes of the body, and thus enters the brain quickly, resulting in a rapid effect on the central nervous system. The mechanism of alcohol overdose and withdrawal is complex. Most of the clinical effects can be explained by the interaction of ethanol with various neurotransmitters and neuroreceptors in the brain.

In ethanol intoxication, serum levels range from 200 mg/dL (mild intoxication) to more than 500 mg/dL (coma). A serum alcohol level of 80 mg/dL is the legal upper limit for driving a car in most of the United States.

In the case of methanol intoxication, serum levels range from 50 mg/dL (mild intoxication) to 100 mg/dL (severe intoxication). Metabolic acidosis manifests as a decreased bicarbonate level on arterial blood gas analysis, and indicates that the generation of hydrogen ions by the liver exceeds the ability of the kidney to excrete them. This excess of systemic hydrogen ions results in compensatory hyperventilation, as the body attempts to make the pH more alkaline. Refer Chapter 5, Airway and Ventilatory Management, for further information on acid-base imbalance.

Ethylene glycol intoxication is characterized by neurologic depression, cardiopulmonary complications, pulmonary edema, and renal tubular degeneration. Serum chemistry reveals metabolic acidosis, as described, and renal toxicity. An aggregation of hydrogen ions can result in increased production and accumulation of lactic acid, which tends to impair renal function. Renal toxicity is suspected when the serum pH is less than 7.35, serum creatinine is more than 2.0 mg/dL, and blood urea nitrogen (BUN) is more than 100 mg/dL.

Isopropyl alcohol intoxication is distinguished from other types of alcohol intoxication by the presence of ketoacids in both the urine and serum. Metabolic acidosis is a reflection of excess ketoacids, requiring buffering by the bicarbonate ions.

Clinical Presentation

Excess ingestion of any type of alcohol may cause central nervous system symptoms such as sluggish reflexes, emotional instability, or out-of-character behavior. Amnesia may result for events that occurred during the period of intoxication. Unconsciousness usually occurs before a person can drink enough for fatal consequences to occur, but the rapid consumption of alcohol can cause death by either respiratory depression or aspiration during vomiting. It is estimated that there are 1.2 million hospital admissions for problems related to alcohol abuse with up to 5% of these patients developing delirium tremens requiring medical treatment. There are signs and symptoms that are specific to each type of alcohol ingested. Descriptions follow:

- *Acute ethanol intoxication:* Muscular incoordination, slurred speech, stupor, hypoglycemia, flushing, seizures, coma, depressed respirations, and hyporeflexia
- *Methanol intoxication:* Neurologic depression, metabolic acidosis, and visual disturbances
- *Ethylene glycol intoxication:* Neurologic depression, cardiopulmonary complications, pulmonary edema, and renal tubular degeneration
- *Isopropyl intoxication:* Neurologic depression, areflexia, respiratory depression, hypothermia, hypotension, and gastrointestinal distress

Diagnostic Tests

A differential diagnosis to rule out other medical conditions, such as hypoglycemia or hyperglycemia, which may mimic overdose or intoxication, is an important component of the initial assessment. Because alcohol ingestion interferes with the liver's ability to produce glucose, alcohol-induced hypoglycemia in the intoxicated patient is fairly common.

Prior to obtaining any diagnostic test, it is extremely important to obtain a history either from the patient,

---

ESSENTIAL CONTENT CASE

Alcohol Overdose

A 19-year-old man is brought to the ED by his roommates who state that he became unresponsive after drinking at a party. Your initial assessment reveals a depressed level of consciousness, with decreased response to stimuli. While reviewing his initial serum chemistry results, you note that the serum alcohol level is 430 mg/dL. Current vital signs are:

T	36.5°C (97.8°F) rectal
HR	120 beats/min

Sinus tachycardia

RR	16 breaths/min
BP	92/70, pulse oximetry 94%

Case Question 1. What are the priority areas for care of this patient?

Case Question 2. What information would help in guiding the treatment?

Answers

1. Maintenance of airway, stabilization of the patient, establish IV access, provide fluids, and provide detoxification.
2. Amount and type of alcohol ingested, time frame since ingestion (gastric lavage is best considered within 1 hour of ingestion).

---

family member, friend, or the person who found the patient to determine the probable substance that was ingested. Once the substance is potentially identified there are diagnostic tests helpful in aiding the treatment of patients following alcohol intoxication. These include:

- *Ethanol and methanol serum levels:* These are elevated if they were ingested. Most laboratories can run these tests. Isopropyl serum levels are not run as commonly as ethanol and methanol levels.
- *Serum creatinine and BUN levels:* These may be elevated due to renal dysfunction.
- *Liver function studies:* The hepatotoxic effects of certain types of alcohol result in abnormal levels.
- *Serum glucose and electrolytes:* These are often abnormal as described previously.

Alcohol Withdrawal Syndrome

Patients who suffer from alcohol abuse of dependence may be admitted to a progressive care unit for an unrelated condition or may be admitted for management of withdrawal symptoms. Symptoms of alcohol withdrawal vary and are documented in Table 11-7. The timing related to the emergence of the symptoms also vary and are influenced by concurrent medical illness, daily heavy alcohol use, older age, and abnormal liver function. As a result it is essential to obtain a complete history from the patient and/or

TABLE 11-7. SYMPTOMS OF ALCOHOL WITHDRAWAL SYNDROME

Symptoms	Time of appearance after cessation alcohol use
Minor withdrawal symptoms: insomnia, tremulousness, mild anxiety, gastrointestinal upset, headache, diaphoresis, palpitations, anorexia	6-12 hours
Alcoholic hallucinosis: visual, auditory, or tactile hallucinations	12-24 hours[a]
Withdrawal seizures: generalized tonic-clonic seizures	24-48 hours[b]
Alcohol withdrawal delirium (delirium tremens): hallucinations (predominately visual), disorientation, tachycardia, hypertension, low-grade fever, agitation, diaphoresis	48-72 hours[c]

[a]Symptoms generally resolve within 48 hours.
[b]Symptoms reported as early as 2 hours after cessation.
[c]Symptoms peak at 5 days.
From: Bayard M, Mcintyre J, Hill KR, Woodside J Jr. Alcohol withdrawal syndrome. Am Fam Physician. 2004. Mar 15;69(6):1443-1450.

family and determine the amount and frequency of alcohol ingested (and last ingested). Use of an alcohol withdrawal symptom assessment form is a helpful way of identifying severity and treatment requirements (Figure 11-3).

Most treatment management regimens include the use of fluid, electrolyte and nutrition repletion as well as the routine administration of thiamine (to prevent Wernicke encephalopathy), multivitamins, folate, and often magnesium. Benzodiazepines are administered on a set schedule to manage the symptoms of withdrawal and delirium tremens, with additional prn doses used as necessary, to decrease hyperexcitability symptoms which may be life-threatening. Intermediate-acting benzodiazepines are commonly preferred in acute and critical care settings. All benzodiazepines appear similarly effective in the treatment of alcohol withdrawal syndrome. In moderate-to-severe withdrawal, long-acting agents are preferred over short-acting drugs. Adjunctive medications may also be used in some cases to treat agitation (ie, haloperidol-caution, as it lowers seizure threshold) and to decrease autonomic symptoms (ie, beta-blockers, dexmedetomidine, and clonidine).

The use of ethanol or preferably fomepizol for alcohol dehydrogenase (ADH) inhabitation is a mainstay in the management of toxicity due to ingestion of methanol, ethylene glycol, or diethylene glycol. Many patients with chronic alcoholism have clinically significant magnesium deficiency because of malnutrition and chronic diuresis from alcohol ingestion, and electrolyte replacement may be indicated. Alcohol withdrawal management in progressive care requires careful nursing assessment, including alcohol usage history, delirium management, and withdrawal assessment symptoms.

Drug Overdose

Drug overdose may involve any type of medication. The majority of overdoses involve analgesics, antidepressants, sedatives, opioids, cough and cold drugs, and street drugs (eg, cocaine, crack cocaine, phencyclidine [PCP], D-lysergic acid diethylamide [LSD]). Acetaminophen is the leading cause of overdose. It can lead to hepatocellular damage and is the most common cause of liver transplant. Street drugs are used to induce a relaxed state, elevate mood, or to produce unusual states of consciousness. Psychoactive drugs often are chemically similar to neurotransmitters such as serotonin, dopamine, and norepinephrine, and act by either directly or indirectly altering neurotransmitter-receptor interactions. Medullary inspiratory neurons are highly sensitive to depression by drugs, especially barbiturates and morphine, and death from an overdose of these agents is often secondary to respiratory arrest. Refer Table 11-8 for presenting signs and symptoms of common agents of drug overdose.

Clinical Presentation

The specific signs and symptoms of drug overdose depend on the substance ingested. However, there are several signs and symptoms that are commonly seen in most patients. These include changes in mental status (typically, decreased level of consciousness), behavioral changes, and respiratory depression. The signs and symptoms of drug overdose for particular drugs are summarized in Table 11-8.

Diagnostic Tests

Diagnostic studies for patients following drug overdose include the following:

- Toxicology screen, which can be either broad-spectrum tests, including testing for the presence of such substances as amphetamines, barbiturates, benzodiazepines, and narcotics, or specific screens, if the substance is known. Generally these are urine studies.
- Arterial blood gas and measurement of anion gap, to evaluate oxygenation, ventilation, and the acid-base status respectively.
- Serum glucose and electrolytes, which can be abnormal.

Principles of Management for Overdose

The principles of management of patients following alcohol intoxication or drug overdose are similar. An initial clinical evaluation is conducted with the priority of resuscitating and stabilizing the patient. The principles of management include maintenance of a patent airway, prevention of complications, elimination of ingested substances or toxic metabolites, and maintenance of hemodynamic stability. Specific treatment depends on the agent, route, and amount of exposure, and the severity of overdose.

Maintenance of Patent Airway

1. Maintain adequate minute ventilation. Stimulate the patient to breathe. If the patient cannot spontaneously maintain minute ventilation, intubation and mechanical ventilation may be required.

Clinical Institute Withdrawal Assessment of Alcohol Scale, Revised (CIWA-Ar)

Patient: _____ Date: _____ Time: _____ (24 hour clock, midnight = 00:00)

Pulse or heart rate, taken for one minute: _____ Blood pressure: _____

NAUSEA AND VOMITNG – Ask "Do you feel sick to your stomach? Have you vomited?" Observation.
0 no nausea and no vomiting
1 mild nausea with no vomiting
2
3
4 intermittent nausea with dry heaves
5
6
7 constant nausea, frequent dry heaves and vomiting

TREMOR – Arms extended and fingers spread apart. Observation.
0 no tremor
1 not visible, but can be felt fingertip to fingertip
2
3
4 moderate, with patient's arms extended
5
6
7 severe, even with arms not extended

PAROXYSMAL SWEATS – Observation.
0 no sweat visible
1 barely perceptible sweating, palms moist
2
3
4 beads of sweat obvious on forehead
5
6
7 drenching sweats

ANXIETY – Ask "Do you feel nervous?" Observation.
0 no anxiety, at ease
1 mild anxious
2
3
4 moderately anxious, or guarded, so anxiety is inferred
5
6
7 equivalent to acute panic states as seen in severe delirium or acute schizophrenic reactions

AGITATION – Observation.
0 normal activity
1 somewhat more than normal activity
2
3
4 moderately fidgety and restless
5
6
7 paces back and forth during most of the interview, or constantly thrashes about

TACTILE DISTURBANCES – Ask "Have you any itching, pins and needles sensations, any burning, any numbness, or do you feel bugs crawling on or under your skin?" Observation.
0 none
1 very mild itching, pins and needles, burning or numbness
2 mild itching, pins and needles, burning or numbness
3 moderate itching, pins and needles, burning or numbness
4 moderately severe hallucinations
5 severe hallucinations
6 extremely severe hallucinations
7 continuous hallucinations

AUDITORY DISTURBANCES – Ask "Are you more aware of sounds around you? Are they harsh? Do they frighten you? Are you hearing anything that is disturbing to you? Are you hearing things you know are not there?" Observation.
0 not present
1 very mild harshness or ability to frighten
2 mild harshness or ability to frighten
3 moderate harshness or ability to frighten
4 moderately severe hallucinations
5 severe hallucinations
6 extremely severe hallucinations
7 continuous hallucinations

VISUAL DISTURBANCES – Ask "Does the light appear to be too bright? Is its color different? Does it hurt your eyes? Are you seeing anything that is disturbing to you? Are you seeing things you know are not there?" Observation.
0 not present
1 very mild sensitivity
2 mild sensitivity
3 moderate sensitivity
4 moderately severe hallucinations
5 severe hallucinations
6 extremely severe hallucinations
7 continuous hallucinations

HEADACHE, FULLNESS IN HEAD – Ask "Does your head feel different? Does it feel like there is a band around your head?" Do not rate for dizziness or lightheadedness. Otherwise, rate severity.
0 not present
1 very mild
2 mild
3 moderate
4 moderately severe
5 severe
6 very severe
7 extremely severe

ORIENTATION AND CLOUDING OF SENSORIUM – Ask "What day is this? Where are you? Who am I?"
0 oriented and can do serial additions
1 cannot do serial additions or is uncertain about date
2 disoriented for date by no more than 2 calendar days
3 disoriented for date by more than 2 calendar days
4 disoriented for place/or person

Total **CIWA-Ar** Score _____
Rater's Initials _____
Maximum Possible Score 67

The **CIWA-Ar** is not copyrighted and may be reproduced freely. This assessment for monitoring withdrawal symptoms requires approximately 5 minutes to administer. The maximum score is 67 (see instrument). Patients scoring less than 10 do not usually need additional medication for withdrawal.

Figure 11-3. Revised Clinical Institute Withdrawal Assessment for Alcohol (CIWA-Ar) scale. (*Adapted from: Sullivan JT, Sykora K, SchneidermanJ, Naranjo CA, Sellers EM. Assessment of alcohol withdrawal: the revised Clinical Institute Withdrawal Assessment for Alcohol Scale (CIWA-AR). Br J Addict. 1989; 84:1353-1357.*)

TABLE 11-8. SIGNS AND SYMPTOMS OF OVERDOSE

Opioids	• Change in LOC • Respiratory depression, aspiration • Hypotension • Miosis • Decreased gastric motility
Barbiturates	• Decreased LOC • Hypothermia
Sedatives	• Respiratory depression • Hypnotics • Shock • Cardiac dysrhythmias • Pulmonary edema
Cocaine	• Hyperexcitability • Headache • Hypertension • Tachycardia • Nausea/vomiting, abdominal pain • Fever • Delirium, convulsions, coma
PCP (phencyclidine)	• Violent behavior • Hallucinations • Seizures • Rhabdomyolysis • Hypertensive crisis
LSD	• Severe agitation • Dilated pupils • Hallucinations
Tricyclics	• Seizures • Coma • Dysrhythmias, ECG changes • Heart failure • Shock
Salicylates	• Tinnitus • Vertigo • Vomiting • Hyperthermia • Altered mental status
Acetaminophen	• GI distress • Hepatotoxicity • Hepatic necrosis

2. Monitor pulse oximetry and blood gas values.
3. Position the patient on their side with the head of the bed elevated > 30° if tolerated.
4. Suction the patient's airway as needed.

Circulation and Maintenance of Hemodynamic Stability

1. Ensure venous access (large-bore peripheral or central access).
2. Administer isotonic fluid to maintain intravascular fluid volume. If hypotension is unresponsive to volume expansion, treatment with vasopressors may be necessary.
3. Obtain a 12-lead ECG and maintain on continuous cardiac monitoring.
4. *Treatment of arrhythmias:* Supraventricular tachycardia with hypertension due to sympathetic nervous system response can be managed with a combination of beta-blocker and vasodilator therapy (eg, esmolol and

nitroprusside), combined alpha- and beta-blocker (labetalol), or a calcium channel blocker (verapamil or diltiazem). Lidocaine or amiodarone may be used for ventricular tachyarrhythmias. This may require transfer to a critical care unit.

Neurologic Depression

1. Measure glucose to rule out hypoglycemia and treat with 50% glucose IV if necessary.
2. Evaluate for carbon monoxide poisoning (carboxyhemoglobin), provide oxygen.
3. Administer thiamine (IV for Wernicke syndrome).
4. Naloxone IV or IM.
5. Flumazenil for benzodiazepine overdose (avoid in those who have potential for seizures).

Catharsis, Clearing Drugs, and Antidotes

1. Ipecac is no longer recommended to induce vomiting. There is little evidence that ipecac prevents drug absorption or systemic toxicity. Ipecac is not used as a first-line treatment for most ingested poisons as there is little evidence that it improves the outcome in poisoning cases. Additionally, side effects from ipecac, such as lethargy, may complicate diagnosis and be confused with the effect of other poisons.
2. *Gastric lavage:* Decreases ingestant absorption and significant amounts of ingested drug can be recovered the closer that lavage is performed to ingestion. Gastric lavage is contraindicated in corrosive ingestions due to risk of gastroesophageal perforation and with hydrocarbons owing to the risk of aspiration-induced hydrocarbon pneumonitis.
3. *Activated charcoal:* Used with most drugs! Charcoal absorbs ingestants within the gut lumen, allowing the charcoal-toxin complex to be eliminated in the stool. Charcoal is not recommended for patients who have ingested caustic acids and alkalis, alcohols, lithium, or heavy metals.
4. *Hemodialysis and hemoperfusion for severe drug intoxication for selected substances:* Hemodialysis can be considered for severe poisoning due to methanol, ethylene glycol, salicylates, and lithium. Hemoperfusion, which involves the passage of blood through an absorptive-containing cartridge (usually charcoal), may be indicated for intoxications with carbamazepine, phenobarbital, phenytoin, and theophylline. Therapeutic plasma exchange has also been used to promote rapid lowering of the toxin level.
5. *Renal dialysis:* Dialysis may be indicated in cases of severe poisoning due to barbiturates, bromide, chloral hydrate, ethanol, ethylene glycol, isopropyl alcohol, lithium, methanol, procainamide, theophylline, salicylates, and possibly heavy metals. Refer Chapter 15, Renal System, for more on renal replacement therapies.

6. *Methanol:* Practice guidelines have been developed by the American Academy of Clinical Toxicology for the treatment of methanol overdose. Folinic acid (leucovorin) in a dose of 1 mg/kg up to 50 mg every 4 to 6 hours for 24 hours is suggested in methanol poisoning to provide the cofactor for formic acid elimination. Gastric lavage may be considered within 1 hour of ingestion. Activated charcoal does not absorb alcohols, but it may be appropriate to administer if other drugs are suspected. To prevent metabolism of alcohols to toxic metabolites, ethanol can be administered orally or intravenously to maintain a blood concentration of 100 to 150 mg/dL. Hemodialysis is often necessary to remove the alcohol and toxic metabolites and is continued until the acidosis is resolved.

7. *Alcohol Withdrawal Syndrome:* Assess patients with an alcohol history with a symptom assessment tool to gauge severity of symptoms and to target treatment appropriately. Treat symptoms of alcohol withdrawal and delirium tremens with benzodiazepines on a regular schedule as clinically dictated. Other drugs may be used as adjuncts for treatment of agitation and management of autonomic symptoms such as haloperidol, clonidine, and selected beta-blockers.

Antidotes

Antidotes help counteract the effects of poisons by neutralizing them or by antagonizing their effects. Poisons or conditions with specific antidotes include the following:

- *Acetaminophen:* *N*-acetylcysteine
- *Opiates:* Naloxone
- *Benzodiazepines:* Flumazenil
- *Digoxin:* Digiband
- *Cyanide:* Kelocyanor
- *Tricyclic antidepressants:* Sodium bicarbonate
- *Beta-blockers or calcium channel blockers:* Glucagon and calcium

Preventing Complications

1. Orient the patient to surroundings.
2. Insert a nasogastric tube for stomach decompression and for the delivery of charcoal or other antidotes.
3. Keep the head of the bed elevated to prevent aspiration.
4. Pad bed side rails and restrain the patient as necessary to prevent self-injury.
5. Institute patient safety measures.
6. Provide support to the patient and family.

COMPLEX WOUNDS AND PRESSURE ULCERS

Complex wounds and pressure ulcers are troubling complications of a hospital stay, especially for acutely ill patients. Complex wounds and pressure ulcers can increase the length of hospitalization, recovery time, and the risk of infection; increase costs of care; and can cause discomfort for patients.

Of significance to clinicians is that pressure ulcers are thought to be preventable in most cases and are seen as a reflection of the quality of care provided.

A *pressure ulcer* is defined by the National Pressure Advisory Panel (NPUAP) as localized injury to the skin and/or underlying tissue usually over a bony prominence, as the result of pressure, or pressure in combination with shear. When a person is immobile the soft tissue is compressed between the skin and the bone. This can lead to ischemia and later tissue death. Typically a pressure ulcer occurs over a bony prominence but can occur anywhere soft tissue is compressed. Pressure ulcer prevalence rates range from 53.2% to 88% and incidence rates vary from 7% to 71.6%, depending on associated risk factors. The most common anatomical sites for pressure ulcers to occur are the sacrum and heels.

There are a number of intrinsic or internal factors related to the risk of pressure ulcer development. Poor nutrition and dehydration contribute to pressure ulcer development because these conditions make tissue more vulnerable to damage. The elderly are at greater risk because of physiologic changes that occur to the skin and tissue with age, such as dermal thinning and the inability of tissue to distribute the mechanical load. Low blood pressure is thought to divert blood away from the skin to more essential organs during critical times. Additionally stress, smoking, surgery, and elevated body temperature are other conditions that can contribute to pressure ulcer development.

According to the NPUAP the six stages of pressures (Table 11-9) are classified as the following:

Pressure Ulcer Stages

Suspected Deep Tissue Injury
Purple or maroon localized area of discolored intact skin or blood-filled blister due to damage of underlying soft tissue from pressure and/or shear. The area may be preceded by tissue that is painful, firm, mushy, boggy, warmer, or cooler

TABLE 11-9. PRESSURE ULCER CLASSIFICATION BRIEF GUIDE

Category/Stage I Pressure Ulcer	Non-blanchable erythema Intact skin
Category/Stage II Pressure Ulcer	Partial thickness tissue loss Wound bed is pink/red
Category/Stage III Pressure Ulcer	Full thickness tissue loss extending into the subcutaneous tissue, slough/eschar may be present in the wound bed but does not obscure depth of the wound
Category/Stage IV Pressure Ulcer	Full thickness tissue loss, the muscle, bone or tendon may be present in the wound bed. Slough/eschar may be present in the wound bed but does not obscure depth of the wound
Unstageable–Unknown depth	Full thickness tissue loss. Unable to visualize base of the wound due to slough or eschar
Deep Tissue Injury	Purple or maroon colored Intact skin

Data from: The international NPUAP/EPUAP pressure ulcer classification system 2009.

as compared to adjacent tissue. Deep tissue injury may be difficult to detect in individuals with dark skin tones. Evolution may include a thin blister over a dark wound bed. The wound may further evolve and become covered by thin eschar. Evolution may be rapid exposing additional layers of tissue even with optimal treatment.

- *Stage I:* Intact skin with non-blanchable redness of a localized area usually over a bony prominence. Darkly pigmented skin may not have visible blanching; its color may differ from the surrounding area. The area may be painful, firm, soft, warmer, or cooler as compared to adjacent tissue. Stage I may be difficult to detect in individuals with dark skin tones. May indicate "at risk" persons (a heralding sign of risk).
- *Stage II:* Partial thickness loss of dermis presenting as a shallow open ulcer with a red pink wound bed, without slough. May also present as an intact or open/ruptured serum-filled blister. Presents as a shiny or dry shallow ulcer without slough or bruising. This stage should not be used to describe skin tears, tape burns, perineal dermatitis, maceration, or excoriation.

Bruising indicates suspected deep tissue injury.

- *Stage III:* Full thickness tissue loss. Subcutaneous fat may be visible but bone, tendon, or muscle is not exposed. Slough may be present but does not obscure the depth of tissue loss. May include undermining and tunneling. The depth of a stage III pressure ulcer varies by anatomical location. The bridge of the nose, ear, occiput, and malleolus do not have subcutaneous tissue and stage III ulcers can be shallow. In contrast, areas of significant adiposity can develop extremely deep stage III pressure ulcers. Bone/tendon is not visible or directly palpable.
- *Stage IV:* Full thickness tissue loss with exposed bone, tendon, or muscle. Slough or eschar may be present on some parts of the wound. Often include undermining and tunneling. The depth of a stage IV pressure ulcer varies by anatomical location. The bridge of the nose, ear, occiput, and malleolus do not have subcutaneous tissue and these ulcers can be shallow. Stage IV ulcers can extend into muscle and/or supporting structures (eg, fascia, tendon or joint capsule) making osteomyelitis possible. Exposed bone/tendon is visible or directly palpable.
- *Unstageable:* Full thickness tissue loss in which the base of the ulcer is covered by slough (yellow, tan, gray, green, or brown) and/or eschar (tan, brown, or black) in the wound bed is difficult to evaluate. Until enough slough and/or eschar is removed to expose the base of the wound, the true depth, and therefore stage, cannot be determined. Stable (dry, adherent, intact without erythema or fluctuance) eschar on the heels serves as "the body's natural (biological) cover" and should not be removed.

Skin assessment, risk assessment, repositioning, nutritional status, and support surfaces are all key pressure ulcer prevention strategies. The two most widely studied and validated risk assessment scales are the Braden and Norton Scales. The Braden scale consists of six subcategories. Each category is scored 1 for the (most at risk) to 4 (least at risk), with the exception of the friction and shear subcategory which is score 1-3. The numbers are added providing a total score that ranges from 4 to 23. If a score falls below 18 the patient is considered at risk for pressure ulcer development. The Norton score includes five parameters: physical condition, mental condition, activity, mobility, and incontinence. The rating for each category is 1-4 with a score potential of 5-20. For both the Braden and Norton scales the lower the score identifies a greater risk of developing a pressure ulcer.

Although the underlying relationship is uncertain, low body weight, poor food intake, and poor nutritional status are all risk factors for the development of pressure ulcers. Patients must have sufficient calories, fluid, and proteins to reduce the risk of development. Patients must also maintain adequate hydration. All patients at nutritional risk should have an evaluation by a registered dietician.

Repositioning should be scheduled for bed and chair bound patients who are at risk of pressure ulcer development. The patient's overall condition needs to be considered when repositioning. If the patient cannot be turned due to a medical condition then an advanced support surface should be used and attempts made for slight adjustments in position. Heels should be suspended off the surface of the bed to prevent pressure on that area. The use of a pillow or a heel elevation device is also recommended. Support surfaces should be used for those individuals at risk for pressure ulcer development. They are used as adjunct therapy and are not to replace turning and repositioning.

HEALTHCARE ACQUIRED INFECTIONS

Nosocomial infections, or hospital associated infections (HAI), are estimated to occur in up to 5% of all acute care hospitalizations, or approximately 2 million cases per year. Hospital associated infections have been identified as one of the most serious patient safety issues in healthcare. Two common HAI's that patients in progressive care units are at risk for include catheter-associated urinary tract infection (CA-UTI) and central line associated blood stream infection (CLA-BSI). Another is hospital acquired pneumonia and ventilator associated events, conditions, and pneumonia (VAE, VAC, VAP, respectively). The pneumonias, their etiology, identification, and management are discussed in Chapter 10 Respiratory System.

Catheter-associated urinary tract infection often results from the presence of an indwelling urinary catheter. Guidelines for the prevention of CA-UTIs issued by the CDC outline several recommendations, including appropriate use of indwelling catheters, education of personnel on

TABLE 11-10. EVIDENCE-BASED STRATEGIES FOR URINARY TRACT INFECTION PREVENTION

- Indwelling urinary catheters should be inserted using aseptic technique and sterile equipment.
- Only hospital personnel who know the correct technique of aseptic insertion and maintenance of the catheter should handle catheters.
- Hospital personnel should be provided with periodic in-service training stressing the correct techniques and potential complications of urinary catheterization.
- Indwelling urinary catheters should be inserted only when necessary and left in place only for as long as necessary.
- Other methods of urinary drainage such as condom catheter drainage, suprapubic catheterization, and intermittent urethral catheterization should be considered as alternatives to indwelling urethral catheterization.
- Hand washing should be done immediately before and after any manipulation of the indwelling urinary catheter site or apparatus.
- Indwelling catheters should be properly secured after insertion to prevent movement and urethral traction.
- A sterile, continuously closed drainage system should be maintained.
- The catheter and drainage tube should not be disconnected unless the catheter must be irrigated, and irrigation should be used only for suspected obstruction.
- If breaks in aseptic technique, disconnection, or leakage occur, the collecting system should be replaced using aseptic technique after disinfecting the catheter-tubing junction.
- Specimen collections should be obtained from the distal end of the catheter, preferably from the sampling port after cleansing with a disinfectant and then the urine specimen aspirated with a sterile needle and syringe.
- Consider the use of antimicrobial catheters for indwelling urinary catheters.

Adapted from: Wong ES, Guideline for prevention of catheter-associated urinary tract infections. http://www.cdc.gov/ncidod/dhqp/gl_catheter_assoc.html. Accessed January 24, 2014.

proper catheter insertion using aseptic technique and sterile equipment, and maintenance to ensure closed sterile drainage (Table 11.10).

A variety of specialized urethral catheters have been designed to reduce the risk of CA-UTI. These include antiseptic-impregnated catheters and catheters coated with silver alloy or nitrofurazone. Several systematic reviews of the use of antimicrobial urinary catheters in the prevention of CA-UTI have demonstrated a reduction in catheter associated bacteriuria, but consensus on the economic benefit compared to standard catheter use has not been reached. Additional strategies for preventing CA-UTI include removal as early as possible, the use of hand held bladder scanners to evaluate retention, computerized order/entry system prompts to remove the catheters, and education on appropriate need for, and use of, indwelling urinary catheters.

Nursing-related care aspects include thorough assessment to determine need for indwelling catheter use, aseptic insertion technique, indwelling catheter care to minimize infection risk, and astute monitoring of patients with urinary catheters for signs of UTI. All of these are important measures to decrease the risk of CA-UTI.

Central venous catheters (CVCs) are frequently used in hospitalized patients and they carry associated risks, the most common being bloodstream infection (BSI). According to the CDC, up to 250,000 hospital-acquired central line associated blood stream infections (CLA-BSI) occur annually in the

US hospitals, with approximately 80,000 of these occurring in ICUs.

A *central line associated blood stream infection* is defined as the presence of bacteremia in a patient with an intravascular catheter with at least one positive blood culture and clinical signs of infections (ie, fever, chills, and/or hypotension), with no apparent source for the BSI except the catheter. Specific criteria for CLA-BSI include a positive culture with the same organism isolated from the catheter and peripheral blood. A BSI is considered to be associated with a central line if the line was in place during the 48-hour period before development of the BSI. Although CVSs account for only a small percentage of all intravenous lines, they cause most BSIs. The most common mechanism of CLA-BSI is migration of the organism from the insertion site along the surface of the catheter and colonization of its distal part. CLA-BSIs can also occur from contamination of the catheter hub or infusate administered through the device.

Several practices have been evaluated in an attempt to reduce the incidence of CLA-BSI. These include using a standardized catheter insertion technique with a skin preparation such as chlorhexidine and careful maintenance of the catheter. In addition, daily review of catheter necessity, the use of antimicrobial-impregnated dressings, and use of antimicrobial catheters have demonstrated reductions in incidence of CLA-BSI. CLA-BSIs often result from contamination of the catheter during insertion, therefore maximum sterile barrier precautions during insertion are indicated to reduce the incidence of CLA-BSI. Effective barrier precautions include the use of sterile gloves, long-sleeved gowns, full-size drape, masks, and head covers by all personnel involved in the central line insertion procedure.

Additional measures advocated for best practices for CVC care include hand hygiene by washing hands with conventional antiseptic-containing soap and water or with waterless alcohol-based gels or foam before and after palpating insertion sites; and before and after insertion, replacing, accessing, or dressing a CVC. Avoidance of antibiotic ointment at insertion sites, which can promote fungal infections and antibiotic resistance, and restricted use of stopcocks on any tubing other than pressure tubing to minimize contamination are also recommended. Table 11.11 outlines evidence-based strategies for CLA-BSI prevention.

Catheters impregnated or coated with antimicrobials or antiseptics have been shown to decrease the risk of CLA-BSI. Chlorhexidine-impregnated dressings have also been found to reduce the rate of CVC colonization. While evidence for the efficacy of CVC catheters coated with antibacterial or antiseptic agents exists, limited information exists related to their cost-effectiveness. Current CDC recommendations include use of CVC catheters coated with antibacterial or antiseptic agents if unable to decrease the rate to less than 3 infections per 1000 catheter days after implementing standards for insertion and care of the catheter.

Nursing-related care aspects include maximal barrier precautions during CVC insertion; maintenance of central

TABLE 11-11. EVIDENCE-BASED STRATEGIES FOR CENTRAL LINE INFECTION PREVENTION

- Education and training should be provided for staff who insert and maintain intravenous lines.
- Maximal sterile barriers should be used during catheter insertion (cap, mask, sterile gown and gloves, and a large sterile drape).
- A 2% chlorhexidine preparation is the preferred skin antiseptic, to be applied prior to insertion.
- Antiseptic- or antibiotic-impregnated catheters should be reserved for very high-risk patients or situations in which catheter-related BSI rates are high despite careful attention to these recommendations.
- Replace peripheral intravenous sites in the adult patient population at least every 96 hours but no more frequently than every 72 hours. Peripheral venous catheters in children should be left in until the intravenous therapy is completed, unless complications such as phlebitis or infiltration occur.
- Replace intravenous tubing no more frequently than every 96 hours but at least every 7 days in patients not receiving blood, blood products or fat emulsions.
- Replace intravenous catheters as soon as possible when adherence to aseptic technique during catheter insertion cannot be ensured (ie, prehospital, code situation).
- Central lines should not routinely be replaced at scheduled intervals.
- Consider use of a central line insertion checklist to ensure that all processes related to central line insertion are executed for each line placement.
- Consider use of a central line insertion cart to avoid the difficulty of finding necessary equipment to institute maximal barrier precautions.
- Replace central line dressings whenever damp, loose, or soiled or at a frequency of every 2 days for gauze dressings and every 7 days for transparent dressings.
- Avoid use of antibiotic ointment at insertion sites because it can promote fungal infections and antibiotic resistance.
- Include daily review of line necessity.
- Assess competency of staff who insert and care for intravascular catheters.

Adapted from: O'Grady NP, Alexander M, Burns LA, et al. *Guidelines for the Prevention of Intravascular Catheter-Related Infections,* Centers for Disease Control and Prevention, 2011.

line site to minimize infection risk; prevention of contamination of CVC ports during blood sampling, infusion of intravenous fluids, or medication administration; maintenance of sterile technique for dressing changes; intravenous tubing changes based on protocol guidelines; and astute monitoring of patients with central lines for signs of infection.

SELECTED INFECTIOUS DISEASES

Multi-drug resistant organisms (MDRO) are bacteria resistant to current antibiotic therapy. MDROs can cause serious local and systemic infections that can be severely debilitating and even life-threatening. The most common MDROs include methicillin-resistant Staphylococcus aureus (MRSA), vancomycin-resistant Enterococcus (VRE), tuberculosis (TB), Acinetobacter, and Clostridium difficile infections (C-diff). According to the CDC the prevalence of infections caused by MDROs is on the rise, making early identification, treatment, and prevention of the transmission of MDROs an important area of focus for healthcare providers.

Methicillin-resistant *Staphylococcus aureus* is a type of staphylococcal organism resistant to traditional antibiotic therapy, including methicillin, oxacillin, amoxicillin, penicillin, and cephalosporins. MRSA can be transmitted by personal contact with contaminated items such as dressings or other infected materials, and can be spread via the hands or equipment of healthcare providers, such as stethoscopes.

Vancomycin-resistant Enterococcus most commonly occurs in hospital and long-term care settings. According to the CDC, persons at-risk for acquiring VRE include those who have been previously treated with the antibiotic vancomycin or other antibiotics for long periods of time, hospitalized persons who have received antibiotics for a long period of time, persons with impaired immune status, those who have had recent surgery or those with invasive catheters. VRE can be passed from person to person by the contaminated hands of caregivers or spread directly to people after they touch surfaces that are contaminated with VRE.

The CDC has identified interventions necessary to control or eradicate MDROs including MRSA and VRE. These categories include administrative support, education, judicious use of antimicrobial agents, MDRO surveillance, infection control precautions, environmental precautions, and decolonization. Additionally, the CDC's Campaign to Prevent Antimicrobial Resistance recommends judicious use of antibiotics and avoiding excessive duration of antibiotic therapy. General measures to prevent MDROs in healthcare settings include infection prevention measures, early detection of infections, appropriate use of antibiotic therapy, and measures to prevent transmission. Nurses in progressive care units play an important role in the prevention of infections, and in instituting measures to prevent transmission of MDROs. The importance of hand hygiene continues to play a significant role in the prevention of infection and in targeting transmission of MDROs. Some organizations have also implemented the use of contact precautions upon admission of high risk patients for MRSA until proven culture negative. Awareness of specific institutional practices for infection prevention and control including the use of standard and contact precautions, along with education of staff, patients and visitors provide the basis for recommendations for control of MDROs in healthcare settings.

SELECTED BIBLIOGRAPHY

SIRS, Sepsis, and MODS

AACN practice alert: Sepsis 2006. www.aacn.org/WD/Practice/Docs/Sepsis-04.2006.pdf. Accessed February 13, 2013.

Aitken LM, Williams G, Harvey M, et al. Nursing considerations to complement the Surviving Sepsis Campaign. *Crit Care Med.* 2011;39:1800-1818.

Balas MC, Vasilevskis EE, Burke WJ, et al. Critical care nurses role in implementing the "ABCDE bundle" into practice. *Crit Care Nurse.* 2012;32:35-47.

Baldwin I, Fealy N. Nursing for Renal Replacement Therapies in the Intensive Care Unit: Historical, Educational, and Protocol Review. *Blood Purif.* 2009;27:174-181 (DOI:10.1159/000190784).

Barr J, Fraser GL, Puntillo K, et al. Clinical practice guidelines for the management of pain, agitation, and delirium in adult patients in the intensive care unit. *Crit Care Med.* 2013;41(1):263-306.

Blackwood B, Wilson-Barnett J. The impact of nurse-directed protocolised-weaning from mechanical ventilation on nursing practice: a quasi-experimental study. *J Int Stud*. 2007;44:209-226.

Bourgault AM, Ipe L, Weaver J, et al. Development of evidence-based guidelines and critical care nurses: knowledge of enteral feeding. *Crit Care Nurse*. 2007;27:17-29.

Carmona Monge FJ, Martinez Lareo M, Garcia Gomez S, et al. Effectiveness and safety of goal directed nurse-led blood glucose control in an intensive care unit: a prospective observational study. *Enferm Intensiva*. 2012;23;11-16.

Chant C, Mustard M, Thorpe KE, Friedrich JO. Nurse vs nomogram-directed glucose control in a cardiovascular intensive care unit. *Am J Crit Care*. 2012;21:270-279.

Davidson J, Powers K, Hedayat K, et al: Clinical practice guidelines for support of the family in the patient-centered intensive care unit: American College of Critical Care Medicine Task Force. *Crit Care Med*. 2007;35:605-622.

Dellinger RP, Levy ML, Opal S, et al. Surviving Sepsis Campaign: International guidelines for management of severe sepsis and septic shock: 2012. *Crit Care Med*. 2013;41:580-637.

Gaieski DF, Edwards JM, Kallan MJ, Carr BG. Benchmarking the incidence and mortality of severe sepsis in the United States. *Crit Care Med*. 2013; 41:1167-1174.

Gupta B, Agrawal P, Soni KD, et al. Enteral nutrition practices in the intensive care unit: understanding of nursing practices and perspectives. *J Anaesthesiol Clin Pharmacol*. 2012;28:41-44.

Institute for Healthcare Improvement. Evaluation for severe sepsis screening tool. http://www.survivingsepsis.org/files/Tools/evaluationforseveresepsisscreeningtool.pdf

Kleinpell R, Aitken L, Schorr CA. Implications of the new international sepsis guidelines for nursing care. *Am J Crit Care*. 2013;22:212-220.

Levy MM, Dellinger RP, Townsend SR, et al. The Surviving Sepsis Campaign: Results of an international guideline-based performance improvement program targeting severe sepsis. *Crit Care Med*. 2010;38:367-374.

Moore LJ, Jones SL, Kreiner LA, et al. Validation of a screening tool for the early identification of sepsis. *J Trauma*. 2009; 66:1539-1546; discussion 1546-1547.

Nguyen HB, Corbett SW, Steele R, et al. Implementation of a bundle of quality indicators for the early management of severe sepsis and septic shock is associated with decreased mortality. *Crit Care Med*. 2007;35:1105-1112.

NICE-SUGAR Study Investigators. Hypoglycemia and risk of death in critically ill patients. *N Engl J Med*. 2012;367:1108-1118.

O'Connor E, Tragen D, Fahey P et al. Improving blood glucose control during critical illness: a cohort study. *J Crit Care*. 2010;25:78-83.

Perel P, Roberts I. Colloids versus crystalloids for fluid resuscitation in critically ill patients. *Cochrane Database Syst Rev*. 2011; (3):CD000567. Review.

Pronovost P, Berenholtz S. Improving sepsis care in the intensive care unit: an evidence-based approach. 2004 VHA Research Series. Available: https://www.vha.com/research/public/sepsis_icu.pdf/. Accessed March 16, 2010.

Rivers EP, Ahrens T. Improving outcomes for severe sepsis and septic shock: tools for early identification of at-risk patients and treatment protocol implementation. *Crit Care Clin*. 2008;23:S1-S47.

Rubinsky M, Clark A. Early enteral nutrition in critically ill patients. *Dimens Crit Care Nurs*. 2012;31:267-274.

Wheeler AP, Bernard GR. Treating patients with severe sepsis. *N Engl J Med*. 1999;340:207-214.

Overdose

Amato L, Minozzi S, Vecchi S, Davoli M. Amato, Laura, eds. Benzodiazepines for alcohol withdrawal. *Cochrane Database Syst Rev* 3(3):2010;CD005063. DOI:10.1002/14651858.CD005063.pub3. PMID 20238336.

Ameres MJ. Acetaminophen (tylenol) poisoning. http://www.emedicinehealth.com/acetaminophen_tylenol_poisoning/article_em.htm. Accessed February 15, 2013.

Anker A. Drug Overdose. http://www.emedicinehealth.com/drug_overdose/page2_em.htm. Accessed February 22, 2013.

Cassidy EM, O'Sullivan I, Bradshaw P, Islam T, Onovo C. Symptom-triggered benzodiazepine therapy for alcohol withdrawal syndrome in the emergency department: a comparison with the standard fixed dose benzodiazepine regimen. *Emerg Med J*. 2011.

Center for Disease Control and Prevention. CDC grand rounds: prescription drug overdoses—a U.S. epidemic. *JAMA*. 2012;307(8):774-776.

Corfee FA. Alcohol withdrawal in the critical care unit. *Aust Crit Care*. 2011;24(2):110-116.

Karch AM. *Nursing 2009 Drug Handbook*. Philadelphia, PA: Lippincott, Williams & Wilkins; 2009.

Marraffa JM, Cohen V, Howland MA. Antidotes for toxicological emergencies: a practical review. *Am J Health-Syst Pharm*. 2012;69(3):199-212.

McKeown NJ, West, PL. Withdrawal syndromes. 2012. http://emedicine.medscape.com/article/819502-overview. Accessed February 25, 2013.

Monte R, Rabunal R, Casariego E, et al. Analysis of the factors determining survival of alcoholic withdrawal syndrome patients in a general hospital. *Alcohol Alcohol*. March-April 2010;45(2):151-158.

Muzyk AJ, Fowler JA, Norwood DK, Chilipko A. Role of a2-agonists in the treatment of acute alcohol withdrawal. *Ann Pharmacother*. May 2011;45(5):649-657.

Schutt RC, Ronco C, Rosner MH. The role of therapeutic plasma exchange in poisonings and intoxications. *Seminars in Dialysis*. 2012;25(2):201-206.

Stewart S, Swain S. Assessment and management of alcohol dependence and withdrawal in the acute hospital: concise guidance. *Clin Med*. 2012;12(3):266-271.

Tetrault JM, O'Connor PG. Substance abuse and withdrawal in the critical care setting. *Crit Care Clin*. 2008;24:767-788.

Complex Wounds and Pressure Ulcers

Agency for Healthcare Research and Quality. Preventing pressure ulcers in hospitals: a toolkit for improving quality of care. http://www.ahrq.gov/research/ltc/pressureulcertoolkit/putool3a.htm. Accessed May 5, 2012.

Bryant N, Nix Denise. *Acute and Chronic Wounds Current Management Concepts*. 4th edition, 2010. Elsevier Mosby, St Louis Missouri.

Cox J. Predictors of pressure ulcers in adult critical care patients. *Am J Crit Care*. 2011;20:364-375.

Guideline for Prevention and Management of Pressure Ulcers, WOCN Clinical Practice Guideline Series, 2010.

Institute for Healthcare (IHI). 5 million lives campaign getting started kit: how to guide. 2008. Cambridge, MA: Author Retrieved February 18, 2013 from http://www.ihi.org/knowledge/Pages/Tools/HowtoGuidePreventPressureUlcers.aspx

Jankowski IM. Tips for protecting critically ill patients from pressure ulcers. *Crit Care Nurse*. 2010;30:S7-S9.

Moore Z, Webster J, Review Group, Cochrane Wounds Group. Dressings and topical agents for preventing ulcers. *Cochrane Database Syst Rev.* 2011.

Niederhauser A, Lukas CV, Parker V, et al. Comprehensive programs for preventing pressure ulcers: a review of the literature. *Adv Skin Wound Care.* 2012;15:167-188.

National Pressure Ulcer Advisory Panel, European Pressure Ulcer Advisory Panel. Pressure ulcer prevention recommendations. In: *Prevention and treatment of pressure ulcers: clinical practice guideline.* Washington (DC): National Pressure Ulcer Advisory Panel; 2009,21-50.

Shanin ES, Dassen T, Halfens RJ. Incidence, prevention and treatment of pressure ulcers in intensive care patients: a longitudinal study. *Int J Nurs Stud.* 2009;46:413-421.

Healthcare Acquired Infections

Brosnahan J, Jull A, Tracy C. Types of urethral catheters for management of short-term voiding problems in hospitalized adults (Cochrane Review). *The Cochrane Database Syst Rev.* 2007;1.

Centers for Disease Control Catheter-associated urinary tract infection. http://www.cdc.gov/HAI/ca_uti/uti.html. Accessed February 16, 2013.

Gould VC, Umscheid C, Agarwal RK, et al. Guidelines for the prevention of catheter-associated urinary tract infection 2009. http://www.cdc.gov/hicpac/pdf/CAUTI/CAUTIguideline2009 final.pdf Accessed February 20, 2013.

Gould VC. Catheter association urinary tract infection (CAUTI) prevention toolkit http://www.cdc.gov/HAI/pdfs/toolkits/CAUTItoolkit_3_10.pdf. Accessed February 20, 2013.

Kleinpell RM, Munro CL, Giuliano KK. Targeting health care acquired infections: evidence based strategies. In: *Patient Safety and Quality: An Evidence Based Handbook for Nurses.* Agency for Healthcare Research and Quality, 2008. http://www.ncbi.nlm.nih.gov/books/NBK2632/. Accessed February 20, 2013.

O'Grady NP, Alexander M, Burns LA, et al. Guidelines for the prevention of intravascular catheter-related infections, 2011. http://www.cdc.gov/hicpac/pdf/guidelines/bsi-guidelines-2011.pdf. Accessed February 20, 2013.

Selected Infectious Diseases

Centers for Disease Control and Prevention. Management of multidrug-resistant organisms in healthcare settings, 2006. http://www.cdc.gov/ncidod/dhqp/pdf/ar/MDROGuideline2006.pdf. Accessed February 20, 2013.

Centers for Disease Control and Prevention. Methicillin resistant Staphylococcus auerus (MRSA) infections http://www.cdc.gov/mrsa/. Accessed February 20, 2013.

Centers for Disease Control and Prevention. Vancomycin-resistant Enterococci in healthcare settings. http://www.cdc.gov/HAI/organisms/vre/vre.html. Accessed February 20. 2013.

Derricott B. Multi-Drug Resistant Organisms (MDROs). 2011. http://www.nursingceu.com/courses/316/index_nceu.html. Accessed February 20, 2013.

Siegel JD, Rhinehart E, Jackson M, et al. The Healthcare Infection Control Practices Advisory Committee (HICPAC). Management of multidrug-resistant organisms. In: Healthcare Settings, 2006. http://www.cdc.gov/hicpac/pdf/MDRO/MDROGuideline2006.pdf. Accessed February 20, 2013.

NEUROLOGIC SYSTEM

Dea Mahanes

KNOWLEDGE COMPETENCIES

1. Correlate neurologic assessments to patient problems and diagnostic findings.

2. Identify indications, complications, and nursing management for commonly used neurodiagnostic tests.

3. Identify causes of increased intracranial pressure and describe strategies for management.

4. Compare and contrast the pathophysiology, clinical presentation, patient needs, and nursing management for:
   - Acute ischemic stroke
   - Hemorrhagic stroke
   - Seizure disorders
   - CNS infections
   - Selected neuromuscular diseases

SPECIAL ASSESSMENT TECHNIQUES AND DIAGNOSTIC TESTS

Although there is no single method of performing a neurologic evaluation, a systematic, orderly approach offers the best results. Knowledge of neurologic disease processes and neuroanatomy allows the progressive care nurse to tailor the assessment to individual patients. Obtaining past medical history and history of present illness or injury is essential and includes preexisting neurologic conditions. The time of symptom onset and mechanism of injury have important implications for diagnostic testing and treatment. The administration of any medications that may potentially alter the neurologic examination, especially sedatives and analgesics, is also noted.

Serial assessments, coupled with accurate documentation, allow for detection of subtle changes in neurologic status. Early detection of changes permits rapid intervention and improves patient outcomes. Neurologic assessment in the progressive care unit can be broken down into the following components: level of consciousness, mental status, motor examination, sensory examination, and cranial nerve examination. A baseline examination is established and subsequent assessments are compared. At a minimum, serial neurologic assessment includes level of consciousness, orientation, motor response, and pupil size and reaction

to light. Whenever a hand-off of care occurs (for example, at shift change), the care providers perform a neurological examination together to provide an accurate baseline for the nurse assuming care of the patient.

Level of Consciousness

There are two components to level of consciousness: arousal and awareness. *Arousal* refers to the state of wakefulness; *awareness* reflects the content and quality of interactions with the environment. Arousal reflects function of the reticular-activating system and brain stem, and awareness indicates functioning of the cerebral cortex. Level of consciousness is assessed on all patients. A change in level of consciousness is the most important indicator of neurologic decline and is immediately acted on by the healthcare team.

Observation of the patient's behavior, appearance, and ability to communicate is the first step in assessing level of consciousness. If the patient responds meaningfully to the examiner without the need for stimulation, then the patient is described as alert. If stimulation is required, auditory stimuli are used first. If the patient does not rouse to auditory stimuli, tactile stimuli such as a gentle touch or shake are used, followed by painful stimuli if necessary to elicit a response. Accepted methods of central painful stimulus include squeezing the trapezius or other large muscle group. Care is taken to avoid causing tissue trauma. Supraorbital pressure is also an acceptable pain stimulus, but is not used if there is any suspicion of facial fracture. Use of a sternal rub may result in a motor response that is difficult to interpret (see Glasgow Coma Scale [GCS]) and often causes bruising. Nail bed pressure is a commonly used peripheral pain stimulus. Response to central stimulus is more indicative of cerebral function than response to peripheral stimulus. Certain responses to peripheral pain, such as the triple flexion response (stereotypical flexion of the ankle, knee, and hip), can result from a spinal reflex arc and thus may remain present even following death by neurologic criteria (brain death).

Glasgow Coma Scale

The GCS (Table 12-1) is often used to monitor neurologic status because it provides a standardized approach to assessing and documenting level of consciousness. Response is determined in three categories: eye opening, motor response, and verbal response. The best response in each category is scored, and the results are added to give a total GCS. Scores range from 3 to 15, with 15 indicating a patient that is alert, fully oriented, and following commands.

The eye opening score reflects the amount of stimulation that must be applied for the patient to open his eyes. Spontaneous eye opening is the best response, followed by eye opening to verbal stimulation, then eye opening to painful stimulation. Scoring of the eye opening section of the scale can be complicated by orbital trauma and swelling, and this is documented accordingly.

The motor portion of the GCS is the most difficult to assess. Response in each extremity is tested, but only the best motor response is used in calculating a total score. The patient is first asked to follow a command such as "Hold up your thumb" or "Wiggle your toes." A patient who does not follow commands with his or her extremities is asked to look up and down. In certain neurologic disorders (such as basilar artery stroke or high cervical spinal cord injury), patients may be unable to follow commands with their extremities but still be awake and aware; assessing the ability to look up and down helps identify these individuals. If the patient does not follow commands, then all four extremities are assessed for response to pain stimuli. Upper extremity response to pain is described as localization, withdrawal, decorticate (flexor) posturing, or decerebrate (extensor) posturing. An attempt by the patient to push the stimulus away is clearly localization, but the response is not always easily apparent. Interpretation of patient's movement is complicated when a sternal rub is used because with both localization and decorticate posturing, the arms move up toward the stimulus. Reaching across the midline of the body to a stimulus (eg, if the right arm comes up to the left shoulder when a left trapezius squeeze is applied) is scored as localization. An easy way to remember decorticate and decerebrate posturing is that decorticate is "into the core," or flexion, and decerebrate is away from the body, or extension (Figure 12-1). Decorticate posturing signifies damage in the cerebral hemispheres or thalamus. Decerebrate posturing indicates damage to the midbrain or pons. The presence of posturing or

TABLE 12-1. GLASGOW COMA SCALE

Behavior	Score[a]
Eye Opening (E)	
Spontaneous	4
To verbal stimuli	3
To pain	2
None	1
Motor Response (M)	
Obeys commands	6
Localizes pain	5
Withdraws to pain	4
Abnormal flexion	3
Extensor response	2
None	1
Verbal Response (V)	
Oriented	5
Confused	4
Inappropriate words	3
Incomprehensible sounds	2
None	1

[a]Coma score = E + M + V (scores range 3-15).

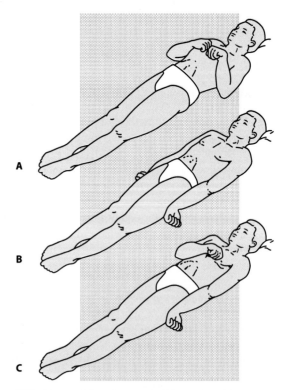

Figure 12-1. Abnormal motor responses. **(A)** Decorticate posturing. **(B)** Decerebrate posturing. **(C)** Decorticate posturing on right side and decerebrate posturing on left side of body. (*Reprinted from: Carlson BA. Neurologic clinical assessment. In: Urden LD, Stacy KM, Lough ME, eds. Thelan's Critical Care Nursing: Diagnosis and Management. St Louis, MO: Mosby; 2002:649.*)

a change from decorticate to decerebrate posturing should be brought to the attention of the physician immediately. Motor response to pain in the lower extremities is usually graded as withdrawal or triple flexion. In triple flexion, pain stimulus results in stereotypical flexion of the ankle, knee, and hip. This response can be differentiated from withdrawal by applying the pain stimulus to a different area of the lower extremity (eg, the medial aspect of the calf). If the response is withdrawal, the patient pulls away from the stimulus. If the response is triple flexion, the response is still stereotypical flexion at the ankle, knee, and hip.

The verbal section of the GCS assesses a patient's ability to speak coherently and with appropriate content. Orientation to person, place, and time is assessed. As mental status declines, orientation to time is lost first, followed by orientation to place. Orientation to person is seldom lost prior to loss of consciousness. Patients with tracheostomies are commonly assigned a verbal score of T and the total GCS is denoted as the sum of the eye opening and motor scores followed by T. Alternatively, the examiner assigns a verbal score based on estimation of the patient's abilities, often determined by noting the patient's response when presented with multiple choices.

Although the GCS is frequently used to monitor hospitalized patients, it is important to remember that only a limited amount of information is provided. Additional assessments are necessary to gain an accurate picture of neurologic functioning; these assessments are based on the type of disease process or injury and the part of the central nervous system (CNS) affected.

Full Outline of UnResponsiveness (FOUR) Score

The *Full Outline of UnResponsiveness* (FOUR) score is another validated tool for the assessment of neurological patients. The FOUR score assigns a value of 0 through 4 in each of four categories: eyes, motor, brain stem reflexes, and respirations. The scores in each category are added together to give a total score of 0 to 16. Table 12-2 provides an overview of the FOUR score, but complete instructions are not included; progressive care nurses who utilize this tool should seek additional information. Because of the inclusion of brain stem reflexes and respiratory pattern, the FOUR score allows the clinician to identify changes in patients with very limited responses.

Mental Status

Although formal measurements of mental status exist, many acutely ill neurologic patients may be unable to complete these assessments because of limited ability to communicate or decreased level of consciousness. Orientation is the component of mental status most often evaluated in the progressive care unit. Other components of mental status assessment include attention/concentration, affect, memory, reasoning, and language function. Attention/concentration, affect, and reasoning are typically assessed informally by simply observing the patient throughout daily care. Short-term memory may be evaluated by giving the patient a list of three items and asking him or her to recall them later. However, deficits are often apparent in informal interactions as well. Difficulty with language can be described as dysarthria (weakness or lack of coordination of the muscles of speech) or aphasia. Aphasia can be either expressive (inability to express thoughts), receptive (inability to comprehend), or global (both expressive and receptive). An individual with expressive aphasia may be able to understand everything that is said but be unable to reply, whereas an individual with receptive aphasia may have nonsensical, fluent speech, but cannot comprehend what is said to him. A patient with dysarthria has slurred speech and is difficult to understand, but the content is appropriate. Dysarthria represents weakness or loss of coordination of the muscles of speech vs a problem with mental status. However, dysarthria often becomes apparent during assessment of mental status and thus is included here.

Delirium is an alteration in mental status that is of particular importance in acutely ill patients, because the development of delirium is associated with worse clinical outcomes and increased hospitalization costs. Delirium is described as hyperactive (restlessness, agitation) or hypoactive (flat affect, apathy, lethargy, decreased responsiveness to the environment). Delirium is characterized by acute changes or fluctuations in mental status, inattention, and

TABLE 12-2. OVERVIEW OF THE FULL OUTLINE OF UNRESPONSIVENESS (FOUR) SCORE

Component	0 Points	1 Point	2 Points	3 Points	4 Points
Eye response	Eyelids remain closed with pain	Eyelids closed but open to pain	Eyelids closed but open to loud voice	Eyelids open but not tracking	Eyelids open or opened, tracking, or blinking to command
Motor response	No response to pain or generalized myoclonus status	Extension to pain	Flexion to pain	Localizing to pain	Thumbs up, fist, or peace sign
Brain stem reflexes	Absent pupil, corneal, and cough reflexes	Pupil and corneal reflexes absent	Pupil or corneal reflexes absent	One pupil wide and fixed	Pupil and corneal reflexes present
Respiration	Breaths at ventilator rate or apnea	Breaths above ventilator rate	Not intubated, irregular breathing	Not intubated, Cheyne-Stokes breathing pattern	Not intubated, regular breathing pattern

Data from: Wijdicks EFM, Bamlet WR, Maramattom BV, et al. Validation of a new coma scale: the FOUR score. Ann Neurol. 2005;58:585-593.)

cognitive changes or perceptual disturbances. Some patients present with a combination of hyperactive and hypoactive delirium. Delirium is usually rapid in onset and reversible. In contrast, dementia is a progressive, irreversible loss of intellectual or cognitive abilities like reasoning, math, or abstract thinking and develops more slowly. Delirium and dementia are not mutually exclusive; a patient with mild to moderate dementia may exhibit delirium in the unfamiliar environment of the hospital.

Contributing factors to the development of delirium include systemic illness (infection, fever, or metabolic dysfunction), inadequate pain control, electrolyte abnormalities, the administration of medications including benzodiazepines or opioids, sleep deprivation, and withdrawal from alcohol or other substances. Delirium is more common in older patients. The first step in treating delirium is to rule out reversible causes. Nursing strategies to prevent delirium and decrease its effects include reorientation, encouraging progressive mobility, modulating stimulation, providing appropriate cognitive activities, promoting normal sleep-wake cycles, ensuring that assistive devices such as hearing aids and glasses are available, treating pain, and family presence. Family members are educated about delirium and provided with guidance in how to interact with the patient (speak clearly and directly, provide frequent reorientation, and avoid multiple simultaneous conversations). Restraints are not used unless patient or staff safety is compromised, because they only add to the patient's confusion and apprehension. In addition to environmental controls, medications can be useful in the management of delirium.

Patients with organic brain disease, regardless of specific diagnosis, often exhibit challenging behaviors. Examples include agitation, emotional lability, and disinhibition. This can be very disconcerting to family members, especially when the patient has not exhibited these behaviors previously. Dealing with agitated, confused patients can be frustrating for staff as well. Although medication administration can be necessary to keep the patient safe, many drugs alter neurologic assessment, delay recovery, or even worsen symptoms. Environmental strategies such as decreasing noise and distractions can be very effective and are always used first. If medications are required to maintain safety, they are combined with environmental strategies and used at the lowest dose possible for the shortest time possible.

Motor Assessment

Motor assessment includes muscle size, tone, strength, and involuntary movements such as tics or tremors. Motor function is assessed in each extremity and evaluated for symmetry. In patients who are able to follow commands, pronator drift is an excellent indicator of upper extremity motor function. To assess pronator drift, instruct the patient to close his or her eyes and raise his or her arms with the palms facing the ceiling. A normal response is for the patient to maintain this

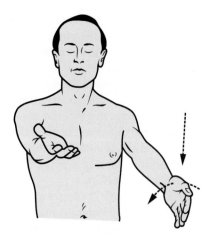

Figure 12-2. Assessment of pronator drift. The patient is asked to hold her or his arms outstretched with the palms supinated and eyes closed. If weakness is present, the weak arm gradually pronates and drifts downward. (*Reprinted from: Lindsay KW, Bone I, Callander R.* Neurology and Neurosurgery Illustrated. *New York, NY: Churchill Livingstone; 1997:19.*)

position until told to stop. Patients with focal motor weakness demonstrate varying degrees of pronator drift. Depending on the severity of weakness, the affected side may drift away from its initial position quickly or slowly, or the palm may simply begin to pronate (Figure 12-2). Further assessment of upper extremity strength involves testing the deltoids, biceps, triceps, and grips. Lower extremity testing includes the hamstrings, quadriceps, dorsiflexion, and plantar flexion. Strength is rated on a 5-point scale (Table 12-3). In patients who do not follow commands, motor assessment consists of first observing the patient for spontaneous movement. If necessary, a pain stimulus is applied and the patient's response is observed. The response is graded numerically as part of the GCS or FOUR score, but may also be described as purposeful, nonpurposeful, or no response.

In an awake, alert patient, complete motor assessment includes testing of coordination, an indicator of cerebellar function. Common testing mechanisms include assessment of rapid alternating movements, finger-to-nose testing, and the heel slide test. To test rapid alternating movements, ask the patient to supinate and pronate his or her hands as quickly as possible. In finger-to-nose testing, the patient is instructed to repeatedly touch his or her nose, then the examiner's finger. To assess the lower extremities, ask the

TABLE 12-3. EVALUATION OF MUSCLE STRENGTH

Grade	Definition
0	No movement
1	Muscle contraction only (palpated or visible)
2	Active movement within a single plane (gravity eliminated)
3	Active movement against gravity
4	Active movement against some resistance
5	Active movement against full resistance (normal strength)

patient to run the heel of his or her foot up and down the shin of the opposite leg as quickly as possible. Patients with cerebellar dysfunction display decreased speed and accuracy on these tests.

Sensation

There are three basic sensory pathways: pain/temperature, position/vibration, and light touch. Light touch is the pathway most often assessed in the progressive care unit, but may be preserved even if lesions of the spinal cord exist because of overlapping innervation. Because most patients with intracranial lesions report altered sensation in an entire extremity or one side of the body, assessment of light touch is likely to identify these patients. Ask the patient to close his or her eyes, and lightly touch each extremity working distal to proximal. Trunk and facial sensation is also assessed.

When a more comprehensive nursing assessment is indicated, testing for pain and position sense provides useful information. A cotton tip applicator with a wooden stem can be broken and used; the end with the cotton is dull and the broken end is sharp. Touch the patient's skin lightly in a random pattern and ask the patient to identify the sensation as sharp or dull. Two seconds should elapse between stimuli. To test position sense, or proprioception, move the patient's index finger or big toe up or down by grasping the digit laterally over the joints. Provide an example of both "up" and "down" positions prior to testing. Repeat these movements in a random order, asking the patient to identify whether the joint is up or down. Always return to the neutral position between movements and carefully grasp the digit to avoid giving the patient clues.

Sensory assessment is performed with the patient's eyes closed. Documentation of comprehensive sensory assessment is best accomplished using a dermatome chart (Figure 12-3). Areas of abnormal sensation can be marked and tracked over time.

Cranial Nerve Assessment and Assessment of Brain Stem Function

Assessment of the cranial nerves provides an indication of the integrity of the nerves themselves and of brain stem function. A screening examination based on pupillary response

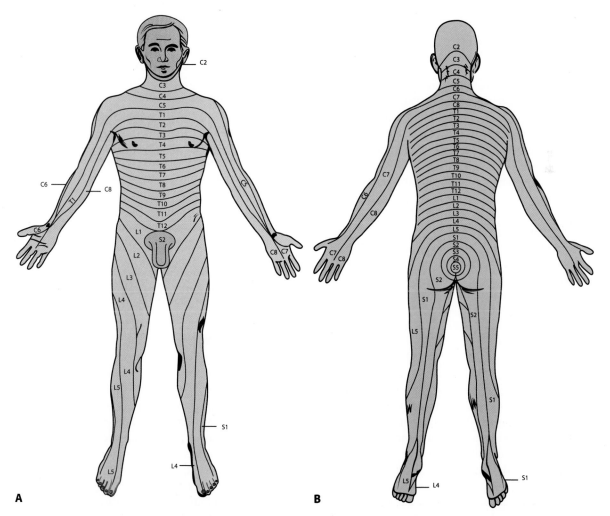

Figure 12-3. Dermatomes. **(A)** Anterior view. **(B)** Posterior view. (*Reprinted from: Carlson BA. Neurologic anatomy and physiology. In: Urden LD, Stacy KM, Lough ME, eds.* Thelan's Critical Care Nursing: Diagnosis and Management. *St Louis, MO: Mosby; 2002:641.*)

TABLE 12-4. CRANIAL NERVE FUNCTION

Nerve	Function
I. Olfactory	Sense of smell
II. Optic	Visual fields, visual acuity
III. Oculomotor	Most extraocular eye movements, ability to elevate eyelid, muscular contraction of the iris in response to light
IV. Trochlear	Eye movement down and toward the nose
V. Trigeminal	Facial sensation, including cornea, nasal mucosa, and oral mucosa; muscles of chewing and mastication
VI. Abducens	Lateral eye movement
VII. Facial	Facial muscles, including eyelid closure; taste in anterior two-thirds of the tongue; secretion of saliva and tears
VIII. Acoustic	Hearing and equilibrium
IX. Glossopharyngeal	Gag reflex, muscles that control swallowing and phonation; taste in posterior third of tongue
X. Vagus (overlapping innervation)	Salivary gland secretion; vagal control of heart, lungs, and gastrointestinal tract
XI. Spinal accessory	Sternocleidomastoid and trapezius muscle strength
XII. Hypoglossal	Tongue movement

and protective reflexes (corneal, gag, cough) is conducted on all patients. Beyond that, the assessment can be customized to the individual based on pathology and the ability to participate in a more comprehensive exam. Patients with brain stem, cerebellar, or pituitary lesions merit more extensive assessment because of the proximity of the cranial nerves to these structures. The assessments noted below are the most commonly performed tests of cranial nerve function in the progressive care unit. Table 12-4 describes the function of all 12 cranial nerves.

Pupil Size and Reaction to Light

Assessment of pupil size and reaction to light is performed in all patients and provides information about the function of cranial nerves II (optic) and III (oculomotor). Pupils are assessed for size, shape, and reaction to light. These are measured in millimeters, not described by words such as large, small, pinpoint, or blown. Reaction to light is described as brisk, sluggish, or fixed/nonreactive. Both eyes are tested for direct and consensual response. To test direct pupillary response, shine a light directly into one eye and observe the response of the pupil in that eye. A normal response is brisk constriction followed by brisk dilation when the light is withdrawn. To test for consensual pupillary response, shine a light into one eye and observe the pupil of the other eye. It should constrict and dilate similarly. Assessing both direct and consensual response provides information about which cranial nerve (optic or oculomotor, and left or right) is affected. Certain medications can affect pupil size and reactivity; for example, atropine can dilate the pupils and narcotics can cause them to become very constricted. Pupillary changes

are often seen late in the course of neurologic decline as increased intracranial pressure (ICP) leads to compression or stretching of cranial nerve III.

Corneal Reflex or Facial Movement/Sensation

The corneal reflex evaluates cranial nerves V (trigeminal) and VII (facial). This test is classically performed with a wisp of cotton lightly drawn across the cornea; a normal response is a blink. A drop of sterile saline can also be used as a stimulus and is less likely to cause corneal abrasions. In alert patients, cranial nerves V and VII can be assessed by testing facial movement and sensation. Movement is assessed by asking the patient to smile, puff out his cheeks with air, and raise his eyebrows. Assessment of facial sensation includes all three branches of cranial nerve V (the trigeminal nerve). The three distributions can be tested by touching the forehead, cheek, and mandible. Patients with cranial nerve VII dysfunction are unable to close the eyelid on the affected side. Strategies to prevent corneal injury include the use of lubricating drops and ointments or taping the lid closed.

Gag and Cough Reflexes

The ability to swallow and the gag reflex are controlled by cranial nerves IX (glossopharyngeal) and X (vagus). To assess the gag reflex in a conscious patient, first explain the procedure and be sure the patient does not have a full stomach. Ask the patient to open his mouth and protrude his tongue (this also provides partial assessment of cranial nerve XII, the hypoglossal nerve). Observe the palate for bilateral elevation when the patient says "ahhh." If the palate does not elevate symmetrically, lightly touch the back of the throat with a tongue blade and observe the response. Both the left and right sides should be tested. To assess the gag reflex in an unconscious patient, use a bite block to keep the patient's teeth separated, then stimulate the back of the throat with a suction catheter or tongue blade. An intact gag reflex is indicated by forward thrusting of the tongue and sometimes the head. The cough reflex is also controlled by cranial nerves IX and X, and can be assessed by noting spontaneous cough or cough in response to suctioning.

Extraocular Eye Movements

Extraocular eye movements are controlled by muscles innervated by cranial nerves III, IV, and VI. To test extraocular movements, the patient is asked to follow an object (usually the examiner's finger) through six positions (Figure 12-4). A normal response consists of the eyes moving in the same direction, at the same speed, and in constant alignment (conjugate eye movement). Abnormal eye movements include nystagmus (a jerking, rhythmical movement of one or both of the eyes) or an extraocular palsy (eye movement in one or both eyes is inhibited in a certain direction). Mild nystagmus with extreme lateral gaze may be normal. Dysconjugate gaze, in which the eyes are not aligned, is an abnormal finding.

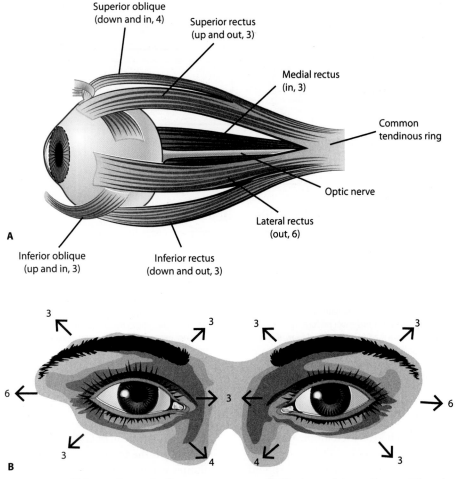

Figure 12-4. Extraocular eye movements. **(A)** Extraocular muscles. The eye movement controlled by the muscle is noted in parentheses, along with the associated cranial nerve supply. **(B)** The six cardinal directions of gaze and associated cranial nerves. (*Reprinted from: Carlson BA. Neurologic clinical assessment. In: Urden LD, Stacy KM, Lough ME, eds. Thelan's Critical Care Nursing: Diagnosis and Management. St Louis, MO: Mosby; 2002:652.*)

Vital Sign Alterations in Neurologic Dysfunction

Vital sign changes due to central nervous system dysfunction occur because of direct brain stem injury, decreased cerebral perfusion, or interruption of nerve pathways. Decreased perfusion causes ischemia and the body's response is to increase the blood pressure in an attempt to provide more nutrients to the brain. Hypotension is rarely seen except in the terminal stages of brain stem dysfunction or as the result of loss of sympathetic tone in patients with spinal cord injury. Abnormalities in heart rate and rhythm are common, and can be a cause of neurologic decline due to clot formation or inadequate cardiac output, or be a symptom of neurologic dysfunction (such as ST-segment abnormalities following subarachnoid hemorrhage). Respiratory patterns vary widely. Some of the more common patterns are shown in Figure 12-5. It is more important to determine if the patient is ventilating adequately than to determine the specific pattern. Temperature is carefully monitored in patients with acute neurologic dysfunction, because hyperthermia (regardless of infectious or noninfectious etiology)

causes increased cerebral metabolic demand. Hypothermia can result from injury to the brain stem or spinal cord.

Cushing response refers to a triad of vital sign changes seen late in the course of neurologic deterioration. The classic triad is marked by widened pulse pressure, bradycardia, and an irregular respiratory pattern. Cushing response is of minimal value in identifying early, significant changes in the patient's condition, but it is useful to be alert for components of Cushing response (eg, systolic hypertension or change in respiratory pattern).

DIAGNOSTIC TESTING

Lumbar Puncture

Lumbar puncture (LP) can be performed for diagnostic or therapeutic purposes. Diagnostic indications for LP include measurement of cerebrospinal fluid (CSF) pressure as an estimation of ICP and sampling of CSF for analysis when central nervous system (CNS) infection, inflammation, or subarachnoid hemorrhage is suspected. Therapeutic indications for

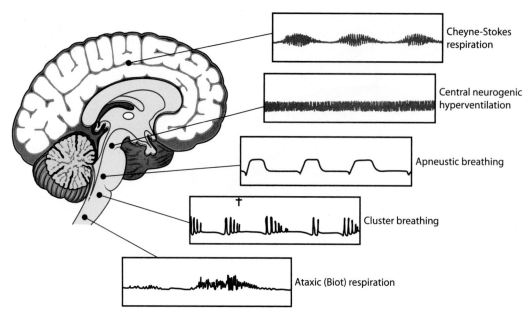

Figure 12-5. Abnormal respiratory patterns associated with increased ICP. Cheyne-Stokes respiration, arising from deep inside the cerebral hemispheres and basal ganglia; central neurogenic hyperventilation, from lower midbrain to middle pons; apneustic breathing, from middle to lower pons; cluster breathing, from upper medulla; and ataxic (Biot) respiration, from medulla. (*Reprinted from: Barker E. Intracranial pressure and monitoring. In: Barker E, ed.* Neuroscience Nursing: A Spectrum of Care. *St Louis, MO: Mosby; 2002:389.*)

LP include drainage of CSF and the placement of tubes for medication administration or ongoing CSF drainage. Examples of disease processes in which LP is used for diagnostic or therapeutic purposes include meningitis, multiple sclerosis, Guillain-Barré syndrome, hydrocephalus, and subarachnoid hemorrhage. Increased ICP is a theoretical contraindication to LP because of the risk for downward herniation of brain tissue due to the pressure gradient created when CSF is removed from the lumbar space. When increased ICP is suspected, a CT scan (described later) may be performed prior to proceeding with the LP. Other contraindications include coagulopathy or infection in the area of skin through which the needle will be introduced. Although recommendations about duration vary based on the specific medication, anticoagulant and antiplatelet medications are often held when LP is planned.

When performing an LP, the clinician locates the L3 to L4 or L4 to L5 intervertebral space and injects a local anesthetic, then inserts a hollow needle with a stylet into the spinal subarachnoid space. The risk of spinal cord injury is minimal because the actual cord ends at L1 and only nerve roots continue below. Proper patient positioning is very important and patients may require sedation if they are unable to remain still. The LP may be performed with the patient sitting up and leaning forward, but a lateral decubitus position is used for most acutely ill patients. The patient lies on his side with his neck flexed forward and his knees pulled up toward the chest. This position widens the intervertebral space, allowing the needle to pass through more easily. The needle is inserted and the stylet is removed. Flow of CSF confirms that the needle is in the spinal subarachnoid space. A manometer is attached to the needle and used to measure an opening pressure. Pressures greater than 20 cm (200 mm) H_2O are considered abnormal. If the purpose of the LP is sampling or removal of CSF, the amount of CSF drained varies based on the indication for the procedure, with smaller volumes needed for laboratory analysis than for treatment of hydrocephalus. If the purpose of the procedure is administration of medications or placement of a lumbar drain, the medications will be given or the drain will be placed once needle placement is confirmed by CSF flow.

Normal CSF is clear and colorless. Infection and blood can change the appearance of CSF. In infection, CSF may be cloudy owing to white blood cells and bacteria. Blood causes the CSF to be pink, red, or brown. Although some blood may be present if a small vessel was traumatized during needle insertion, this blood clears as more CSF is drained. Blood due to CNS hemorrhage does not clear. Common tests performed on CSF include analysis of cell counts with differential, glucose, protein, lactate, Gram stain, and culture with sensitivities. Special assays may be requested to look for specific inflammatory or demyelinating disease processes. Once the needle is removed, a small self-adhesive bandage is placed over the insertion site.

Postprocedure care varies with physician preference, hospital protocol, and whether or not the patient complains of headache, but always includes monitoring the insertion site for bleeding, drainage, or hematoma development. Patients may complain of headache (due to loss of CSF), local pain at the insertion site, or pain radiating to the thigh (if a nerve root was hit during the procedure). Flat positioning and increased fluid intake are sometimes recommended after LP but have not been shown to reduce the incidence of post-LP headache. If headache does occur, these strategies are used in combination with analgesic administration. If the headache persists, an autologous blood patch may be used to stop continued CSF leakage.

Computed Tomography

Computed tomography (CT) is a common diagnostic tool when neurologic dysfunction is suspected. An x-ray beam moves in a 360° arc and a detector measures penetration of the x-ray beam into tissue. Penetration of the x-ray beam varies based on tissue density. The computer translates the collected x-ray beams into images. The result is a series of finely cut pictures showing bony structures, CSF, and brain tissue. Bone is visualized as white because it is most dense. CSF and air are black because of their low density. Brain tissue is seen in varying shades of gray. The appearance of recent intracranial bleeding is white; over time the color darkens as the blood breaks down. CT scans are quick, noninvasive, and easy to perform, and can identify most causes of acute neurologic deterioration, including bleeding, significant edema, and hydrocephalus.

Computed tomography scanning can be performed with a contrast medium to allow for better visualization of lesions such as tumors, abscesses, or vascular abnormalities. CT angiography (CTA) uses scanning during intravenous contrast administration to allow visualization of cerebral blood vessels. CTA is useful in the diagnosis of cerebral vascular anomalies, such as aneurysms or narrowed vessels. A three-dimensional reconstruction of the cerebrovasculature can be created from the images by using a special computer program.

During CT, the patient is placed on a narrow table that is moved up into a donut-shaped gantry. Because the table is narrow, the patient is positioned carefully and secured with padding or straps. Patient movement causes blurry images. Sedation may be required for patients who are unable to cooperate. In patients who receive contrast, assessment of renal function (blood urea nitrogen, creatinine, glomerular filtration rate) is essential because the contrast agent can cause acute kidney injury, especially if the patient is dehydrated or has pre-existing renal compromise, or if given in combination with other nephrotoxic agents. Because the administration of iodinated contrast medium has been associated with lactic acidosis, metformin is discontinued if contrast administration is anticipated.

The primary risks of CT scans result from the use of contrast. Patients with a history of allergic reaction to contrast or iodine require premedication. If contrast dye is administered, intravenous fluids are given before and after the study to decrease the risk of contrast-induced nephropathy (CIN). For more on CIN see Chapter 15, Renal System.

Magnetic Resonance Imaging

Magnetic resonance imaging (MRI) offers greater anatomic detail than CT scanning without using ionized radiation. The patient is placed in a strong magnetic field and controlled bursts of radio pulse waves are delivered, causing protons within atomic nuclei to resonate. The radiofrequency signals emitted by the resonating nuclei are measured and used to construct images. Cross-sectional images can be obtained in coronal, sagittal, and oblique planes. A contrast agent is sometimes administered, and highlights areas where the blood-brain barrier is disrupted. MRI scans are useful in diagnosing disorders of the brain stem, posterior fossa, and spinal cord, areas that are difficult to fully evaluate with CT. MRI also offers an advantage over CT in the identification of demyelinating disorders such as multiple sclerosis or neuro-degenerative diseases. Specific MRI sequences can be used to detect suspected lesions that cannot be seen on CT, such as early cerebral infarction and intramedullary tumors. Magnetic resonance angiography (MRA) uses a specialized computer program to highlight the cerebral vasculature. MRA is useful in the evaluation of suspected arteriovenous malformations (AVMs), aneurysms, and cavernous angiomas. Acute bleeding and bony abnormalities such as fractures can be better visualized using CT. The time requirement for MRI scans is typically longer than that of CT scans, which can be a disadvantage when needing to make treatment decisions based on diagnostic results. In addition, access to the patient is significantly limited during the scan.

All patients must be screened for the presence of implanted or embedded metal prior to MRI. Metallic objects inside the body may become dislodged or slip in the large magnetic tube and can cause patient injury. Most aneurysm clips are now made of nonferrous material and are safe for MRI; it is important to obtain additional information about the device, including when and where it was placed. Orthopedic hardware may also be safe, depending on the part of the body being imaged and the length of time since the hardware was placed. Patients who are either unable to reliably complete the MRI screening or who have a history of impaled metal fragments or shrapnel must have radiographs taken prior to MRI. The MRI magnet can also damage internally magnetized units, such as cardiac pacemakers, causing them to malfunction. An MRI-safe pacemaker is now available but many patients have older devices. Programmable shunts, frequently used for long-term management of hydrocephalus, are affected by the MRI and must be reprogrammed following the procedure. Devices such as medication pumps and nerve/spinal cord stimulators may or may not be MRI safe. At minimum, they need to be turned off before and reprogrammed after the procedure. With all devices and implants, it is important to obtain as much information as possible about the device type and when it was placed, and to report this information to the MRI technologist. Many IV pumps and other types of medical equipment contain metal and cannot be taken into the room where the MRI machine is located. Of note, the same screening precautions apply to the staff member who accompanies the patient to MRI. Any card with a magnetic strip, such as a credit card or even an employee ID, will be damaged by the MRI magnet and is removed. Patient education is important prior to scanning. Patients must be screened closely for any contraindications. In addition, all metal objects, such as jewelry, nonpermanent dentures, prostheses, hairpins, clothing with snaps or zippers, and ECG electrodes with metal snaps must be removed. Transdermal medication patches may also need to be removed. Patients should be advised of the loud "booming" noise of the scanner. Inform patients that the nurse or technician is in full view of them in the scanner and that they can talk to them if they feel uncomfortable on the table. Ensure the safety and comfort of the patient with safety belts and blankets for positioning. Patients who are claustrophobic may need sedation. Open-sided MRI machines are available at some institutions and decrease feelings of claustrophobia. There are no postprocedure interventions associated with MRI. Gadolinium-based contrast agents are sometimes administered in MRI and have been associated with nephrogenic systemic fibrosis (NSF) when given to patients with severe renal insufficiency, so renal function is assessed prior to administration. NSF causes fibrotic changes in the skin and other organs.

Cerebral (Catheter) Angiography

Although CTA and MRA are commonly used to assess the cerebrovasculature, catheter angiography remains the gold standard. Cerebral (catheter) angiography is similar to cardiac catheterization. Angiography can be performed for both diagnostic purposes and therapeutic intervention. Blockages or abnormalities of the cerebral circulation can be visualized, aiding in the diagnosis of vascular malformations (such as aneurysms or AVMs) and arterial stenosis. Angioplasty (with or without stent placement) can be performed for narrowed cerebral vessels. Blood vessels can also be therapeutically embolized; this is sometimes done to decrease blood supply to a tumor prior to surgical resection or as treatment for an aneurysm.

During cerebral angiography, a catheter is placed in the femoral or brachial artery and threaded up into the carotid or vertebral arteries, and a radiopaque contrast material is injected. The flow of the contrast material is tracked using radiographic films and fluoroscopy. Patients are kept NPO for 6 hours prior to nonemergent angiography. Coagulation studies are checked on all patients because coagulopathy is a relative contraindication to cerebral angiography. Many patients require sedation during the procedure. General anesthesia may be needed for uncooperative patients because the risk of vessel injury is increased if the patient moves her or his head during the procedure.

Potential complications include neurologic deficit due to injury to an intracranial vessel, allergic reaction to contrast, hematoma formation at the site of catheter insertion, vessel injury (dissection), retroperitoneal hematoma, and vessel spasm following injection of contrast. All patients undergoing cerebral angiography receive hydration because of the large amount of contrast agent used.

Following angiogram, patients are typically kept on bed rest with the head of bed flat for 4 to 6 hours to help prevent hematoma formation at the puncture site. In some cases, a special arterial closure device is used to promote clot formation and allow quicker mobilization, typically after about 2 hours. The amount of time the patient must remain flat is reflected in the postangiography orders. The arterial puncture site is monitored frequently for development of a hematoma, and the neurovascular status of the limb is also checked. Careful monitoring of vital signs and neurologic examination aid in the detection of intra- or extracranial emboli or hemorrhage.

Transcranial Doppler Ultrasound

Transcranial Doppler (TCD) ultrasound studies allow visualization of the blood flow through major cerebral blood vessels by directing ultrasonic waves through the thinner parts of the skull bone. A probe that emits ultrasonic waves is placed on the skin. Structures are differentiated based on how much of the wave is reflected back to the probe. A Doppler effect is created when the probe detects moving structures, like red blood cells in a blood vessel. The velocity of blood flow can be calculated. TCDs are noninvasive and can be done at the patient's bedside. TCDs are used at many institutions to aid in the detection of vasospasm after aneurysmal subarachnoid hemorrhage.

Electroencephalography

The electroencephalogram (EEG) is a measurement of the brain's electrical activity. EEG is performed by attaching a number of electrodes to standard locations on the scalp. These electrodes are attached to a recorder, which amplifies and records the activity. EEG is useful in evaluating causes of coma (structural vs metabolic), identifying seizure disorders, and determining the anatomic origin of seizures.

A routine EEG usually lasts 40 to 60 minutes with a portable machine for bedside use. The patient is instructed to lie still with his or her eyes closed. A mild sedative may be prescribed for restless or uncooperative patients, but the interpreter of the EEG must be aware of this because medications may cause changes in the recording. Documentation during the study is done by the technician and may include changes in blood pressure, changes in level of consciousness, medications the patient is currently taking or has taken within 48 hours, patient movement or posturing, and any noxious stimuli introduced. It is best to plan nursing care around the time of the test so that no interventions are done during this examination. When the EEG is complete, the electrodes are removed and any medications that were held prior to the study are resumed. In patients with symptoms concerning for seizure, such as intermittent twitching or fluctuating mental status, a prolonged EEG may be ordered in an attempt to correlate the symptoms with EEG findings. This type of EEG often lasts up to 24 hours, and requires the nurse to note any occurrences of the symptom or behavior thought to represent possible seizure activity.

Continuous EEG monitoring is used to guide treatment in patients with status epilepticus. Patients with status epilepticus are transferred to the intensive care unit for management because invasive airway management and continuous infusions of medications are typically required. Continuous EEG monitoring is also used in the diagnosis and management of intractable or difficult-to-control seizures, usually in conjunction with video monitoring. Continuous monitoring can also be helpful in identifying non-epileptic seizures.

Electromyography/Nerve Conduction Studies

Electromyography (EMG) evaluates the electrical activity of skeletal muscle during movement and rest. Nerve conduction studies (NCS) evaluate peripheral nerve function by measuring the transmission of electrical impulses after stimulation. Conditions in which EMG may aid diagnosis include myopathies and neuropathies, myasthenia gravis (in which the neuromuscular junction is affected), and Guillain-Barré syndrome. The patient may experience some pain related to insertion of the needle electrodes.

INTRACRANIAL PRESSURE

The skull in adults is a closed, nondistensible compartment that contains three components: brain parenchyma (80%), blood (10%), and CSF (10%). The Monro-Kellie hypothesis states that to maintain a constant intracranial volume, an increase in any of the three components must be accompanied by a decrease in one or both of the other components. If this reciprocal decrease does not occur, ICP rises. The body is able to compensate for a limited amount of increased intracranial volume by displacement of intracranial venous blood, decreased production of CSF, or displacement of CSF into the spinal subarachnoid space. ICP rises when these compensatory mechanisms have been exceeded (Figure 12-6). Compliance refers to the change in volume needed to result in a given change in pressure and reflects the effectiveness of the compensatory mechanisms. With decreased compliance, a small increase in volume results in a large increase in ICP. Compliance is based on several factors, including the amount of volume increase and the time over which the increase occurs. Smaller increases in volume result in less increase in pressure. Increases in volume that occur over a long period of time are better tolerated than rapid increases because there is time for compensation to occur. Older adults typically have increased compliance because of cerebral atrophy. Increased ICP can result in cerebral hypoperfusion, ischemia, herniation, and eventually death.

Cerebral Blood Flow

The brain cannot store oxygen or glucose in significant quantities. Therefore, constant blood flow is required to maintain cerebral metabolism. If cerebral blood flow (CBF) is insufficient, brain cells do not receive sufficient substrate

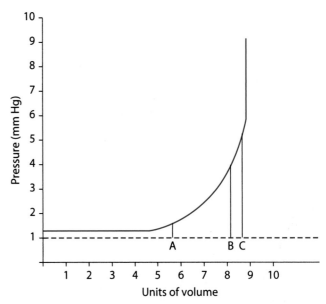

Figure 12-6. Intracranial volume-pressure curve. **(A)** Pressure is normal, and increases in intracranial volume are tolerated due to compensatory mechanisms. **(B)** Increases in volume may cause increases in pressure. **(C)** Small increases in volume may cause large increases in pressure (compensatory mechanisms have been exceeded). (*Reprinted from: Mendez KA. Neurologic therapeutic management. In: Urden LD, Stacy KM, Lough ME, eds. Thelan's Critical Care Nursing: Diagnosis and Management. St Louis, MO: Mosby; 2002:702.*)

to function and will eventually die. CBF is determined by blood pressure and cerebral vascular resistance.

Autoregulation refers to the ability of cerebral blood vessels to maintain consistent CBF by dilating or constricting in response to changes in blood pressure. Vasodilation occurs in response to decreased blood pressure; increased blood pressure results in vasoconstriction. In persons without neurologic disease, autoregulation allows consistent cerebral perfusion when mean arterial pressure is 60 to 160 mm Hg. In the injured brain, the autoregulatory response becomes less predictable. When autoregulation is impaired, CBF becomes dependent on systemic arterial pressure.

Cerebral vascular resistance can also be altered through chemoregulatory processes. An increase in the pressure of arterial carbon dioxide ($PaCO_2$) produces a lower extracellular pH and causes dilation of cerebral vessels. Conversely, a decrease in $PaCO_2$ raises pH and results in cerebral vasoconstriction. Vasodilation also results from PaO_2 levels less than 50 or a buildup of metabolic by-products such as lactic acid. Other factors can decrease cerebral vascular resistance and thus alter CBF, including certain anesthetic agents (halothane, nitrous oxide), sodium nitroprusside, and some histamines.

Causes of Increased Intracranial Pressure

Increased ICP occurs as a result of cerebral edema, mass lesions, increased intracranial blood volume, or increased amounts of CSF. These factors often occur in combination. Pain, suctioning, or an overstimulating environment can also increase ICP.

Cerebral Edema

Cerebral edema is an abnormal accumulation of water or fluid in the intracellular or extracellular space, resulting in increased brain volume. Vasogenic edema results from increased capillary permeability of the vessel walls, which allows plasma and protein to leak into the extracellular space. Cytotoxic edema occurs when fluid collects inside the cells due to failure of cellular metabolism. This causes further breakdown of the cell membrane. Cytotoxic edema can lead to capillary damage, which then results in vasogenic edema.

Mass Lesion

Mass lesions in the brain parenchyma include brain tumors, hematomas, and abscesses. In addition to raising ICP, mass lesions contribute to ischemia by compression of cerebral vessels.

Increased Blood Volume

Venous outflow obstruction can result from compression of the jugular veins (neck flexion, hyperextension, rotation), causing an increase in intracranial blood volume. Increased intrathoracic pressure or increased intra-abdominal pressure (Trendelenburg position, prone position, extreme hip flexion, Valsalva maneuver, coughing, tracheal suctioning) also results in venous outflow obstruction. As discussed previously, cerebral vasodilation occurs as the result of hypoxia, hypercapnia, increased metabolic demands, drug effects, or increased systemic blood pressure combined with autoregulatory failure; these factors cause an overall increase in intracranial blood volume.

Increased Cerebrospinal Fluid Volume

Approximately 500 mL of CSF is produced every day. CSF normally flows through the ventricular system into the subarachnoid space where it is absorbed by the arachnoid granulations (Figure 12-7). Obstruction of CSF flow, decreased reabsorption of CSF, or increased production leads to increased intracranial CSF volume (hydrocephalus). Hydrocephalus is referred to as communicating or noncommunicating

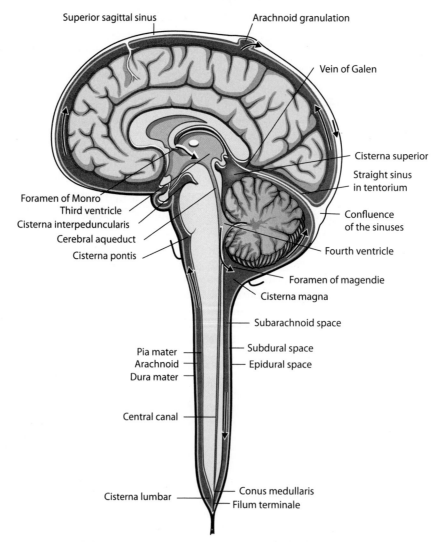

Figure 12-7. Flow of CSF/ventricular system. Drawing illustrates the ventricular system and other structures involved in CSF production, flow, and reabsorption. Arrows indicate the normal direction of flow of CSF. (*Reprinted from: Novack CR, Demarest RJ. Meninges, ventricles, and cerebrospinal fluid. In: The Nervous System: Introduction and Review. New York, NY: McGraw-Hill;1986:46.*)

(also called obstructive). In meningitis or subarachnoid hemorrhage, the arachnoid granulations become clogged with cellular debris and cannot absorb CSF normally, which leads to communicating hydrocephalus. An example of noncommunicating hydrocephalus is obstruction of CSF flow due to a tumor or cyst in the third ventricle of the brain.

Clinical Presentation

Early signs of increased ICP include confusion, restlessness, lethargy, disorientation, headache, nausea or vomiting, and visual abnormalities such as diplopia. Change in level of consciousness is the most important indicator of elevated ICP. The patient may become unable to follow commands and develop motor deficits; abnormal posturing is an ominous sign. Changes in vital signs may occur. Increased systolic blood pressure is the body's attempt to maintain cerebral perfusion. As ICP worsens, alterations in heart rate or respiratory pattern may also emerge. Pupillary changes are usually late signs of increased ICP. Any of these signs and symptoms requires immediate physician notification. Unless the cause of elevated ICP is known, a CT scan is ordered to evaluate for mass lesions (tumor, blood clot) or hydrocephalus. Invasive ICP monitoring devices are discussed in Chapter 20, Advanced Neurologic Concepts.

Herniation

Prolonged elevation of ICP may result in cerebral herniation. Folds in the dura mater divide the intracranial cavity into several compartments. Herniation is the distortion and displacement of the brain from one compartment to another, which damages structures and decreases CBF through compression. Classic signs associated with herniation reflect pressure on the brainstem and surrounding structures. Level of consciousness deteriorates, and the patient may demonstrate decorticate or decerebrate posturing. Compression or stretching of the oculomotor nerves (cranial nerve III) causes pupil changes; typically, pupil asymmetry is noted first, followed by a large non-reactive pupil on one side. As compression continues, the other pupil also becomes large and non-reactive and vital sign changes (Cushing response, altered respiratory pattern) occur. When any of these classic signs are noted, emergency action is needed to prevent brain death from occurring.

Principles of Management of Increased ICP

Management focuses on early recognition of increased ICP, avoiding activities known to elevate ICP, and aggressive treatment if changes in neurologic examination occur. Principles of management of increased ICP follow.

Monitoring Neurologic Status

Assess baseline neurologic signs, then reassess frequently and compare to previous findings. Include level of consciousness, coma score, pupillary size and reaction to light, eye movement, and motor and sensory function. Assess vital signs and compare with previous findings to identify trends. Close monitoring of neurologic status facilitates the identification and treatment of complications, such as the development of an epidural or subdural hematoma. In these cases, surgical evacuation of the hematoma may be required. In cases of diffuse cerebral edema, a portion of the skull may be removed to increase compliance and allow the brain to swell outside the contained area of the skull. This procedure is referred to as a craniectomy.

Adequate Oxygenation and Ventilation

Both hypoxemia and hypercarbia can result in cerebral vasodilation and increased ICP. Hyperventilation is not routinely used to decrease ICP because the resulting decrease in $PaCO_2$ may lead to vasoconstriction and worsen cerebral ischemia. Controlled hyperventilation can be used in the setting of impending herniation to "buy time" for other measures to be implemented and take effect.

Blood Pressure and Fluid Management

In the absence of invasive monitoring, blood pressure and fluid management varies based on the underlying disease process. Hypotension is avoided. If the patient is hypotensive, nonglucose-containing fluids are infused to ensure euvolemia; vasopressors may also be required.

Positioning

Because the venous system of the brain is valveless, increased intrathoracic or intra-abdominal pressure reduces venous return and increases ICP. In general, the head of the bed is elevated to 30°. Hip flexion is minimized. A bowel regimen is used to avoid constipation.

Neck positioning affects venous drainage and can raise ICP. The head and neck are maintained in a neutral position, avoiding flexion, hyperextension, or rotation. Cervical collars are carefully applied to avoid decreasing jugular venous return.

Preventing Increased Cerebral Metabolic Demand

Seizure activity increases cerebral metabolic demand and ICP. The prophylactic use of anticonvulsants is common in neurologically impaired patients at risk for seizures. Additional information on the management of seizures is included later in this chapter.

Fever increases ICP by increasing metabolic demand. For each elevation of 1°C, cerebral metabolic demand increases by approximately 6%. Methods to normalize temperature include antipyretics and air-or water-filled cooling blankets. Shivering increases metabolic demand and is avoided.

Agitation also increases cerebral metabolic demand. Work with other healthcare providers and the patient's family to maintain a clam, quiet environment. Agitation due to pain is avoided through the use of analgesics. If analgesics or sedatives are used, short-acting agents are preferred because of the importance of on-going neurological assessment. Careful monitoring of respiration is indicated due to the effect of these medications on ventilation; hypoventilation can cause increased ICP.

Cerebrospinal Fluid Drainage

Cerebrospinal fluid drainage via an intraventricular catheter can be used to lower ICP. Additional information on the use of intraventricular catheters for CSF drainage can be found in Chapter 20, Advanced Neurologic Concepts.

Medications to Decrease Cerebral Edema

Osmotic diuretics reduce cerebral edema by pulling extracellular fluid from brain tissue into the blood vessels. Mannitol is the most commonly used agent and is given as a bolus dose of 0.25 to 1 g/kg body weight. Mannitol is administered using a filter because it crystallizes easily. Euvolemia is maintained and electrolytes are closely monitored. Some practitioners also use hypertonic saline to increase serum osmolality and pull water into the vascular space.

Corticosteroids (eg, dexamethasone) are useful in decreasing cerebral edema associated with intracranial tumors. Steroids are generally not useful in the management of cerebral edema related to traumatic brain injury or stroke. Potential complications of steroid therapy include gastric irritation or hemorrhage and hyperglycemia.

Additional Treatments for Elevated Intracranial Pressure

Other measures to decrease ICP include continuous infusion of analgesics, sedatives, and/or anesthetic agents, the use of neuromuscular blocking agents, and induced barbiturate coma. Patients requiring these interventions are transferred to the intensive care unit for management.

ESSENTIAL CONTENT CASE

Acute Ischemic Stroke

A 64-year-old algebra teacher recently admitted to the progressive care unit for treatment of new onset atrial fibrillation. She has a history of diabetes controlled with diet and oral medications. At 7:15 in the morning, during bedside hand-off of care, the nurses find the patient slumped against the bedrail. She looks at them when they call her name, but is unable to speak, follow commands, or move her right side.

The patient's blood glucose is 142. Her vital signs are: HR 110 beats/min and irregular, BP 158/92, RR 16 breaths/min, oxygen saturation 96% on room air. The night shift nurse last checked on the patient about an hour ago, at 6:15 AM. After obtaining a stat head CT which revealed no bleeding and reviewing inclusion/exclusion criteria, the acute stroke team determines that the patient is an appropriate candidate for recombinant tissue plasminogen activator (rtPA). The initial bolus is administered at 8:00 AM, followed by the infusion.

About 30 minutes after the rtPA is given, a bed becomes available in the ICU and the patient is transferred for continued monitoring. She continues to have right arm weakness (strength 2/5) and aphasia, but her leg weakness and aphasia are resolving.

Case Question 1: What actions should the nurses take?

Case Question 2: How often should VS and neurological assessment be performed for a patient who has received rtPA for acute ischemic stroke?

Answers
1. The patient appears to be breathing well and is alert, so the first step is to follow institutional guidelines for summoning the acute stroke team. Other priorities include checking a blood glucose level, taking vital signs, and determining the last time that the patient was seen normal.
2. Every 15 minutes for 2 hours after rtPA is administered, then every 30 minutes for an additional 6 hours, then every hour until 24 hours have passed since rtPA was given.

ACUTE ISCHEMIC STROKE

Etiology, Risk Factors, and Pathophysiology

Stroke is the leading cause of death and disability in the United States and worldwide. The brain cannot store oxygen or glucose and therefore requires a constant flow of blood to supply these nutrients. The blood supply to the brain can be altered through several different processes. These include embolism, thrombosis, hemorrhage, and compression or spasm of the vessels. Ischemic stroke due to embolism or thrombus formation accounts for approximately 85% of all strokes. Edema occurs in the area of ischemic or infarcted tissue and contributes to further neuronal cell death. If ischemia is not reversed, neuronal cell death and infarction of brain tissue occurs. The penumbra is an area of tissue that surrounds the core ischemic area. The penumbra receives some blood flow from adjacent vessels but perfusion is marginal. If CBF is improved, the penumbra may recover.

Risk factors for stroke include hypertension, cardiac disease (coronary artery disease, heart failure, atrial fibrillation, endocarditis, patent foramen ovale, myocardial infarction, carotid artery disease), diabetes, increased age, race (African American), male gender, prior stroke, family history, dyslipidemia, hypercoagulability (cancer, pregnancy, high RBCs, sickle cell disease), smoking, obesity, physical inactivity, alcohol or illicit drugs, and some forms of hormone therapy. Transient ischemic attack (TIA) is an important warning sign for stroke. With a TIA, the patient develops stroke symptoms that resolve without tissue infarction. Although most resolve within minutes, an extensive workup to identify treatable causes is warranted with any TIA.

The pathophysiology of stroke varies based on the precipitating event. Thrombosis and embolism formation, described below, result in acute ischemic stroke.

Thrombosis

Thrombosis is the most common cause of ischemic stroke and is usually due to atherosclerosis and the formation of plaque within an artery. A thrombus then forms at the site of the plaque and causes brain tissue ischemia along the course of the affected vessel, which results in infarct if not quickly reversed.

Thrombosis because of atherosclerosis of large cerebral vessels results in large areas of infarct. Considerable edema often develops, further increasing ischemia by compressing areas surrounding the infarct. Significant functional deficits are common. If thrombus forms in a smaller branching artery, a lacunar infarct develops. Lacunar infarcts result in smaller areas of neuronal cell death. Deficits are less apparent, unless the infarct is in a crucial area, such as the internal capsule. Patients with a history of atherosclerosis or arteritis are at highest risk for thrombotic strokes. Thrombotic strokes tend to develop during periods of sleep or inactivity, when blood flow is less brisk.

Embolism

Embolism refers to the occlusion of a cerebral vessel, most often by a blood clot but also by infectious particles, fat, air, or tumor fragments. Embolism is often associated with heart disease that results in bacterial vegetations or blood clots; these vegetations or clots are easily detached from the wall or valves of the heart and then travel to the brain, lodging in a cerebral vessel. Chronic atrial fibrillation, valvular disease, prosthetic valves, cardiomyopathy, and atherosclerotic lesions of the proximal aorta are common causes of embolism. Less common causes include atrial myxomas, patent foramen ovale, and bacterial endocarditis. The fragmented substance easily lodges at the bifurcation of the middle cerebral artery, sometimes breaking apart and traveling further into the cerebral vascular system. The onset of an embolic occlusion is rapid, with symptoms that develop without warning.

Clinical Presentation

Symptoms of stroke range from very mild to significant loss of functional abilities. Common signs and symptoms include weakness in an extremity or on one side of the body, sensory changes, difficulty speaking or understanding speech, facial droop, headache, and visual changes. Clinical presentation of stroke varies based on the area of ischemia or infarction. The National Institute of Health Stroke Scale (NIHSS) is often used to evaluate and monitor patients after stroke. An overview of the NIHSS scoring system is presented in Table 12-5. Additional training is needed to accurately perform this assessment.

Stroke in a Cerebral Hemisphere

Signs and symptoms occur on the side of the body contralateral to the stroke. Weakness or paralysis occurs in one or both extremities, and sensory loss may be noted. Visual field deficits are also contralateral to the lesion. The patient often displays an ipsilateral gaze preference, in effect "looking to the lesion." The left hemisphere is dominant in right-handed individuals and many left-handed patients. As the dominant hemisphere, it controls language functions and language-dependent memory. Dominant hemisphere strokes often produce receptive, expressive, or global aphasia. Nondominant hemisphere strokes often cause neglect syndromes in which the patient becomes unaware of the environment and even his or her own body on the contralateral side.

TABLE 12-5. NATIONAL INSTITUTES OF HEALTH STROKE SCALE (NIHSS)

Tested Item	Title	Response and Scores
1A	Level of Consciousness	0—Alert 1—Drowsy 2—Obtunded 3—Coma/unresponsive
1B	Orientation Questions (2)	0—Answers both correctly 1—Answers 1 correctly 2—Answers neither correctly
1C	Response to Commands (2)	0—Performs both tasks correctly 1—Performs 1 task correctly 2—Performs neither
2	Gaze	0—Normal horizontal movements 1—Partial gaze palsy 2—Complete gaze palsy
3	Visual Fields	0—No visual field defect 1—Partial hemianopia 2—Complete hemianopia 3—Bilateral hemianopia
4	Facial Movement	0—Normal 1—Minor facial weakness 2—Partial facial weakness 3—Complete unilateral palsy

5	Motor Function (arm)
	  a. Left
	  b. Right
		0—No drift
		1—Drift before 5 seconds
		2—Falls before 10 seconds
		3—No effort against gravity
		4—No movement

6	Motor Function (leg)
	  a. Left
	  b. Right
		0—No drift
		1—Drift before 5 seconds
		2—Falls before 5 seconds
		3—No effort against gravity
		4—No movement

7	Limb Ataxia	0—No ataxia 1—Ataxia in 1 limb 2—Ataxia in 2 limbs
8	Sensory	0—No sensory loss 1—Mild sensory loss 2—Severe sensory loss
9	Language	0—Normal 1—Mild aphasia 2—Severe aphasia 3—Mute or global aphasia
10	Articulation	0—Normal 1—Mild dysarthria 2—Severe dysarthria
11	Extinction or Inattention	0—Absent 1—Mild (loss 1 sensory modality lost) 2—Severe (loss 2 modalities lost)

Additional information is available at http://www.ninds.nih.gov/disorders/stroke/strokescales.htm. (From Jauch EC, Saver JL, Adams HP, et al. Guidelines for the early management of patients with acute ischemic stroke: a guideline for healthcare professionals from the American Heart Association/American Stroke Association. Stroke. 2013:44: published on-line January 31, 2013. Accessed February 22, 2013.)

Cerebellar or Brain Stem Stroke

Motor and sensory function may be impaired on one or both sides of the body. Loss of equilibrium, decreased fine motor abilities, and nausea/vomiting are typical. Cranial nerve deficits are common and include dysarthria, nystagmus, dysphagia, and decreased cough reflex. Careful evaluation of airway protection and swallowing ability is essential to determine aspiration risk. Patients with severe deficits often require a feeding tube and potentially a tracheostomy. Because cortical injury is not present, patients maintain a normal mental status and level of alertness unless pressure in the posterior fossa leads to disruption of the reticular activating system.

In patients with cerebellar stroke, obstructive hydrocephalus may occur due to occlusion of the ventricular drainage system by edema. Surgical decompression of the posterior fossa may be necessary and an external ventricular drain may be placed.

Brain stem stroke owing to basilar artery occlusion results in quadriplegia and loss of facial movements (locked-in syndrome). Cognition is intact, and vertical gaze is maintained. These patients will be able to follow commands to look up or down. Early consultation with a speech language pathologist is recommended to help with the development of alternative communication strategies.

Diagnostic Tests

The goal of initial diagnostic testing in acute stroke is to rule out intracranial hemorrhage, because treatments for hemorrhagic and ischemic stroke differ significantly. This is typically accomplished by obtaining a noncontrast head CT, which can be quickly and easily obtained, although some centers use MRI for initial testing. Specialized MRI scans (diffusion-weighted imaging, perfusion-weighted imaging) can detect areas of ischemia before they are apparent on CT. MRA detects areas of vascular abnormality, as might be seen with clot due to arterial dissection. Other tests that may be done acutely include cerebral angiography and carotid ultrasound. Transthoracic or transesophageal echocardiography is used to assess cardiac causes of stroke. Hypercoagulable states are detected through laboratory work. All patients who present with stroke receive an ECG, are placed on cardiac monitoring for at least 24 hours, and undergo laboratory evaluation of cardiac biomarkers because of the correlation between cerebrovascular and cardiovascular disease. In addition, conditions that mimic stroke, such as hypoglycemia, must be ruled out.

Principles of Management of Acute Ischemic Stroke

Stroke is a medical emergency and is treated with the same urgency as acute myocardial infarction. Just as "time is muscle" when the heart is ischemic, "time is brain" when cerebral ischemia occurs. The goals of treatment are to restore circulation to the brain when possible, stop the ongoing ischemic process, and prevent secondary complications. Management principles include the following:

Evaluation of Conditions That Mimic Acute Ischemic Stroke

Other conditions may mimic acute ischemic stroke and must be ruled out. Hypoglycemia may cause stroke-like symptoms and is easily detected by using a bedside monitor to check

blood glucose. Radiologic tests are performed on all patients with signs and symptoms of stroke to rule out intracranial bleeding. Other conditions that may mimic acute ischemic stroke include toxic or metabolic disorders, migraines, seizures, mass lesions such as brain tumors or abscesses, and psychological disorders.

Fibrinolytic Therapy

Fibrinolytic therapy is administered in an attempt to restore perfusion to the affected area. IV administration of rtPA is considered in all patients who meet the inclusion/exclusion criteria (Table 12-6) and can be treated within 3 hours of the onset of symptoms. Patients who can be treated between 3 and 4.5 hours after symptom onset can also receive rtPA,

TABLE 12-6. INCLUSION AND EXCLUSION CRITERIA FOR TREATMENT WITH rtPA AFTER ACUTE ISCHEMIC STROKE

Inclusion criteria:
- Diagnosis of ischemic stroke causing measurable neurological deficit
- Aged ≥ 18 years

Exclusion criteria:
- Significant head trauma or prior stroke in previous 3 months
- Symptoms suggest subarachnoid hemorrhage
- Arterial puncture at noncompressible site in previous 7 days
- History of previous intracranial hemorrhage
- Intracranial neoplasm, arteriovenous malformation, or aneurysm
- Recent intracranial or intraspinal surgery
- Elevated blood pressure (systolic > 185 mm Hg or diastolic > 110 mm Hg)
- Active internal bleeding
- Acute bleeding diathesis, including but not limited to
- Platelet count < 100 000/mm³
- Heparin received within 48 hours, resulting in abnormally elevated aPTT
- Greater than the upper limit of normal
- Current use of anticoagulant with INR > 1.7 or PT > 15 seconds
- Current use of direct thrombin inhibitors or direct factor Xa inhibitors with elevated sensitive laboratory tests (such as aPTT, INR, platelet count, and ECT, TT, or appropriate factor Xa activity assays)
- Blood glucose concentration < 50 mg/dL (2.7 mmol/L)
- CT demonstrates multilobar infarction (hypodensity > 1/3 cerebral hemisphere)

Relative exclusion criteria
- Only minor or rapidly improving stroke symptoms (clearing spontaneously)
- Pregnancy
- Seizure at onset with postictal residual neurological impairments
- Major surgery or serious trauma within previous 14 days
- Recent gastrointestinal or urinary tract hemorrhage (within previous 21 days)
- Recent acute myocardial infarction (within previous 3 months)

ADDITIONAL relative exclusion criteria for patients considered for treatment 3 to 4.5 hours after symptom onset:
- Aged > 80 years
- Severe stroke (NIHSS > 25)
- Taking an oral anticoagulant regardless of INR
- History of both diabetes and prior ischemic stroke

ECT, ecarin clotting time; TT, thrombin time

Adapted from: Jauch EC, Saver JL, Adams HP, et al. Guidelines for the early management of patients with acute ischemic stroke: a guideline for healthcare professionals from the American Heart Association/American Stroke Association. Stroke. 2013:44: published on-line January 31, 2013. Accessed February 22, 2013.

although there are several additional exclusion criteria. The recommended dose for rtPA is 0.9 mg/kg, with 10% of the total dose given as a bolus over 1 to 2 minutes followed by the remainder of the dose as an infusion over 1 hour. The maximum dose recommended is 90 mg. In a large-scale study, rtPA administration resulted in improved outcomes at 3 months poststroke. There is an increased risk of intracerebral hemorrhage (ICH) following rtPA administration so frequent neurologic assessments are essential. Vital signs and neurologic checks are done every 15 minutes for the first 2 hours, then every 30 minutes for 6 hours, and then hourly until 24 hours following initial treatment. If neurologic deterioration occurs, rtPA is stopped if still infusing, the physician is notified, and a head CT is performed to assess for bleeding. Following rtPA administration, antiplatelet or anticoagulant medicines are avoided for 24 hours. Placement of nasogastric tubes, bladder catheters, and invasive lines is delayed to decrease the risk of hemorrhage.

Endovascular Treatment

Endovascular treatment is an option for the management of acute ischemic stroke at some centers. However, the possibility of intra-arterial treatment should not delay the use of intravenous rtPA in patients who are eligible to receive it. Available endovascular therapies include intra-arterial fibrinolysis and mechanical clot extraction or disruption. These treatments, guided by cerebral angiography, must be performed by a physician specially trained in interventional neuroradiology and are not available at all centers. Although rtPA is not FDA-approved for intra-arterial administration, it is sometimes used for patients with middle cerebral artery occlusion who can be treated within 6 hours of the onset of symptoms and are not able to receive intravenous rtPA. Because medication can be infused directly into the thrombus, smaller doses can be used, making this a treatment option for certain patients with exclusion criteria for intravenous rtPA (eg, major surgery in the previous 14 days). Mechanical thrombectomy using a special device may improve recanalization rates when used alone or in combination with fibrinolysis. Care of the patient following endovascular treatment for stroke includes standard postangiogram monitoring, stroke-specific care, and other interventions as ordered by the physician.

Blood Pressure Management

Careful blood pressure management is essential after acute ischemic stroke because a marked or sudden decrease in blood pressure can significantly decrease cerebral perfusion. The physician may elect to hold the patient's home antihypertensive medications to maximize cerebral blood flow, especially in the first 24 hours after stroke. For patients who are not eligible for fibrinolytic therapy, blood pressure is not treated emergently unless the systolic blood pressure exceeds 220 mm Hg or the diastolic blood pressure exceeds 120 mm Hg. Because of the risk of hemorrhage, blood pressure management is more stringent in patients who are eligible for or who have received fibrinolytic therapy (Table 12-7).

TABLE 12-7. APPROACH TO BLOOD PRESSURE MANAGEMENT AFTER ACUTE ISCHEMIC STROKE IN PATIENTS WHO ARE CANDIDATES FOR REPERFUSION THERAPY

Patient otherwise eligible for acute reperfusion therapy except that BP is > 185/110 mm Hg
- Labetalol 10-20 mg IV over 1-2 minutes, may repeat 1 time; or
- Nicardipine 5 mg/h IV, titrate up by 2.5 mg/h every 5-15 minutes, maximum 15 mg/h; when desired BP reached, adjust to maintain proper BP limits; or
- Other agents (hydralazine, enalaprilat, etc) may be considered when appropriate

If BP is not maintained at or below 185/110 mm Hg, do not administer rtPA.

Management of BP during and after rtPA or other acute reperfusion therapy to maintain BP at or below 180/105 mm Hg

Monitor BP every 15 minutes for 2 hours from the start of rtPA therapy, then every 30 minutes for 6 hours, and then every hour for 16 hours.
If systolic BP > 180-230 mm Hg or diastolic BP > 105-120 mm Hg:
- Labetalol 10 mg IV followed by continuous IV infusion 2-8 mg/min; or
- Nicardipine 5 mg/h IV, titrate up to desired effect by 2.5 mg/h every 5-15 minutes, maximum 15 mg/h

If BP not controlled or diastolic BP > 140 mm Hg, consider IV sodium nitroprusside

Adapted from: Jauch EC, Saver JL, Adams HP, et al. Guidelines for the early management of patients with acute ischemic stroke: a guideline for healthcare professionals from the American Heart Association/American Stroke Association. Stroke. 2013: 44: published on-line January 31, 2013. Accessed February 22, 2013.

Management of Increased Intracranial Pressure

Cerebral edema occurs in the area of infarct and may lead to increased ICP. For further discussion of treatment options, refer to the section on ICP. Hemicraniectomy may be used to alleviate increased ICP in patients with large infarcts, particularly in the distribution of the middle cerebral artery. Aggressive treatment of fever is warranted to avoid increases in cerebral metabolic demand.

Glucose Management

Hyperglycemia is associated with worse outcomes after stroke and is treated; lowering blood glucose to 140 to 180 mg/dL is a common goal. Hypoglycemia is deleterious and must be avoided.

Preventing and Treating Secondary Complications

Patients are at significant risk for decreased airway maintenance and aspiration following stroke. Decreased level of consciousness, facial weakness, and cranial nerve deficits contribute. Intubation is sometimes necessary during the acute phase, and some patients may need a tracheostomy. Dysphagia is very common after stroke, so careful assessment of swallowing ability is indicated before any oral intake. Many hospitals have dysphagia screening protocols in place, but consultation with the speech language pathologist is often indicated. Placement of a feeding tube may be necessary if the patient is unable to swallow safely.

Deep venous thrombosis is a common complication in stroke patients and may lead to pulmonary embolism. Strategies to decrease risk include elastic compression stockings, intermittent pneumatic compression devices, subcutaneous administration of low-dose anticoagulants, and early progression in activity.

In addition to pneumonia and DVT, patients with stroke are at risk for urinary tract infection (UTI). Indwelling catheters are used only when accurate output is medically necessary and cannot be obtained using alternate methods. When an indwelling catheter is used, it is removed as soon as possible. In patients without indwelling catheters, urinary retention may occur; methods of evaluation include bedside bladder scanning or catheterization for postvoid residual volumes.

Preventing Recurrent Stroke

The use of antiplatelet and anticoagulant medications varies depending on the size of the infarct, presumed etiology, and whether or not the patient received fibrinolytic therapy. Patients are commonly placed on aspirin within 24 to 48 hours after the initial event and the decision to use other antiplatelet or anticoagulant medications is made on an individual basis. Anticoagulation is typically not used in the acute phase of treatment because it increases the risk of hemorrhagic conversion (development of bleeding within the infarcted tissue), but may be used in certain circumstances.

Carotid endarterectomy is the most common surgical procedure to prevent further ischemic strokes, but is not typically performed in the time period immediately following a stroke due to the risk of reperfusion injury and hemorrhage. Stenosis may also be treated with angioplasty, with or without stent placement.

Other strategies to prevent recurrent stroke include statins for dyslipidemia and behavior modification to address risk factors.

HEMORRHAGIC STROKE

Etiology, Risk Factors, and Pathophysiology

Approximately 15% of all strokes are hemorrhagic. In subarachnoid hemorrhage, bleeding into the subarachnoid space occurs, usually as the result of a ruptured aneurysm. Although subarachnoid hemorrhage is a type of stroke, management issues differ significantly. Subarachnoid hemorrhage is discussed in Chapter 20, Advanced Neurologic Concepts. Here, hemorrhagic stroke refers to intraparenchymal bleeding (also called intracerebral hemorrhage or ICH).

Hypertension is the most common cause of ICH. Other causes include vascular malformations (AVMs or cavernous malformations), coagulopathy, amyloid angiopathy, tumor, vasculitis, venous infarction, and illicit drug abuse. Amyloid angiopathy is most common in patients older than the age of 70. It is a presumed diagnosis in older patients with repeated ICH, but can only be definitively diagnosed by deposits of beta-amyloid protein found in the vessel walls (usually on autopsy). AVM is a common cause of ICH in younger patients (ages 20-40). AVMs are congenital abnormalities in which a tangled mass of blood vessels is present.

Within the AVM, the arterial circulation and venous circulation connect without going through a capillary system. Following resolution of the acute ICH, AVMs are treated with endovascular embolization, surgical resection, or stereotactic radiosurgery.

In addition to direct tissue injury, the hematoma formed by ICH displaces nearby brain tissue and causes ischemia through compression. Edema occurs around the site of hemorrhage. If the ICH occurs deep within the cerebral hemispheres, it can rupture into the ventricle (intraventricular hemorrhage). The mortality rate is higher in hemorrhagic stroke than ischemic stroke.

Clinical Presentation

Intracerebral hemorrhage presents with an acute onset of neurologic deficits often associated with a severe headache, nausea/vomiting, decreased consciousness, and sometimes seizures. Neurologic deficits vary based on the area of the brain affected and are similar to the focal deficits experienced by patients with acute ischemic stroke.

Diagnostic Tests

Intracerebral hemorrhage is diagnosed using CT scanning or, less commonly, MRI. Tests that may be performed to determine the etiology of the hemorrhage include CTA, MRA, and cerebral angiography.

Principles of Management of Intracerebral Hemorrhage

Initial priorities of care for the patient with ICH include blood pressure control and correction of coagulopathy. Bleeding can continue or recur for several hours after the initial event, so prompt action is essential. Intermittent or continuous intravenous medications are commonly used to keep the systolic blood pressure below 140 to 160 mm Hg. Treatment of coagulopathy is based on the underlying cause of abnormal clotting. Fresh frozen plasma, platelets, vitamin K, or prothrombin complex concentrate may be ordered; regardless of the agent used, the goal is rapid correction of coagulopathy.

Operative management may or may not be indicated based on size and location of hemorrhage. Cerebellar hemorrhage may require a suboccipital craniectomy to evacuate the clot and decrease pressure on vital structures. Intraventricular hemorrhage may cause hydrocephalus, which is treated by placement of an external ventricular drain. Antiepileptic drugs (AEDs) are recommended for patients who experience a seizure or who show electrographic evidence of seizure on EEG. AEDs may also be administered to prevent seizures if the hemorrhage is in a part of the brain associated with seizure risk such as the temporal or frontal lobe.

Similar to patients with acute ischemic stroke, prevention of secondary complications is an essential element of nursing care for patients with ICH. Patients are at risk of aspiration and require careful monitoring of airway clearance, as well as assessment for dysphagia. Meticulous skin care, attention to bowel and bladder management, and prevention of hospital-acquired infections are all important to good outcomes.

SEIZURES

Etiology, Risk Factors, and Pathophysiology

Seizures are rapid, repeated bursts of abnormal electrical activity within the brain that result from an imbalance of excitatory and inhibitory impulses. Signs and symptoms depend on the location of the abnormal activity. A seizure is often a symptom or consequence of an underlying neurologic problem, such as a tumor, hemorrhage, trauma, or infection. Systemic disturbances such as hypoxia, hypoglycemia, drug overdose, and drug or alcohol withdrawal may also cause seizures. Many seizures are considered idiopathic, but treatable causes must be ruled out.

During a seizure, the metabolic demands of the brain for oxygen and glucose increase dramatically. The body tries to keep up with these increased requirements by increasing cerebral blood flow (CBF). If CBF does not keep up with demand, neurons revert to anaerobic metabolism, which leads to secondary ischemia and brain injury.

Clinical Presentation

Clinical presentation varies based on the origin and extent of the brain's abnormal electrical activity. Seizures can be described as focal (starting in one area of the cerebral cortex and limited to one hemisphere) or generalized (rapidly affecting both cerebral hemispheres).

Focal Seizures

Focal seizures may or may not affect consciousness. Focal seizures that do not impact consciousness (also called simple partial seizures) present with motor activity such as twitching or jerking in an extremity or one side of the face, sensory symptoms such as an unusual taste or smell, or autonomic sensations such as sweating or vomiting.

Focal seizures that alter consciousness (also called complex partial seizures) present with automatisms (smacking the lips, chewing motions, or fidgeting), purposeless activity such as running or arm jerking, or change in affect such as elation or fear. A focal seizure can progress into a bilateral generalized convulsive seizure.

Generalized Seizures

Generalized seizures are characterized by abnormal electrical discharge that rapidly affects both hemispheres. There are several types of generalized seizures:

- *Absence:* Sudden lapse of consciousness and activity that lasts 3 to 30 seconds. Commonly described as a staring spell.
- *Myoclonic:* Sudden, brief muscle jerking of one or more muscle groups. Commonly associated with metabolic, degenerative, and hypoxic causes.
- *Atonic (also called drop attacks):* Sudden loss of muscle tone.

ESSENTIAL CONTENT CASE

Seizures

A 52-year-old man with a history of seizures is admitted to the progressive care unit for close monitoring after he presented to the ED with an increase in seizure frequency. His seizures started after a traumatic brain injury (TBI) 4 years prior. They have been well-controlled on levetiracetam until a few days ago, when he ran out of his medication. This morning 911 was called when he experienced a seizure at the post office. He had two more brief tonic-clonic seizures in the ED. Soon after admission to the progressive care unit, he has another tonic-clonic seizure.

Generalized tonic-clonic seizure activity continues for 8 minutes and stops after lorazepam is administered. The physician orders a loading dose of fosphenytoin.

The patient does not have any more seizure activity. He is continued on levetitacetam and phenytoin, and transferred to the acute care floor the next day.

Case Question 1: What are the initial priorities of care for this patient?

Case Question 2: What is the primary adverse effect associated with fosphenytoin?

Answers
1. The first priority is to keep the patient safe by clearing objects out of the area and positioning the patient to allow drainage of oral secretions. The physician is contacted immediately.
2. Fosphenytoin, similar to phenytoin, can cause cardiovascular side effects, especially hypotension.

- *Clonic:* Rhythmic muscle jerking.
- *Tonic:* Sustained muscle contraction.
- *Tonic-clonic:* Muscle activity varies between sustained contraction and jerking.

Patients are more likely to be injured during a generalized seizure than during a focal seizure and may complain of generalized muscle aches after the seizure stops if convulsions led to sustained muscle activity.

Status Epilepticus

Status epilepticus indicates prolonged or recurring seizures without a return to baseline mental status. The classic definition of *status epilepticus* is a seizure or series of seizures lasting longer than 30 minutes, but treatment is typically instituted much sooner and recent guidelines suggest a definition of seizure activity longer than 5 minutes. Status epilepticus is a medical emergency with a significant mortality rate, higher in the elderly or when the seizure is a symptom of an underlying acute process. There are two primary types of status epilepticus: convulsive status epilepticus and nonconvulsive status epilepticus. In convulsive status epilepticus, seizure activity is readily apparent using clinical observation. In nonconvulsive status epilepticus, no outward clinical seizures may be noted but consciousness is impaired and seizure activity is apparent on EEG.

Diagnostic Testing

Diagnostic testing for patients with seizures may include:

- Laboratory work to identify electrolyte abnormalities, metabolic disorders, or anti-epileptic drug levels.
- CT to assess for intracranial processes such as an ICH or tumor.
- MRI to look for structural lesions that may indicate a seizure focus.
- LP when an infectious process (eg, meningitis) is the suspected source of seizure activity.
- EEG to evaluate for seizure activity. One normal EEG does not rule out seizure. Prolonged EEG monitoring may be required.
- Continuous video monitoring in conjunction with continuous EEG recordings to correlate clinical phenomena with electrical activity in the brain.
- Intracranial electrodes with continuous EEG monitoring in the evaluation of patients with intractable seizures to identify a focus or foci prior to surgical resection. Intracranial electrodes are inserted via burr holes or a craniotomy.

Principles of Management of Seizures

Management of the patient with seizures focuses on controlling the seizure as quickly as possible, preventing recurrence, maintaining patient safety, and identifying the underlying cause. Observation of seizure type, duration, and any precipitating factors is essential. Following a seizure, patients may experience a period of confusion and altered mental status that slowly resolves. They may complain of a headache or muscle aches. Todd's paralysis describes continued focal symptoms that can persist for up to 36 hours after a seizure. Because of the risk of missing underlying intracranial pathology, patients with focal neurologic deficits following a seizure are diagnosed with Todd's paralysis only after other causes have been ruled out.

Maintaining Patient Safety and Airway Management

From a nursing perspective, the first priority is to protect the patient from injury. Ensure a safe environment during the seizure by clearing objects out of the area. Padded side rails are indicated for patients at high risk for seizures. During a seizure, attempting to restrain patient movement may result in injury and is avoided.

Airway management assists with maintaining adequate cerebral oxygenation. Maintaining the airway may depend on stopping the seizure. Positioning the patient on his or her side decreases aspiration. Supplemental oxygen is provided. Nothing should be placed in the patient's mouth during a seizure. ECG monitoring, continuous pulse oximetry, and blood pressure monitoring are required in patients with prolonged seizures. Hypoglycemia can induce seizure activity, so a glucose level is checked immediately and treated as appropriate.

Medication Administration for Prolonged Seizures and Status Epilepticus

The average seizure stops within 2 minutes without requiring medication. Patients with prolonged seizures or status epilepticus receive a benzodiazepine such as lorazepam. The second medication given is typically phenytoin or fosphenytoin. Fosphenytoin is converted to phenytoin in the blood and is preferred because it causes less tissue injury should extravasation occur. Both agents can cause cardiovascular side effects, predominately treatment-resistant hypotension. Cardiac and respiratory status should be closely monitored. If seizure activity continues, the patient will require transfer to the intensive care unit for continuous intravenous medications.

The prolonged muscle activity that occurs with prolonged convulsive seizure activity may cause tissue breakdown and lead to rhabdomyolysis. Serum creatine phosphokinase is elevated and myoglobin may be present in the urine. Hydration is essential to avoiding renal dysfunction.

Treatment Options for Patients With Seizures

Many patients require ongoing medication for seizure control. Some common medications include levetiracetam, phenytoin, carbamazepine, oxcarbazepine, valproic acid, lamotrigine, and lacosamide. Approximately two-thirds of patients treated with medication are able to attain good seizure control.

Some patients with seizures uncontrolled by medications may be helped by surgery to remove the seizure focus. These patients most often have seizures originating from the temporal lobe. Selection criteria include intractable seizures that significantly impact quality of life and are uncontrolled by medication, an identifiable unilateral focus of seizure activity, and seizure focus in an area where removal will cause no major neurologic deficit. A craniotomy is used to access and excise the seizure focus. The primary complications are hemorrhage and infection. Patients are kept on their previous seizure medications during the postoperative period. About 50% of patients become seizure free after surgery and an additional 30% experience a significant improvement in seizure control.

For patients with intractable seizures who do not have an identifiable focus, placement of a vagus nerve stimulator may be considered. Vagal nerve stimulation reduces seizure duration, frequency, or intensity by providing intermittent electrical stimulation of the vagus nerve. The exact mechanism of action has not been determined.

INFECTIONS OF THE CENTRAL NERVOUS SYSTEM

Meningitis

Meningitis is an acute inflammation of the meninges of the brain and spinal cord. Meningitis can be caused by bacteria, viruses, fungi, or parasites. Risk factors include immunocompromise, trauma, surgery that disrupts the meninges, and crowded living conditions. Signs and symptoms include fever, headache, neck stiffness, irritability, vomiting, photophobia, altered level of consciousness, seizures, weakness, and cranial nerve deficits. Other signs of meningitis include Kernig sign (severe pain in the hamstring with knee extension when the hip is flexed 90°) and Brudzinski sign (involuntary flexion of the knees and hips when the neck is flexed). Many patients with meningococcal meningitis have a characteristic rash (petechial rash that progresses to purple blotches). Diagnostic testing includes LP for opening pressure and CSF analysis, blood cultures, and other laboratory tests to look for infection. CT scanning is performed prior to LP in patients with papilledema or focal neurologic findings. Complications of meningitis include hydrocephalus, cerebral edema, and vasculitis. Nursing priorities include management of elevated ICP, implementation of seizure precautions, and prompt administration of antimicrobial therapy. Delays in antimicrobial therapy are associated with worse outcomes. Isolation may be required until the causative organism is identified and treated; notify the infection control practitioner and follow institutional guidelines.

Encephalitis

Encephalitis is inflammation of the brain parenchyma. There are many causes of encephalitis, including arboviruses such as West Nile, but the most common type seen in the United States is encephalitis due to the herpes simplex virus (HSV). HSV encephalitis can result from a new infection, or can represent a reactivation of a preexisting infection. Signs and symptoms include fever, focal or diffuse neurologic changes, headache, and seizures. HSV encephalitis predominately affects the inferior frontal and temporal lobes. Diagnostic testing includes MRI, EEG, and CSF analysis. The diagnosis is often presumed pending specialized testing of the CSF. Empiric therapy is started with an antiviral agent.

Intracranial Abscess

An intracranial abscess is a collection of pus in the brain and can be extradural, subdural, or intracerebral. The infective agent enters the brain through the bloodstream, via an opening in the dura (as may occur with a basilar or open skull fracture or following a neurosurgical procedure), or by direct migration from chronic otitis media, poor dentition, frontal sinusitis, or mastoiditis. Signs and symptoms typically develop over a few weeks and may include headache, seizures, fever, neck pain, focal neurologic signs such as hemiparesis, cranial nerve deficits, and change in level of consciousness. Diagnostic testing includes CT with contrast administration, MRI, EEG, and potentially aspiration of the lesion for culture. Treatment includes prolonged antibiotic therapy (usually 6 weeks) and surgical drainage of the abscess.

NEUROMUSCULAR DISEASES

Although there are a variety of neuromuscular diseases that may result in hospitalization, only a small number of these patients require admission to the progressive care unit.

Myasthenia gravis (MG) and Guillain-Barré syndrome (GBS) often cause respiratory muscle weakness and decreased airway clearance. These patients may be admitted to the progressive care unit for close monitoring of respiratory status. They may also be admitted to ventilator weaning units after initial stabilization in the ICU. In addition, patients with chronic progressive neuromuscular diseases such as amyotrophic lateral sclerosis (ALS) may be admitted to the progressive care unit for management of respiratory failure or other complications.

Myasthenia Gravis

In MG, autoimmune-mediated destruction of acetylcholine receptors results in decreased neuromuscular transmission and muscle weakness. Myasthenia gravis is a chronic disease with periodic exacerbations. Diagnostic testing includes laboratory testing for acetylcholine receptor antibodies, EMG, CT scanning of the chest to evaluate for abnormalities of the thymus, and "Tensilon testing."

Edrophonium chloride (Tensilon) is a short-acting acetylcholinesterase inhibitor that can be administered intravenously. Improvement in symptoms following edrophonium chloride injection is highly suggestive of MG. Adverse effects of edrophonium chloride include bradycardia, asystole, increased oral and bronchial secretions, and bronchoconstriction.

Treatment for acute MG exacerbation includes plasma exchange or IV immunoglobulin in addition to supportive care. Long-term management may include the administration of anticholinesterase medications, thymectomy, or immunosuppression. Priorities of nursing management during an acute exacerbation include close monitoring of respiratory status and prevention of secondary complications.

Guillain-Barré Syndrome

Guillain-Barré syndrome causes progressive muscle weakness, sensory loss, and areflexia due to peripheral nerve demyelination. Symptoms generally start in the lower extremities and ascend. Diagnostic studies include LP and nerve conduction studies. Approximately 25% to 40% of patients require mechanical ventilation. Some patients experience autonomic instability characterized by variations in heart rate and blood pressure. Neuropathic pain related to inflammation and demyelination occurs and requires both pharmacologic and nonpharmacologic treatment. In addition to supportive therapy, patients may receive plasma exchange or IV immunoglobulin. Most patients recover with minimal deficits, but may require weeks to months of hospitalization. Nursing priorities include close monitoring of respiratory status and prevention of complications related to prolonged immobility.

Amyotrophic Lateral Sclerosis

Amyotrophic lateral sclerosis is a progressive disease that affects the motor neurons, causing muscle weakness without affecting sensation or cognition. Patients most commonly present with extremity weakness that is asymmetric and more pronounced distally. Bulbar symptoms such as dysarthria and dysphagia may be present initially, or may develop as the disease progresses. The rapidity of progression varies widely among patients. Eventually, ALS causes respiratory failure due to muscle weakness and decreased airway protection.

Patients with ALS may be admitted to the progressive care unit when airway protection becomes problematic and complications such as pneumonia develop, or if they use assisted ventilation (BiPAP or mechanical ventilation) at home and require admission for other complications or procedures. Nursing care focuses on decreasing respiratory complications and other complications of immobility, controlling pain, and providing psychological support.

SELECTED BIBLIOGRAPHY

Assessment and Diagnostic Testing

Alexandrov AW. Transcranial Doppler monitoring. In: Weigand DL, ed. *AACN Procedure Manual for Critical Care*. 6th ed. St. Louis, Missouri: Saunders, 2011.

Balas MC, Rice M, Chaperon C, et al. Management of delirium in critically ill older adults. *Crit Care Nurse*. 2012;32:15-26.

Bleck TP. Levels of consciousness and attention. In: Goetz CG, ed. *Textbook of Clinical Neurology* [electronic version]. 3rd ed. Philadelphia, PA: Saunders; 2007.

Bruno M, Ledoux D, Lambermont B, et al. Comparison of the full outline of UnResponsiveness and Glasgow Liege Scale/Glasgow Coma Scale in an intensive care unit population. *Neurocrit Care*. 2011;15:447-453.

Brust JCM. Coma. In: Rowland LP, Pedley TA, eds. *Merritt's Neurology* [electronic version]. 12th ed. Philadelphia, PA: Lippincott Williams and Wilkins; 2010.

Daroff RB, Fenichel GM, Jankovic J, Mazzioatta JC. Bradley's neurology in clinical practice, Volume I: *Principles of Diagnosis and Management* [electronic version]. 6th ed. Philadelphia, PA: Saunders; 2012.

Delapaz R. CT and MRI. In: Rowland LP, Pedley TA, eds. *Merritt's Neurology* [electronic version]. 12th ed. Philadelphia, PA: Lippincott Williams and Wilkins; 2010.

Ely EW, Shintai A, Truman B, et al. Delirium as a predictor of mortality in mechanically ventilated patients in the intensive care unit. *JAMA*. 2004;291:1753-1762.

Fletcher JJ, Nathan BR. Cerebrospinal fluid and intracranial pressure. In: Goetz CG, ed. *Textbook of Clinical Neurology* [electronic version]. 3rd ed. Philadelphia, PA: Saunders; 2007.

Hickey JV, Murphy KP. Neurodiagnostic tests. In: Bader MK, Littlejohns LR, eds. *AANN Core Curriculum for Neuroscience Nursing*. 5th ed. Glenview, IL: American Association of Neuroscience Nurses; 2010.

Kanal E, Barkovich AJ, Bell C, et al. ACR guidance document for safe MR practices: 2007. *AJR*. 2007;188:1-27.

Koenigsberg RA, Bianco BA, Faro SH, et al. Neurodiagnostic tools. In: Goetz CG, ed. *Textbook of Clinical Neurology* [electronic version]. 3rd ed. Philadelphia, PA: Saunders; 2007.

Kramer AA, Wijdicks EFM, Snavely VL, et al. A multicenter prospective study of interobserver agreement using the Full Outline of Unresponsiveness score coma scale in the intensive care unit. *Crit Care Med*. 2012;40:2671-2676.

Lee K, Fishman RA. Lumbar puncture and cerebrospinal fluid examination. In: Rowland LP, Pedley TA, eds. *Merritt's Neurology* [electronic version]. 12th ed. Philadelphia, PA: Lippincott Williams and Wilkins; 2010.

Mohr JP, Delapaz R, Rundek T. Neurovascular imaging. In: Rowland LP, Pedley TA, eds. Merritt's Neurology [electronic version]. 12th ed. Philadelphia, PA: Lippincott Williams and Wilkins; 2010.

Neto AS, Nassar AP, Cardoso SO, et al. Delirium screening in critically ill patients: a systematic review and meta-analysis. *Crit Care Med*. 2012;1946-1951.

Stewart-Amidei C, Blissitt PA, Brooks L. Assessment. In: Bader MK, Littlejohns LR, eds. *AANN Core Curriculum for Neuroscience Nursing*. 5th ed. Glenview, IL: American Association of Neuroscience Nurses; 2010.

Website for information on delirium and assessment methods: www.icudelirium.org (ICU Delirium and Cognitive Impairment Study Group; Vanderbilt University Medical Center, Veterans Affairs TN Valley Geriatric Research Education and Clinical Center). Accessed February 23, 2013.

Wijdicks EFM, Bamlet WR, Maramottom BV, Manno EM, McClelland RL. Validation of a new coma score: the FOUR score. *Ann Neurol*. 2005;58:585-593.

Intracranial Pressure

Madden LK, March K. Intracranial pressure management. In: Bader MK, Littlejohns LR, eds. *AANN Core Curriculum for Neuroscience Nursing*. 5th ed. Glenview, IL: American Association of Neuroscience Nurses; 2010.

March K. Intracranial pressure concepts, cerebral blood flow, and metabolism. In: Bader MK, Littlejohns LR. eds. *AANN Core Curriculum for Neuroscience Nursing*. 5th ed. Glenview, IL: American Association of Neuroscience Nurses; 2010.

March K, Olson D, Arbour R. Technology. In: Bader MK, Littlejohns LR, eds. *AANN Core Curriculum for Neuroscience Nursing*. 5th ed. Glenview, IL: American Association of Neuroscience Nurses; 2010.

Acute Ischemic Stroke and Hemorrhagic Stroke

Elijovich L, Patel PV, Hemphill JC. Intracerebral hemorrhage. *Sem in Neurol*. 2008;28(5):657-667.

Hinkle JL, Guanci MM, Stewart-Amidei C. Cerebrovascular events of the nervous system. In: Bader MK, Littlejohns LR, eds. *AANN Core Curriculum for Neuroscience Nursing*. 5th ed. Glenview, IL: American Association of Neuroscience Nurses; 2010.

Seizures

Berg AT, Berkovic SF, Brodie MJ, et al. Revised terminology and concepts for organization of seizures and epilepsies: report of the ILAE Commission on Classification and Terminology, 2005-2009. *Epilepsia*. 2010;51(4):676-685.

Buelow JM, Dean P, Miller W, Plueger M. Epilepsy. In: Bader MK, Littlejohns LR, eds. *AANN Core Curriculum for Neuroscience Nursing*. 5th ed. Glenview, IL: American Association of Neuroscience Nurses; 2010.

Engel J, Jr, Weibe S, French J, et al. Practice parameter: temporal lobe and localized neocortical resections for epilepsy: report of the Quality Standards Subcommittee of the American Academy of Neurology, in association with the American Epilepsy Society and the AANS. *Neurology.* 2003;60:538-547.

Huff JS, Fountain NB. Pathophysiology and definitions of seizures and status epilepticus. *Emerg Med Clin N Am.* 2011;29:1-13.

Infections of the Central Nervous System

Kennedy PGE. Viral encephalitis. *J Neurol.* 2005;252:268-272.

Pass M. Central nervous system infections. In: Barker E, ed. *Neuroscience Nursing: A Spectrum of Care.* 3rd ed. St Louis, MO: Mosby, Inc; 2008.

van de Beek D, Brouwer MC, Thwaites GE, Tunkel AR. Advances in treatment of bacterial meningitis. *Lancet.* 2012;380:1693-1702.

VanDemark MV, Neatherlin JS, Stewart-Amidei C, Bautista C, Omert T. Infectious and autoimmune processes. In: Bader MK, Littlejohns LR, eds. *AANN Core Curriculum for Neuroscience Nursing.* 5th ed. Glenview, IL: American Association of Neuroscience Nurses; 2010.

Neuromuscular Diseases

Burns TM. Guillain-Barré syndrome. *Semin Neurol.* 2008;28:152-167.

Chiu A, Cocito D, Leone M, et al, and the Piedmonte and Valle d'Aosta Register for Guillain-Barré Syndrome. Guillain-Barré syndrome: a prospective, population-based incidence and outcome survey. *Neurology.* 2003;60(7):1146-1150.

Polak M, Lorimer M, Koopman W, De Sepulveda LB. Neuromuscular disorders of the nervous system. In: Bader MK, Littlejohns LR, eds. *AANN Core Curriculum for Neuroscience Nursing.* 5th ed. Glenview, IL: American Association of Neuroscience Nurses; 2010.

Sharshar T, Chevret S, Bourdain F, Raphaël J, for the French Cooperative Group on Plasma Exchange in Guillain-Barré Syndrome: early predictors of mechanical ventilation in Guillain-Barré syndrome. *Crit Care Med.* 2003;31(1):278-283.

Evidence-Based Practice

American Association of Critical Care Nurses. Practice alert: delirium assessment and management. Issued November 2011. Available at www.aacn.org. Accessed February 23, 2013.

Barr J, Fraser GL, Puntillo K, et al. Clinical practice guidelines for the management of pain, agitation, and delirium in adult patients in the intensive care unit. *Crit Care Med.* 2013;41:263-306.

Brophy GM, Bell R, Claassen J, et al. Guidelines for the evaluation and management of status epilepticus. *Neurocrit Care.* 2012; 17(1):3-23.

Eaton JD, Saver JL, Albers GW, et al. Definition and evaluation of transient ischemic attack. *Stroke.* 2009;40:2276-2293.

Jauch EC, Saver JL, Adams HP, et al. Guidelines for the early management of patients with acute ischemic stroke: a guideline for healthcare professionals from the American Heart Association/American Stroke Association. *Stroke.* 2013: 44: published on-line January 31, 2013. Accessed February 22, 2013.

March K, Madden L. Intracranial pressure management. In: Littlejohns LR, Bader MK, eds. *AACN-AANN Protocols for Practice: Monitoring Technologies in Critically Ill Neuroscience Patients.* Sudbury, MA: Jones and Bartlett Publishers; 2009.

Morgenstern LB, Hemphill JC, Anderson C, et al. Guidelines for the management of spontaneous intracerebral hemorrhage: a guideline for healthcare professionals from the American Heart Association/American Stroke Association. *Stroke.* 2010;41:2108-2129.

Pugh S, Mathiesen C, Meighan M, Summers D, Zrelak P [electronic version]. *Guide to the Care of the Hospitalized Patient With Ischemic Stroke: AANN Clinical Practice Guideline.* 2nd ed. Glenview, IL: American Association of Neuroscience Nurses; 2011. Available at http://www.aann.org/pubs/content/guidelines.html. Accessed June 1, 2013.

Slazinski T, Anderson TA, Catell E, et al. Care of the patient undergoing intracranial pressure monitoring/external ventricular drainage or lumbar drainage: AANN Clinical Practice Guideline Series. Glenview, IL: American Association of Neuroscience Nurses; 2011.

Summers D, Leonard A, Wentworth D, et al. Comprehensive overview of nursing and interdisciplinary care of the acute ischemic stroke patient. *Stroke.* 2009;40 2911-2944.

Tunkel AR, Glaser CA, Bloch KC, et al. The management of encephalitis: clinical practice guidelines by the Infectious Diseases Society of America. *Clin Infect Dis.* 2008;47:303-327.

Tunkel AR, Hartman BJ, Kaplan SL, et al. Practice guidelines for the management of bacterial meningitis. *Clin Infect Dis.* 2004;39:1267-1284.

HEMATOLOGIC AND IMMUNE SYSTEMS

Diane K. Dressler

13

KNOWLEDGE COMPETENCIES

1. Analyze laboratory test results used to assess the status of the hematologic and immune systems:
   - Complete blood count
   - White blood cell differential
   - International normalized ratio
   - Activated partial thromboplastin time
   - D-dimer

2. Describe the etiology, pathophysiology, clinical manifestations and collaborative management for common hematological problems in acutely ill patients.

3. Provide comprehensive management for immuno-suppressed patients in the acute care setting.

The hematologic and immune systems play a major role in the body's response to illness. Organs and tissues require a continuous supply of oxygen from the red blood cells (RBC), while the white blood cells (WBC) mount an immune response. The platelets and other coagulation components are essential for hemostasis. Assessment of these processes and treatment of hematologic and immune problems are an important part of patient management.

SPECIAL ASSESSMENT TECHNIQUES, DIAGNOSTIC TESTS, AND MONITORING SYSTEMS

A complete patient assessment guides the selection of screening tests for hematologic and immune problems. Historical data are particularly important and should include family history, occupational exposures, lifestyle behaviors, diet, allergies, past medical problems, surgeries, co-morbid conditions, transfusion of blood or blood components, and current medications. Abnormal physical assessment data from each body system collectively assist in the identification of risk factors or acute abnormalities pertinent to hematologic and immune function. In addition, a variety of laboratory tests assist the clinician to evaluate problems in these systems (Table 13-1).

Complete Blood Count

The complete blood count (CBC) is a primary assessment tool for evaluation of the hematologic and immune status. The RBC count and RBC indices, along with the hemoglobin and hematocrit levels, provide valuable information regarding the oxygen-carrying capability of the blood. The total WBC count and the WBC differential reveal the body's ability to provide an immune response against foreign substances and to participate in the normal inflammatory process required for tissue restoration. Important information concerning hemostasis is obtained from the platelet count, with additional studies required to fully evaluate the coagulation process.

Red Blood Cell Count

The RBC count is determined by the number of erythrocytes per cubic millimeter of blood. Normal values for men are higher than for women. A decrease in the number of RBC or in the amount of hemoglobin indicates anemia. Anemia can be due to many factors, including decreased production or increased destruction of RBC, loss of RBC by hemorrhage, vitamin B_{12} deficiency, and/or iron deficiency. An increase in the total number of RBC occurs as a compensatory mechanism in persons with chronic hypoxia or as an adaptation to

TABLE 13-1. NORMAL VALUES FOR HEMATOLOGIC AND IMMUNE SCREENING TESTS[a]

Laboratory Test	Normal Value
RBC	Males: 4.7-6.1 million/mm³ Females: 4.2-5.4 million/mm³
Hgb	Males: 14-18 g/dL Females: 12-16 g/dL
Hct	Males: 42%-52% Females: 37%-47%
RBC indices	
MCV	80-95 fL
MCH	27-31 pg
MCHC	32%-36%
RDW	11%-14.4%
Reticulocyte count	0.5%-2%
WBC	5000-10000/mm³ (5000-10000/μL)
WBC differential (% of total)	
Neutrophils	55%-70%
Segmented	56%
Bands	3%-6%
Eosinophils	1%-4%
Basophils	0.5%-1.0%
Monocytes	2%-8%
Lymphocytes	20%-40%
T-cells	800-2500 cells/μL
T-helper (CD4) cells	600-1500 cells/μL
T-suppressor (CD8) cells	300-1000 cells/μL
Platelet count	150,000-400,000/mm³
Bleeding time	1-9 minutes
Prothrombin time	11-12.5 sec
Therapeutic anticoagulation	1.5-2 times normal
INR	0.8-1.1
Therapeutic anticoagulation	2.0-3.0
aPTT	30-40 sec
Therapeutic anticoagulation	1.5-2.5 times normal
ACT	70-120 sec
Therapeutic anticoagulation	150-210 sec
Fibrinogen	200-400 mg/dL
D-dimer	< 0.4 mcg/mL

ACT, activated clotting time; aPTT, activated partial thromboplastin time; Hct, hematocrit; Hgb, hemoglobin; INR, International Normalized Ratio; MCH, mean corpuscular hemoglobin; MCHC, mean corpuscular hemoglobin concentration; MCV, mean corpuscular volume; RBC, red blood cell count; RDW, red blood cell distribution width; WBC, white blood cell count

[a]*Normal values vary between laboratories. Refer to local laboratory standard values when interpreting test results.*

high altitudes. Further assessment of the ability of the bone marrow to produce RBC is obtained by a reticulocyte count.

Hemoglobin

Hemoglobin is the primary carrier of oxygen to body tissues. As the number of RBCs change, so does the hemoglobin content. A decline in hemoglobin to a level as low as 7 g/dL may be well tolerated, in some patients, while in others a decline can result in significant symptoms. The rate at which the decline in hemoglobin level occurs often influences the symptoms and tolerance of the patient. A decline that occurs gradually over time is often tolerated, whereas a rapid decline frequently results in poor tolerance by the patient. Elderly patients and those with underlying cardiac or pulmonary disorders may become symptomatic with even small changes in the hemoglobin content of the blood.

Hematocrit

Hematocrit measures the RBC mass in relationship to a volume of blood and is expressed as the percentage of cells per 100 mL of blood. Multiplying the hemoglobin value by 3 gives an estimate of hematocrit. The hematocrit is particularly sensitive to changes in the volume status of the patient. It increases with fluid losses (hemoconcentration) and decreases with increased plasma volume (hemodilution). Interpretation of hemoglobin and hematocrit results must take into account the time the values were obtained in relationship to blood volume loss, fluid loss, and/or fluid administration; for example, values obtained immediately after an acute hemorrhage may appear normal, because compensatory mechanisms have not had time to restore plasma volume. Restoration of plasma volume by compensation or crystalloid resuscitation lowers the hemoglobin and hematocrit.

Red Blood Cell Indices

The RBC indices (mean corpuscular volume, mean corpuscular hemoglobin, mean corpuscular hemoglobin concentration, and RBC distribution width) are measurements of the size, weight, and hemoglobin concentration of the individual RBCs also known as erythrocytes. These indices are useful in determining the etiology of anemia.

Total White Blood Cell Count

Leukocytes, or WBCs circulating in the blood, are measured as an indicator of the total amount of WBCs in the body. Most WBCs are not sampled in a CBC because they are marginated along capillary walls, circulating in the lymphatic system, or residing in lymph nodes and other body tissues.

Increased WBCs, or *leukocytosis*, is usually caused by an elevation in one type of WBC. It is most often associated with a normal immune system response to an acute infection, but is also an expected result of an inflammatory process. WBCs are known to have both positive and negative effects. Positive effects include phagocytosis of microorganisms. Potentially destructive effects include the release of oxygen-free radicals from neutrophils and excessive amounts of cytokines from macrophages. An abnormal production of leukocytes in the bone marrow occurs during leukemia.

Leukopenia refers to a decrease in the total WBC number. This occurs when bone marrow production is inhibited or during certain infections when rapid consumption of WBCs takes place. The life span of a circulating WBC is only hours to days; therefore, a constant replacement process is necessary to prevent leukopenia and immune compromise, which can result in infection and harm to the patient.

White Blood Cell Differential

The differential is a measure of five different categories of leukocytes, with each type reported as a percentage of the total WBC count. The absolute count for each category of white cell (also referred to a cell line) is calculated by multiplying the percentage of each type of cell by the total WBC count. Increases or decreases in any one cell line help evaluate normal immune response and predict impaired immunity.

Neutrophils, or segmented neutrophils (also called "segs"), are the primary responders to infection and inflammation in the body. They also are an accurate indicator of how the immune system is functioning. With active infections the bone marrow also releases an immature form of neutrophil called a band. Bands quickly mature into segmented neutrophils with greater phagocytic properties to respond to infection. Leukocytosis is usually caused by an increased number of segmented neutrophils and is called neutrophilia. A "left shift" refers to leukocytosis with an increased percentage of bands. Neutropenia, or a decreased number of circulating neutrophils, places the body at increased risk for infection. An absolute neutrophil count (ANC = WBC × [% neutrophils + % bands]) of less than 1000 cells/mm^3 severely compromises immune system response, particularly to bacterial infections.

Monocytes are large phagocytic cells that circulate briefly in the blood before maturing into macrophages. These leukocytes are important scavengers of microorganisms and other foreign material. They also activate lymphocytes by presenting antigens to T cells.

Lymphocytes are the WBCs responsible for the body's adaptive (specific) immune responses. Subsets of T and B lymphocytes are assessed by specific cell counts. Lack of properly functioning lymphocytes or inadequate numbers of these cells places the body at risk for bacterial, viral, and fungal infections and certain malignancies. The CD4 cell is a subset of lymphocytes. It is the target of HIV infection leading to the development of acquired immunodeficiency syndrome (AIDS).

Eosinophils increase in numbers and activity during parasitic infections and allergic responses. They attach to parasites and use enzymes to kill them. Increased percentages of these cells are also seen during an allergic response. Basophils are another WBC associated with allergy. They break down during allergic reactions, releasing their intracellular contents such as heparin and histamine.

Platelet Count

The platelet count is determined by the number of platelets per cubic millimeter of blood. Platelets are called *thrombocytes* because of their role in the initiation of blood coagulation at the site of damaged blood vessel walls. Two-thirds of the body's platelets are circulating in the blood, with the remaining one-third sequestered within the spleen. Thrombocytopenia (decreased number of platelets) is associated with increased risk of spontaneous bleeding and is caused by decreased production, increased consumption, or increased destruction of platelets. Hypercoagulability of the blood can result from increased circulating platelets caused by proliferative disorders, malignancies, and inflammation. Qualitative assessment of platelet function is determined by the bleeding time.

Coagulation Studies

Prothrombin Time and International Normalized Ratio

The prothrombin time (PT) evaluates the extrinsic pathway and final common pathway of fibrin clot formation. Because of different reagents used in testing, PT values from different facilities are not standardized, so comparing results may lead to discrepancies. The International Normalized Ratio (INR) is a calculation developed to standardize interpretation of PT results. The PT and INR may be reported together, but the INR is now the recommended parameter for establishing the therapeutic range for oral anticoagulant therapy. The INR is a general test of coagulation, and will be elevated in patients with liver disease, biliary tract disease, and those who are therapeutically anticoagulated with warfarin. It is also elevated in patients with coagulopathies such as disseminated intravascular coagulation (DIC).

Activated Partial Thromboplastin Time

The activated partial thromboplastin time (aPTT) is reported in seconds and is used to evaluate fibrin clot formation stimulated by the intrinsic and common pathways of coagulation. This test is used to screen for congenital coagulation disorders and for monitoring anticoagulation with unfractionated (IV) heparin therapy. Prolonged aPTT is noted in persons with liver disease, vitamin K deficiency, and DIC.

Activated Coagulation Time

The activated coagulation time (ACT) is reported in seconds. The test is used most commonly to monitor effects of unfractionated heparin during and following cardiovascular procedures such as cardiopulmonary bypass and percutaneous coronary interventions. It is generally performed at the point of care.

Fibrinogen

The fibrinogen level is tested during evaluation for bleeding disorders. Fibrinogen is the plasma protein that becomes the fibrin clot. Plasma levels of fibrinogen may be increased during an inflammatory response, pregnancy, or acute infection. Decreased levels are present with liver disease and DIC.

D-Dimer

D-dimer is a very specific indicator of fibrinolysis, the natural process that breaks down fibrin clots. Levels of D-dimer are elevated in thrombotic disorders such as deep venous thrombosis (DVT) and pulmonary emboli (PE). Levels are also elevated during thrombolytic drug therapy and in DIC.

Additional Tests and Procedures

After obtaining basic laboratory screening tests, additional laboratory and diagnostic testing is necessary to identify specific etiologies for hematologic and immune function. For patients with hematologic disorders, a bone marrow aspiration, or further studies of specific clotting factor assays may be performed.

Blood, sputum, urine, and wound specimens for gram stain and culture help identify sources of infection. Molecular diagnostic techniques such as polymerase chain reaction (PCR) detect infectious agents not readily cultured, such as viruses. Noninvasive studies such as ultrasound may determine liver, spleen, or lymph node abnormalities. Radiologic procedures (radiographs, CT scans, arteriograms) may be needed to identify areas of infection or hemorrhage.

PATHOLOGIC CONDITIONS

Critically and acutely ill patients often have combined abnormalities involving the hematologic and immune systems. Anemia, immune compromise, and coagulopathy are three distinct problems that may be seen together in a critical or acute care patient. Each of these problems pose major threats to the patient's potential outcome and is evaluated separately.

Anemia

Etiology, Risk Factors, and Pathophysiology

Anemia is defined as a hemoglobin count less than 12 g/dL and is the most common hematologic disorder. Its etiology may be classified into disorders of RBC production, increased destruction of RBC, or acute blood loss.

A patient history gives important clues to the etiology of anemia. Decreased production may result from nutritional deficiencies in substrates necessary for RBC production such as iron, folic acid, or vitamin B_{12}. Those at high risk for iron deficiency anemia include children, adolescents, pregnant women, elderly, and patients with malabsorption syndromes. Folic acid deficiency is common in alcoholics. Dietary vitamin B_{12} deficiency may occur in strict vegetarians and also occurs due to a lack of intrinsic factor (postgastrectomy or with pernicious anemia) or Crohn disease. Another common cause of anemia is chronic blood loss from the gastrointestinal (GI) tract or from heavy menstruation. Daily blood testing in hospitalized patients may also contribute to anemia, because the patient's bone marrow cannot keep up with the loss.

Anemia may be associated with chronic illness, such as chronic inflammation, infection, cancer, hepatitis, and renal failure. Patients with renal failure experience anemia owing to the reduced production of the hormone erythropoietin. The life span of the RBC is also decreased in some chronic disease states, and the bone marrow is unable to compensate adequately, resulting in anemia. Cancer that specifically involves the bone marrow may replace normal bone marrow with malignant cells, disturb the development and maturation process of blood cells and fill the marrow with immature cells that prevent RBC generation.

Anemia can also occur in cancer patients as a result of bone marrow suppression due to their specific treatment. Here the bone marrow fails to produce cells, sometimes causing a drop in all three types of blood cells (WBC, RBC, and platelets) known as pancytopenia. Medications such as chemotherapeutic agents often suppress the bone marrow and cause anemia. Other causes of anemia include radiation therapy to marrow-producing bones such as the sternum and other long bones in the body.

Hemolytic anemia results from excessive destruction of RBCs. This can occur episodically or chronically. Abnormalities intrinsic to the RBC are usually the result of hereditary causes of hemolytic anemia, such as sickle cell disease. Extrinsic sources of hemolysis include immune destruction from a transfusion reaction, splenic disorders, damage by artificial heart valves, cardiopulmonary bypass, or use of an intra-aortic balloon pump.

Sickle cell anemia is an inherited abnormality of hemoglobin which results in chronic hemolytic anemia and occlusion of blood vessels. The problem mainly affects the African American population and can manifest itself as sickle cell trait, or the more serious sickle cell disease beginning in early childhood. During episodes of low oxygen tension, the RBCs change their shape (to a sickle rather than rounded shape) and adhere to the endothelial lining of blood vessels where they activate coagulation. This results in hemolytic anemia, blood vessel occlusion, and ischemic pain in organs and tissues. Other complications include bone disorders, injury to the spleen, and stroke. Hydroxyurea is a cytotoxic drug that may be prescribed to help prevent complications. Stress, infection, and illness can precipitate an acute exacerbation. Patient management includes hydration, blood transfusion, and pain management during acute episodes.

Acute hemorrhage also leads to anemia. Trauma, surgical blood loss, coagulopathy, GI bleeding, and bleeding from excessive anticoagulation are frequently encountered as causes of anemia in critically and acutely ill patient populations. With acute hemorrhage, both cellular components and plasma are lost simultaneously. The remaining cells are normal (normocytic, normochromic) and the main problem is an insufficient number of RBC. Until volume replacement from fluid resuscitation or mobilization of fluids from extracellular sources occurs, a drop in hematocrit may not be appreciated. Following an episode of blood loss, the reticulocyte count will generally rise as newly produced immature RBCs are released into the circulation.

Regardless of the etiology of an anemia, the critical effect of decreased RBCs and hemoglobin is a decrease in the oxygen-carrying capacity of the blood and a reduction in oxygen content. This may be tolerated if anemia develops slowly and the body can compensate, but may be life threatening if sudden blood loss occurs. Rapid loss of blood volume results in hypovolemic shock and cardiovascular instability, further reducing delivery of oxygen to body tissues.

Clinical Signs and Symptoms

Clinical manifestations are related to the body's compensatory mechanisms that attempt to maintain perfusion of oxygen to vital tissues. Clinical manifestations may not be obvious until the hemoglobin level is less than 7 g/dL. As compensatory mechanisms are overwhelmed, serious signs and symptoms occur. Patients with underlying pathology involving the pulmonary and cardiovascular system have less of an ability to tolerate the effects of anemia and become symptomatic more quickly.

Cardiovascular

- Tachycardia, palpitations
- Angina
- Decreased capillary refill
- Orthostatic hypotension
- ECG abnormalities (arrhythmias, ischemic changes)
- Hypovolemic shock (hypotension, tachycardia, decreased cardiac output, increased systemic vascular resistance)

Respiratory

- Increased respiratory rate
- Dyspnea on exertion, progressing to dyspnea at rest

Skin/Musculoskeletal

- Pallor of skin and mucous membranes
- Dusky nail beds
- Decreased skin temperature

Neurologic

- Headache
- Light-headedness
- Syncope
- Irritability/agitation
- Restlessness
- Severe fatigue

Abdominal

- Enlarged liver and/or spleen
- Anorexia, nausea, vomiting

Principles of Management of Anemia

Management of the anemic patient must be guided by the severity of symptoms. The level of concern for decreases in hemoglobin and hematocrit is determined by the patient's signs and symptoms and if active bleeding is suspected. Restoration of adequate blood to assure oxygen delivery to the tissues is a priority in critically and acutely ill patients. Identification of the etiology of anemia and resolution of the underlying cause is done simultaneously.

Improving Oxygen Delivery

Oxygen delivery is a product of the amount of hemoglobin in the blood, the saturation of the hemoglobin with oxygen, and

TABLE 13-2. SUMMARY OF CURRENT GUIDELINE RECOMMENDATIONS ON RED BLOOD CELL TRANSFUSION

1. For hospitalized patients who are stable, transfusions should be restricted to patients with a hemoglobin below 7 to 8 g/dL.
2. In hospitalized patients with preexisting cardiovascular disease, transfusions should be limited to patients with symptoms or hemoglobin levels of 8 g/dL or less.
3. Transfusion decisions should be made according to patient symptoms as well as hemoglobin levels.

Carson JL, Grossman BJ, Kleinman S, et al. Red blood cell transfusion: a clinical practice guideline from the AABB. *Ann Int Med.* 2012. Available at: http://www.annals.org/content/early/2012/03/26. Accessed March 10, 2012.

the cardiac output. Management strategies focus on optimizing each of those components.

1. Administration of supplemental oxygen can enhance oxygen saturation. Use of oxygen, particularly during activity, may minimize desaturation and dyspnea.
2. Adequate hemoglobin can be replaced in acute situations only by transfusion of RBCs. Transfusion of packed red blood cells (PRBC) is considered when blood loss is severe, the patient is actively bleeding, or when the patient is very symptomatic (Table 13-2).
3. Cardiac output can be optimized with volume replacement, including PRBCs, in situations of bleeding and hypovolemia. Other manipulations of cardiac output may be guided by hemodynamic monitoring and calculations to assess oxygen delivery and utilization.
4. Monitoring vital signs, oxygen saturation, and subjective patient data before, during, and after a change in therapy or activity identifies the patient's ability to tolerate anemia.
5. Limiting strenuous activity and planning periods of rest are important nursing interventions for the anemic patient.

Identifying and Treating Underlying Disease State

Further diagnostic testing may be indicated to determine the etiology of anemia. Radiologic and endoscopic studies to locate sites of bleeding, particularly in the GI tract, may be necessary. Treatment of the underlying cause of anemia may include the following:

1. Administer recombinant human erythropoietin to restore bone marrow production of RBCs in chronic anemia. The response may take several weeks, so it is not appropriate in situations in which acute correction of anemia is necessary. Chronic renal failure patients and patients receiving chemotherapy may benefit from this treatment.
2. Supplemental oral ferrous sulfate or IV iron-sucrose may be indicated if iron deficiency anemia is present.
3. Vitamin B_{12} and folic acid–related anemia may also require supplementation.
4. Dietary consultation may be needed prior to discharge to help patients and families plan meals with foods high in iron.

Minimizing Blood Loss and Reducing the Need for Transfusion

1. Use small volume collection tubes and microanalysis techniques.
2. Assess the need for routine and additional blood testing to decrease diagnostic blood loss.
3. Use blood salvage systems in surgical patients.
4. Use prophylactic agents to reduce the risk of GI bleeding.
5. Screen all patients for anticoagulants and bleeding risk prior to procedures.
6. Accept normovolemic anemia in stable patients.

Immunocompromise

Etiology, Risk Factors, and Pathophysiology

All critically and acutely ill patients may be considered compromised hosts because their defense mechanisms are inadequate due to a combination of factors, such as underlying disease, medical therapy, nutritional status, age, or stress. Patients in critical care units and acute or progressive care units are considered to be at high risk for infection. The term *immunocompromise* is applied to patients whose immune mechanisms are defective or inadequate. The patient with immunocompromise is more likely to develop an opportunistic infection. Once infection develops, it may quickly progress to systemic inflammatory response syndrome (SIRS) and sepsis.

Immune system protection from infection is categorized into three levels: natural defenses, innate (general) immunity, and adaptive (specific) immunity. Natural defenses include having intact epithelial surfaces (skin and mucous membranes) with normal chemical barriers (pH, secretions) present and all protective reflexes (blink, swallow, cough, gag, sneeze) intact. The invasive catheters and tubes used in critical and acute care units bypass these protective barriers and allow an introduction of pathogens.

The innate response to infection includes activation of the phagocytic WBC (neutrophils and monocytes) to attack the foreign microorganisms (antigens) that have entered the body, bypassing or overwhelming the natural defenses. The macrophages play a key role in processing the invading antigen and presenting it to the lymphocytes involved in the adaptive immune response.

Lymphocytes (B cells and T cells) are responsible for the orchestration of an immune response specific to each foreign protein or antigen. B lymphocytes create antigen-specific antibodies or immunoglobulins to aid in the destruction of the antigen and to protect the body from future encounters with the antigen. This is called *humoral immunity*. T lymphocytes have different subsets of cells created to modulate the immune system response (including CD4 helper T cells) and cells that have cytotoxic properties, the CD8 cytotoxic T cells. The immune response of the T lymphocytes is called *cell-mediated immunity*. Both types of lymphocytes work closely together in a specific immune response. However, humoral immunity is the primary protection against

bacterial invasion and cell-mediated immunity is primarily directed against infection by viral and fungal organisms, and some malignancies. Additionally, T cells are most responsible for the rejection of foreign tissue and for delayed hypersensitivity reactions.

Deficiencies in immune system function can be categorized into primary, or congenital, immune system defects and secondary, or acquired, immune system dysfunction. Immune deficiencies may be pinpointed to a specific cell type or may involve abnormalities in multiple components of the immune system. Secondary or acquired immunodeficiencies are the most likely type encountered in critical and acute care patients. Acquired immunodeficiency may be secondary to age, malnutrition, stress, chronic disease states, drugs with immunosuppressive effects, cancer and its treatment, HIV infection, and other factors.

Today, an increased number of patients are undergoing organ transplantation and receiving immunosuppressive agents. Patients who receive organ transplants require lifelong immunosuppressive drug therapy to prevent recognition and rejection of the transplanted tissue by the immune system. Patients typically receive a combination of drugs that affect various components of the immune response. Higher doses are required during the first weeks and months after the transplant, and doses are decreased over time to minimize the risk of infection and other complications. Acute cellular rejection may be diagnosed by evidence of failure of the transplanted organ (such as elevated serum creatinine and decreased urine output in a kidney recipient) or by obtaining a biopsy diagnostic of rejection. Rejection is commonly treated by augmented immunosuppression, such as a series of doses of IV methylprednisolone. During and following treatment, these patients are at high risk for infection. Immunosuppressive drugs also may be used in the management of other disorders such as autoimmune diseases like rheumatoid arthritis and lupus.

As new regimens and new chemotherapy agents are used to treat cancer, many of these agents have the potential to produce significant bone marrow suppression. More aggressive chemotherapeutic treatment of cancer has led to higher numbers of patients with bone marrow suppression. These patients are at high risk for the development of complications, including neutropenia and risk of serious infection.

Neutropenia is a term used to describe the state where the absolute neutrophil count is less than 1000 cells/mm^3 with an increased susceptibility to infection and sometimes neutropenic fever and sepsis. Many factors contribute to the susceptibility of the neutropenic patient to develop an infection. The duration of neutropenia, functional capability of the existing neutrophils, the patient's defense mechanisms and natural barriers to infection, and endogenous and exogenous flora all are influential in the development of infection. The key to preventing sepsis and infection is early detection and intervention.

Detection of infection in the immunocompromised patient may be difficult since the body's defense mechanisms are suppressed. Due to the lack of neutrophils, the patient may not be able to mount a vigorous inflammatory response and classic signs and symptoms of infection may be diminished or absent. Therefore redness, febrile response, or even the development of pus may not occur because purulent drainage is largely the result of dying neutrophils at the site of infection. Since the neutropenic patient can be severely infected and on the verge of becoming septic, while lacking the usual paramount signs of infection, malaise or pain may be the patient's only complaint.

Fever in this patient population is another key sign of infection and warrants aggressive investigation. Since development of fever may not be possible, the nurse must be keenly aware of other signs of sepsis including alterations in blood pressure, pulse, and respiratory rate that are the result of compensatory mechanisms. The rapid onset of sepsis in a neutropenic patient requires diligent and meticulous assessment skills with early intervention, as these patients do not present or respond as those with a functional, normal immune system.

Human immunodeficiency virus (HIV) is another disorder which leads to immunocompromise. It primarily affects helper T cells, decreasing their number and function. This in turn has a profound effect on adaptive immunity. Following diagnosis, the CD4 cells are monitored, and a CD4 count of $< 400/mm^3$ is associated with a poor prognosis. Viral load testing is also performed to measure the amount of viral particles per cubic millimeter of blood. Patients with HIV are susceptible to opportunistic infections and certain malignancies, and as these develop they may progress to a diagnosis of AIDS. HIV is managed with antiretroviral drugs and effective treatment of infections. Patients are surviving longer, and may develop disorders requiring hospitalization. They are most likely to require critical care if they acquire a serious opportunistic infections or experience an adverse reaction to antiretroviral therapy. They may also be admitted with conditions not directly related to HIV or AIDS.

Clinical Signs and Symptoms*

Local Evidence of Inflammation and Infection

- Redness
- Edema
- Warmth
- Pain
- Purulent drainage

General Evidence of Infection

- Fever or hypothermia
- Rigors or shaking chills
- Fatigue and malaise

- Changes in level of consciousness
- Lymphadenopathy
- Tachycardia
- Tachypnea

System-Specific Evidence

Neurologic

- Headache
- Nuchal rigidity
- Changes in mental status, agitation

Respiratory

- Cough
- Change in color, amount of sputum
- Dyspnea, orthopnea

Genitourinary

- Dysuria
- Urgency
- Frequency
- Flank pain
- Abdominal pain
- Cloudy and/or bloody urine

Gastrointestinal

- Nausea
- Vomiting
- Diarrhea
- Cramping abdominal pain
- Enlarged liver or spleen

Principles of Management for Immunocompromised Patients

Patients with high risk for the development of infection must be identified on admission to the unit. Measures to protect and strengthen immune system function should be included in the plan of care. All healthcare team members must utilize measures to prevent the development of hospital-acquired infections. Close monitoring for signs and symptoms of a local or systemic inflammatory response is especially important to detect infection early. Identification of the source and likely organisms causing infection allows for initiation of broad-spectrum, empiric antimicrobial coverage. Culture and sensitivity reports guide the choice of drugs specific to the organisms isolated from the patient. Care is planned in a way that risks for introduction of pathogens and infection are minimized. Hand washing is the main intervention for the prevention of infection. Additionally, the number of lines, tubes, and drains is minimized when possible. Although utilization of central lines, indwelling catheters, and other devices is commonplace in critical and acute care settings, the nurse must be vigilant to constantly evaluate the ongoing need for such devices.

Identification of Patients With High Risk of Infection

Immunocompromised risk factors are as follows:

1. Neonates and the elderly
2. Malnutrition

---

*As noted earlier, immune-compromised patients may not show any of these clinical signs and symptoms. They may have some, they may have none. The neutropenic patient may have very subtle, suppressed signs of sepsis; thus heightened vigilance is necessary so that essential treatment is provided.

3. Use of medications with known immunosuppressive effects such as steroids, cancer chemotherapeutic agents, and transplant immunosuppressive agents
4. Recent radiation therapy to areas of the body that impact bone marrow production
5. Chronic systemic diseases such as renal or hepatic failure or diabetes
6. Diseases involving the immune system such as HIV infection
7. Loss of protective epithelial barriers through:
   - Oral or nasogastric intubation
   - Presence of decubitus ulcers
   - Burns
   - Surgical wounds
   - Skin and soft tissue trauma
   - Mucositis
8. Invasive catheters or prosthetic devices in place such as:
   - Intravascular catheters, including peripheral, central, and arterial lines
   - Indwelling urinary catheters
   - Endotracheal intubation and mechanical ventilation
   - Heart valve replacements
   - Orthopedic hardware such as artificial joints, pins, plates, or screws
   - Dialysis, apheresis catheters, shunts, fistulas, or grafts
   - Cardiovascular devices such as ventricular-assist devices, pacemakers, or implantable defibrillators
   - Synthetic vascular grafts
   - Ventricular shunts

Implementing Measures to Protect and Strengthen Immune System Function

1. Take meticulous care of the skin and mucous membranes to prevent loss of barrier protection.
2. Use the enteral route for feeding when possible to maintain caloric intake and normal gut function.
3. Avoid the use of indwelling urinary catheters or remove them as early as possible.
4. Minimize patient stress and the release of endogenous glucocorticoids by relieving pain or using alternative methods such as guided imagery or music for relaxation, and other comfort measures (positioning, massage).
5. Administer colony-stimulating factors (G-CSF or GM-CSF) to stimulate bone marrow production of neutrophils and monocytes when appropriate.

Implementing Measures to Prevent Hospital-Acquired Infections

1. All personnel and visitors are to wash their hands before and after contact with the patient. Hand washing remains the number one method to prevent hospital-acquired infection.
2. Patients at high risk should have a private room.
3. Institute respiratory hygiene/cough etiquette for patients with signs of respiratory infection and appropriate isolation for known or suspected patient infection.
4. Adhere to strict aseptic technique for all care of intravascular catheters and any invasive procedures performed at the patient's bedside.
5. Eliminate environmental sources of infection (eg, leftover fluids used for irrigations). Clean surfaces frequently with recommended disinfectant, including bedside table, equipment, and any surfaces where contamination is likely.
6. Track the date and time fluids, tubings, and catheters and change them at the prescribed intervals.
7. Review facility protocol regarding use of filtered water, restriction of fresh fruits and vegetables, and other neutropenic precautions.
8. Encourage use of incentive spirometry, turning, deep breathing, and mobility with ambulation if possible.

Early Detection of Local or System Inflammatory Response and Sepsis

1. Monitor the patient closely for signs and symptoms consistent with infection and sepsis and communicate abnormal findings to the healthcare team.
2. Initiate sepsis protocol when signs of SIRS are present.
3. Collect specimens for culture and sensitivity from potential sources of infection (eg, urine, sputum, blood, stool, wound drainage).
4. Institute antibiotic therapy as directed. See Chapter 11 Multisystem Problems, for more information on the management of sepsis.

Coagulopathies

Etiology, Risk Factors, and Pathophysiology

Critically and acutely ill patients with coagulopathy may have a problem involving platelets, hemostasis, fibrinolysis, or a combination of these abnormalities. Acquired disorders of coagulation, as opposed to inherited disorders, are seen most frequently in critical and acute care units.

Thrombocytopenia

Platelets initiate the coagulation process at the site of blood vessel injury. Quantitative platelet disorders are associated with bleeding when the platelet count drops to less than $50,000/mm^3$, especially if there is tissue trauma. Spontaneous bleeding is possible at counts of $< 20,000/mm^3$, and counts that reach 5000 to $10,000/mm^3$ predict high risk for hemorrhage. Four general mechanisms are responsible for thrombocytopenia: (1) decreased production of platelets by the bone marrow, (2) shortened survival due to platelet utilization and destruction, (3) sequestration of platelets in the spleen, and (4) intravascular dilution of platelets during massive transfusion.

Thrombocytopenia may also be related to immune mechanisms. Drug-induced thrombocytopenia occurs when a drug induces an antigen-antibody reaction that results in the formation of immune complexes that destroy platelets by complement-mediated lysis. There are several types of

ESSENTIAL CONTENT CASE

Chronic Immunosuppression

A 35-year-old African American man is admitted to the progressive care unit with dyspnea and altered mental status. The patient's history includes diabetes mellitus and chronic renal failure treated by kidney transplantation 3 months ago. Recent kidney function testing suggested possible rejection, and the patient received a course of augmented steroids. Current medications include tacrolimus, mycophenolate mofetil, prednisone, metoprolol, and insulin. Significant findings on admission include the following:

Blood pressure	90/60 mm Hg
Heart rate	116 beats/min
Respiratory rate	28 breaths/min
Temperature	102°F
WBC	12,500/mm^3 with 15% bands
Hemoglobin	11.2 g/dL
Hematocrit	32%
Platelets	89,000/mm^3
Serum glucose	320 mg/dL
Serum creatinine	1.9 mg/dL
Chest x-ray	Infiltrates left lower lobe

During the admission interview, the patient appears dyspneic, tachypneic, and complains of thirst. He has a dry cough, and crackles are heard over the left lung field. The physician arrives on the unit and discusses the patient with the progressive care nurse, who knows this patient from previous hospitalizations. Following analysis of the patient's history, physical examination, and diagnostic data, a multidisciplinary care plan is developed.

Case Question 1. What are this patient's risk factors for hematologic and immune problems?

Case Question 2. What should the nursing assessment focus on?

Case Question 3. What therapeutic interventions should be carried out immediately?

Case Question 4. Analyze the diagnostic test results and outline how the values provide diagnostic information.

Case Question 5. Analyze the assessment data and explain how it will be used to direct patient care.

Case Question 6. What are the most likely working diagnoses?

Case Question 7. What types of consultations should be ordered?

Case Question 8. What are your priority nursing interventions during these first few hours of hospitalization?

Answers
1. Risk factors include chronic immunosuppression, recently augmented immunosuppression, and diabetes.
2. Assessment should focus on the evaluation of potential sources of infection and indicators of hyperglycemia, electrolyte imbalance, and renal insufficiency.
3. Initial interventions should include IV fluids, antibiotics, supplemental oxygen, and respiratory therapy.
4. The elevated WBC and band cells indicate acute infection. The low platelet count can indicate sepsis and potential clotting problems. The serum glucose suggests poorly controlled blood sugar, and frequent testing is indicated. The elevated serum creatinine indicates renal insufficiency in the transplanted kidney. The chest x-ray suggests pneumonia.
5. The cough, respiratory distress and crackles suggest possible pneumonia. The elevated respiratory rate can be indicative of respiratory distress and diabetic ketoacidosis. The thirst may be due to fever and hyperglycemia.
6. Pneumonia, hyperglycemia, renal insufficiency.
7. An infectious disease consultation and consultation with the diabetic management team are indicated. The renal transplant team needs to be notified of the admission.
8. Nursing priorities include frequent assessment of respiratory status, blood sugar, and kidney function. Collaborative interventions such as fluids, antibiotics, and insulin are administered. Consultants are notified promptly regarding the patient's admission and condition.

immune-related thrombocytopenia that are seen in critical and acute care. Heparin-induced thrombocytopenia (HIT) is an immune-mediated reaction to heparin that results in the formation of antiplatelet antibodies which activate platelets and form clots. This then leads to platelet consumption and a precipitous drop in the platelet count. The patient may develop intravascular clotting resulting in clinical thrombosis. Venous thrombosis is most common and may result in limb ischemia and pulmonary emboli. When this syndrome is suspected, all heparin is stopped, and confirmatory testing for HIT antibodies is performed. Treatment options include administration of direct thrombin inhibitors such as argatroban. Patients diagnosed with HIT should not receive heparin again.

Immune thrombocytopenia purpura (ITP) is an autoimmune disorder that results in the destruction of platelets in the spleen and a platelet count of less than 20,000/mm^3. This disorder was formerly called idiopathic thrombocytopenia, but was renamed when it was identified as an immune process. In adults ITP may occur as a primary disorder or may be secondary to medications or autoimmune disorders such as systemic lupus erythematosus. For some the cause may never be determined. Patients develop petechiae, purpura, and epistaxis. Splenomegaly may develop as platelets are destroyed in the spleen. Treatment options include steroids, intravenous immunoglobin, administration of monoclonal antibody treatment, and, in some cases, splenectomy.

Thrombotic thrombocytopenic purpura (TTP) is a syndrome characterized by thrombocytopenia, hemolytic anemia, renal failure, fever, and neurologic changes. The cause of this disorder is unclear, but is thought to involve dysfunction of an enzyme which leads to abnormal platelet aggregation. Patients with TTP may develop widespread vascular occlusion in organs, as well as jaundice, purpura, petechiae, and bleeding. Acutely ill individuals may be treated with plasmapheresis.

Hemolytic-uremic syndrome is characterized by thrombocytopenia, hemolytic anemia, and renal failure. It is most often the result of infectious colitis and the toxin released from *E coli* 0157:H7. Children are most often affected by this syndrome, and will require hospitalization for supportive care including dialysis.

Patients may have adequate numbers of platelets but still have a bleeding tendency due to qualitative platelet disorders. Drug-induced suppression of platelet function is commonly associated with use of aspirin and nonsteroidal anti-inflammatory agents (NSAIDs). In addition to many of the medications used, critically and acutely ill patients may have many factors that predispose them to the potential impairment of platelet function, including renal failure and uremia.

Disorders of Hemostasis

Disorders of hemostasis may be caused by inherited abnormalities of coagulation factors. Hemophilia types A and B are congenital deficiencies in factors VIII and IX. Von Willebrand disease represents a deficiency or dysfunction of the plasma protein of the same name. Replacement of the deficient factor keeps these chronic diseases under control. Patients with these disorders may be monitored in critical or progressive care units when undergoing routine surgical procedures or when hospitalized for other medical problems.

Acquired coagulation disorders can be associated with deficient coagulation factor production. This may be caused by a decreased intake of vitamin K, the vitamin essential for the formation of clotting factors II, VII, IX, and X. Deficiencies in vitamin K as a result of dietary deficiency, intestinal malabsorption, liver disease, use of warfarin, or antibiotic therapy are also common. Vitamin K deficiency prolongs the PT/INR. Because most coagulation factors are produced in the liver, patients with liver disease have deficiencies of fibrinogen and other factors in addition to deficiencies of the vitamin K–dependent factors.

Many of the drugs used routinely in hospitalized patients have anticoagulant and antiplatelet effects (Table 13-3). Therapeutic anticoagulation using heparin, warfarin, and other agents interferes directly with the clotting process. The intrinsic pathway and the final common pathway are affected by the administration of heparin. If bleeding from heparin is minimal, it can be controlled by decreasing the dose or temporarily stopping its administration. If bleeding is severe, the antidote to reverse heparin, protamine sulfate, may be administered intravenously. Low-molecular-weight heparin is associated with fewer bleeding and immunological complications.

Warfarin acts by inhibiting the production of vitamin K–dependent clotting factors. Effects from warfarin take several days to be observed after initiation of the drug, but may persist for many days following administration. If significant bleeding occurs while on warfarin, replacement of vitamin K–dependent factors by use of fresh frozen plasma may be necessary. Giving replacement vitamin K may also be helpful, but its effectiveness depends on the time needed by the liver to synthesize new clotting factors.

Use of thrombolytic agents (alteplase, reteplase) to dissolve thrombi (pathologic clots) may result in patient bleeding from sites where a protective clot previously formed. These agents are used in combination with other anticoagulants, and may precipitate obvious or occult bleeding. Patients who receive anticoagulants are monitored for any sign of bleeding complications.

Disseminated intravascular coagulation is a complex coagulopathy which can develop in patients already critically ill from a wide variety of disorders (Table 13-4). The underlying condition triggers the release of proinflammatory cytokines, which activate the coagulation cascade and result in the formation of micro clots. The micro clots obstruct the capillaries of organs and tissues. This initiates a series of events which result in both bleeding and thrombosis (Figure 13-1). DIC can be seen in patients who are seriously ill with

TABLE 13-3. ANTICOAGULANTS COMMONLY USED IN ACUTE CARE

Classification	Drug
Indirect thrombin inhibitor	Heparin sodium
Direct thrombin inhibitor	Argatroban
	Bivalirudin
	Lepirudin
Factor Xa inhibitor	Fondaparinux (Atrixtra)
Vitamin K–dependent factor inhibitor	Warfarin (Coumadin)
Glycoprotein IIb/IIIa inhibitors	Abciximab (Reopro)
	Eptifibatide (Integrilin)
	Tirofiban (Aggrastat)
Thrombolytic agents	Alteplase (Activase)
	Reteplase
Antiplatelet agents	Aspirin
	Clopidogrel (Plavix)
	Dipyridamole (Persantine)
	Prasugrel (Effient)

TABLE 13-4. ETIOLOGIES OF DIC

Infection and Sepsis
- Acute bacterial
- Acute viral

Trauma
- Head injury
- Crushing injury
- Burns
- Snake venom

Cardiovascular
- Shock
- Extracorporeal circulation

Obstetrical
- Eclampsia and pre-eclampsia
- Amniotic fluid embolism
- Abortion

Immunological
- Blood transfusion reaction

Neoplastic Disease
- Acute leukemia
- Metastatic cancer

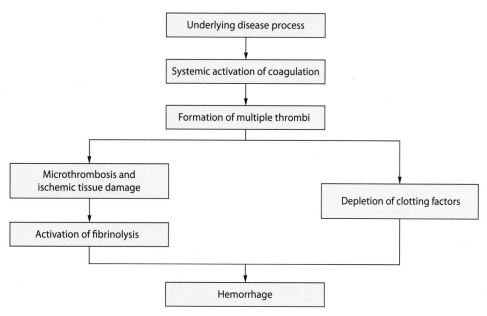

Figure 13-1. Clinical consequences of DIC.

sepsis, traumatic injury, and extensive surgery. It is also seen in patients newly diagnosed with acute forms of leukemia and as a complication in cancer treatment.

During the process of DIC, stimulation of the clotting cascade rapidly depletes existing platelets and coagulation factors, consuming them faster than the body can replace them. Depletion of substrates of the coagulation process leaves the body at risk for spontaneous bleeding or hemorrhage from surgical sites, or even minimal trauma.

Multiple tiny clots are formed within the blood and flow to the small vessels where they are trapped. Microcirculatory thrombosis then leads to tissue ischemia, infarction, and organ dysfunction. Single or multisystem organ dysfunction may occur.

Simultaneous activation of fibrinolysis releases the enzyme plasmin. Plasmin breaks down some of the fibrin in a physiologic attempt to open the microcirculation, and this produces fibrin degradation products, including D-dimer. Anticoagulant pathways are impaired, further interfering with the balance needed for appropriate hemostasis. Clots are unable to form at new sites of injury, and existing clots are dissolved, leading to bleeding from both old and new sites. Because of the complex pathophysiology, clinical manifestations of DIC are likely to include bleeding from multiple sites and evidence of organ ischemia, including the skin, which may show ischemic changes in the hands and feet.

Laboratory diagnosis of DIC requires careful interpretation of coagulation panel results (Table 13-5). In many cases absolute certainty regarding a diagnosis of DIC may not be possible. With or without a clear diagnosis of DIC, a primary goal of therapy is to treat the underlying condition. In addition, supportive care is provided with volume replacement and support of vital organ systems, including ventilatory

assistance. Significant bleeding is managed with blood and component therapy.

Clinical Signs and Symptoms

Coagulopathy may be a subtle, occult process or a massive, obvious emergency. Assessment must encompass each body system, looking for evidence of abnormality in single or multiple components of the coagulation process.

Abnormal Platelet Numbers or Function

- Petechiae of skin or mucous membranes
- Spontaneous bleeding from gums or nose
- Thrombocytopenia
- Prolonged bleeding time

Abnormal Coagulation Factors

- Hemorrhage into subcutaneous tissue, muscle, or joints
- Ecchymosis, purpura
- Bleeding which responds slowly to local pressure
- Prolonged PT/INR, aPTT
- Decreased fibrinogen
- Decrease in level of specific coagulation factors

TABLE 13-5. LABORATORY RESULTS SUGGESTING DIC

Test	Abnormality
INR	Elevated
aPTT	Elevated
Platelet count	Decreased
Fibrinogen	Decreased
D-dimer	Increased

General Assessment for Bleeding or Decreased Organ Perfusion as a Result of Microthrombosis

Skin/Musculoskeletal

- Oozing of blood from multiple sites, including incisions, intravascular catheters
- Petechiae
- Purpura
- Ecchymosis
- Ischemic changes in toes, fingers, nose, lips, ears
- Pain, swelling, and limited joint mobility
- Increased size of body part, increased girth

Neurologic

- Any change in level of consciousness, pupils, movement or sensation may indicate intracranial bleeding.
- Impaired vision with retinal hemorrhage.
- Headache

Gastrointestinal

- Blood in gastric aspirate
- Coffee ground emesis or gastric aspirate
- Melena or frank bloody stool
- Abdominal pain
- Enlarged liver or spleen

Genitourinary

- Hematuria
- Decreased urine output
- Vaginal bleeding

Cardiovascular

- Hypotension or labile blood pressure
- Hypovolemia and/or shock (with rapid loss of large volume of blood)

Principles of Management of Coagulopathies

The management of coagulopathy varies with the type and severity of the disorder. The overall goal of therapy is to restore normal hemostasis and prevent/treat hypovolemic shock. Supportive care focuses on the control and prevention of further bleeding associated with activities of daily living and therapeutic interventions.

Restoration of Normal Hemostasis

1. Treatment of quantitative platelet disorders may include transfusion of platelets. Transfusion is recommended for patients who are actively bleeding or prior to invasive procedures or surgery.
2. Destruction of platelets by immune mechanisms may be treated with steroids or IV immunoglobulin infusion. If related to use of heparin, then heparin is discontinued. Splenectomy may be performed for severe persistent problems where spleen sequestration is suspected.
3. Dysfunctional platelets may be treated by stopping the offending agent, such as aspirin or NSAIDs. Dialysis improves platelet function in patients with renal failure.
4. Acute replacement of coagulation factors can be accomplished with transfusion of fresh frozen plasma. Cryoprecipitate replaces fibrinogen, factor VIII, and von Willebrand factor. Recombinant factor VIIa may be used for persistent hemorrhage. For hemophiliac patients, factor VIII or factor IX concentrates are used to replace the specific factor deficiency.
5. Intravenous vitamin K may be used to treat warfarin-related bleeding or vitamin K deficiency.
6. Heparin therapy may be stopped, or the dosage decreased or reversed with IV protamine sulfate.

Controlling and Preventing Bleeding

1. Modify nursing care measures to minimize trauma and prevent skin and mucous membrane breakdown:
   - Provide gentle oral care.
   - Use electric razor or refrain from shaving.
   - Minimize use of automatic blood pressure cuffs to prevent skin trauma and subcutaneous bleeding; use manual cuffs.
   - Minimize peripheral blood sampling.
   - Avoid IM injections.
   - Use specialty mattress, pad side rails; avoid restraint use.
   - Handle patients gently when turning or moving.
   - Remove adhesive dressings with care.
   - Use low-suction setting to suction endotracheal tube and pharynx.
2. Modify nursing care procedures to control bleeding:
   - Minimize traumatic procedures; apply direct pressure afterward for at least 5 to 10 minutes or until bleeding has stopped.
   - Use ice packs on new hematomas or hemarthrosis.
   - Do not dislodge or attempt to remove blood clots from areas of bleeding.
   - Control environment to prevent hypothermia.

SELECTED BIBLIOGRAPHY

Anemia

Carson JL, Grossman BJ, Kleinman S, et al. Red blood cell transfusion: a clinical practice guideline from the AABB. *Ann Int Med;* 2012. http://www.annals.org/content/early/2012/03/26. Accessed March 10, 2012.

Collins TA. Packed red blood cell transfusions in critically ill patients. *Crit Care Nurse.* 2011;31(1):25-34.

Field JJ, Vichinsky EP, DeBaun MR. Overview of the management of sickle cell disease. In: Tirnauer JS, ed. *Up-To-Date.* www.uptodate.com. Accessed January 30, 2013.

Gaspard KJ. Disorders of red blood cells. In: Porth CM and Matfin G, eds. *Pathophysiology: concepts of altered health states*, 8th ed. Philadelphia, PA: Wolters Kluwer Health; 2009.

George JN. Clinical manifestations and diagnosis of immune (idiopathic) thrombocytopenia purpura in adults. In: Tirnauer JS, ed. *Up-To-Date.* www.uptodate.com. Accessed January 30, 2013.

Kessler D, Shaz B, Grima K. Advances in blood transfusion. *Am Nurse Today*. 2012;7(3):8-12.

Kyles DM. Blood conservation and blood component replacement. In: Carlson KK, ed. *Advanced Critical Care Nursing*. St. Louis, MO: Saunders Elsevier; 2009.

Munro N. Hematologic complications of critical illness, anemia, neutropenia, thrombocytopenia and more. *AACN Adv Crit Care*. 2009;20(2):145-154.

Pagana KD, Pagana TJ. *Mosby's Manual of Diagnostic and Laboratory Tests*, 4th ed. St. Louis, MO: Mosby Elsevier; 2010.

Rauen CA. Beyond the blood mess: hematologic assessment. *Crit Care Nurse*. 2012;32(5):42-46.

Rote NS, McCance KL. Structure and function of the hematologic system. In: Huether SE, McCance KL, eds. *Pathophysiology: The Biologic Basis for Disease in Adults and Children*, 6th ed. St. Louis, MO: Elsevier Mosby; 2010.

Schrier SL. Approach to the adult patient with anemia. In: Landaw SA, ed. *Up-To-Date*. www.uptodate.com. Accessed January 30, 2013.

Vichinsky EP. Overview of the clinical manifestations of sickle cell disease. In: Tirnauer JS, ed. *Up-To-Date*. www.uptodate.com. Accessed January 30, 2013.

Immunocompromised Patient

Bonilla FA. Secondary immune deficiency due to miscellaneous causes. In: Feldweg AM, ed. *Up-To-Date*. www.uptodate.com. Accessed January 30, 2013.

Centers for Disease Control and Prevention. Guideline for isolation precautions: preventing transmission of infectious agents in healthcare settings. 2007. Access at www.cdc.gov.

Fishman JA. Approach to the immunocompromised patient with fever and pulmonary infiltrates. In: Thorner AR. ed. *Up-To-Date*. www.uptodate.com. Accessed January 30, 2013.

Freifeld AG, Bow EJ, Sepkowitz MJ, et al. Clinical practice guideline for the use of antimicrobial agents in neutropenic patients with cancer: 2010 update by the Infectious Diseases Society of America. *Clin Infec Dis*. 2011;52(4): e56-e93.

Kaplan JE, Benson C, Holmes KH, et al. Guidelines for the prevention and treatment of opportunistic infections in HIV-infected adults and adolescents. Recommendations from CDC, the National Institutes of Health, and the HIV Medicine Association of the Infectious Diseases Society of America. *MMWR Recomm Rep*. 2009;58(RR-4):1-207. Accessed 11/1/13

Porth CM. Disorders of white blood cells and lymphoid tissue. In: Porth CM, Matfin G, eds. *Pathophysiology: Concepts of Altered Health States*, 8th ed. Philadelphia, PA: Wolters Kluwer Health; 2009.

Relf MV, Shelton BK, Jones KM. Common immunological disorders. In: Morton PG, Fontaine DK, eds. *Critical Care Nursing*, 10th ed. Philadelphia, PA: Wolters Kluwer, Lippincott Williams & Wilkins, 2013.

Shelton BK. Caring for the immunocompromised patient. In: Carlson KK, ed. *Advanced Critical Care Nursing*. St. Louis, MO: Saunders Elsevier; 2009.

Wolff PB. Hematological and immune disorders. In: Sole ML, Klein DG, Moseley MJ. *Introduction to Critical Care Nursing*. 5th ed. St. Louis, MO: Saunders Elsevier; 2009.

Coagulopathy

Dressler DK. Coagulopathy in the ICU. *Crit Care Nurse*. 2012; 32(5):48-59.

Ferraris VA, Brown JR, Despotis GJ, et al. 2011 update to the Society of Thoracic Surgeons and the Society of Cardiovascular Anesthesiologists blood conservation clinical practice guideline. *Ann Thorac Surg*. 2011;91(3):944-982.

Greenlaw D. Common hematological disorders. In: Morton PG, Fontaine DK, eds. *Critical Care Nursing*, 10th ed. Philadelphia, PA: Wolters Kluwer, Lippincott Williams & Wilkins; 2013.

James SH. Clots kill: hematologic pharmacology for ST-segment elevation myocardial infarction. *Crit Care Nurse*. 2012;32(6): 35-41.

Karch AM. Drugs that alter blood coagulation. *Am Nurse Today*. 2012;7(11):26-31.

Landaw SA, George JN. Approach to the adult patient with thrombocytopenia. In: Tirnauer JS, ed. *Up-To-Date*. www.uptodate. com. Accessed January 30, 2013.

Linkins LA, Dans AL, Moores LK, et al. Treatment and prevention of heparin-induced thrombocytopenia: antithrombotic therapy and prevention of thrombosis, 9th ed. American College of Chest Physicians evidence-based practice guidelines. *Chest*. 2012:141(2 suppl): e495S-e530S.

Mayer, B. Hematologic disorders and oncologic emergencies. In: Urden, LD, Stacy KM, Lough ME, eds. *Critical Care Nursing*. 6th ed. St. Louis, MO: Elsevier Mosby, 2010.

Rice TW, Wheeler AP. Coagulopathy in critically ill patients: part 1. *Chest*. 2009;136:1631-1643.

Warkentin TE. Heparin-induced thrombocytopenia in critically ill patients. *Crit Care Clin*. 2011;27(4):805-823.

Wheeler AP, Rice TW. Coagulopathy in critically ill patients: part 2. *Chest*. 2010;137:185-194.

GASTROINTESTINAL SYSTEM

14

Deborah A. Andris, Elizabeth Krzywda,
Carol Rees Parrish, and Joe Krenitsky

KNOWLEDGE COMPETENCIES

1. Describe the etiology, pathophysiology, clinical
   presentation, patient needs, and principles of
   management for:
   - Acute upper gastrointestinal bleeding
   - Liver failure
   - Acute pancreatitis
   - Bowel ischemia

   - Bowel obstruction
   - Bariatric (gastric bypass surgery)
2. Identify nutritional requirements for enterally fed
   acutely ill patients.
3. List important interventions to decrease the risk for
   aspiration pneumonia during enteral feeding.

PATHOLOGIC CONDITIONS

Acute Upper Gastrointestinal Bleeding

Life-threatening gastrointestinal (GI) bleeding originates most commonly in the upper GI tract and requires immediate therapy to prevent complications. Although bleeding stops spontaneously in 80% to 90% of cases, patients presenting with sudden blood loss are at risk for decreased tissue perfusion and oxygen-carrying capability. There can be effects on every organ system in the body. Acute upper GI bleeding has a mortality of 6%-13%. Bleeding that originates distal to the ligament of Treitz is considered to be lower GI bleeding which, unlike upper GI bleeding, is not associated with the same morbidity and mortality. Lower GI bleeding is generally a disease of the elderly patient and may be associated with cancer. A poor prognosis with upper GI bleeding is related to age above 65, shock, overall poor health, active bleeding at the time of presentation, elevated creatinine or transaminases, onset of bleeding during hospitalization, and initial low hematocrit. Death is not a direct result of blood loss, but is related to age and comorbidities.

Etiology, Risk Factors, and Pathophysiology

A variety of abnormalities within the GI tract can be the source of upper GI bleeding (Table 14-1). The most common cause of upper GI bleeding is peptic ulcer disease, accounting for 31%-67% of all cases followed by erosive disease, variceal bleeding, esophagitis, cancer, and Mallory-Weis tears. The pathogenesis of peptic ulcer disease is related to hypersecretion of gastric acid, coupled with impaired GI tract mucus secretion. Normally, mucus protects the gastric wall from the erosive effects of acid. Peptic ulcers occur in the stomach and the duodenum, and are characterized by a break in the mucosal layer that penetrates the muscularis mucosa (innermost muscular layer), resulting in bleeding. Infection of the mucosa by *Helicobacter pylori,* an organism naturally found in the GI tract, also has been implicated in the pathogenesis of peptic ulcer disease.

Gastroesophageal varices develop when there is increased pressure in the portal venous system of the liver. If blood cannot flow easily through the liver because of obstructive disease, it is diverted to collateral channels. These channels are normally low-pressure vessels found in the distal esophagus (esophageal varices), the veins in the proximal stomach (gastric varices), and in the rectal vault (hemorrhoids) (Figure 14-1). Acute upper GI hemorrhage occurs when esophageal and/or gastric varices rupture from increased portal vein pressure (portal hypertension). Esophagogastric varices do not bleed until the portal pressure exceeds 12 mm Hg. Portal hypertension is most commonly caused by primary liver disease

TABLE 14-1. COMMON SOURCES OF UPPER GASTROINTESTINAL BLEEDING

Peptic Ulcer Disease
- Gastric ulcer
- Duodenal ulcer

Varices
- Esophageal
- Gastric

Pathologies of the Esophagus
- Tumors
- Mallory-Weiss syndrome
- Inflammation
- Ulcers

Pathologies of the Stomach
- Cancer
- Erosive gastritis
- Stress ulcer
- Tumors

Pathologies of the Small Intestine
- Peptic ulcers
- Angiodysplasia

(see next section), liver trauma, or thrombosis of the splenic or portal veins. Massive upper GI hemorrhage is associated with these variceal bleeds.

Mallory-Weiss syndrome is a linear, nonperforating tear of the gastric mucosa near the gastroesophageal junction.

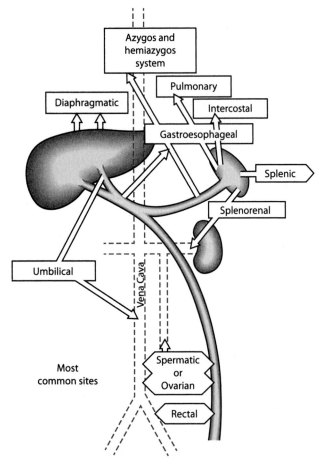

Figure 14-1. The liver with collateral circulation.

ESSENTIAL CONTENT CASE

Upper GI Bleeding

A 45-year-old white man is admitted with reports of an 8-hour history of nausea and vomiting of large amounts of "coffee-ground secretions" and frequent "maroon-colored" stools. He reports a previous history of peptic ulcer disease diagnosed at age 35. He has been hospitalized twice in the past for active GI bleeding. A duodenal ulcer near the pylorus on the posterior wall of the stomach is diagnosed by upper endoscopy. Significant findings on his admission profile are:

Vital Signs

Blood pressure	96/60 mm Hg lying; 90/58 mm Hg sitting
Heart rate	120 beats/min; sinus tachycardia
Respiratory rate	32 breaths/min, deep
Temperature	37.3 °C (oral)

Respiratory
- Breath sounds clear in all lung fields

Cardiovascular
- S_1/S_2, no murmurs
- Extremities cool, diaphoretic; pulses present but weak

Abdomen
- Distended with hyperactive bowel sounds (BSs) in all four quadrants
- Tender right upper quadrant, no rebound tenderness

Neurologic
- Alert, oriented
- Anxious

Genitourinary
- 50 mL of amber cloudy urine following Foley catheter insertion
- Stools liquid maroon, guaiac positive

Arterial Blood Gases
- pH 7.49
- $Paco_2$ 28 mm Hg
- HCO_3 19 mEq/L
- Pao_2 61 mm Hg on room air
- Sao_2 89%

Laboratory

Hematocrit	25%
Hemoglobin	7.0 g/dL
White blood cell count	17,000/mm^3
Prothrombin time	11 seconds
Activated partial Thromboplastin time	30 seconds
Platelet count	110,000/mm^3
Serum potassium	3.5 mEq/L (decreased)
Serum sodium	150 mEq/L
Serum glucose	210 mg/dL
Serum blood urea nitrogen	40
Serum creatinine	0.9
Liver function testing	Within normal limits

Case Question 1. Initial management of the patient with upper GI bleeding would include:

(A) Volume resuscitation

(B) Hemodynamic stabilization

(C) Identification of the site of bleeding

(D) Initiation of treatment to control bleeding within 24 hours of admission

Case Question 2. After the bleeding site is identified and bleeding is controlled, the drug of choice to treat a non-variceal bleed is:

(A) Histamine receptor antagonists

(B) Proton pump inhibitors (PPIs)

(C) Antacids

(D) Anti-spasmodics

Answers

1. The correct answer is A. The fundamental goal for initial management of the patient is volume resuscitation. However, hemodynamic stabilization, identification of the bleeding site, and control of bleeding are all key points for managing the patient with upper GI bleeding. Assessment of vital signs is the most reliable reflection of blood loss. If the patient is hemodynamically stable, resuscitation begins with the administration of 2 to 3 liters of crystalloid. Blood products are considered if the response is poor.

2. The correct answer is B. PPIs are the drug of choice in this patient population as they have a more durable and sustained acid suppression. In randomized controlled clinical trials, PPIs were shown to decrease recurrent bleeding.

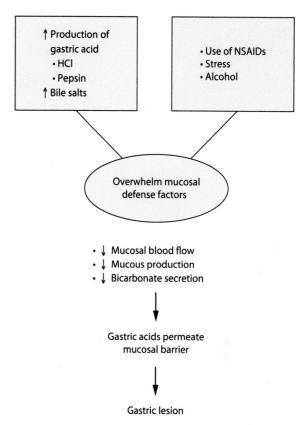

Figure 14-2. Pathogenesis of gastritis.

The tear is the result of pressure changes in the stomach that occur with forceful vomiting. Alcohol abuse and inflammatory conditions of the stomach and esophagus are also associated with this disorder. Classically, these tears occur in alcoholic patients who experience intense retching and vomiting associated with binge drinking. However, they may also occur in any patient with a history of repeated emesis.

Hemorrhagic gastritis describes gastric lesions that do not penetrate the muscularis mucosa. These are also referred to as stress ulcers. Onset of bleeding is sudden and is often the first symptom. The causes of gastritis are multifactorial (Table 14-2), but are most commonly associated with nonsteroidal anti-inflammatory drug (NSAID) use, alcohol abuse, and physiologic conditions that cause severe stress (eg, trauma, surgery, burns, severe medical problems).

TABLE 14-2. CAUSES OF GASTRITIS

Alcohol Abuse
NSAID use
Aspirin
Ascriptin
Ecotrin
Severe Physiologic Stress
Burns (Curling ulcer)
CNS disease (Cushing ulcer)
Trauma
Surgery
Medical complications
Sepsis
Acute renal failure
Hepatic failure
Long-term mechanical ventilation

Alcohol and NSAIDs are known to directly disrupt the mucosal defense mechanisms of the stomach (Figure 14-2). Use of NSAIDs is particularly problematic in the elderly and contributes to increased incidence of symptomatic acute upper GI bleeding in this population.

Regardless of the etiology, upper GI bleeding resulting in a sudden loss of blood volume is associated with decreased venous return to the heart and subsequently cardiac output (CO). The decrease in CO triggers the release of epinephrine and norepinephrine, causing intense vasoconstriction and tissue ischemia (Figure 14-3). In addition, aldosterone and antidiuretic hormones are released, resulting in sodium and water retention. The clinical signs and symptoms of upper GI hemorrhage are directly related to the effects of the decrease in CO and the vasoconstriction response typically seen in hypovolemic shock.

Clinical Presentation

History

Individuals may have a history of peptic ulcer disease, tobacco abuse, alcohol abuse, liver disease, severe physiologic stress, NSAID use, anticoagulation or antiplatelet therapy, and/or are older or elderly.

Signs and Symptoms

The response of an individual to blood loss will depend on the rate and amount of blood loss, patient's age, overall health

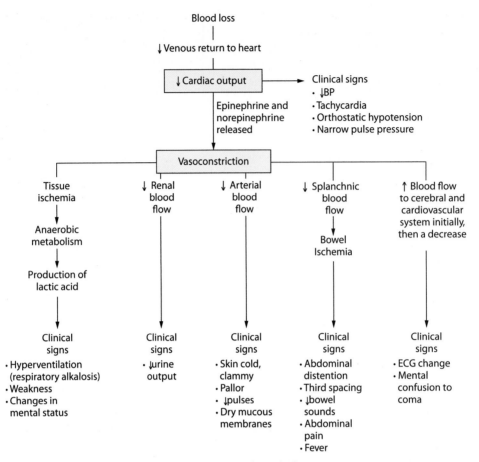

Figure 14-3. Hypovolemic shock.

status, and the timing of the initial resuscitation. Specific signs and symptoms include:

- *Hematemesis:* Bright red blood or coffee ground emesis
- Melena or maroon-colored stools
- Hematochezia
- Nausea
- Epigastric pain
- Abdominal distention
- Bowel sounds increased or decreased
- If blood loss is greater than 25% of blood volume, hypotension (orthostatic), altered hemodynamic values (decreased central venous pressure [CVP], pulmonary capillary wedge pressure [PCWP], mean arterial pressure [MAP], CO)
- Rapid, deep respirations
- Tachycardia
- Fever
- Cold, clammy skin
- Dry mucous membranes
- Decreased pulses
- Weakness
- Decreased urine output
- Anxiety
- Mental status changes
- Restlessness
- Electrocardiographic (ECG) changes consistent with ischemia (eg, ST-segment elevation, arrhythmias)

Diagnostic Tests

- Hematocrit may be normal initially, then decreased with fluid resuscitation and blood loss. It is important to note that the hematocrit may not accurately reflect the actual volume of blood loss due to hemodilution and movement of extravascular fluid. The hematocrit decreases as extravascular fluid enters the vascular space in an attempt to restore volume. This process continues for 24 to 72 hours.
- Hemoglobin may also be normal initially, then decreased with fluid resuscitation and blood loss.
- White blood cell count is elevated.
- Platelet count may be decreased depending on amount of blood loss.
- Serum sodium is usually elevated initially due to hemoconcentration.
- Serum potassium is usually decreased with vomiting.
- Serum blood urea nitrogen (BUN) is mildly elevated.
- Serum creatinine is elevated.
- Serum lactate is elevated with severe bleeding.

- Prothrombin time (PT) is usually decreased.
- Activated thromboplastin time (aPTT) is usually decreased.
- Arterial blood gases show respiratory alkalosis (early), then later metabolic acidosis with severe shock and hypoxemia.
- Gastric aspirate shows normal or acidotic pH and is guaiac positive.

Principles of Management for Upper GI Bleeding

The fundamental goal of initial treatment is volume resuscitation. The management of the patient with acute upper GI bleeding focuses on hemodynamic stabilization, identification of the bleeding site, and initiation of definitive medical or surgical therapies to control or stop the bleeding. Measures to decrease anxiety in this patient population are also indicated owing to the severity and sudden onset of GI bleeding.

Hemodynamic Stabilization

The initial assessment of the patient with GI bleeding begins with assessment of vital signs, the most reliable reflection of the amount of blood lost. In the presence of hemodynamic instability, resuscitation begins. Risk criteria for patients with acute GI bleed include ongoing bleeding, hemoglobin less than 8 g/dL, transfusion requirement, systolic blood pressure less than 100 mm Hg on presentation, elevated prothrombin time, and alteration in mental status.

1. Monitor and record cardiovascular status (blood pressure, heart rate including orthostatic changes), hemodynamics (CVP, PCWP, CO, MAP), and peripheral pulses.
2. Insert at least two large-bore intravenous (IV) catheters and begin fluid resuscitation with crystalloid solution (eg, normal saline or lactated ringer solution). Administer fluids to maintain MAP at 60 mm Hg or higher.
3. Obtain blood for measurement of hematocrit, hemoglobin, and clotting studies, as well as for a type and cross-match for packed red blood cells (PRBC). Usually 6 units (U) at a minimum are ordered. The initial hematocrit is rarely useful for estimating transfusion requirements. Estimates for the amount of blood loss are most reliably guided by vital sign values (Table 14-3).
4. Administer prescribed IV colloids, crystalloids, or blood products until the patient is stabilized. After the administration of 2 to 3 liters of crystalloid fluids, blood products may be considered during the initial resuscitation if the hemodynamic response is poor. PRBC are used to rapidly increase the hematocrit while providing less volume compared to when whole blood is used. Each unit of PRBC increases the hematocrit by 2% to 3% and improves gas exchange. It may take up to 24 hours after blood is administered for changes to be reflected in the

TABLE 14-3. ESTIMATING BLOOD LOSS FROM ACUTE GI BLEEDING

Clinical Signs	Estimated Blood Loss
Systolic BP > 90 mm Hg Orthostatic hypotension Heart rate < 110 beats/min	20%-25% total blood volume (approximately 1000 mL)
Systolic BP 70-90 mm Hg Heart rate 110-130 beats/min	25%-40% total blood volume (approximately 1500-2000 mL)

Signs of moderately decreased tissue
  perfusion:
   Anxiety
   Cool, clammy skin
   Decreased urine output
   Hyperventilation
   Diminished pulses	

Systolic blood pressure < 70 mm Hg
Mean arterial pressure < 60 mm Hg
Signs of severely decreased tissue
  perfusion:
   Impaired mental status
   Cold, clammy, diaphoretic skin
   Thready pulses
   Decreased urine output
   Metabolic acidosis
   ECG changes
   Heart failure
   Respiratory failure
	> 40% total blood volume

hematocrit values, especially if large amounts of crystalloid solutions were administered during the resuscitation period. In addition to blood, platelets and clotting factors may also be given.
5. Monitor coagulation studies (eg, PT/PTT, platelet count).
6. Monitor fluid balance and renal function (intake and output, daily weight, BUN, creatinine, and hourly urine output).
7. Insert a nasogastric tube if bleeding is massive (> 40% of blood volume) to assess for the rate of bleeding. Placement of a gastric tube in the presence of varices is somewhat controversial and practices vary between institutions. Use of gastric lavage is also controversial. Proponents believe that removing blood clots by gastric lavage is useful in that it allows the stomach to contract and tamponade bleeding vessels. Removal of blood may give some indication of the rate of bleeding and may minimize the chance of pulmonary aspiration. If lavage is ordered, room temperature saline usually is used.
8. Position the patient in the left lateral decubitus position to minimize aspiration associated with hematemesis.
9. Monitor temperature and maintain normothermia. Rapid fluid resuscitation, particularly with blood products, can lead to hypothermia, with interference of normal coagulation. Warming of fluids may be required to prevent hypothermia if traditional measures are insufficient.

10. Prepare for urgent endoscopic therapy if estimated blood loss is greater than 3 U of blood, bright red blood is found in emesis or nasogastric aspirate, or if a variceal bleed is suspected. Usually all other patients will complete endoscopy within 24 hours of admission.

11. Administer supplemental oxygen. Monitor respiratory function. Airway protection with endotracheal intubation to prevent aspiration is indicated in patients with ongoing hematemesis or altered mental status.

Identify the Bleeding Site

Although the history and physical examination are used to differentiate between upper and lower GI bleeding, endoscopic examination is required to determine the exact site of bleeding and will direct future therapy. Endoscopic visualization at the bedside is preferred to allow for early direct visualization of the upper tract during resuscitation measures.

1. The presence of blood in the upper GI tract can make it difficult to identify the bleeding source and deliver treatment. Prokinetic agents facilitate gastric emptying of retained blood and may be administered prior to endoscopy. A recent meta-analysis has shown that when either erythromycin or metoclopramide is given pre-endoscopy, the need for a repeat procedure to identify the bleeding source is reduced.

2. Administer sedation (eg, midazolam [Versed]) as ordered and institute monitoring protocol.

3. Position patient in a left lateral decubitus position to prevent aspiration of GI contents during endoscopy. Have oral-tracheal suction available at the bedside before the procedure begins.

4. Monitor for cardiac ischemia during the examination (eg, ST-segment changes [see Chapter 18, Advanced ECG Concepts], arrhythmias).

Institute Therapies to Control or Stop Bleeding

Definitive therapies to treat the bleeding differ depending on the cause. A general approach for treatment is summarized in Figure 14-4. In nonvariceal upper GI bleeding, endoscopic treatment is widely accepted as the most effective method to control acute ulcer bleeding and has become the standard for prevention of ulcer rebleeding. Although individual studies have been too small to show significant advantage for endoscopic therapy in reducing mortality, a meta-analysis indicates endoscopic therapy prevents not only rebleeding but also death. Administration of PPIs prior to endoscopy is now routine for patients in whom an ulcer is suspected. The PPIs

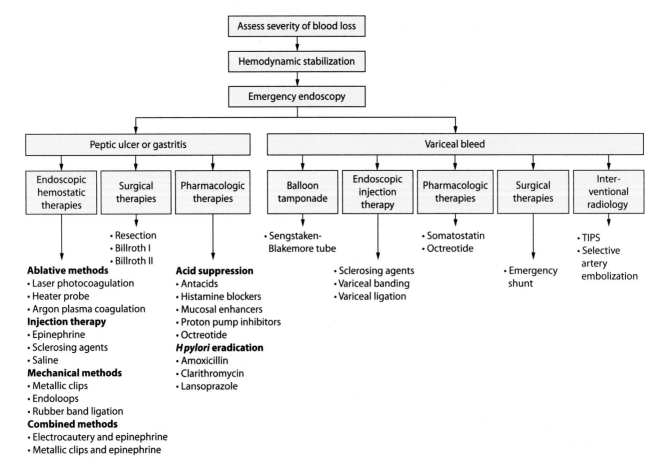

Figure 14-4. Upper GI bleeding treatment guide.

quickly neutralize acid, which results in stabilization of the blood clot. An acidic environment will inhibit platelet aggregation and lyse an already formed clot. Several therapeutic interventions are available for the endoscopist and include ablative or coagulation therapy (laser, monopolar, bipolar, or multipolar electrocoagulation, and heater probe), pharmacologic therapy also known as *sclerotherapy,* and mechanical and combination therapies. Pharmacologic treatments are easy to use, inexpensive, and available in most settings. The goal of this treatment is to control bleeding by tamponade, vasoconstriction, and/or an inflammatory reaction after the injection of a variety of agents. Saline alone will compress the vessels. Sclerosants such as alcohol, ethanolamine, and polidocanol cause greater vascular thrombosis, but can result in tissue injury and necrosis and are used less frequently. Epinephrine (1:10,000-1:20,000) provides local tamponade, vasoconstriction, and improved platelet aggregation to promote hemostasis. It is the agent of choice in the United States. Its effects will only last for 20 minutes and therefore requires it be used with an additional more durable treatment.

Electrocautery and argon plasma coagulation are examples of ablative treatments and are equally effective. Bleeding vessels can also be mechanically compressed using metallic clips, endoloops, or rubber band ligation. Metallic clips are the mechanical treatment of choice and have been shown to be as effective as other endoscopic techniques. Combination therapy with epinephrine injection has become the standard treatment for actively bleeding ulcers. Adding a second endoscopic treatment, either an ablative therapy or endoclips, significantly reduces the rate of recurrence, need for surgery, and mortality. It is no longer recommended to use epinephrine alone. If the patient rebleeds, a second attempt with endoscopic control is advocated before surgical intervention. Rebleeding is more common in patients with variceal bleeds and is highest initially after admission and for the first 24 hours.

Endoscopy rarely causes serious complications. Risks include GI perforation, precipitation of bleeding, aspiration, respiratory or cardiac compromise, and missed lesions.

Treatment of a Mallory-Weiss tear is supportive therapy. Bleeding episodes are self-limited and the mucosa will heal within 72 hours in 90% of patients.

Today significant bleeding from stress gastritis is rarely encountered. This is due to improvements in the management of shock and sepsis, as well as the prophylactic use of acid-suppressive therapy.

Pharmacologic treatment to reduce portal hypertension may be considered as preparations are underway for emergent upper endoscopy in the patient admitted with variceal upper GI bleeding. In the past, vasopressin was used in combination with nitroglycerin. Somatostatin or its analogue octreotide are now the vasoactive agents of choice. They can induce splanchnic vasoconstriction without the cardiac side effects of vasopressin. Continuous intravenous infusion of these agents results in temporary control of bleeding so that resuscitation, diagnostic, and therapeutic measures can

TABLE 14-4. PHARMACOLOGIC THERAPIES FOR ULCER DISEASE/GASTRITIS

Agent	Action
Antacids	Acid neutralizers

Histamine blockers
  Cimetidine
  Ranitidine
  Famotidine
  Nizatidine
	Block production of gastric acid (pepsin, HCl) by inhibiting the action of histamine

Cytoprotective agent Sucralfate	Forms protective barrier over ulcer site

Proton pump inhibitors
  Omeprazole (Prilosec)
  Lansoprazole (Prevacid)
  Rabeprazole (Aciphex)
  Pantoprazole (Protonix)-IV
	Suppress secretion of gastric acid

Mucosal barrier enhancers
  Colloidal bismuth
  Prostaglandins
	Protect mucosa from injurious substances

be completed. Pharmacologic treatments are summarized in Table 14-4. At the time of endoscopy, both sclerotherapy and variceal banding or ligation have been shown to control bleeding. Currently, balloon tamponade (Sengstaken-Blakemore tube) is reserved for patients with massive hemorrhage. Once bleeding is controlled, more definitive therapies can be used. Treatment of esophagogastric varices will also include antibiotic prophylaxis for spontaneous bacterial peritonitis. A third-generation cephalosporin is indicated as bacteremia is often present in patients on admission for variceal bleeding.

1. Monitor for complications of endoscopic therapy and/or the sclerosing agents used to treat the ulcer or varix. Complications may include fever and pain because of esophageal spasm, motility disturbances of the esophageal sphincter, and perforation. Systemic complications of endoscopic therapy and/or sclerosing agents also may occur and predominantly affect the cardiovascular and respiratory systems. Cardiovascular effects include heart failure, heart block, mediastinitis and pericarditis. Respiratory effects include aspiration pneumonia, atelectasis, pneumothorax, embolism, and acute respiratory distress syndrome.

2. Institute pharmacologic therapies as prescribed to treat peptic ulcer disease or gastritis (stress ulcers). The most common pharmacologic agents and their actions are reviewed in Table 14-4. PPIs are the drug of choice in patients who have had nonvariceal bleeding. They provide a more durable and sustained acid suppression than histamine receptor antagonists. The use of PPIs has been shown in randomized clinical trials to lead to a decrease in recurrent bleeding due to ulcer disease, need for transfusions, surgery, and the length of hospital stay. The use of high dose IV PPIs for 3 days after successful endoscopic treatment has been recommended

TABLE 14-5. PHARMACOLOGIC THERAPIES FOR VARICEAL UPPER GI BLEEDING

Drug	Action	Administration
Somatostatin	Inhibits splanchnic blood flow	Administered by continuous IV infusion at 250 mcg/h
Octreotide	Vasodilates splanchnic vessels to decrease blood flow	IV infusion at 25 mcg/h
Nonselective beta-adrenergic blockers: propranolol, nadolol	Decreases cardiac output and reduces splanic flow (decreases portal hypertension)	Administered orally to reduce resting pulse by 20% or to 55-60 beats/min

(80 mg esomeprazole bolus, 8 mg/h continuous infusion). Oral PPIs are recommended for 6-8 weeks after an upper GI bleeding episode to allow for healing of the mucosa. Their use is especially beneficial in patients who use chronic NSAIDs or who have had *Helicobacter pylori* infection.

3. Administer pharmacologic therapies as prescribed to treat variceal bleeding (Table 14-5). Pharmacologic agents exert their effect by constricting splanchnic blood flow and thereby reducing portal pressure.

4. Intra-aortic balloon pump therapy may be instituted to achieve temporary vascular control in patients in shock. This therapy optimizes blood pressure, increases aortic diastolic pressure, increases coronary flow, and allows time for rapid resuscitation.

5. A tamponade tube, most commonly the Sengstaken-Blakemore tube (Figure 14-5), may be used to emer-

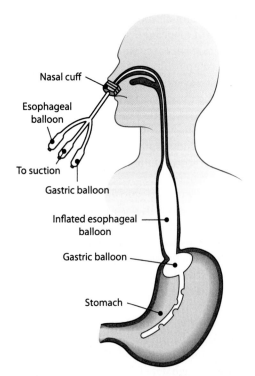

Figure 14-5. Placement of a Sengstaken-Blakemore tube.

gently decrease blood flow through the varix and to control bleeding so that endoscopy can be performed. Rebleeding is common after deflation or removal. Monitor for complications of this tube, including pulmonary aspiration, rupture of the esophagus, asphyxia, and erosion of the esophageal or gastric wall.

Maintain esophageal suction to prevent aspiration. Keep scissors at the bedside to cut and remove the tube if it becomes malpositioned and the tamponade balloon occludes the airway. Endotracheal intubation is usually recommended to prevent pulmonary complications. Release pressure of the esophageal and or gastric balloons at regular intervals to prevent erosions. Administer frequent mouth care and monitor the skin around the tube to prevent necrosis from pressure of the tube.

Interventional Radiologic Technique to Control Bleeding

When variceal bleeding is severe and cannot be controlled endoscopically, emergent portal decompression is achieved with the percutaneous transjugular intrahepatic portosystemic shunt (TIPS).

In the TIPS procedure, a long needle is passed from the right transjugular vein to the hepatic vein into a branch of the portal vein and a stent is placed. This decreases the pressure in the portal vein (decreases portal pressure) and subsequently on the varices to prevent rupture and bleeding.

The advantage of the TIPS procedure is that it can be performed in the interventional radiology department. Complications of the TIPS procedures include puncture of the biliary system, bleeding, infection, and clotting of the stent. Postprocedural systemic failure (septic shock, renal failure) and hepatic encephalopathy (see next section) are also associated complications.

1. Monitor blood pressure, ECG, and pulse oximetry throughout the procedure.
2. Administer preprocedure antibiotic coverage for gram-negative organisms as prophylaxis for sepsis.
3. Provide moderate IV sedation to treat anxiety.
4. Provide pain medication (eg, fentanyl). Certain parts of the procedure, such as balloon dilation of the intrahepatic tract, can be painful.
5. Have lidocaine and atropine available to manage potential complications of the procedure. The vasopressin infusion can cause bradyarrhythmias. Due to the proximity of the hepatic vein to the right ventricle of the heart, ventricular ectopy can be induced during the procedure.
6. Have crystalloids, vasopressors, PRBCs, and fresh frozen plasma readily available to manage hypotension from sepsis, bleeding, or sedation.
7. Have continuous and intermittent suction ready to manage bleeding and airway patency.

Surgical Therapies to Stop Bleeding

Surgery is considered for patients who have massive bleeding that is immediately life threatening and for patients who

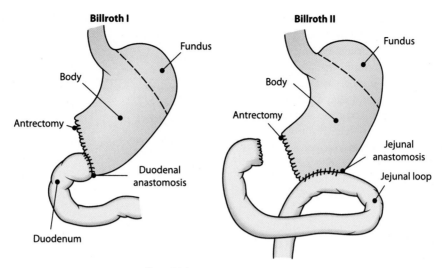

Figure 14-6. Billroth I and II procedures.

continue to bleed despite aggressive medical therapies. Surgical therapies for peptic ulcer disease or stress ulcers include gastric resections such as antrectomy, gastrectomy, vagotomy, or combination procedures. An antrectomy or gastrectomy may be performed to decrease the acidity of the duodenum or stomach by removing gastric-acid secreting cells. A vagotomy decreases acid secretion in the stomach by dividing the vagus nerve along the esophagus. Combination procedures are common and one example is the Billroth I, which is a vagotomy and antrectomy with anastomosis of the stomach to the duodenum. A Billroth II consists of a vagotomy, resection of the antrum, and anastomosis of the stomach to the jejunum (Figure 14-6). The latter is preferred over the Billroth I because it does not present the risk for dumping syndrome. Gastric perforations can be treated by simple closure.

Surgical decompression of portal hypertension can be accomplished by a procedure called a portacaval shunt. This procedure connects the portal vein to the inferior vena cava, diverting blood from the liver into the vena cava to decrease portal pressure. With the newer interventional radiology techniques this surgery is seldom performed. Liver transplantation can also relieve portal hypertension, but must be considered by weighing the risks vs the benefits in this patient population.

1. Monitor for fluid and electrolyte imbalances postoperatively due to intraoperative fluid loss and the drains inserted to decompress the stomach or to drain the surgical site.
2. Provide for adequate nutrition to promote wound healing.
3. Monitor the appearance of the incision and surrounding tissue.
4. Document and report all wound drainage (color, amount, odor) and complaints of pain or tenderness.
5. Culture any suspicious drainage.
6. Monitor white blood cell count and temperature trends.

Interventional Radiologic Technique to Control Bleeding

When variceal bleeding is severe and cannot be controlled endoscopically, emergent portal decompression is achieved with the percutaneous TIPS.

Reducing Anxiety

1. Encourage communication with a calm, interested, and centered approach; for example, "Mr. B, you look nervous (worried) to me. Can you tell me what is bothering you?"
2. Assess the patient's previous coping skills that were used in similar difficult situations (eg, did family presence, watching TV, listening to music, or using relaxation techniques alleviate anxiety?).
3. Offer appropriate reassurance, facts, and information as requested by the patient. Explain the ICU routine and procedures to the patient. Present information in terms that the patient can understand. Repeat and rephrase the information as necessary. Allow the patient to ask questions.
4. Help the patient to establish a sense of control. Assist the patient to make distinctions among those things he or she can (and should) control (eg, bath time, working on reducing anxiety level) and those things that cannot be controlled (eg, need for vasopressors and monitoring equipment).
5. Guide the patient in discovering that he or she has some control over anxiety and fear. Encourage the patient to participate in breathing and relaxation exercises as a strategy to control the current situation.

Liver Failure

Pathogenesis

The liver has a central role in the body's metabolism. Metabolic functions include the synthesis of carbohydrates, fats, proteins, and vitamins for nutrition, energy, and key metabolic pathways. Additional processes performed by the liver include the formation of bile, bilirubin metabolism, synthesis of coagulation factors, and detoxification of drugs and toxins. Liver failure may be acute or chronic. Irrespective of the cause of liver injury, inflammation results in damage to hepatocytes, known as "hepatitis." Injured areas are surrounded by scar tissues leading to fibrosis, and after a period of time progressive fibrosis results in cirrhosis or replacement of the normal hepatic tissue with fibrotic tissue. Chronic liver failure is a slow deterioration that evolves over years leading to cirrhosis. Liver dysfunction potentially can be reversed early as the liver has a regenerative capability; however, fibrotic changes are irreversible resulting in chronic dysfunction and eventual end-stage liver disease.

Acute failure, also known as fulminant hepatic failure, results in a rapid deterioration of liver function in a person without prior liver disease. This cellular insult results in massive cell necrosis leading to a multiorgan dysfunction. Acute liver failure is rare and defined by a coagulation abnormality (usually an INR > 1.5) and encephalopathy without previous liver disease. The time between presentation of either encephalopathy or coagulopathy is usually defined as within 26 weeks.

Etiology and Risk Factors

The leading causes of acute liver failure in the United States and Europe are acetaminophen overdose and idiosyncratic drug reactions, while other causes include viral hepatitis, autoimmune disease, and shock (Table 14-6). Survival in acute liver failure can be categorized into patients in whom intensive care enables recovery of hepatic function and patients who require liver transplantation. Common causes of chronic liver disease include nonalcoholic fatty liver disease, nonalcoholic steatohepatitis, alcoholic liver disease, chronic hepatitis B and C, and hemochromatosis.

TABLE 14-6. COMMON CAUSES OF LIVER FAILURE

Inflammatory Liver Disease
Viruses
Hepatitis A, B, C, D, and E
Herpes simplex
Epstein-Barr
Cytomegalovirus
Adenovirus
Parasites
Liver tumors
Toxic ingestion of drugs
Acetaminophen
Halothane
Methyldopa
Toxic ingestion of chemicals and poisons
Chlorinated hydrocarbons
Phosphorus
Cirrhosis of the Liver
Nonalcoholic fatty liver disease
Alcohol ingestion
Biliary disease
Cardiac disease
Hepatitis

TABLE 14-7. CHILD-PUGH CRITERIA FOR HEPATIC FUNCTIONAL RESERVE

Clinical and Laboratory Measurement	Patient Score for Increasing Abnormality		
	1	2	3
Encephalopathy (grade)	None	1 or 2	3 or 4
Ascites	None	Mild	Moderate
Bilirubin (mg/dL)	–1-2	2.1-3	≥ 3.1
Albumin (g/dL)	≥3.5	2.8-3.4	≤ 2.7
Prothrombin time (increase, in seconds)	1-4	4.1-6	≥ 6.1

Grade A, 5-6; grade B, 7-9; grade C, 10-15

Nonalcoholic fatty liver disease is one of the most common causes of chronic liver disease in the Western world. It is associated with obesity, type 2 diabetes, and metabolic syndrome. The spectrum of liver disease associated with this syndrome can range from simple steatosis to advanced fibrosis and cirrhosis. Alcoholic liver injury results from the toxic effects of ethanol on the hepatocytes.

The Child-Pugh classification has served as a longstanding assessment tool to score hepatic function. This classification is based on two clinical variables and three biochemical tests (Table 14-7). Classes A to C are used to define patients from well-compensated disease (Class A) to advanced decompensated disease (Class C).

Clinical manifestations are directly related to failure of the liver to perform important metabolic processes (Table 14-8). Complications of liver failure include ascites, hepatic encephalopathy, acute respiratory distress syndrome, electrolyte imbalance, hepatorenal syndrome, and spontaneous bacterial peritonitis.

Jaundice

Jaundice is secondary to excessive deposition of bilirubin in tissues including skin, mucous membranes, and sclera, resulting in the characteristic yellow discoloration. This deposition of bilirubin represents failure of the liver to adequately uptake, conjugate, and excrete bilirubin. Pruritus is a common associated symptom that can cause much discomfort to patients.

Ascites

Ascites is the abnormal collection of fluid in the peritoneal cavity. Cirrhosis is the most common cause of ascites and is theorized to be a result of portal hypertension. Increased pressure in the portal system occurs secondary to fibrosis in the liver, causing an obstruction to venous flow. This results in increased nitric oxide, vasodilatation, and renal function compromise, resulting in sodium and water retention. Fluid shifts from the intravascular space into the peritoneal space.

Hepatic Encephalopathy

Hepatic encephalopathy defines a spectrum of neuropsychiatric abnormalities that occur with liver failure. Most theories

TABLE 14-8. SEQUELAE OF LIVER FAILURE

Sequelae	Outcome	Clinical Manifestations
Impaired splanchnic hemodynamics	Portal hypertension	Varices, acute upper GI bleeding
	Hyperdynamic circulation	Increased CO, decreased SVR, decreased perfusion
Reduced liver metabolic processes	Altered fat, protein, and carbohydrate metabolism	Malnutrition, impaired healing
	Decreased phagocytic function of Kupffer cells	Infection
	Decreased synthesis of blood clotting components	Bleeding
	Decreased removal of activated clotting factors	Emboli
	Decreased metabolism of vitamins and iron	Impaired skin integrity
	Impaired detoxification	Increased ammonia, mental status changes, increased drug levels
Impaired bile formation and flow	Impaired bilirubin metabolism	Jaundice

support the pathogenesis that decreased hepatic clearance of certain cerebral toxins results in psychiatric manifestations. Serum ammonia is most often implicated. Ammonia is produced by bacteria in the bowel and in the liver it is converted to urea for excretion. In liver failure, this function of the liver is impaired, allowing ammonia to directly enter the central nervous system. Because ammonia is neurotoxic, as serum ammonia levels rise, the patient often exhibits signs of impaired cerebral functioning or encephalopathy. These signs can range from minor sensory-perceptual changes such as muscle tremors, slurred speech, or slight mental status changes to marked confusion or profound coma.

Classifications of deterioration in brain function have been used, from grade I (mild or episodic drowsiness, impaired concentration/intellect, but arousable and coherent); grade II (increased drowsiness, confusion, and disorientation, but able to arouse); grade III (very drowsy, agitated, disoriented, but able to respond to simple verbal commands); to grade IV (unresponsive except to painful stimuli). Cerebral edema can occur in up to 80% of patients with grade IV encephalopathy. The cause of cerebral edema is poorly understood but recognized as a leading cause of death. Patients with hepatic encephalopathy need to be carefully assessed for other causes of encephalopathy such as sepsis, uremia, acidosis, alcohol withdrawal, hypoxia, and intracerebral bleed.

Acute Respiratory Distress Syndrome

The major pulmonary complication in liver failure is arterial hypoxemia. The cause has been linked to vascular dilatation in the lung and acute respiratory distress syndrome. Pulmonary edema is also a common finding.

Electrolyte Imbalance

A variety of electrolyte imbalances occur in liver failure. Hypoglycemia develops due to massive hepatic cell necrosis, leading to loss of glycogen stores and diminished glucose release. Hypokalemia may occur from inadequate oral intake, increased potassium losses from vomiting, or from medical interventions (eg, nasogastric suction or diuretic therapy). Hypomagnesemia commonly occurs in conjunction with hypokalemia as there is a close relationship between the movement of these electrolytes. Hypocalcemia is a complication of blood transfusions because the citrate used to anticoagulate stored blood causes calcium depletion. Hypophosphatemia is also commonly associated with acute liver failure. The exact mechanisms remain unknown. Alkalosis and acidosis may both occur.

Hepatorenal Syndrome

Hepatorenal syndrome is a unique form of renal failure associated with severe liver disease. This syndrome represents the most frequent fatal complication of liver failure. The pathogenesis is thought to be related to portal hypertension and eventual sustained renal vasoconstriction, resulting in decreased renal perfusion.

Esophageal and Gastric Varices

Esophageal and gastric varices result from portal hypertension and develop in most patients with advanced cirrhosis. Mortality is significant and prevention with measures including beta-blockers and endoscopic band ligation is employed (see previous section addressing GI bleeding). Similar prominent veins in the abdominal wall and around the umbilicus (caput medusa) may develop.

Spontaneous Bacterial Peritonitis

Spontaneous bacterial peritonitis is defined as an infected ascitic fluid collection without an evident intra-abdominal source. This represents the most common bacterial infection seen and occurs approximately in a quarter of patients admitted with chronic liver failure and ascites. A single microbial organism is usually responsible, such as E coli, and is theorized to be caused by intestinal translocation of organisms that are able to seed the ascitic fluid.

Malnutrition

The liver has a multitude of functions including metabolism of carbohydrates, fats, and proteins. The liver also stores essential minerals such as iron, copper, and vitamins A, B$_{12}$, D, and K.

Malnutrition occurs frequently in patients with hepatic failure due to decreased oral intake and alterations in the metabolism and storage of nutrients. In advanced hepatic

ESSENTIAL CONTENT CASE

Liver Failure

A 54-year-old man is admitted with a 3-day history of shortness of breath, increased confusion, vomiting, and weakness. He was hospitalized in the past year with upper GI bleeding from esophageal and gastric varices. He was diagnosed at that time as having Laînnec cirrhosis, liver failure due to alcohol abuse. Significant findings on his admission profile were:

History
Complaints of decreased appetite for the past 2 months; also complaints of nausea and weakness.

Vital Signs
Blood pressure   98/50 mm Hg lying; 90/54 mm Hg sitting
Heart rate   Sinus tachycardia with frequent PVCs
Respiratory rate 28 breaths min; shallow
Temperature   100° F, orally

Cardiopulmonary
- Rales and coarse rhonchi throughout all lung fields
- Dyspneic; using accessory muscles
- S_3/S_4; no murmurs
- Extremities cool, weak pulses
- 3+ edema lower extremities

Neurologic
- Alert, but disoriented to time and place
- Irritable

Abdomen
- Marked ascites, dull to percussion
- Hyperactive BSs in all four quadrants

Genitourinary
- Urine dark, amber, and cloudy
- Large hemorrhoid protruding from rectal vault
- Liquid stool; black; guaiac positive

Laboratory data
Arterial blood gases on 2 L O_2 per nasal cannula

Ph	7.49
Paco$_2$	30 mm Hg
Pao$_2$	54 mm Hg
Sao$_2$	87%
HCO$_3^-$	28
Hematocrit	30%
AST	80 IU/L
ALT	84 IU/L
Bilirubin	Total 10 mg/dL
PT	18 seconds
aPTT	> 45 seconds
Fibrinogen	158 mg/dL
Albumin	3.0
Potassium	3.2 mEq/L
Sodium	130 mEq/L
Creatinine	2.8 mg/dL
BUN	40 mg/dL
Glucose	80 mg/dL
Urine electrolytes	
Sodium	5 mEq/L/day
Potassium	10 mEq/L/day

Case Question 1. Based on your initial assessment of this patient which complication/s of liver failure would you be most concerned about?

(A) Hepatorenal syndrome
(B) GI bleeding
(C) Hepatic encephalopathy
(D) Fluid and electrolyte abnormalities
(E) All of the above.

Case Question 2. Which factor/s contribute/s to malnutrition in the patient with renal failure?

(A) Decreased oral intake
(B) Altered metabolism and storage of nutrients
(C) Altered mental status
(D) All of the above

Answers
1. The correct answer is E. The most common complications of liver failure are hepatorenal syndrome, GI bleeding, hepatic encephalopathy, and fluid and electrolyte abnormalities. It is important to assess for changes in mental status which could be indicative of hepatic encephalopathy. The patient has a low BP, is tachycardic, and has a low hematocrit—all of which could be signs of GI bleeding. He certainly has fluid and electrolyte abnormalities. All of these complications put the patient at risk for hepatorenal syndrome.
2. The correct answer is D. The liver metabolizes carbohydrates, fats, and proteins and also plays a key role in the storage of essential minerals, vitamins, and glycogen. When the liver is not able to synthesize and store glycogen, rapid muscle loss will occur. Altered mental status may lead to a decrease in oral intake which will further compromise nutritional status.

failure, the impaired ability to synthesize and store glycogen results in rapid muscle loss even during brief periods of decreased nutrient intake. Patients frequently require vitamin K to normalize PT and PTT, and those with recent ethanol intake should receive intravenous thiamine.

Clinical Presentation
History
- Exposure to contaminated food, water
- Exposure to blood, body fluids
- Alcohol abuse

Signs and Symptoms

Impaired Thought Processes
- Mental status changes (confusion, lethargy)
- Behavioral changes
- Delirium
- Seizures
- Coma

Impaired Gas Exchange
- Hypoxemia
- Pulmonary edema

Fluid Volume Deficit or Excess

- Hypotension
- Skin cool, pale, and dry
- Urine output < 30 mL/h
- Tachycardia
- Dry mucous membranes

Hyperdynamic Circulation

- Arrhythmias
- Fever
- Palmar erythema (flushed palms)
- Jugular vein distension
- Rales
- Murmur
- Increased CO
- Decreased systemic vascular resistance

Altered Nutrition

- Decreased appetite
- Muscle wasting
- Nausea and vomiting

Impaired Liver Metabolism

- Jaundice
- Dry skin
- Ascites

Diagnostic Tests

- Total bilirubin > 1 mg/dL
- AST >36 IU/L
- ALT >24 IU/L
- PT >13 seconds
- aPTT > 45 seconds
- Fibrinogen < 200 mg/dL
- Albumin < 3.2 g/dL
- Ammonia > 45 mg/dL
- Ultrasound, endoscopy, endoscopic retrograde cholangiopancreatography (ERCP), liver angiography/biopsy

Principles of Management for Liver Failure

The management of the patient with liver failure is centered on decreasing the metabolic requirements of the liver, supporting cardiopulmonary status, supporting hematologic and nutritional functions of the liver, and preventing and treating complications.

Decrease Metabolic Requirements of the Liver

1. Place the patient on bed-rest to decrease the metabolic needs of the liver. Position the head of the bed at 45° at all times to minimize complications related to ascites. Institute measures to prevent skin breakdown.
2. Monitor drugs that are metabolized or detoxified by the liver, especially narcotics and sedatives.

Support Cardiopulmonary Status

1. Monitor fluid balance. The patient may have a fluid volume deficit related to portal hypertension, ascites, GI bleeding, or coagulation abnormalities. Fluid overload may be a problem related to sodium excess and hypoalbuminemia.
2. Assist with paracentesis that may be instituted to reduce ascites. Fast removal of fluid via paracentesis requires IV colloid replacement to prevent dehydration. Administer diuretics such as furosemide and spironolactone as prescribed. Weigh patient daily. Monitor abdominal girth when ascites is present.
3. Monitor respiratory status and correlate with arterial blood gas results. Administer oxygen as ordered. Administer sedatives and analgesics cautiously. Assist the patient with maneuvers to improve oxygenation.

Support Hematologic, Nutritional, and Metabolic Functions of the Liver

1. Monitor for signs of bleeding (eg, gastric contents, stools, urine) and test for occult blood. Observe for petechiae and bruising. Monitor hematologic profile.
2. Administer blood and blood products as ordered.
3. Institute measures for variceal bleeding as needed, including beta blockers.
4. Institute measures to provide for safety and to minimize tissue trauma. Provide for frequent mouth care. Avoid use of rectal tubes.
5. Provide frequent small meals and a bedtime snack containing carbohydrate to prevent muscle wasting. Normal amounts of protein are tolerated in patients who have received appropriate medications for encephalopathy. Consider enteral nutrition (EN) if oral intake is insufficient.
6. Monitor for signs and symptoms of infection. Maintain sterility of invasive lines and tubes. Maintain aseptic technique when performing procedures.

Preventing and Treating Complications

The most common complications of liver failure are hepatic encephalopathy, fluid and electrolyte imbalances, hepatorenal syndrome, and variceal hemorrhage.

1. Observe for changes in mental status. Institute safety measures during periods of mental status changes. Rule out other causes of encephalopathy. Treat precipitating causes.
2. Administer cleansing enemas and cathartics to keep the bowel empty. Lactulose has been a first line treatment to decrease gut ammonia production. Recent research has demonstrated the efficacy of Rifaximin in maintaining remission from hepatic encephalopathy. Monitor patient response to therapy through neurologic assessments and serum ammonia levels. Monitor the use of medications metabolized by the liver.

3. Institute protocols for acute upper GI hemorrhage due to variceal rupture (see previous section).

4. The first and only definitive treatment for hepatorenal syndrome has been liver transplant. Some response has been demonstrated with the use of albumin as an intravascular expander in combination with a vasoconstrictor Terlipressin, another vasopressin analogue.

Artificial Liver Support Systems

Efforts to find ways to assist patients with acute liver failure until organ transplantation have led to research in devices that support the liver until an organ is available, or the liver's regenerative systems recover. All artificial liver support systems involve extracorporeal circulation of the patient's blood through filters that remove waste products normally filtered by the liver. Currently available liver support systems are not recommended outside of clinical trials.

Liver Transplantation

Liver transplantation has changed the survival of patients with liver failure. The decision to proceed with transplantation requires a detailed assessment and multidisciplinary review. The model for end-stage liver disease, or MELD, is a scoring system that uses serum creatinine, bilirubin, and INR to predict mortality in end-stage liver disease. In 2002, the MELD was adopted as the index to determine transplant priority.

Acute Pancreatitis

Acute pancreatitis is inflammation of the pancreas resulting from premature activation of pancreatic exocrine enzymes, such as trypsin, phospholipase A, and elastase within the pancreas. The disease ranges in severity from a mild self-limiting form to severe acute pancreatitis. Severe acute pancreatitis is seen in approximately one-fifth of patients with pancreatitis and has a mortality rate of 30%. In the severe acute form, autodigestion and necrosis of the pancreas can occur. This results in the release of inflammatory mediators, which can lead to multisystem failure (see Chapter 11, Multisystem Problems).

The diagnosis of acute pancreatitis is based on at least two of the three following criteria: characteristic abdominal pain or epigastric pain that may radiate to the back; serum amylase or lipase values greater than 3 times the normal range; and characteristic findings on imaging, most often CT imaging. In general, serum lipase is thought to be more sensitive than serum amylase as a marker of pancreatitis. Organ failure and pancreatic necrosis are the two most important markers of severity. To accurately identify the severity of acute pancreatitis, scoring systems have been used such as the acute physiology and chronic health evaluation (APACHE–II).

Recent scoring systems that offer an assessment of disease severity within the first 24 hours have demonstrated clinical usefulness. The bedside index of severity of acute pancreatitis (BISAP) is one example. This tool has demonstrated both accuracy as well as simplicity. The score is calculated on five variables:

1. Blood urea nitrogen greater than 25 mg/dl
2. Impaired mental status with a Glasgow Coma Score greater than 15
3. Presence of systemic inflammatory response syndrome
4. Age greater than 60 and
5. Pleural effusion on imaging

Each variable provides one point and scores of 3, 4, and 5 are associated with hospital mortality of 5.3%, 12.7%, and 22.5% respectively.

Etiologies, Risk Factors, and Pathophysiology

The leading causes of acute pancreatitis are alcohol disease and biliary tract disease (stones). Drug-induced causes have been linked to metronidazole, tetracycline, azathioprine, and estrogens. Other less common etiologies are hyperlipidemia, hypercalcemia, infectious, autoimmune, vascular, genetic, pancreatic neoplasms, and idiopathic.

The pathogenesis of acute pancreatitis is not completely clear. The pancreas normally has a protective mechanism, an enzyme called trypsin inhibitor, to prevent activating enzymes before they reach the duodenum, thereby preventing inflammation of pancreatic cells. Regardless of the etiology, the process of premature activation of pancreatic enzymes is characteristic of pancreatitis, leading to local inflammation and potential necrosis of the pancreas. The activated enzymes can also enter the systemic circulation via the portal vein and lymphatics. This is thought to stimulate platelet-activating factor and humoral systems (kinin, complement, fibrinolysis). This results in multisystem failure with a variety of complications (Table 14-9; see also Chapter 11, Multisystem Problems). Pancreatic abscess, pseudocyst, and necrosis are not uncommon with fulminant forms of the disease.

TABLE 14-9. COMMON MULTISYSTEM COMPLICATIONS OF ACUTE PANCREATITIS

Pulmonary
Atelectasis
Acute respiratory distress syndrome
Pleural effusions

Cardiovascular
Cardiogenic shock

Neurologic
Pancreatic encephalopathy

Metabolic
Metabolic acidosis
Hypocalcemia
Altered glucose metabolism

Hematologic
Disseminated intravascular coagulation
GI bleeding

Renal
Prerenal failure

Clinical Presentation

Signs and Symptoms

Pancreatic Inflammation

- *Acute pain:* Severe, relentless, knifelike; midepigastrium or periumbilical
- Abdominal guarding
- Nausea
- Rebound tenderness
- Vomiting
- Abdominal distention
- Hypoactive BSs

Fluid Volume Deficit

- Hypotension
- Tachycardia
- Mental status changes
- Cool, clammy skin
- Decreased urine output

Impaired Gas Exchange

- Decreasing Pao_2 (< 60 mm Hg) and Sao_2 (< 90%)

Diagnostic Tests

- Serum amylase > 100 IU/L
- Serum pancreatic isoamylase > 50%
- Serum lipase > 24 IU/dL
- Serum triglycerides > 150 mg/dL
- Urine amylase > 14 IU/h
- Serum calcium < 8.5 mg/dL
- Serum sodium < 135 mEq/L
- Serum potassium < 3.5 mEq/L
- Serum magnesium < 1.5 mg/dL
- Increased ALT (> 120 U/L), in gallstone pancreatitis
- C-reactive protein (> 120 mg/L)

Imaging Studies

- Computed tomography (CT)
- ERCP
- MRI

Principles of Management of Acute Pancreatitis

The management of the patient with acute pancreatitis centers on disrupting the cycle of enzyme release of the pancreas and treating complications that can occur with multisystem disease. Interventions within the first 24 hours have been identified as essential to positive outcomes including increased survival. These interventions include scoring severity with BISAP or an alternative scoring system and aggressive fluid resuscitation. Additional principles of management include preventing hypoxemia, resting the pancreas, pain management, and supporting other organ systems that may fail because of mediators released during the inflammatory process.

Fluid Resuscitation

Patients with acute pancreatitis experience significant hypovolemia as a result of third space losses, vomiting, and vascular permeability related to inflammatory mediators. Hypovolemia can compromise pancreatic circulation and has been linked to pancreatic necrosis. Aggressive fluid and electrolyte replacement is viewed as the key element in the initial management. In severe acute pancreatitis, blood vessels in and around the pancreas may also become disrupted, resulting in hemorrhage.

1. In adults, infusion of intravenous fluids is begun with rates between 250 and 300 mL/h. High-dose fresh frozen plasma is indicated to replace lost circulating proteins. Monitor outcomes of fluid replacement therapy, including blood pressure, heart rate, intake and output, preload indicators (CVP, PCWP), skin turgor, capillary refill, mucous membranes, and urine output (goal of at least 0.5 mL/kg/h).
2. Monitor for signs and symptoms of hemorrhage (low hematocrit and hemoglobin levels). Cullen sign is a bluish discoloration around the umbilical area, and Grey Turner sign is a bluish discoloration around the flanks, indicating blood in the peritoneum. Monitor for increasing abdominal girths.
3. Monitor electrolytes for imbalances related to prolonged vomiting or fluid sequestration. Calcium, sodium, magnesium, and potassium are most commonly affected. Monitor QT intervals on the electrocardiogram and implement seizure precautions with severe hypocalcemia. Hyperglycemia also may be present due to the stress response and impaired secretion of insulin by the islet cells in the inflamed pancreas. Administer an insulin infusion, then sliding scale insulin to obtain a normoglycemic state.

Pain Management

Acute pain is the only universal sign of acute pancreatitis. It is caused by peritoneal irritation from activated pancreatic exocrine enzymes, edema or distention of the pancreas, or interruption of the blood supply to the pancreas. Treatment of pain is a priority because it causes increased exocrine enzyme release by the pancreas, which may worsen the pathologic process.

1. Assess the degree of pain by having the patient use a pain-rating scale.
2. Administer pain analgesics. There is controversy about the use of opiate analgesics (eg, morphine) because they may cause spasm of the sphincter of Oddi, which may worsen the pain. Use a pain rating scale to assess patient outcomes regardless of what is prescribed. Consider scheduled doses or continuous infusion of pain medication for severe pain. Consider epidural analgesia for unrelieved acute pain.
3. Assess patient anxiety and administer sedatives with analgesics.
4. Assist the patient to a position which promotes comfort. The knee-to-chest position often decreases the intensity of the pain.

Preventing Pancreatic Stimulation

Preventing stimulation of pancreatic exocrine secretion is a priority to interrupt the cycle of pancreatic inflammation.

1. In the past, avoiding the use of the upper GI tract with oral or gastric feeding was recommended until the patient no longer reported abdominal pain and the serum amylase has returned to normal. That recommendation has been changed.
2. Enteral nutrition with jejunal feedings is often preferred to prevent pancreatic stimulation and enzyme secretion. New research suggests that gastric feedings may be feasible as well.
3. Administer pharmacologic agents as prescribed to block the secretion of pancreatic enzymes. These include anticholinergic agents, cimetidine, and somatostatin.

Treat Local Complications in the Pancreas

Local complications in the pancreas include peripancreatic fluid collections, pancreatic pseudocyst, and necrotic collections. In an effort to standardize the recognition and definition of these complications, scoring systems have emerged; one of the most recognized is the Atlanta Classification. Percutaneous or stent therapies to drain the fluids in and around the pancreas and/or surgical resection or debridement may be required, especially if the pancreas becomes infected. Biliary ERCP and laparoscopic cholecystectomy are indicated for gallstone pancreatitis.

Treat Multisystem Failure

Cardiopulmonary complications are the most common multisystem problems. As mentioned, they are thought to be due to pancreatic enzyme–induced mediators. Pancreatic ischemia is also known to promote the release of myocardial depressant factor. This causes decreased myocardial contractility and CO. Surgical therapies such as a pancreatic resection may be performed to prevent systemic complications of acute necrotizing pancreatitis by removing necrotic or infected tissue. In some cases, a pancreatectomy may be performed, but it is associated with considerable mortality.

1. Administer oxygen therapy to maintain arterial oxygen tension and oxygen saturation. Mechanical ventilation with adjunct therapies to promote maximal alveolar gas exchange is often used to manage acute respiratory failure (see Chapter 10, Respiratory System).
2. Administer low-dose dopamine to support myocardial contractility. Dobutamine may also be considered if sepsis is not a complication. Avoid alpha constrictors.
3. Institute measures to prevent infection. Monitor for signs and symptoms of sepsis and initiate appropriate treatment if indicated.
4. Manage coagulopathies (see Chapter 13, Hematologic and Immune Systems).
5. Treat acute tubular necrosis if a complicating factor (see Chapter 15, Renal System).

Intestinal Ischemia

Major disorders of the intestine include intestinal ischemia. Vascular occlusion of the mesenteric vessels is rare but catastrophic and will result in profound illness. Intestinal ischemia may present as intestinal angina, ischemic colitis, or intestinal infarction. Ischemic colitis is the most common ischemic injury. Ischemia may be acute or chronic. Acute forms are due to sudden and complete arterial occlusion by emboli, thrombosis of atherosclerotic stenosis, small vessel occlusion, or venous thrombosis. Gradual occlusion is better tolerated as there is time for collateral circulation to form. Sudden or acute ischemia is poorly tolerated because the bowel is not protected by collateral circulation. There is an extensive mesenteric collateral circulation which protects against ischemic insults. The colon is particularly susceptible to low-flow states; in particular, the splenic flexure, ileocecal junction, and rectosigmoid.

Etiology, Risk Factors, and Pathophysiology

Intestinal ischemia develops from a compromise in blood flow to the intestine, which is inadequate to meet metabolic demands. It is the result of both hypoperfusion and reperfusion injury. Both the small intestine and the large bowel can be affected. Ischemic colitis will affect segments of the colon with normal colon on either side of the affected area. The right colon is affected 25% of the time, transverse 10%, left 33%, distal colon 25%, and the entire colon 7%. Disease involving the right side of the colon is usually more severe with the patient at risk for having involvement of the small intestine. Three major arterial trunks—the celiac axis, superior mesenteric artery, and inferior mesenteric artery comprise the splanchnic (intestinal) circulation. Ischemic colitis is the most common form of intestinal ischemia. The colon is perfused by the superior mesenteric artery, the inferior mesenteric artery, and branches of the internal iliac arteries.

An acute occlusion is usually the result of a cardiogenic embolus with the superior mesenteric artery most frequently affected. The tissue injury that occurs will result in the release of cellular contents and the by-products of anaerobic metabolism into the general circulation. The ischemic bowel loses protein, electrolytes, and fluid into the lumen and wall of the bowel. The third-space extracellular fluid loss decreases the circulating blood volume. Full-thickness necrosis leads to bowel perforation and peritonitis.

The underlying causes of intestinal ischemia are diverse and include decreased CO, hypovolemia, arrhythmias, hypercoagulable states, mechanical obstruction, vascular disease, and trauma. Predisposing medications include cocaine, cardiac glycosides, and alpha-stimulating sympathomimetic amines (epinephrine, norepinephrine). The elderly patient with systemic atherosclerosis is particularly at risk. In a retrospective study, hyperthyroidism, stroke, and chronic obstructive pulmonary disease were statistically significant independent predictors of mortality.

Clinical Presentation

Signs and symptoms will vary depending on the severity of the ischemia and area and length of intestine affected. The most common signs on admission to the hospital are hematochezia, abdominal pain, and diarrhea.

History

- Obstruction
- Diabetes mellitus
- Dyslipidemia
- Smoking
- Heart failure
- Aortic or coronary artery bypass surgery
- Shock
- Atrial fibrillation
- Atherosclerosis
- Medications: digitalis, diurectics, NSAIDs, catecholamines, and neurolyptics
- Recurrent indistinct abdominal symptoms

Signs and Symptoms

- Anorexia
- Fever
- Tachycardia
- Leukocytosis
- Metabolic acidosis
- Elevated lactate
- Elevated LDH
- Peritoneal signs (abdominal guarding and rebound tenderness)
- Acute onset, colicky, left lower abdominal pain
- Urgent desire to defecate
- Diarrhea
- Cramping
- Abdominal distention
- Decreased BSs
- Hematochezia (bloody stools)
- Abdominal tenderness
- Ileus
- Nausea and vomiting
- Post-prandial pain
- Muscle rigidity
- Fluid volume deficit

Diagnostic Tests

Diagnosis is based on clinical findings and supported by radiographic corroboration and colonoscopic evaluation. The use of a barium enema to diagnose acute colonic ischemia is no longer implemented. A CT scan is useful in supporting clinical suspicion and for identifying potential complications. Colonoscopy is the diagnostic modality of choice. It should be performed on an unprepped colon within 48 hours of presentation.

Colonoscopy will identify mucosal abnormalities and biopsies can be obtained. Findings will depend on the stage and severity of the ischemia. The finding of hemorrhagic, dusky mucosa with patches of inflammation is typical.

Arteriography is indicated if acute mesenteric ischemia involving the small intestine is suspected. Arteriography can identify the site of occlusion and in addition can facilitate treatment. A cardiac work-up (ECG, holter monitor, transthoracic echocardiogram) are done to exclude a cardiac source for an embolism.

Principles for Management of Intestinal Ischemia

Patient priorities revolve around treating the intravascular fluid volume deficit maximizing and avoiding the use of vasopressors. Most patients will respond to conservative supportive therapy.

Medical treatment for intestinal ischemia will depend on the presentation and severity of the insult. Supportive care is provided with patients placed on bowel rest, antibiotics, and intravenous fluids. Hemodynamic status is optimized and vasoconstrictive drugs are avoided. The patient is monitored for signs of bowel necrosis such as persistent fever, leukocytosis, peritoneal irritation, or protracted pain or bleeding.

In the case of nonocclusive mesenteric insufficiency, a continuous infusion of a vasodilator, such as papaverine, into the superior mesenteric artery can be given intra-arteriorly at the time of arteriography.

Exploratory laparotomy with thromboembolectomy or bypass of the occlusion can be performed if the diagnosis is an acute mesenteric occlusion due to clot or an atherosclerotic plaque. Surgery is also indicated for peritonitis or clinical deterioration (increasing abdominal tenderness, guarding, rebound tenderness, rising temperature, and/or paralytic ileus) with 20% of patients needing surgical intervention for resection of the involved bowel. Current advances in endovascular treatments are increasingly used in patients with chronic mesenteric ischemia. The option for percutaneous transluminal angioplasty with stent placement avoids the risks associated with an open repair.

Bowel Obstruction

Bowel obstruction is a common cause for hospitalization and results in 15% of all emergency admissions for abdominal pain and 1.9% of all hospital admissions. Intestinal transit can be affected by either a mechanical or functional obstruction. Mechanical obstructions can be due to lesions which block the internal lumen (luminal or intrinsic) or by lesions which compress the bowel lumen from the outside of the intestine (extrinsic). Mechanical obstructions can be further classified as either a small-bowel obstruction (SBO) or a large-bowel obstruction (LBO); and complete or partial. Complete obstruction always requires surgical management, whereas a partial obstruction can be managed conservatively with serial examinations. Ileus and colonic pseudo-obstruction are categorized as functional obstructions.

Etiology, Risk Factors, and Pathophysiology
Small-Bowel Obstruction

Adhesions due to previous surgery are the most common cause of an SBO followed by malignant tumors (peritoneal implants), hernias, and inflammatory bowel disease.

Adhesions account for more than 70% of all SBO. Studies have demonstrated that the incidence of SBO is lower in patients who have minimally invasive procedures vs open surgery.

Large-Bowel Obstruction

Colorectal cancer is the most common cause of an LBO in the United States with the descending colon and rectosigmoid the most common sites of obstruction. Other causes of a mechanical obstruction owing to intrinsic causes include fecal impaction and foreign bodies. Inflammation (diverticulitis or inflammatory bowel disease), ischemia, intussusception, and anastomotic stricture are also intrinsic etiologies. Extrinsic causes include hernias, abscess, volvulus, or tumors in adjacent organs. Adhesions rarely lead to obstruction of the large bowel.

Early in the course of the obstruction, bowel motility and contractions will increase as the bowel attempts to push contents past the point of obstruction. This can account for diarrhea in the initial presentation. The intestine becomes fatigued, dilates, and contractions are less frequent and intense. Water and electrolytes accumulate in the bowel lumen and lead to dehydration and hypovolemia. Hypochloremia, hypokalemia, and metabolic alkalosis are not uncommon especially if the patient is vomiting or has high nasogastric tube losses. Abdominal distention can compromise respiratory function. In general, with either an SBO or LBO, a segment of the intestine can become trapped and the blood supply can become compromised or strangulated. The blood supply can also be compromised by the increasing tension related to the abdominal distention. Ischemia could result and, if not treated, can lead to bowel necrosis. The cecum is the most common site of colonic ischemia or perforation.

Ileus

An ileus is intestinal distention and the slowing or absence of the passage of intestinal contents. It is a functional obstruction, so a mechanical cause cannot be identified. Common causes of an ileus are drug induced (anticholinergics, psychotropics, or opiates), metabolic derangements, neurogenic, and infections. Ileus is most common after abdominal operations and persists the longest after colon surgery.

Acute Colonic Pseudo-Obstruction

Pseudo-obstruction, also called Ogilvie syndrome, is a condition of distention of the colon with signs and symptoms of obstruction, in the absence of a physical or mechanical cause. Acute colonic pseudo-obstruction (ACPO) is characterized by the absence of intestinal contractility. The exact cause remains unknown. It is commonly seen in hospitalized or institutionalized patients, the elderly, and patients with chronic renal failure, respiratory, cerebral, or cardiovascular disease. It has an unknown prevalence and incidence, and as its name implies, it primarily affects the colon. It is diagnosed only after excluding mechanical LBO. Patients may have a history of unnecessary repeated laparotomy.

Clinical Presentation

Signs and symptoms will vary depending on the cause and location of the obstruction.

History

- Prior abdominal surgery
- Ischemia
- Hernia
- Abdominal cancer
- Abdominal radiation
- Inflammatory bowel disease

Signs and Symptoms

- Failure to pass stool or flatus
- Diarrhea
- Crampy or colicky abdominal pain; sometimes localized to periumbilical and epigastric regions, but usually diffuse
- Abdominal distention
- Generalized tenderness
- Nausea and vomiting
- Bowel sounds may be hyperactive with rushes or may be absent
- Visible peristalsis
- Tympany
- Tachycardia
- Hypotension
- Fever
- Localized tenderness, rebound, guarding (suggest peritonitis)

Diagnostic Tests

Plain films of the abdomen will demonstrate whether an obstruction is present. Dilated loops of bowel with air fluid levels are characteristic in the proximal bowel; distal bowel is collapsed. A CT scan of the abdomen and pelvis with oral contrast will show where the obstruction is, identify the transition zone, and demonstrate the etiology. It has become the diagnostic exam of choice. A small-bowel follow-through or water-soluble contrast enema may be necessary. Electrolyte disorders are common due to vomiting and lack of oral intake. The most common electrolyte abnormality is hypokalemia. The patient will exhibit either a metabolic or contraction alkalosis (renal sodium reabsorption in exchange for H^+) or metabolic acidosis (GI bicarbonate loss and hypovolemic tissue hypoperfusion).

Principles for Management of Bowel Obstruction

Treatment options will vary depending on the diagnosis. Initially, a nasogastric tube is placed to decompress the bowel, the intravascular fluid volume deficit is treated with isotonic fluids, electrolyte abnormalities are corrected, bowel rest is initiated, and antiemetics and antibiotics are administered.

Long intestinal tubes are no longer indicated and are associated with longer hospital stays and prolonged ileus. A rectal tube can be used to decompress the distal colon in patients with LBO.

Treatment of an ileus is entirely supportive therapy. The most effective treatment is to address the underlying cause. Metabolic or electrolyte abnormalities are corrected and medications which may be producing the ileus are discontinued.

Acute colonic pseudo-obstruction is treated with the administration of neostigmine, a parasympathomimetic agent. It is important that mechanical causes for the obstruction have been excluded before administering the drug. In the treatment of ACPO, 2.5 mg of neostigmine is given intravenously over 3 minutes. The pseudo-obstruction will resolve within less than 10 minutes with the patient passing stool and flatus. If no response occurs, the dose can be repeated 4 hours later. Bradycardia, bronchospasm, and hypotension are side effects of neostigmine and patients must be monitored with telemetry. Atropine should be readily available. Patients with cardiac disease are not the candidates for this treatment. Patients who do not respond to neostigmine should undergo a colonoscopy for decompression. Surgery is only reserved for patients with signs of ischemia, perforation, or whose clinical status deteriorates.

Approximately 90% of all SBOs will resolve spontaneously with supportive therapy. Surgical therapy is required to treat an LBO and may be needed to treat an SBO. Procedures indicated may include lysis of adhesions, reduction of hernias, bypass of obstructions, and resection of affected intestine. Self-expandable metallic colon stents may be placed at the time of colonoscopy to decompress the colon and can be a bridge to elective surgery in patients with a malignancy. A permanent or temporary diverting ileostomy or colostomy may be performed. A flexible sigmoidoscopy can be used initially to decompress a sigmoid volvulus; definitive surgery follows.

1. Administer colloids and crystalloids to treat the fluid volume deficit. Normal saline with potassium supplementation is the replacement fluid of choice. Monitor patient response to fluid resuscitation—hemodynamic parameters (MAP, heart rate), body weight, and intake and output. A Foley catheter is placed to monitor urine output.
2. Administer antimicrobial therapy to treat intra-abdominal infection. Few practitioners will administer antibiotics while the patient is being observed.
3. Position with head of bed elevated to promote lung expansion to relieve pressure from the distended abdomen. Assist with deep breathing exercises to promote lung expansion, mobilization of secretions, and relaxation.
4. Administer analgesics and sedatives for pain management. Avoid excess use of opiates to promote the return of peristalsis. The use of narcotics in the patient in whom a decision has not been made to operate and the diagnosis is uncertain is controversial.
5. Insert a nasogastric tube and apply and maintain suction to drain and decompress the upper GI tract.
6. Monitor and report signs and symptoms of ongoing infection, peritoneal signs, or deterioration in status. Multiple follow-up abdominal radiographs and serial clinical examinations are indicated. Classic symptoms associated with strangulated bowel are leukocytosis, fever, tachycardia, and severe abdominal pain.
7. Provide nutrition as prescribed. Total parenteral nutrition (PN) may be required early in the course of therapy. Enteral therapy should be initiated as early as possible because it promotes the return of peristalsis and may assist in maintaining the gut mucosal barrier function. Enteral nutrition should be used with caution if bowel ischemia is suspected.

Bariatric (Weight Loss) Surgery

Bariatric surgery is increasingly becoming an option for weight reduction for obese individuals who have not been successful with conservative weight loss strategies such as diet, exercise, and pharmacologic therapy. Candidates for bariatric surgery include those patients with a body mass index (BMI) of 40, or a BMI between 35 and 40 in the presence of certain comorbidities, such as diabetes, hypertension, obstructive sleep apnea, and cardiovascular disease.

Because all patients who have bariatric surgery are obese, and many have comorbid diseases, surgical recovery can be particularly challenging. Obesity, diabetes mellitus, coronary artery disease, sleep apnea, and other conditions more common among the obese patients require careful postoperative monitoring.

Surgical Procedures

There are three main types of weight loss surgery: restrictive, malabsorptive, and combined restrictive and malabsorptive. These procedures can be performed via either the laparoscopic or open approach. The majority are done laparoscopically because there is less pain, fewer wound complications, a shorter hospital stay, and quicker recovery. All procedures limit the volume of food eaten and alter gastric emptying. The risk for nutritional deficiencies will vary depending on the surgery performed. The restrictive procedures include the vertical banded gastroplasty (VBG), the laparoscopic adjustable gastric band (LAGB), and more recently the laparoscopic sleeve gastrectomy (LSG). There has been a recent change in the make-up of bariatric surgeries being performed in the United States. The number of laparoscopic sleeve gastrectomies being performed has increased with a reduction seen in the use of the LAGB. The LSG originated as a part of the duodenal switch operation. The laparoscopic Roux-en-Y (LRYGB) is categorized as both restrictive and malabsorptive, and has become the most commonly performed bariatric operation in the United States.

The VBG is done infrequently today, but was popular in the 1980s. The upper stomach near the esophagus is stapled vertically to create a small pouch. A band is placed to restrict the outlet from the pouch. With the LAGB, restriction is accomplished by placing an inflatable silicone band around the antrum of the stomach thereby creating a small pouch. The band is connected to an implanted reservoir under the skin, usually just below the rib cage. The pouch opening can be made smaller or larger by inflating or deflating the band via the reservoir.

The LSG has become an acceptable primary bariatric surgery. The procedure reduces the stomach to about 25% of its original size. A large portion of the stomach is removed following the major curve. The open edges are stapled to form a sleeve or tube with a "banana" shape. The procedure permanently reduces the size of the stomach. Although it is described as a restrictive procedure, recent studies have identified similar metabolic effects as seen with the LRYGB. These effects could potentiate a sense of satiety for patients. Studies demonstrate that weight loss after the LSG to be between that seen with the LAGB and LRYGB. It is a safe surgery which is easy to perform.

The biliopancreatic diversion (BPD), biliopancreatic diversion with duodenal switch (BPD-DS), and duodenal switch (DS) are malabsorptive procedures. These surgeries carry the highest risk for nutritional deficiencies as they result in significant alteration in digestion and malabsorption of protein, vitamins, and minerals. In general, there are three main components of these surgeries: a partial gastrectomy, the common or nutrient limb, and biliopancreatic limb. The common limb is a 50 to 100 cm portion of distal small bowel where limited digestion and absorption occur, while the biliopancreatic limb is created from the remainder of the proximal small bowel and functions to divert digestive juices to the nutrient or common limb.

The laparoscopic Roux-en-Y results in both restriction and malabsorption and is the gold standard surgery for treating obesity. The stomach is separated with a stapler and a 15-mL pouch is created. The small intestine is divided and the distal stomach, duodenum, and first part of the jejunum are bypassed. The distal end of the jejunum is anastomosed to the pouch (gastrojejunostomy) to allow for emptying while the proximal end is connected side to side to the jejunum (jejunojejunostomy) creating a 75- to 150-cm roux limb. The surgery also has a hormonal effect. Removing the gastric fundus, the primary site of ghrelin production, enhances weight loss by reducing appetite.

Principles for Management of Postoperative Bariatric Surgery

Standard nursing care of the postoperative patient, including assessment of vital signs and incisions, management of pain, pulmonary exercise, and deep vein thrombosis (DVT) prophylaxis is always implemented. In addition to standard postoperative care, assessment for, and prevention of, complications inherent to bariatric surgery are essential.

Respiratory Insufficiency

Airway obstruction and oxygenation problems are important postoperative concerns following bariatric surgery. A large number of these patients have documented obstructive sleep apnea preoperatively, which places them at higher risk for postoperative respiratory problems. Patients with sleep apnea will use their CPAP or BiPAP machine while in the hospital to help minimize this risk. The increased risk of postoperative oxygenation problems from anesthesia and postoperative analgesics in this vulnerable group requires careful respiratory monitoring for 24 to 48 hours after surgery.

Assessment for Anastomotic Leaks

Leakage of gastric contents at the site of anastomosis is a potentially life-threatening complication and if not recognized early can lead to overwhelming sepsis. Signs and symptoms of an anastomotic leak include fever, left shoulder pain, tachypnea, and tachycardia. Thirst and hypotension are typically appreciated in progressive sepsis. Abdominal pain may occur, but the absence of it does not preclude the possibility of an anastomotic leak. The only sign of a leak may be unexplained tachycardia.

A leak is diagnosed with either a limited upper GI radiograph or a CT scan. A contained leak can be treated with percutaneous drainage. If the leak is not contained, the patient is returned to the operating room for definitive treatment. A leak could result in an intra-abdominal abscess. The key to treating a leak is to identify it early.

Nausea and Vomiting

Nausea and vomiting should not be considered an expected consequence of bariatric surgery. The cause may be mechanical or behavioral. Vomiting should be very short lived as patients adjust to eating and drinking. Behavioral causes include eating too quickly, overeating, not chewing food well, drinking while eating, or a poor food choice. Dehydration may present as nausea. Anastomotic stricture or another mechanical cause of obstruction must be ruled out. Antiemetics are usually not helpful. If the nausea is due to dehydration, the symptoms will resolve with the administration of intravenous fluids. Counseling the patient will address the behavioral etiologies.

Prevention of Pulmonary Embolus

Patients having bariatric procedures are at high risk for pulmonary embolus (PE). Early ambulation postoperatively, which is particularly challenging in this patient population, is important in terms of reducing risk for DVT and PE. Preventing DVT and PE requires a combination of pharmacologic prophylaxis, use of sequential compression devices, and a program of ambulation for the patient. Optimal pain management is important not just for comfort, but to promote mobility. In patients with a prior history of DVT or PE or a history of a clotting disorder, an inferior vena cava filter may be placed preoperatively.

Skin Care

The bariatric surgery patient is at high risk for skin breakdown and poor wound healing. Skin folds harbor moisture, bacteria, and yeast; in addition, the blood supply to adipose tissue is poor. The best skin care is prevention and includes daily inspection of the skin, frequent turning, early ambulation, and special attention to the positioning of catheters and drainage tubes so that they are not hidden with skin folds. Skin care needs to be thorough, paying special attention to the folds under the breasts, back, abdomen, and perineum.

Postoperative Medication Alterations

Another important consideration in the care of patients after bariatric surgery is the administration of medications. Because a portion of small bowel has been bypassed, absorption of medications will be impacted. Medications previously given as sustained-released formulations should be given in regular-release form to compensate for the changes in absorption. Tolerance of the gastrointestinal effects of some medications may be altered, and patients should be carefully monitored for a new or changing side effect profile.

Resumption of preoperative diabetic medications, both insulin and oral agents, should also be carefully monitored. Requirements for glucose control change dramatically immediately after surgery and resumption of preoperative doses may lead to significant hypoglycemia. Postoperatively, glucose management should be done with short-acting sliding scale insulin. Many patients will be able to completely discontinue the use of diabetic medications, including insulin, after surgery.

Patient Education

Recovery from bariatric surgery is a lengthy and involved process, extending beyond surgical healing. Patient education is a critical part of acute nursing care. Because anastomotic leak and PE can occur up to 2 weeks after surgery, patients should understand the signs and symptoms to be watchful for at home. Nutritional instruction and dietary progression is an important part of the process, and advancing diet properly is a significant component of reducing nausea, vomiting, and other discomfort for weeks and months after operation. Patients having malabsorptive procedures remain at long-term risk for vitamin and mineral deficiencies, and are best served by a sure understanding of long-term follow-up and dietary supplementation.

NUTRITIONAL SUPPORT FOR ACUTELY ILL PATIENTS

The negative consequences of malnutrition have been known for centuries, and there is substantial evidence that malnourished, hospitalized patients have increased morbidity, compromised surgical outcomes, slower ventilator weaning, and increased mortality rates. However, the science of nutrition support for the acutely ill patient is still young. In recent years, several large randomized studies have investigated the timing of nutrition, nutrient needs, and specific nutrients that best affect outcomes, but many important questions related to progressive care nutrition remain unanswered.

There is accumulating evidence that the route of nutrition support can affect morbidity in the acutely ill patient. In addition, protocols and care bundles for the proper initiation and monitoring of patients on nutrition support may reduce complications.

Nutrition Requirements

The advent of routine use of PN in the 1970s allowed the provision of large quantities of calories, and protein in an attempt to improve nutrition status. This ill-advised notion of providing supraphysiologic levels of nutrition, or "hyperalimentation," led to widely published case reports of respiratory failure and hepatic compromise associated with overfeeding. Controlled trials have demonstrated that overfeeding does not provide increased nutritional benefits, and actually has detrimental effects (Table 14-10).

Current recommendations for feeding acutely ill patients suggest approximately 25 total calories/kg/day based on the patient's ideal body weight, or 27.5 total calories/kg/day in the presence of systemic inflammatory response syndrome. A total of 1.2 to 1.5 g/kg/day of protein is also recommended. In severely malnourished patients, reduced calories (15-20 kcals/kg) are initiated to minimize electrolyte shifts from refeeding. When electrolytes are stable, progression to 30 or more calories/kg may be attempted to improve nutrition status. Close monitoring for tolerance is indicated.

Nutritional Case: Special Populations

Bariatric Surgery

The management of postoperative nutrition begins preoperatively with a comprehensive assessment of nutritional status, identification of psychosocial barriers, and a strong educational component and a plan for consistent follow-up to reinforce principles and measurement of success. Eighty percent of gastric bypass procedures today are malabsorptive or combined restrictive and malabsorptive procedures.

TABLE 14-10. POTENTIAL CONSEQUENCES OF OVERFEEDING OF MACRONUTRIENTS[a]

Carbohydrate	Fat
Hyperglycemia	Impaired immune response
Synthesis and storage of fat Hepatic steatosis	Fat overload syndrome with neurologic, cardiac, pulmonary, hepatic, and renal dysfunction
Increased carbon dioxide production increasing minute ventilation	Thrombocyte adhesiveness
	Accumulation of lipid in the reticuloendothelial system (RES), leading to RES dysfunction

[a]Remember to look for additional sources of dextrose and fat, such as propofol, intravenous fluids (IVF), continuous venovenous hemodialysis (CVVHD), peritoneal dialysis.
Reprinted with permission from the University of Virginia Health System from Nutrition Support Traineeship Syllabus, University of Virginia Health System, Charlottesville, VA; Updated June 2013.

As experience and number of surgeries increase, other less well-known deficiencies are starting to emerge. Nutritional supplementation is standard therapy for all bypass operations. Ongoing monitoring and reinforcement of compliance is essential. It is important to note that medication absorption is also altered in these patients. Ethyl alcohol (EtOH) absorption is enhanced, while sustained release and enteric-coated tablets may pass through undissolved, or unutilized. Efficacy of drugs requiring a large volume of food or high-fat meal may be compromised (antifungals, antipsychotics). In addition, reports of increased pregnancies while on birth control have surfaced.

Postgastrectomy Syndromes

Gastric resection can predispose patients to both nutritional intolerances and deficiencies. Intolerances include dumping syndrome, fat maldigestion, gastric stasis, and lactose intolerance. Combinations of these are most likely responsible for acute postoperative weight loss, the most frequent complication of gastrectomized patients. Nutrient deficiencies can develop months to years after gastric resections and can result in deleterious clinical consequences. Patients are at higher risk of developing osteoporosis and iron- and vitamin B_{12}-deficiency anemia. Decreased acid production and small bowel bacterial overgrowth most likely play a role in the later two. Ongoing nutritional monitoring of these patients will prevent deficiencies and identify those in need of intervention.

Parenteral Nutrition

Parenteral nutrition is indicated for patients who are malnourished, are at risk for becoming malnourished, and who are unable to receive EN (Table 14-11). PN can be life saving in some cases, but is not without complications and should be used only when necessary (Table 14-12). Prospective trials have demonstrated that the metabolic and infectious complications of PN outweigh the benefits in patients who do not have significant malnutrition. Studies have demonstrated that even short-term PN, used to supplement enteral nutrition in the ICU, has not enhanced benefits and is associated with increased infectious complications and length of stay. The need for PN should be evaluated daily in the inpatient setting, and patients who regain GI function are transitioned to enteral feeding.

Enteral Nutrition

Current evidence suggests that EN is the preferred method of feeding the acutely ill patient. It is associated with less infectious complications, expense, and confers some gut protection in terms of immunity, attenuation of systemic response, and atrophy (Table 14-13). Patients who do not receive full amounts of EN have a greater need for rehabilitation services compared to patients receiving full feedings.

Unfortunately, the delivery of EN is impeded by various situations that occur in progressive care units; for example,

TABLE 14-11. INDICATIONS FOR PARENTERAL NUTRITION

Parenteral nutrition is usually indicated in the following situations:
• Documented inability to absorb adequate nutrients via the gastrointestinal tract. This may be due to: 　Massive small-bowel resection/short-bowel syndrome (at least initially) 　Radiation enteritis 　Severe diarrhea 　Steatorrhea
• Complete bowel obstruction, or intestinal pseudo-obstruction
• Persistent ileus
• Severe catabolism with or without malnutrition when gastrointestinal tract is not usable within 5-7 days
• Inability to obtain enteral access
• Inability to provide sufficient nutrients or fluids enterally
• Pancreatitis accompanied by abdominal pain with jejunal delivery of nutrients
• Persistent GI hemorrhage
• Acute abdomen
• Lengthy GI work-up requiring NPO status
• High-output enterocutaneous fistula (> 500 mL) if feeding ports cannot be distally placed
• Trauma requiring repeat surgical procedures
Parenteral nutrition may be indicated as above in the following situations:
• Enterocutaneous fistula (<500 mL)
• Inflammatory bowel disease not responding to medical therapy
• Hyperemesis gravidarum when nausea and vomiting persist longer than 5-7 days and EN is not possible
• Partial small bowel obstruction
• Intensive chemotherapy/severe mucositis
• Major surgery/stress when EN is not expected to resume within 7-10 days
• Intractable vomiting when jejunal feeding is not possible
• Chylous ascites or chylothorax

Reprinted with permission from the University of Virginia Health System from Nutrition Support Traineeship Syllabus, University of Virginia Health System, Charlottesville, VA; Updated June 2013.

TABLE 14-12. CONTRAINDICATIONS FOR PARENTERAL NUTRITION

• Functioning gastrointestinal tract
• Treatment anticipated for < 5 days in patients without severe malnutrition
• Inability to obtain venous access
• A prognosis that does not warrant aggressive nutrition support
• When the risks of PN are judged to exceed the potential benefits

Reprinted with permission from the University of Virginia Health System from Nutrition Support Traineeship Syllabus, University of Virginia Health System, Charlottesville, VA; Updated June 2013.

TABLE 14-13. BENEFITS OF ENTERAL FEEDING

• Stimulates immune barrier function
• Physiologic presentation of nutrients
• Maintains gut mucosa
• Attenuates hypermetabolic response
• Simplifies fluid/electrolyte management
• More "complete" nutrition than PN
• Less infectious complications (and costs associated with these complications)
• Stimulates return of bowel function
• Less expensive

Reprinted with permission from the University of Virginia Health System from Nutrition Support Traineeship Syllabus, University of Virginia Health System, Charlottesville, VA; Updated June 2013.

TABLE 14-14. COMMON BARRIERS TO OPTIMIZING ENTERAL NUTRITION DELIVERY

- Diagnostic procedures (feedings are stopped)
- Propofol (Diprivan) (calories from the lipid preparation must be calculated as part of the total kcal provided to prevent overfeeding—1.1 cal/mL infused)
- Enteral access issues (clogged/dislodged tubes or obtaining postpyloric access if needed)
- Feedings held due to drug-nutrient interactions
- Hypotensive episodes (patient is often flat in bed necessitating that feedings be turned off)
- Miscalculation of EN requirements
- "NPO" at midnight for tests, surgery, or procedures
- Conditioning regimes and/or therapies that require the feedings to be turned off
- Transportation off the unit
- Hemodialysis (EN is often stopped during hemodialysis if the patient is deemed unstable by the nurse, often after the patient experiences hypotension)
- Perceived or real "GI intolerance or dysfunction"
  - Nausea/vomiting
  - Complaints of fullness
  - Abdominal distention
  - Lack of bowel sounds (see Bowel Sounds)
  - Diarrhea (see Table 14-21)
  - Aspiration risk/no gag (see Aspiration)
  - Gastric residual volume (see Gastric Residual Volume)

A note on checking GRV with jejunal tubes: There is no need to check a GRV with a jejunal tube; there is no "reservoir" to hold EN, hence the flow of EN distally begins immediately.

Reprinted with permission from the University of Virginia Health System from Nutrition Support Traineeship Syllabus, University of Virginia Health System, Charlottesville, VA; Updated June 2013.

EN may be stopped for diagnostic or therapeutic procedures in patients who are unstable, or have clogged or dislodged enteral tubes (Table 14-14). Successful EN is also commonly thwarted by misguided perceptions and beliefs related to the definition of GI "intolerance." Many clinical responses are based on experiential assumptions and practices, as well as beliefs about how the GI tract functions in acute illness. The following sections review these myths and present facts related to GI tolerance or intolerance of enteral feeding.

Gastric Residual Volume

Little evidence exists to support the practice of checking gastric residual volume (GRV, the volume of fluid in the stomach), as an indicator of GI tolerance and potential adverse clinical outcomes in enterally fed patients. One of the physiologic functions of the stomach is to act as a reservoir and to control delivery of nutrients into the small bowel. This allows for maximal assimilation with bile salts and pancreatic enzymes. A number of factors contribute to the GRV: endogenous secretions, normal gastric emptying, exogenous fluids, and the cascade effect (Table 14-15).

Endogenous Secretions and Exogenous Additions

Two to four liters per day of saliva and gastric secretions are produced above the pylorus. Conservatively, this translates into 3 L of fluid that pass through the pylorus every 24 hours

TABLE 14-15. ABSORPTION AND SECRETION OF FLUID IN THE GI TRACT

GASTROINTESTINAL FLUID MOVEMENT	
Additions	**mL**
Diet	2000
Saliva	1500
Stomach	2500
Pancreas/Bile	2000
Intestine	1000
Subtractions	
Colointestinal	8900
NET STOOL LOSS	**100**

(an average of 125 mL/h). Once gastric access is obtained, exogenous medications, water flushes, and EN add to this volume. Commonly in acute care, clinicians expect the stomach to be empty or only contain a very small amount of tube feeding or other liquid upon checking. However, one study demonstrated that 40% of healthy volunteers have an average GRV greater than 100 mL.

The Cascade Effect

The predominant position of progressive care unit patients is supine, preferably with backrest elevation > 30° or higher. In this position, the stomach partially splits over the spine and is mechanically divided into two parts, the fundus (proximal) and the antrum (distal). Because the fundus is the noncontractile portion of the stomach, contents fill the fundus until they "cascade over" the spine into the antrum and finally exit through the pylorus. Thus, if the patient's feeding port is in the proximal stomach or fundus when the GRV is checked, the aspirated GRV may be erroneous. The GRV in this case may be a function of the patient's supine positioning rather than decreased GI motility.

Checking Gastric Residual Volume

The routine practice of checking GRV has not been validated. Some of the factors that make the routine assessment of GRV questionable are listed below:

1. Type of tube (Salem sump vs Dobbhoff-like feeding tube vs a gastrostomy)
2. Location of the gastrostomy on the patient's abdominal wall (fundus, antrum)
3. Position of the patient when GRV is checked (supine, right or left lateral decubitus, prone)
4. Method of aspiration (20-, 35-, 50-, 60-mL syringe vs gravity drainage vs low constant suction)
5. The volume of the aspirate obtained
6. Disposition of the aspirate (ie, reinfused or discarded)
7. The effects of GI stress prophylaxis medications (proton pump inhibitors) on the production and volume of gastric secretions
8. Lack of data linking elevated GRV to pulmonary aspiration

TABLE 14-16. SUGGESTED APPROACHES TO EVALUATE GASTRIC RESIDUAL VOLUME

- Confirm that the BRE is > 30°-40°. Maintain a semi-recumbent position with the backrest elevation (shoulders) elevated ≥ 30°-45°, or place patient in reverse Trendelenburg at 30°-45° if no contraindication exists for that position. Patients with femoral lines can be elevated up to 30°.
- Do not consider automatic cessation of EN until a second high GRV is demonstrated at least 4 hours after the first.
    Clinically assess patient for:
    Abdominal distention/discomfort
    Bloating/fullness
    Nausea/vomiting
- Place patient on their right side for 15-20 minutes before checking a GRV again (to take advantage of the effect of gravity and to avoid the cascade effect).
- Consider diverting the level of infusion of EN lower in the GI tract (postpyloric).
- Switch to a more calorically dense product to decrease the total volume infused.
- Avoid constipation.
- Review and minimize all fluids given enterally, including medications and water flushes.
- Minimize use of narcotics, or consider use of a narcotic antagonist to promote intestinal contractility.
- Verify appropriate placement of feeding tube.
- Switch from bolus feeding to continuous infusion.
- Initiate prokinetic therapy (or leave standing orders to allow nurse to initiate Rx prn). Typical doses for available prokinetics:
    Metoclopramide—5-20 mg qid (may need to give IV initially)
    Erythromycin—125-250 mg qid
    Domperidone—10-30 mg qid (non–FDA-approved drugs; have to obtain from Canada)
- Consider raising the threshold level or "cut-off" value for GRV for a particular patient.
- Consider stopping the GRV checks if the patient is clinically stable, has no apparent tolerance issues, and has shown relatively low GRVs for 48 hours. Should the clinical status change, GRV checks can be resumed.
- If consideration is given to increase the time interval between GRV checks to > 6-8 hours, the clinical situation may warrant cessation of GRV checks.
- Consider a proton pump inhibitor (PPI) in order to decrease volume of endogenous gastric secretions (eg, omeprazole, lansoprazole, esomeprazole, pantoprazole, rabeprazole).
- Initiate oral hygiene regimen.

Reprinted with permission from the University of Virginia Health System from Nutrition Support Traineeship Syllabus, University of Virginia Health System, Charlottesville, VA; Updated June 2013.

The practice of measuring GRV is poorly standardized. Furthermore, GRV as a valid measure of EN tolerance or whether the amount of GRV is even linked to the risk of aspiration pneumonia events has yet to be proven. Until more evidence is available, good clinical judgment is needed when evaluating GRV (Table 14-16).

Aspiration

Aspiration is the passage of materials into the airway below the level of the vocal cords. The aspirated material may be saliva, nasopharyngeal secretions, bacteria, food, beverage, gastric contents, or any other liquid or substance. The incidence of aspiration pneumonia from EN is unclear, because it is difficult to identify an aspiration event, and definitions of aspiration vary. Commonly quoted aspiration pneumonia rates in EN patients, however, are between 5% and 36%.

Detection

Several methods of evaluating patients for aspiration risk have been popularized through "conventional wisdom." These include the routine monitoring of GRV (discussed above), evaluation of gag reflex, testing tracheal secretions for the presence of glucose, and the addition of blue food color to feeding formulas.

The gag reflex is the least-reliable protective reflex in ensuring that aspiration does not occur. More important to airway protection are reliable cough and swallow reflexes. The presence of glucose in tracheal secretions is not a specific or sensitive method of detecting aspiration of EN. Tracheal glucose can be positive in patients who are not receiving EN. Finally, some tube-feeding formulas have low glucose concentrations and do not result in a positive test when aspirated.

Several studies have demonstrated that adding blue dye to feeding formulas is not a sensitive method for detecting aspiration and should not be used to indicate aspiration of gastric contents. In addition, some food dyes are mitochondrial toxins leading the Food and Drug Administration to release a Public Health Advisory Report noting the toxicity associated with the use of FD&C Blue No. 1 added to EN solutions.

Reducing Aspiration Risk
Body Position

The position of the patient is one of the primary factors influencing aspiration risk (Table 14-17). Studies have confirmed that aspiration and pneumonia are significantly more likely when patients are supine with the backrest elevation at less than 30°. While the semirecumbent position with backrest elevation of more than 30° cannot guarantee absolute protection against aspiration, it is a method that is inexpensive

TABLE 14-17. RISK REDUCTION FOR ASPIRATION PNEUMONIA

- Maintain a semi-recumbent position with the head (shoulders) elevated > 30°-45° or placing patient in reverse Trendelenburg at 30°-45° if no contraindication is present to that position. Patients with femoral lines can be at 30°.
- Good oral care.
- Minimize use of narcotics.
- Verify appropriate placement of feeding tube.
- Clinically assess GI tolerance:
    Abdominal distention
    Fullness/discomfort
    Vomiting
    Excessive residual volumes (see gastric residual volume section)
- Use guided feeding tube placement (CO_2 monitor).
- Use prokinetic medications or place jejunal tube if elevated gastric residual volumes persist of if the patient is at increased risk of reflux and spiration.
- Tracheal glucose or blue color is not helpful.
- Evaluate for use of orogastric feeding tubes in mechanically ventilated patients.
- Remove nasoenteric or oroenteric feeding tubes as soon as possible.

Reprinted with permission from the University of Virginia Health System from Nutrition Support Traineeship Syllabus, University of Virginia Health System, Charlottesville, VA; Updated June 2013.

and relatively easy to accomplish and monitor. Strict use of semirecumbent position is the most consistent and potent means to reduce the likelihood of aspiration.

Tube Size and Placement Issues

The incidence of aspiration, and subsequently pneumonia, are not affected by the feeding tube size. However, radiographic confirmation of accurate placement is essential. Moreover, there is evidence that pulmonary injury during beside placement of feeding tubes occurs more frequently than is generally appreciated. Using a method to provide feedback that the airway has been inadvertently intubated with the feeding tube can decrease the incidence of injury that may occur before the confirmatory radiograph is obtained. Several studies have reported that use of CO_2 detection, electromagnetic guidance, or a preliminary radiograph during placement decreases the incidence of inadvertent pulmonary intubation and injury. It is commonly believed that placing the tip of the feeding tube beyond the pylorus decreases the incidence of aspiration events. However, despite numerous studies and a meta-analysis on the topic, it remains unclear if a properly positioned jejunal tube can reduce aspiration risk. The majority of acutely ill patients in these studies received gastric tube feedings safely and effectively. In studies that used protocols for the prevention of aspiration, very low rates of aspiration pneumonia were demonstrated. From a purely evidence-based standpoint, then the question of jejunal placement of feeding tubes and aspiration risk remains unanswered.

Considering the time and expense associated with jejunal placement of feeding tubes, it is reasonable to use the gastric route unless intolerance is evident. Exceptions to this approach include patients known to be at increased risk for aspiration due to altered anatomy (eg, esophagectomy) or motility (eg, scleroderma, severe gastroparesis). These patients may benefit from jejunally placed tubes.

Feeding Rate

The delivery rate of the feeding formula may influence aspiration and pneumonia. Bolus administration of 350 mL reduces lower esophageal sphincter pressure, which may precipitate reflux. Continuous EN (transpyloric-duodenal feeds) has been associated with more rapidly attained feeding tolerance, but no significant change in aspiration incidence. In one study, reduced aspiration events were associated with cyclic infusion feedings (16-hour cycle), compared to continuous feedings. The authors postulated that cyclic EN resulted in a reduction of gastric pH and subsequently prevented colonization of gastric contents. However, randomized trials have failed to demonstrate associations between gastric pH, gastric colonization, or pneumonia incidence in patients fed with cyclic vs continuous feedings.

Pharmacologic Interventions

Prokinetic medications have been evaluated to determine whether they improve EN tolerance. Metoclopramide and erythromycin improve gastric emptying, and a combination of these two medications may be superior to either drug alone. However, prokinetic medications do not appear to reduce the incidence of aspiration pneumonia.

Bowel Sounds

Auscultating the abdomen to determine the presence of BS, and thus GI tract function, is a well-entrenched practice yet has never been validated as a marker of GI tract function. However, from a theoretical perspective, if BS were related to peristalsis, the absence of BS may suggest that a functional ileus exists. If nothing is moving through the GI tract (unlikely as 7 L of secretions are produced daily; see Table 14-15), the patient will require gastric decompression. In fact, initiating EN in patients without BS may stimulate the bowel to function normally and BS may emerge in some patients.

Studies that have investigated the effectiveness of auscultation for BS reported that the practice did not improve diet management in postoperative abdominal surgery patients, nor did flatus and bowel movements predict ability to tolerate oral intake. In addition, studies suggest that enteral feeding initiated within the first 24-48 hours of ICU admission with or without the presence of BS is safe.

Auscultation of BS practices in the clinical setting varies. Clinician assessment practices include how the quadrants are auscultated, the frequency of auscultation, time spent listening for sounds, and the interpretation of the sounds. BS are nonspecific and hence are best used in conjunction with the overall clinical assessment of the patient. Suggested approaches to assessment of GI function when BS are absent are found in Table 14-18.

Nausea and Vomiting

Many factors contribute to nausea and vomiting in the progressive care setting such as medications, the disease process, surgery, procedures, and bedside interventions (eg, during placement of a feeding tube or endotracheal suctioning). After careful assessment and treatment of the underlying cause (Table 14-19), antiemetic coverage may allow the continuation of EN while making the patient more comfortable. It is important that when ordering antiemetics and/or prokinetics, they be scheduled until clinical symptoms abate. Because PRN orders are often not administered for a variety of reasons (eg, patient unable or unaware that the medications may be requested, off floor for procedure, dose is not given), scheduled antiemetics may improve efficacy. However, it is important that the medications be discontinued when no longer necessary to prevent undesirable side effects.

Osmolality or Hypertonicity of Formula

Hypertonic or hyperosmolar formulas are often assumed to be responsible for diarrhea in the EN-fed patient, although no data exists to support this concept. As a result, some

TABLE 14-18. SUGGESTED APPROACHES FOR GI ASSESSMENT OF GI FUNCTION WHEN BOWEL SOUNDS ARE ABSENT

- Assess need for, and volume of, gastric decompression (ie, compare volume aspirated to normal secretions above the pylorus expected over time frame between aspirations).
- Distinguish significance by differentiating those patients requiring:
  Low constant suction
  Gravity drainage
  An occasional gastric residual check every 4-6 hours (small bowel aspirates should not be checked)
- Abdominal examination—firm, distended, tympanic.
- Presence of nausea, bloating, feeling full, vomiting.
- Evaluate whether patient is passing gas or stool.
- Compare clinical examination with the differential diagnosis, specifically high suspicion for abdominal process.
- Finally, after determining low risk from above, consider a trial of EN at low rate of 10-20 mL/h and clinically observe for any of the symptoms listed above.

Reprinted with permission from the University of Virginia Health System from Nutrition Support Traineeship Syllabus, University of Virginia Health System, Charlottesville, VA; Updated June 2013.

TABLE 14-20. OSMOLALITY OF SELECTED LIQUIDS AND MEDICATIONS

Typical Liquids	(mOsm/kg)	Drug	(mOsm/kg)
EN formulas	250-710	Acetaminophen elixir	5400
Milk/eggnog	275/695	Diphenoxylate suspension	8800
Gelatin	535	KCl elixir (sugar-free)	3000
Broth	445	Ferrous sulfate liquid	4700
Sodas	695	Furosemide (oral)	3938
Popsicles	720	Metoclopramide	8350
Juices	~ 990	Multivitamin liquid	5700
Ice cream	1150	Na phosphate	7250
Sherbet	1225	Docusate sodium syrup	3900

Reprinted with permission from the University of Virginia Health System from Nutrition Support Traineeship Syllabus, University of Virginia Health System, Charlottesville, VA; Updated June 2013.

believe that diluting formula is an essential step. Diluting formula increases nursing time and the potential for contamination as well as decreasing the nutrient content of the feeding. The GI tract dilutes all foods and fluids ingested (or infused) by secreting saliva, and gastric and pancreatobiliary juices (including bicarbonate) to ensure isotonicity. This occurs whether it is delivered gastrically or jejunally. A clear or full liquid diet is more hypertonic or hyperosmolar than most commercial EN products available in the market as are many medications (Table 14-20). Yet, these are not ordered at one-quarter or half-strength. Because jejunal feedings circumvent the first step in food processing by bypassing the stomach, controversy exists related to how they should be managed. Some believe they should be managed differently than gastric feedings. However, as learned from patients with gastrectomies, where all the food they eat is delivered directly from the esophagus into the jejunum, normal feedings (albeit smaller portions)

TABLE 14-19. SUGGESTED APPROACHES TO REDUCE NAUSEA AND VOMITING IN ENTERALLY FED PATIENTS

1. Review medication profile; change suspected agents to an alternative.
2. Try a prokinetic agent or antiemetic—review orders for "prn" vs scheduled doses as well as delivery method.
3. Switch to a more calorically dense product to decrease the total volume infused.
4. Seek transpyloric access of feeding tube.
5. Tighten glucose control to avoid gastroparesis from hyperglycemia.
6. Consider analgesic alternatives to opiates.
7. Vent gastric port, if available–if feeding into small bowel, vent gastric port (if available).
8. Consider a proton pump inhibitor in order to decrease sheer volume of endogenous gastric secretions (eg, omeprazole, lansoprazole, esomeprazole, pantoprazole, rabeprazole).
9. If bacterial overgrowth is a possibility, treat with enteral antibiotics.

Reprinted with permission from the University of Virginia Health System from Nutrition Support Traineeship Syllabus, University of Virginia Health System, Charlottesville, VA; Updated June 2013.

are consumed without adverse consequences. In those patients requiring frequent or large water boluses, dilution of formula may help, but the flow rate will need to be increased in order to deliver the same amount of nutrition. With this exception, dilution of EN should be avoided.

Diarrhea

Diarrhea occurs in patients in the hospital setting regardless of oral, EN, or IV nutrition. The assumption that EN is a major cause of diarrhea is a myth. Although definitive evidence is needed to put this notion to rest, numerous studies have suggested other compelling reasons for diarrhea such as concurrent medications, especially those containing sorbitol, and infectious agents (*Clostridium difficile* in particular). Other commonly cited, but unfounded assumptions for the origin of diarrhea include low serum albumin level, strength, and osmolality of the formula, formula composition, rate of infusion, use of fiber-free EN, and disuse of the GI tract. Recent study on the effects of "fermentable, oligo-, di-, mono-saccharides and polyols" (FODMAPs) suggest that they may adversely affect bowel activity. Found in many enteral formulas, FODMAPs are highly osmotic and fermentable by gut bacteria and have been associated with gas, bloating, cramping, and diarrhea in some patients receiving EN. After potential causes for diarrhea have been ruled out (Table 14-21), medications to slow GI motility may be warranted.

Flow Rates and Hours of Infusion

Typical infusion rates for the initiation of EN range from 10 to 50 mL/h with increases of 10 to 25 mL every 4 to 24 hours. Unfortunately, like other EN-support practices, little science exists to confirm or refute such regimens. There is limited evidence from work done with healthy volunteers or from studies using faster advancement rates of EN. Only one study has demonstrated that continuous enteral feeding may be started at the final goal rate in acutely ill patients without negative consequences. In the study, feedings started

TABLE 14-21. SYSTEMATIC APPROACH WHEN ADDRESSING DIARRHEA IN ENTER-ALLY FED PATIENTS

- Quantify stool volume—determine if it is really diarrhea (> 250 mL/d).
- Review medication list—look for elixirs or suspensions with sorbitol (not always listed on the ingredient list—may need to contact manufacturer)
- Try and correlate timing of diarrhea in relation to start of new medication(s) or switch off medications to enteral route once enteral access is obtained; common offenders include:
  - Acetaminophen and Guaifenesin elixir
  - Neutra-Phos
  - Lactulose
  - Standing orders for stool softeners/laxatives
- Check for *Clostridium difficile* or other infectious etiologies.
- Try a fiber-containing formula or add a fiber powder (not in poorly perfused or dysmotile gut):
  - Few clinical studies
  - Supports the health of colonocytes
- Added fructooligosaccharide (FOS) and fermentable, oligo-, di-, monosaccharides and polyols (FODMAPs) in some patients may precipitate or aggravate diarrhea.
- Once infectious causes are ruled out:
  - Consider an antidiarrheal agent such as Imodium (may need standing order vs " prn" to be effective)
- Check for fecal impaction.
- Check total hang time of EN (should not exceed 8 hours) (open systems only).
- Consider providing protein powders by bolus vs adding directly to formulas to decrease contamination risk.
- Check fecal fat as last resort; if negative it does not mean patient is not malabsorbing; if positive however, there is need to evaluate further.
- Continue to feed.

Reprinted with permission from the University of Virginia Health System from Nutrition Support Traineeship Syllabus, University of Virginia Health System, Charlottesville, VA; Updated June 2013.

TABLE 14-22. EXAMPLE OF EN PROGRESSION REGIMEN

Continuous

Initiation: Full strength at 50 mL/h and increase by 20 mL every 4 hours to goal rate (all products except a 2 cal/mL product). A 2 cal/mL product is started at 25 mL/h (as few patients need ≥ 50 mL/h to meet needs). The final goal rate is dependent on the patient's caloric requirements and GI comfort.

Postop patients: surgeons may want to start slower at 20-25 mL/h and advance once tolerance is achieved.

Intermittent/bolus

Initiation: 125 mL, full strength (regardless of product) every 3 hours for two feedings; increase by 125 mL every two feedings to final goal volume per feeding during waking hours.

Reprinted with permission from: University of Virginia Health System from Nutrition Support Traineeship Syllabus, University of Virginia Health System, Charlottesville, VA; Updated June 2013.

are marketed. Many believe that adequate outcome data are not available to warrant the use of these expensive products. Prospective, randomized trials have not demonstrated advantages of specialized "pulmonary" or "glucose control" feeding formulas. In fact, in a large randomized multicenter trial of a specialized enteral formula with fish oil and antioxidants for patients with acute lung injury, mortality increased with the specialized feeding compared to standard products. The majority of acutely ill patients may be fed with standard polymeric tube-feeding formulas.

SELECTED BIBLIOGRAPHY

Upper GI Bleeding

Alhazzani W, Alenezi F, Jaeschke RZ, et al. Proton pump inhibitors versus histamine 2 receptor antagonists for stress ulcer prophylaxis in critically ill patients: a systematic review and meta-analysis. *Crit Care Med.* 2013;41(3):1-13.

Andreyev HJN, Davidson SE, Gillespie C, et al. Practice guidance on the management of acute and chronic gastrointestinal problems arising as a result of treatment for cancer. *Gut.* 2012;61:179-192.

Cappell MS, Friedel D. Acute nonvariceal upper gastrointestinal bleeding: endoscopic diagnosis and therapy. *Med Clin N Am.* 2008;92:511-550.

Cappell MS, Friedel D. Initial management of acute upper gastrointestinal bleeding: from initial evaluation up to gastrointestinal endoscopy. *Med Clin N Am.* 2008;92:491-509.

Conrad SA. Acute upper gastrointestinal bleeding in critically ill patients: causes and modalities. *Crit Care Med.* 2002;30(suppl 6): S365-S368.

D'Amico G, Pietrosi G, Tarantino I, et al. Emergency sclerotherapy versus vasoactive drugs for variceal bleeding in cirrhosis: a Cochrane meta-analysis. *Gastroenterology.* 2003;124(5):1277-1291.

Dhamija N, Pousman R, Bajwa O, Marik PE. Management of gastrointestinal bleeding. In: Vincent J, Abraham E, Kochanek P, Moore FA, and Fink MP, eds. *Textbook of Critical Care*, 6th ed, St Louis, MO: Saunders Elsevier; 2011:86-91.

Dworzynski K, Pollit V, Kelsey A, et al. Management of acute upper gastrointestinal bleeding: summary of NICE guidance. *BMJ.* 2012;344:1-5.

El-Tawil AM. Management of non-variceal upper gastrointestinal tract hemorrhage: controversies and areas of uncertainty. *World J Gastroenterol.* 2012;18(11):1159-1165.

at goal-flow rate did appear to reduce the calorie deficit that frequently accrues in the hospitalized patient. Whether EN runs continuously, nocturnally, during the day, or is given as a bolus, is often institution specific. However, with the increased use of insulin infusions to ensure "tight glucose control," and thus improve outcomes in acutely ill patients, continuous infusions of EN may protect the patients from hypoglycemic episodes.

It is difficult to achieve goal volumes of EN in acutely ill patients. Frequent interruptions in the delivery of EN are common (see Table 14-14). As a result, it is reasonable to consider "padding" flow rates by basing calculations on < 24 hours to improve delivery of the desired dose. Sample tube-feeding protocols for EN initiation and progression are described in Table 14-22.

Formula Selection

A vast array of EN products are available, including specialty formulas marketed for patients with diabetes, pulmonary, hepatic, and renal failure. Other formulas contain nutrients that may modulate immune function, or have nutrients in their most basic (elemental) form for patients with malabsorptive syndromes. It is important to remember that medical nutrition products are not required to meet the same level of scientific scrutiny as medications before they

Green BT, Rockey DC. Acute gastrointestinal bleeding. *Semin Gastrointest Dis*. 2003;14:44-65.

Holster IL, Kuipers EF. Management of acute nonvariceal upper gastrointestinal bleeding: current policies and future perspectives. *World J Gastroenterol*. 2012;18(11):1202-1207.

Jairath V, Barkun AN. Improving outcomes from acute upper gastrointestinal bleeding. *Gut*. 2012;61(9):1246-1249.

Kryzwda E, Andris D, eds. AACN Advanced Critical Care Symposium, Gastroenterology in Critically Ill Patients. April-June 2010; 21(2):165-219.

Peter A, Wilcox M. Modern endoscopic therapy of peptic ulcer bleeding. *Dig Dis*. 2008;26:291-299.

Proctor DD. Critical issues in digestive diseases. *Clin Chest Med*. 2003;24:623-632.

Rossle M. When endoscopic therapy or pharmacology fails to control variceal bleeding: what should be done? Immediate control of bleeding by TIPS? *Langenbecks Arch Surg*. 2003;388:155-162.

Schuetz A, Jauch KW. Lower gastrointestinal bleeding: therapeutic strategies, surgical techniques and results. *Curr Concepts Clin Surg*. 2001;386:17-25.

Sorbi D, Gostout CJ, Peura D, et al. An assessment of the management of acute bleeding varices: a multicenter prospective member-based study. *Am J Gastroenterol*. 2003;98:2424-2434.

Targownik L, Gralnek IM. A risk score to predict the need for treatment of upper GI hemorrhage. *Gastrointest Endoscopy*. 2001;54: 797-799.

Toubia N, Sanyal A. Portal hypertension and variceal hemorrhage. *Med Clin N Am*. 2008;92:551-574.

Zhu LL, Xu LC, Chen Y, et al. Poor awareness of preventing aspirin-induced gastrointestinal injury with combined protective medications. *World J Gastroenterol*. 2012;18(24):3167-3172.

Zuckier L. Acute gastrointestinal bleeding. *Semin Nuclear Med*. 2003;33:297-311.

Liver Failure

Bachir NM, Larson AM. Adult liver transplantation in the United States. *Am J Med Sci*. June 2012;343(6):462-469.

Bari K, Garcia-Tsao G. Treatment of portal hypertension. *World J Gastroenterol*. Mar 21, 2012;18(11):1166-1175.

Bass NM, Mullen KD, Sanyal A, et al. Rifaximin treatment in hepatic encephalopathy. *N Engl J Med*. 2010;362:1071-1081.

Dasher K, Trotter JF. Intensive care unit management of liver-related coagulation disorders. *Crit Care Clin*. July 2012;28(3):389-398.

Foston TP, Carpentar D. *Crit Care Nurse N Am*. Sept 2010; 22(3):395-402.

Koffron A, Stein JA. Liver transplantation: indications, pretransplant evaluation, surgery, and posttransplant complications. *Med Clin N Am*. 2008;92:861-888.

Lata J. Hepatorenal syndrome. *World J Gastroenterol*. Sept 28, 2012; 18(36):4978-4984.

Lee WM. Recent developments in acute liver failure. *Best Practice Res Clin Gastroenterology*. Feb 2012;26(1):3-16.

Munoz SJ. Hepatic encephalopathy. *Med Clin N Am*. 2008;92:795-812.

Munoz SJ. The hepatorenal syndrome. *Med Clin N Am*. 2008;92:813-837.

Polson J, Lee WM. AASLD position paper: the management of acute liver failure. *Hepatology*. 2005;41:1179-1197.

Rahimi RS, Rockey DC. Complications and outcomes in chronic liver disease. *Curr Opin Gastroenterol*. 2011;27:204-209.

Rahimi RS, Rockey DC. Complications of cirrhosis. *Curr Opin Gastroenterol*. 2012;223-229.

Rikkers LF. Surgical complications of cirrhosis and portal hypertension. In: Townsend CM, Beauchamp RD, Evers BM, Mattox KL, eds. *Sabiston Textbook of Surgery*. Philadelphia, PA: Saunders Elsevier; 2008:1524-1546.

Rose CF. Ammonia-lowering strategies for the treatment of hepatic encephalopathy. *Clin Pharmacol Ther*. Sept 2012;92(3):321-331.

Sagi SV, Mittal S, Kasturi KS, Sood GK. Terlipressin therapy for reversal of type 1 hepatorenal syndrome: a meta-analysis of randomized controlled trials. *J Gastroenterol Hepatol*. 2010;25: 880-885.

Sibae A, Cappell MS. Accuracy of MELD scores in predicting mortality in decompensated cirrhosis from variceal bleeding, hepatorenal syndrome, alcoholic hepatitis or acute liver failure as well as mortality after non-transplant surgery or TIPS. *Dig Dis Sci*. April 2011;56(4):977-987.

Vuppalanchi R, Chalasani N. Nonalcoholic fatty liver disease and nonalcoholic steatohepatitis: selected practical issues in their evaluation and management. *Hepatology*. 2009;49:306-317.

Wong F. Recent advances in our understanding of hepatorenal syndrome. *Nat Rev Gastroenterology Hepat*. May 2012;9(7):381-391.

Acute Pancreatitis

AGA Institute. AGA institute medical position statement on acute pancreatitis. *Gastroenterology*. 2007;132:2019-2021.

Anans N, Park JJ, Wu BU. Modern management of acute pancreatitis. *Gastroenterol Clin N Am*. Mar 2012;41(1):1-8.

Bollen T. Imaging of acute pancreatitis: update of the revised Atlanta classification. *Radiol Clin N Am*. 2012;50:429-445.

Brisinda G, Vanellla S, Crocco A, et al. Severe acute pancreatitis: advances and insights in assessment of severity and management. *Eur J Gastroentel Hepatol*. 2011;23:541-551.

Cappell MS. Acute pancreatitis: etiology, clinical presentation, diagnosis, and therapy. *Med Clin N Am*. 2008;92:889-923.

Cruz-Santamaria DM, Taxonera G, Giner M. Update on pathogenesis and clinical management of acute pancreatitis. *World J Gastroint Pathophys*. June 2012;15(3):67-70.

Fischer JM, Gardner TB. The "golden hours" of management in acute pancreatitis. *Am J Gastroenterology*. Aug 2012;(107):1146-1150.

Mirtallo JM, Forbes A, McClave SA, et al. International consensus guideline for nutrition therapy in pancreatitis. *J Parenter Enteral Nutr*. May 2012;36(3):284-289.

Singh VK, Wu BU, Bollen TL, et al. A prospective evaluation of the bedside index for severity in acute pancreatitis score in assessing mortality and intermediate markers of severity in acute pancreatitis. *Am J Gastroenterol*. 2009;104:966-971.

Talukdar R, Vege SS. Early management of severe acute pancreatitis. *Curr Gastroenterol Rep*. 2011;13:123-130.

Warndorf MG, Kurtznab JT, Bartel MJ, et al. Early fluid resuscitation reduces morbidity among patients with acute pancreatitis. *Clin Gastroenterol Hepatol*. 2011;9:705-709.

Wu BU, Bakker OJ, Papachristou GI, et al. Blood urea nitrogen in the early assessment of acute pancreatitis. *Arch Intern Med*. 2011;171:669-676.

Intestinal Ischemia/Bowel Obstruction

Batke M, Cappell MS. Adynamic ileus and acute colonic pseudo-obstruction. *Med Clin N Am*. 2008;92:649-670.

Berland T, Oldenburg A. Acute mesenteric ischemia. *Curr Gastroenterol Rep*. 2008;10:341-346.

Brandt LJ, Feuerstadt P, Blaszka MC. Anatomic patterns, patient characteristics, and clinical outcomes in ischemic colitis: a study of 313 cases supported by histology. *Am J Gastroenterol.* 2010;105:2245-2252.

Cappell MS, Batke M. Mechanical obstruction of the small bowel and colon. *Med Clin N Am.* 2008;92:575-597.

Dayton MT, Dempsey DT, Larson GM, Posner AR. New paradigms in the treatment of small bowel obstruction. *Curr Prob Surg.* 2012;49(11):642-717.

De Giorgio R, Cogliandro RF, Barbara G, et al. Colonic intestinal pseudo-obstruction: clinical features, diagnosis, and therapy. *Gastroenterol Clin N Am.* 2011;40:787-807.

Diaz JJ, Bokhari F, Mowery, NT, et al. Guidelines for management of small bowel obstruction. *J Trauma.* 2008;64:1651-1664.

Edwards MS, Cherr GS, Craven TE, et al. Acute occlusive mesenteric ischemia: surgical management and outcomes. *Ann Vasc Surg.* 2003;17:72-79.

Feuerstadt P, Brandt LJ. Colon ischemia: recent insights and advances. *Curr Gastroenterol Rep.* 2010;12:383-390.

Georgescu EF, Carstea D, Dumitrescu D, et al. Ischemic colitis and large bowel infarction: a case report. *World J Gastroenterol.* 2012;18(39):5640-5644.

Green BT, Tendler DA. Ischemic colitis: a clinical review. *Southern Med J.* 2005;98:217-222.

McConnell EA. What's behind intestinal obstruction? *Nursing.* 2001;31(10):58-63.

McNamara I, Tremelling M, Dunkley I, et al. Management of intestinal obstruction in malignant disease. *Clin Med.* 2003;3:311-314.

Potluri V, Zhukovsky DS. Recent advances in malignant bowel obstruction: an interface of old and new. *Curr Pain Headache Rep.* 2003;7:270-278.

Sotiriadis J, Brandt LJ, Behin DS, et al. Ischemic colitis has a worse prognosis when isolated to the right side of the colon. *Am J Gastroenterol.* 2007;102:2247-2252.

Nutrition

ACOG Practice Bulletin No. 105. Bariatric surgery and pregnancy. *Obstet Gynecol.* 2009;113:1405-1413.

Aills L, Blankenship J, Buffington C, Furtado M, Parrot J. ASMBS allied health nutritional guidelines for the surgical weight loss patient. *Surg Obes Relat Dis.* 2008;4:S73-S108.

Bankhead R, Boullata J, Brantley S, et al. Enteral nutrition practice recommendations, Enteral Nutrition Practice Recommendations Task Force and the A.S.P.E.N. Board of Directors. *JPEN.* 2009;33(2):122-167.

Barr J, Hecht M, Flavin KE, et al. Outcomes in critically ill patients before and after the implementation of an evidence-based nutritional management protocol. *Chest.* April 2004;124(4):1446-1457.

Barrett JS, Gearry RB, Muir JG, et al. Dietary poorly absorbed, short-chain carbohydrates increase delivery of water and fermentable substrates to the proximal colon. *Aliment Pharmacol.* 2010;31:874-882.

Booth CM, Heyland DK, Paterson WG. Gastrointestinal promotility drugs in the critical care setting: a systematic review of the evidence. *Crit Care Med.* 2002;30:1429-1435.

Braunschweig CL, Levy P, Sheean PM, Wang X. Enteral compared with parenteral nutrition: a meta analysis. *Am J Clin Nutr.* 2001;74:534-542.

Brozovich M, Read T, Andujar J, et al. Bowel sounds, flatus, and bowel movement do not correlate with tolerance of oral intake following major abdominal surgery: a prospective study (abstract). *Dis Colon Rectum.* 2005;48(3):625.

Burns SM, Carpenter R, Blevins C, et al. Detection of inadvertent airway intubation during gastric tube insertion: capnography versus a colorimetric carbon dioxide detector. *Am J Crit Care.* 2006;15(2):188-195.

Casaer MP, Mesotten D, Hermans G, et al. Early versus late parenteral nutrition in critically ill adults. *N Engl J Med.* 2011;365(6):506-517.

Cerra FB, Benitez MR, Blackburn GL, et al. Applied nutrition in ICU patients. A consensus statement of the American College of Chest Physicians. *Chest.* 1997;111:769-778.

Chan L. Drug therapy-related issues in patients who received bariatric surgery (part I). *Prac Gastroenterol.* 2010;XXXIV(7):28-32. Available at www.ginutrition.virginia.edu. Accessed March 4, 2013.

Chan L. Drug therapy-related issues in patients who received bariatric surgery (part II). *Prac Gastroenterol.* 2010;XXXIV(8):24-32. Available at www.ginutrition.virginia.edu. Accessed March 4, 2013.

Dark DS, Pingleton SK, Kerby GR. Hypercapnia during weaning. A complication of nutritional support. *Chest.* 1985;88:141-143.

Davies AR, Morrison SS, Bailey MJ, et al. A multicenter, randomized controlled trial comparing early nasojejunal with nasogastric nutrition in critical illness. *Crit Care Med.* 2012;40(8):2342-2348.

de Aguilar-Nascimento JE, Kudsk KA. Clinical costs of feeding tube placement. *JPEN J Parenter Enteral Nutr.* 2007;31(4):269-273.

Desachy A, Clavel M, Vuagnat A, et al. Initial efficacy and tolerability of early enteral nutrition with immediate or gradual introduction in intubated patients. *Intensive Care Med.* 2008;34(6):1054-1059.

Drover JW, Dhaliwal R, Heyland DK. Small bowel versus gastric feeding in the critically ill patient: results of a meta-analysis. *Crit Care Med.* 2003;30:A44.

FDA Public Health Advisory FDA/Center for Food Safety & Applied Nutrition. Reports of blue discoloration and death in patients receiving enteral feedings tinted with the dye, FD&C blue NO. September 29, 2003.

Grap MJ, Munro CL, Hummel RS, et al. Effect of backrest elevation on the development of ventilator-associated pneumonia. *Am J Crit Care.* 2005;14(4):325-332.

Heymsfield SB, Head CA, McManus CB, 3rd, Seitz S, Staton GW, Grossman GD. Respiratory, cardiovascular, and metabolic effects of enteral hyperalimentation: influence of formula dose and composition. *Am J Clin Nutr.* 1984;40:116-130.

Holzapfel L, Chevret S, Madinier G, et al. Influence of long-term oro- or nasotracheal intubation on nosocomial maxillary sinusitis and pneumonia: results of a prospective, randomized, clinical trial. *Crit Care Med.* 1993;21(8):1132-1138.

Kostadima E, Kaditis AG, Alexopoulos EI, et al. Early gastrostomy reduces the rate of ventilator-associated pneumonia in stroke or head injury patients. *Eur Respir J.* 2005;26(1):106-111.

Krenitsky J. Gastric versus jejunal feeding: evidence or emotion? *Prac Gastroenter.* 2006;30(9):46. Available at www.ginutrition.virginia.edu. Accessed March 4, 2013.

Krenitsky J. Immunonutrition—fact, fancy or folly? *Prac Gastroenterol.* 2006;30(5):47. Available at www.ginutrition.virginia.edu. Accessed March 4, 2013.

Lansford T, Moncure M, Carlton E, et al. Efficacy of a pneumonia prevention protocol in the reduction of ventilator-associated pneumonia in trauma patients. *Surg Infect (Larchmt).* 2007; 8(5):505-510.

Mackenzie SL, Zygun DA, Whitmore BL, et al. Implementation of a nutrition support protocol increases the proportion of mechanically ventilated patients reaching enteral nutrition targets in the adult intensive care unit. *J Parenter Enteral Nutr.* 2005;29:74-80.

Madsen D, Sebolt T, Cullen L, et al. Listening to bowel sounds: an evidence-based practice project. *Am J Nurs.* 2005;105(12):40-49.

Marik PE, Zaloga GP. Gastric versus post-pyloric feeding: a systematic review. *Crit Care.* 2003;7:R46-R51.

Martindale RG, McClave, SA, Vanek VW, et al. Guidelines for the provision and assessment of nutrition support therapy in the adult critically ill patient: Society of Critical Care Medicine and American Society for Parenteral and Enteral Nutrition: Executive Summary. *Crit Care Med.* 2009;37(5):1757-1761.

McClave SA, Sexton LK, Spain DA, et al. Enteral tube feeding in the intensive care unit: factors impeding adequate delivery. *Crit Care Med.* 1999;27:1252-1256.

Metheny NA, Clouse RE. Bedside methods for detecting aspiration in tube fed patients. *Chest.* 1997;111:724-731.

Miller AD, Smith KM. Medication and nutrient administration considerations after bariatric surgery. *Am J Health Syst Pharm.* 2006;63(19):1852-1857.

Montejo JC, Minambres E, Bordeje L, et al. Gastric residual volume during enteral nutrition in ICU patients. The REGANE study. *Intensive Care Med.* 2010;36(8):1386-1393.

Munera-Seeley V, Ochoa JB, Brown N, et al. Use of a colorimetric carbon dioxide sensor for nasoenteric feeding tube placement in critical care patients compared with clinical methods and radiography. *Nutr Clin Prac.* Jun-Jul 2008;23(3):318-321.

Nguyen NQ, Chapman M, Fraser RJ, et al. Prokinetic therapy for feed intolerance in critical illness: one drug or two? *Crit Care Med.* 2007;35(11):2561-2567.

O'Donnell K. Small but mighty: selected micronutrient issues in gastric bypass patients. *Prac Gastroenterol.* 2008;XXXII(5):37. Available at www.ginutrition.virginia.edu. Accessed March 4, 2013.

O'Donnell, K. Severe micronutrient deficiencies in RYGB patients: rare but potentially devastating. *Prac Gastroenterol.* 2011;XXXV(11):13. Available at www.ginutrition.virginia.edu. Accessed March 4, 2013.

O'Keefe-McCarthy, Santiago C, Lau G. Ventilator-associated pneumonia bundled strategies: an evidence-based practice. *World-Views Evid Based Nurs.* 2008;193-204.

Parrish CR. Enteral feeding: the art and the science. *Nutr Clin Pract.* 2003;18:76.

Parrish CR, Krenitsky J, McCray S. University of Virginia Health System Nutrition Support Traineeship Syllabus. Charlottesville, VA: University of Virginia Medical Center Nutrition Services Department; Updated June 2013.

Parrish CR, McClave S. Checking gastric residual volumes: a practice in search of science? *Prac. Gastroenterol.* 2008;32(10):33. Available at www.ginutrition.virginia.edu. Accessed March 4, 2013.

Poulard F, Dimet J, Martin-Lefevre L, et al. Impact of not measuring residual gastric volume in mechanically ventilated patients receiving early enteral feeding: a prospective before-after study. *J Parenter Enteral Nutr.* 2010;34(2):125-130.

Rassias AJ, Ball PA, Corwin HL. A prospective study of tracheopulmonary complications associated with the placement of narrow-bore enteral feeding tubes. *Crit Care.* 1998;2(1):25-28.

Reignier J, Mercier E, Le Gouge A, et al. Effect of not monitoring residual gastric volume on risk of ventilator-associated pneumonia in adults receiving mechanical ventilation and early enteral feeding: a randomized controlled trial. *JAMA.* 2013;309(3):249-256.

Rice T, Wheeler AP, Thompson BT, et al. Initial trophic vs. full enteral feeding in patients with acute lung injury: the EDEN randomized trial. *JAMA.* 2012;307(8):795-803.

Rice TW, Swope T, Bozeman S, et al. Variation in enteral nutrition delivery in mechanically ventilated patients. *Nutrition.* 2005; 21(7-8):786-792.

Rice TW, Wheeler AP, Thompson BT, et al; NHLBI ARDS clinical trials network enteral omega-3 fatty acid, gamma-linolenic acid, and antioxidant supplementation in acute lung injury. *JAMA.* 2011;306(14):1574-1581.

Rogers C. Postgastrectomy nutrition. *Nutr Clin Pract.* 2011;26(2): 126-136.

Saalwachter Schulman A, Sawyer RG. Have you passed gas yet? Time for a new approach to feeding patients postoperatively. *Prac Gastroenterol.* 2005;32(10):82. Available at www.ginutrition. virginia.edu. Accessed March 4, 2013.

Salord F, Gaussorgues P, Marti-Flich J, et al. Nosocomial maxillary sinusitis during mechanical ventilation: a prospective comparison of orotracheal versus the nasotracheal route for intubation. *Intensive Care Med.* 1990;16(6):390-393.

Singer P, Anbar R, Cohen J, et al. The tight calorie control study (TICACOS): a prospective, randomized, controlled pilot study of nutritional support in critically ill patients. *Intensive Care Med.* 2011;37(4):601-619.

Sorokin R, Gottlieb JE. Enhancing patient safety during feeding-tube insertion: a review of more than 2,000 insertions. *JPEN J Parenter Enteral Nutr.* 2006;30(5):440-445.

Talpers SS, Romberger DJ, Bunce SB, Pingleton SK. Nutritionally associated increased carbon dioxide production. Excess total calories vs high proportion of carbohydrate calories. *Chest.* 1992;102:551-555.

van den Berghe G, Wouters P, Weekers F, et al. Intensive insulin therapy in critically ill patients. *N Engl J Med.* 2001;345: 1359-1367.

van den Broek PWJH, Rasmussen-Conrad EL, Naber AHJ, et al. What you think is not what they get: significant discrepancies between prescribed and administered doses of tube feeding. *Brit J Nutr.* 2009;101(1):68-71.

van Nieuwenhoven CA, Vandenbroucke-Grauls C, van Tiel FH, et al. Feasibility and effects of the semirecumbent position to prevent ventilator-associated pneumonia: a randomized study. *Crit Care Med.* 2006;34:396-402.

van Zanten AR, Dixon JM, Nipshagen MD, et al. Hospital-acquired sinusitis is a common cause of fever of unknown origin in orotracheally intubated critically ill patients. *Crit Care.* 2005; 9(5):R583-R590.

Willcutts K. Pre-op NPO and traditional post-op diet advancement: time to move on. *Prac Gastroenterol.* 2010;XXXIV(12):16. Available at www.ginutrition.virginia.edu. Accessed March 4, 2013.

Yavagal DR, Karnad DR, Oak JL. Metoclopramide for preventing pneumonia in critically ill patients receiving enteral tube feeding: a randomized controlled trial. *Crit Care Med.* 2000;28(5): 1408-1411.

On-Line References of Interest

http://www.ginutrition.virginia.edu. Accessed March 4, 2013.

da Silva L, McCray S. Vitamin B$_{12}$: no one should be without it. *Practic Gastroenterol.* 2008;XXXIII(1):34. Accessed March 4, 2013.

DiBaise JK. Small intestinal bacterial overgrowth: nutritional consequences and patients at risk. *Prac Gastroenterol.* 2008; XXXII(12):15. Accessed March 4, 2013.

McCray S. Lactose intolerance: considerations for the clinician. *Prac Gastroenterol.* 2003;XXVII(2):21. Accessed March 4, 2013.

Parrish CR, Yoshida C. Nutrition intervention for the patient with gastroparesis: an update. *Prac Gastroenterol.* 2005;XXIX(8):29. Accessed March 4, 2013.

Radigan A. Post-gastrectomy: managing the nutrition fall-out. *Prac Gastroenterol.* 2004;XXVIII(6):63. Accessed March 4, 2013.

Ukleja A. Dumping syndrome. *Prac Gastroenterol.* 2006; XXX(2):32. Accessed March 4, 2013.

Bariatric (Gastric Bypass) Surgery

Andris DA. Surgical treatment for obesity—ensuring success. *J WOCN.* 2005;32:393-401.

Boza C, Gamboa C, Salinas J, et al. Laparoscopic roux-en-Y gastric bypass versus laparoscopic sleeve gastrectomy: a case-control study and 3 years of follow-up. *SOARD.* 2012;8:243-249.

Buchwalk H. Overview of bariatric surgery. *J Am Coll Surg.* 2002; 194(3):367-375.

Doolen JL, Miller SK. Primary care management of patients following bariatric surgery. *J Am Acad Nurse Pract.* 2005;17(11):446-450.

Mitka M. Surgery for obesity. *JAMA.* 2003;289(14):1761-1762.

National Institute of Diabetes, Digestive, and Kidney Diseases (NIDDK) of the National Institutes of Health. *Gastric surgery for severe obesity.* Retrieved March 15, 2013 from http://win.niddk.nih.gov/publications/PDFs/gasurg12.04bw.pdf.

Nguyen NT, Nguyen B, Gebhart A, et al. Changes in the makeup of bariatric surgery: anational increase in use of laparoscopic sleeve gastrectomy. *J Am Coll Surg.* 2013;216(2):252-257.

Parikh M, Issa R, McCrillis A, et al. Surgical strategies that may decrease leak after laparoscopic sleeve gastrectomy. A systematic review and meta-analysis of 9991 cases. *Ann Surg.* 2013;257(2): 231-237.

Rusch MD, Andris DA. Maladaptive eating and poor dietary compliance after weight loss surgery. *NCP.* 2007;22(1):41.

Rusch MD, Andris D, Wallace JR. Reasons for failed weight loss surgery. *Clin Nutr Insight.* 2009;35(1):1.

Sakran N, Goitein D, Raziel A, et al. Gastric leaks after sleeve gastrectomy: a multicenter experience with 2,834 patients. *Surg Endosc.* 2013;27:240-245.

Saul D, Stephens D, de Cassia Hofstatter R, et al. Preliminary outcomes of laparoscopic sleeve gastrectomy in a veterans affairs medical center. *Am J Surg.* 2012;204:e1-e6.

Still CD. Before and after surgery: the team approach to management. *J Fam Prac.* 2005;54(3). Retrieved March 13, 2013 from http://www.findarticles.com/p/articles/mi_m0689/is_3_54/ai_n13783681

Vidal P, Ramon JM, Goday A, et al. Laparoscopic gastric bypass versus laparoscopic sleeve gastrectomy as a definitive surgical procedure for morbid obesity. Midterm results. *Obes Surg.* 2012:e1-e8.

von Drygalski A, Andris DA. Anemia after bariatric surgery: more than just iron deficiency. *NCP.* 2009;24(2).

von Drygalski A, Andris DA, Nuttleman PR, et al. Anemia after bariatric surgery cannot be explained by iron deficiency alone: results of a large Cohort study. *SOARD.* 2011;7:151-156.

Watkins BM, Montgomery KF, Ahroni JH, et al. Adjustable gastric banding in an ambulatory surgery center. *Obes Surg.* 2005;15(7):1045-1049.

RENAL SYSTEM

15

Carol Hinkle

KNOWLEDGE COMPETENCIES

1. Describe the etiology, pathophysiology, clinical presentation, patient needs, and principles of management of acute renal failure (ARF).

2. Differentiate between the three types of ARF:
   - Prerenal
   - Intrarenal
   - Postrenal

3. Compare and contrast the pathophysiology, clinical presentation, patient needs, and management approaches of life-threatening electrolyte imbalances:
   - Sodium (Na^+)
   - Potassium (K^+)

   - Calcium (Ca^{++})
   - Magnesium (Mg^{++})
   - Phosphorus (PO_4^{--})

4. Differentiate between the indications for and the efficacy of the different types of renal replacement therapies.

5. Describe the nursing interventions for patients undergoing renal replacement therapy.

SPECIAL ASSESSMENT TECHNIQUES, DIAGNOSTIC TESTS, AND MONITORING SYSTEMS

There are a wide variety of diagnostic tests available for use in determining the cause and location of renal dysfunction. The creatinine and blood urea nitrogen (BUN) levels are monitored closely, because these levels and their relationship to each other (BUN:creatinine ratio) provide valuable information about the kidney's filtering ability. The BUN level provides valuable information about the state of renal perfusion, whereas the creatinine level is more precise in evaluating actual tubular function. Creatinine clearance is useful for assessing the glomerular filtration rate. Urine Na^+ values vary as the kidneys attempt to retain or excrete water. Urine volume, specific gravity (SG), and osmolality are useful in identifying the kidney's ability to excrete and concentrate fluid. Comparisons of these test values as found in prerenal and intrarenal failure are shown in Table 15-1. These tests help establish a firm diagnosis.

Radiologic tests also give important information about the kidneys. A kidney ultrasound may be used to look for stones or injuries. Both CT and MRI are able to identify tumors, hemorrhage, trauma, and perfusion of the kidney. An arteriogram identifies the vascular system of the kidney and renal artery stenosis.

Physical assessment related to the kidneys includes monitoring of the intake and output, daily weights, and noting a positive or negative fluid balance. Observation of the patient's urine for color, clarity, and odor adds to the assessment. Signs of volume overload may include pulmonary crackles, peripheral edema, jugular venous distention, or an S_3 heart sound. Volume deficit may be denoted by the presence of dry mucus membranes and weak peripheral pulses. The kidneys help control the internal environment of the body, therefore, when kidney function decreases, the progressive care nurse may see changes in most, if not all, body systems.

PATHOLOGIC CONDITIONS

Acute Renal Failure

The most common renal problem seen in acutely ill patients is the development of acute renal failure (ARF), also now called

TABLE 15-1. DIAGNOSTIC TESTS USED IN DIFFERENTIAL DIAGNOSIS OF ARF

Test	Normal Values	Prerenal	Intrarenal
Urine			
Volume	1.0-1.5 L/d	< 400 mL/d	< 400 mL/d
Specific gravity	1.10-1.20	> 1.020	< 1.010
Osmolality	500-1200 mOsm/kg	> 500 mOsm/kg	< 350 mOsm/kg
Sodium	40-220 mEq/L/24 hours	< 20 mEq/L	> 30 mEq/L
Fe Na	1%-2%	< 1%	>2%-3%
Serum			
BUN	7-18 mg/dL	> 25 mg/dL	> 25 mg/dL
Creatinine	0.5-1.5 mg/dL	Normal	> 1.2 mg/dL
BUN: creatinine ratio	10-20:1	> 20:1	10:1[a]

[a]Both values elevated but ratio constant.

acute kidney injury (AKI). ARF/AKI is the abrupt decrease of renal function with progressive retention of metabolic waste products (eg, creatinine and urea). Oliguria, urine output of less than 400 mL/day, is a common finding in ARF. The development of ARF in the acutely ill patient has an estimated mortality of 30%-80%. Patients who develop ARF due to sepsis have a higher mortality. A history of chronic renal failure (CRF) complicates the clinical course of any illness.

A classification system (Figure 15-1) for the AKI spectrum is Risk of renal dysfunction, Injury to the kidney, Failure of kidney function, Loss of kidney function, and End-stage kidney disease (RIFLE). This system allows patients to be classified by changes in serum creatinine and/or urine output.

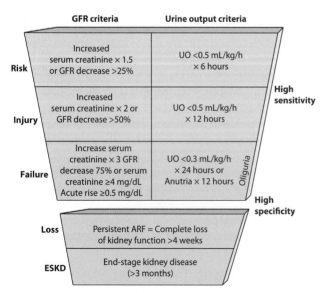

Figure 15-1. Defining characteristics of RIFLE criteria. (*From: Bellomo R, Ronco C, Kellum JA, et al. Acute Renal Failure-Definition, outcome measures, animal models, fluid therapy and information technology needs. Available at: http://ccforum .com/content/8/4/R206. Page R206. Accessed April 1, 2013.*)

Etiology, Risk Factors, and Pathophysiology

Acute renal failure is best understood when the condition is considered in terms of the location of damage to the renal system: prerenal, intrarenal, or postrenal causes of failure. Each type of ARF has different etiologies, pathophysiology, laboratory findings, and clinical presentation.

Prerenal Failure

Physiologic conditions that lead to decreased perfusion of the kidneys, without intrinsic damage to the renal tubules, are identified as prerenal failure (Table 15-2). The decrease in renal arterial perfusion causes a decrease in the rate of filtration of blood through the glomerulus. When perfusion pressure falls less than 70 mm Hg, the protection of autoregulation is lost, further decreasing glomerular filtration.

Renal tubular function, at this point, is still completely normal. As a result of the decreased glomerular filtration rate (GFR), the kidneys are unable to adequately filter waste products from the blood. Consequently, more Na^+ and water are reabsorbed by the kidneys, resulting in oliguria. If the decreased perfusion state persists, irreversible damage to the renal tubules may occur, resulting in intrarenal failure. Most forms of prerenal failure are easily reversed by treating the cause and increasing renal perfusion.

Intrarenal Failure

Physiologic conditions that damage the renal tubule, nephron, or renal blood vessels are identified as intrarenal failure (see Table 15-2). Following prolonged decreases in renal perfusion, the kidneys gradually suffer damage that is not readily reversed with the restoration of renal perfusion. Acute tubular necrosis is the most common form of intrarenal failure.

When the insult to the kidney is nephrotoxic (from drugs or substances that cause direct damage to the kidney), the nephron damage occurs primarily at the epithelial layer. Because this layer has the ability to regenerate, rapid healing often occurs following nephrotoxic insults. When the insult is ischemic or inflammatory, the nephron's basement membrane is also damaged and regeneration is not possible. Ischemic and inflammatory insults are more likely to cause CRF than nephrotoxic insults.

The underlying pathophysiologic abnormality in intrarenal failure is renal cellular damage. In healthy kidneys, the glomerulus normally acts as a filter, preventing the passage of large molecules into the glomerular filtrate. Damage to the glomerulus allows protein and cellular debris to enter the renal tubules, leading to intraluminal obstruction.

Contrast-induced nephropathy (CIN) is seen in about 10% of patients receiving contrast media. It is thought that the contrast media causes renal vasoconstriction. *CIN* is defined as a 25% increase in creatinine or an absolute increase of 0.5 mg/dL. Patients who are at increased risk for CIN include diabetics, the elderly, or those with underlying renal insufficiency. Also, using greater amounts of the media increases the risk of CIN. The rise in creatinine occurs within 24 hours but

TABLE 15-2. CAUSES OF ARF

PRERENAL FAILURE

Hypovolemia
- Burns
- Excessive use of diuretics
- GI losses
- Hemorrhage
- Third spacing
- Shock

Altered Peripheral Vascular Resistance
- Anaphylactic reaction
- Antihypertensive medications
- Neurogenic shock
- Septic shock

Decreased Cardiac Output
- Arrhythmias
- Cardiac tamponade
- Cardiogenic shock
- Heart failure
- Myocardial infarction
- Pulmonary embolism

INTRARENAL FAILURE

Ischemic
- Prolonged decreased renal perfusion
- Septic shock
- Transfusion reaction
- Trauma/crush injury

Nephrotoxic
- Antibiotics
- Fungicides
- Gram-negative toxins
- Pesticides
- Radiographic dyes

Inflammatory
- Acute glomerulonephritis
- Acute vasculopathy
- Acute interstitial nephritis

POSTRENAL FAILURE

Mechanical
- Clots
- Stones
- Strictures
- Tumors

Functional
- Medications
- Neurologic disorders

frequently resolves in 3-5 days. The patient may be oliguric or may have no decrease in urine output.

Postrenal Failure

Physiologic conditions that partially or completely obstruct urine flow from the kidney to the urethral meatus can cause postrenal failure (see Table 15-2). Partial obstruction increases renal interstitial pressure, which in turn increases Bowman capsule pressure and opposes glomerular filtration. Complete obstruction leads to urine backup into the kidney, eventually compressing the kidney. With complete obstruction, there is no urine output from the affected kidney. Postrenal failure is an uncommon cause of ARF in acutely ill patients. The treatment for postrenal failure is focused on removing the obstruction.

Clinical Phases

There are three clinical phases of ARF, seen primarily in intrarenal failure. The first, the oliguric phase, begins within 48 hours of the insult to the kidney. In intrarenal failure, the oliguric phase is accompanied by a significant rise in BUN and creatinine. The degree of elevation of these waste products is less pronounced in prerenal failure. The most common complications seen in this phase of renal failure are fluid overload and acute hyperkalemia. The oliguric phase may last from a few days to several weeks. The longer the oliguric phase continues, the poorer the patient's prognosis.

The diuretic phase follows the oliguric phase. During this phase, there is a gradual return of renal function. Although the BUN and creatinine continue to rise, there is an increase in urine output. The patient's state of hydration prior to the diuretic phase determines the amount of urine output. A patient who is fluid overloaded may excrete up to 5 L of urine a day and have marked Na^+ wasting. The average time in this phase is 7 to 10 days. Patients must be observed carefully for risk of complications from fluid and electrolyte deficits. If the patient receives dialysis during the oliguric phase, the diuretic phase may be decreased or absent.

The recovery phase marks the stabilization of laboratory values and can last 3 to 12 months. Some degree of residual renal insufficiency is common following ARF. Some patients never recover renal function and progress to CRF.

Clinical Presentation

The diverse causes of renal failure determine the clinical presentation of the patient. Renal failure can cause multiple organ dysfunction and, therefore, manifests itself in a variety of ways. Uremia describes the clinical syndrome that accompanies the detrimental effects of renal dysfunction on the other organ systems. The clinical presentation of the patient in uremia reflects the degree of nephron loss and, correspondingly, the loss of renal function.

Signs and Symptoms

- Oliguria (< 400 mL/day) or anuria (< 100 mL/day)
- Tachycardia
- Hypotension (prerenal)
- Hypertension (intrarenal)
- Flat neck veins (prerenal)
- Distended neck veins (intrarenal)
- Dry mucous membranes
- Cool, clammy skin
- Lethargy
- Deep, rapid respirations
- Vomiting
- Nausea
- Confusion

Diagnostic Tests

Laboratory tests are extremely important in diagnosing and evaluating the effectiveness of interventions in the ARF patient. Table 15-1 presents the usual laboratory values seen in prerenal and intrarenal failure.

Principles of Management of Renal Failure

A collaborative approach of the healthcare team to the treatment of patients in renal failure begins with early recognition of patients at risk for renal failure. The focus is on maintaining adequate renal perfusion and avoiding renal compromise.

Much has changed in the prevention and treatment of ARF over the past several decades. These advances have focused on prompt correction of hypotension and the early use of renal replacement therapies (RRTs) before the development of uremia. Once the patient develops ARF, the goal is to quickly reestablish homeostasis by elimination of the underlying cause. Management of ARF also includes correction of fluid imbalance, prevention and correction of life-threatening electrolyte imbalances, treatment of acidosis, prevention of further renal damage, prevention and treatment of infection, and the improvement of nutritional status.

Prevention of CIN involves the use of extensive hydration before and after any procedure using contrast media. There is debate about whether IV normal saline or sodium bicarbonate is best for hydration. Patients who are considered to be at risk for CIN may also receive oral acetylcysteine with their hydration. Diuretics should be avoided during this time. Also, stopping nephrotoxic drugs such as aminoglycoside antibiotics, non-steroidal anti-inflammatory drugs, and chemotherapeutic agents prior to the procedure may be helpful.

Correction of Fluid Imbalance

Maintaining fluid balance in the renal failure patient is a challenge. A fine balance must be achieved in providing the fluid necessary for adequate renal perfusion while preventing fluid overload. It is often difficult to assess if the patient is volume depleted or overloaded. In these cases the patient may be transferred to a critical care unit for placement of a pulmonary artery catheter to assess the patient's fluid status.

1. Calculate daily fluid needs. In prerenal disease, fluid replacement must be matched with fluid loss, both in amount and composition. Insensible fluid losses must be considered in this calculation (Table 15-3). Normal saline volume loading (before a potential insult) of the patient at risk for renal dysfunction is a widely accepted practice. Additionally, volume expansion is beneficial in preventing a volume-depleted patient from progressing to intrarenal failure. In contrast, oliguric patients can rarely tolerate more than 1000 mL of fluid per day. It is often necessary to place constraints on other therapies (eg, IV drug administration, nutritional support) during

---

ESSENTIAL CONTENT CASE

Contrast-Induced Nephropathy

A 74-year-old woman was admitted for substernal chest pain, shortness of breath, and weakness. She has a history of type II diabetes mellitus. She underwent diagnostic cardiac catheterization with successful angioplasty and placement of two stents. She is now 4 hours post-procedure and receiving normal saline at 200 mL/hour. Vital signs are stable and she has had 50 mL urine output.

The next morning, serum creatinine has increased from a baseline of 1.2 mg/dL to 1.8 mg/dL. Urine output has remained marginal at 25-30 mL/h. Normal saline is continuing at 125 mL/h. The physician decides to keep her one more day to monitor her renal status. On the second post-procedure day, serum creatinine remains at 1.8 mg/dL but urine output has increased to 35-40 mL/h. She is discharged to follow up in the office in 3 days.

Case Question 1: What puts this patient at risk of CIN?

Case Question 2: Why is the patient being discharged when the creatinine has not returned to baseline?

Answers
1. The risk of developing CIN includes a history of diabetes, increased age, lack of pre-hydration prior to using contrast medium, and the use of increased amounts of contrast media (ie, related to the length of two procedures done at the same time).
2. The patient is discharged to be followed up as an outpatient because research demonstrates that creatinine returns to baseline within 3-5 days in most patients that develop CIN. However, patients with pre-existing renal insufficiency prior the CIN may develop into CRF.

---

this phase. During the diuretic phase, the patient may require 1 to 4 L of fluid per day to prevent hypovolemia. The patient is frequently allowed to lose more fluid than is replaced in an effort to facilitate fluid movement from the interstitial and intracellular spaces into the vascular space.

2. Obtain accurate intake and output measurements. All insensible losses should be included in the

TABLE 15-3. MINIMAL VOLUMES OF FLUID ASSOCIATED WITH INSENSIBLE FLUID LOSSES

Situation/Condition	Volume
Respiratory losses	500-850 mL/d (dependent on minute ventilation rate)
Fever (loss/°C elevation >38.0)	200 mL
Diaphoresis	500 mL
Diarrhea	50-200 mL/stool

measurements. Fluid therapy decisions are often based on the patient's output.

3. Obtain daily weights. Body weight should be allowed to decrease by 0.2 to 0.3 kg/day as a result of catabolism. If the patient's weight is stable or increasing, volume expansion is suspected. If weight loss exceeds these recommendations, volume depletion or hyper-catabolism is investigated.

4. Administer diuretics when the patient's response is hypervolemic only. Increasing dosages may be used in an attempt to determine the optimal dose. Once the diagnosis of renal failure is established, diuretics may be used to avoid fluid overload and to potentiate the effects of antihypertensive medications. Potassium-sparing diuretics are typically avoided because K^+ elimination is diminished in renal failure. Two commonly used diuretics are mannitol and furosemide. Mannitol, an osmotic diuretic, is used in an attempt to prevent ARF. It causes vasodilation of the renal vessels and expands vascular volume by enhancing movement of fluid from the interstitial space. The benefit of using mannitol once ARF is established is unclear. Mannitol can contribute to fluid overload without excretory renal function and should be used cautiously. Furosemide, a loop diuretic, is the most common diuretic used in ARF. It works by blocking Na^+ reabsorption in the renal tubules, thereby enhancing excretion of Na^+ and water. It is often used to reduce fluid overload and dialysis frequency in ARF. Furosemide is used cautiously in patients receiving aminoglycoside antibiotics because it potentiates the nephrotoxic effects of these medications.

5. Institute RRT as needed. There are three types of RRT available. These include intermittent hemodialysis (IHD), peritoneal dialysis (PD), or the newer continuous renal replacement therapy (CRRT), which includes several varieties of therapy. These are discussed later in this chapter. Sustained low efficiency dialysis (SLED) is considered one of the continuous therapies. These newer therapies may be better tolerated in hemodynamically-unstable patients than peritoneal dialysis or hemodialysis but generally are only done in the critical care unit because of the intensity of monitoring required. However, because some progressive care units (PCUs) may use these therapies, they are included in this chapter.

Preventing and Treating Life-Threatening Electrolyte Imbalances

There are a number of electrolyte imbalances that can occur in renal failure, the most common being hyperkalemia, hypocalcemia, hypermagnesemia, and hyperphosphatemia. In ARF, the electrolyte status guides decisions about the type of fluid replacement and RRT. The management of these electrolyte disorders is detailed later in this chapter.

Treating Acidosis

Renal failure patients often develop metabolic acidosis, with mild respiratory alkalosis compensation.

1. Administer sodium bicarbonate ($NaHCO_3$) as indicated. Treatment is usually not instituted until the serum bicarbonate level drops to less than 15 mEq/L. Even then, replacement of only half the base deficit is made to avoid overcorrection of the pH. Excessive administration of $NaHCO_3$ can cause metabolic alkalosis, tetany, and pulmonary edema.

2. If a patient is being dialyzed, using a dialysate-containing bicarbonate will facilitate buffering of the patient's acidotic state. Dialysates containing bicarbonate are preferred to those with lactate.

Preventing Additional Kidney Damage

In ARF, drugs metabolized or excreted by the kidney require adjustment to avoid excessive blood levels and potential nephrotoxicity. Particular attention must be given to medication scheduling related to RRT schedules. Medications may be eliminated or have their actions potentiated by these therapies. As a result, selected medications, such as antibiotics, are often monitored with peak and trough levels. A clinical pharmacist is a helpful resource on appropriate medication selection, dosing, and monitoring during ARF.

1. Modify medication dosing. Because many medications are eliminated by the kidney, drug administration (dose and schedule) must be altered in the patient with renal failure. Medication dose and schedule decisions are based on the drug and the patient's degree of renal dysfunction. The phase of renal failure and other concomitant treatments help determine the appropriate dose of medication.

2. Administer antihypertensive agents as needed. Hypertension is a major problem for many renal failure patients, often requiring concomitant use of several antihypertensive agents. Most antihypertensive agents are not removed by RRT. During hemodialysis, it is important to adjust the dosage schedule of antihypertensive agents to avoid hypotensive episodes during dialysis. Some antihypertensive agents, however, are eliminated by the kidney. Therefore, dialysis patients receiving these medications require alterations in their dose or dosing schedule.

Preventing and Treating Infection

Renal failure patients are at high risk for infection and are commonly treated with antimicrobial agents. These antimicrobial agents need to be carefully selected and monitored, and often require dosage adjustment. Careful monitoring of both renal function and drug levels during antimicrobial therapy is necessary to avoid further renal damage. Assessment of surgical and line placement sites for signs of inflammation is imperative.

Improving Nutritional Status

The challenge in the management of the renal failure patient's nutritional status is to provide a balance between sufficient calories and protein to prevent catabolism, yet not create problems, such as fluid and electrolyte imbalances or increase the requirement for RRT. The clinical dietician is an important resource for the healthcare team. The typical renal failure patient is hypermetabolic, with caloric needs potentially twice normal. Additional stresses, related to being ill, can further elevate caloric requirements. Nausea and vomiting, common in uremia, further decrease oral caloric intake. Adequate nutrition is also important in preventing infection by helping maintain the integrity of the immune system. Hyperglycemia should be avoided in the patient aiming for a target plasma glucose of 110-149 mg/dL.

1. Restrict the patient's fluid, K^+, Na^+, and protein intake. Because these patients cannot eliminate wastes, fluid, or electrolytes, their dietary intake of these substances is typically restricted. The degree of restriction depends on the cause and severity of their disease; for example, the level of Na^+ restriction is determined by the cause of the renal failure and the serum Na^+ level. Some causes lead to Na^+ wasting and others to Na^+ retention. Phosphorus may need to be restricted and Ca^{++} supplemented if the Ca^{++} level is low in conjunction with normal PO_4^{--} levels.

2. Administer necessary vitamin supplementation. Supplementation of folic acid, pyridoxine, and the water-soluble vitamins is most frequently necessary.

3. Consult a dietitian for a diet plan. Dietary requirements change for patients depending on their renal status and the severity of their underlying condition. Although the precise role of nutrition in ARF is controversial, malnutrition is thought to increase morbidity and mortality. Nutrition, enteral or parenteral, used in conjunction with daily RRT, is thought to improve survival and promote healing of renal tubular cells though enteral nutrition is the preferred route.

The usual approach to hypercatabolic states is to provide adequate proteins and carbohydrates to provide for resynthesis of damaged or lost tissue elements. Protein requirements may range initially from 0.8 to 1 g/kg/day and increase with RRT to 1 to 1.5 g/kg/day to a maximum of 1.7 g/kg/day for patients on CRRT. Nonprotein calories, usually in the form of fat, are given for nonanabolic metabolic needs.

Life-Threatening Electrolyte Imbalances

The kidneys play a major role in the regulation of fluid and electrolyte balance in the body. Regulation of body fluids and electrolytes helps ensure a stable internal environment, resulting in maximal intracellular function. Any renal dysfunction results in abnormalities in both fluid and electrolyte balance.

For all of the electrolyte disorders, the indications for treatment vary from patient to patient. The signs and symptoms of any electrolyte imbalance are not necessarily determined by the degree of abnormality. Rather, the signs and symptoms are determined by the cause of the condition, as well as the magnitude and rapidity of onset. For many of the electrolyte imbalances, it is difficult to determine at precisely what level signs or symptoms may occur.

Sodium Imbalance: Hyperosmolar Disorders
Etiologies, Risk Factors, and Pathophysiology

Serum osmolality, a measure of the number of particles in a unit of blood volume, is an important indicator of fluid status. Because serum osmolality is determined primarily by the serum Na^+ level, evaluation of Na^+ levels provides valuable information on serum osmolality and potential excesses or deficits of total body water. A quick estimate of serum osmolality can be calculated by simply doubling the serum Na^+ value. Normal serum osmolality values are 285 to 295 mOsm/kg. Abnormal serum Na^+ levels are classified as disorders of osmolality, with hyperosmolality referring to high Na^+ levels, which may be indicative of water deficit, or hypo-osmolality referring to low sodium levels, which may be indicative of water excess.

Acutely ill patients often are at risk for disorders of osmolality, with children and the elderly at highest risk. As a person ages, the hypothalamus becomes less sensitive to changes in osmolality and is, therefore, less able to alert the body to abnormalities through normal mechanisms. Additionally, the neurologic signs indicative of osmolality disorders are often ignored or assessed as being related to age rather than to a physiologic abnormality.

Hyperosmolar disorders are the result of a deficit of water. The causes of hyperosmolality include inadequate intake of water, excessive loss of water, or conditions that cause an inhibition of antidiuretic hormone (ADH). In acutely ill patients, hyperosmolar disorders develop because of inadequate intake, usually related to loss of consciousness or endotracheal intubation, and ADH inhibition, as manifested by diabetes insipidus in a patient with a head injury. The signs and symptoms seen are the result of the ensuing cerebral dehydration. Water is pulled from the intracellular space to enhance intravascular volume, leaving the cells dehydrated.

Clinical Presentation
Signs and Symptoms
- Lethargy
- Restlessness
- Disorientation
- Delusions
- Seizures
- Oliguria
- Hypotension
- Thirst

- Tachycardia
- Dry mucous membranes
- Coma

Diagnostic Tests

- Serum Na^+ > 145 mEq/L
- Serum osmolality > 295 mOsm/kg
- Urine SG > 1.030

Sodium Imbalance: Hypo-Osmolar Disorders

Hypo-osmolality disorders are the result of an excess of water. The causes of hypo-osmolality include excess intake or impaired secretion of water, excess ADH as in the syndrome of inappropriate ADH, replacement of volume loss with pure water, and salt-wasting disorders. Hypo-osmolar disorders are extremely common in acutely ill patients, most often related to the use of D_5W IV solutions. Because these patients have often lost some volume, balanced fluid replacement is extremely important. The signs and symptoms seen with hypo-osmolar disorders are related to cerebral intracellular swelling, as water moves from the intravascular to the intracellular spaces.

Clinical Presentation

Signs and Symptoms

- Confusion
- Delirium
- Seizures
- Muscle twitching
- Nausea
- Weight gain
- Headache
- Personality changes
- Coma
- Anorexia
- Vomiting

Diagnostic Tests

- Serum Na^+ < 135 mEq/L
- Serum osmolality < 280 mOsm/kg
- Urine SG < 1.010

Potassium Imbalance: Hyperkalemia

Etiologies, Risk Factors, and Pathophysiology

There are three primary causes of hyperkalemia: increased intake, decreased excretion, and redistribution of K^+ from intracellular to extracellular fluid. Rarely is increased intake a sole cause of hyperkalemia, but it is commonly found in combination with decreased K^+ excretion. The most common causes of hyperkalemia in the acutely ill are ARF, cellular destruction (eg, from crush injuries), and excess supplementation. Because cardiac tissue is sensitive to K^+ levels, hyperkalemia often manifests first as changes in the electrical conduction, demonstrated by changes on ECG tracings. Elevated serum K^+ levels alter the conduction of electrical impulses, particularly in cardiac and muscle tissue.

These conduction abnormalities can lead to serious cardiac arrhythmias and death.

Clinical Presentation

Because K^+ impacts normal neuromuscular and cardiac function, these systems are carefully evaluated when hyperkalemia is suspected. It is important to note that a patient may be experiencing hyperkalemia and may have no ECG or rhythm changes.

Signs and Symptoms

- Vague muscle weakness
- Decreased deep tendon reflexes
- Flaccid paralysis
- Mental confusion
- Nausea
- Diarrhea
- Cramping

ECG Changes

- Tall, tented T waves
- QT interval may shorten
- Intraventricular conduction is slowed
- Widened QRS
- Wide P waves
- Bradycardia
- First-degree atrioventricular (AV) block
- Advanced AV block with ventricular escape rhythms, ventricular fibrillation, or asystole

Diagnostic Tests

- Serum K^+ > 5.5 mEq/L

Potassium Imbalance: Hypokalemia

Etiologies, Risk Factors, and Pathophysiology

The causes of hypokalemia include decreased intake, increased excretion or impaired conservation of potassium, excess or abnormal loss, and increased movement of K^+ into the cells. In the acutely ill patient, hypokalemia is often related to the use of diuretics and excess losses through the gastrointestinal tract. Muscle weakness, including cardiac muscle, is the hallmark sign of hypokalemia. Asystole can result from severe hypokalemia. Depressed levels of serum K^+ lead to increased irritability of cardiac muscle and neuromuscular cells. Serious cardiac arrhythmias, and death, may result from hypokalemia.

Clinical Presentation

Signs and Symptoms

- Weakness
- Respiratory muscle weakness, hypoventilation
- Paralytic ileus
- Abdominal distention
- Cramping
- Confusion, irritability
- Lethargy

ECG Changes

- Ventricular ectopy and flat, inverted T waves
- QT interval prolongation
- U-wave development
- ST-segment shortening and depression

Diagnostic Tests

- Serum K^+ < 3.5 mEq/L

Calcium Imbalance: Hypercalcemia
Etiologies, Risk Factors, and Pathophysiology

The causes of hypercalcemia are threefold: increased Ca^{++} release from the bone, increased Ca^{++} absorption from the gastrointestinal tract, and decreased Ca^{++} excretion.

Clinical Presentation

Signs and Symptoms

- Somnolence
- Stupor
- Nausea
- Anorexia
- Polyuria
- Lethargy
- Coma
- Vomiting
- Constipation
- Renal calculi

ECG Changes

- Arrhythmias
- Shortened QT interval
- Shortened ST segment
- Flat, inverted T waves

Diagnostic Tests

- Serum Ca^{++} > 10.5 mg/dL

Calcium Imbalance: Hypocalcemia
Etiologies, Risk Factors, and Pathophysiology

True hypocalcemia is rare. The causes of hypocalcemia are classified into three categories: decreased absorption of Ca^{++}, increased loss of Ca^{++}, and decreased amounts of physiologically active Ca^{++}. Acutely ill patients may develop hypocalcemia most often related to either gastrointestinal losses or malabsorption. The low Ca^{++} levels result in muscle contraction, seen as tetany, and bronchospasm.

Clinical Presentation

Signs and Symptoms

- Positive Chvostek sign (twitching of the upper lip in response to tapping of the facial nerve)
- Positive Trousseau sign (carpopedal spasm in response to occlusion of circulation to the extremity for 3 minutes)
- Tetany

- Seizures
- Respiratory arrest
- Bronchospasms
- Stridor
- Wheezing
- Paralytic ileus
- Diarrhea

ECG Changes

- Arrhythmias
- Lengthened QT interval
- ST-segment sagging and prolongation
- T-wave inversion

Diagnostic Tests

- Serum Ca^{++} < 8.5 mg/Dl

Magnesium Imbalance: Hypermagnesemia
Etiologies, Risk Factors, and Pathophysiology

Hypermagnesemia is most commonly seen in renal failure patients with an inability to excrete Mg^{++} or with increased intake of Mg^{++} from antacid. ARF is the most common etiology of hypermagnesemia in acutely ill patients. Both neuromuscular and cardiac depressions are observed. Hypermagnesemia may also develop in nonrenal failure situations when Mg^{++} intake is increased, excretion is decreased, or adrenal insufficiency or hyperparathyroidism causes increased Mg^{++}.

Clinical Presentation

Signs and Symptoms

- Respiratory depression
- Hypotension
- Diminished deep tendon reflexes
- Flaccid paralysis
- Drowsiness
- Lethargy

ECG Changes

- Cardiac arrest
- Prolonged PR and QT intervals
- Widened QRS
- Increased T-wave amplitude
- Bradycardia

Diagnostic Tests

- Serum Mg^{++} > 2.1 mEq/L

Magnesium Imbalance: Hypomagnesemia
Etiologies, Risk Factors, and Pathophysiology

Hypomagnesemia frequently occurs in alcoholic and acutely ill patients and is often associated with hypocalcemia and hypokalemia. Hypomagnesemia can be caused by decreased intake, increased excretion, such as with diuretic therapy, and excessive loss of body fluids. The hypomagnesemia seen in the acutely ill is most often the manifestation of a compromised nutritional status, secondary to starvation and malabsorption.

Clinical Presentation

Signs and Symptoms

- Hyperreflexia
- Positive Chvostek and Trousseau signs
- Nystagmus
- Seizures
- Tetany

ECG Changes

- Prolonged PR and QT intervals
- Broad, flat T waves
- Ventricular arrhythmias

Diagnostic Tests

- Serum Mg^{++} < 1.3 mEq/L

Phosphate Imbalance: Hyperphosphatemia
Etiologies, Risk Factors, and Pathophysiology

The most common cause of hyperphosphatemia in all patients, including the acutely ill, is renal failure; the regulation of phosphate in the body is done by the kidneys. Hyperphosphatemia is also seen in hypoparathyroidism, excessive intake of alkali or vitamin D, Addison disease, and with bone tumors or fractures. Hyperphosphatemia is often associated with hypocalcemia.

Clinical Presentation

Signs and Symptoms

- Muscle cramps
- Joint pain
- Seizures

Diagnostic Tests

- Serum phosphate > 4.5 mg/dL

Phosphate Imbalance: Hypophosphatemia
Etiologies, Risk Factors, and Pathophysiology

Hypophosphatemia is caused by hyperparathyroidism, hyperinsulinism, administration of IV glucose, and conditions that cause bone deterioration, such as osteomalacia. This condition is not often seen in acutely ill patients. When seen, it is frequently in conjunction with hypercalcemia.

Clinical Presentation

Signs and Symptoms

- Muscle weakness and wasting
- Fatigue
- Confusion
- Oliguria
- Tachycardia
- Anorexia
- Dyspnea
- Cool skin

Diagnostic Tests

- Serum phosphate < 3.0 mg/dL

Principles of Management of Electrolyte Imbalances
Hyperosmolar Disorders

1. Administer free water. Fluid replacement can be given orally, if feasible, or with intravenous administration of D_5W. The goal is to normalize the serum Na^+ level over a 48- to 72-hour period. A gradual return to normal avoids cellular overhydration.
2. Monitor Na^+ and serum osmolality level frequently. Care must be taken to correct the Na^+ and osmolality level gradually. Correcting these levels too quickly may precipitate hypo-osmolar conditions and seizures.
3. Administer desmopressin (nasally) or vasopressin (IV, IM, subcutaneously) in diabetes insipidus. These medications inhibit the action of ADH.

Hypo-Osmolar Disorders

1. Restrict water intake. Mild, asymptomatic hyponatremia often is not treated or is treated only with a water restriction.
2. Institute RRT. RRT is indicated for severe fluid overload in the presence of renal failure.
3. Administer hypertonic saline. Hypertonic saline may be needed to correct Na^+ levels less than 115 mEq/L when the patient is symptomatic. Careful, slow administration of hypertonic saline is important to avoid sudden shifts in serum osmolality and subsequent hyperosmolality.
4. Monitor Na^+ and serum osmolality levels frequently. Care must be taken to correct these levels gradually. Rapid correction can precipitate hyperosmolar conditions and seizures.

Hyperkalemia

Of all the potential electrolyte disorders, hyperkalemia is considered the most life-threatening because of potassium's profound impact on the electrophysiology of the heart. Hyperkalemia is also the most common reason for initiation of dialysis in the ARF patient.

1. Initiate cardiac monitoring. Because hyperkalemia does affect cardiac tissue, continuous ECG monitoring assists in recognizing cardiac manifestations of altered K^+ levels.
2. Restrict dietary intake of K^+ to 40 mEq/d. A dietary restriction is considered conservative management and is usually instituted in conjunction with other therapies aimed at removing K^+ from the body.
3. Administer cation-exchange resins. Sodium polystyrene sulfonate (Kayexalate) is used to increase K^+ excretion and is administered by mouth or enema with sorbitol. Sorbitol acts to draw fluid into the bowel where the polystyrene causes an exchange

between Na^+ and K^+ ions. The K^+ is then eliminated from the body through feces.

4. Administer hypertonic (50%) glucose and regular insulin. Insulin acts to drive K^+ into the cells on a temporary basis, thereby protecting the heart from the effect of the elevated serum (extracellular) K^+ level.

5. Administer $NaHCO_3$. Its administration causes movement of K^+ temporarily into the cell, encouraging the exchange of hydrogen (H^+) ion inside the cells with the excess K^+ ion outside the cell.

6. Administer calcium salts, such as calcium gluconate. Calcium elevates the stimulation threshold, protecting the patient from the negative myocardial effects of hyperkalemia. The administration of calcium does not change the level of K^+ in the extracellular fluid.

7. Institute RRT. Hemodialysis may be necessary for rapidly removing K^+ when the patient's K^+ level cannot be controlled by other methods.

Hypokalemia

1. Administer K^+ supplementation. Depending on the severity of the deficit, oral or IV replacements can be utilized. Ideally, IV supplementation of K^+ is given through a central line due to the irritating nature of K^+ to the tissues. Potassium replacement is given in at least 50 mL of fluid with no more than 20 mEq replaced per hour. It is common for patients to be unable to tolerate more than 10 mEq/h if the supplementation is given peripherally. Because K^+ is primarily an intracellular cation, allow at least 1 hour after administration for the movement of the K^+ into the cells before evaluating the serum K^+ level. A level obtained too quickly after supplementation is completed may reflect an artificially high serum value. Also, hemolysis may occur during blood draws resulting in an artificially high level.

2. Evaluate the patient's diuretic therapy.

Hypercalcemia

1. Administer normal saline IV and diuretics. In the presence of normal renal function, normal saline infusions given with diuretics increase the GFR and enhance Ca^{++} excretion from the kidneys.

2. Administer corticosteroids. Corticosteroids decrease absorption of Ca^{++} from the gastrointestinal tract.

3. Administer plicamycin. Plicamycin increases the bone uptake and storage of Ca^{++}.

4. Administer oral phosphate (PO_4^{--}) supplementation. PO_4^{--} binds Ca^{++} so that it is excreted in stool.

Hypocalcemia

1. Administer Ca^{++} supplementation. Calcium-containing antacids may be used. Often Ca^{++} supplementation is done concurrently with the administration of PO_4^{--}

binders, such as aluminum hydroxide. There is a reciprocal relationship between Ca^{++} and PO_4^{--} levels in the body. Calcium may be given orally in the form of antacids or intravenously as calcium gluconate or calcium chloride when symptoms are serious.

2. Administer vitamin D supplementation. Vitamin D is necessary for Ca^{++} to be absorbed from the gastrointestinal tract.

3. Institute seizure precautions. Patients with hypocalcemia are at risk for developing tetany and seizures.

Hypermagnesemia

1. Institute RRT. See later under Hyperphosphatemia.

2. Discontinue use of Mg^{++}-containing antacids.

3. Administer normal saline and diuretics. If the patient has normal renal function, the administration of saline and diuretics increases GFR and enhances excretion of Mg^{++}.

4. Administer calcium gluconate intravenously.

Hypomagnesemia

1. Administer Mg^{++} supplementation. Oral administration or Mg^{++} sulfate IM or IV may be used. IV Mg^{++} should not be given faster than 150 mg/min. Total daily replacement should not exceed 30 to 40 g.

2. Reduce auditory, pressure, and visual stimuli.

Hyperphosphatemia

1. Administer aluminum hydroxide-binding gels. These gels bind with phosphate in the intestine, limiting the absorption, promoting excretion, and decreasing the serum level.

2. Institute RRT. If the patient is symptomatic, hemodialysis is the most effective choice to rapidly decrease the serum levels.

3. Administer acetazolamide. Acetazolamide increases the urinary excretion of phosphate.

Hypophosphatemia

1. Administer phosphate supplementation. Supplementation can be administered by mouth or IV.

2. Discontinue use of phosphate-binding gels.

RENAL REPLACEMENT THERAPY

For many years, hemodialysis and peritoneal dialysis were the only therapies available to manage renal failure or situations in which the patient becomes volume overloaded. Many acutely ill patients cannot tolerate the rapid fluid and electrolyte shifts associated with traditional hemodialysis because of hemodynamic instability and cardiac arrhythmias. Peritoneal dialysis, an option for patients who cannot tolerate the hemodynamic changes associated with hemodialysis, is limited to patients without recent abdominal incisions, respiratory distress, or bowel perforations.

Several alternative therapies to manage acute fluid and electrolyte problems have been introduced during the past 25 years, beginning with continuous arteriovenous hemofiltration (CAVH). A number of additional CRRTs have been introduced, offering more treatment options for the acutely ill patient with renal failure or fluid overload. These therapies include using a double-lumen venous access and a pump for continuous venovenous hemofiltration (CVVH) and the addition of dialysate for continuous venovenous hemodialysis (CVVHD). Continuous venovenous hemodiafiltration (CVVHDF) combines the principles of CVVH and CVVHD. Some patients may benefit from high-volume hemofiltration to promote even higher clearances of substances from the bloodstream. Using CRRT, many of the desirable outcomes of hemodialysis can be accomplished without the associated hemodynamic instability. Slow low efficiency dialysis (SLED) involves using hemodialysis at lower flow rates usually over a 12-hour period at night. This therapy decreases the large fluid shifts problematic for the hemodynamically-unstable patient.

The goal of any type of RRT is the removal of excess fluid and uremic toxins and correction of electrolyte imbalances. Each of the RRT methods is able to accomplish that goal, with varying levels of success. These homeostatic corrections are accomplished through the processes of diffusion, osmosis, filtration, or convection. Diffusion, the process by which substrates move from an area of high concentration to one of a lesser concentration, provides for movement of fluids and electrolytes from the body into the filtrate. Through osmosis, water from an area of lesser solute concentration moves to an area of greater solute concentration, becoming part of the filtrate. Filtration also occurs, allowing for movement of water and solute as a result of a difference in hydrostatic pressure. Convection involves the movement of fluids and solutes being pushed through a membrane by pressure and creating a drag, which pulls larger particles along with the fluid.

Renal replacement therapies are grouped into three general categories: those requiring arteriovenous access, those requiring venous access only, or those requiring a peritoneal access (Table 15-4). RRT is applied for periods of 4 hours or more, with some requiring continuous use. Except for peritoneal dialysis, all of the RRT devices require extracorporeal blood flow. This flow is accomplished through the use of two catheters, one arterial and one venous, or through a single venous catheter with two lumens. Filtration and dialysis occur as the blood moves through a dialyzer or hemofilter.

Access

Before any type of RRT can be performed, access to the bloodstream or peritoneum is necessary. The type of access is determined by the reason for initiation and method of renal replacement. It can be either temporary or permanent.

Permanent Vascular Access

Permanent access is achieved by placement of either an arteriovenous fistula or graft. A fistula is a surgically created anastomosis between an artery, usually the radial, brachial, or femoral, and an adjacent vein. This anastomosis allows arterial blood to flow through the vein, causing venous enlargement and engorgement. Permanent access is necessary for patients requiring chronic dialysis.

Arteriovenous grafts are placed in patients who do not have adequate vessels to create a fistula. A prosthetic graft is implanted subcutaneously and used to anastomose an artery to a vein. A period of maturation, usually 2 to 3 weeks, is necessary before the access can be used. This maturation time allows for the venous side to dilate and the vessel wall to thicken, permitting repeated insertion of dialysis needles.

TABLE 15-4. SUMMARY OF RENAL REPLACEMENT THERAPIES

Type	Indications	Contraindications	Complications
Hemodialysis	Life-threatening fluid/electrolyte imbalances Renal failure Poisoning/drug overdose	Hemodynamic instability Hypovolemia Coagulation disorders	Blood loss
Peritoneal dialysis	Fluid/electrolyte imbalances Renal failure	Recent abdominal surgery Abdominal adhesions Peritonitis Respiratory distress Pregnancy	Peritonitis
Continuous renal replacement therapy SCUF CVVH CVVHD CVVHDF SLED	Fluid/electrolyte imbalances Renal failure Fluid overload	Need for emergent therapy	Filter clotting Worsening uremia for SCUF

Abbreviations: CVVH, continuous venovenous hemofiltration; CVVHD, continuous venovenous hemodialysis; CVVHDF, continuous venovenous hemodiafiltration; SCUF, slow continuous ultrafiltration; SLED, slow low efficiency dialysis

Temporary Vascular Access

Temporary access to the bloodstream is obtained through cannulation of an artery and/or a large-diameter vein, with a large-bore, double- or single-lumen catheter specifically designed for dialysis. These catheters are inserted and maintained similar to other arterial and central venous devices, but are generally larger and used primarily for dialysis treatments. A single double-lumen catheter is more commonly used than a single-lumen, single-vessel catheter to maximize the filtration and dialysis capabilities of the renal replacement devices. These catheters can be used for extended periods of time with meticulous attention to sterile technique. The location for catheter placement is chosen to maximize blood flow and prevent kinking of the catheter with patient movement. To initiate hemofiltration (CVVH), hemodialysis (CVVHD), or hemodiafiltration (CVVHDF), a single 14- to 16-gauge double-lumen catheter is placed in the subclavian, jugular, or femoral vein. The jugular is the preferred site and the subclavian is the least preferred site.

Peritoneal Access

Peritoneal catheters are made of silastic tubing, with multiple perforations to allow for fluid exchange, and an attached cuff, soft disk, or balloon to anchor the catheter. When peritoneal dialysis needs to be initiated immediately, a rigid stylet, designed for single acute use only, is inserted. Both types of catheters are inserted through small incisions in the abdomen and threaded into the peritoneal space.

Dialyzer/Hemofilters/Dialysate

There are a variety of dialyzers and hemofilters available for use. The type of dialyzer or hemofilter chosen is determined by the patient's condition and desired outcomes of the RRT. All dialyzers have a blood and dialysate compartment, separated by a semipermeable membrane. The dialyzer has two inlet ports and two outlet ports, one each for blood and dialysate. During dialysis, blood and dialysate are pumped through the dialyzer in opposite directions.

Hemofilters are made of highly permeable hollow fibers or plates. These fibers or plates are surrounded by an ultra-filtrate space and have arterial and venous blood ports. Plasma water and certain solutes are separated from the blood by the hemofilter and drain into a collection device.

Dialysate solution, used in any therapy that has dialysis as a component, is specifically designed to create concentration gradients so that optimal removal of wastes, acid-base and electrolyte balance, and maintenance of extracellular fluid balance can be achieved. The specific solution is determined by the patient's condition and desired outcomes. Although standard solutions may initially be used, they can be tailored to meet the individual patient's needs and contain varying concentrations of Na^+, K^+, Mg^+, Ca^{++}, Cl^-, glucose, and buffers.

Procedures

Hemodialysis and Sustained Low Efficiency Dialysis

Initiation of hemodialysis or SLED through a temporary access is accomplished using a procedure called *coupling*. During coupling, the dialysis catheter and the dialysis circuitry are connected, using sterile technique. To initiate dialysis through a permanent access, two 14- or 16-gauge needles are inserted into the dilated vein of the fistula or the graft portion of the synthetic graft. One needle is considered arterial, used for blood outflow, and the other is considered venous, used for blood return.

The basic components of a hemodialysis system are shown in Figure 15-2. Blood, leaving the patient through the arterial needle, is pumped through the circuitry and returned to the patient through the venous needle. A blood pump moves the blood through the dialysis circuitry and dialyzer, allowing for different flow rates. Both arterial and venous pressures are monitored in the circuitry.

Peritoneal Dialysis

Peritoneal dialysis is accomplished through a series of cycles or exchanges. The dialysate, administered into the peritoneal cavity, remains in the cavity for a preset amount of time (dwell time) and then is drained. Each set of these activities is called a cycle or exchange. Dialysate flows into the peritoneal cavity by gravity, taking approximately 10 minutes for 2 L of fluid to infuse. During the dwell time, diffusion, osmosis, and ultrafiltration occur. Dwell times are based on patient need. With an optimally functioning catheter, it takes 10 minutes for 2 L of fluid to drain from the abdomen. Other forms of peritoneal dialysis include continuous ambulatory peritoneal dialysis (CAPD) and continuous cyclic peritoneal dialysis (CCPD), although these forms are generally not used in the PCU. However, if the patient uses this type of therapy at home for CRF, it is possible that it will be continued in the PCU.

Continuous Renal Replacement Therapy

In CRRT, the blood lines are primed with a saline solution with or without unfractionated heparin as an anticoagulant and then attached to the appropriate vascular access catheter arm (one for outflow and one for inflow). Blood is pumped from the outflow side and passes through the hemofilter. The use of anticoagulation (ie, unfractionated heparin or citrate) assists with blood flow and prolongs the filter life. The blood returns to the body via the inflow tubing after fluid and electrolytes are moved into the ultrafiltrate. The ultrafiltrate is collected in a bag after removal. In CVVHD, blood leaves the patient through the outflow catheter and is pumped through a dialyzer rather than a hemofilter. Wastes and fluid are removed and drained into an ultrafiltrate bag. The blood is then returned to the body through the inflow catheter. The dialysate is pumped through the dialyzer countercurrent to blood flow. Figure 15-3 shows the basic setup of CVVHD. In

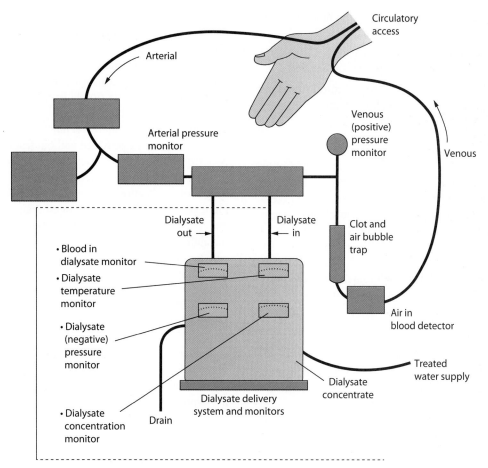

Figure 15-2. Components of a hemodialysis system. (*Reprinted from Thompson JM, McFarland GK, Hirsch JE, et al, eds. Mosby's Manual of Clinical Nursing. St Louis, MO: Mosby; 1989:592, with permission from Elsevier.*)

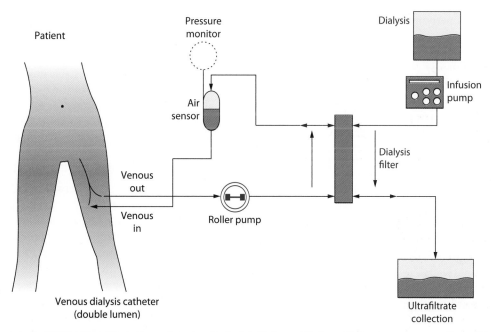

Figure 15-3. Components of a CVVHD system. (*Used with permission from Strohschein BL, Caruso DM, Greene KA. Continuous venovenous hemodialysis. Am J Crit Care. 1994;3:95.*)

CVVHDF, both dialysis fluid and replacement fluids are used to make the system more efficient.

Indications for and Efficacy of Renal Replacement Therapy Modes

Each type of RRT is indicated for different clinical situations and achieves different goals. The goals of therapy are clearly delineated before selection of the type of therapy.

Hemodialysis

Hemodialysis is implemented when aggressive therapy is indicated in acute situations. Hemodialysis is contraindicated in patients with hemodynamic instability (although hypotension may be a relative contraindication), hypovolemia, coagulation disorders, or vascular access problems.

Considered the gold standard for the treatment of ARF and CRF, hemodialysis is the most effective of all of the RRTs. Fluid and uremic wastes can be eliminated from the body during a 4- to 6-hour treatment. Approximately 200 mL of blood is utilized in the circuit, which can add to a patient's unstable condition.

Peritoneal Dialysis

Today, peritoneal dialysis is rarely used for acutely ill patients who need dialysis but are unable to tolerate the hemodynamic changes associated with hemodialysis. CRRT is used instead. Peritoneal dialysis may be performed in a PCU for a patient who is on chronic peritoneal dialysis and presently hospitalized with an acute illness. Utilizing the peritoneal membrane as the dialyzer, effective elimination of fluid and waste products can be achieved. Peritoneal dialysis is slower and less effective than hemodialysis.

Peritoneal dialysis is contraindicated in patients who have had recent or extensive abdominal surgery; who have abdominal adhesions, peritonitis, or respiratory distress; or who are pregnant.

Continuous Renal Replacement Therapy

Patients appropriate for CRRT are chosen after evaluating their clinical diagnosis, hemodynamic parameters, and metabolic status. The specific type of CRRT is selected after considering the patient's fluid and electrolyte status, metabolic needs, and severity of uremia. The most commonly used forms of CRRT are CVVH, CVVHD, or CVVHDF.

Slow Continuous Ultrafiltration

When a slow, continuous ultrafiltration is desired, slow continuous ultrafiltration (SCUF) is the therapy of choice. This therapy is primarily for use in patients with a fluid volume excess and some degree of renal function. Because fluid removal is the primary goal, this procedure is performed without simultaneous fluid replacement. There is a minimal impact on the urea and creatinine levels.

Continuous Venovenous Hemofiltration

The main objective of CVVH is fluid removal. Although large changes in blood chemistries are not expected, it is possible for a patient to achieve and maintain a stable volume and composition of electrolytes in his or her extracellular fluid. The higher the blood flow rate achieved in CVVH, the more solutes that can be removed. Because large volumes of fluid can be removed, the healthcare team has more flexibility in treating patients. Nutrition, a problem in many acutely ill patients, can often be enhanced in these patients because nutrition (even total parenteral nutrition when enteral cannot be tolerated) can be provided without fear of fluid overload.

Continuous venovenous hemofiltration, in some institutions, has become the treatment of choice when patients have contraindications to hemodialysis or peritoneal dialysis. Fluid shifts in CVVH are less rapid than with hemodialysis, making the therapy attractive when persistent hemodynamic instability, especially hypotension, is present. Other patients who may benefit from CVVH are patients with uncontrolled heart failure, pulmonary edema, or hepatorenal syndrome. Patients can be maintained on CVVH for several weeks until either long-term hemodialysis can be initiated or there is return of renal function. There are no absolute contraindications for CVVH. Unfortunately, the therapy has to be discontinued for transportation off the unit such as for selected diagnostic tests (eg, computed tomographic scans) and the continuous nature of the therapy limits mobility, particularly if a femoral access is used (eg, out of bed to chair).

Continuous Venovenous Hemodialysis

Continuous venovenous hemodialysis combines the principles of hemofiltration with a slow form of dialysis (see Figure 15-3). More aggressive removal of fluid and solute is possible than with CVVH. Dialysate is infused through a dialyzer, countercurrent to the patient's blood flow.

The indications for CVVHD are similar to those for hemodialysis. Selection of CVVHD is generally made because a patient is unstable and not able to tolerate the rapid fluid and electrolyte shifts that occur with hemodialysis. CVVHD provides an avenue for these hemodynamically unstable patients to achieve a stable fluid and electrolyte balance without further compromise of their status. There are no absolute contraindications for CVVHD. Maintaining patency of the dialyzer is key to successful CVVHD. Patients with coagulopathies require special monitoring.

General Renal Replacement Therapy Interventions

The frequency of RRT as a therapy in PCUs is on the rise. Some practitioners feel CRRT will replace hemodialysis as the therapy of choice for ARF in the more unstable patient.

Although each therapy has unique characteristics, all require similar interventions. Careful observations and interventions are essential, as is accurate fluid management. Close monitoring of mean arterial pressure, urine output, central venous pressure, daily weights, and state of anticoagulation are critical. Careful monitoring of acid-base and serum chemistries is mandatory. The progressive care nurse assumes a primary responsibility for early recognition and initial interventions for patient and system problems.

SELECTED BIBLIOGRAPHY

General Renal and Electrolyte

Alspach JG, ed. *Core Curriculum for Critical Care Nursing*. 6th ed. Philadelphia, PA: Saunders; 2006.

Candela L, Yucha C. Renal regulation of extracellular fluid volume and osmolality. *Nephrol Nurs J*. 2004;31(4):397-406.

Hinkle C. Electrolye disorders in the cardiac patient. *Crit Care Nurs Clin North Am*. 2011; 23(4): 635-643.

McCance K, Huether S, ed. *Pathophysiology: The Biologic Basis for Disease in Adults and Children*. 6th ed. Maryland Heights, MO: Mosby Elsevier; 2010.

Molzhan A, Butera E, eds. *Contemporary Nephrology Nursing: Principles and Practice*. 2nd ed. Pittman, NJ: American Nephrology Nursing Association; 2007.

Morton P, Fontaine, D, eds. *Critical Care Nursing: A Holistic Approach*. 9th ed. Philadelphia, PA: Wolters Kluwer/Lippincott Williams & Wilkins; 2009.

Schrier RW, ed. *Renal and Electrolyte Disorders*. 7th ed. Philadelphia, PA: Wolters Kluwer/Lippincott Williams & Wilkins; 2010.

Urden LD, Stacy KM, Lough ME, ed. *Thelan's Critical Care Nursing: Diagnosis and Management*. 5th ed. St Louis, MO: Mosby; 2006.

Yucha C. Renal regulation of acid-base balance. *Nephrol Nurs J*. 2004;31(2):201-208.

Renal Failure

Bellomo R, Ronco C, Kellum JA, Mehta RL, Palevsky P, Acute Dialysis Quality Initiative Work Group. Acute renal failure—definition, outcome measures, animal models, fluid therapy and information technology needs: the Second International Consensus Conference of the Acute Dialysis Quality Initiative (ADQI) Group. *Crit Care*. 2004;8:R204-R212.

Broden CC. Acute renal failure and mechanical ventilation: reality or myth? *Crit Care Nurse*. 2009;29(2):62-76.

Cotton AB. Medical nutrition therapy in acute kidney injury. *Nephrol Nurs J*. 2007;34(4):444-445.

Dirkes S. Acute kidney injury: not just acute renal failure anymore? *Crit Care Nurse*. 2011;31(1):37-49.

Druml W. Nutritional management of acute renal failure. *J Ren Nutr*. 2005;15(1):63-70.

Isaac S. Contrast-induced nephropathy: nursing implications. *Crit Care Nurse*. 2012;32(3):41-48.

KDIGO clinical practice guideline for acute kidney injury: acute kidney injury work group. *Kidney Int Suppl*. 2012;2(1):1-138.

Russell T. Acute renal failure related to rhabdomyolysis: pathophysiology, diagnosis and collaborative management. *Nephrol Nurs J*. 2005;32(4):409-417.

Uchino S, Kellum JA, Bellomo R, et al. Beginning and ending supportive therapy for the kidney investigators. Acute renal failure in critically ill patients: a multinational, multicenter study. *JAMA*. 2005;294(7):813-838.

Wood S. Contrast-induced nephropathy in critical care. *Crit Care Nurse*. 2012;32(6):15-23.

Renal Replacement Therapy

Acute Dialysis Quality Initiative. Guidelines for Practice. *Crit Care*. 2004;8:204-212. www.adqi.net. 2004.

ANNA. *Continuous Renal Replacement Therapy: Nephrology Nursing Guidelines for Care*. Pittman, NJ: Anthony Janeppi, Inc; 2005.

Bernardini J. Peritoneal dialysis: myths, barriers and achieving optimal outcomes. *Nephrol Nurs J*. 2004;31(5):494-498.

Dirkes S, Hodge K. Continuous renal replacement therapy in the adult intensive care unit: history and current trends. *Crit Care Nurse*. 2007;27(2):61-81.

Golestaneh L, Richter B, Amato-Hayes, M. Logistics of renal replacement therapy: relevant issues for critical care nurses. *AJCC*. 2012; 21(2):126-130.

Kelman E, Watson D. Preventing and managing complications of peritoneal dialysis. *Nephrol Nurs J*. 2006;33(6):647-657.

Oudemans-van Straaten HM, Wester JP, de Pont AC, et al. Anticoagulation strategies in continuous renal replacement therapy: Can the choice be evidence based? *Intensive Care Med*. 2006;32: 188-202.

Palevsky PM, Baldwin I, Davenport A, Goldstein S, Paganini E. Renal replacement therapy and the kidney: minimizing the impact of renal replacement therapy on the recovery of acute renal failure. *Curr Opin Crit Care*. 2005;11:548-554.

Wooley JA, Btaiche I, Good KL. Metabolic and nutritional aspects of acute renal failure in critically ill patients requiring continuous renal replacement therapy. *Nut Clin Practice*. 2005;20(2):176-191.

Online References

American Society of Nephrology (www.asn-online.org). Accessed April 1, 2013.

National Institute of Diabetes, Digestive, and Kidney Diseases (www.niddk.nih.gov). Accessed April 1, 2013.

U.S. Renal Data Systems (www.usrds.org). Accessed April 1, 2013.

ENDOCRINE SYSTEM | 16

Christine Kessler

KNOWLEDGE COMPETENCIES

1. Outline the nursing management of patients receiving blood glucose monitoring.

2. Describe the etiology, pathophysiology, clinical presentation, patient needs, and principles of management for:
   - Hyperglycemic states

- Diabetic ketoacidosis
- Hyperosmolar hyperglycemic states
- Acute hypoglycemia
- Syndrome of inappropriate antidiuretic hormone secretion
- Diabetes insipidus

SPECIAL ASSESSMENT TECHNIQUES, DIAGNOSTIC TESTS, AND MONITORING SYSTEMS

Blood Glucose Monitoring

Good glycemic control is paramount to improved morbidity and mortality in critically and acutely ill patients. Frequent assessments of blood glucose levels in these patients are commonly performed at the bedside using small quantities of blood obtained from finger sticks, or via arterial lines or central venous catheters. A drop of blood is placed onto a chemical reagent strip and inserted into a portable glucometer (Figure 16-1). This point-of-care (POC) glucometer bedside analysis allows for more rapid interventions of glycemic disorders than is possible from laboratory glucose analysis. Newer technologies have greatly enhanced both the usability and accuracy of bedside glucometers.

Despite the obvious benefits of glucometers and improved technology, inaccuracies of glucose measurements can occur. However, recent studies have found discrepancies of 10% to 36% between glucometer values and laboratory glucose values. While nationally an acceptable discrepancy between glucometer values and laboratory values is +/− 20%, such a variance range may be detrimental. Any large discrepancies between laboratory and the bedside glucometers

should be investigated. This is particularly true when blood glucose values are in the lower ranges. In this instance, a blood glucose reading of 70 mg/dL may actually be closer to 54 mg/dL—a range that may require immediate action. There are many reasons for these discrepancies, but one important reason is that these glucometers were not originally developed or intended for use in critically ill and/or unstable patients. The FDA is currently weighing new, stricter industry guidelines for glucometer efficacy and an acceptable range for POC and laboratory glucose value discrepancies.

Equipment- and Procedure-Related Discrepancies

While POC glucometers were not specifically designed for potentially unstable patients, they do provide timely and reasonably accurate glucose monitoring. One common source of errors in glucose measurement is the incorrect operation of the glucometer device. Other causes may include the use of expired glucose reagent strips or insufficient blood application on the strip. Exogenous glucose contamination of blood samples for testing can also impair testing accuracy. This can happen as a result of an incorrectly withdrawn blood sample from arterial or central venous line. Some researchers have found that arterial sampling may overestimate glucose levels. Also, laboratory glucose analysis errors may occur if venous

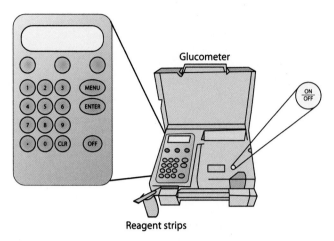

Figure 16-1. Reagent strip and glucometer for bedside testing of blood glucose levels.

sampling is obtained at a site above an intravenous (IV) infusion of a glucose-containing solution. If any doubt exists about the accuracy of the glucometer value, a repeat measurement should be done or a laboratory analysis obtained. Tips for glucometer use are reviewed in Table 16-1.

Patient-Related Discrepancies

Several clinical conditions may influence POC glucose measurements. Shock or hypotensive states, along with vasopressor use, can lead to inadequate tissue perfusion in fingers thereby increasing inaccuracies of fingerstick glucometer analysis (usually overestimation of the blood glucose). Hematocrit levels may also adversely affect glucose levels. A hematocrit value of less than 34% can result in overestimation of blood glucose, while hematocrit values of greater than 55% may lead to underestimation of the blood glucose. Other naturally occurring blood substances can also interfere with glucose measurement accuracy, such as high triglycerides, which are associated with higher glucose levels.

TABLE 16-1. TIPS FOR BLOOD GLUCOMETER (BGM) USE

- Review the manufacturer's guidelines for specific procedures related to the use of your BGM device. User error is the most common reason for inaccurate readings.
- Ensure that the BGM device is calibrated and clean before using.
- Do not use alcohol to clean the machine.
- For patients with cold hands, let the hand hang down below the level of the heart so that blood can flow to the fingertips.
- Obtain a drop of blood and let it be drawn completely onto the reagent pad. Do not smear the blood.
- Use the side of the finger rather than the underpad as it has fewer nerve endings (therefore is less painful) and more capillaries (will get larger drop of blood).
- Correlate the BGM device reading with the clinical assessment of the patient.
- Use universal precautions during the entire procedure.

TABLE 16-2. CLINICAL SITUATIONS THAT MAY AFFECT THE ACCURACY OF POC BLOOD GLUCOSE MEASUREMENTS

Blood glucose levels > 500 mg/dL *(variable error)*
Inadequate tissue perfusion (hypovolemia and shock) *(variable error)*
Vasoactive drugs *(variable error)*
Low blood and skin temperature *(variable error)*
Hct < 30% *(false high reading)* or > 55% *(false low reading)*
High blood triglycerides *(false low reading)*
High uric acid *(false low reading)*
High blood oxygen *(false low reading)*
Acetaminophen use *(false low reading)*
L-dopa use *(variable error)*
Ascorbic acid use *(variable error)*
Icodextrin in peritonea dialysis fluids *(significant false high readings)*

Oxygenation and uric acid levels may result in erroneously low blood glucose levels. Finally, patients receiving certain drugs, such as acetaminophen, L-dopa, and ascorbic acid, may yield erroneous results because the drug may chemically affect some reagent strips. Manufacturers of reagent strips are currently endeavoring to develop strips impervious to drug interference. Clinical situations that may affect the accuracy of POC glucose monitoring are listed in Table 16-2.

Several options may help provide greater accuracy in bedside glucose monitoring. Studies suggest that glucose levels obtained from standing unit-based blood gas and chemistry analyzers, are more accurate than those from glucometers. Because these unit analyzers provide essential chemistry values such as potassium simultaneously with glucose values, they may quickly alert the nurse to critical values; for example, insulin induces a shift of potassium from the extracellular to the intracellular compartment, which can lead to hypokalemia and subsequently life-threatening arrhythmias. Knowing the potassium in conjunction with the glucose level may potentially avert serious patient decline. In cases of instability and/or rapidly changing interventions and treatments, it may be especially important to use a standing POC unit versus a standalone bedside glucometer.

It is possible that continuous glucose monitoring (CGM) devices that are currently used by millions of people with insulin-dependent diabetes in the outpatient setting may one day be accurately used in critically and acutely ill patient populations as well. These devices use subcutaneous glucose sensors and have demonstrated that they optimize insulin therapy, metabolic control, and safety in the outpatient setting. Data from the CGM can be downloaded to a computer for a visual display of the patient's continuous glucose levels, as well as daily and weekly glucose trends. These devices also provide safety benefits as they come with hypo- and hyperglycemia alarms. Currently, only the subcutaneous CGM is FDA-approved; however, in future, intravenous glucose sensors are likely to be developed and available for use in hospitalized patients as well.

Patient Teaching

Prior to hospital discharge, patients requiring ongoing glucose monitoring should be evaluated for competency using the glucometer. It is important to first determine the patient's fasting glycemic goal. Underlying patient morbidities, cognitive skills, frailty, and age affect glycemic target goals. In a relatively healthy outpatient, a target fasting glucose between 85 and 140 mg/dL is usually acceptable. Two-hour postprandial, blood glucose levels should be kept less than 180 mg/dL whenever possible. These goals are achieved through the use of oral hypoglycemic agents, insulin, and in outpatients, injectable incretins (ie, GI hormones that increase the release of insulin from beta cells and enhance proper glucose metabolism). Accurate glucometer measurements are essential to safely achieve glycemic targets.

Ideally, patients should test their blood glucose levels before each meal and at bedtime to evaluate the effectiveness of their therapy, especially if on insulin therapy. This can also improve safety if ongoing insulin dose adjustments are necessary. However, frequent glucose-monitoring schedules may not be feasible, and some patients may struggle with adherence to rigid self-monitoring schedules. In these instances, patients are encouraged to test at least once in a day at alternating times to track glucose patterns. Fasting and preprandial glucose levels, as well as bedtime, postexercise, and 2-hour postprandial glucose measurements are recommended. At the very least, "paired testing" performed once or twice a week can effectively trend blood glucose levels. Paired tests are performed by checking blood glucose just prior to a meal and repeated 2 hours after the meal.

PATHOLOGIC CONDITIONS

Hyperglycemic States

Diabetes is the fourth most common comorbidity plaguing hospitalized patients. This disease, along with the specter of hyperglycemia, carries a legacy of vascular compromise and is associated with a three- to fourfold increase in hospital morbidity and mortality. A more troubling fact is that 12% of patients, without a history of diabetes, will develop hyperglycemia during hospitalization. Unfortunately, these patients have a nearly 18-fold increased risk of in-hospital mortality—far greater than those with known diabetes. This increase in mortality is believed to be related to the patients' exaggerated response to physiologic stress and lack of physiologic resiliency.

Hyperglycemia occurs in hospitalized patients due to natural metabolic responses to acute injury and stress. During acute illness, the liver produces and releases glucose in response to glucocorticoids, catecholamines, growth hormone, and various cytokines (interleukin-6 [1L-6], interleukin-1a [1L-1a], and tumor necrosis factor-alpha). As a result, fat and protein are catabolized and blood glucose surges.

Conditions such as myocardial infarction, stroke, surgery, trauma, pain, and sepsis may cause the release of these biological mediators and counter-regulatory hormones. In essence, the greater the stress response, the higher the blood glucose will be. To help minimize the adverse outcomes associated with hyperglycemia, rigorous glucose monitoring and effective management of blood glucose is essential. This is usually accomplished in critically ill patients utilizing frequent blood glucose testing paired with continuous insulin infusion. Standard infusion protocols, or standing order sets, are often used to maintain glucose values in the targeted range.

Insulin Infusions

A great deal of controversy exists related to how tightly glucose should be controlled in the hospitalized patient. Some studies have shown that tight glucose control using insulin infusions (pre- and postprandial blood glucose target near 110 mg/dL) can improve morbidity and mortality and reduce infections in the critically ill, postsurgical cardiovascular patient population, despite an increased risk of hypoglycemia. Unfortunately, this mortality benefit has not been demonstrated in medical ICU patients or patients in the general wards or progressive care units. In fact, intensive insulin therapy in medical ICU population has been found to slightly increase mortality due to the associated increase in hypoglycemia. Based on these recent findings, the American Diabetes Association and American Association of Clinical Endocrinologists (AACE) have jointly recommended a revised glucose target of 140 to 180 mg/dL in the ICU setting, and between 100 and 180 mg/dL for most patients admitted to general medical-surgical units. In the medical-surgical population, it is advised that preprandial sugars be less than 140 mg/dL and random or postprandial sugars be less than 180 mg/dL.

An insulin infusion is preferable in all hyperglycemic, critically and acutely ill patients, not just those experiencing diabetic ketoacidosis (DKA) and hyperosmolar hyperglycemic states (HHS). Patients at greatest risk are those undergoing major cardiovascular surgery and organ transplants, those with decompensated diabetes (such as DKA and HHS), those in cardiogenic shock or renal failure, and in those receiving high-steroid doses (Table 16-3). These patients often have

TABLE 16-3. COMMON INDICATIONS FOR IV INSULIN INFUSIONS

DKA and nonketotic hyperosmolar state
Critical care illness
Myocardial infarction, cardiogenic shock, and stroke
Postoperative cardiac surgical care
General perioperative care, intra-abdominal surgery, and organ transplantation
Prolonged NPO status in patients with type 1 diabetes
Total parenteral nutrition
Hyperglycemia during high-dose corticosteroid therapy
Labor and delivery
To determine an insulin requirement before initiation of subcutaneous insulin therapy

increased hepatic glucose production, impaired insulin release and sensitivity, and widely fluctuating insulin needs.

IV insulin infusions are also preferred over subcutaneous insulin injections due to erratic tissue absorption in the presence of hypotension, generalized edema, and use of vasopressors. Many hospitals have adopted insulin infusion protocols for use in critical and acute care areas. An effective insulin infusion protocol should incorporate an algorithm that easily adapts to individual patient responses, attains the glucose goal quickly with minimal hypoglycemic risk, and may be used hospital wide. Infusion rates should be increased, decreased, or stopped temporarily based on blood glucose readings and the prescribed algorithm. Whatever protocol is used, it is important to consider the degree of insulin resistance. Patients who are highly insulin resistant may require a much higher hourly infusion rate.

Along with an insulin infusion, hyperglycemic patients will require a tandem infusion of 0.9% normal saline or 5% dextrose and 0.45% normal saline, at a rate commensurate with the patients' fluid requirements. A dextrose solution is always preferred in patients with type 1 diabetes. Most patients will also require simultaneous infusion of potassium as insulin is known to drive potassium into cells, especially into liver and muscle cells, which may increase the risk of hypokalemia.

When the infusion is discontinued, subcutaneous insulin is often started using a basal insulin to cover glucose produced endogenously by the liver. Bolus insulin, also called correctional insulin, is used to cover food intake and intermittent surges of blood glucose. It is essential that all type 1 diabetics receive basal insulin or DKA will ensue. If the patient is to receive subcutaneous, multi-dose insulin (MDI) following the infusion, then both basal and bolus insulin should be provided a minimum of 30 minutes prior to discontinuing the IV as IV insulin disappears from the bloodstream within 5 minutes after discontinuation of IV insulin therapy. It is important to note that the effects of long-acting, basal insulin, such as glargine and detemir, do not appear for several hours after injection and should be administered 2 hours prior to discontinuing the insulin infusion. Insulin actions by type of insulin are listed in Table 16-4. After discontinuation of the insulin infusion POC blood glucose testing should continue before meals and at bedtime in patients who are eating, or every 4-6 hours in patients who are NPO or receiving continuous enteral feeding.

Hyperglycemic Emergencies

Diabetes ketoacidosis (DKA) and hyperglycemic hyperosmolar (HHS) are two extremes in the spectrum of decompensated diabetes. The incidence of DKA is defined as acute hyperglycemia with acidosis, and HHS is classified as acute hyperglycemia without acidosis (nonketotic).

Diabetes is a metabolic disease that results in inadequate uptake of glucose by cells, resulting in hyperglycemia. There are 13 forms of diabetes mellitus (DM) that fall

TABLE 16-4. INSULIN ACTION CHART BY TYPE

Type	Onset	Peak	Duration
Rapid Acting (Bolus)			
Humalog (lispro)	<15 minutes	30-90 minutes	<5 hours
Novolog (aspart)	10-20 minutes	1-2 hours	3-5 hours
Apidra (glulisine)	10-15 minutes	.5-1.5 hours	<3 hours
Humulin R (regular)	40-60 minutes	2-3 hours	4-6 hours
Novolin R (regular)	30 minutes	2-5 hours	8 hours
Intermediate (Basal)			
Humulin N (NPH)	2-4 hours	4-10 hours	14-18 hours
Novolin N (NPH)	90 minutes	4-12 hours	up to 24 hours
Long, "Peakless" (Basal)			
Lantus (glargine)	3-5 hours	minimal	22-26 hours
Levemir (detemir)	2-4 hours	minimal	13-20 + hours

within one or both main diabetes classifications: types 1 and 2 diabetes. Type 1 DM is an autoimmune disorder and often has a juvenile or early adulthood onset, although it can occur at any age. When it occurs in middle or old age, type 1 DM is referred to as latent autoimmune diabetes in adults (LADA). The key disorder in type 1 DM is minimal or absent insulin secretion by the pancreatic beta islet cells. Type 2 diabetes usually occurs in older adults, but can be seen in youth, and is associated with impaired insulin receptor sensitivity. Insulin production in type 2 diabetes may initially be high or normal, then falls dramatically as the disease progresses. Although hyperglycemia is a shared feature, the etiology, risk factors, pathophysiology, and management priorities vary considerably for each classification of diabetes.

Etiology, Risk Factors, and Pathophysiology

Insulin is normally released from the pancreas by beta islet cells (Islets of Langerhans) in response to an increase in blood glucose. Insulin is necessary for cellular uptake of glucose by most cells in the body (except brain and liver cells). Without insulin, the glucose fails to enter cells and accumulates in the blood, resulting in hyperglycemia and a vascular inflammatory state. Cells deprived of glucose begin to starve, triggering a mobilization of stored glucose via the breakdown of protein and fat (gluconeogensis) and release of stored glucose from the liver (glycogenolysis). This triggers a complex series of physiologic processes that account for the major signs and symptoms associated with DKA and HHS.

Diabetic Ketoacidosis

The most common scenarios associated with DKA are underlying or concomitant infection (40%), missed insulin treatments (25%), and newly diagnosed, previously unknown diabetes (15%). Other associated causes make up roughly 20% in the various series. Among the other causes are myocardial infarction, stroke, trauma, and pancreatitis. Although DKA is primarily a complication of type 1 diabetes,

TABLE 16-5. CAUSES OF DKA

Infections (Especially Bladder Infections)
Missed or Inadequate Doses of Insulin (Primarily in Type 1 Diabetes)
Initial Presentation of Type 1 Diabetes
Various Stressors
- Trauma
- Surgery
- Pregnancy
- Acute illness
- Renal failure
- Myocardial infarction/ischemia

Drug Impairment of Glucose Metabolism
- Thiazide diuretics
- Phenytoin
- Beta-blockers
- Calcium channel blockers
- Steroids
- Epinephrine
- Psychotropics
- Salicylate poisoning

it can occur (rarely) in some forms of type 2 diabetes under conditions of extreme stress, including "ketone-prone" type 2 diabetes a disorder found in African American males (Table 16-5).

In general, DKA consists of the biochemical triad of hyperglycemia, ketonemia, and metabolic acidosis (with a large anion gap). This disorder is typically characterized by hyperglycemia (> 300 mg/dL), low bicarbonate level (< 15 mEq/L), and acidosis (pH < 7.30) with ketonemia and ketonuria. While definitions vary, moderate DKA can be categorized by pH of less than 7.2 and serum bicarbonate less than 10 mEq/L, whereas severe DKA has pH of less than 7.1 and bicarbonate less than 5 mEq/L.

DKA can develop in less than 24 hours. The initiating event in DKA is an insufficient or absent level of circulating insulin. This insulin deficiency results in increased fatty acid metabolism, increased liver gluconeogenesis (formation of glucose from amino acids and proteins), and increased secretion of counterregulatory hormones, including glucagon and the stress hormones (catecholamines, cortisol, and growth hormone). These hormones counteract the glucose-lowering effects of insulin and are released in response to stress and other stimuli. The pathophysiology of DKA can be organized into two main components: fluid volume deficit and acid-base imbalance (Figure 16-2).

Fluid Volume Deficit With Associated Electrolyte Imbalance
Because of the insulin deficiency, there is both hyperglycemia and increased amino acid release from cells. The stress response in the body leads to metabolic decompensation, and stress hormones further trigger a rise in plasma glucose and ketones. The hyperglycemia causes an osmotic diuresis and hypotonic losses leading to fluid volume deficits (intracellular and extracellular) and electrolyte losses. As serum glucose exceeds the renal threshold, glycosuria results. In the absence of insulin, protein stores are also broken down by the liver into amino acids and then into glucose for energy. This further increases serum blood glucose, increases urine glucose, and worsens the osmotic diuresis and ketonemia. Urinary losses of water, sodium, magnesium, calcium, and phosphorus cause an increase in serum osmolality and decreased electrolyte levels. Potassium levels may be increased or decreased, depending on the amount of nausea and vomiting, acid-base balance, and fluid status of the patient. This hyperosmolality causes additional fluid shifts from the intracellular to the extracellular space, increasing dehydration. Hypovolemic shock can result from severe fluid losses in DKA. Volume depletion decreases glomerular filtration of glucose and creates a cycle of progressive hyperglycemia. The increase in serum osmolarity also is thought to further impair insulin secretion and promote insulin resistance. The altered neurologic status frequently seen in these patients is due primarily to brain cell dehydration and serum hyperosmolarity.

Acid-Base Imbalance
Cells without glucose starve and begin to use existing stores of fat and protein to provide energy for body processes (gluconeogenesis). Fats are broken down faster than they can be metabolized in the liver, which results in an accumulation of ketone acids. These ketone acids are usually cleared in peripheral tissues. If the ketogenic pathway is overwhelmed ketone acids accumulate in the blood stream where hydrogen ions (H^+) dissociate, causing a profound metabolic acidosis. Acetone is formed during this process and is responsible for the "fruity breath" found in these patients.

Metabolic acidosis may be worsened with severe fluid volume deficits because hypovolemia results in tissue hypoperfusion and production of lactic acids from anaerobic metabolism. Excess lactic acid results in what is called *increased anion gap* (increased body acids). Sodium, potassium, chloride, and bicarbonate are responsible for maintaining a normal anion gap in the body which is normally less than 12 to 14 mEq/L (Table 16-6). The anion gap represents the difference between the cations (Na^+, K^+) and anions (Cl^-, HCO_3^-). Ketone accumulation, a by-product of gluconeogenesis, causes an increase in the anion gap more than 14 mEq/L.

The normal physiologic response to metabolic acidosis is to produce bicarbonate to buffer the ketones and H^+ ions. The patient with DKA often has diminished bicarbonate levels because of the osmotic diuresis. The respiratory system attempts to compensate by blowing off carbon dioxide to restore normal blood pH. This explains the deep rapid breathing, called "Kussmaul respirations," often seen in these patients.

Metabolic acidosis also results in potentially life-threatening electrolyte imbalances. Serum potassium is elevated initially in DKA probably due to potassium shifts from the intracellular to the extracellular space because of the acidosis. Later, hypokalemia is common because of insulin-induced transfer of plasma potassium into cells and increased urinary excretion of potassium with the osmotic diuresis.

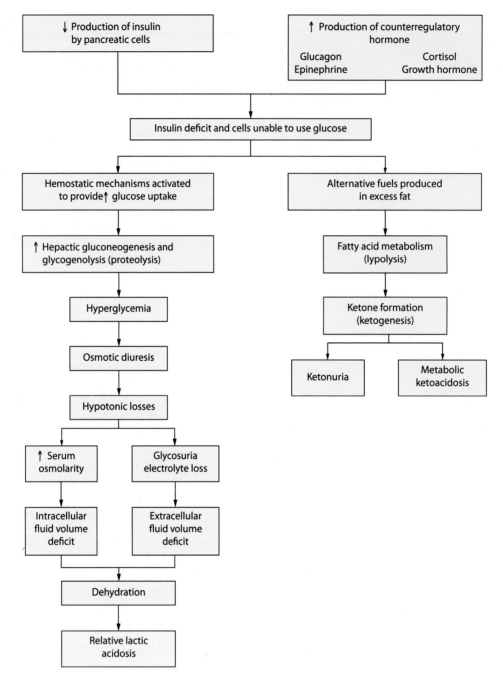

Figure 16-2. Pathogenesis of DKA.

TABLE 16-6. CALCULATION OF ANION GAP (NORMAL <12 MEQ/L)[a]

$Na^+ - (Cl^- + HCO_3^-)$ = anion gap
Example from DKA case study:
    $130 - (94 + 11) = 25$ mEq/L (anion gap acidosis)
Example from HHS case study:
    $152 - (121 + 22) = 9$ mEq/L (no anion gap)

[a]Note: Potassium is often added to the sodium but because it is generally a small number, it is often excluded in the calculation.

Hyperosmolar Hyperglycemic States

The pathogenesis of HHS is similar to the pathogenesis of DKA with the following differences. HHS is classified as hyperglycemia with profound dehydration in the absence of ketosis. The onset of hyperglycemia in HHS is progressive. Many of these patients have a history of type 2 DM with some circulating insulin levels. The extremely severe hyperglycemia in HHS results in profound extracellular fluid volume contraction, marked intracellular dehydration, and excessive loss of electrolytes. In addition, because there is some insulin,

ESSENTIAL CONTENT CASE

Diabetic Ketoacidosis

An 18-year-old woman was admitted to the MICU with a diagnosis of DKA. She was stressed about numerous school examinations, had run out of her basal insulin, glargine, and was only taking random, short-acting insulin to cover her meals, as she neglected to check her blood sugars. During the past 2 days she had been experiencing flu-like symptoms (vomiting, abdominal cramping). On arrival in the ED, she was flushed and vaguely confused, clutching an extralarge cup of diet soda. Significant findings on her admission profile were:

Respiratory rate	38 breaths/min, deep ("fruity" breath)
Blood pressure	98/50 mm Hg
Heart rate	110 beats/min; sinus tachycardia
Skin	Warm and flushed
Arterial blood gases	pH 7.09
$Paco_2$	24 mm Hg
Pao_2	88 mm Hg
HCO_3	11 mEq/L
SaO_2	94%
Serum glucose	440 mg/dL
Serum acetone	4+
Serum ketones	4+
Serum osmolality	310 mOsm/kg
Anion gap	22 mEq/L
Serum potassium	5.2 mEq/L
Serum BUN	28 mg/dL
Serum creatinine	1.5 mg/dL
Serum sodium	130 mEq/L
Serum magnesium	1.1 mg/dL
Serum phosphate	2.2 mg/dL
Serum chloride	94 mEq/L
White blood cell count	14,000/mm³
Urine glucose	2+ (large)
Urine ketone	3+ (large)

Case Question 1. True or False—Intravenous hydration should be given prior to insulin administration.

Case Question 2. True or False—Sodium bicarbonate IV is indicated in this case.

Case Question 3. True or False—Despite a mildly-elevated serum potassium, a tandem IV with potassium should still be added after hydration and an insulin infusion have been initiated.

Answers
1. True
2. False (used if pH is < 7.0)
3. True

ESSENTIAL CONTENT CASE

Hyperosmolar Hyperglycemic State

A 72-year-old man was admitted to the MICU with a diagnosis of hyperglycemic crisis. He lives alone with his small dog. His daughter dialed 911 after finding her father unresponsive at his home. She reported that he had complained of flulike symptoms 3 weeks earlier. His history is significant for heart failure and type 2 DM. His daily medications include carvedilol 6.25 mg orally twice a day, lipitor 40 mg once a day, lisinopril 20 mg orally once a day, furosemide (Lasix) 20 mg orally twice a day, KCl 20 mEq/d orally, and glipizide 10 mg orally twice a day. On arrival in the ED he was comatose. Significant findings on his admission profile were:

Blood pressure	82/44 mm Hg; MAP 56 mm Hg
Heart rate	121 beats/min
Respiratory rate	14 breaths/min, shallow
Skin	Dry, poor turgor; dry mucous membranes
Arterial blood gases on cannula	pH 7.34 2 L/min O_2 per nasal
$Paco_2$	49 mm Hg
Pao_2	56 mm Hg
HCO_3^-	22 mEq/L
Sao_2	88%
Serum glucose	1040 mg/dL
Serum osmolality	362 mOsm/kg
Serum potassium	3.6 mEq/L
Serum BUN	41 mg/dL
Serum creatinine	2.2 mg/dL
Serum sodium	152 mEq/L
Serum phosphate	2.0 mg/dL
Serum chloride	121 mEq/L

Case Question 1. True or False—Because of the extremely high blood sugar, insulin administration should precede IV hydration.

Case Question 2. True or False—The relative metabolic acidosis is related to ketone acid accumulation.

Case Question 3. True or False—The mortality of HHS exceeds that of DKA.

Answers
1. False (Hydration more effectively lowers blood sugar and reduces stroke risk)
2. False (It is due to lactic acid accumulation related to dehydration)
3. True

secretion lipolysis is suppressed. Therefore, there is no overproduction of ketones and no specific physical signs and symptoms of ketosis (no Kussmaul respiration, renal excretion of ketones, abdominal pain, nausea, vomiting, or anorexia). The lack of these emergent signs and symptoms may cause these patients to not seek early treatment. Sustained osmotic diuresis results, leading to massive volume losses, electrolyte imbalance, and central nervous system (CNS) dysfunction. Mortality rates, therefore, are higher with HHS, because of the severe volume loss and because it occurs more frequently in a chronically ill patients. Death results from CNS depression of vital body functions (cardiac and respiratory centers in the brain are depressed), cerebral edema, cardiovascular collapse, renal shutdown, and vascular embolism.

Clinical Presentation

DKA	HHS
History	
Younger with history of type 1 DM or previously undiagnosed; preexisting infection common	Elderly with history of type 2 DM, and preexisting chronic illness which are associated with decreased renal glucose excretion, concurrent illness frequently precipitates viral infections or pneumonia
Signs and Symptoms	
Nonspecific: Polyuria, polydipsia, weakness, abdominal cramping, stupor, coma	Nonspecific: Polyuria, polydipsia, weakness confusion, coma
Specific: Nausea, vomiting, anorexia, Kussmaul respiration, fruity breath	Specific: None
Diagnostic Tests	
Serum glucose 250 to 800 mg/dL (usually < 500)	Serum glucose At least 600 mg/dL often > 1000 mg/dL
Serum osmolality < 330 mOsm/kg/H_2O	Serum osmolality > 350 mOsm/kg/H_2O
Ketoacidosis	Ketoacidosis
↓ pH	Not a feature
Mild: < pH 7.20-7.30	pH > 7.30
Moderate: pH 7.10-7.19	
Severe: pH < 7.09	
HCO_3 < 15 mEq/L	HCO_3^- > 15 mEq/L
Serum ketones > 2+	Serum ketones below 2+
Positive urine ketones	Minimal urine ketones
Positive anion gap > 12	Variable anion gap
Dehydration	Dehydration
Volume depletion (decrease intracellular and extracellular)	Severe volume depletion (intracellular and extracellular)
Renal function	Renal function
Increased BUN: creatinine ratio	Marked increase in BUN: creatinine ratio
Urine ketones +2	↓ GFR
Electrolyte depletion	Electrolyte depletion
Potassium, magnesium, phosphate, calcium	Potassium, magnesium, phosphate, sodium

Principles of Management for Hyperglycemic Emergencies

The management of the patient in acute DKA and HHS revolves around six primary areas: fluid replacement, treatment of hyperglycemia, electrolyte replacement, treatment of any underlying disorders, prevention and management of complications, and patient/family teaching.

Fluid Replacement

Treatment of intracellular and extracellular fluid volume deficits is a priority for both DKA and HHS to restore

TABLE 16-7. CORRECTION OF SERUM SODIUM LEVELS IN THE PRESENCE OF HYPERGLYCEMIA

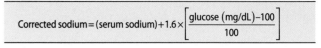

$$\text{Corrected sodium} = (\text{serum sodium}) + 1.6 \times \left[\frac{\text{glucose (mg/dL)} - 100}{100} \right]$$

intravascular volume and prevent cardiovascular collapse. Initial volume replacement is based on assessment of vascular status.

1. Administer normal saline (0.9%). The choice of IV fluid depends on the initial blood pressure readings and the serum sodium level. The presence of hyperglycemia and dehydration masks the true serum sodium level, requiring a correction of serum sodium levels prior to IV fluid selection (Table 16-7). IV fluids are generally infused at rapid rates (1000 to 2000 mL in the first hour, 1000 mL in the second hour, and then at 500 mL/h) until fluid volume is restored or initially around 15 to 20 mL/kg/h.

2. Titrate the rate of infusion based on urine output, mean arterial blood pressure, and central venous pressure measurements. Typically, the patient with HHS has more profound fluid volume deficits, but because the patient is older and often has other underlying medical problems, the rate of fluid replacement needs to be carefully titrated. Serum glucose falls with initiation of fluids alone. It is critical that insulin therapy not be started without simultaneously correcting the fluid deficit. Otherwise, the result is an acute loss of vascular volume, worsening of the hypernatremia, shock, and increased risk of mortality.

3. Change IV fluid to 5% dextrose with 0.45 NaCl at 150 to 200 mL/h when serum glucose reaches 250 mg/dL. Maintain insulin therapy.

Treating Hyperglycemia

In both DKA and HHS some insulin replacement is needed, although the requirements in DKA are typically lower than HHS.

1. Regular insulin 0.15 U/kg as IV bolus.

2. Initiate low-dose IV insulin at a rate of 0.1 U/kg/h. If serum glucose does not fall by 50 to 70 mg/dL in the first hour, double insulin infusion on an hourly basis until glucose falls by 50 to 70 mg/dL.

3. Monitor serum glucose levels closely and titrate insulin infusion accordingly. Once the serum glucose reaches 250 mg/dL, the insulin infusion should be decreased to a rate of 2 to 4 U/h and the IV fluids changed to half normal saline with glucose (D5-1/2NS). This ensures that hypoglycemia does not occur during ongoing treatment of the acute condition. It is essential that insulin infusion continues in the patient with DKA

until the serum pH is corrected to avoid intracellular hypokalemia. Additional glucose may be needed to achieve this outcome. Glucose-containing solution should also be started in the patient with HHS when serum glucose reaches 250 to 300 mg/dL to protect against cerebral edema.

Electrolyte Replacement

Electrolyte deficits are usually present in both DKA and HHS due to the osmotic diuresis. Hypokalemia may be masked by acidosis. Potassium levels rise 0.6 mEq/L for every 0.1 drop in pH.

1. Administer potassium supplements according to serum levels:
   - If serum K^+ is < 3.3 mEq/L, hold insulin and administer 40 mEq K^+/h (2/3 KCl and 1/3 KPO_4^-) until K^+ is > 3.3 mEq/L.
   - If serum K^+ is > 5.0, hold K^+ and check K^+ every 2 hours.
   - If serum K^+ is > 3.3 mEq/L or < 5.0 mEq/L give 20 to 30 mEq K^+ in each liter of volume replacement.

   Replacement of potassium is a priority during the correction of hyperglycemia to avoid hypokalemia during rehydration, when potassium moves into the cell along with glucose. To avoid cardiac arrhythmias associated with hypokalemia, delay insulin administration until serum potassium levels are greater than 3.3 mEq/L. The rate of potassium chloride infusion should be adjusted according to frequently monitored serum potassium levels and the urine output.

2. Monitor magnesium, calcium, and phosphate levels every 2 hours during rehydration. Hemodilution may further decrease serum levels of these electrolytes. Magnesium and calcium replacements are given based on serum levels. Total body phosphorous levels are depleted due to osmotic diuresis. This may result in impaired cardiac and respiratory functions. Phosphate deficiencies are usually corrected with volume replacement. If needed, the administration of potassium phosphate 20 mEq/L is the best method of phosphate replacement as it replaces both potassium and phosphate simultaneously. Phosphate replacements should not be administered in patients with renal failure. If hypokalemia is refractory to potassium replacement, magnesium replacement should be considered.

3. Assess need for bicarbonate therapy:
   - If pH is < 6.9, dilute $NaHCO_3^-$ (100 mmol) in 400 mL H_2O. Infuse at 200 mL/h.
   - If pH is 6.9 to 7.0, dilute $NaHCO_3^-$ (50 mmol) in 200 mL H_2O. Infuse at 200 mL/h.
   - If pH is > 7.0, hold $NaHCO_3^-$.

   Repeat HCO_3 administration every 2 hours until pH is > 7.0. Monitor serum K^+ closely.

Treating Underlying Disorders

The precipitating cause for the hyperglycemic emergency needs to be determined. Underlying infection is a common precipitating factor in both DKA and HHS.

1. Investigate precipitating factors utilizing the following tests: urinalysis, complete blood count, ECG, chest x-ray, and appropriate cultures. Administer antibiotics as appropriate if infection is suspected.
2. Obtain history from patient and family about the possibility of missed insulin doses.

Preventing and Managing Complications

1. Monitor serum glucose, electrolytes (sodium and potassium), and arterial blood gases every 1 to 2 hours until normal levels are attained.
2. Measure serum phosphate and magnesium initially and repeat as necessary.
3. Monitor temperature, blood pressure, pulse, respiratory rate, pulse oximetry, urinary output, and central venous pressure at frequent intervals.
4. Evaluate neurologic status at frequent intervals. Institute seizure precautions if cerebral edema is suspected. Institute measures to avoid aspiration in patients with altered mental status. Administer dexamethasone and mannitol if appropriate.
5. Titrate fluid replacement carefully to prevent heart failure. Auscultate lung sounds frequently during fluid replacement.
6. Administer anticoagulants as ordered. Hyperosmolar patients are at great risk for developing thrombosis.

Patient and Family Education

Particularly in type I DM, the key to prevention of recurrent DKA is adequate patient education regarding diabetes management. Contact the diabetes educator (if available) to help teach the skills needed to manage diabetes once the patient is stable and ready to receive information. Table 16-8 outlines the required skills for diabetic management. Return demonstrations by the patient or designated caregiver are essential.

TABLE 16-8. SKILLS FOR DIABETIC MANAGEMENT

Blood glucose monitoring
Insulin administration
Diet therapy
Meal planning
Exercise therapy
Urine ketone testing
Sick day management
Recognition of signs and symptoms of hypoglycemia and hyperglycemia
Proper treatments for hypoglycemia and hyperglycemia

Expected Outcomes
1. The patient or caregiver will be able to verbalize essential aspects of diet therapy, meal planning, exercise therapy, sick day management, signs and symptoms of hypoglycemia and hyperglycemia, and proper treatments for hypoglycemia and hyperglycemia.
2. The patient or caregiver will be able to demonstrate blood glucose monitoring, insulin administration, and urine ketone testing.

Instruction regarding the need for routine medical follow-up and the availability of hospital and community resources is also an important component of the diabetes management plan. The patient is typically discharged on the inpatient insulin doses (via multiple dose insulin or insulin pump). Sometimes a patient who was on pre-admission insulin may resume the pre-admission doses unless an adjusted dose is required due to weight loss, decreased renal function, or marked increase in exercise (typically less insulin is required with those conditions).

Patients with type 2 diabetes treated for HHS are typically discharged with basal or basal/bolus insulin. This may be a temporary mode of therapy until the effects of glucose toxicity abate. In the presence of good renal function, these patients may also be discharged on metformin for its insulin sensitizing effects. All hospitalized patients treated for hyperglycemia need follow up with their primary care provider and/or an endocrinologist soon after discharge.

Acute Hypoglycemia

Hypoglycemia is a blood glucose level less than 60 mg/dL and is a common endocrine emergency. Hypoglycemia results from the imbalance between glucose production and glucose utilization. Of the acute complications, hypoglycemia is most common in insulin-dependent (types 1 and 2) diabetics. It also can occur with type 2 diabetics who are treated with oral hypoglycemic agents, especially sulfonylureas like glipizide, glyburide, and glimepiride.

Etiology, Risk Factors, and Pathophysiology

Hypoglycemia can be divided into two categories: fasting hypoglycemia (> 5 hours after a meal) and postprandial hypoglycemia (1-2 hours after a meal) (Table 16-9). *Fasting hypoglycemia* occurs when the normal physiologic response (gluconeogenesis and glycogenolyisis) to a falling glucose level is altered and there is an imbalance in glucose production and utilization. Hypoglycemia in a diabetic person is most commonly caused by excessive insulin or oral hypoglycemic agent,

TABLE 16-9. CAUSES OF HYPOGLYCEMIA (PARTIAL LISTING)

Fasting Hypoglycemia
Excessive insulin dosage
Decreased need for insulin
  Decreased food intake
  Increased exercise
  Renal failure/dialysis
  Liver failure
  Heart failure
Drugs
  Oral hypoglycemic agents
  Alcohol and alcohol binges
  Salicylates
  Beta-adrenergic blockers

Postprandial Hypoglycemia
Excessive insulin effect
Postgastric surgery

too much exercise, or not enough caloric intake. Exercise can lead to increased insulin sensitivity immediately or hours later as sugar moves readily into muscles. One cause of postprandial hypoglycemia is gastric bypass surgery because surgical alterations cause smaller amounts of foods to be ingested and this food passes more rapidly through the small intestine. In addition, the resultant rapid weight loss decreases insulin resistance further, increasing the risk of hypoglycemia.

Glucose is the obligate fuel for the brain and CNS. The brain is unable to synthesize or store glucose and must rely on circulating plasma blood glucose levels for survival. As blood glucose declines rapidly, epinephrine, glucagon, glucocorticoids, and growth hormones are released. Patients exhibit adrenergic symptoms—tachycardia, anxiety, sweating, trembling, and hunger. These symptoms can occur even if the blood glucose is normal but there is a sudden acute decline (ie, blood glucose level rapidly decreases to 80-90 mg/dL). In moderate to severe hypoglycemic reactions, the CNS is affected, signifying that the brain is being deprived of the glucose it needs.

Hypoglycemic unawareness is an autonomic neuropathy with potentially serious consequences. Hypoglycemic unawareness is defined as the loss of adrenergic symptoms of hypoglycemia that prompt a patient to act to prevent the progression of severe hypoglycemia and it results from altered counterregulation systems as described. Both type 1 and 2 diabetics may have deficiencies in counterregulation systems.

Clinical Presentation
Signs and Symptoms

- Mild hypoglycemic symptoms (adrenergic response)
  - Diaphoresis (most common)
  - Tremors
  - Shakiness
  - Tachycardia
  - Paresthesias
  - Pallor
  - Excessive hunger
  - Anxiety
- Moderate to severe hypoglycemic symptoms (CNS or neuroglycopenic symptoms)
  - Headache
  - Inability to concentrate
  - Mood changes
  - Drowsiness
  - Irritability
  - Confusion
  - Impaired judgment
  - Slurred speech
  - Staggering gait
  - Double or blurred vision
  - Morning headaches
  - Nightmares
  - Psychosis (late)
  - Seizures
  - Coma

Diagnostic Tests

- Serum blood glucose level for fingerstick glucose < 60 mg/dL

Principles of Management for Acute Hypoglycemia

The management of the patient with acute hypoglycemia depends on the severity of the reaction. Principles of management include normalization of blood glucose concentrations and patient teaching.

Normalization of Blood Glucose Concentrations

Treatment of the hypoglycemia depends on its severity as described below.

Mild Reaction

1. Administer 10- to 15-g carbohydrate (Table 16-10). Follow in 10 minutes with another 10 to 15 g if the condition does not improve.
2. Obtain a blood glucose measurement.
3. If the next meal is more than 2 hours away, provide the patient with a complex carbohydrate (ie, 4-oz milk).
4. If patient is not alert enough to swallow or unable to do so, inject 1 to 2 mg glucagon. If the patient cannot swallow and has a feeding tube, administer a liquid source of glucose (regular, non-diet soda).

Moderate and Severe Reactions

1. Administer IV glucose. The initial bolus is 50% dextrose (equivalent of 25-g glucose) followed by a continuous IV infusion until oral replacement is possible.
2. Glucagon Hcl 1 to 2 mg IV/IM/SC may be given in the hospital or at home and repeated every few hours.
3. Provide for patient rest.
4. Monitor glucose levels frequently for several hours.

Patient Teaching

The best treatment for hypoglycemia is prevention.

1. Teach the early signs and symptoms of hypoglycemia. Instruct the patient to always carry a source of fast-acting carbohydrate (see Table 16-10).
2. Advise the patient not to skip or delay meals and to limit alcohol to no more than 2-oz hard liquor, 8-oz wine, or 24-oz beer per day. It is advisable to never drink on an empty stomach. When an alcoholic beverage is consumed, it is prudent to ingest some protein-rich calories.
3. Evaluate the patient's pattern of blood glucose self-monitoring.
4. Teach the patient and family or friends how to give glucagon for severe reactions.
5. Stress the importance of wearing visible diabetes identification.
6. Assess the patient's pattern of activity and alert the patient to the risk of hypoglycemia within minutes to five hours following exercise.

Syndrome of Inappropriate Antidiuretic Hormone Secretion

Antidiuretic hormone (ADH), also known as arginine vasopressin (AVP), is produced by the hypothalamus and is stored in the posterior pituitary gland. ADH exerts its primary effects in the distal collecting tubules of the kidneys where it decreases water excretion, conserving body water, thereby increasing urine concentration (osmolality) and hemodilution. Osmoreceptors in the hypothalamus monitor changes in blood osmolality. An increase of osmolality by 2% leads to ADH release by the posterior pituitary. In high concentration, usually via exogenous administration, ADH has potent vasopressor effects along with pro-coagulant (platelet aggregation) properties. The syndrome of inappropriate antidiuretic hormone (SIADH) and diabetes insipidus (DI) are the most common disorders associated with ADH secretion in the critically ill.

Etiology, Risk Factors, and Pathophysiology

The syndrome of inappropriate antidiuretic hormone is characterized by excessive release of ADH unrelated to the plasma osmolality, or the concentration of electrolytes and other osmotically active particles. Normal mechanisms that control ADH secretion fail, causing impaired water excretion and profound hyponatremia. SIADH is a syndrome of water intoxication.

There are many causes of SIADH (Table 16-11). Vasopressin can be produced by a variety of malignancies, most commonly oat cell carcinoma of the lung. Therefore, patients who develop "idiopathic" SIADH are screened for malignant tumors. SIADH is also commonly associated with pulmonary conditions, metabolic and traumatic CNS disorders, and drugs, particularly chlorpropamide, thiazide diuretics, opiates, and barbiturates. Surgical patients are also at risk because of increased vasopressin secretion due to perioperative surgical stress and the use of opiate analgesics such as morphine.

Clinically, SIADH is distinguished by hyponatremia and water retention that progresses to water intoxication. The seriousness of the patient's signs and symptoms depends on how fast the serum sodium falls. As water intoxication progresses and the serum becomes more hypotonic, brain cells swell, causing neurologic impairment. Without treatment, irreversible brain damage and death can occur.

TABLE 16-10. EXAMPLES OF FOODS WITH 10 TO 15 G OF CARBOHYDRATE EQUIVALENTS FOR TREATMENT OF MILD HYPOGLYCEMIC REACTIONS

4 oz orange juice
6 oz regular (non-diet) cola
3 glucose tablets
6-8 oz skim milk or milk with 2% fat
3 graham cracker squares
6-8 lifesavers
6 jelly beans
2 tbsp raisins
1 small (2-oz) tube of cake icing

TABLE 16-11. ETIOLOGIES OF SIADH (PARTIAL LISTING)

Malignancies
Lung
Lymphoma
Gastrointestine

Pulmonary Diseases/Conditions
Positive pressure ventilation
Asthma
Pneumonia
Chronic obstructive pulmonary disease
Acute respiratory failure
Tuberculosis

CNS Disorders
Head trauma
Meningitis, encephalitis
Cerebrovascular accidents
Brain tumors
Guillain-Barré syndrome

Drugs
Vasopressin
Desmopressin
Thiazide diuretics
Narcotics
Barbiturates
Nicotine
Antineoplastic drugs
Tricyclic antidepressants

Others
AIDS
Senile atrophy

Clinical Presentation

Signs and Symptoms

EARLY

- Urine volume decreased and concentrated
- Nausea
- Vomiting
- Headache
- Impaired taste
- Dulled sensorium
- Muscle weakness and cramps
- Anorexia
- Weight gain
- Crackles
- Dyspnea
- Increased CVP, PCWP
- Weakness/fatigue

LATE

- Confusion
- Hostility
- Aberrant respirations
- Hypothermia
- Coma
- Convulsions

DIAGNOSTIC TESTS

- Serum Na$^+$ < 130 mEq/L
- Serum osmolality < 280 mOsm/kg

- Increased urine osmolality > 500 mOsm/kg
- Urine sodium > 20 mEq/L
- Blood urea nitrogen and creatinine decreased (hemodilution)

Principles of Management for SIADH

Principles of management depend on the severity and duration of the hyponatremia. Recognition of early clinical manifestations of SIADH is key to prevent life-threatening complications. Continued assessment of neuromuscular, cardiac, gastrointestinal, and renal systems is important. Generally, treatment focuses on restricting fluids, replenishing sodium deficits, and in severe cases of hyponatremia, inhibiting antidiuretic actions. Treatment of the underlying disorder is also a priority.

Fluid Restriction and Treating Hyponatremia

Fluid restriction is the mainstay of treatment and, to be effective, a negative water balance must be achieved.

1. Treatment of mild hyponatremia (sodium level > 125 and < 135 mEq/L) includes fluid restriction of 800 to 1000 mL/d. This allows sodium level to correct over 3 to 10 days. If fluid restriction alone is not effective, demeclocycline (Declomycin) can be administered. Demeclocycline allows excretion of water because it inhibits the effect of ADH on the renal tubules.
2. If severe neurologic symptoms of SIADH are present along with severe hyponatremia (< 125 mEq/L), administer 3% saline infusion over 2-3 hours. Furosemide is also given to increase urinary water excretion.
3. Assess cardiovascular and respiratory functions closely to evaluate the effects of the excess volume on these systems. Right and left ventricular volumes may increase, causing heart failure. Tachypnea, reports of shortness of breath, and fine crackles are indicators of fluid overload and impending heart failure.
4. Provide for patient comfort with limited fluid intake. Provide for frequent mouth care. Explain why fluid is being restricted and allow the patient to develop the schedule for allotted fluid intake. If the patient complains of nausea, administer an antiemetic prior to meals.

Replenish Sodium Deficits

1. In severe symptomatic hyponatremia, infuse 3% saline at a rate of 0.1 mL/kg/min for 2 hours to raise plasma sodium. Monitor closely for signs of hypernatremia, fluid overload, and heart failure because this treatment causes a transient increase in the serum sodium.
2. Monitor neurologic status closely and protect the patient from harm. Institute seizure precautions as necessary. Monitor respiratory status closely.

Inhibit Antidiuretic Hormone Actions

In cases where SIADH does not resolve within 1 to 2 weeks, drugs that interfere with the renal effect of vasopressin, such

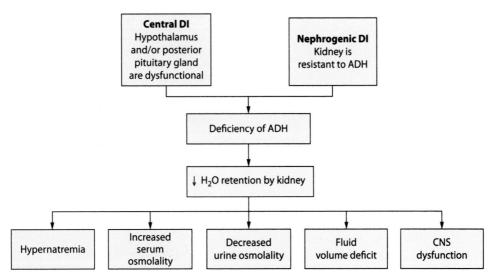

Figure 16-3. Pathogenesis of DI.

as demeclocycline, may be ordered. The full effect of these drugs makes them unsuitable for acute management of the syndrome.

Diabetes Insipidus

Etiology, Risk Factors, and Pathophysiology

Diabetes insipidus (DI) results from a group of disorders in which there is an absolute or relative deficiency of ADH (called *central DI*) or an insensitivity to its effects on the renal tubules (called *nephrogenic DI*) (Figure 16-3). Diabetes insipidus may complicate the course of critically and acutely ill patients and can result in acute fluid and electrolyte disturbances.

There are many causes of DI (Table 16-12). Central or neurogenic DI results from damage to the hypothalamic/pituitary system. An absolute deficiency of ADH results in an impaired ability to concentrate urine, polyuria, and a subsequent risk for dehydration. Patients with head trauma or those who have had neurosurgery must be watched closely for at least 7 to 10 days after the injury for evidence of DI as DI does not present for at least 48 to 72 hours after the initial hypothalamic or hypophyseal (system of blood vessels that link the hypothalamus and the anterior pituitary) trauma.

Nephrogenic DI is characterized by renal tubule insensitivity to ADH and develops because of structural or functional changes in the kidney. This results in impaired urine-concentrating ability and free water conservation. Nephrogenic DI is less dramatic than neurogenic DI in its onset and appearance.

Regardless of the etiology, in DI the ability of the body to increase ADH secretion or respond to ADH is impaired. A persistent output of dilute urine and increasing hemoconcentration is the hallmark of DI. Signs and symptoms of dehydration are present in those patients in whom the thirst mechanism has been impaired (neurogenic DI) or in whom there is inadequate fluid replacement. In addition, if a hyperosmolar state exists, intracellular brain volume depletion occurs as water moves from within the brain cells to the plasma. Typically, symptoms manifest when serum sodium levels exceed 155 mEq/L.

TABLE 16-12. CAUSES OF DI

ADH Insufficiency (Neurogenic DI)
Familial (hereditary)
Trauma
Neoplasms
Infections
Tuberculosis
Cryptococcosis
Syphilis
CNS infections
Vascular
Cerebrovascular hemorrhage
Aneurysm (circle of Willis)
Cerebral thrombosis
ADH Insensitivity (Nephrogenic DI)
Familial (hereditary)
Drug induced
Lithium
Demeclocycline
Glyburide
Colchicine
Amphotericin B
Gentamicin
Furosemide
Electrolyte disorders
Hypokalemia
Hypercalcemia
Renal disease
Excessive Water Intake (Secondary DI)
Excessive IV fluid administration
Psychogenic polydipsia (lesion in thirst center)

Clinical Presentation

Signs and Symptoms

ADH DEFICIENCY

- Polydipsia (if alert)
- Polyuria (5-20 L in 24 hours)

FLUID VOLUME DEFICIT

- Orthostatic hypotension
- Weight loss
- Tachycardia
- Decreased CVP, PCWP
- Poor skin turgor
- Dry mucous membranes

INTRACELLULAR BRAIN VOLUME DEPLETION

- Confusion
- Restlessness
- Lethargy
- Irritability
- Seizures
- Coma

Diagnostic Tests

- Water deprivation test
- Serum sodium > 155 mEq/L
- Serum osmolality > 295 mOsm/kg/L
- Urine osmolality inappropriately low with high serum osmolality (< 150 mOsm/kg/L)
- Urine specific gravity decreased
- BUN and creatinine increased (hemoconcentration)

Principles of Management for Diabetes Insipidus

The management of the patient in DI is directed at correcting the profound fluid volume deficit and electrolyte imbalances associated with this condition. If fluid losses are not replaced, hypovolemic shock can rapidly develop (see Chapter 9, Cardiovascular System). In some cases of DI, vasopressin or agents that simulate ADH release and renal response to ADH are prescribed to treat the disorder. As with other disorders, diagnosis and treatment of the cause of DI are priorities.

Fluid Volume Replacement

If the patient is alert and the thirst mechanism is not impaired, allow the patient to drink water to maintain normal serum osmolality. In many critically ill patients, this is not possible.

1. Administer hypotonic volume, such as dextrose 5% in water, quarter-strength or half-strength saline, IV as prescribed to restore the hypotonic fluid lost through osmotic diuresis. The administration of normal saline to replace volume is usually contraindicated because it presents an added renal load, promoting osmotic diuresis and worsening dehydration. In severe DI, where large amounts of fluid replacement are required, the IV intake is usually titrated to urine output; for example, 400 mL of

TABLE 16-13. EXPECTED OUTCOMES FOR THE PATIENT WITH DI

Adequate fluid balance is maintained/restored as evidenced by
- Blood pressure within 10 mm Hg of patient baseline
- Heart rate 60-100 beats/min
- Normal skin turgor
- Peripheral pulses return to baseline
- CVP and PCWP within patient norms
- Serum osmolality 275-295 mOsm/kg
- Serum sodium 135-145 mEq/L
- Urine osmolality appropriate for serum osmolality

urine output for 1 hour is replaced with 400 mL IV fluid the next hour. Hypotonic saline solutions are preferred (quarter-strength or half-strength saline). A good rule of thumb is to reduce serum sodium by 0.5 mEq/L every hour but no more than 12 mEq/L per day.

2. Monitor fluid status: Hourly urine outputs along with measurements of urine specific gravity every 1-2 hours should be done along with daily weight and strict intake and output. Monitor for signs of continuing fluid volume deficit. If the serum Na is > 155 mEq/L, rehydration should occur over 48 hours. A serum Na + > 170 necessitates ICU care. Expected outcomes for the patient with DI are listed in Table 16-13.

3. Monitor neurologic status continuously. An altered level of consciousness indicates intracellular dehydration of the brain and hypovolemia.

4. Frequent electrolyte monitoring is recommended during the initial phase of treatment.

ADH Administration or Enhancement

In central DI, desmopressin (DDAVP), an ADH analogue, is the drug of choice and is available in subcutaneous, IV, intranasal, and oral preparations. Desmopressin acts on the distal tubules and collecting ducts of the kidney to increase water reabsorption and has very specific actions with little or no ADH-like activity elsewhere in the body, most notably vasopressor effects that are prominent in another vasopressin analogue, aqueous (arginine) vasopressin (Pitressin). Vasopressin is only given intramuscularly or IV and is useful only for very short duration in unconscious patients in whom recovery of ADH secretion is expected. However, aqueous vasopressin is less specific than DDAVP and can cause profound vasoconstriction in splanchnic, portal, coronary, cerebral, peripheral, pulmonary, and intrahepatic vessels—thus it is not preferred for DI therapy in critically and acutely ill patients unless DDAVP is ineffective. Adjunctive therapy to enhance ADH release includes nonhormonal agents such as chlorpropamide, carbamazepine, thiazides, and nonsteroidal anti-inflammatory drugs (NSAIDs).

1. If the patient is unconscious, injectable DDAVP is given IV or IM 1 to 4 µg every 12 hours until therapeutic goals are achieved, such as a urine output of

2-3 ml/kg/hour, urine specific gravity 1.010-1.020 and serum sodium 140-145 mEq/l. In conscious patients, the nasal replacement route is given 10 to 20 µg by spray 2 to 3 times a day. It is important that DDAVP or other ADH analogues not be administrated unless serum sodium is at least above 145 mmol/L, as serious hyponatremia may result. Oral formulations of ADH have a slower onset and duration of action and are not useful in acute situations. Major side effects to watch for include headache, abdominal cramps, or allergic reactions such as facial flushing. Monitor for overmedication, which may precipitate hypervolemia. Signs and symptoms of fluid volume excess include dyspnea, hypertension, weight gain, and angina. Hyponatremia is another serious consequence and if it develops rapidly can cause extreme cerebral edema and osmotic demyelination syndrome. Therefore, close monitoring of serum sodium is necessary.

3. For nephrogenic DI, DDAVP intranasal or oral agents may be adminstered or alternative drugs such as chlorpropamide or NSAIDs (such as indomethacin) may be given. Volume excess remains a risk from treatment. Chlorpropamide, an older antidiabetic agent, may also result in hypoglycemia.

SELECTED BIBLIOGRAPHY

Blood Glucose Monitoring

American Diabetes Association. Clinical practice recommendations. *Diabetes Care.* 2013;36:S1-S110.

Endocrine Society. Management of hyperglycemia in hospitalized patients in non-critical care setting: an endocrine society clinical practice guideline. January 2012. Accessed February 18, 2013.

Karon BS, Gandhi GY, Nuttall GA, Bryant SC. Accuracy of Roche Accu-Chek from whole blood capillary, arterial, and venous glucose values in patients receiving intensive intravenous insulin therapy after cardiac surgery. *Am J Clin Pathol.* 2007;127(6):919-926.

Klonoff DC. The Food and Drug Administration is now preparing to establish tighter performance requirements for blood glucose monitors. *J Diabetes Sci Technol.* 2010;4(3):499-504.

Malone B. Blood glucose meters: is FDA ready to tighten up accuracy standards? *Clin Lab News.* 2010;36(5):1-4.

Vaddiraju S, Burgess DJ, Tomazos I, Jain FC, Papadimitrakopoulos F. Technologies for continuous glucose monitoring: current problems and future promises. *J Diabetes Sci Technol.* 2010;4(6):1540-1562.

Hyperglycemia, DKA, and HHS

American Diabetes Association. Standards of medical care in diabetes 2012 (Position Statement). *Diabetes Care.* 2012;35 (suppl 1): S11-S63.

Blouin D. Too much of a good thing: management of diabetic ketoacidosis in adults. *Can Fam Physician.* January 1, 2012;58:55-57.

Inzucchi SE, Siegel MD. Glycemic control in the ICU—how tight is too tight? *N Engl J Med.* 2009;360:1346-1349.

Management of Hyperglycemia in Hospitalized Patients in Non-Critical Care Setting: An Endocrine Society Clinical Practice Guideline. *J Clin Endocrinol Metab.* January 1, 2012;97:16-38.

Moghissi ES, Korytkowski MT, DiNardo M, et al. American Association of Clinical Endocrinologists and American Diabetes Association Consensus Statement on Inpatient Glycemic Control. *Endocrine Practice*;2009;15:1-17 and *Diabetes Care.* 2009;Jun;32(6):1119-1131.

Rajesh G, Hurwitz S. Hypoglycemia, with or without insulin therapy, is associated with increased mortality among hospitalized patients. *Diabetes Care.* December 17, 2012, doi: 10.2337/dc12-1296. Accessed February 18, 2012.

Sato H, Carvalho G, Sato T, et al. The Association of Preoperative Glycemic Control, Intraoperative Insulin Sensitivity, and Outcomes after Cardiac Surgery. *J Clin Endocrinol Metab.* September 2010;95(9):4338-4344.

Bui H, To T, Stein R, Fung K, Daneman D. Is diabetic ketoacidosis at disease onset a result of missed diagnosis? *J Pediatr.* 2010;Mar;156(3):472-477.

The NICE-SUGAR Study Investigators. Intensive versus conventional glucose control in critically ill patients. *N Engl J Med.* 2009;360:1283-1297.

The NICE-SUGAR Study Investigators. Hypoglycemia and risk of death in critically ill patients. *N Engl J Med.* 2012; 367:1108-1118.

Umpierrez G. Randomized study of basal-bolus insulin therapy in the inpatient management of patients with type 2 diabetes undergoing general surgery (RABBIT 2 surgery). *Diabetes Care.* 2011;34:256-261.

Van den Berghe G, Wilmer A, Hermans G, et al. Intensive insulin therapy in the medical ICU. *N Engl J Med.* 2006;354:449-461.

Van den Berghe G, Wouters P, Weekers F, et al. Intensive insulin therapy in the critically ill patients. *N Engl J Med.* 2001;345:1359-1367.

SIADH and Diabetes Insipidus

Crawford A, Harris H. Waterworld, part 2: understanding diabetes insipidus in adults. *Nurs Crit Care.* 2012;7(1):12-16.

Ellison DH, Berl T. Clinical practice. The syndrome of inappropriate antidiuresis. *N Engl J Med.* 2007;356:2064-2072.

Gross P. Clinical management of SIADH. *Ther Adv in Endo and Metab.* 2012;3(2):61-73.

Loh JA, Verbalis JG. Disorders of water and salt metabolism associated with pituitary disease. *Endocrinol Metab Clin North Am.* Mar 2008;37(1):213-234.

Mavrakis AN, Tritos NA. Diabetes insipidus with deficient thirst: report of a patient and review of the literature. *Am J Kidney Dis.* May 2008;51(5):851-859.

Thornton SN. Thirst and hydration: physiology and consequences of dysfunction. *Physiol Behav.* 2010;100:15-20.

Tomky D. Detection, prevention, and treatment of hypoglycemia in the hospital. *Diabetes Spectr.* 2005;18(1):39-44.

TRAUMA

Allen C. Wolfe and Benjamin C. Hughes

KNOWLEDGE COMPETENCIES

1. Describe the mechanisms of traumatic injury and relate them to accurate assessment of overt and covert injuries.

2. Discuss the common physiologic and psychosocial effects on the patient and family because of major traumatic injury.

3. Identify the unique needs of the trauma patient in the progressive care unit.

4. Apply selected management principles to treat trauma patients with thoracic, abdominal, and musculoskeletal injuries.

SPECIALIZED ASSESSMENT TECHNIQUES, DIAGNOSTIC TESTS, AND MONITORING SYSTEMS

Trauma is an increasing healthcare problem in the United States. The cost of treating trauma exceeds $400 billion annually. For Americans between the ages of 1 and 44, trauma is the leading cause of death, surpassing cancer and atherosclerosis. Although the death rate is high for this patient population, the disability rate is even greater. This chapter focuses on thoracic, abdominal, musculoskeletal, and pelvic trauma. Although traumatic brain injury and spinal cord injury account for approximately 50% of all trauma deaths, these topics are covered in Chapter 20, Advanced Neurologic Concepts.

Acutely ill trauma patients are unlike other hospitalized patients and require specialized assessment and monitoring. For the trauma victim, admission to the progressive care setting is sudden and unplanned, without time for psychological preparation or the stabilization of chronic conditions. Trauma patients are often young; however, trauma among the elderly is an increasing problem because of the population's longer life span. Traumatic injuries may be subtle, and complications are common (Table 17-1). Alcohol or drug abuse plays a major role in the cause of the trauma and subsequent treatment. Rehabilitation is often needed after

injury, and a trauma victim's quality of life may never return to pre-injury status. This is especially true for traumatic brain and spinal cord injuries; however, even in lower extremity trauma, it may take a full year for an individual to return to work. Trauma takes a significant emotional and financial toll on the patient, family, and society.

Management of traumatic injury in the initial phases of care occurs in tandem with assessment; for example, the control and insertion of an airway, the administration of fluids, and pain medication may all be provided before the site of bleeding is identified and controlled. One of the most important aspects of assessing the traumatically injured patient is to determine the mechanism of injury, whether blunt or penetrating trauma. Based on this information, an "index of suspicion" regarding specific injuries is developed to ensure that no injuries are overlooked and a trauma patient plan of care is developed.

Primary and Secondary Trauma Survey Assessment

The life-threatening nature of trauma often requires that traditional assessment priorities be changed to address other more serious physical findings (Tables 17-2 and 17-3). The primary and secondary surveys reveal immediate life-threatening injuries and direct the trauma team toward an

TABLE 17-1. **MAJOR COMPLICATIONS IN TRAUMA**

Complication	Associated Conditions	What to Look for	Nursing Interventions
Hypovolemia	Internal hemorrhage Multiple-system injuries Fractures of major bones Coagulopathies	Decreased blood pressure Tachycardia, tachypnea Cool, clammy skin Pallor Decreased urine output Frank hemorrhage Anxiety Obtunded sensorium	Notify physician immediately. Type and cross-match patient's blood Check amount of blood on hand in blood bank. Administer transfusion as ordered. Administer medications as ordered. Monitor vital signs every 15 minutes.
Sepsis	Systemic infection Peritonitis	Increased WBCs Increased or decreased temperature Tachycardia Sudden hypotension Increased serum glucose Decreased platelets, decreased Pao_2 Confusion/disorientation Diaphoresis/flushed face	Monitor ABGs, electrolytes, and CBC. Notify physician. Monitor vital signs every 15 minutes. Administer fluid replacement and medications as ordered. Maintain normothermia.
Neurogenic shock	Spinal cord injury	Hypotension Hypothermia with absence of sweating below injury level Flaccid paralysis below injury level Bradycardia	Notify physician. Administer fluid replacement and medications as ordered. Monitor vital signs every 15 minutes. Insert Foley catheter and nasogastric tube as ordered.
Pulmonary embolism	Immobility Fracture of the long bones, pelvis, or ribs Improper handling of fractures before and during admission	Chest pain Shortness of breath Sudden disorientation Petechiae over axillae and chest Decreased Pao_2 Tachycardia	Notify physician. Assist with transport to lung scan. Monitor ECG. Administer O_2.
ARDS	Chest trauma Sepsis Multiple transfusions Brain injuries Multiple-system injuries	Decreased $Paco_2$, decreased Pao_2 Decreased lung compliance Decreased tidal volume Increased airway pressures Increased WBC	Assess chest, monitor lung volumes and compliance. Draw serial ABGs. Administer O_2 or ventilator therapy as ordered. Suction as needed. Administer medications as ordered. Monitor ECG.
Pneumonia	Blunt chest trauma Immobility Atelectasis Endotracheal intubation	Increased temperature Increased WBC Decreased breath sounds Rales on auscultation Radiologic changes Positive sputum cultures	Assess chest, monitor lung volumes and compliance Suction as needed Supplemental O_2 as needed. Serial chest x-rays as ordered.
Wound dehiscence	Abdominal surgery Wound infection Poor nutritional status	Pink serous wound exudate Poor wound approximation	Notify physician. Have sterile saline and dressings on hand. Prevent/correct abdominal distention.
Gastrointestinal fistula	Penetrating abdominal trauma Sepsis	Bile, fecal, or pancreatic drainage from wounds or drain sites	Monitor amount, odor, and color of drainage. Meticulous skin care around drainage sites. Perform dressing changes as necessary.
Pneumothorax	Mechanical ventilation PEEP Improper central line placement	Decreased or absent breath sounds Radiologic evidence Decreased Pao_2, cyanosis, restlessness Unequal chest expansion Hyperresonance over affected area Decreased tidal volume Tracheal deviation Increased airway pressures Hemodynamic instability	Notify physician STAT Administer supplemental O_2. Assist with chest tube insertion or thoracentesis. Insert 18-gauge needle into second intercostal space, mid clavicle line, if trained to do so. Assist with chest tube insertion. If chest tubes in place, check for patency and suction. Monitor vital signs every 15 minutes.

(continued)

TABLE 17-1. MAJOR COMPLICATIONS IN TRAUMA (CONTINUED)

Complication	Associated Conditions	What to Look for	Nursing Interventions
Renal failure	Prolonged hypotension	Increased serum BUN/creatinine	Record hourly intake and output.
	Sepsis	Decreased urine output, decreased specific gravity	Foley catheter care daily.
	Ruptured aorta	Increased serum potassium	Monitor laboratory values.
	Toxic drug reaction	Increased confusion	Administer hemodialysis or peritoneal dialysis as ordered.
	ARDS	Uremic frost	
Bronchoesophageal fistula	Prolonged tracheostomy	Gastric contents suctioned through tracheostomy	Maintain NPO status.
	Overinflation of cuff balloon	Radiologic confirmation	Maintain proper positioning of endotracheal tube to maintain ventilation.
	Prolonged need for NG tube	Respiratory distress	Administer feedings as ordered via gastrostomy or jejunostomy tube.
Diabetes insipidus	Brain injuries	Increased urine output	Record hourly intake and output, check urine specific gravity every 4 hours.
		Decreased urine specific gravity	Maintain fluid balance.
		Decreased urine osmolality	Replace urine output as ordered.
		Severe thirst	Administer vasopressin (Pitressin) as ordered.
Atelectasis	Immobility	Radiologic changes	Provide pulmonary hygiene.
	Prolonged anesthesia	Decreased Pao$_2$	Turn and position every 1-2 hours.
	Blunt chest trauma	Inability to cough	Kinetic therapy.
	Pain	Decreased breath sounds	Encourage coughing and deep breathing.
	Endotracheal intubation		Draw and monitor serial ABGs.
			Administer O$_2$ as needed.
			Incentive spirometer.
Empyema	Blunt chest trauma	Purulent chest drainage	Monitor amount and consistency of chest tube drainage as ordered.
	Pneumonia	Increased temperature	Culture chest tube drainage as ordered.
	Prolonged atelectasis	Increased WBC	Maintain chest tube patency.
	Pleural effusion	Generalized malaise	Provide pulmonary hygiene and chest physiotherapy.
	Open chest wound	Radiologic confirmation	
		Sepsis	
Aspiration	Unconscious patients	Suctioning of gastric contents from tracheal tube or ET tube	Notify physician immediately.
	Spinal cord injury	Radiologic confirmation	Take chest x-ray STAT.
	Sudden vomiting	Increased temperature and WBCs	Turn patient to side or suction if vomits.
	Malfunctioning NG tube	Decreased Pao$_2$	Elevate head of bed when giving tube feedings.
	Decreased gag reflex		
	Prolonged endotracheal intubation		
Meningitis	Brain injury	Increased temperature	Administer medications as ordered.
	Skull fracture	Increased WBC	Monitor vital signs and neurologic checks every hour.
	Maxillofacial trauma	Positive spinal fluid cultures	Assist with spinal tap.
	Intraventricular catheter placement	Changes in neurologic status	Draw serial WBCs.
Sensory deprivation/ ICU psychosis	Prolonged stay in ICU	Confusion	Arrange for psychiatric consult if necessary.
	Sleep deprivation	Disorientation	Provide quiet environment.
		Hallucinations	Plan nursing care in blocks of time to promote sleep.
		Restlessness	Administer medications as ordered.
		Combativeness	Use consistent approach to orient to reality.

From: Cardona VD, Hurn PD, Mason PJB, Scanlon AM, Veise-Berry SW, eds. Trauma Nursing From Resuscitation Through Rehabilitation. Philadelphia, PA: WB Saunders; 1994:840-841.

individualized resuscitation. This approach ensures that common causes of tissue injury are rapidly identified so that appropriate therapeutic interventions can begin. If the patient's status changes at any time during the secondary survey, the practitioner must return to the primary survey to again review airway, breathing, circulation, disability, and environment/exposure to determine if there has been any physiologic decompensation.

Diagnostic Studies

Diagnostic Peritoneal Lavage, Ultrasound, and Computed Axial Tomography

Hemorrhage is of major concern during the primary survey of the trauma patient. Both external and occult bleeding must be considered. Secondary survey diagnostic studies may include diagnostic peritoneal lavage (DPL), ultrasound, and computed axial tomography (CAT) to diagnose occult hemorrhage.

TABLE 17-2. PRIMARY SURVEY

Airway and C-Spine	**Assessment** • Assess patency and airway obstruction **Management** • Basic airway maneuvers–jaw thrust or chin lift accompanied by assessment for foreign bodies in the airway • Insert nasopharyngeal airway or oral pharyngeal airway • Establish a definitive airway if necessary • Maintain C-spine in neutral position with an appropriate device while maintaining airway patency
Breathing	**Assessment** • Assess respiratory rate and depth after exposure of chest and neck area • Assure C-spine immobilization is maintained • Assess for injury to neck to include but not limited to deformity, tracheal deviation, sub-Q emphysema, etc • Assess for chest wall motion and use of accessory muscle **Management** • Apply high flow oxygen • Maintain airway by definite airway if necessary • Assure CO_2 and pulse oximetry monitoring with intubation • Alleviate tension pneumothorax or seal open pneumothorax

Circulation	**Assessment**
	• Identify source of hemorrhage–internal or external
	• Assess vital signs to include skin color, capillary refill, and pulses
	Management
	• Stop the bleeding
	  • external direct pressure
	  • internal locate source and need for operative intervention
	• Establish large bore IV access and obtain blood samples during this process
	• Initiate warmed isotonic (LR or NS) or colloid fluid resuscitation
	• Initiate warming measures to combat hypothermia

Disability	**Assessment** • Assess neurological status to include mental status, pupillary size, and response
Exposure	**Assessment** • Completely disrobe patient but avoid hypothermia

Diagnostic peritoneal lavage is a fast and inexpensive procedure performed to detect free blood in the peritoneal cavity. The test is especially important in the blunt, multisystem trauma patient who is unconscious or those unable to verbalize abdominal pain palpation.

Under local anesthetic, a lavage catheter is percutaneously places into the abdomen. The physician, physician assistant, or nurse practitioner instills and removes sterile fluid from the patient's peritoneal cavity. A positive tap is defined as the aspiration of greater than 10 mL of blood. If that initial tap is negative, 1 L of saline is instilled and the abdomen is drained by gravity. A minimal fluid return of 250 mL is needed for a sufficient laboratory sample. Hence, only 25 mL of blood must accumulate for DPL to be positive. The lavage is considered positive, and thus the need for surgical intervention is indicated, by 100,000 red blood cells (RBCs)/mm^3 or more, greater than 500 white blood cells (WBCs)/mm^3, or a positive gram stain for food fibers or bacteria. However, retroperitoneal injuries, such as pancreatic injury, do not show up as positive with a lavage, so

vigilant observation of abdominal expansion is required by the nurse.

Ultrasound is used increasingly to diagnose hemorrhage in the trauma patient. Commonly known as the focused abdominal sonograph for trauma (FAST), it can be completed in less than 3 minutes. This noninvasive technique may quickly show injury in the hemodynamically unstable patient. However, the usefulness of ultrasound depends on the experience and expertise of the person performing the study; a DPL may have to be performed for confirmation of hemoperitoneum that was observed by ultrasound.

Focused abdominal sonograph for trauma alone is not acceptable for questionable or borderline findings. For these situations, serial physical examinations coupled with FAST are recommended to better evaluate abdominal injuries. CAT is a good alternative to DPL in the stable trauma patient. CAT scanning continues to be the gold standard for diagnosis of injury if the patient is hemodynamically stable. For a comparison of DPL, ultrasound, and CAT, refer Table 17-4.

Cervical Spine Radiograph

A cervical spine (C-spine) x-ray is one of the first priorities of assessment after the primary survey. All trauma patients are presumed to have a C-spine injury until all seven cervical vertebrae have been cleared or visualized as intact on x-ray or CAT scan. A cervical collar to immobilize the neck is applied until the C-spine has been evaluated and found to be free of injuries.

Radiographic Studies

Radiographic studies are performed after the primary survey. These studies should not delay resuscitation, but may be essential in determining the extent of injury. Depending on the mechanism of injury, common x-rays may include chest, pelvis, and musculoskeletal studies.

Serial Examinations

Trauma patients require frequent reexamination to ensure that all injuries are identified and that the patient's status is not deteriorating. Missed injuries may lead to pain, disability, and increased mortality for the patient. Examples of trauma where repeated assessments by the same provider are recommended include traumatic brain injury and abdominal injuries. Intercranial or occult abdominal bleeding may not be evident initially. Having a high degree of suspicion for traumatic injuries comes from knowledge of mechanism of injury and the specific injuries created by destructive blunt or penetrating forces.

Mechanism of Injury

The principles of mechanism of injury give the trauma team insight into the possible injuries sustained by the patient. How an injury occurred, the nature of the forces involved, and suspected tissue and organ damage are all important

TABLE 17-3. SECONDARY SURVEY

Item to Assess	Establishes/Identifies	Assess	Finding	Confirm By
Level of consciousness	• Severity of head injury	• GCS score	• 8, severe head injury • 9-12, moderate head injury • 13-15, minor head injury	• CT scan • Repeat without paralyzing agents
Pupils	• Type of head injury • Presence of eye injury	• Size • Shape • Reactivity	• Mass effect • Diffuse brain injury • Ophthalmic injury	• CT scan
Head	• Scalp injury • Skull injury	• Inspect for lacerations and skull fractures • Palpable defects	• Scalp laceration • Depressed skull fracture • Basilar skull fracture	• CT scan
Maxillofacial	• Soft tissue injury • Bone injury • Nerve injury • Teeth/mouth injury	• Visual deformity • Malocclusion • Palpation for crepitation	• Facial fracture • Soft tissue injury	• Facial bone x-ray • CT scan or facial bones
Neck	• Laryngeal injury • C-spine injury • Vascular injury • Esophageal injury • Neurologic deficit	• Visual inspection • Palpation • Auscultation	• Laryngeal deformity • Subcutaneous emphysema • Hematoma • Bruit • Platysmal penetration • Pain, tenderness of C-spine	• C-spine x-ray or CT • Angiography/duplex exam • Esophagoscopy • Laryngoscopy
Thorax	• Thoracic wall injury • Subcutaneous emphysema • Pneumo-hemothorax • Bronchial injury • Pulmonary contusion • Thoracic aortic disruption	• Visual inspection • Palpation • Auscultation	• Bruising, deformity, or paradoxical motion • Chest wall tenderness, crepitation • Diminished breath sounds • Muffled heart tones • Mediastinal crepitation • Severe back pain	• Chest x-ray • CT scan • Angiography • Bronchoscopy • Tube thoracostomy • Pericardiocentesis • TE ultrasound
Abdomen/flank	• Abdominal wall injury • Intraperitoneal injury • Retroperitoneal injury	• Visual inspection • Palpation • Auscultation • Determine path of penetration	• Abdominal wall pain/tenderness • Peritoneal irritation • Visceral injury • Retroperitoneal organ injury	• DPL/ultrasound • CT scan • Laparotomy • Contrast GI x-ray studies • Angiography
Pelvis	• Genitourinary (GU) tract injuries • Pelvic fracture(s)	• Palpate symphysis pubis for widening • Palpate bony pelvis for tenderness • Determine pelvic stability only once • Inspect perineum • Rectal/vaginal exam	• GU tract injury (hematuria) • Pelvic fracture • Rectal, vaginal, and/or perineal injury	• Pelvic x-ray • GU contrast studies • Urethrogram • Cystogram • IVP • Contrast-enhanced CT
Spinal cord	• Cranial injury • Cord injury • Peripheral nerve(s) injury	• Motor response • Pain response	• Unilateral cranial mass effect • Quadriplegia • Paraplegia • Nerve root injury	• Plain spine x-rays • CT scan • MRI
Vertebral column	• Column injury • Vertebral instability • Nerve injury	• Verbal response to pain, lateralizing signs • Palpate for tenderness • Deformity	• Fracture vs dislocation	• Plain x-rays • CT scan • MRI
Extremities	• Soft tissue injury • Bony deformities • Joint abnormalities • Neurovascular deficits	• Visual inspection • Palpation	• Swelling, bruising, pallor • Malalignment • Pain, tenderness, crepitation • Absence/diminished pulses • Tense muscular compartments • Neurologic deficits	• Specific x-rays • Doppler examination • Compartment pressures • Angiography

Reproduced with permission from: Advanced Trauma Life Support Student Course Manual. 9th ed. American College of Surgeons. 2012. Chapter 1. 27-28.

TABLE 17-4. INDICATIONS, ADVANTAGES, AND DISADVANTAGES OF COMMON DIAGNOSTIC TESTS FOR BLUNT ABDOMINAL TRAUMA

Procedure	Indications	Advantages	Disadvantages
DPL	Decreased BP with suspicion of internal hemorrhage	Easy, rapid, inexpensive	Invasive, unable to pinpoint location of injury, cannot evaluate retroperitoneum
Ultrasound (FAST)	Decreased BP with suspicion of internal hemorrhage	Easy, rapid, inexpensive, noninvasive, can be repeated	Sensitive to operator experience, unable to pinpoint location of injury, cannot evaluate retroperitoneum
CT scan	Normal BP with suspicion of internal hemorrhage	Can pinpoint which organ is damaged, including the retroperitoneum	Time consuming, costly, must lie flat

aspects of mechanism of injury. This knowledge is required when assessing a trauma patient at the scene of the accident and in the emergency department, as well as in the progressive care unit. Knowing this information helps anticipate potential complications.

Injuries result when a body is exposed to an uncontrolled outside source of energy that disrupts the body's integrity or functional ability. This energy can come from a variety of sources, and can be kinetic, penetrating, chemical, thermal, electrical, or radiating energy. The severity of the resultant injury is determined by several factors: the force or speed of impact, the length of the impact or exposure, the total surface area exposed, and related risk factors such as age, gender, preinjury health, and alcohol/drug ingestion.

Mechanisms of injury are typically divided into two major categories: blunt and penetrating. *Blunt trauma* is defined as injuries that are not open to the atmosphere, and *penetrating injuries* are those in which the body has been pierced. Blunt trauma usually results from motor vehicle or motorcycle collisions, assaults, falls, contact sports injuries, pedestrian/vehicle collisions, or blast injuries. Assessment strategies useful in diagnosing blunt traumatic injuries include physical assessment, ultrasound, DPL, CAT scanning, radiographic studies angiography, and blood count, and blood chemistry analysis. Penetrating trauma is commonly caused by bullets or knives in urban areas and by farm or industrial equipment in rural areas.

Knowledge of mechanism of injury provides clinicians with information to determine patterns of injury. These common patterns are helpful when assessing trauma patients who cannot speak to indicate areas of pain. Patterns of injury offer the trauma team an index of suspicion and direction to focus the primary and secondary surveys. Such injury patterns help determine which tests and the sequence of the diagnostic tests needed to identify each of the patient's injuries; for example, in motor vehicle crashes, the common pattern of injury for the unrestrained driver include head, pelvis, chest, and musculoskeletal areas (eg, hip, ankle, and foot trauma) (Figure 17-1A). Thoracic trauma is often owing to impact with a steering wheel. Other patterns of injuries to unrestrained passengers demonstrate an increased incidence of craniofacial trauma resulting from hitting the head on the windshield (Figure 17-1B). Fractures of the clavicle and humerus are more frequent among passengers, possibly due to the defensive reflex action of raising the arms prior to impact. Similar patterns of injury have been identified for victims of falls and pedestrians struck by motor vehicles (Figure 17-2). Knowledge of these patterns of injuries also helps prevent further damage or complications during the resuscitation efforts; for example, if a patient has sustained a head injury with a high suspicion of basilar skull fracture, a nasogastric tube should not be inserted because it could be passed through the fracture directly into the brain. It should be inserted orally as alternative. A Foley catheter should not

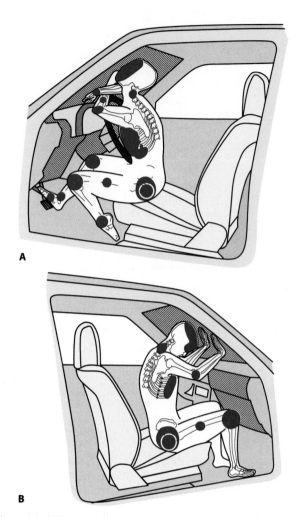

Figure 17-1. Major areas of impact injuries (solid dark areas). The "hostile" contact areas are striped (windshield, steering column, dashboard, and foot pedals). **(A)** Unrestrained drivers. **(B)** Unrestrained front seat passengers. (*From: Daffner R, Deeb Z, Lupetin A, Rothfus W. Patterns of high speed impact injuries in motor vehicle occupants.* J Trauma. *1988;28:499-500.*)

be inserted if the mechanism of injury suggests bladder rupture or trauma. A more definitive examination such as the urethrogram or cystogram is warranted.

Physiologic Consequences of Trauma

Traumatic injury unleashes a cascade of vasoactive mediators, such as various neurohormones, prostaglandins, and cytokines that serve a protective function through the stress response. However, in severe multisystem trauma, these same mediators that help the trauma patient survive the initial injury may prolong the stress response and contribute to complications and even death. This response is best limited by enhancing the patient's healing ability through attention to physiologic and psychosocial care. Priorities include supporting tissue oxygenation through with the use of oxygen, ventilatory support, and hemodynamic support if necessary. The trauma patient undergoes continuous vital sign moni-

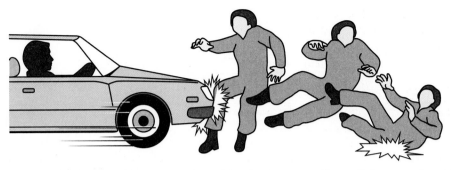

Figure 17-2. With an impact to the lower leg from the car bumper or hood, the adult pedestrian rotates and is propelled onto lower leg or hip causing additional injury. (*Illustration reprinted with permission from: Weigelt J, Brasel KJ, Klein J. Mechanism of injury. In: McQuillan KA, Makic MBF, Whalen E, eds. Trauma nursing: from resuscitation through rehabilitation, 4th ed. St Louis, MO: Saunders Elsevier; 2009:180.*)

toring, including pulse oximetry. Pain and anxiety are treated at the same time as injuries are assessed.

Traumatic injury creates fractures, wounds, and crushed tissues that may not be readily visible. Once the ABCs or primary trauma survey has been completed and management begins, the head-to-toe, in-depth assessment, known as the secondary survey, is initiated. In the secondary survey, evidence is accumulated for the detailed diagnosis of multiple trauma and definitive care is planned. A high index of suspicion is needed to link patterns of trauma, mechanism of injury, and physiologic consequences to the traumatic injuries. The progressive care nurse assists in stabilizing the patient with fluids, ventilatory and circulatory support, while also providing emotional support during diagnostic tests. Many times the nurse is responsible for addressing pain control for the patient and the psychosocial needs of the patient and family.

Consequences of traumatic injury include blood loss, tissue destruction, intense pain due to damaged tissues, and altered oxygenation and ventilation. Fluid balance, airway management, aggressive pain control, and wound care are priorities. Stabilization of fractures and surgical repair of injured organs are accomplished in the early operative period. The priority for care in the early phases of trauma is to optimize tissue oxygenation (see Chapter 19, Advanced Cardiovascular Concepts). Although patients in progressive care settings frequently have more than one injured system, a focus on one body system at a time assists in providing an organized management plan.

COMMON INJURIES IN THE TRAUMA PATIENT

Thoracic Trauma

Etiology and Pathophysiology

Thoracic trauma accounts for approximately 25% of all trauma-related deaths and may include injuries created by fractured ribs, blunt cardiac injury, vascular injury, and contused or punctured lung tissue. The most common mechanisms of injury to the chest include blunt trauma (motor vehicle-related injuries) and penetrating trauma from

gunshots and stabbings. Common injuries associated with thoracic trauma include tension pneumothorax, hemothorax, open pneumothorax, pulmonary contusion, rib fractures/flail chest, cardiac tamponade, cardiac contusion, or aortic disruption (Figure 17-3).

Injury to the lung parenchyma may cause a tension pneumothorax, which may result in hemodynamic collapse and is therefore a medical emergency. Air collects under positive pressure in the pleural space, collapses the lung, and shifts the heart and great vessels to the opposite side of the chest from the injury causing hemodynamic collapse. Management consists of early detection of the tension pneumothorax and insertion of a chest tube. In emergent situations, if a chest tube insertion is not an option, a large bore angiocath can be inserted into the chest wall at the midclavicular line, second intercostal space to relieve the pressure and tension. Another alternate location is the lateral approach at the midaxillary line. These procedures are known as needle decompressions.

A hemothorax is defined as blood in the pleural space. Fractures to the first and second ribs are considered most serious. If these ribs are broken, one can assume significant force was sustained in the traumatic event, therefore damage to the underlying vessels is possible. An initial chest x-ray demonstrating a widened mediastinum often confirms this suspicion of hemothorax. If the hemothorax is large enough and the patient is experiencing respiratory difficulty, a chest tube is placed to drain the hemothorax. If the patient is hemodynamically unstable, the physician may need to perform an open thoracotomy to control the bleeding.

An open pneumothorax is present when there is passage of air in and out of the pleural space. This usually occurs when there is a penetrating injury to the chest wall by either a gunshot or stab wound. A dressing may be applied to the open sucking chest wound with careful attention to taping only three sides of the dressing. If the dressing is made occlusive, a tension pneumothorax may occur. The patient needs a chest tube placed in the affected side.

Pulmonary contusion is injury to the lung parenchyma, which commonly occurs after blunt injury to the chest.

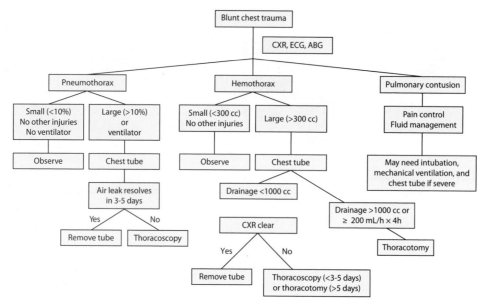

Figure 17-3. Algorithm: Therapeutic approach to the patient with blunt chest trauma. (*From: Mattox K, Feliciano D, Moore F, eds. Trauma. 4th ed. New York, NY: McGraw Hill; 2000:525.*)

A pulmonary contusion may lead to alveolar capillary membrane disruption. Depending on the severity of the contusion, hypoxemia occurs, which may worsen several days after the injury, progressing to respiratory failure and acute respiratory distress syndrome (ARDS). Pulmonary contusions are difficult to identify and diagnose during the initial trauma resuscitation because clinical findings may not occur until several hours after the injury. This injury is an example of when an index of suspicion and knowing the mechanism of injury assists the progressive care nurse to anticipate pulmonary complications such as hypoxemia progressing to respiratory failure and ARDS.

Fractured ribs are also common in blunt trauma. Fractured lower ribs can damage the liver or spleen, and upper rib fractures may puncture lung tissue. All patients with rib fractures are suspected of having a pulmonary contusion. A flail chest may occur when three or more adjacent ribs are fractured in two segments, creating a "floating segment" that may puncture the lung and compromise effective ventilation efforts. Diagnosis of a flail chest is made by observing inward movement of the chest during inspiration and outward movement during expiration. This injury is best assessed when the patient is breathing spontaneously. With this kind of injury there is a paradoxical motion of the chest wall which results in hypoxemia. Due to pain, the patient is often unable to take a deep breath leading to atelectasis and further compromising oxygenation and ventilation. Pneumonia and/or respiratory failure may ensue if not treated.

Blunt cardiac injury may result in damage to the myocardium, coronary arteries, or structures of the heart (septum or valves) as a result of blunt force to the chest. These injuries might be subtle and difficult to diagnose but should always be a matter of concern when a patient has sustained chest trauma. The transthoracic echocardiography, 12-lead ECG and biochemical markers (troponin levels) are used to assist in the identification of myocardial injuries. Dysrhythmias are common in these patients. Sinus tachycardia, atrial fibrillation, and premature ventricular contractions are most common. In contrast ventricular tachycardia and fibrillation are unfortunately more common if the area of myocardial damage is large.

Cardiac tamponade is a potentially life-threatening complication of both blunt and penetrating chest trauma. The pericardial membrane (sac) is normally stiff and noncompliant. Bleeding into the pericardial sac (effusion) causes compression of the heart, which then compromises cardiac function and cardiac output. The rate at which fluid accumulates around the heart in the pericardial sac determines whether the effusion will lead to cardiac tamponade or compensation (stretching of the sac and accommodation). A rapid accumulation of blood does not allow the pericardial sac to stretch and the tamponade may lead to pulseless electrical activity and/or cardiogenic shock.

Traumatic aortic disruption is a surgical emergency and the most common cause of immediate death in the thoracic trauma patient population. A clinician with a high index of suspicion and knowledge of mechanism of injury, such as high-speed motor vehicle collision, will identify this injury earlier and potentially improve the outcome. Historically, the gold standard for diagnosis was angiography. But with the modern advances in bedside echocardiography and the quickness of the CAT and MRI imaging, these tests frequently allow for a confident diagnosis without the need for angiography. A widened mediastinum is typically seen on chest x-ray. The survival rate of the patient is directly related to how quickly this injury is diagnosed and the patient is taken to the operating room.

Principles for Management of Thoracic Trauma

Management of the patient with trauma to the chest must be individualized to the patient and includes several basic principles: ventilatory support to prevent hypoxemia; monitoring chest tubes for drainage; providing optimal pain control and positioning to promote adequate oxygenation/ventilation, to decrease complications of immobility, and to promote wound healing; and limiting the risks of infection.

Ventilatory Support

The goals for ventilatory support of the trauma patient are the same as the ventilatory goals for any patient in the progressive care unit. Management focuses on improving oxygenation, correcting acidosis, easing the work of breathing and decreasing the risk of ventilator associated conditions (VAC). Ventilatory therapy may be definitive or supportive, depending on the patient's injury and requirements. Definitive care for a flail chest may include the use of the ventilatory support to stabilize the chest wall. Supportive ventilatory care is imperative in the patient with a pulmonary contusion who exhibits signs of ARDS. The nurse caring for the trauma patient must be comfortable with the modes of conventional mechanical ventilation and have an awareness of some of the nonconventional ventilatory techniques (see Chapter 5, Airway and Ventilatory Management).

Monitoring Chest Tubes

Chest tubes are inserted for patients with chest wall injuries and punctured lung tissue and those requiring thoracotomy. Care of the patient with chest tubes includes observing for drainage characteristics, signs of a resolving air leak, and prevention of infection. Meticulous sterile technique, insertion site care, and drainage system set up are key components of chest tube management. Trauma patients may have draining wounds and suture lines adjacent to the chest tube site, which can make dressing changes more complicated. Infection surveillance, prevention, and assessment are essential nursing functions for all trauma patients.

Pain Control

Pain control, both systemic and local, is needed and may even preempt the need for mechanical ventilation in patients with milder degrees of thoracic trauma; for example, when patients are able to breathe deeply and cough effectively, smaller airways remain open, atelectasis is avoided, and healing can occur. Patient-controlled analgesia (PCA), epidural narcotic infusions, or local anesthetics can be used for aggressive pain control in the trauma patient to allow for enhanced pulmonary function exercises and avoid the need for mechanical ventilation.

Patients report that chest tubes, suctioning, and turning are all extremely painful. Managing a patient's pain aggressively is not only a humane concern, but it also allows the patient to focus mental and physical energy on healing. Pain can be controlled through narcotics that act centrally, locally, or regionally, and through drugs that act at the periphery to interrupt the painful stimulus (see Chapter 6, Pain, Sedation, and Neuromuscular Blockade Management and Chapter 7, Pharmacology). Nonpharmacologic approaches can also operate at the central level through cognitive distraction or relaxation, and peripherally by using positioning or application of heat and cold.

Patient-controlled analgesia gives the patient control to request pain medication at a preset time interval. Epidural PCA is used with success in patients with rib fractures and may decrease the need for mechanical ventilation, an important benefit in older trauma patients. Vigilant nursing care is essential because the epidural catheter may migrate and not provide adequate pain relief. A patient's report of pain relief needs to be requested by the nurse at hourly intervals initially; it is the only reliable measurement for pain.

The progressive care nurse will have to rely on assessment data to determine the need for antianxiety and analgesic medication administration. If there is a perception, the nurse perceives the injury as painful, and the patient is unable to communicate or physiologically respond to painful stimuli due to drugs (beta-blockers, etc) pain medication should be encouraged based on that perception.

A variety of nonpharmacologic pain-reducing strategies are useful in patients with trauma, and the nurse needs to combine these with drug therapy for maximal gain. Because narcotics have side effects, combining them with a nonsteroidal anti-inflammatory agent and a cognitive intervention may offer the patient the best pain reduction possible. Cognitive interventions for pain includes relaxation, guided imagery, music therapy, pet therapy, or hypnosis. Clear documentation of what strategies or combinations work best for the individual is needed. This approach requires an established communication system between patient, nurse, nurse practitioner, and/or physician. Anxiety and sleeplessness contribute to the pain response and should be addressed by asking the patients how they typically try to relax and by eliminating as much environmental noise as possible. Encouraging rest and sleep and limiting patient interruptions provides better pain management.

Positioning

Early mobilization of the trauma patient assists in promoting oxygenation and ventilation, and other complications of immobility. This includes positioning the patient in and out of bed. Information obtained from daily chest x-ray results is essential for accurate positioning of the patient. Positions to be considered include: sitting, prone, and lateral decubitus. The lateral decubitus position with the good lung down is especially important to maximize oxygenation if there is unilateral lung disease or injury to one side of the chest. An example of how the concept of therapeutic positioning can be used by the nurse is to position the patient and observe chest excursion, respiratory rate, pulse oximetry, peak inspiratory pressures, and if applicable, hemodynamic data for improvement. Continuous lateral rotation and/or prone positioning beds may be helpful for selected injuries and or conditions.

Abdominal Trauma

Etiology and Pathophysiology

Trauma to the abdomen may occur to organs in three distinct abdominal regions: peritoneal cavity, retroperitoneum, and pelvis. The trauma will be directly related to the mechanism of injury and the anatomical location that was impacted. The organs most affected by blunt abdominal trauma are the spleen, liver, and kidneys. From penetrating mechanisms, the liver and intestines are more commonly injured (most penetrating trauma is anterior). The types of injuries sustained could be organ contusions, lacerations, fractures, vascular disruption and hemorrhage, and crush-type tissue damage. Abdominal trauma is frequently not as overt on primary and secondary assessments as other injuries, but it is frequently more life threatening. Physical examination, the presence of pain, FAST, and the abdominal CAT scan are the main methods used to diagnose potential injuries and are the primary tools used to determine if the patient needs to go directly to the operating room or should be closely monitored. Vigilance in nursing assessment for overt changes and observance of trends are the keys to identifying abdominal injuries. The MRI, DPL, and angiography also might be used for assessment.

The FAST and the abdominal CAT scan are two diagnostic tools used in conventional trauma assessment. FAST exams are rapid, noninvasive, and can be repeated multiple times throughout the resuscitation period. Abdominal CAT scanning requires a hemodynamically normal patient and is more costly than FAST exams. Historically, if the patient was unable to reliably confirm or deny the presence of abdominal pain, a DPL would be performed. For patient safety during a DPL a decompressed bladder and stomach is necessary. The entry into the abdomen with the needle increases the likelihood of injury.

To perform a DPL, a catheter is inserted just below the umbilicus and normal saline is infused. The bag is then lowered below the abdomen and the fluid allowed to drain out. If the fluid does not come out or it is bloody or cloudy, there is a high probability of abdominal trauma. A DPL cannot discover a retroperitoneal bleed.

Damage to the spleen is one of the most frequently encountered blunt abdominal trauma injuries. Depending on severity of splenic injury, interventions range from nonoperative observation, embolization angiography, and bedrest for mild lacerations to removal of a massively ruptured spleen. Liver trauma runs the spectrum from minor injury to severe laceration, requiring operative repair and packing. The bowel, pancreas, and kidneys can be directly injured or sustain secondary injury as a result of poor perfusion and/or inflammation during the trauma, resuscitation, or critical care phase of recovery.

Typically, presenting signs and symptoms in abdominal trauma include pain and hypovolemia. Complications from abdominal trauma are directly linked to the function of the gastrointestinal tract and include metabolic/nutritional alterations, infections such as peritonitis, and pancreatitis. Patients may require extensive dressing changes if the wound is open or requires frequent surgeries for staged repair of the abdominal organs.

Principles of Abdominal Trauma Management

Selected principles of caring for the patient with abdominal trauma include monitoring for bleeding, infection prevention and management, and initiating early (within 24-48 hours) nutritional support.

Monitoring for Bleeding

Acute hemorrhage is commonly addressed during the primary survey and frequently requires surgery. Occult bleeding may not be initially evident and later be discovered by the acute care nurse. Common abdominal injuries that may not initially exhibit signs and symptoms of bleeding include liver laceration, splenic fractures, and slow retroperitoneal bleeds.

Spleen injuries were historically treated with splenectomy. The conventional wisdom is to preserve the spleen if possible. Splenorrhaphy, embolization repair of the spleen, or watchful waiting is increasing in popularity. The goal is to allow the spleen to heal and preserve the valuable immunoprotective function. If splenectomy is indicated due to massive injury, patients are given polyvalent pneumococcal vaccine within 72 hours after surgery to prevent infection with pneumococci. These patients will have immune compromise the rest of their lives. Management also includes a minimum of 3 days of bedrest, monitoring for rebleeding, and interventions to prevent the complications of immobility.

Infection Prevention and Management

Abdominal trauma victims are at high risk for infection even when surgery has not been performed. One of the major nursing care priorities (after airway and bleeding) in all trauma patients is prevention, assessment, and management of infections. Traumatic wounds can be simple lacerations or abrasions from a motor vehicle crash or complex open abdominal surgical wounds that require packing and frequent trips to the operating room. Care for the patient with a large abdominal wound is directed by the type of wound (open or closed) and the degree of intracompartment contamination due to the injury and surgery. Careful consideration of antimicrobial therapy must also be considered with contaminated wounds. The dressing changes are frequently performed by the acute care nursing staff, so assessment for signs of infection as well as wound healing is essential during these dressing changes. Premedicating the patient or timing dressing changes around pain medication administration is another important role of the nurse providing holistic care. These patients frequently may have multiple sources of infection. The presence of a central line, Foley catheter, ET tube, nasogastric tube, chest tube, and peripheral IV all increase the risk of hospital-acquired infection. Sepsis is always a risk for any trauma patient and that risk is increased with abdominal trauma victims.

Nutritional Support

Nutritional support in the trauma patient is multifactorial and an integral part of trauma care. Management focuses on the route and timing of nutritional support. Other considerations include composition of nutrient formulation, assessment of laboratory tests that measure nutrition, and enteral verses parenteral feedings. Trauma patients have increased metabolic needs due to a hypermetabolic stress response caused by severe injuries, wound healing, and/or sepsis.

Enteral nutrition is encouraged whenever possible at the earliest time after injury. Even a small amount of nutrition delivered via tube feeding to the gut is believed to be beneficial. A variety of metabolic derangements in the hypermetabolic trauma patient make nutritional support an early imperative. Insertion and maintenance of a small-bowel feeding tube, percutaneous gastrostomy tube, or jejunostomy tube is often required after injury until the patient can be orally fed. Total parenteral nutrition is recommended only if the gastrointestinal tract is unable to tolerate adequate nutrients. Accurate nutritional assessment conducted in collaboration with the nutritionist is essential, as trauma patients are at risk of complications from overfeeding as well as underfeeding. Diarrhea, inappropriate withholding of tube feedings, and the potential for increased aspiration are issues that need to be addressed for trauma patients (see Chapter 14, Gastrointestinal System).

Musculoskeletal Trauma

Etiology and Pathophysiology

Trauma to the musculoskeletal system accounts for approximately 70% to 85% of polytrauma injuries. Patients in the progressive care setting with extremity or pelvic fractures often have other injuries due to the significant physical impact to the body. Motor vehicle trauma, falls, sports injuries, and industrial trauma are all frequent causes of musculoskeletal trauma. Victims of motorcycle crashes frequently have severe fractures with extensive soft tissue damage. Massive blood loss, edema of tissues, tissue destruction, and pain accompany musculoskeletal injuries.

Compartment syndrome is a serious complication of extremity trauma as a result of contused tissue swelling in a specific muscle compartment (Figure 17-4). This may lead to lack of perfusion and nerve compression in the area. Muscle compartments are located in the forearm, leg, hand, foot, thigh, abdomen, and chest. The nurse assesses for signs of compartment syndrome and performs early and repeated neurovascular checks. However, neurovascular assessment of the five P's (pain, pallor, pulselessness, paresthesia, paralysis) may not provide accurate early assessment of rising compartment pressures. Nursing management consists of immobilization and extremity level with the heart or below. Elevation of the extremity can worsen condition. Assessment of compartment pressures requires the use of a specialized needle that is inserted directly into the tissue compartment. The needle/catheter is attached to a transducer and the compartment pressures are evaluated and monitored. Even open fractures may have significantly increased compartment pressures (normal pressure 0-8 mm Hg). If the compartment pressures are found to be high, a fasciotomy will be preformed to relieve the pressure. A fasciotomy entails surgically opening the skin and fascia to relieve the pressure in a muscle compartment and is the treatment of choice for compartment syndrome. The primary goal of fasciotomy

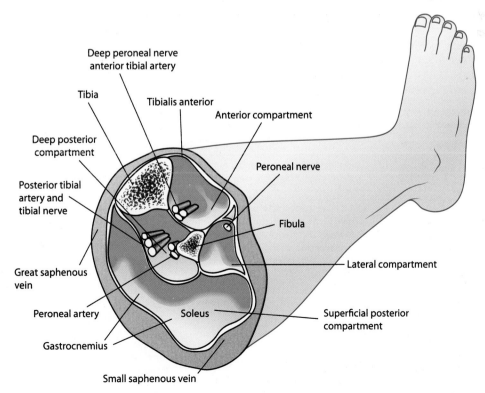

Figure 17-4. Compartments of the lower leg. (*Illustrated and used with permission by David Hayes, Fultan, MD, 2009.*)

is to improve perfusion and minimize distal tissue damage from ischemia.

Principles of Management of Musculoskeletal Trauma
Management of extremity trauma focuses on early stabilization of fractures to prevent further tissue damage, infection, bleeding, and disability. Complications from musculoskeletal trauma include immobility, which can lead to increased incidence of pulmonary emboli, fat emboli, deep venous thrombosis, and pressure ulcers. Pain control to promote mobility, and assessment of neurovascular status are key components to managing these patients (Table 17-5).

TABLE 17-5. PHYSICAL COMPLICATIONS RELATED TO IMMOBILITY COMMONLY SEEN IN TRAUMA PATIENTS

Body System	Complications	Pathophysiology	Prevention
Neurologic	Potentially affects all body systems	Caused by decreased level of consciousness; injury to cortex, motor, or sensory systems.	• Neurologic assessment. • Specific focus on the effects seen in other body systems. • Understand neurologic basis of complication.
Respiratory	Fatigue, decreased productivity; infection, pneumonia, respiratory acidosis	Decreased respiratory movement, unable to mobilize secretions, alterations in blood gases.	• Assessment of respiratory status and changes in level of consciousness. • Mobilization of secretions by turning, coughing, and deep breathing; postural drainage, percussion, vibration, early ambulation, humidification, and hydration.
Cardiovascular	Orthostatic hypotension, fatigue, increased cardiac workload, thrombosis, embolus	Increased heart rate, CVP, cardiac output, stroke volume in supine position; loss of supporting muscle tone resulting in venous stasis; orthostatic neurovascular receptors cannot adjust to position changes; hypercoagulability and external pressure to vessels.	• Cardiovascular assessment. • Encourage mobilization, exercise, range of motion, positioning. • Antiembolic devices. • Provide adequate hydration. • Avoid Valsalva maneuver.
Gastrointestinal	Anorexia, fatigue, malnutrition, constipation, impaction, bowel obstruction, diarrhea, dehydration	Negative nitrogen balance and protein deficiency; stress; decreased appetite creates bowel intolerance; muscle weakness; diminished ability to apply abdominal pressure needed for evacuation; psychological factors and position for defecation may increase difficulty.	• Assessment of GI functioning, including baseline history of nutrition, exercise, and bowel habits. • Coordinate bowel plan with nutrition specialist. • Adequate hydration. • Positioning and privacy. • Gastrocolic reflex timing factors; use of digital stimulation. • Stool softeners and suppositories as, bowel stimulants. • Adjust tube feedings to avoid constipation or diarrhea. • Small, frequent feedings to increase tolerance and decrease anorexia. • Encourage intake of protein, fluids, bulk foods.
Urinary	Urinary reflux, incontinence, urinary stasis, renal calculi, urinary tract infection	Loss of effect of gravity, urinary stasis in renal pelvis; increased calculi formation from urine sediment in renal pelvis; diminished coordination of sphincters and muscles in supine position; bladder distention, overflow incontinence.	• Assess urinary tract function. • Promote movement and exercise. • Maintain fluid intake. • Decrease calcium intake, increase loss from bones. • Monitor distention and voiding patterns. • Prevent incontinence. • Use upright or sitting position for voiding if possible. • Intermittent catheters preferred to indwelling.
Musculoskeletal	Muscle atrophy, contractures	Muscles shorten and atrophy; loss of ROM as supporting ligaments, tendons, and capsule lose mobility; loss of ROM becomes permanent; spasticity of antagonistic muscle with weakness of opposing muscle creates contracture.	• Ongoing assessment • Passive, active, and active-assisted ROM exercises • Appropriate positioning and body alignment in both bed and chair
	Osteoporosis, stress fractures, heterotrophic ossification	Normal bone-building activities depend on weight bearing and movement; increased destruction of bone, release of calcium; bone becomes porous and fragile; abnormal calcification over large joints may also occur.	• Calcium supplement to diet is not recommended. • Promote weight bearing.
Integumentary	Skin breakdown; stages I-IV skin ulcers; secondary infection of skin ulcers, sepsis enter body.	Prolonged pressure to skin diminishes capillary blood supply and stops flow of nutrients to cells; necrosis of cells results in skin breakdown, allowing infection to occur.	• Assessment of skin integrity, nutritional status, and risk factors for breakdown. • Reposition; shift pressure and patient weight frequently. • Check for changes in blanching, sustained redness. • Keep off all red areas. • Massage at-risk areas to promote circulation. • Teach patient to inspect own skin and shift weight. • Increase protein in diet, monitor hydration status. • Take immediate, consistent action on any areas of breakdown.

Fractures are repaired early after a traumatic injury to decrease bleeding and to limit immobility and its complications (eg, pulmonary embolism). Guidelines for the management of venous thromboembolism for trauma patients include thromboprophylaxis and mechanical prophylactic devices, such as sequential compression devices (Tables 17-6 and 17-7).

TABLE 17-6. EVIDENCE-BASED PRACTICE: MANAGEMENT OF VENOUS THROMBO-EMBOLISM IN TRAUMA PATIENTS[a,b]

Risk Factors
- Patients with major trauma, spinal cord or spinal fractures are at high risk for venous thromboembolism (VTE) following trauma.
- Older age is an increased factor for venous thromboembolism but it is not clear at which exact age the risk increases substantially.

The Role of Low-Molecular-Weight Heparin (LMWH)
- There are insufficient data to make recommendations for general use of LMWH as VTE prophylaxis in trauma patients.
- LMWH could be used for VTE prophylaxis in trauma patients with the following patterns: (1) pelvic fracture requiring operative fixation or prolonged bed rest (> 5 days); (2) complex lower extremity fractures (defined as open fractures or multiple fractures in one extremity) requiring operative fixation or prolonged bed rest (>5 days); (3) spinal cord injury with complete or incomplete motor paralysis. The use of LMWH is predicted on the fact that these patients do not have other injuries that put them at high risk for bleeding.
- The use of LMWH or oral anticoagulants for several weeks postinjury should be considered in patients who remain at high risk for VTE (ie, elderly pelvic fracture patients, spinal cord injury patients, patients who remain at prolonged bed rest [>5 days], and patients who require prolonged hospitalization or rehabilitation).

The Use of Low-Dose Heparin
- There is little evidence to support a benefit of low-dose heparin as a sole agent for prophylaxis in the trauma patient at high risk for VTE.
- For patients in whom bleeding could exacerbate their injuries, the safety of low-dose heparin has not been established and an individual decision should be made when considering anticoagulant prophylaxis.

The Use of Sequential Compression Devices (SCD)
- There are insufficient data to support a standard on this topic.
- In the subset of spine-injured, head-injured patients, SCD may have some benefit.
- For patients in whom the lower extremity is inaccessible to place SCDs at the calf level, foot pumps may act as an effective alternative to lower the rate of DVT formation.

The Role of A-V Foot Pumps
- There are insufficient data to suggest recommendations for this topic.
- Foot pumps are less effective than SCD for prevention of DVT.
- A-V foot pumps may be used as a substitute for SCDs in those high-risk trauma patients who cannot wear SCDs due to external fixators or casts.

The Role of the Vena Cava Filter
A vena cava filter should be inserted in patients with:
- Recurrent PE despite full anticoagulation
- Proximal DVT and contraindications to full anticoagulation
- Proximal DVT and major bleeding while on full anticoagulation
- Progression of iliofemoral clot despite anticoagulation (rare)
Extended indications for prophylactic vena cava filter placement in a patient with established DVT or PE include:
- Large free-floating thrombus in the iliac vein or IVC
- Following massive PE in which recurrent emboli may prove fatal
- During and after surgical embolectomy

Data compiled from: [a]Eastern Association for the Surgery of Trauma: Practice Management Guidelines for Venous thromboembolism in Trauma Patients. Available: www.east .org or www.guidelines.gov. Accessed June 26, 2013; and [b]Geerts W, Bergquist D, Pineo G, et al (2008).

TABLE 17-7. AACN PRACTICE ALERT GUIDELINES FOR DEEP VEIN THROMBOSIS PREVENTION

Expected Practice
- Assess all patients upon admission to the ICU for risk factors of deep vein thrombosis (DVT) and anticipate orders for DVT prophylaxis based on risk assessment. Clinical regimens for DVT prophylaxis based on risk are as follows:
  - Moderate-risk patients including medically ill and postoperative patients—on low-dose, unfractionated heparin or low-molecular-weight heparin (LMWH).
  - Higher-risk patients including major trauma or orthopedic surgery—LMWH.
  - Patients with high risk for bleeding—on mechanical prophylaxis including graduated compression stockings and/or intermittent pneumatic compression devices.
  - Mechanical prophylaxis may also be anticipated in conjunction with anticoagulant-based prophylaxis regimens.
  - Review each patient's current DVT risk factors including clinical status, necessity for central venous catheter (CVC), current status of DVT prophylaxis, risk for bleeding, and response to treatment daily with the physician and during multidisciplinary rounds.
  - Maximize patient mobility whenever possible and take measures to reduce the amount of time the patient is immobile because of the effects of treatment (eg, pain, sedation, neuromuscular blockade, mechanical ventilation).
  - Ensure that mechanical prophylaxis devices are fitted properly and in use at all times except when being removed for cleaning and/or inspection of skin.

www.aacn.org/clinical practice/practice alerts:pdf 2010. Accessed January 28, 2014.

Stabilizing Fractures

Fractures are repaired early after a traumatic injury to decrease further bleeding and to limit pulmonary embolism complications. External fixation is used for pelvic fractures and lower limb fractures. Frequent sensation, movement, and vascular checks on affected extremities are essential. If the presence of pulses is in doubt, Doppler ultrasound should be used at the bedside.

Pain Control

Pain control is best achieved with an individualized strategy of medications and nonpharmacologic therapies. Patients respond best when strict attention is paid to pain control and their own unique coping style is used. Patients are expected to move in the bed and get out of the bed as soon as possible after an injury. Titrated pain medication is required to achieve this goal using PCA or continuous infusion. Nurses need to determine patient anxieties regarding the trauma and promote adequate sleep and rest. Sleep deprivation from a noisy environment, constant worry, and needless pain only makes the patient perceive a more intense pain.

COMPLICATIONS OF TRAUMATIC INJURY IN SEVERE MULTISYSTEM TRAUMA

The key to survival for patients with multiple trauma is to limit the extent of complications experienced and increase the delivery of oxygen to the tissues during the initial phase of resuscitation. In the history of trauma as a clinical specialty this has been called the "golden hour." The resuscitation goal is to prevent tissue oxygen deprivation due to hypoperfusion and identify and eliminate the cause of problem. Shock, by definition, occurs when cellular oxygen delivery does not meet oxygen demands, which leads to cellular hypoxia. When adequate oxygen and blood flow are provided during the resuscitative phase of trauma, the likelihood of shock and hypoperfusion complications decrease. Heart rate and blood pressure are not considered adequate parameters to judge the effectiveness of resuscitation, because they indicate only the body's compensation for the stress of trauma and not real-time tissue oxygenation. Appropriate measures to evaluate resuscitation should focus on assessing tissue oxygen delivery, including oxygen transport, delivery, and utilization. Evaluation of base deficit as an indicator of oxygen delivery at the cellular level is invalid. Base deficit is a good prognostic indicator of the effects of the general resuscitation efforts but not at the cellular level. Therefore, as the base deficit rises, a lactic acid test should also be done to assess perfusion at the cellular level (see Chapter 19, Advanced Cardiovascular Concepts). Serum lactate rises with inadequate oxygenation and is an additional diagnostic indicator of the adequacy of reperfusion and oxygen delivery. To preserve adequate blood flow in the acutely injured trauma patient, permissive hypertension may be used. In contrast, permissive hypotension is based on the concept that resuscitation to attain normal blood pressures may increase bleeding from a site that has already "clotted" through the normal clotting cascade process. In this case large volumes of blood are not encouraged.

Common complications of trauma are infection/sepsis, ARDS, and systemic inflammatory response syndrome (SIRS) (see Chapter 10, Respiratory System, and Chapter 11, Multisystem Problems). Patients with sepsis and SIRS experience a persistent inflammatory response, which can lead to acute lung injury and multiple organ dysfunction syndrome (MODS). Multiple organ dysfunction or failure begins during hypoperfusion and shock phase, and if reperfusion is not quick or adequate enough, the organs sustain ischemia, inflammation, injury, and possibly infarction. The clinical presentation of organ dysfunction may have a rapid onset or take days to weeks to present. It can be assessed by the critical care nurse as signs and symptoms of ARDS, pancreatitis, ARF, hepatic insufficiency, or any organ failure. Delivering oxygen to the tissues by maintaining increased blood flow during resuscitation and early acute care phases is believed to decrease the length of hypoperfusion and anaerobic metabolism and these often lethal complications.

Achieving adequate oxygen delivery to the tissues requires oxygen, hemoglobin, and sufficient cardiac output to deliver them to the organs and cells. This is typically accomplished with massive fluid and or blood resuscitation. Massive transfusion is defined as the administration of more than 10 U of blood (whole blood or packed red blood cells) within 24 hours, replacing the patient's total blood volume. Trauma patients are at risk of experiencing significant complications after massive fluid/blood administration. Hypothermia coagulopathy, acidosis, electrolyte imbalances, transfusion-related acute lung injury (TRALI), transfusion-associated circulatory overload (TACO), transfusion-associated immunomodulation (TRIM–a down regulation of immune function or immunosupression), and the cause of posttransfusion infections have all been attributed to massive fluid or blood replacement. Monitoring for and treating these complications are essential during the critical care phase of trauma patient care.

Acute Respiratory Distress Syndrome

Patients with trauma have an increased incidence of ARDS (see Chapter 10, Respiratory System). Precipitating factors for ARDS in the trauma patient include direct or indirect injury to the lungs. Examples of direct injury include smoke inhalation, rib fractures, or large pulmonary contusions. Indirect injury may be due to sepsis, massive fluid resuscitation, and prolonged hypoperfusion states (shock) which may all lead to an inflammatory insult and alveolar infiltration.

Standard treatment for ARDS includes mechanical ventilation, oxygen titrated to maintain Pao_2 above 60 mm Hg, and ventilatory modes and methods to recruit closed alveoli and decrease lung injury. In addition to mechanical ventilation, another method to improve oxygenation is positioning for optimal ventilation and perfusion. This is a unique challenge for acutely ill trauma patients because their traumatic injuries may preclude many positions; for example, the patient with an unstable pelvic fracture, a spinal cord injury, or lower extremity fractures may be difficult or impossible to turn. Meticulous nursing care to prevent ventilator associated complications (VAC) is a priority for all trauma patients receiving mechanical ventilation.

Infection/Sepsis

Trauma patients are at high risk of developing an infection and potentially sepsis. This is because of the nature of the injury, the environment in which the injury occurred, the nonsterile conditions in which invasive devices may have been initially placed, and the multiple invasive procedures, including surgery, necessary for trauma resuscitation and management. The procedures preformed during resuscitation are at best undertaken under clean conditions.

The classic signs and symptoms of infection are sometimes difficult to isolate in a recovering trauma patient. Fever, tachycardia, elevated white blood cell count, hypoglycemia inflammation, pain, and a hyperdynamic state are classic indicators of infection and sepsis. These assessment parameters are also common after injury, resuscitation, and during the healing process due to the stress response on the immune system. The classic rule in trauma care is that there is an infection—it just needs to be found and treated.

When clear identification of an infectious source is elusive, a finding of elevated C-reactive protein and procalcitonin levels are sometimes considered confirmation that an infectious source exists. Meticulous attention to sterile technique and hand washing is essential in this vulnerable patient population.

Systemic Inflammatory Response Syndrome

Identification and management of SIRS requires knowledge of the underlying inflammatory process (see Chapter 11, Multisystem Problems). Assessment criteria for SIRS includes two or more of the following: temperature greater than 38°C or less than 36°C, heart rate greater than 90 beats/min, respiratory rate greater than 20 breaths/min, $Paco_2$ less than 32 mm Hg, and white blood cell count greater than 12,000/mm^3 or less than 4000/mm^3. The systemic inflammatory response has occurred because of direct injury to tissues/organs and lack of oxygen delivery (hypoperfusion) during the shock state. These circumstances lead to the release of biological mediators from injured tissue/cells, which cause an intense systemic inflammation, vasodilatation, and increased membrane permeability (edema, leaky tissue). The cardiopulmonary changes typical in SIRS include high cardiac output, decreased systemic vascular resistance, and elevated oxygen requirements and consumption.

Goals for managing the patient with SIRS are to provide the essentials such as oxygenation and nutrition, limit known stressors such as pain and fever, and support organ system function. The delivery of oxygen and nutrients requires an adequate cardiac output, oxygen-saturated hemoglobin, and an environment (pH) in which the cells can extract and utilize the delivered oxygen. Fluid resuscitation, vasoactive and inotropic drug administration may be necessary to maximize oxygen delivery during the SIRS phase.

The individual's response to SIRS may be prolonged and destructive, leading to MODS. As organs begin to dysfunction and fail, treatments such as maximal ventilatory support and hemodialysis may be necessary. Mortality remains high for MODS, requiring increased attention to prevention of early following trauma hypoperfusion. Limiting the initial shock (hypoperfusion) state decreases the likelihood of SIRS and therefore MODS. In trauma care, the multidisciplinary team's interventions in the first 24 hours of injury often determine survival.

PSYCHOLOGICAL CONSEQUENCES OF TRAUMA

Acute illness places many stresses on patients and families, resulting in unique psychosocial implications. Trauma injury is by nature unexpected. It typically affects young, healthy individuals and can launch both the patient and family into a cycle of chaos and crisis. Common responses to trauma include anxiety, fear, grief, loss, guilt, depression, denial, sleeplessness, and hopelessness.

Fear begins immediately as the awake trauma patient is transported from the scene. Fear is related to the unknown, the specifics of the injuries, and impact on the patient's future, including body image, family, and career. Loss typifies the experience of trauma and can be characterized as loss of physical functioning, loss of quality of life, or even loss of significant others due to the traumatic event. Guilt may ensue as the patient may perceive responsibility for the event (directly or indirectly) and this can be overwhelming. Depression and denial are common coping mechanisms used during personal crises and may be exhibited in a variety of ways by trauma victims. It should be noted that although the injuries were sustained by the patient, the family members, and family structure frequently are also traumatized.

Monitoring the patient's response to injury is as much the responsibility of the nurse as monitoring the patient's blood pressure. As there are long-term physiologic effects of a low blood pressure (shock), so are there long-term psychological effects of unmet or unidentified emotional needs. There are also psychoneuroimmunologic in responses that can impact the physical recovery. The emotional response to injury should be assessed. Talk to the patient and listen to their responses and perceptions. Help them to identify and articulate their concerns and fears.

Fear creates anxiety in the trauma patient, and unrelieved pain may worsen anxiety. With the intense monitoring and frequent care interruptions in the progressive care environment, sleep may be impossible. A vicious cycle is thus initiated whereby sleeplessness leads to an increased perception of pain, which in turn creates needless anxiety and inhibits sleep. The importance of viewing these responses as cyclical emphasizes that the progressive care nurse may intervene anywhere in the cycle of responses and make a major impact on all three; for example, providing pain-relieving strategies that permit sleep automatically decreases anxiety. A focus on information sharing may ease the patient's mind so that sleep can occur and pain perception decreases. The nurse has a significant role in intervening to stop this vicious cycle through a variety of holistic strategies.

All families of trauma patients experience a crisis. Families may have no idea of how to act or what the healthcare team expects of them. Clinicians have a key role in providing the right amount of support and information to meet family needs, and in identifying family-coping mechanisms. Knowing the phases of family emotional response and suggested interventions is useful (Table 17-8). Early assessment of family system structure, relationship process, and family functioning are keys to effective management of the psychosocial needs of the patient and family. Getting to know and work with family members in trauma care is essential and can be best facilitated with flexible visiting policies, family presence during rounds, procedures, and codes when appropriate, and where family members are wanted and expected by the patient, the nurse, and the entire team.

TABLE 17-8. PHASES AND MANIFESTATIONS OF STRESS AND NURSING INTERVENTIONS FOR FAMILIES OF TRAUMA PATIENTS

Phase	Manifestations	Interventions
High anxiety	Restlessness Fainting Nausea High-pitched voice	Encourage ventilation of feelings Provide accurate information
Denial	Families commonly state, "Everything will be all right"	Reiterate the facts of the situation
Anger	Verbal abuse directed toward healthcare staff	Active listening Allow ventilation of angry feelings Help to refocus on the real cause of anger
Remorse	Elements of guilt and sorrow "If only" stage	Listen to family's expressions of remorse Interject reality
Grief	Intense period of sadness Crying	Encourage flow of tears Provide empathetic gestures such as silent physical closeness, holding a trembling hand, embracing limp shoulders

From: Hopkins AG. The trauma nurse's role with families in crisis. Crit Care Nurse. 1994;14(2):37.

SELECTED BIBLIOGRAPHY

General Trauma

AACP-SCCM Consensus Conference Committee. Definitions for sepsis and organ failure and guidelines for the use of innovative therapies in sepsis. *Chest.* 1992;101:1644-1655.

American College of Surgeons Committee on Trauma. *Advanced Trauma Life Support for Doctors.* 9th ed. Chicago, IL: ACS; 2012.

Aresco C. Trauma. In: Morton P, Fontaine D, eds. *Critical Care Nursing: A Holistic Approach,* 9th ed. New York, NY: Lippincott Williams & Wilkins; 2008.

Boswell S, Scalea T. Initial management of traumatic shock. In: McQuillan K, Makic M, Whalen E. *Trauma Nursing: From Resuscitation Through Rehabilitation.* 4th ed. St Louis, MO: Saunders Elsevier; 2009.

Branney SW, Wolfe RE, Moore EE, et al. Quantitative sensitivity of ultrasound in detecting free intraperitoneal fluid. *J Trauma.* 1995;39:375.

Cunnenn J, Cartwright M. The puzzle of sepsis: fitting the pieces of inflammatory response with treatment. *AACN Clin Iss.* 2004;15:18-44.

Emergency Nurses Association. *Trauma Nursing Core Course-Provider Manual.* 6th ed. Chicago, IL: ENA; 2007.

Feliciano DV, Mattox KL, Moore, EE. *Trauma.* 6th ed. New York, NY: McGraw-Hill Co; 2008.

Frawley P. Thoracic trauma. In: McQuillan K, Makic M, Whalen E, eds. *Trauma Nursing: From Resuscitation Through Rehabilitation.* 4th ed. St Louis, MO: Saunders Elsevier; 2009.

Goldstein AS, Scalfani SJA, Kupterstein NH, et al. The diagnostic superiority of computed tomography. *J Trauma.* 1985;25:939.

Jones K, Abdominal injuries. In: McQuillan K, Makic M, Whalen E, eds. *Trauma Nursing: From Resuscitation Through Rehabilitation.* 4th ed. St Louis, MO: Saunders Elsevier; 2009.

Levy M, Fink M, Marshall J, et al. 2001 SCCM/ESICM/ATS/SIS International sepsis definitions conference. *CCM.* 2003;31:1250-1256.

Mattox K, Feliciano D, Moore E, ed. *Trauma.* 4th ed. New York, NY: McGraw Hill; 2000.

McKinney MG, Lentz K, Nunez D, et al. Can ultrasound replace diagnostic peritoneal lavage in the assessment of blunt trauma? *J Trauma.* 1994;37:439.

McQuillan K, Makic M, Whalen E. *Trauma Nursing: From Resuscitation Through Rehabilitation.* 4th ed. St Louis, MO: Saunders Elsevier; 2009.

Otomo Y, Henmi H, Mashiko K, et al. New diagnostic peritoneal lavage criteria for diagnosis of intestinal injury. *J Trauma.* 1998;44:991.

Ruggiero M. Effects of vasopressin in septic shock. *AACN Advance Crit Care.* 2008;19:281-290.

Rushton C, Reina M, Reina D. Building trustworthy relationships with critically ill patients and families. *AACN Adv Crit Care.* 2007;18:19-30.

Saunders CJ, Battistella FD, Whetzel TP, Stokes RB. Percutaneous diagnostic peritoneal lavage using a Veress needle versus an open technique: a prospective randomized trial. *J Trauma.* 1998;44:883.

VonRueden K, Bolton P, Vary T. Shock and multiple organ dysfunction syndrome. In: McQuillan K, Makic M, Whalen E, eds. *Trauma Nursing: From Resuscitation Through Rehabilitation.* 4th ed. St Louis, MO: Saunders Elsevier; 2009.

Wiegand D, Carlson K. *AACN Procedure Manual for Critical Care.* 5th ed. St Louis, MO: Elsevier Saunders; 2005.

Selected Online References

http//:www.aacn.org. Accessed June 29, 2013.

http//:www.east.org. Accessed June 29, 2013.

http//:www.trauma.org. Accessed June 29, 2013.

http//:www.facs.org. Accessed June 29, 2013.

http//:www.sccm.org. Accessed June 29, 2013.

http//:www.ena.org. Accessed June 29, 2013.

Evidence-Based Practice

Dellinger P, Levy MM, Carlet JM, Bion J, et al. Surviving sepsis campaign guidelines: international guidelines for management of severe sepsis and septic shock. *Crit Care Med.* 2008;36(1):296-327.

Geerts W, Bergqvist D, Pineo G, et al. Prevention of venous thromboembolism. *Chest.* 2008;133:381S-453S.

Advanced Concepts in Caring for the Critically Ill Patient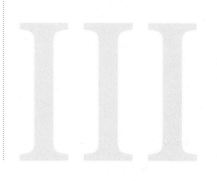

ADVANCED ECG CONCEPTS

Carol Jacobson

KNOWLEDGE COMPETENCIES

1. Identify electrocardiogram (ECG) characteristics and treatment approaches for each of the following advanced arrhythmias:
   - Supraventricular tachycardias
   - Wide QRS beats and rhythms
2. Using the 12-lead ECG, determine the following:
   - Bundle branch blocks
   - QRS axis

- Patterns of myocardial ischemia, injury, and infarct
3. Identify ECG characteristics of single- and dual-chamber pacemakers during normal and abnormal functioning.
4. Identify ECG characteristics of Brugada syndrome and long QT syndromes.

THE 12-LEAD ELECTROCARDIOGRAM

The 12-lead ECG records electrical activity as it spreads through the heart from 12 different leads, which are in turn recorded by electrodes placed on the arms and legs, and in specific spots on the chest. Each lead represents a different "view" of the heart and consists of two electrodes. A bipolar lead has two poles—one positive and one negative. A unipolar lead has one positive pole and a reference pole that is a point in the center of the chest that is mathematically determined by the ECG machine. The standard 12-lead ECG consists of six frontal plane limb leads that record electrical activity traveling up/down and right/left in the heart, and six precordial leads that record electrical activity in the horizontal plane traveling anterior/posterior and right/left. Limb leads are recorded by electrodes placed on the arms and legs, and precordial leads are recorded by electrodes placed on the chest (Figure 18-1).

A camera analogy makes the 12-lead ECG easier to understand. Each lead of the ECG represents a picture of the electrical activity in the heart taken by the camera. In any lead, the positive electrode is the recording electrode or the camera lens. The negative electrode tells the camera which way to "shoot" its picture and determines the direction in which the positive electrode records. When the positive electrode sees electrical activity traveling toward it, it records an upright deflection on the ECG. When the positive electrode sees electrical activity traveling away from it, it records a negative deflection (Figure 18-2). If the electrical activity travels perpendicular to a positive electrode, no activity is recorded. The standard 12-ECG records three bipolar frontal plane leads (leads I, II, and III) and three unipolar frontal plane leads (aVR, aVL, and aVF). In addition, there are six unipolar precordial leads: V_1, V_2, V_3, V_4, V_5, and V_6.

The three bipolar frontal plane leads are illustrated in Figure 18-3A. In each lead, the camera represents the positive pole of the lead. In lead I, the positive electrode is on the left arm and the negative electrode is on the right arm. Any electrical activity in the heart that travels toward the positive electrode (camera lens) on the left arm is recorded as an upright deflection and any activity traveling away from it is recorded as a negative deflection. In lead II, the positive electrode is on the left leg and the negative electrode is on the right arm. Any electrical activity traveling toward the left leg electrode (camera lens) is recorded as an upright deflection and any activity traveling away from it toward the right arm

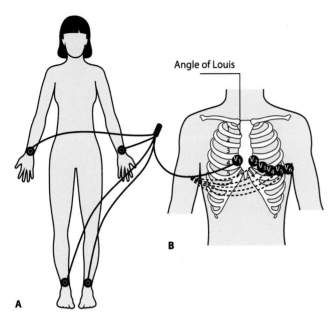

Figure 18-1. **(A)** Limb electrodes can be placed anywhere on arms and legs. Standard placement is shown here on wrists and ankles. **(B)** Chest electrode placement. V_1 = fourth intercostal space to right of sternum; V_2 = fourth intercostal space to left of sternum; V_3 = halfway between V_2 and V_4 in a straight line; V_4 = fifth intercostal space at mid clavicular line; V_5 = same level as V_4 at anterior axillary line; V_6 = same level as V_4 at midaxillary line.

reference spot in the center of the chest that is mathematically determined by the ECG machine. The same principles apply to unipolar leads: any electrical activity traveling toward the positive electrode is recorded as an upright deflection and any traveling away from it is recorded as a negative deflection. The six unipolar precordial leads are recorded from their locations on the chest as shown in Figure 18-3C. The view of the heart by unipolar leads can be compared to a telephoto lens on the camera, "zooming in" on the electrical activity in the heart.

The hexaxial reference system (or axis wheel) is formed when the six frontal plane leads are moved together in such a way that they bisect each other in the center (Figure 18-4A). Each lead is labeled at its positive end to make it easy to remember where the positive electrode is. In Figure 18-4B, the hexaxial reference system is superimposed over a drawing of the heart to illustrate how each lead views the heart.

The normal sequence of depolarization through the heart begins with an electrical impulse originating in the sinus node, high in the right atrium, and spreading leftward through the left atrium and downward toward the AV node, low in the right atrium (Figure 18-5A). Leads I and aVL, with their positive electrodes (camera lens) on the left side of the body, record this leftward electrical activity as an upright P wave, and leads II, III, and aVF, with their positive electrodes at the bottom of the heart, record the downward spread of activity as upright P waves. Lead aVR, with its positive electrode on the right shoulder, sees the electrical activity moving away from it and records a negative P wave.

As the impulse spreads through the AV node, no electrical activity is recorded because the AV node is too small to be recorded by surface leads. As the impulse exits the AV node, it moves through the bundle of His and enters the right and left bundle branches. The left bundle branch sprouts some Purkinje fibers high on the left side of the septum that carry the impulse into the septum and cause it to depolarize first in a left-to-right direction. The electrical impulse then enters

electrode is recorded as a negative deflection. In lead III, the positive electrode is on the left leg and the negative electrode is on the left arm. Any electrical activity coming toward the left leg electrode (camera lens) is recorded upright and any traveling away from it toward the left arm is recorded negative. The view of the heart by the bipolar leads can be compared to a wide-angle camera lens.

The three unipolar frontal plane leads, aVR, aVL, and aVF, are illustrated in Figure 18-3B. The camera represents the location of the positive electrode: on the right shoulder for aVR, on the left shoulder for aVL, and at the foot (left leg) for aVF. The "negative end" of the unipolar lead is a

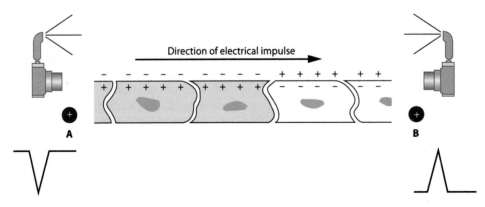

Figure 18-2. A strip of cardiac muscle depolarizing in the direction of the arrow. A positive electrode at **B** sees depolarization coming toward it and records an upright deflection. A positive electrode at **A** sees depolarization going away from it and records a negative deflection.

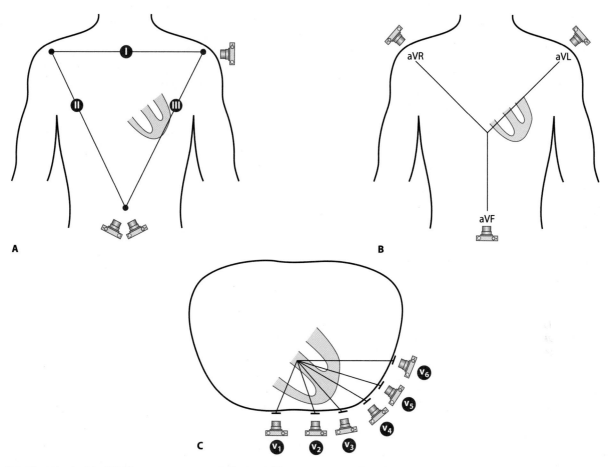

Figure 18-3. The 12 leads of the ECG. The camera represents the location of the positive, or recording, electrode in each lead. **(A)** Bipolar frontal plane leads I, II, and III. **(B)** Unipolar frontal plane leads aVR, aVL, and aVF. **(C)** Unipolar precordial leads V_1 to V_6.

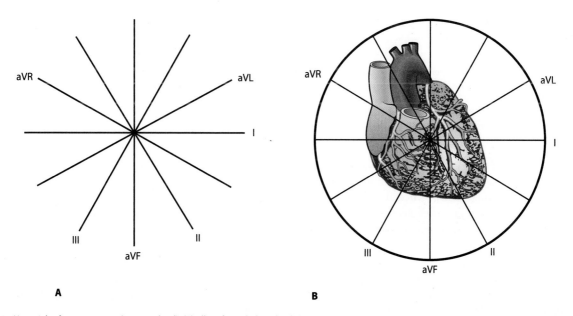

Figure 18-4. Hexaxial reference system (or axis wheel). **(A)** All six frontal plane leads bisecting each other. Each lead is labeled at its positive end. **(B)** The axis wheel superimposed on the heart to demonstrate each lead's view of the heart. Leads I and aVL face the left lateral wall; leads II, III, and aVF face the inferior wall.

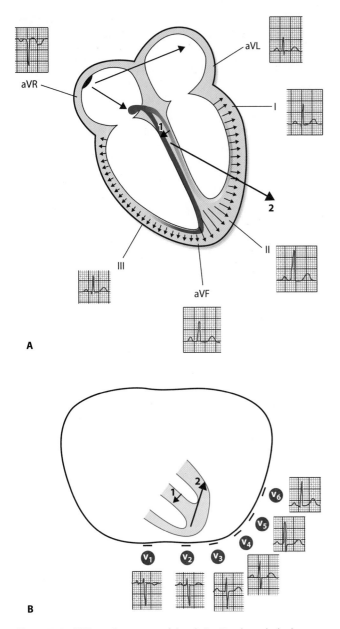

Figure 18-5. (A) Normal sequence of depolarization through the heart as recorded by each of the frontal plane leads. **(B)** Cross-section of the thorax illustrating how the six precordial leads record normal electrical activity in the ventricles. The small arrow (1) shows the initial direction of depolarization through the septum, followed by the direction of ventricular depolarization, indicated by the larger arrow (2).

the Purkinje system of both ventricular free walls simultaneously and depolarizes them from endocardium to epicardium, as shown by the small arrows through the ventricular wall in Figure 18-5A. The millions of electrical forces travel through the heart in three dimensions simultaneously, but if averaged together they move downward, leftward, and posteriorly toward the large left ventricle, as indicated by the large arrow in the same figure. This large arrow represents the mean axis, which is the net direction of electrical depolarization through the ventricles when all the smaller arrows are averaged together.

The QRS complex is recorded as the ventricles depolarize. Leads I and aVL, with their positive electrodes on the left side of the body, see the septum depolarizing away from them and record a small negative deflection (Q wave). These leads then see the large left ventricular free wall depolarizing toward them and record an upright deflection (R wave). Leads II, III, and aVF, with their positive electrodes at the bottom of the heart, may not see septal activity at all and record no deflections. However, if these leads see septal electrical activity coming slightly toward them, they record a positive deflection. As the forces continue moving downward toward leads II, III, and aVF, an upright deflection (R wave) is recorded. Lead aVR, positive on the right shoulder, sees all activity moving away from it and records a negative deflection (QS complex). Figure 18-5A illustrates how the six frontal plane leads record normal electrical activity as it spreads through the atria and ventricles.

The six precordial leads record electrical activity traveling in the horizontal plane. Figure 18-5B illustrates the position of the precordial leads and how they record electrical activity as it spreads through the ventricles. Lead V_1 is located on the front of the chest and records a small R wave as the septum depolarizes toward it from left to right. It then records a deep S wave as depolarization spreads away from it through the thick left ventricle. As the positive electrode is moved across the precordium from the V_1 to the V_6 position, it records progressively more left ventricular forces and the R wave gets progressively larger. Lead V_6 is located on the left side of the chest and may record a small Q wave as the septum depolarizes from left to right away from the positive electrode, and it records a large R wave as electrical activity spreads toward the positive electrode through the thick left ventricle.

In addition to P waves and QRS complexes, the ECG records T waves as the ventricles repolarize. Normal T waves are slightly asymmetrical with an ascending limb that is more gradual than the descending limb. T waves are usually upright in leads I, II, and V_{3-6}, and negative in lead aVR. T waves can vary in other leads. A normal T wave is not taller than 5 mm in a limb lead or 10 mm in a chest lead. Tall T waves can indicate hyperkalemia or myocardial ischemia or infarction.

The ST segment begins at the end of the QRS complex (the J point) and ends at the beginning of the T wave. It is normally at the baseline (the isoelectric segment between the T wave and the next P wave), and should not stay on the baseline for longer than 0.12 second (Figure 18-6). The ST segment should gently curve upward into the T wave without forming a sharp angle. Normal ST-segment elevation and depression is discussed under "ST-Segment Monitoring" later in this chapter.

The U wave is sometimes seen following the T wave, and when present it should be smaller than the T wave and point in the same direction as the T wave. U waves are thought to represent repolarization of the midmyocardial cells (M-cells)

Lead II   Lead V$_1$

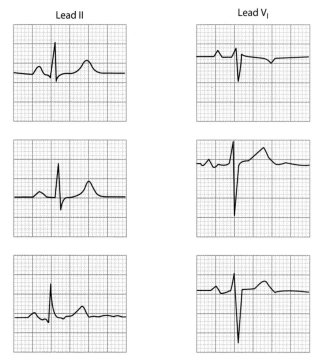

Figure 18-6. Normal ST segment and T waves.

in the ventricles. Large U waves can be seen in hypokalemia and with certain drugs, like quinidine. Inverted U waves can indicate myocardial ischemia.

Figure 18-7 shows a normal 12-lead ECG. Normal sinus rhythm is present, and the QRS axis is +45°. P waves are normal (they are flat in V$_2$, but this is not necessarily abnormal), and T waves are normal. The QRS complex is normal (0.08-second wide), there are no abnormal Q waves, and R-wave progression is normal across the precordium. The ST segment is at baseline in all leads. This ECG is used for comparison as abnormalities are discussed throughout this chapter.

Axis Determination

The *hexaxial reference system* (axis wheel) forms a 360° circle surrounding the heart that by convention is divided

into 180 positive degrees (+180°) and 180 negative degrees (−180°) (Figure 18-8). The normal QRS axis is defined as −30° to +90° because most of the electrical forces in a normal heart are directed downward and leftward toward the large left ventricle. Left axis deviation is defined as an axis of −31° to −90° and occurs when most of the forces move in a leftward and superior direction, as can happen in a variety of conditions, such as left ventricular hypertrophy, left anterior fascicular block, inferior myocardial infarction (MI), or left bundle branch block (LBBB) (Table 18-1). Right axis deviation is defined as +91° to +180° and occurs when most of the forces move rightward, as can happen in conditions such as right ventricular hypertrophy, left posterior fascicular block, and right bundle branch block (RBBB) (see Table 18-1). When most of the forces are directed superior and rightward between −90° and −180°, the term *right superior axis* is used. This axis can occur with ventricular tachycardia and occasionally with bifascicular block.

The mean frontal plane QRS axis can be determined in a number of ways. The most accurate method is to average the forces moving right and left with those moving up and down because this represents the frontal plane, lead I is the "pure" right/left lead and lead aVF is the "pure" up/down lead; it is easiest to use these two perpendicular leads to calculate the mean axis. Figure 18-9A shows the frontal plane leads of a 12-lead ECG. Leads I and aVF are shown enlarged along with the axis wheel with small dash marks along the axes of lead I and lead aVF (Figure 18-9B). These dash marks represent the small, 1-mV boxes on the ECG paper. To determine the mean QRS axis, follow these steps:

1. Look at the QRS complex in lead I and count the number of positive and negative boxes. Mark the net vector along the appropriate end of lead I on the axis wheel. In Figure 18-9B, the QRS complex in lead I is five boxes positive and two boxes negative, resulting in a net three boxes positive, or + 3. Count three dash marks toward the positive end of lead I and put a mark on the axis wheel at that spot.

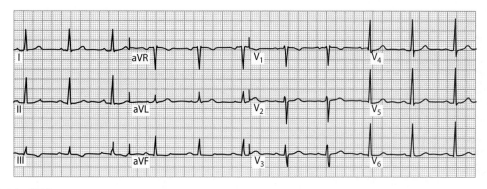

Figure 18-7. Normal 12-lead ECG.

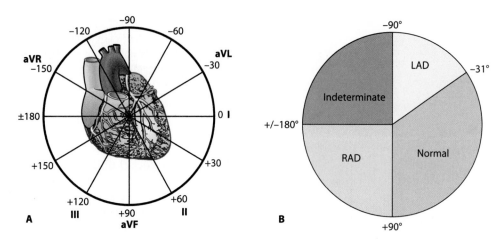

Figure 18-8. (A) Degrees of the axis wheel. **(B)** Normal axis = −30° to + 90°; left axis deviation = −31° to −90°; right axis deviation = +91° to +180°; right superior axis = −90° to −180°.

2. Look at the QRS complex in aVF and follow the same procedure as above. In this example, the QRS complex in aVF is eight boxes positive and has two very small negative deflections that equal approximately one box when combined, resulting in a net +7. Count seven dash marks along the positive end of aVF's axis and place a mark at that spot.

3. Draw a perpendicular line down from the mark on lead I's axis and a perpendicular line across from the mark on aVF's axis.

4. Draw a line from the center of the axis wheel to the spot where the two perpendicular lines meet. This line represents the mean QRS axis. In the example in Figure 18-9B, the axis is about +65°.

A quick but less precise method of axis determination is to place the axis in its proper quadrant of the axis wheel by looking at leads I and aVF, because these leads divide the

wheel into four quadrants. As illustrated in Figure 18-10, if both of these leads are positive, the axis falls in the normal quadrant, 0° to +90°. If lead I is positive and aVF is negative, the axis falls in the left quadrant, 0° to −90°. If lead I is negative and aVF is positive, the axis falls in the right quadrant, +90° to +180°. If both leads are negative, the axis falls in the right superior quadrant or "no-man's-land" −90° to −180°. Locating the correct quadrant is sometimes adequate, but because 30° of the left quadrant is considered normal, it is necessary to be more precise in describing the axis when it falls in the left quadrant. To "fine-tune" the axis when it is in the left quadrant, look at lead II. If lead II has a positive QRS, the axis is in the normal part of the left quadrant (0° to −30°); if it has a negative QRS, the axis is left deviated (−31° to −90°).

Using the ECG in Figure 18-11A, first place the axis in the appropriate quadrant by using leads I and aVF. Lead I is upright and aVF is negative, placing the axis in the left quadrant. However, because 30° of the left quadrant is considered normal, we need to fine-tune the axis to determine where within the left quadrant it actually falls. Since lead II is mostly negative, the axis is deviated to the left. The axis wheel shows how to count boxes in this example. The axis is −60°.

Using the ECG in Figure 18-11B, place the axis in the appropriate quadrant. Because lead I is negative and aVF is positive, the axis is in the right quadrant. The axis wheel shows how boxes are counted in this example. The axis is +130°.

Bundle Branch Block

When one of the bundle branches is blocked, the ventricles depolarize asynchronously. Bundle branch block is characterized by a delay of excitation to one ventricle and an abnormal spread of electrical activity through the ventricle whose bundle is blocked. This delayed conduction results in widening of the QRS complex to 0.12 second or more and a characteristic pattern best recognized in precordial leads V_1 and V_6 and limb leads I and aVL.

TABLE 18-1. SUMMARY OF CAUSES OF AXIS DEVIATIONS

Axis: −30° to +90°
- Normal

Left Axis Deviation: −31° to −90°
- Left ventricular hypertrophy
- Left anterior fascicular block
- Inferior myocardial infarction
- Left bundle branch block
- Congenital defects
- Ventricular tachycardia
- Wolff-Parkinson-White syndrome

Right Axis Deviation: +91° to +180°
- Right ventricular hypertrophy
- Left posterior fascicular block
- Right bundle branch block
- Dextrocardia
- Ventricular tachycardia
- Wolff-Parkinson-White syndrome

Right Superior Axis: −90° to −180°
- Ventricular tachycardia
- Bifascicular block

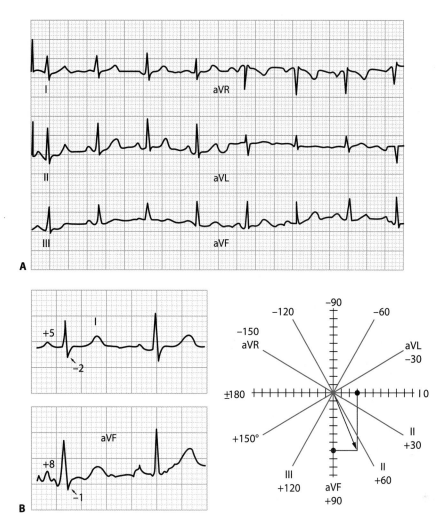

Figure 18-9. Calculating the mean QRS axis. **(A)** The six frontal plane leads of an ECG. **(B)** Leads I and aVF enlarged. See the text for instructions on calculating the axis using leads I and aVF on the axis wheel.

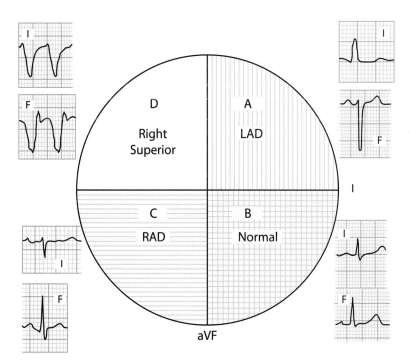

Figure 18-10. The four quadrants of the axis wheel. **(A)** Left axis deviation quadrant; lead I is positive and lead aVF is negative. **(B)** Normal axis quadrant; leads I and aVF are both positive. **(C)** Right axis deviation quadrant; lead I is negative and lead aVF is positive. **(D)** Right superior quadrant; leads I and aVF are both negative. (*With permission from: Marriott HJL:* Practical Electrocardiography. *8th ed. Baltimore, MD: Williams & Wilkins; 1988:35.*)

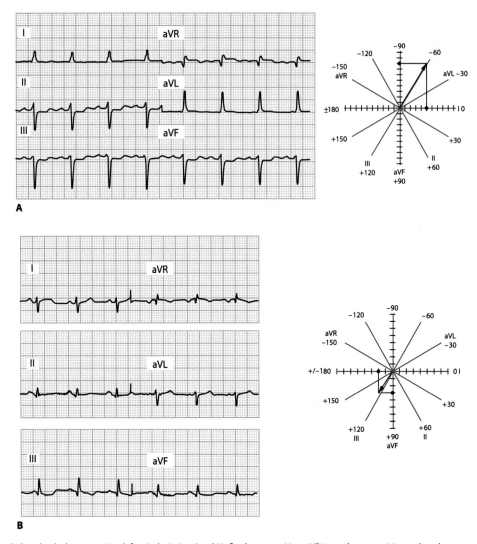

Figure 18-11. **(A)** Frontal plane leads demonstrating left axis deviation. Lead I is five boxes positive; aVF is two boxes positive and ten boxes negative for a net of −8. The axis is −60°. **(B)** Frontal plane leads demonstrating right axis deviation. Lead I is two boxes positive and four boxes negative for a net of −2; lead aVF is one box negative and four boxes positive for a net of +3. The axis is +120°.

Normal ventricular depolarization as recorded by leads V$_1$ and V$_6$ is illustrated in Figure 18-12. The positive electrode for V$_1$ is located on the front of the chest at the fourth intercostal space to the right of the sternum, close to the right ventricle. The positive electrode for V$_6$ is located in the left midaxillary line at the fifth intercostal space, close to the left ventricle. Lead V$_1$ records a small R wave as the septum depolarizes from left to right toward the positive electrode. It then records a negative deflection (S wave) as the main forces travel away from the positive electrode toward the left ventricle, resulting in the normal rS complex in V$_1$. Lead V$_6$ may record a small Q wave as the septum depolarizes left to right away from the positive electrode. It then records a tall R wave as the main forces travel toward the left ventricle, resulting in the normal qR complex in V$_6$. When both ventricles depolarize together, the QRS width is less than 0.12 second.

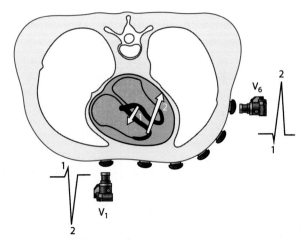

Figure 18-12. Normal ventricular depolarization as recorded by leads V$_1$ and V$_6$.

Right Bundle Branch Block

The presence of a block in the right bundle branch causes a different spread of electrical forces in the ventricles and thus a different pattern to the QRS complex. Three separate forces occur, as seen in Figure 18-13A.

1. Septal activation occurs first from left to right (*arrow 1*), resulting in the normal small R wave in V_1 and small Q wave in V_6.
2. The left ventricle is activated next through the normally functioning left bundle branch. Depolarization spreads normally through the Purkinje fibers in the left ventricle (*arrow 2*), causing an S wave in V_1 as the impulse travels away from its positive electrode and an R wave in V_6 as the impulse travels toward the positive electrode in V_6.
3. The right ventricle depolarizes late and abnormally as the impulse spreads via cell-to-cell conduction

through the right ventricle (*arrow 3*). This abnormal activation causes a wide second R wave (called R prime [R′]) in V_1 as it travels toward the positive electrode in V_1 and a wide S wave in V_6 as it travels away from the positive electrode in V_6 because muscle cell-to-cell conduction is much slower than conduction through the Purkinje system, the QRS complex widens to 0.12 second or greater.

Right bundle branch block can be recognized by a wide rSR′ pattern in V_1 and a wide qRs pattern in V_6, I, and aVL, because the positive electrode in these two limb leads is located on the left side of the body. The ECG in Figure 18-13B illustrates RBBB.

Left Bundle Branch Block

Figure 18-14 illustrates the spread of electrical forces through the ventricles when the left bundle branch is blocked.

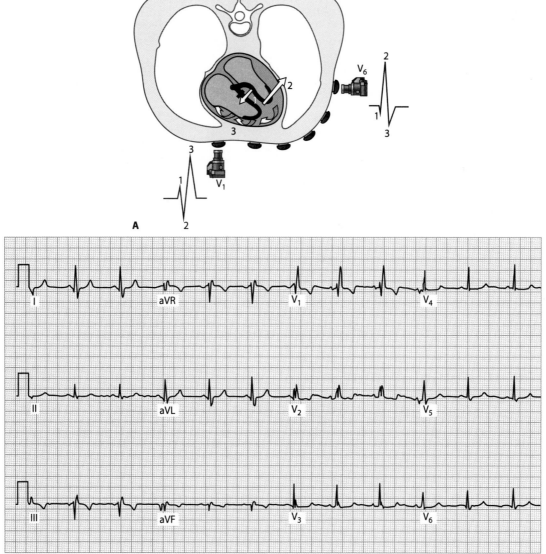

Figure 18-13. **(A)** Ventricular depolarization with RBBB as recorded by leads V_1 and V_6. **(B)** 12-lead ECG illustrating RBBB.

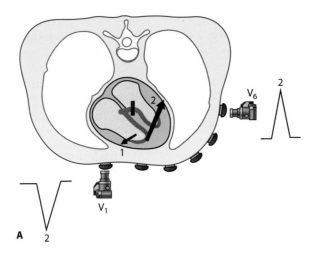

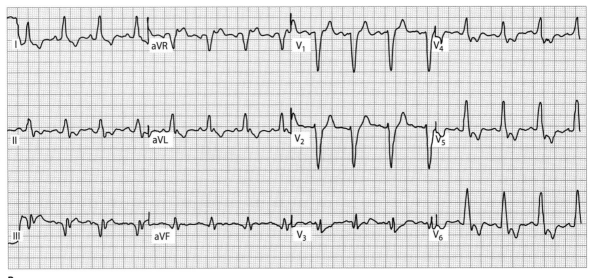

Figure 18-14. **(A)** Ventricular depolarization with LBBB as recorded by leads V_1 and V_6. **(B)** 12-lead ECG illustrating LBBB.

In LBBB, the septum does not depolarize in its normal left-to-right direction because the block occurs above the Purkinje fibers that normally activate the left side of the septum. This results in the loss of the normal small R wave in V_1 and loss of the Q wave in V_6, I, and aVL. Two main forces occur in LBBB:

1. The right ventricle is activated first through the Purkinje fibers (*arrow 1*). Because the right ventricular free wall is so much thinner than that of the left ventricle, forces traveling through it are often not recorded in V_1. Sometimes a small, narrow R wave is recorded in V_1 during LBBB, and this wave is most likely the result of forces traveling through the right ventricular free wall.

2. The left ventricle depolarizes late and abnormally as the impulse spreads via cell-to-cell conduction through the thick left ventricle (*arrow 2*).

This causes V_1 to record a wide negative QS complex as the impulse travels away from its positive electrode. The lateral leads V_6, I, and aVL record a wide R wave as the impulse travels through the large left ventricle toward their positive electrodes. The QRS widens to 0.12 second or greater due to the slow cell-to-cell conduction in the left ventricle.

Left bundle branch block can be recognized by a wide QS complex in V_1 and wide R waves with no Q waves in V_6, I, and aVL. The ECG in Figure 18-14B illustrates LBBB.

Acute Coronary Syndrome

The term *acute coronary syndrome* (ACS) is used to refer to the pathophysiologic continuum that begins with plaque rupture in a coronary artery and ultimately results in cell necrosis (infarction) if the process is not arrested. ACS encompasses three distinct phases of this continuum: (1) unstable angina

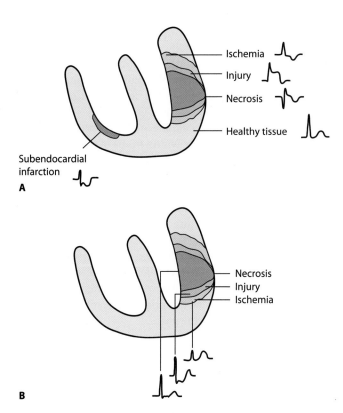

Figure 18-15. Zones of myocardial ischemia, injury, and infarction with associated ECG changes. **(A)** Indicative changes of ischemia, injury, and necrosis seen in leads facing the injured area. **(B)** Reciprocal changes often seen in leads not directly facing the involved area.

(UA), (2) non–ST-elevation MI (NSTEMI), and (3) ST-elevation MI (STEMI). The terms STEMI and NSTEMI refer to the presence or absence of ST elevation on the admission ECG in a patient who is having an MI as diagnosed by elevated biochemical markers in the blood. Once an infarction has occurred, the terms Q-wave or non–Q-wave MI indicate the ultimate presence or absence of Q waves on the ECG.

Myocardial infarction can occur because of blockage of a coronary artery with thrombus or from severe and prolonged ischemia due to coronary artery spasm or unrelieved obstruction of a coronary artery. When infarction does occur, there are three "zones" of tissue damage, each of which produces characteristic changes on the ECG (Figure 18-15).

Myocardial ischemia can result in several changes on the ECG (Figure 18-16). The most familiar patterns of ischemia are horizontal or downsloping ST-segment depression of 0.5 mm or more, and T-wave inversion. Other indicators of ischemia include an ST segment that remains on the baseline longer than 0.12 second; an ST segment that forms a sharp angle with the upright T wave, tall, wide-based T waves; and inverted U waves.

Myocardial injury is most often indicated by ST-segment elevation of 1 mm or more above the baseline in leads facing the infarcted area (Figure 18-17). Other signs of

acute injury include a straightening of the ST segment that slopes up to the peak of the T wave without spending any time on the baseline, tall, peaked T waves, and symmetric T-wave inversion.

Necrosis or death of myocardial tissue is indicated on the ECG by development of Q waves that are greater than 0.03 second wide or 25% of the ensuing R-wave amplitude (see Figures 18-5A and 18-9 for normal Q waves and Figures 18-18 and 18-19 for abnormal Q waves). Q waves can develop transiently with severe ischemia and with subendocardial MI, and transmural infarction can occur without the development of Q waves. Therefore, the newer terms *Q-wave*

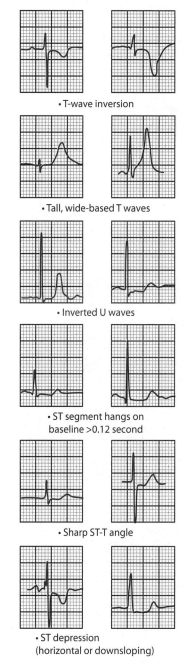

• T-wave inversion

• Tall, wide-based T waves

• Inverted U waves

• ST segment hangs on baseline >0.12 second

• Sharp ST-T angle

• ST depression (horizontal or downsloping)

Figure 18-16. ECG patterns associated with myocardial ischemia.

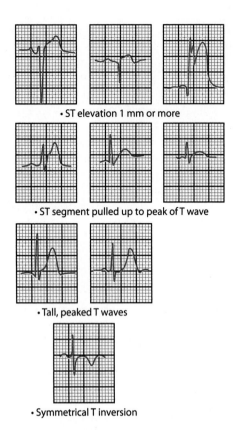

- ST elevation 1 mm or more

- ST segment pulled up to peak of T wave

- Tall, peaked T waves

- Symmetrical T inversion

Figure 18-17. ECG patterns associated with acute myocardial injury.

and *non–Q-wave* MI are preferred over the older terms *transmural* and *subendocardial* infarction. In any case, the presence of abnormal Q waves is still considered to be ECG evidence of myocardial necrosis.

The ECG reflects the evolution of the infarction from the acute stage through the fully evolved stage. Very early MI often causes peaking and widening of the T waves followed within minutes by ST-segment elevation. ST-segment elevation can persist for hours to several days, but resolves more quickly with successful reperfusion. Once the ST segment has returned to baseline, ECG evidence of the acute infarction stage is lost. Q waves appear within hours of pain onset and usually remain forever, although sometimes Q waves disappear over the years after infarction. T-wave inversion occurs within hours after infarction and can last for months. T waves often return to their previous upright position within a few months after acute MI. Thus, an *evolving infarct* is one in which serial ECGs show ST segments returning toward baseline, the development of Q waves, and T-wave inversion. The term *old infarction* or *infarct of undetermined age* is used when the first ECG recorded shows Q waves, ST segment at baseline, and T waves either inverted or upright, indicating that an MI occurred at some point in the past.

Locating the Infarction From the ECG

ST-segment elevation, Q waves, and T-wave inversion are recorded in leads facing the damaged myocardium and are called the *indicative changes of infarction*. Leads not facing the involved tissue often show changes related to the loss of electrical forces (depolarization and repolarization) in the damaged tissue. These leads record mirror-image changes that are called *reciprocal changes*. Figure 18-15 illustrates indicative and reciprocal changes associated with MI, and Table 18-2 lists leads in which indicative and reciprocal changes are found in each of the major types of MI.

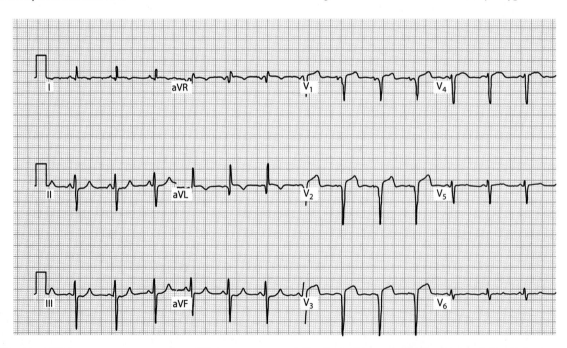

Figure 18-18. 12-lead ECG demonstrating acute anterior wall MI. Q waves are present in V$_1$ to V$_3$ and ST-segment elevation is present in V$_1$ to V$_4$. An abnormal Q wave is also present in aVL.

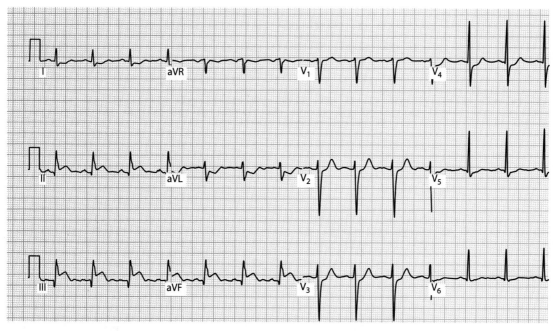

Figure 18-19. 12-lead ECG demonstrating acute inferior wall MI. ST elevation is present in II, III, and aVF; reciprocal ST depression is present in I, aVL, and V$_2$ to V$_4$. Q waves can be seen in III and aVF.

Anterior wall MI is recognized by indicative changes in leads facing the anterior wall precordial leads V$_1$ to V$_4$ (see Figure 18-18). Reciprocal changes are often recorded in the inferior leads II, III, and aVF, and sometimes in V$_5$ with proximal left anterior descending (LAD) artery stenosis. Inferior wall MI is diagnosed by indicative changes in leads II, III, and aVF (see Figure 18-19), and reciprocal changes are often seen in leads I and aVL. Lateral wall MI presents with indicative changes in leads I, aVL, and/or V$_5$ and V$_6$, with reciprocal changes in leads II, III, and aVF (Figure 18-20). Posterior wall MI is less obvious because in the standard 12-lead ECG there are no leads that face the posterior wall, and therefore there are no indicative changes recorded (Figure 18-21). The diagnosis is suspected when ST segment depression is present in the anterior leads, especially V$_1$ and V$_2$ but often all the way to V$_4$. Reciprocal changes seen in these leads include a taller R wave than normal (mirror image of the Q wave that would be recorded over the posterior wall), ST-segment depression (mirror image of the ST elevation from the posterior wall), and upright, tall T waves (mirror image of the T-wave inversion from the posterior wall). Posterior leads V$_7$, V$_8$, and V$_9$ should be recorded whenever posterior wall MI is suspected (Figure 18-23B).

Right ventricular MI occurs in up to 45% of inferior MIs; therefore, it usually is associated with indicative changes in the inferior leads II, III, and aVF (Figure 18-22). In addition, it is not uncommon to see ST elevation in V$_1$ as well, because V$_1$ is the chest lead that is closest to the right ventricle. ST elevation in V$_1$, together with ST elevation in the inferior leads, is suspicious for right ventricular MI. Another clue is discordance between the ST segment in V$_1$ and the ST segment in V$_2$. Normally, when the ST segment in V$_1$ is elevated, it is related to anterior or septal MI, in which case the ST in V$_2$ is also elevated. *Discordance* means that the ST segments do not point in the same direction—V$_1$ shows ST elevation while V$_2$ is either normal or shows ST depression. This finding is suspicious for right ventricular MI. The American Heart Association (AHA) and the American College of Cardiology (ACC) have recommended that right-sided chest leads V$_3$R and V$_4$R be recorded in all patients presenting with ECG evidence of acute inferior wall infarction. Leads V$_3$R through V$_6$R develop ST elevation when acute right ventricular MI is present. Lead V$_4$R is the most sensitive and specific lead for recognition of right ventricular MI. Figure 18-23A shows location of right sided chest leads and Figure 18-23B shows location of posterior leads.

TABLE 18-2. ECG CHANGES ASSOCIATED WITH MYOCARDIAL INFARCTION

Location of MI	Indicative Changes (ST elevation)	Reciprocal Changes (ST depression)
Anterior	V$_1$-V$_4$ (not necessarily all of these leads) AVR with proximal LAD occlusion	II, III, AVF, V5 with proximal LAD occlusion
Septal	V$_1$, V$_2$	V5 with proximal LAD occlusion
Anterolateral	V$_1$-V$_6$, I, AVL	II, III, AVF
Inferior	II, III, AVF	I, AVL
Posterior	Posterior leads V$_8$, V$_9$	V1-V3
Lateral	I, AVL, V$_5$, V$_6$	II, III, AVF
Right ventricle	Right side leads V$_3$R-V$_6$R	

ESSENTIAL CONTENT CASE

Acute MI

You are caring for a patient who is admitted with acute chest pain. His VS are stable but he is complaining of 8/10 chest pain which began 2 hours ago and has steadily increased. This is his initial ECG:

    The cath lab is not yet ready for this patient, so while waiting to transport him you initiate ST segment monitoring.

    The ST segment alarm rings and when you check the patient you see higher ST elevation on the monitor. You get another ECG:

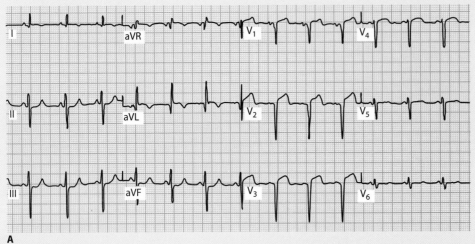

A

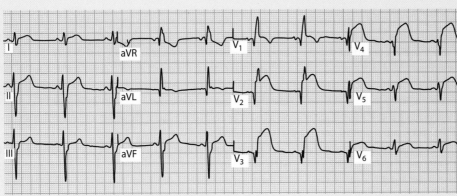

B

Case Question 1. What is your interpretation of this ECG, rhythm, QRS axis, Bundle branch block and ST segments?

Case Question 2. What would be a good lead for ST segment monitoring in this patient? Describe how to initiate ST segment monitoring.

Case Question 3. What is your interpretation of this ECG, rhythm, QRS axis, Bundle branch block, and ST segments?

Case Question 4. What is the significance of these changes and what complications can result?

Answers

1. The rhythm is sinus rhythm in the 80s. The QRS axis is about −45°. There is no bundle branch block present. There is ST segment elevation in leads V_2-V_4 and slight ST depression in leads II, III, and AVF. The interpretation is anterior wall STEMI.

2. Since this is an anterior wall MI, lead V_3 is the best lead for ST segment monitoring. If you only have one V lead available then you will lose your best arrhythmia monitoring lead (V_1), but V_3 would be a good choice for ST segment monitoring. The ST baseline reference point should be the patient's current ST segment levels (not the isoelectric line) so that if there is any change from the current ST position the monitor will alarm. The ST measuring point is 0.06 sec (60 msec) after the J point (the point where the QRS ends and the ST segment begins).

3. The rhythm is sinus rhythm. The QRS axis has shifted even more leftward and is now about −70°. There is now RBBB. The combination of significant left axis deviation and RBBB indicates probably bifascicular block: RBBB and left anterior hemiblock. The ST segments are even higher now and ST elevation extends all the way from V_2 to V_6.

4. The higher ST segment elevation indicates extension of the MI. Bifascicular block means that two of the three pathways of conduction into the ventricle are blocked, creating a high potential for third degree AV block. This patient needs to get to the cath lab and get his artery opened!

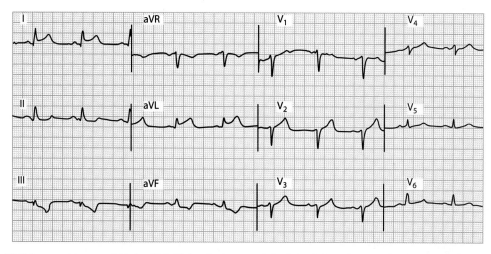

Figure 18-20. 12-lead ECG demonstrating acute lateral wall MI. ST elevation is present in leads I and aVL, and reciprocal ST depression is seen in leads II, III, and aVF.

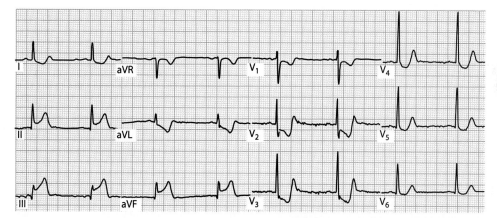

Figure 18-21. 12-lead ECG demonstrating acute inferior and posterior MI. ST elevation is present in leads II, III, and aVF (inferior leads), and ST depression is present in all of the V leads. ST depression in V_1-V_3 is indicative of posterior MI. The ST depression in V_4-V_6 is reciprocal to the inferior MI.

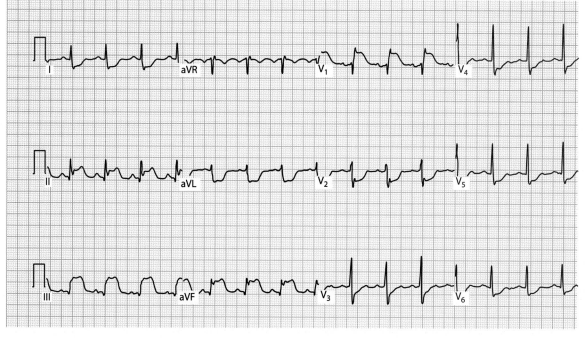

Figure 18-22. 12-lead ECG demonstrating acute right ventricular MI. ST elevation is present in II, III, aVF, and V_1; reciprocal ST depression is present in all other leads. Note the discordant ST elevation in V_1 and ST depression in V_2.

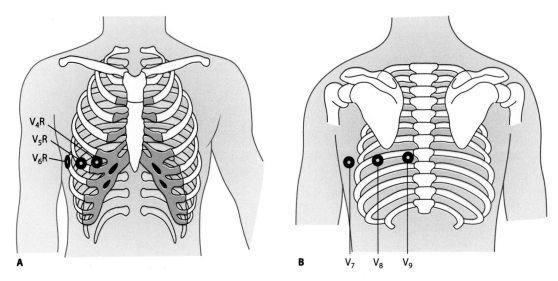

Figure 18-23. **(A)** Right side chest leads. V$_4$R at right fifth intercostal space, mid clavicular line; V$_5$R at right fifth intercostal space, anterior axillary line; V$_6$R at right fifth intercostal space, midaxillary line. **(B)** Posterior leads: V$_7$ at posterior axillary line; V$_8$ at tip of scapula; V$_9$ next to spine.

Preexcitation Syndromes

Preexcitation means early activation of the ventricle by supraventricular impulses that reach the ventricle through an accessory conduction pathway faster than they travel through the AV node. Many people have tracts of tissue, often referred to as "bypass tracts" or "accessory pathways," that can carry electrical impulses directly from atria to ventricles, bypassing the delay in the AV node and causing early and abnormal depolarization of the ventricles. These accessory pathways can be found anywhere around the tricuspid or mitral valve rings. The most common type of preexcitation syndrome is the Wolff-Parkinson-White syndrome, in which the impulse travels down the accessory pathway from the atria directly into the ventricles, completely bypassing AV node delay. Other anatomic connections exist that can bypass the normal AV node delay or create connections between different parts of the conduction system and the ventricles and cause variations of the preexcitation pattern. Fibers originating in the atria and inserting into the bundle of His have been demonstrated anatomically and can result in a short PR interval and normal QRS complex (formerly called Lown-Ganong-Levine syndrome).

Wolff-Parkinson-White Syndrome

In Wolff-Parkinson-White syndrome, the ventricle is stimulated prematurely by an electrical impulse traveling through the accessory pathway while the impulse simultaneously descends normally through the AV node (Figure 18-24A). Impulses travel faster through the accessory pathway because they bypass the normal AV node delay. Part of the ventricle receives the impulse early via the accessory pathway and begins to depolarize before the rest of the ventricle is activated through the His-Purkinje system. Early stimulation of the ventricle results in a short PR interval and a widened QRS

complex as the impulse begins to depolarize the ventricle via muscle cell-to-cell conduction. Premature stimulation of the ventricle causes a characteristic slurring of the initial part of the QRS complex, called a delta wave. The remainder of the QRS complex is normal because the rest of the ventricle is depolarized normally through the Purkinje system. This preexcitation results in ventricular fusion beats as the ventricles are depolarized simultaneously by the impulse coming through the accessory pathway and through the normal AV node. The degree of preexcitation varies, depending on the relative rates of conduction down the accessory pathway and through the AV node, and it determines the length of the PR interval and size of the delta wave (Figure 18-24A to 18-24C).

Wolff-Parkinson-White syndrome is recognized on the ECG by the presence of a short PR interval (< 0.12 second) and delta waves in many leads. Figure 18-25A, B show two examples of this type of pattern. Preexcitation syndromes are clinically significant because the presence of two pathways into the ventricle is a setup for reentrant tachycardias, which occur frequently in people with accessory pathways and are a part of the "syndrome" of Wolff-Parkinson-White. See the section Supraventricular Tachycardias later in this chapter for more information on arrhythmias associated with accessory pathways.

Treatment

Wolff-Parkinson-White syndrome does not require treatment unless it is associated with symptomatic tachycardias. Specific therapy depends on the mechanism of the tachyarrhythmia, the effect of drugs on conduction through the AV node and the accessory pathway, and on the patient's tolerance of the arrhythmia. The section on supraventricular tachycardias later in this chapter discusses drug treatment of tachycardias associated with accessory pathways.

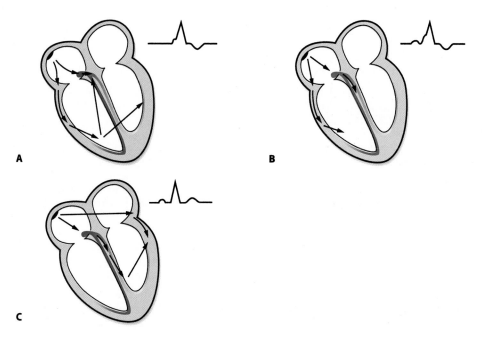

Figure 18-24. Varying degrees of preexcitation. **(A)** Maximal preexcitation when the ventricles are activated totally by the accessory pathway. **(B)** Less-than-maximal preexcitation when the ventricles are activated by the impulse traveling through both the accessory pathway and the normal AV conduction system. **(C)** Concealed accessory pathway. The ventricles are activated through the normal AV conduction system with no participation of the accessory pathway, resulting in a normal PR interval and normal QRS complex.

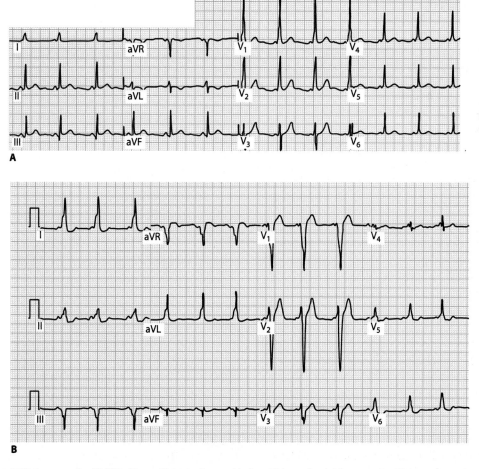

Figure 18-25. **(A)** 12-lead ECG demonstrating Wolff-Parkinson-White syndrome with short PR interval and delta waves. Lead V_1 is positive, indicating a posterior accessory pathway. **(B)** Wolff-Parkinson-White syndrome with short PR and delta waves with a negative V_1, indicating an anterior or right-sided accessory pathway.

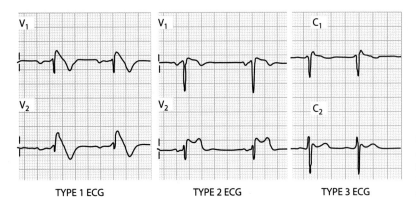

Figure 18-26. Three ECG patterns of Brugada syndrome. Type I shows the coved ST segment elevation and T wave inversion and is considered the diagnostic pattern. Type 2 shows the saddle-back type ST elevation with an inverted T wave in V_1 and upright T wave in V_2. Type 3 shows minimal ST elevation but an elevated J point creating a RBBB-type pattern in V_1.

Radio-frequency (RF) catheter ablation of the bypass tract provides a cure for the tachyarrhythmias associated with accessory pathways in many patients. RF ablation is an invasive procedure that requires the introduction of several catheters into the heart through the venous and sometimes arterial systems. An electrophysiology study is done first to record intracardiac signals and determine the mechanism of the tachycardia. The electrophysiology study confirms the presence and location of the accessory pathway, participation of the pathway in maintaining the tachycardia, and conduction characteristics of the accessory pathway. A special ablation catheter is then positioned next to the bypass tract and RF energy is delivered through the catheter to the tract, destroying the tissue and preventing it from being able to conduct. Permanent tissue damage in the accessory pathway is the goal of RF ablation, and when successful, it prevents further episodes of tachycardia.

Brugada Syndrome

Brugada syndrome (BS) is an inherited channelopathy involving mutations of the SCN5A gene that participates in regulation of cardiac sodium channels. It is associated with a high incidence of VT/VF and sudden cardiac death (SCD) in people with structurally normal hearts. BS is estimated to be responsible for at least 4% of all sudden deaths and at least 20% of sudden deaths in patients with structurally normal hearts. It is seen worldwide but is most prevalent in Southeast Asia, occurs most often in men (8:1 male to female ratio), and typically manifests in the third or fourth decade of life.

Brugada syndrome is characterized by ST-segment elevation and a RBBB-type QRS pattern in leads V_1-V_3, typically without the dominant S waves in the lateral leads that is seen with true RBBB. Three patterns of ST elevation have been identified (Figure 18-26): (1) type 1 ECG pattern with a coved ST segment elevation > 2 mm, followed by a negative T wave; (2) type 2 ECG pattern with a saddle-back shaped ST elevation followed by a positive or biphasic T wave; and (3) type 3 ECG pattern with ST elevation < 1 mm with coved or saddle-back pattern. All three patterns can be seen in BS but only the type 1 pattern is considered diagnostic (Figure 18-27). BS is diagnosed by the presence of a type 1 or coved-type ST-segment elevation in > 1 right precordial lead (V_1-V_3) plus one of the following conditions: documented VF or polymorphic VT, a family history of SCD at a young age (< 45 years), a type 1 ECG in family members, otherwise unexplained syncope, nocturnal agonal respiration, or inducibility of VT/VF with programmed electrical stimulation. The diagnosis is also considered positive when a type 2 or type 3 ECG pattern present at baseline converts to the diagnostic type 1 pattern after sodium channel blocker administration, along with one or more of the above clinical criteria.

The mainstay of therapy for BS is an implantable cardioverter defibrillator (ICD). ICD implantation is a class I recommendation for survivors of cardiac arrest due to VF or hemodynamically unstable sustained VT not because of a reversible cause, and a class IIa recommendation for patients with BS who have had syncope or documented VT.

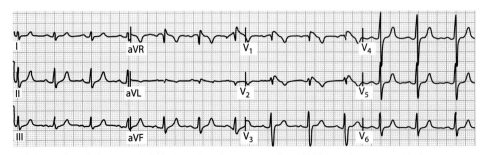

Figure 18-27. 12-lead ECG showing Type I Brugada pattern in a young man with syncope.

Quinidine is the only drug that has been shown to be effective in preventing ventricular arrhythmias in patients with BS. The best way to manage asymptomatic BS patients is still debated.

The QT Interval and Long-QT Syndromes

The QT interval is measured from the beginning of the QRS complex to the end of the T wave and is used clinically as a reflection of ventricular repolarization time. The QT interval is heart rate dependent; it shortens at faster heart rates and lengthens at slower heart rates, therefore, the measured QT interval must be corrected for heart rate (QTc = QT corrected for heart rate). A normal QTc is < 0.46 second (460 msec) in women and < 0.45 second (450 msec) in men. A prolonged QTc indicates abnormally prolonged ventricular repolarization and is associated with torsades de pointes (TdP) and SCD. The most commonly used method of correcting the measured QT interval for heart rate is the Bazett formula:

QTc = measured QT interval divided by the square root of the preceding R-R interval (all measurements in seconds).

Figure 18-28 illustrates how to use the Bazett formula. A QTc > 500 msec increases the risk of developing TdP.

Long-QT syndrome (LQTS) can be acquired or congenital. The acquired type is usually due to drugs that prolong ventricular repolarization or to electrolyte abnormalities, especially hypokalemia or hypomagnesemia. The congenital type is owing to gene mutations that affect ion channels on the cardiac cell membrane and is hereditary. Both types of QT-interval prolongation increase the risk of TdP and can be a cause of sudden cardiac death.

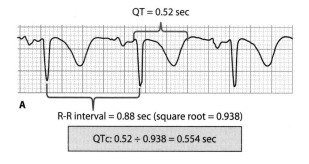

QT = 0.52 sec

A

R-R interval = 0.88 sec (square root = 0.938)

QTc: 0.52 ÷ 0.938 = 0.554 sec

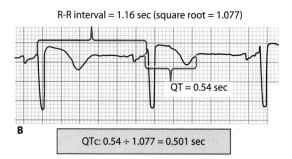

R-R interval = 1.16 sec (square root = 1.077)

QT = 0.54 sec

B

QTc: 0.54 ÷ 1.077 = 0.501 sec

Figure 18-28. Two examples showing Bazett correction for measured QT intervals.

The AHA's practice standards for ECG monitoring in hospital settings lists the following indications for QT-interval monitoring:

1. Initiation of a drug known to cause TdP
2. Overdose from potentially proarrhythmic agents
3. New-onset bradyarrhythmias and
4. Severe hypokalemia or hypomagnesemia.

Each facility should develop a protocol that defines a single consistent method of QT-interval monitoring that is used by all practitioners responsible for cardiac monitoring. The protocol should define the equipment used (manual or electronic), the method for determining the end of the T wave, the formula for heart rate correction, criteria for lead selection, and require that whichever lead is chosen should be used for serial measurements in the same patient.

Acquired Long-QT Syndrome

The most common cause of acquired LQTS is drug therapy. Many drugs prolong the QT interval by inhibiting potassium channels that are responsible for repolarization of cardiac cells. The most common classes of drugs that prolong the QT interval and cause TdP include antiarrhythmics, antibiotics, antipsychotic and antidepressant drugs, antihistamines, and gastric motility agents. A list of drugs commonly associated with Tdp is available at www.qtdrugs.com. Episodes of TdP in the acquired form of LQTS are most commonly precipitated by short-long RR intervals, such as those caused by a ventricular premature beat (short cycle) followed by a compensatory pause (long cycle). Episodes of TdP are also associated with bradycardia or frequent pauses in the rhythm, thus, the acquired type is commonly referred to as pause-dependent LQTS.

The risk of developing TdP from drugs increases in the presence of hypokalemia or hypomagnesemia, high doses or rapid IV infusion of QT prolonging drugs, or consumption of other drugs that also prolong the QT interval or slow drug metabolism. Other risk factors for TdP include heart failure (HF) or myocardial ischemia, liquid protein weight-loss diets or starvation, bradycardia or sudden pauses in rhythm, acute neurological events (eg, subarachnoid hemorrhage), older age, female sex, and genetic predisposition to QT prolongation. Significant changes in QTc after initiation of a drug known to be associated with TdP include an increase in QTc of > 60 msec from the predrug baseline QTc, or a QTc > 500 msec. Other warning signs of TdP during drug administration include widening or distortion of the T wave, development of enlarged U waves or T-U waves, exaggerated T-U wave distortion on beats terminating pauses, T wave alternans (alternating T wave amplitude from beat to beat), and PVC couplets or short runs of polymorphic VT occurring on the T wave of the beat terminating a pause.

Treatment of TdP includes identifying and managing the cause, discontinuing any causative drugs, and correcting electrolyte imbalances. IV magnesium can be administered to control episodes of TdP until the cause is corrected. Overdrive atrial or ventricular pacing at a rate of 80 beats/min or faster can prevent the pauses that may precipitate episodes of TdP and cause the QT interval to shorten as the heart rate is increased. Pacing and magnesium are temporary management strategies until the cause is eliminated. If TdP becomes sustained or degenerates into VF, defibrillation with an unsynchronized shock is required to terminate the episode.

Congenital Long-QT Syndromes

Congenital LQTS involves mutations in several genes that control potassium or sodium channels on cardiac cells. Thirteen different genes causing genetic LQTS have been identified and are named LQT1 through LQT13. The three most common are LQT1, LQT2, and LQT3, which are responsible for up to 90% of genotyped cases of LQTS. LQT1 and LQT2 are due to mutations of genes that affect potassium channel function (KCNQ1 and KCNH2), and LQT3 is because of mutations of the SCN5A gene that affects sodium channel function. The three main types all present with long QT intervals but differ from each other in several ways. The ECG in LQT1 often has wide, broad-based T waves that cause the prolonged QT interval, and arrhythmia events often occur during physical activity, especially swimming or diving. In LQT2, the ECG often shows notched T waves in multiple leads, and arrhythmia events are typically triggered by emotional upset or loud noises, such as alarm clocks or telephones. LQT3 usually shows long-ST segments, which are responsible for the long-QT interval, and arrhythmia events commonly occur at rest or during sleep. T wave abnormalities are often present in all three types. There is overlap between these types in terms of ECG and clinical presentation. Figure 18-29 illustrates the three main types of congenital LQTS.

Patients with congenital LQTS often present in childhood or in their teens. They may be asymptomatic and their LQTS is incidentally discovered when they are screened after a syncopal episode or when a family member is diagnosed with LQTS. Symptoms can range from palpitations and dizziness to seizures to cardiac arrest. The diagnosis is made by family history and a careful review of symptoms, triggering events if they can be identified, and the ECG. Genetic testing can identify the genotype and help direct therapy.

Treatment depends on severity of symptoms and risk stratification. Lifestyle modifications include avoiding competitive sports and extreme exertion, especially swimming in LQT1 patients. Patients with LQT2 should avoid startling loud noises such as alarm clocks or telephones. Hypokalemia and hypomagnesemia must be avoided, and electrolyte loss due to vomiting, sweating, etc, should be replaced. All LQTS patients should avoid drugs known to prolong the QT interval. Beta-blockers are the mainstay of medical therapy for all patients with LQTS and are especially effective in decreasing the incidence of exercise-induced events and SCD in LQT1 and LQT2 patients. They are less effective in LQT3. ICD implantation is a class I recommendation for any patient who has had a cardiac arrest owing to VT or VF in which no reversible cause is identified. ICD is a class IIa recommendation for patients with long-QT syndrome who have syncope and/or VT while receiving beta-blockers.

ADVANCED ARRHYTHMIA INTERPRETATION

The study of cardiac rhythms provides a never-ending challenge to those interested in learning about arrhythmias. In most basic ECG classes the content presented is limited to basic rhythms originating in the sinus node, atria, AV junction, and ventricles, and to basic AV conduction abnormalities. Rarely does time permit the inclusion of more advanced concepts. This section discusses some of these more advanced concepts of arrhythmia interpretation and provides clues to aid in recognition of selected arrhythmias not usually covered in a basic course.

Supraventricular Tachycardias

Supraventricular tachycardia (SVT) describes a rapid rhythm that arises above the level of the ventricles (atria or AV junction) or utilizes the atria or AV node as part of the circuit that maintains the tachycardia but whose exact origin is not known. Usually, SVT is used to describe a narrow QRS tachycardia where atrial activity (P waves) cannot be identified, and therefore the origin of the tachycardia cannot be determined from the surface ECG. The presence of the narrow QRS indicates the supraventricular origin of the rhythm and conduction through the normal His-Purkinje system into the ventricles.

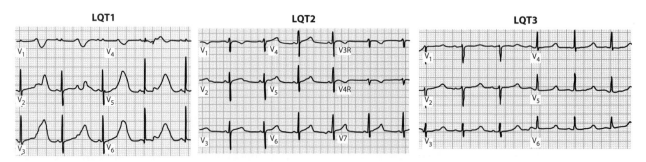

Figure 18-29. Representative V leads from the three major types of LQTS. The LQT1 patient is a 2-year-old girl who is in second-degree AV block with 2:1 conduction. The LQT2 patient is a 13-year-old girl who had a cardiac arrest at a slumber party. The LQT3 patient is a 17-year-old boy who had a "seizure."

Sometimes SVT conducts with bundle branch block, which results in a wide QRS but does not change the fact that the rhythm is supraventricular in origin. Thus, *SVT* can be used for narrow QRS tachycardias whose mechanism is uncertain or for wide QRS tachycardias that are known to be coming from above the ventricles.

Supraventricular tachycardias can be classified into those that are AV nodal passive and those that are AV nodal active. *AV nodal passive SVTs* are those in which the AV node is not required for the maintenance of the tachycardia but serves only to passively conduct supraventricular impulses into the ventricles. Examples of AV nodal passive arrhythmias include atrial tachycardia, atrial flutter, and atrial fibrillation, all of which originate within the atria and do not need the AV node to sustain the atrial arrhythmia. In these rhythms, the AV node passively conducts the atrial impulses into the ventricles but does not participate in the maintenance of the arrhythmia itself. *AV nodal active tachycardias* require participation of the AV node in the maintenance of the tachycardia. The two most common causes of a regular, narrow QRS tachycardia are AV nodal reentry tachycardia and circus movement tachycardia using an accessory pathway, both of which require the active participation of the AV node in maintaining the tachycardia.

Atrial fibrillation is a supraventricular rhythm that is usually easily recognized because of its irregularity, but atrial tachycardia, atrial flutter, junctional tachycardia, AV nodal reentry tachycardia, and circus movement tachycardia can all present as regular, narrow QRS tachycardias whose mechanism often cannot be determined from the ECG. Because AV nodal reentry tachycardia and circus movement tachycardia are the most common causes of a regular, narrow QRS tachycardia, they are discussed in detail here.

Atrioventricular Nodal Reentry Tachycardia

In people with AV nodal reentry tachycardia (AVNRT), the AV node has two pathways that are capable of conducting the impulse into the ventricles. One pathway conducts more rapidly and has a longer refractory period than the other pathway (Figure 18-30A). In AVNRT, a reentry circuit is set, usually using a slowly conducting pathway just outside the body of the AV node as the antegrade limb into the ventricle and the faster conducting pathway in the AV node as the retrograde limb back into the atria (Figure 18-30C).

The sinus impulse normally conducts down the fast pathway into the ventricles, resulting in a normal PR interval of 0.12 to 0.20 second. If a PAC occurs and enters the AV node before the fast pathway with its longer refractory period has recovered its ability to conduct, the impulse conducts down the slow pathway into the ventricle because of its shorter refractory period (Figure 18-30B). This slow conduction causes the PR interval of the PAC to be longer than the PR interval of sinus beats. The long conduction time through the slow pathway allows the fast pathway time to recover, making it possible for the impulse to conduct backward through the fast pathway into the atria. This returning impulse may

then reenter the slow pathway, which is again ready to conduct antegrade because of its short refractory period, thus setting up a reentry circuit within the AV node and resulting in AVNRT. Figure 18-30C illustrates the mechanism of the most common type of AVNRT in which antegrade conduction occurs over the slow pathway and retrograde conduction over the fast pathway. The resulting rhythm is usually a narrow QRS tachycardia because the ventricles are activated through the normal His-Purkinje system. P waves are either not seen at all or are barely visible peeking out at the tail end of the QRS complex because the atria and ventricles depolarize almost simultaneously (Figure 18-31A and B). In the presence of preexisting bundle branch block or rate-dependent bundle branch block, the QRS in AVNRT is wide.

In about 4% of cases of AVNRT, the impulse conducts antegrade into the ventricle through the fast pathway and retrograde into the atria through the slow pathway, reversing the circuit within the AV node. This reversal of the circuit in the AV node results in P waves that appear immediately in front of the QRS because atrial activation is delayed because of slow conduction backward through the slow pathway. These P waves are inverted in inferior leads because the atria depolarize in a retrograde direction.

Treatment

AV nodal reentry tachycardia is an AV nodal active SVT because the AV node is required for the maintenance of the tachycardia. Therefore, anything that causes block in the AV node, such as vagal stimulation or drugs like adenosine, beta-blockers, or calcium channel blockers, can terminate the rhythm. AVNRT is usually well tolerated unless the rate is extremely rapid. Episodes can become frequent and, if not controlled with drugs, can interfere with lifestyle. Many people learn to stop the rhythm by coughing or breath holding, which stimulates the vagus nerve. Acute medical treatment involves administering any drug that blocks AV node conduction, but adenosine is usually used first because of its rapid effect, short duration of action, and lack of significant side effects. RF ablation can destroy the slow pathway and prevent recurrence of the arrhythmia. Refer to Table 3-4 in Chapter 3 for recommendations on management of AVNRT.

Circus Movement Tachycardia

Circus movement tachycardia is an SVT that occurs in people who have accessory pathways (see the section Preexcitation Syndromes earlier). *AV reentrant tachycardia* (AVRT) is also used to describe this arrhythmia, but to avoid confusion between AVRT and AVNRT, *circus movement tachycardia* is used here.

In circus movement tachycardia, an impulse travels a reentry circuit that involves the atria, AV node, ventricles, and accessory pathway. *Orthodromic* is used to describe the most common type of circus movement tachycardia, in which the impulse travels antegrade through the AV node into the ventricles and retrograde back into the atria through the accessory pathway (Figure 18-32A). The result

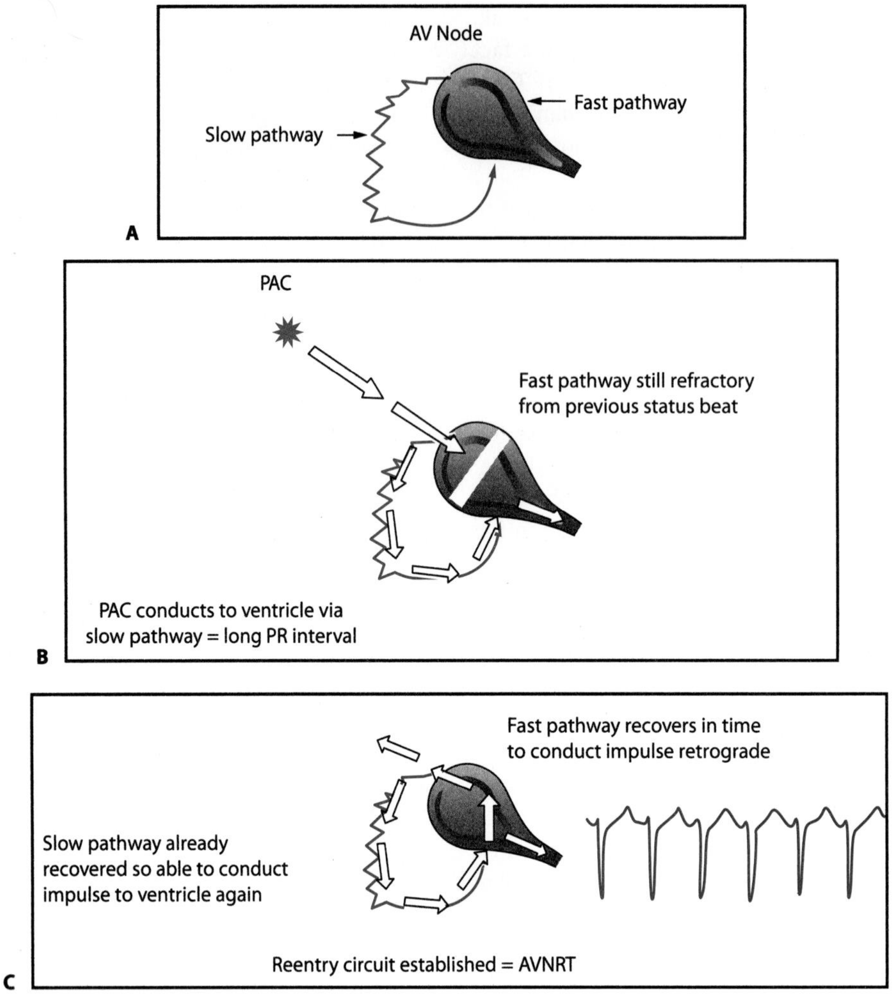

Figure 18-30. Mechanism of AVNRT. **(A)** Illustrates the dual AV nodal pathways responsible for AVNRT. The normal AV node is the fast-conducting pathway with a long refractory period; the slow-conducting pathway lies outside the AV node and has a shorter refractory period. **(B)** A PAC finds the fast pathway still refractory but is able to conduct through the slow pathway. **(C)** When the impulse arrives at the end of the slow pathway, it finds the AV node recovered and ready to conduct retrograde to the atria. The slow pathway has already recovered due to its short refractory period and is able to conduct the same impulse back into the ventricle. This sets up the reentry circuit and causes AVNRT.

is a regular, narrow QRS tachycardia because the ventricles are activated through the normal His–Purkinje system. In the presence of bundle branch block, a wide QRS pattern is present. Because the atria and ventricles depolarize separately, P waves, if visible at all, are seen following the QRS complex in the ST segment or between two QRS complexes, usually closest to the first QRS.

Antidromic describes the rare form of circus movement tachycardia in which the accessory pathway conducts the impulse from atria to ventricles and the AV node conducts it retrograde back to the atria (Figure 18-32B). Antidromic circus movement tachycardia is a regular wide QRS tachycardia because the ventricles depolarize abnormally through the accessory pathway. This form of SVT is often indistinguishable from ventricular tachycardia on the ECG.

Treatment
Circus movement tachycardia is an AV nodal active tachycardia because the AV node is necessary for maintenance

of the arrhythmia. Vagal maneuvers and drugs that block AV conduction can be used to terminate an episode of tachycardia. Acute treatment is aimed at slowing conduction through the AV node with a vagal maneuver or drugs such as adenosine, beta-blockers, or calcium channel blockers, or at slowing accessory pathway conduction with drugs like procainamide or amiodarone. Catheter ablation of the accessory pathway is the only class I recommendation for long-term management of CMT. Class IIa recommendations include flecainide, propafenone, sotalol, amiodarone, and beta-blockers.

Atrial Fibrillation in Wolff-Parkinson-White Syndrome
Atrial fibrillation occurs more frequently in people with accessory pathways than in the general population and can be life threatening. Atrial flutter and fibrillation are especially dangerous in the presence of an accessory pathway because the pathway can conduct impulses rapidly and without delay into the ventricles, resulting in dangerously

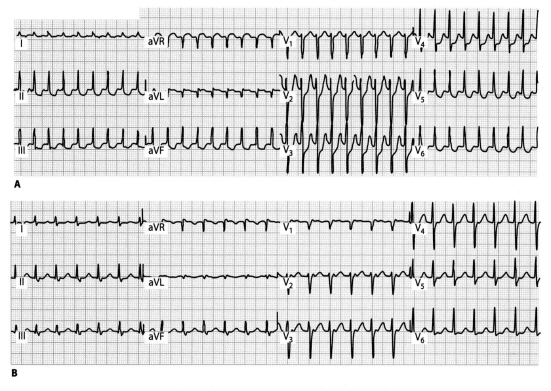

Figure 18-31. **(A)** AVNRT, rate 214. No P waves are visible. **(B)** AVNRT, rate 150. P waves distort the end of the QRS complex in leads II, III, aVF, and V$_1$ to V$_3$. *(From: Jacobson C. Arrhythmias and conduction disturbances. In: Woods SL, Froelicher ES, Motzer SA, Bridges EJ, eds. Cardiac Nursing. 3rd ed. Philadelphia, PA: JB Lippincott; 1995:341.)*

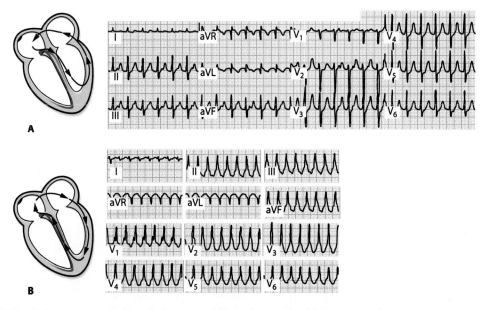

Figure 18-32. **(A)** Orthodromic circus movement tachycardia. P waves are visible on the upstroke of the T wave in leads II, III, aVF, and V1 to V3. *(From: Jacobson C. Arrhythmias and conduction disturbances. In: Woods SL, Froelicher ES, Motzer SA, Bridges EJ, eds. Cardiac Nursing. 3rd ed. Philadelphia, PA: JB Lippincott; 1995:342.)* **(B)** Antidromic circus movement tachycardia.

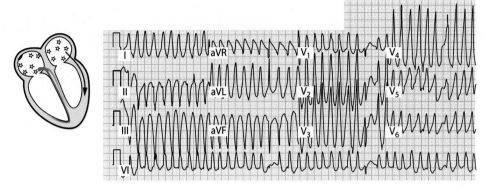

Figure 18-33. Atrial fibrillation conducting into the ventricle through an accessory pathway. Note the extremely short RR intervals in the V leads. QRS is fast, wide, and irregular.

fast ventricular rates (Figure 18-33). These rapid ventricular rates can degenerate into ventricular fibrillation and result in sudden death. When atrial fibrillation is the mechanism of the tachycardia in Wolff-Parkinson-White syndrome, the QRS complex is wide and bizarre due to conduction of the impulses into the ventricle through the bypass tract. The ventricular response to the atrial fibrillation is irregular and very rapid, often approaching rates of 300 beats/min or more because of lack of delay in conduction through the accessory pathway. Atrial fibrillation with accessory pathway conduction must be recognized and differentiated from atrial fibrillation conducting through the AV node because treatment is different for the two situations. When accessory pathway conduction is known or suspected, flecainide, ibutilide, or procainamide are recommended because they prolong the refractory period of the accessory pathway and slow ventricular rate, and they may convert the atrial fibrillation to sinus rhythm.

Verapamil often is used to slow AV conduction in atrial fibrillation conducting into the ventricles through the AV node, but can be very dangerous and even lethal when used in the presence of an accessory pathway. Digitalis, verapamil, and diltiazem can shorten the refractory period in the accessory pathway, resulting in even faster ventricular rates and degeneration into ventricular fibrillation. In addition, the hypotensive effects of these agents may intensify the hypotension related to the arrhythmia's rapid ventricular rate.

Polymorphic Ventricular Tachycardias

Polymorphic ventricular tachycardia (PVT) refers to VT with unstable, continuously varying QRS morphology often occurring at rates of approximately 200 beats/min. It can occur in short repetitive runs, longer sustained runs, or can degenerate into VF and cause sudden cardiac death. PVT can be classified based on whether it is associated with a normal or prolonged QT interval.

Polymorphic VT with a normal QT interval can occur in the presence of ventricular ischemia during acute coronary syndrome or following MI, although it is not a common arrhythmia. Figure 18-34 shows PVT in a patient during acute anterior-wall MI. Therapy of PVT associated with ischemia should be directed toward relieving the ischemia by either surgery or angioplasty. Beta-blockers are recommended for PVT if ischemia is suspected. For recurrent PVT in the absence of a long-QT interval, IV amiodarone is useful and lidocaine may be helpful. If PVT becomes sustained or degenerates to VF, defibrillation with an unsynchronized shock is necessary. Table 3-6 in Chapter 3 summarizes recommendations for managing PVT.

Torsades de pointes means "twisting of the points" and describes polymorphic VT that occurs with abnormal ventricular repolarization. This abnormal repolarization presents on the ECG as an abnormally prolonged QT or QTU interval. See the section on long-QT syndromes in this chapter for more information on long-QT syndromes.

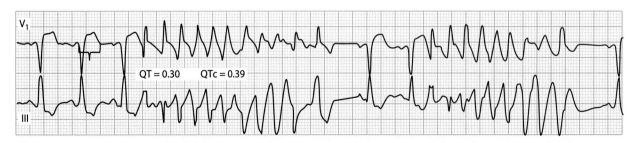

Figure 18-34. Polymorphic VT with a normal QT interval. This patient was having an acute MI (note ST elevation in lead V₁).

ESSENTIAL CONTENT CASE

Patient with Syncope

Your 20-year-old patient was admitted with a head laceration after an episode of syncope with seizure. He had one previous episode of "fainting" about a month ago but did not seek medical care. His BP is 126/72 mm Hg, heart rate 50 beats/min, and complains of pain at the laceration site but is awake, oriented, and cooperative. This is the 12-lead ECG obtained as part of his workup for syncope:

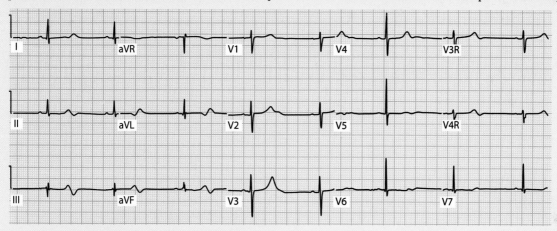

Case Question 1. What is your interpretation of this ECG, rhythm, QRS axis, and Bundle branch block?

Case Question 2. Is there anything on the ECG that might indicate a cause of his "seizure?"

You put him on the bedside monitor and set the alarms. He remains stable for the next few hours, then you hear his monitor alarm. When you enter the room he is complaining of extreme dizziness and says he feels like he might pass out. This is his rhythm on the monitor:

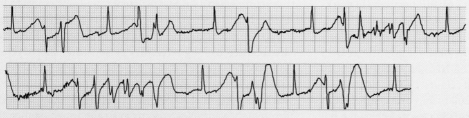

Case Question 3. What is this rhythm?

Case Question 4. What treatment is indicated for this rhythm acutely and long term?

In the next minute the rhythm does this:

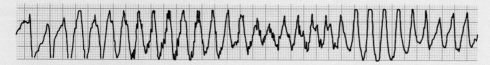

Case Question 5. What is the treatment now?

Answers
1. The rhythm is sinus bradycardia. The QRS axis is normal. There is no bundle branch block.
2. The QT interval is long, about 0.58 sec (580 ms) in lead II and 0.60 sec (600 ms) in lead V$_2$. The T waves are biphasic or notched. This is a form of congenital long-QT syndrome which increases the risk of TdP and sudden cardiac death. Patients often present with syncope, or seizures that are due to episodes of TdP that last long enough to result in loss of consciousness.
3. The basic rhythm appears to be sinus (narrow QRS beats) with PVC couplets and short runs of TdP.
4. Treatment of short runs of TdP includes IV magnesium or overdrive pacing to shorten the QT interval. Any drugs that might contribute to QT interval prolongation should be discontinued, and any electrolyte imbalances need to be corrected. Beta-blockers are the mainstay of long-term treatment of congenital long-QT syndrome. Patients who continue to have significant ventricular arrhythmias on beta-blockers or who experience a SCD event should receive an ICD implant.
5. This strip represents a sustained run of TdP. Long runs that don't terminate spontaneously cause loss of consciousness and usually degenerate into VF. Defibrillation is the treatment for sustained TdP.

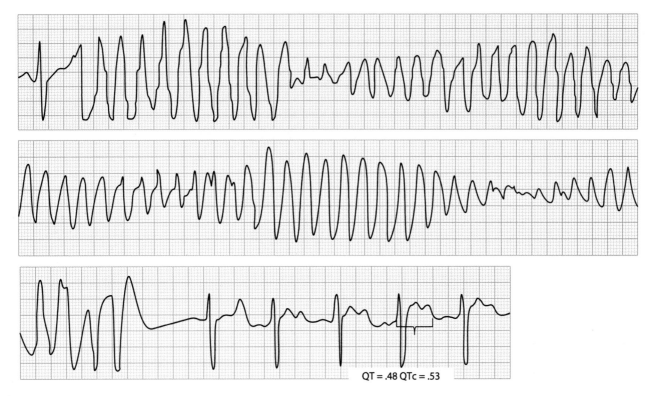

QT = .48 QTc = .53

Figure 18-35. Torsades de pointes. Note characteristic "twisting" appearance during VT and the long-QT interval during sinus rhythm.

Characteristic ECG findings of TdP include: (1) markedly prolonged QT intervals with wide TU waves; (2) initiation of the arrhythmia by an R-on-T PVC with a long coupling interval; and (3) wide, bizarre, multiform QRS complexes that change direction frequently, appearing to twist around the isoelectric line (Figure 18-35). Ventricular rate during TdP is commonly 200 to 250 beats/min. TdP is usually self-terminating and occurs in repeated episodes, but it can deteriorate into ventricular fibrillation.

Differentiating Wide QRS Beats and Rhythms

Determining the origin of a wide QRS beat or a wide QRS tachycardia is one of the most common problems encountered when caring for monitored patients. A supraventricular beat with abnormal, or aberrant, conduction through the ventricles, can look almost identical to a beat that originates in the ventricle. The problem with aberration is that it can mimic ventricular arrhythmias, which require different therapy and carry a different prognosis than aberrancy. Aberrancy is always secondary to some other primary disturbance and does not itself require treatment. Nurses must be able to identify accurately which mechanism is responsible for the wide QRS rhythm being observed whenever possible, initiate appropriate treatment when needed, and avoid inappropriate treatment.

Mechanisms of Aberration

Aberrancy is the temporary abnormal intraventricular conduction of supraventricular impulses. Aberration occurs whenever the His-Purkinje system or ventricle is still partly refractory when a supraventricular impulse attempts to travel through it. The refractory period of the conduction system is directly proportional to preceding cycle length. Long cycles are followed by long refractory periods, and short cycles are followed by short refractory periods. An early supraventricular beat, such as a PAC, may enter the conduction system during a portion of its refractory period, forcing conduction through the ventricles to occur in an abnormal manner. Beats that follow a sudden lengthening of the cycle may conduct aberrantly because of the increased length of the refractory period that occurs when the cycle lengthens (Figure 18-36). The right bundle branch has a longer refractory period than the left; therefore, aberrant beats tend to conduct most often with an RBBB pattern, although LBBB aberration is common in people with cardiac disease.

Electrocardiographic Clues to the Origin of Wide QRS Beats and Rhythms
P Waves

If P waves can be seen during a wide QRS tachycardia, they are very helpful in making the differential diagnosis of aberration vs ventricular ectopy. Atrial activity, represented by the P wave on the ECG and preceding a wide QRS beat or run of tachycardia, strongly favors a supraventricular origin of the arrhythmia. Figure 18-37 shows three wide QRS beats that could easily be mistaken for PVCs if not for the obvious presence of the early P wave initiating the run.

An exception to the preceding P-wave rule occurs with end-diastolic PVCs. *End-diastolic PVCs* occur at the end of diastole, after the sinus P wave has been recorded but before it has a chance to conduct through the AV node into the ventricle.

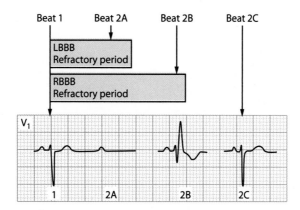

Figure 18-36. Diagram of refractory periods in the bundle branches and the effect of cycle length on conduction. The right bundle has a longer refractory period than the left. Beat 2A occurs so early that it cannot conduct through either bundle branch. Beat 2B encounters a refractory right bundle and conducts with RBBB. Beat 2C falls outside the refractory period of both bundles and is able to conduct normally.

Figure 18-38 shows sinus rhythm with an end-diastolic PVC occurring immediately after the sinus P wave. Here, the P wave preceding the wide QRS is merely a coincidence and does not indicate aberrant conduction. The PR interval is much too short to have conducted that QRS complex. In addition, the P wave preceding the wide QRS is not early; it is the regularly scheduled sinus beat coming on time. Thus, early P waves that precede early wide QRS complexes are usually "married to" those QRSs and indicate aberrant conduction, while "on-time" P waves in front of end-diastolic PVCs are not early and do not cause the wide QRS.

P waves seen during a wide QRS tachycardia also can be very helpful in making the differential diagnosis between SVTs with aberration and ventricular tachycardia. If P waves are seen associated with every QRS, the rhythm is supraventricular in origin (Figure 18-39A). P waves that occur independently of the QRS and have no consistent relationship to QRS complexes indicate the presence of AV dissociation, which means that the atria and the ventricles are under the control of separate pacemakers and strongly favors ventricular tachycardia (Figure 18-39B).

QRS Morphology

The shape of the QRS complex is very helpful in determining the origin of a wide QRS rhythm. When using QRS morphology clues, it is extremely important to examine the correct leads and apply the criteria only to leads that have been proven helpful. Many practitioners prefer to monitor with lead II because usually it shows an upright QRS complex and clear P wave. Lead II, however, has no value in determining the origin of a wide QRS rhythm. The single best arrhythmia monitoring lead is V_1, followed by V_6 and V_2 in certain situations.

When applying QRS morphology criteria for wide QRS rhythms, it is helpful to first decide whether the QRS complexes have an RBBB morphology or an LBBB morphology. RBBB morphology rhythms have an upright QRS in lead V_1, while LBBB morphology rhythms have a negative QRS complex in V_1.

When dealing with a wide QRS rhythm of RBBB morphology (upright in V_1), follow these steps to evaluate QRS morphology (Figures 18-40 and 18-41A):

1. Look at V_1 and determine if the upright QRS complex is monophasic (R wave), diphasic (qR), or triphasic (rsR'). Monophasic and diphasic complexes favor a ventricular origin, if the left peak ("rabbit ear") is taller. A taller right rabbit ear does not favor either diagnosis. A triphasic rsR' is typical of RBBB aberration in V_1.
2. Look at V_6 and determine whether the QRS is monophasic (all negative QS), diphasic (rS), or triphasic

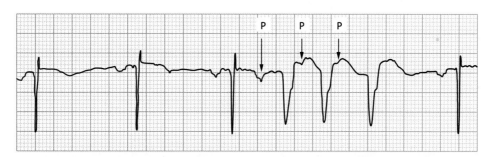

Figure 18-37. Sinus rhythm with PACs and three wide QRS beats that could be mistaken for ventricular tachycardia. Note the P waves preceding the wide QRS complexes, indicating aberrant conduction. *(From: Jacobson C. Arrhythmias and conduction disturbances. In: Woods SL, Froelicher ES, Motzer, SA, Bridges EJ, eds. Cardiac Nursing. 3rd ed. Philadelphia, PA: JB Lippincott; 1995:346.)*

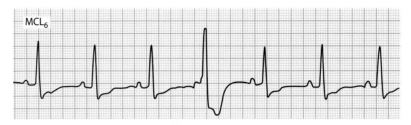

Figure 18-38. Sinus rhythm with an end-diastolic PVC. The P wave preceding the PVC is the sinus P wave that coincidentally occurs just before the PVC. *(From: Jacobson C. Arrhythmias and conduction disturbances. In: Woods SL, Froelicher ES, Motzer SA, Bridges EJ, eds.* Cardiac Nursing. *3rd ed. Philadelphia, PA: JB Lippincott; 1995:347.)*

(qRs). A monophasic or diphasic complex in V_6 favors a ventricular origin, and the triphasic qRs complex is typical of RBBB aberration in V_6.

If the QRS has an LBBB morphology (negative in V_1), follow these steps to evaluate morphology (Figures 18-40 and 18-41B):

1. Look at V_1 or V_2 (both are helpful in this case) and determine if the R wave (if present) is wide or narrow. A wide R wave of more than 0.03 second favors a ventricular rhythm, and a narrow R wave favors a supraventricular origin with LBBB aberration.
2. Next look at the downstroke of the S wave in V_1 or V_2. Slurring or notching on the downstroke favors a ventricular origin. LBBB aberration typically slurs on the upstroke if it slurs at all.
3. Measure from the onset of the QRS complex to the deepest part of the S wave in V_1 or V_2. A measurement of more than 0.06 second favors a ventricular rhythm and a narrower measurement favors LBBB aberration. Note that this measurement can be prolonged due to either a wide R wave or slurring on the downstroke of the S wave, either one of which favors the ventricular origin of the rhythm.

4. Look at V_6 and determine whether a Q wave is present. Any Q wave (either a QS or qR complex) favors a ventricular origin.

Concordance

Concordance means that all the QRS complexes across the precordium from V_1 through V_6 point in the same direction; positive concordance means they are all upright, and negative concordance means they are all negative (Figure 18-42A). Negative concordance favors a diagnosis of ventricular tachycardia when it occurs in a wide QRS tachycardia, and positive concordance favors ventricular tachycardia as long as Wolff-Parkinson-White syndrome can be ruled out.

FUSION AND CAPTURE BEATS

Ventricular fusion beats occur when the ventricles are depolarized by two different wavefronts of electrical activity at the same time. Fusion often results when a supraventricular impulse travels through the AV node and begins to depolarize the ventricles at the same time that an impulse from a ventricular focus depolarizes the ventricles. When two different impulses contribute to ventricular depolarization, the resulting QRS shape and width are determined by the relative contributions of both the supraventricular and the

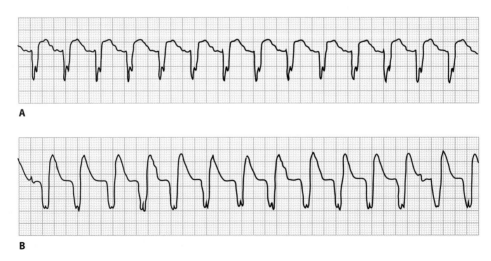

Figure 18-39. Two very similar, wide QRS tachycardias. **(A)** Sinus tachycardia, rate 115. P waves can be seen on the downslope of the T wave preceding each QRS, indicating a supraventricular origin of the tachycardia. **(B)** P waves are independent of QRS complexes, indicating AV dissociation, which favors ventricular tachycardia. *(From: Jacobson C. Arrhythmias and conduction disturbances. In: Woods SL, Froelicher ES, Motzer SA, Bridges EJ, eds.* Cardiac Nursing. *3rd ed. Philadelphia, PA: JB Lippincott; 1995:347.)*

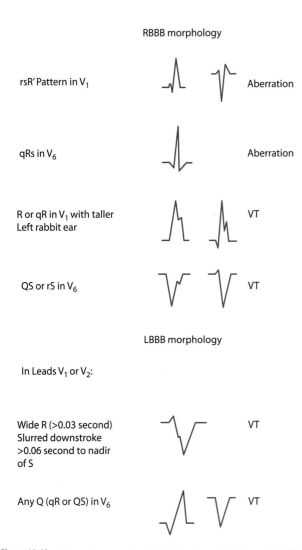

RBBB morphology

rsR' Pattern in V₁   Aberration

qRs in V₆   Aberration

R or qR in V₁ with taller
Left rabbit ear   VT

QS or rS in V₆   VT

LBBB morphology

In Leads V₁ or V₂:

Wide R (>0.03 second)
Slurred downstroke
>0.06 second to nadir
of S   VT

Any Q (qR or QS) in V₆   VT

Figure 18-40. Morphology clues for wide QRS beats and rhythms with RBBB and LBBB patterns. *(From: Jacobson C. Arrhythmias and conduction disturbances. In: Woods SL, Froelicher ES, Motzer SA, Bridges EJ, eds. Cardiac Nursing. 3rd ed. Philadelphia, PA: JB Lippincott; 1995:348.)*

ventricular impulses. In the presence of a wide QRS tachycardia, the presence of fusion beats indicates AV dissociation, which means that the atria and ventricles are under the control of separate pacemakers. Capture beats occur when the supraventricular impulse manages to conduct all the way into and through the ventricle, depolarizing ("capturing") the ventricle and resulting in a normal QRS in the midst of the wide QRS tachycardia. The presence of fusion and capture beats in a wide QRS tachycardia is strong evidence supporting the diagnosis of ventricular tachycardia, but they occur rarely and cannot be counted on to make the diagnosis. Figure 18-42B shows fusion beats in a wide QRS tachycardia. Helpful ECG clues for differentiating aberrancy from ventricular ectopy are summarized in Table 18-3.

ST-SEGMENT MONITORING

Many bedside monitors have software programs that allow for continuous monitoring of the ST segment in addition to routine arrhythmia monitoring. Continuous ST-segment monitoring can detect ischemia related to reocclusion of the involved artery in patients with acute MI who have received thrombolytic therapy, angioplasty, or other interventional cardiologic procedures aimed at opening occluded coronary arteries. ST-segment monitoring is also useful in detecting silent ischemia (ischemic episodes that occur in the absence of chest pain or other symptoms) that would otherwise go unnoticed with symptom and arrhythmia monitoring alone. Early detection of ischemic changes is critical in identifying patients who need interventions to reestablish blood flow to myocardium before permanent damage occurs.

ST elevation in leads facing damaged myocardium is the ECG sign of myocardial injury. ST depression is often recorded as a reciprocal change in leads that do not directly face involved myocardium (see Table 18-2). In addition, ST depression can be recorded in leads facing ischemic tissue. Therefore, either ST elevation or ST depression indicates myocardium at risk for infarction and a patient potentially at risk for complications related to infarction. The sooner the artery is opened and blood flow reestablished to ischemic or injured tissue, the more myocardium is salvaged and the fewer complications and deaths occur.

Measuring the ST Segment

Clinically significant ST-segment deviation is defined as ST elevation or depression 1 mm or more from the baseline, or isoelectric line, measured 60 msec (0.06 second) after the J point. The J point is the point at which the QRS ends and the ST segment begins. Figure 18-43A illustrates a normal ST segment, and Figure 18-43B illustrates ST-segment elevation and depression.

ST-segment monitoring software in newer bedside monitors defines the baseline and the ST-segment measuring point. It also sets default alarm parameters so the equipment can audibly notify the nurse when the patient's ST segment falls outside the defined parameters. Most monitors allow the user to redefine the baseline, reset the J point, choose where the ST segment is measured, and change the alarm parameters to account for individual patient variations. The monitor then displays the ST-segment measurement in millimeters on the screen, and most monitors also allow for trending of the ST segment over specified time intervals.

Choosing the Best Leads for ST-Segment Monitoring

Some monitoring systems offer continuous 12-lead ECG monitoring, which eliminates the need to select the "best" leads to monitor for a given clinical situation. Most younger generation bedside monitors offer at least two leads for simultaneous ECG monitoring and some offer three leads. The single best lead for arrhythmia monitoring is V₁, with V₆ being next best. Using two or three leads for ST-segment monitoring is optimal because a single lead may miss significant ST-segment deviations. Since current bedside

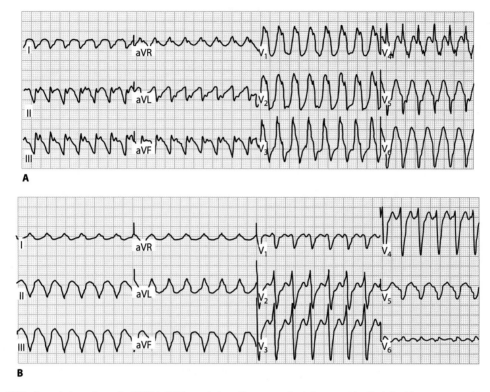

Figure 18-41. 12-lead ECG of ventricular tachycardia. **(A)** With RBBB morphology. Note monophasic R wave with taller left rabbit ear in V$_1$ and QS complex in V$_6$. **(B)** With LBBB morphology. Note wide R wave in V$_1$ and V$_2$, and qR pattern in V$_6$.

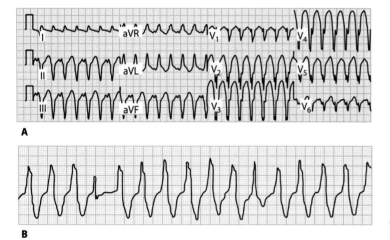

Figure 18-42. **(A)** 12-lead ECG of ventricular tachycardia with negative concordance. **(B)** Rhythm strip of ventricular tachycardia with fusion beats.

TABLE 18-3. ECG CLUES FOR DIFFERENTIATING ABERRATION FROM VENTRICULAR ECTOPY

	Aberrancy	Ventricular Ectopy
P waves	Precede QRS complexes	Dissociated from QRS or occur at rate slower than QRS; if 1:1 V-A conduction is present, retrograde P waves follow every QRS
Precordial QRS concordance	Positive concordance may occur with WPW	Negative concordance favors VT; positive concordance favors VT if WPW ruled out
Fusion or capture beats		Strong evidence in favor of VT
QRS axis	Often normal; may be deviated to right or left	Right superior axis favors VT; often deviated to left or right
RBBB QRS morphology	Triphasic rsR′ in V$_1$: triphasic qRs in V$_6$	Monophasic R wave or diphasic qR complex in V$_1$: left "rabbit ear" taller in V$_1$: monophasic QS or diphasic rS in V$_6$
LBBB QRS morphology	Narrow R wave (< 0.04 second) in V$_1$; straight downstroke of S wave in V$_1$ (often slurs or notches on upstroke); usually no Q wave in V$_6$	Wide R wave (> 0.03 second) in V$_1$ or V$_2$; slurring or notching on downstroke of S wave in V$_1$; delay of greater than 0.06 second to nadir of S wave in V$_1$ or V$_2$; any Q wave in V$_6$

Normal ST segment

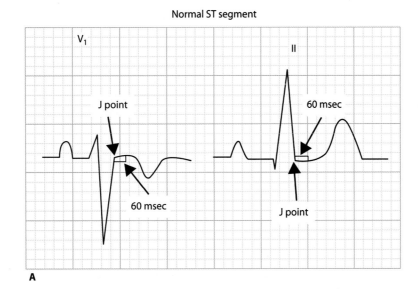

A

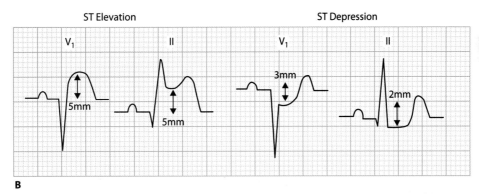

B

Figure 18-43. **(A)** Normal ST segment on the baseline in leads V_1 and II. **(B)** ST-segment elevation and ST-segment depression.

monitors allow for the use of only one V lead at a time, using V_1 as the arrhythmia monitoring lead (or V_6 if V_1 is not available because of dressings, etc) means that limb leads must be used for ST-segment monitoring. The best limb leads are discussed below.

The best way to choose leads for ST-segment monitoring is to know the patient's "ischemic fingerprint." To determine the patient's ischemic fingerprint, obtain a 12-lead ECG during a pain episode or with inflation of the balloon during angioplasty and note which leads show the most ST-segment displacement (either elevation or depression) during the acute ischemic event. Choose the lead or leads with the most ST-segment displacement as the bedside ST-segment monitoring leads.

If no ischemic fingerprint is available, use a lead or leads that have been determined through research to be best for the artery involved (Table 18-4). The limb leads that have been shown to best detect ischemia related to all three major coronary arteries (right coronary, left anterior descending, and circumflex) are leads III and aVF. In the case of the right coronary artery (RCA), leads III and aVF directly face the inferior wall supplied by this artery and record ST elevation with inferior wall injury. The left anterior descending and

circumflex artery supply the anterior and lateral walls, respectively. Because these walls are not directly faced by leads III and aVF, ST-segment depression is recorded as a reciprocal change when anterior or lateral wall injury occurs. Table 18-5 summarizes critical elements of ST-segment monitoring.

CARDIAC PACEMAKERS

Chapter 3, Interpretation and Management of Basic Cardiac Rhythms, describes the components of a temporary pacing system and basic pacemaker operation. This section discusses single-chamber and dual-chamber pacemaker

TABLE 18-4. RECOMMENDED LEADS FOR CONTINUOUS ECG MONITORING

Purpose	Best Leads
Arrhythmia detection	V_1 (V_6 next best)
RCA ischemia, inferior MI	III, aVF
LAD ischemia, anterior MI	V_3 (III, aVF best limb leads)
Circumflex ischemia, lateral MI	I, aVL (III, aVF good reciprocal leads)
RV infarction	V_4R
Axis shifts	I and aVF together

TABLE 18-5. EVIDENCE-BASED PRACTICE: ST-SEGMENT MONITORING

Patient Selection

Class I: ST-segment monitoring recommended for the following types of patients:

- Patients in the early phase of acute coronary syndromes (unstable angina, "rule-out MI, ST elevation MI, non–ST-elevation MI").[a,c]
- Patients presenting to emergency department with chest pain or anginal equivalent symptoms.[a,c]
- Patients who have undergone nonurgent percutaneous coronary intervention and who have suboptimal angiographic results.[a,c]
- Patients with possible variant angina due to coronary vasospasm.[a,c]

Class II: ST-segment monitoring may be of benefit in some patients but is not considered essential for all:

- Patients with post-acute MI (after 24-48 hours).[a]
- Patients who have undergone nonurgent, uncomplicated percutaneous coronary intervention 1.
- Patients at high risk for ischemia after cardiac or noncardiac surgery.[a]
- Pediatric patients at risk of ischemia or infarction due to congenital or acquired conditions.[a]

Electrode Application

- Make sure skin is clean and dry before applying monitoring electrodes.[a,b,c]
- Place electrodes according to manufacturer recommendations when using a derived 12-lead ECG system.[a]
- When using a 3- or 5-wire-monitoring system, place electrodes as follows:
  – Place arm electrodes in infraclavicular fossa close to shoulder[a] or on top or back of shoulder as close to where arm joins torso as possible.
  – Place leg electrodes at lowest point on rib cage or on hips.[a,b]
  – Place V_1 electrode at the fourth intercostal space at right sternal border.[b]
  – Place V_6 electrode at the fifth intercostal space at left midaxillary line.[b]
- Mark electrode placement with indelible ink.[a,c]
- Replace electrodes every 48 hours or more often if skin irritation occurs.[b]

Lead Selection

- Monitor all 12 leads continuously if using a 12-lead monitoring system.[b]
- Use V_1 (or V_6 if V_1 is not possible due to dressings, etc) for arrhythmia monitoring in all multilead combinations.[b]
- Choose the ST-segment monitoring lead according to the patient's "ischemic fingerprint" obtained during an ischemic event whenever possible.[b,c] Use the lead with the largest ST-segment deviation (elevation or depression).[b]
- If no ischemic fingerprint is available, use either lead III[b,c] or aVF (whichever has tallest QRS complex)[b] for ST-segment monitoring.
- Lead V_3 is the best lead for detecting anterior wall ST-segment deviation,[c] but can only be used if the chest lead is not being used for arrhythmia monitoring in lead V_1.

Alarm Limits

- Establish baseline ST level with patient in the supine position.[a,c]
- Set ST alarm parameters at 1 mm above and below the patient's baseline ST level in patients at high risk for ischemia.[a]
- Set ST alarm parameters at 2 mm above and below the patient's baseline ST level in more stable patients.[a]

[a]Data compiled from Drew BJ, Califf RM, Funk M. Practice standards for electrocardiographic monitoring in hospital settings. *Circulation*, 2004; 110: 2721-2746; [b]Jacobson C, Marzlin K, Webner C. *Cardiovascular Nursing Practice: a comprehensive resource manual and study guide for clinical nurses.* [c]Burien, WA: Cardiovascular Nursing Education Associates, 2007; [c]AACN Practice Alert: ST Segment Monitoring. American Association of Critical Care Nurses. 2009. http://www.aacn.org/WD/Practice/Docs/PracticeAlerts/ ST_Segment_Monitoring_05-2009.pdf.

function and evaluation of pacemaker rhythm strips for appropriate capture and sensing.

Cardiac pacemakers are classified by a standardized five-letter pacemaker code that describes the location of the pacing wire(s) and the expected function of the pacemaker. Table 18-6 illustrates the five-letter code. The first letter in the pacemaker code describes the chamber that is paced (A = atrium, V = ventricle, D = dual [atrium and ventricle], 0 = none). The letter in the second position describes the chamber where intrinsic electrical activity is sensed (A = atrium, V = ventricle, D = dual, 0 = none). The letter in the third position describes the pacemaker's response to sensing of intrinsic electrical activity (I = inhibited, T = triggered, D = dual [inhibited or triggered], 0 = none). The fourth letter indicates the presence or absence of rate modulation, and the fifth letter describes multisite pacing functions. To know how a pacemaker should function, it is necessary to know at a minimum the first three letters of the code, which describe where the pacemaker is supposed to pace, where it is supposed to sense, and what it should do when it senses. The last two letters representing advanced pacemaker function are not covered in this text; see the recommended references at the end of the chapter.

Three types of temporary pacing are commonly used in critical care or telemetry settings. The first is transvenous pacing through a wire introduced into the apex of the right ventricle via a peripheral or central vein and set in the demand mode (sensitive to intrinsic ventricular activity). Ventricular pacing is always done in the demand mode to avoid the delivery of pacing stimuli into the vulnerable period of the cardiac cycle, which could induce ventricular tachycardia or fibrillation (see Chapter 3, Interpretation and Management of Basic Cardiac Rhythms). This type of pacing is described by the pacemaker code as a VVI pacemaker—it paces the ventricle, senses intrinsic ventricular electrical activity, and inhibits its output when sensing occurs.

The second type of pacing done in critical care or telemetry is temporary epicardial pacing (either atrial, ventricular, or dual chamber) via pacing wires attached to the atria and/or ventricles during cardiac surgery. If atrial pacing is done with no sensing of atrial electrical activity, also called asynchronous mode, the pacemaker operates as an A00 pacemaker—it paces the atria, does not sense, and therefore does not respond to intrinsic atrial activity. If atrial pacing is done with sensing of atrial electrical activity, also called the demand mode, the pacemaker operates as an AAI pacemaker—it paces the atria, senses atrial activity, and inhibits its output when it senses. Dual-chamber pacing can be done in several modes involving pacing and sensing functions in one or both chambers and described by the pacemaker code according to the mode chosen. The two most common dual-chamber modes used with temporary epicardial pacing (and occasionally with temporary transvenous pacing) are DVI (paces atria and ventricles, senses only in the ventricle, and inhibits pacing output when sensing occurs) and DDD (paces both chambers, senses both chambers, and either triggers or inhibits pacing output in response to sensing). The common dual-chamber pacing modes are listed in Table 18-7.

The third type of temporary pacing is external (transcutaneous) pacing. External pacing is done in emergency situations requiring immediate pacing when placement of a temporary transvenous pacing wire is not feasible. External pacing is not as reliable as transvenous or epicardial pacing and is used as a temporary measure until transvenous pacing can be

TABLE 18-6. PACEMAKER CODES

First Letter: Chamber Paced	Second Letter: Chamber Sensed	Third Letter: Response to Sensing	Fourth Letter: Rate Modulation	Fifth Letter: Multisite Pacing[a]
0 = None	0 = None	0 = None	0 = None	0 = None
A = Atrium	A = Atrium	I = Inhibited	R = Rate modulation	A = Atrial
V = Ventricle	V = Ventricle	T = Triggered		V = Ventricular
D = Dual (A&V)	D = Dual (A&V)	D = Dual (I&T)		D = Dual

[a] *Multisite indicates either pacing in both atria or both ventricles or pacing multiple sites within a chamber.*

instituted. External pacing is briefly described in Chapter 3, Interpretation and Management of Basic Cardiac Rhythms.

Evaluating Pacemaker Function

Evaluating pacemaker function requires knowledge of the mode of pacing expected (VVI, AAI, etc); the minimum rate of the pacemaker, or pacing interval; and any other programmed parameters in the pacemaker. The basic functions of a pacemaker include stimulus release, capture, and sensing. *Stimulus release* refers to pacemaker output, or the ability of the pacemaker to generate and release a pacing impulse. *Capture* is the ability of the pacing stimulus to result in depolarization of the chamber being paced. *Sensing* is the ability of the pacemaker to recognize and respond to intrinsic electrical activity in the heart. Pacemaker operation is evaluated according to these three functions. Single-chamber pacemaker evaluation is much less complicated than dual-chamber evaluation. Because single-chamber ventricular pacing is a very common type of temporary pacing in critical care and telemetry units, VVI pacemaker evaluation is discussed here.

VVI Pacemaker Evaluation

Stimulus release, capture, and sensing must all be assessed when evaluating VVI pacemakers. A VVI pacemaker is expected to pace the ventricle at the set rate unless spontaneous ventricular activity occurs to inhibit pacing. The set rate of the pacemaker, or *pacing interval*, is measured from one pacing stimulus to the next consecutive stimulus. Pacemakers have a *refractory period*, which is a period following either pacing or sensing in the chamber, during which the pacemaker is unable to respond to intrinsic activity. During the refractory period, the pacemaker in effect has its eyes closed and is not able to see spontaneous activity. In a normally functioning VVI pacemaker, pacing spikes occur at the set pacing

interval and each spike results in a ventricular depolarization (capture). If spontaneous ventricular activity occurs (either a normally conducted QRS or a PVC), that activity is sensed and the next pacing stimulus is inhibited. Figure 18-44A and B shows normal VVI pacemaker function.

Stimulus Release

Stimulus release depends on a pacemaker with enough battery power to generate the electrical impulse, and on an intact pacemaker lead system to deliver the electrical stimulus to the heart. The presence of a pacer spike on the rhythm strip or monitor indicates that the stimulus was released from the generator and entered the body. The presence of the spike does not indicate where the stimulus was delivered (eg, atria or ventricles), only that it entered the body somewhere. Total absence of pacing stimuli, when they should be present, can indicate a faulty pulse generator or battery, or a break or disconnection in the lead system. Pacing stimuli also can be absent when pacing is inhibited by the sensing of intrinsic electrical activity. Figure 18-45 illustrates total loss of stimulus release in a patient whose pacemaker battery was depleted.

Capture

Capture is indicated by a wide QRS complex immediately following the pacemaker spike and represents the ability of the pacing stimulus to depolarize the ventricle. Loss of capture is recognized by the presence of pacer spikes that are not followed by paced ventricular complexes (Figure 18-46). Causes of loss of capture include:

- Inadequate stimulus strength, which can be corrected by increasing the electrical output of the pacemaker (turning up the milliampere level).
- Pacing wire out of position and not in contact with myocardium, which can be corrected by repositioning the wire and sometimes the patient.

TABLE 18-7. DUAL-CHAMBER PACING MODES

Mode	Chamber(s) Paced	Chamber(s) Sensed	Response to Sensing
DVI	Atrium and ventricle	Ventricle	Inhibited
VDD	Ventricle	Atrium and ventricle	Atrial sensing triggers ventricular pacing Ventricular sensing inhibits ventricular pacing
DDI	Atrium and ventricle	Atrium and ventricle	Inhibited
DDD	Atrium and ventricle	Atrium and ventricle	Atrial sensing inhibits atrial pacing, triggers ventricular pacing Ventricular sensing inhibits atrial and ventricular pacing

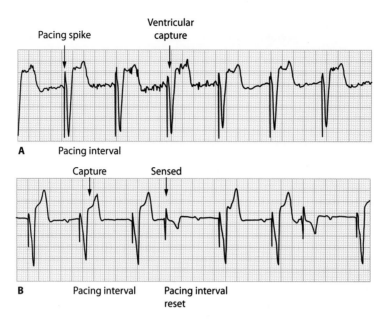

Figure 18-44. Normal VVI pacemaker function. **(A)** Pacing electrical activity ("pacer spike") followed by a wide QRS complex indicating ventricular capture. Pacemaker sensing cannot be evaluated because no intrinsic QRS complexes are present. **(B)** Pacemaker capture and sensing both normal. Intrinsic QRS complexes are sensed, inhibiting ventricular pacing output, and resetting the pacing interval. Absence of intrinsic ventricular electrical activity causes pacing to occur with capture.

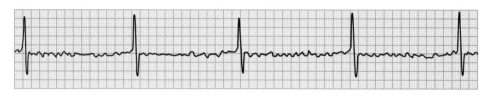

Figure 18-45. Absence of stimulus release in a patient with a permanent pacemaker. Underlying rhythm is atrial fibrillation with complete AV block and a very slow ventricular rate. The battery in the pacemaker generator was depleted.

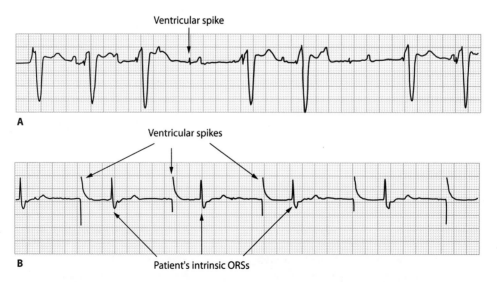

Figure 18-46. **(A)** VVI pacemaker with intermittent loss of capture. **(B)** VVI pacemaker with total loss of capture.

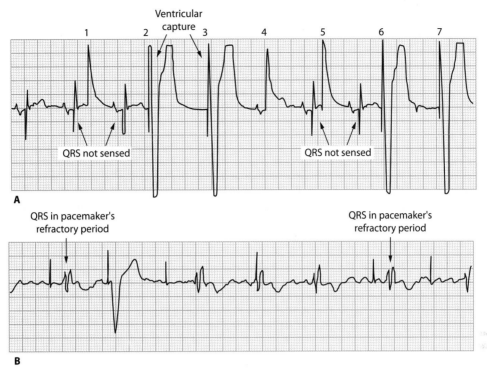

Figure 18-47. **(A)** Intermittent loss of sensing in a VVI pacemaker. Delivery of the pacing stimulus during the heart's refractory period makes it appear that capture is lost as well. Because the heart is physiologically unable to respond to the pacing stimulus when it falls in the refractory period, this is not a capture problem. Pacer spikes 1, 2, 5, and 6 should not have occurred; their presence is due to loss of sensing. Pacer spike 4 occurred coincident with the normal QRS complex, resulting in a "pseudofusion" beat, and does not represent loss of sensing. **(B)** Loss of capture in a VVI pacemaker. Only one pacer spike captures the ventricle. Two QRS complexes occur during the pacemaker's refractory period and thus are not sensed. This does not represent loss of sensing because the pacemaker has its "eyes closed" during the time intrinsic ventricular activity occurred.

- Pacing lead positioned in infarcted tissue, which can be corrected by repositioning the wire to a place where the myocardium is not injured and is capable of responding to the stimulus.
- Electrolyte imbalances or drugs that alter the ability of the heart to respond to the pacing stimulus.
- Delivery of a pacing stimulus during the ventricles refractory period when the heart is physiologically unable to respond to the stimulus. This problem occurs with loss of sensing (undersensing) and can be corrected by correcting the sensing problem (Figure 18-47A).

Sensing

Sensing of intrinsic ventricular electrical activity inhibits the next pacing stimulus and resets the pacing interval. Sensing cannot occur unless the pacemaker is given the opportunity to sense. It must be in the demand mode and there must be intrinsic ventricular activity that occurs for the pacemaker to have an opportunity to sense. In Figure 18-44A, sensing cannot be evaluated because there is no intrinsic ventricular activity that occurs, and therefore the pacemaker is not given an opportunity to sense. In Figure 18-44B, the occurrence of two spontaneous QRS complexes provides the pacemaker with an opportunity to

sense. In this example, sensing occurred normally, as indicated by the absence of the next expected pacing stimulus and resetting of the pacing interval by the intrinsic QRS complex.

Two sensing problems can occur: undersensing (Figure 18-47A and 18-48A) and oversensing (Figure 18-48B). Undersensing, also called "failure to sense" or "loss of sensing," can be caused by:

- Asynchronous (fixed rate) mode in which the sensing circuit is off. This problem can be corrected by turning the sensitivity control to the demand mode.
- Pacing catheter out of position or lying in infarcted tissue, which can be corrected by repositioning the wire. Pacing wire repositioning must be done by a physician; however, turning the patient onto his or her side sometimes temporarily works when the pacing wire loses contact with the ventricle.
- Intrinsic QRS voltage too low to be sensed by the pacemaker. Turning the sensitivity control clockwise or decreasing the sensitivity number increases the sensitivity of the pacemaker and makes it able to "see" smaller intrinsic electrical signals. Repositioning the wire sometimes helps.
- Break in connections, battery failure, or faulty pulse generator. Check and tighten all connections along

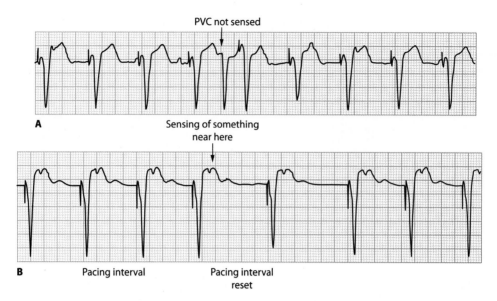

Figure 18-48. **(A)** Undersensing in a VVI pacemaker. The PVC is not sensed and pacing occurs at the programmed pacing interval, resulting in a pacemaker spike on the T wave of the PVC. **(B)** Oversensing in a VVI pacemaker. The pacing rate slows for two intervals, presumably due to sensing of something near the T wave, which resets the pacing interval from the point where sensing occurred.

the pacing system, and replace the battery if it is low. A chest x-ray may detect wire fracture. Change the pulse generator if problems cannot be corrected any other way.

- Intrinsic ventricular activity falling in the pacemaker's refractory period. If a spontaneous QRS complex occurs during the time the pacemaker has its eyes closed, the pacemaker cannot see it. This event occurs when the pacemaker fails to capture, which can allow an intrinsic QRS to occur during the pacemaker's refractory period. This problem is due to loss of capture and does not reflect a sensing malfunction (see Figure 18-47B).

Oversensing means that the pacemaker is so sensitive that it inappropriately senses internal or outside signals as QRS complexes and inhibits its output. Common sources of outside signals that can interfere with pacemaker function include electromagnetic or RF signals, or electronic equipment in use near the pacemaker. Internal sources of interference can include large P waves, large T-wave voltage, local myopotentials in the heart, or skeletal muscle potentials (see Figure 18-48B). Because a VVI pacemaker is programmed to inhibit its output when it senses, oversensing can be a dangerous situation in a pacemaker-dependent patient, resulting in ventricular asystole. Oversensing is usually due to the sensitivity control being set too high, which can be corrected by turning the sensitivity dial counterclockwise and reducing the pacemaker's sensitivity. It is recommended that the sensitivity control be set between the 1 and 3 o'clock positions on the dial (about 2 mV) rather than all the way to the right, unless a higher sensitivity is required to make the pacemaker sense QRS complexes.

Stimulation Threshold Testing

The stimulation threshold is the minimum output of the pacemaker necessary to capture the heart consistently. The stimulation threshold changes over time; when the pacing lead is first placed, the stimulation threshold is usually very low. Over time, the threshold increases and it takes more output to result in capture. When caring for a patient with a temporary pacemaker, stimulation threshold testing should be done every shift until a stable threshold is reached. Once the threshold has been determined, set the output 2 to 3 times higher than threshold to ensure an adequate safety margin for capture. To determine the stimulation threshold, follow these steps:

- Verify that the patient is in a paced rhythm. The pacing rate may need to be temporarily increased to override an intrinsic rhythm.
- Watch the monitor continuously while slowly decreasing output by turning the output control counterclockwise.
- Note when the pacing stimulus no longer captures the heart (a pacing spike not followed by a paced beat).
- Slowly increase the output until 1:1 capture resumes. This is the stimulation threshold.
- Set the output 2 to 3 times higher than threshold (ie, if threshold is 2 mA, set output between 4 and 6 mA).

DDD Pacemaker Evaluation

Dual-chamber pacemakers have become very complicated, with multiple programmable parameters and varying functions depending on the manufacturer. It is impossible to present dual-chamber pacemaker function in detail in a single chapter. To understand dual-chamber pacemaker function, it is necessary to understand the timing cycles involved in dual-chamber pacing. More detailed information on dual chamber pacemaker function is available in the references at the end of this chapter. In this section, the major timing cycles are defined and basic DDD pacemaker evaluation is covered in a very generic manner, because each pacemaker is different depending on the manufacturer. Dual-chamber pacemakers can function in a variety of modes (see Table 18-7). Because the DDD mode is most commonly used, basic DDD function is described here.

According to the pacemaker code, DDD means that both chambers (atria and ventricles) are paced, both chambers are sensed, and the mode of response to sensed events is either inhibited or triggered, depending on which chamber is sensed. When atrial activity is sensed, pacing is triggered in the ventricle after the programmed AV delay. When ventricular activity is sensed, all pacemaker output is inhibited.

The following timing cycles determine dual-chamber pacemaker function:

- *Pacing interval* (or lower rate limit): The base rate of the pacemaker, measured between two consecutive atrial pacing stimuli. The pacing interval is a programmed parameter.
- *AV delay* (or AV interval): The amount of time between atrial and ventricular pacing, or the "electronic PR interval." This is measured from the atrial pacing spike to the ventricular pacing spike and is a programmed parameter.
- *Atrial escape interval* (or VA interval): The interval from a sensed or paced ventricular event to the next atrial pacing output. The VA interval represents the amount of time the pacemaker waits after it paces in the ventricle or senses ventricular activity before pacing the atrium. The atrial escape interval is not a programmed parameter, but is derived by subtracting the AV delay from the pacing interval. Its length can be estimated by measuring from a ventricular spike to the next atrial pacing spike.
- *Total atrial refractory period* (TARP): The period of time following a sensed P wave or a paced atrial event during which the atrial channel will not respond to sensed events (ie, "has its eyes closed"). The TARP consists of the AV delay and the PVARP (see below).
- *Postventricular atrial refractory period* (PVARP): The period of time following an intrinsic QRS or a paced ventricular beat during which the atrial channel is refractory and will not respond to sensed atrial activity. PVARP is a programmable parameter but is not evident on a rhythm strip.
- *Blanking period:* The very short ventricular refractory period (VRP) that occurs with every atrial pacemaker output. The ventricular channel "blinks its eyes" so it does not sense the atrial output and inappropriately inhibits ventricular pacing. The blanking period is a programmable parameter but is not evident on a rhythm strip.

- *Ventricular refractory period*: The period of time following a paced ventricular beat or a sensed QRS during which the ventricular channel ignores intrinsic ventricular activity (ie, "has its eyes closed"). VRP is a programmable parameter but is not evident on a rhythm strip.
- *Maximum tracking interval* (or upper rate limit): The maximum rate at which the ventricular channel will track atrial activity. The upper rate limit prevents rapid ventricular pacing in response to very rapid atrial activity, such as atrial tachycardia or atrial flutter. The maximum tracking interval is a programmable parameter and usually is set according to how active a patient is expected to be and how fast a ventricular rate is likely to be tolerated.

Because a dual-chamber pacemaker has both atrial and ventricular pacing and sensing functions, evaluation includes assessing atrial capture, atrial sensing, ventricular capture, and ventricular sensing. To evaluate dual-chamber pacemaker function accurately, it is necessary to know the following information: mode of function (DDD, DVI, etc), minimum rate, upper rate limit, AV delay, PVARP, and VRPs. In the real world of bedside nursing, this information is not always available, so we do the best we can with what we have. The following sections briefly discuss the issues of assessing atrial and ventricular capture and sensing in a dual-chamber pacing system.

Atrial Capture

Atrial capture, unlike ventricular capture, is not always easy to see. Often, the atrial response to pacing is so small that it cannot be seen in many monitoring leads, so we cannot rely on the presence of a P wave following every atrial pacer spike as evidence of atrial capture. If a clear P wave is present after every atrial pacemaker spike, atrial capture can be assumed. In the absence of a clear P wave, atrial capture can only be assumed when an atrial pacer spike is followed by a normally conducted QRS complex within the programmed AV delay. If the atrial spike captures the atrium and there is intact AV conduction, the presence of the normal QRS indicates that the atrium must have been captured for conduction to have occurred into the ventricles before the ventricular pacing stimulus was delivered. Because a DDD pacemaker paces the ventricle at a preset AV interval following atrial pacing, the presence of a ventricular paced beat following an atrial paced beat does not verify capture, because the ventricle paces at the end of the AV delay whether atrial capture occurs or not. Therefore, atrial capture can only be assumed when there is an obvious P wave after every atrial pacing spike or when an atrial pacing spike is followed by a normal QRS within the programmed AV delay.

Atrial Sensing

Atrial sensing is verified by the presence of a spontaneous P wave that is followed by a paced ventricular beat at the end of the programmed AV delay. If a P wave is sensed, it starts

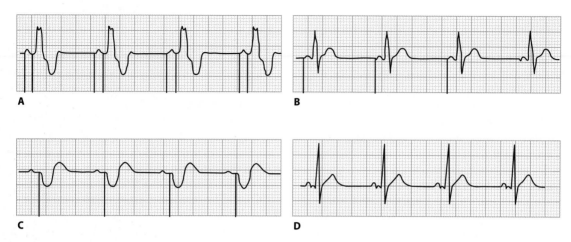

Figure 18-49. Four states of DDD pacing. **(A)** Atrial and ventricular pacing (AV sequential pacing state). **(B)** Atrial pacing, ventricular sensing. **(C)** Atrial sensing, ventricular pacing (atrial tracking state). **(D)** Atrial and ventricular sensing (inhibited pacing state).

the AV delay and ventricular pacing is triggered at the end of the AV delay unless AV conduction is intact and results in a normal QRS. The presence of a normal P wave followed by a normal QRS only proves that AV conduction is intact, not that the P wave was sensed by the pacemaker. Therefore, atrial sensing is verified by a spontaneous P wave followed by a paced QRS.

Ventricular Capture

Ventricular capture is recognized by a wide QRS immediately following a ventricular pacing spike. Ventricular capture is much easier to recognize than atrial capture and is no different than with single-chamber ventricular pacing.

Ventricular Sensing

Ventricular sensing can only be verified if there is spontaneous ventricular activity present for the pacemaker to sense. Ventricular sensing is verified by an atrial pacer spike followed by a normal QRS that inhibits the ventricular pacing spike, which is the same event that proves atrial capture. If a QRS is sensed before the next atrial pacing spike is due, both the atrial and ventricular pacing stimuli are inhibited and the VA interval (atrial escape interval) is reset.

Dual-chamber pacemakers are capable of operating in four states of pacing: atrial and ventricular pacing, atrial pacing with ventricular sensing, atrial sensing with ventricular pacing, and atrial and ventricular sensing. All four states of pacing can occur within a short period of time, and the timing cycles determine which state of pacing is done. Figure 18-49 shows the four states of dual-chamber pacing, and Figure 18-50 illustrates the basic principles of dual-chamber pacemaker evaluation.

Cardiac Resynchronization Therapy (CRT) With Biventricular Pacing

Patients with chronic HF often have intraventricular conduction delays (especially LBBB) that result in ventricular dyssynchrony and impair cardiac function. This intraventricular conduction delay causes electrical and mechanical abnormalities in ventricular function that interfere with ventricular filling, impair cardiac output, worsen mitral regurgitation, and contribute to mortality in patients with HF. LBBB causes both electrical and mechanical abnormalities that result in ventricular dyssynchrony. Interventricular dyssynchrony refers to the time delay between right and left ventricular contraction, where the RV depolarizes and contracts before the LV. Intraventricular dyssynchrony refers to the abnormal segmental contraction within the LV as it depolarizes late and abnormally in LBBB.

When the RV contracts before the LV, the septum depolarizes and contracts with the RV instead of with the LV. Since the septum normally contributes to LV ejection by

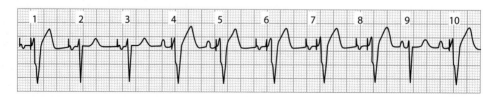

Figure 18-50. DDD pacemaker operating in all four states of pacing. Beats 1, 6, 7, and 8 illustrate AV sequential pacing (A pace and V pace); beats 2 and 3 illustrate atrial pacing and ventricular sensing; beats 4, 5, and 10 illustrate atrial sensing and ventricular pacing; beat 9 is an intrinsic beat with normal P wave and normal conduction to the ventricle. Atrial capture is proven evident in beats 1, 2, 3, 6, 7, and 8; atrial sensing is verified by beats 4, 5, and 10; ventricular capture is evident in beats 1, 4, 5, 6, 7, 8, and 10; ventricular sensing is verified by beats 2, 3, and 9.

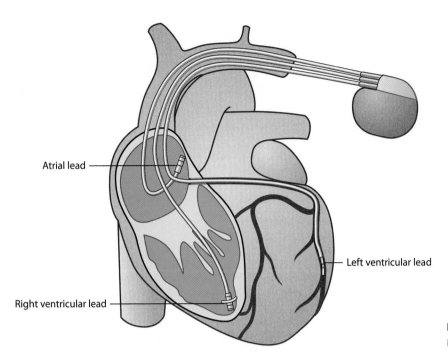

Figure 18-51. Lead placement for biventricular pacing.

contracting with the LV, normal septal function is lost in LBBB. Since the septum contracts with the RV, it is relaxed by the time the LV begins contracting, and increasing pressure in the LV causes paradoxical septal motion by pushing the septum into the RV. In LBBB the papillary muscles that are responsible for holding the mitral valve leaflets tight depolarize late and fail to keep valve leaflets from everting into the atria during LV systole, resulting in mitral regurgitation. The combination of paradoxical septal wall motion and mitral regurgitation contribute to the already reduced LV stroke volume that occurs in HF. Portions of the LV that are activated first contract before those portions that are activated late, creating mechanical dyssynchrony that reduces systolic function by about 20%, reduces stroke volume, increases wall stress, and delays relaxation.

Cardiac resynchronization therapy (CRT) is biventricular pacing aimed at improving electromechanical activity in the failing heart. The goals of CRT are to improve hemodynamics by restoring ventricular synchrony, and improve quality of life via symptom relief. CRT devices can be stand-alone pacemakers or combination ICD and biventricular pacemakers (CRT-D). Class I recommendations for CRT include patients with the following characteristics: heart failure with NYHA class II, III, or ambulatory IV symptoms; left ventricular ejection fraction < 35%; presence of significant intraventricular conduction delay (QRS duration > 150 msec); sinus rhythm; symptomatic in spite of optimal goal directed medical therapy for heart failure. Class IIa indications include patients with LVEF < 35% and NYHA class II, III, or ambulatory IV symptoms with QRS duration between 120 and 149 msec; those with non-LBBB pattern wide QRS of > 150 msec; those with atrial fibrillation who are likely to be near 100% ventricular paced; and those undergoing new

or replacement device implantation with anticipated requirement for > 40% ventricular pacing.

Cardiac resynchronization therapy is accomplished by placing standard pacing leads in the right atrium and into the right ventricular apex as is done for normal dual chamber pacing. A third lead is advanced through the coronary sinus and into a lateral or posterior left ventricular vein for pacing of the LV (Figure 18-51).

The goal in biventricular pacing is to cause both ventricles to depolarize and contract simultaneously, thus eliminating the interventricular and intraventricular dyssynchrony that occurs during LBBB. The AV interval is often programmed shorter than intrinsic AV conduction in order to force the ventricles to pace rather than allowing intrinsic conduction to occur. Biventricular pacing causes both ventricles to contract simultaneously and allows the septum to contract with the LV. Controlling the AV delay restores the normal timing between left atrial and left ventricular contraction, allowing the LV papillary muscles to contract earlier and put tension on the mitral valve leaflets to reduce or prevent mitral regurgitation. Biventricular pacing allows the LV to complete contraction and begin relaxation earlier, which increases filling time and improves "atrial kick."

Electrocardiographic evaluation of biventricular pacemaker function is more complicated than single ventricle pacing from the right ventricular apex. Pacing from the RV apex creates a LBBB pattern with a wide negative QRS complex in lead V1. Left ventricular pacing is more complicated due to the fact that the LV lead can be placed in either a lateral or posterior LV vein and can be located in an apical or a basal site within the vein. The resulting QRS varies in morphology, depending on the location of

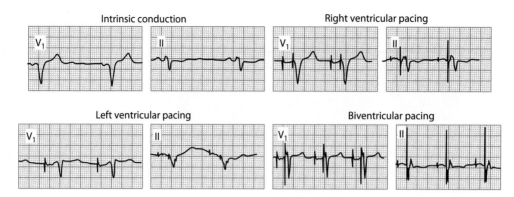

Figure 18-52. ECG in biventricular pacing.

the LV lead, but, in general, LV pacing produces a RBBB pattern with a wide upright QRS complex in lead V1. It makes logical sense that pacing both ventricles simultaneously would result in a narrow QRS complex preceded by a pacemaker spike, but this narrowing is not always obvious with biventricular pacing. Loss of capture in one or the other ventricle should cause a change in the morphology of the paced QRS that would indicate single chamber pacing from the ventricle that is still being captured. A shift in the frontal plane axis may also occur with loss of capture in one ventricle.

Some experts recommend recording four 12-lead ECGs at the time of implant: during intrinsic conduction, in the course of RV pacing with capture, in LV pacing with capture, and during biventricular pacing with capture in both ventricles. These ECGs should be examined to determine which lead best demonstrates an obvious difference between the four pacing states recorded, then the best lead should be used as the monitoring lead for pacemaker evaluation. Figure 18-52 shows leads V1 and II recorded during intrinsic conduction, RV pacing, LV pacing, and bi-ventricular pacing. Note the similarity between the intrinsic QRS with LBBB and the RV paced QRS which produces an "iatrogenic" LBBB pattern. The ventricular pacing spike is not visible in lead V1 in the course of LV pacing, and the QRS is negative during LV pacing in this patient as opposed to the more common upright QRS during LV pacing. The QRS during Bi-V pacing is narrower than the intrinsic beats and the single chamber paced beats. Lead V1 would be a good monitoring lead for this patient due to the differences in QRS morphology among these four examples.

SELECTED BIBLIOGRAPHY

Abraham WT, Fisher WG, Smith AL, et al. Cardiac resynchronization in chronic heart failure. *N Eng J Med.* 2002;346(24): 1845-1853.

Antzelevitch C, Brugada P, Borggrefe M. Brugada syndrome: report of the Second Consensus Conference. *Circulation.* 2005;111: 659-670.

Antzelevitch C, Nof E. Brugada syndrome: recent advances and controversies. *Curr Cardiol Rep.* 2008;10(5):376-383.

Barold SS, Herweg B, Giudici M. Electrocardiographic follow-up of biventricular pacemakers. *Ann Noninvasive Electrocardiol.* 2005;10(2):231-255.

Brenyo AJ, Huang DT, Aktas MK. Congenital long and short QT syndromes. *Cardiology.* 2012;122:237-247.

Castellanos A, Interian I, Myerburg RJ. The resting electrocardiogram. In: V Fuster, RAO' Rourke, RA Walsh, P Poole-Wilson (eds.), *Hurst's The Heart* (12th ed). New York, NY: McGraw-Hill, 2008.

Elizari M, Acunzo RS, Ferreiro M. Hemiblocks revisited. *Circulation.* 2006;115:1154-1163.

Fowler SJ, Priori SG. Clinical spectrum of patients with a Brugada ECG. *Curr Opin Cardiol.* 2008;24:74-81.

Goldberger AL. Clinical electrocardiography: a simplified approach. Philadelphia, PA: Mosby Elsevier, 2006.

Haji SA, Movahed A. Right ventricular infarction–diagnosis and treatment. *Clin Cardiol.* 2000;23:473-482.

Jacobson C, Marzlin K, Webner C. Cardiovascular Nursing Practice: a comprehensive resource manual and study guide for clinical nurses. Burien, WA: Cardiovascular Nursing Education Associates, 2007.

Kenny T. *The Nuts and Bolts of Cardiac Pacing.* Malden, MA: Blackwell Futura, 2005.

Leclercq C, Kass DA. Retiming the failing heart: principles and current clinical status of cardiac resynchronization. *J Am Coll Cardiol.* 2002;39:194-201.

Mirvis DM, Goldberger AL. Electrocardiography. In: RO Bonow, DL Mann, DP Zipes, P Libby, eds., *Braunwald's Heart Disease—A Textbook of Cardiovascular Medicine.* 9th ed. pp. 126-167. Philadelphia, PA: Elsevier. 2011.

Pugazhendhi V, Ellenbogen KA. Bradyarrhythmias and pacemakers. In: V Fuster, RA Walsh, RA Harrington, eds., *Hurst's The Heart.* 13th ed. pp. 1025-1057. New York, NY: McGraw Hill, 2011.

Seslar SP, Zimetbaum PJ, Berul CI, Josephson ME. (2012). Diagnosis of congenital long QT syndrome. In: DS Basow, ed., Uptodate. Waltham, MA: Uptodate.

Sgarbossa EB, Pinski SL, Barbagelata A, et al. Electrocardiographic diagnosis of evolving acute myocardial infarction in the presence of left bundle-branch block. *N Engl J Med.* 1996;334:481-487.

Wilde AM, Antzelevitch C, Borggrefe M. Proposed diagnostic criteria for the Brugada syndrome. *Circulation.* 2002;106: 2514-2519.

Evidence Based Practice

AACN Practice Alert: ST Segment Monitoring. American Association of Critical Care Nurses. 2009. http://www.aacn.org/WD/Practice/Docs/PracticeAlerts/ ST_Segment_Monitoring_05-2009.pdf.

Drew BJ, Ackerman MJ, Funk M. Prevention of Torsade de Pointes in hospital settings. *J Am Coll Cardiol.* 2010;55:934-947.

Drew BJ, Califf RM, Funk M. Practice standards for electrocardiographic monitoring in hospital settings. *Circulation,* 2004;110:2721-2746.

Epstein AE, DiMarco JP, Ellenbogen KA. ACC/AHA/HRS 2008 guidelines for device-based therapy of cardiac rhythm abnormalities: a report of the American College of Cardiology/American Heart Association Task Force on Practice Guidelines. *Circulation.* 2008;117:e350-e408.

Hancock EW, Deal BJ, Mirvis DM. AHA/ACCF/HRS recommendations for the standardization and interpretation of the electrocardiogram part V: electrocardiogram changes associated with cardiac chamber hypertrophy. A scientific statement from the American Heart Association Electrocardiography and Arrhythmias Committee, Council on Clinical Cardiology; the American College of Cardiology Foundation; and the Heart Rhythm Society. *Circulation.* 2009;119:e251-e261.

Jacobson C. Bedside cardiac monitoring. In: Burns S, ed. *AACN Protocols for Practice: Noninvasive Monitoring.* 2nd ed. Boston: Jones and Bartlett; 2006.

Rautaharju PM, Surawicz B, Gettes LS. AHA/ACCF/HRS recommendations for the standardization and interpretation of the electrocardiogram part IV: the ST segment, T and U waves, and the QT interval. A scientific statement from the American Heart Association Electrocardiography and Arrhythmias Committee, Council on Clinical Cardiology; the American College of Cardiology Foundation; and the Heart Rhythm Society. *Circulation.* 2009;119:e241-e250.

Surawicz B, Childers R, Deal BJ, Gettes LS. AHA/ACCF/HRS recommendations for the standardization and interpretation of the electrocardiogram part III: intraventricular conduction disturbances: a scientific statement from the American Heart Association Electrocardiography and Arrhythmias Committee, Council on Clinical Cardiology; the American College of Cardiology Foundation; and the Heart Rhythm Society. *Circulation.* 2009;119:e235-e240.

Tracy CM, Epstein AE, Darbar D. 2012 ACCF/AHA/HRS focused update of the 2008 guidelines for device-based therapy of cardiac rhythm abnormalities: a report of the American College of Cardiology Foundation/American Heart Association Task Force on Practice Guidelines. *Circulation.* 2012;126:1784-1800.

Wagner GS, Macfarlane P, Wellens H, et al. AHA/ACCF/HRS recommendations for the standardization and interpretation of the electrocardiogram: part VI: acute ischemia/infarction: a scientific statement from the American Heart Association Electrocardiography and Arrhythmias Committee, Council on Clinical Cardiology; the American College of Cardiology Foundation; and the Heart Rhythm Society. *Circulation.* 2009;119:e262-e270.

ADVANCED CARDIOVASCULAR CONCEPTS

Barbara Leeper

KNOWLEDGE COMPETENCIES

1. Describe the etiology, pathophysiology, clinical presentation, patient needs, and principles of management of:
   - Cardiomyopathy
   - Valvular disease
   - Pericarditis
   - Aortic aneurysm
   - Cardiac transplantation

2. Compare and contrast the pathophysiology, clinical presentation, patient needs, and management approaches of:

   - Cardiomyopathy
   - Valvular disease
   - Pericarditis
   - Aortic aneurysm
   - Cardiac transplantation

3. Identify indications for, complications of, and nursing management of patients receiving intra-aortic balloon pump and ventricular assist device therapy.

PATHOLOGIC CONDITIONS

Cardiomyopathy

Cardiomyopathy is a disease involving destruction of the cardiac muscle fibers, causing impairment of myocardial function and decreased cardiac output (CO). The body responds to this with initiation of several neuroendocrine responses including activation of the sympathetic nervous system and renin-angiotensin-aldosterone chain. The prevailing result is marked vasoconstriction, retention of sodium and water, and further myocyte injury. This process contributes to remodeling of ventricular myocytes and the downward spiral of cardiomyopathy. The cause of cardiomyopathy is often unknown. Cardiomyopathies are commonly classified into three types: dilated, hypertrophic, and restrictive (Figure 19-1).

Dilated cardiomyopathy, the most common type of cardiomyopathy, is commonly caused by coronary artery disease and is associated with impaired myocardial contractility and increased ventricular filling pressures. Coronary artery disease contributes to ventricular remodeling thereby reducing

ejection fraction. The two case studies presented later in this chapter involve patients with dilated cardiomyopathy. Hypertrophic cardiomyopathy may occur in both the young and the elderly. Hypertrophic cardiomyopathy is often categorized as obstructive or nonobstructive. Ventricular hypertrophy occurs in both types. The diagnosis of obstructive hypertrophic cardiomyopathy is made if hypertrophy of the intraventricular septum is also present. This is the congenital form and is often referred to as hypertrophic obstructive cardiomyopathy (HOCM). In the past other terms used to describe this type of cardiomyopathy were idiopathic hypertrophic subaortic stenosis (IHSS), and asymetric septal hypertrophy (ASH). The hypertrophied septum obstructs left ventricular outflow tract just below the aortic valve, thereby limiting ejection. Blood volume is "trapped" within the left ventricular chamber.

Restrictive cardiomyopathy is the least common of the three types. A classic finding for this type of cardiomyopathy is ventricular fibrosis caused by infiltration of the cardiac myocytes with abnormal cells such as sarcoid or amyloid disease.

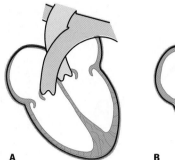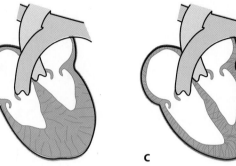

Figure 19-1. Types of cardiomyopathies. **(A)** Dilated (cardiac dilatation and impaired contractility). **(B)** Hypertrophic (decreased size of ventricular chambers and increased ventricular muscle mass). **(C)** Restrictive (decreased ventricular compliance).

The fibrotic muscle tissue becomes very rigid with decreased compliance, thus limiting distention during diastole.

Etiology and Pathophysiology

A variety of conditions may cause or contribute to the development of cardiomyopathy (Table 19-1). As noted previously,

TABLE 19-1. ETIOLOGY OF CARDIOMYOPATHY

Dilated Cardiomyopathy
- Idiopathic
- Toxins, such as lead, alcohol, cocaine
- Muscle dystrophy
- Myotonic dystrophy
- Hypophosphatemia
- Hypocalcemia
- Hypokalemia
- Viral, bacterial, or fungal infections
- Lupus erythematosus
- Peripartum or postpartum status
- Rheumatoid disease
- Scleroderma
- Hypertension
- Thiamine deficiency
- Microvascular spasm

Hypertrophic Cardiomyopathy
- Idiopathic
- Genetic transmission
- Friedreich ataxia
- Hypoparathyroidism
- Amyloidosis

Restrictive Cardiomyopathy
- Idiopathic
- Myocardial fibrosis
- Infiltration
- Hypertrophy
- Amyloidosis
- Hemochromatosis
- Glycogen deposition
- Scleroderma

coronary artery disease is the most common cause of dilated cardiomyopathy in the United States.

Pathophysiology of Dilated Cardiomyopathy

Dilated cardiomyopathy begins with gradual destruction of the myocardial fibers impairing myocardial contraction. As the disease progresses, left ventricular dilatation occurs with increased blood volume in the left ventricle at the end of diastole. Additionally, ventricular compliance is reduced, which contributes to an increase in filling pressures (ie, left ventricular end diastolic pressure) and a decrease in CO. Left atrial volume and pressure eventually increase as the atrium struggles to overcome the higher LVEDP and eject blood into the left ventricle. The increased left atrial pressure often leads to an increased pulmonary capillary pressure as the higher filling pressures are reflected back into the pulmonary vascular bed. Right ventricular failure will eventually occur as the right ventricle has a limited capacity to increase its force of contraction against the higher pressures in the pulmonary vascular bed. Eventually, the right ventricle will dilate along with the left ventricle. In addition the atrioventricular valves (mitral and tricuspid) may develop insufficiency due to the dilated chambers stretching the papillary muscle and interfering with the closure of the valves.

Pathophysiology of Hypertrophic Cardiomyopathy

Patients with hypertrophic cardiomyopathy have a greatly thickened ventricular wall (see Figure 19-1). It is not uncommon for the ventricular chamber size to be dramatically reduced due to hypertrophy. In obstructive cardiomyopathy, the intraventricular septum is also involved in the hypertrophic process, whereas in nonobstructive cardiomyopathy the septum is relatively normal. Common causes of the nonobstructive form include aortic stenosis and hypertension. The hypertrophied ventricle becomes rigid, causing a reduced ventricular compliance and distensibility. Myocardial contractility becomes impaired, resulting in a decreased stroke volume and CO.

If HOCM is present, left ventricular systolic ejection will be further compromised by obstruction of the outflow tract as the anterior leaflet of the mitral valve presses against an enlarged intraventricular septum.

ESSENTIAL CONTENT CASE

Cardiomyopathy

A 56-year-old man was admitted to the emergency room with shortness of breath. His chest x-ray revealed an enlarged heart and pulmonary congestion. His 12-lead ECG was consistent with left ventricular hypertrophy and his rhythm was AF with a ventricular rate of 102. Clinical findings included bilateral crackles auscultated one-third up from the bases, bilateral lower extremity, +41 pitting edema to the midcalf, JVD, an S_3, and a systolic murmur heard best at the apex. An emergency echocardiogram showed impaired contractility of a dilated left ventricle.

Case Question 1. After the patient is admitted to your unit and your assessment concurs with the findings in the ED, you anticipate the initial priority for the medical management of this gentleman will be:

(A) Initiate inotropic support
(B) Obtain electrophysiology consult for a biventricular pacemaker workup
(C) Administer a diuretic to reduce fluid overload
(D) Administer carvedilol to control the ventricular rate

Case Question 2. When auscultating his heart sounds you know the most likely cause of his systolic murmur is:

(A) Aortic stenosis
(B) Mitral insufficiency
(C) Tricuspid stenosis
(D) Pulmonic insufficiency

Answers: 1. C; 1. B

ESSENTIAL CONTENT CASE

Cardiomyopathy

A 32-year-old woman was admitted to the progressive care unit at 31 weeks' gestation with dyspnea and fatigue. She had bilateral, basilar crackles, and her oxygen saturation via pulse oximetry was 88%. An echocardiogram showed a markedly dilated left ventricle with diffuse hypokinesis and an ejection fraction of 20% to 25%.

A pulmonary artery catheter was placed and the following parameters obtained:

RA	12 mm Hg
PA	48/26 mm Hg
PAOP	24 mm Hg
CO	3.7 L/min
CI	1.8 L/min/m^2

A dobutamine infusion was initiated at 5 mcg/kg/min and oxygen was applied at 6 L/min via nasal cannula.

Case Question 1. The most likely medical diagnosis for this patient is:

(A) HOCM
(B) Restrictive cardiomyopathy
(C) Peripartum cardiomyopathy
(D) Idiopathic cardiomyopathy

Case Question 2. Her hemodynamic profile indicates a low CI with possible volume overload as evidenced by:

(A) PA pressure 48/26 mm Hg
(B) Elevated RAP (12 mm Hg) and PAOP (24 mm Hg)
(C) EF 20%-25%
(D) Spo$_2$ 88%

Case Question 3. Your plan of care for this patient includes which of the following:

(A) Improve oxygen delivery to the tissues
(B) Increase myocardial contractility
(C) Careful management of preload as blood volume is normally 1.5 times higher during pregnancy
(D) Education about self-management of heart failure and coping strategies
(E) All of the above

Answers: 1. C; 2. B; 3. E

Stress is placed on the left atrium as it attempts to propel blood forward into the stiff left ventricle. It is not uncommon for left atrial enlargement to develop as the left atrium is forced to contract against high left ventricular resistance.

Pathophysiology of Restrictive Cardiomyopathy

The ventricles of patients with restrictive cardiomyopathy become rigid as fibrotic tissue infiltrates the myocardium. The stiffness of the ventricles decreases the compliance, or distensibility, of the ventricles, thus limiting ventricular filling and increasing end-diastolic pressures. Myocardial contractility is impaired, leading to decreases in CO. As with the other types of cardiomyopathy, atrial workload is increased as the atria attempt to propel blood forward into stiff ventricles. It is common for the atrioventricular valves to become insufficient and for the pressures in the pulmonary vascular bed and peripheral venous bed to increase, leading to the development of edema.

Clinical Presentation

Patients may be asymptomatic for lengthy periods of time (months to years) prior to being diagnosed with a cardiomyopathy. By the time patients develop symptoms myocardial contractility may be significantly impaired. The heart rate increases initially as the heart attempts to maintain an

adequate CO. As the disease progresses and/or during physical exertion, the impaired myocardium is no longer able to maintain an adequate CO to meet the metabolic demands of the tissues in spite of the increased heart rate.

Dilated Cardiomyopathy

1. Inability to maintain adequate CO:
   - Fatigue
   - Weakness
   - Sinus tachycardia
   - Pulses alternans
   - Narrowed pulse pressure
   - Decreased CO

2. Increased left ventricular filling pressures (LVEDP)
   - Dyspnea
   - Orthopnea
   - Paroxysmal nocturnal dyspnea
   - Crackles
   - S_3/S_4
   - Arrhythmias (atrial fibrillation, ventricular tachycardia or fibrillation)
   - Systolic murmur associated with mitral valve insufficiency
   - Abnormal hemodynamic profile:
     - Increased pulmonary artery systolic (PAS) and pulmonary artery diastolic (PAD) pressures
     - Elevated pulmonary artery occlusion pressure (PAOP)
     - Increased systemic vascular resistance (SVR)
     - Elevated V wave on PAOP waveform with mitral valve insufficiency
3. Increased right ventricular filling pressures:
   - Peripheral edema
   - Jugular vein distention (JVD)
   - Hepatomegaly
   - Elevated V wave on the right atrial (RA) waveform and systolic murmur associated with tricuspid valve insufficiency
4. Increased atrial pressures:
   - Palpitations
   - S_4 may develop as the atria attempt to eject blood into stiff ventricles.
   - Atrial arrhythmias may occur, such as premature atrial complexes (PACs) or atrial fibrillation (AF), due to increased atrial pressure
   - Elevated A wave on PAOP waveform
   - Elevated RA pressures
   - Elevated A wave on the RA waveform

Hypertrophic Cardiomyopathy

1. Inability to maintain adequate CO:
   - Angina
   - Syncope
   - Fatigue
   - Sinus tachycardia
   - Ventricular fibrillation
   - CO is initially normal, then decreases
2. Increased ventricular filling pressures:
   - Dyspnea
   - Orthopnea
   - Arrhythmias, such as premature ventricular contractions or ventricular tachycardia
   - Abnormal hemodynamic profile:
     – Elevated PAS and PAD pressures
     – Elevated PAOP pressure
     – Increased SVR
3. Increased atrial pressure:
   - S_4 may develop as the atria attempt to eject blood into rigid ventricles.

- Atrial arrhythmias may occur (eg, PAC, AF) due to the increased atrial pressure.
- Palpitations.
- Elevated A wave on PAOP waveform.
- Elevated RA pressure.
4. Left outflow tract obstruction:
   - Systolic murmur as blood flows through a narrowed outflow tract due to septal hypertrophy; heard at apex

Restrictive Cardiomyopathy

Signs and symptoms of restrictive cardiomyopathy and pericarditis are similar. Diagnosis can usually be made after an echocardiogram.

1. Inability to maintain adequate CO:
   - Activity intolerance
   - Weakness
   - Sinus tachycardia
   - Arrhythmias
   - Decreased CO/cardiac index (CI)
2. Increased left ventricular filling pressures:
   - Dyspnea
   - JVD
   - S_3
   - Narrowed pulse pressure
   - Systolic murmur with mitral valve insufficiency
   - Abnormal hemodynamic profile:
     - Elevated PAS, PAD, and PAOP pressures
     - Elevated SVR
     - Elevated V wave on PAOP waveform with mitral valve insufficiency
3. Increased right ventricular pressures:
   - Peripheral edema
   - Hepatomegaly
   - Jaundice
   - JVD
   - Systolic murmur with tricuspid valve insufficiency
   - Kussmaul sign (increased neck vein distention with inspiration)
   - Elevated V wave on the RA waveform if tricuspid valve insufficient
4. Increased atrial pressures:
   - Palpitations.
   - S_4 may develop as the atria attempt to eject blood into rigid ventricles.
   - Atrial arrhythmias may occur (eg, PACs, AF) due to the increase in atrial pressure.
   - Elevated A wave on PAOP waveform.
   - Elevated RA pressure.
   - Elevated A wave on the RA waveform.

Diagnostic Tests

Dilated Cardiomyopathy

- *Chest x-ray:* Left ventricular dilation with potential enlargement and dilatation of all four cardiac chambers

- *12-lead ECG:* ST-segment and T-wave changes; left axis deviation; left ventricular hypertrophy and bundle branch block (left bundle branch block most common)
- *Echocardiography:* Dilated left ventricle with an increase in chamber size (other chambers may be enlarged also); diminished ventricular contractility; decreased septal wall movement; elevated ventricular volumes and decreased ejection fraction

Hypertrophic Cardiomyopathy

- *Chest x-ray:* Normal or left atrial and ventricular hypertrophy
- *12-lead ECG:* ST-segment and T-wave changes; septal Q waves due to septal hypertrophy; left ventricular hypertrophy
- *Echocardiography:* Thickened ventricular walls with a decrease in chamber size; left ventricular outflow obstruction created by thickened ventricular septum and motion of mitral valve leaflet

Restrictive Cardiomyopathy

- *Chest x-ray:* Normal or slight enlargement of left atria and ventricle
- *12-lead ECG:* ST-segment and T-wave changes; low QRS amplitude
- *Echocardiography:* Thickened ventricular walls; enlarged atria; diminished ventricular contractility; decreased ventricular volumes; elevated ventricular end-diastolic pressures

Principles of Management of Cardiomyopathy

The primary objectives in the management of cardiomyopathy are to treat the underlying cause (if known); maximize cardiac function; assist the patient and family members to cope with a debilitating, chronic disease; and prevent complications associated with cardiomyopathy.

Improvement of Cardiac Function

Dilated Cardiomyopathy

1. Improve myocardial oxygenation: As ventricular dilatation occurs, ventricular wall tension increases, increasing the myocardial workload and oxygen consumption. Oxygen therapy should be initiated as necessary to increase oxygenation delivery. Pulse oximetry, mixed venous oxygenation saturation (Svo_2), and arterial blood gases are helpful in guiding sufficient oxygen therapy. If the patient has an Svo_2 catheter or PA catheter, monitoring the Svo_2 is also a very accurate means of assessing oxygenation status.
2. Increase myocardial contractility: Inotropic agents including β1 receptor stimulating agents (eg, dobutamine) and phosphodiesterase inhibitors (eg, milrinone) produce a positive inotropic effect (eg, strengthen myocardial contractility) and cause mild vasodilation, thereby reducing the workload of the failing ventricle.

3. Decrease preload and afterload: Diuretics decrease excess fluid and ventricular end-diastolic volumes; fluid and sodium restrictions also may be necessary. Vasodilators (eg, isosorbide dinitrate, hydralazine) dilate arterial and venous vessels, decreasing venous return and resistance to ventricular systolic ejection (afterload).
4. Administer beta blockers (eg, metoprolol, carvedilol) to reduce risk/prevent sudden cardiac death (VF, VT), as well as prevent further deterioration of the myocytes.
5. Administer ACE inhibitors or ARBs to block the negative effects of angiotensin II on the cardiac cells, as well as reduce ventricular afterload.
6. Mechanical cardiac assist devices (eg, intra-aortic balloon therapy, ventricular assist device [VAD] therapy), and in some critical situations extracorporeal membrane oxygenation (ECMO), may be instituted to assist with improving CO/CI and oxygen delivery to the tissues.
7. Dual-chamber biventricular pacemaker/implantable cardioverter defibrillator: Refer to Chapter 9, Cardiovascular System (section Improvement of Left Ventricular Function).
8. Ventricular reconstruction procedure: This is a surgical procedure focusing on removal of a ventricular aneurysm and scar tissue on the left ventricle, usually a result of a myocardial infarction (MI). The left ventricle is returned to its normal shape and is able to contract more efficiently.
9. Cardiac transplantation may be necessary if medical therapy does not relieve patient symptoms.

Hypertrophic Cardiomyopathy

The management of the patient with hypertrophic cardiomyopathy focuses on promoting myocardial relaxation and decreasing left ventricular obstruction.

1. *Decrease myocardial contractility:* Use beta-blockers to decrease heart rate, contractility, and myocardial oxygen consumption.
2. *The following medications are usually contraindicated in patients with hypertrophic cardiomyopathy:*
   - Diuretics, because a decrease in fluid volume decreases ventricle filling pressures and CO.
   - Inotropes (eg, dobutamine, milrinone), because an increase in contractility contributes to an increase in the left ventricular outflow obstruction.
   - Vasodilators (eg, nitroglycerin, nitroprusside), because they decrease end-diastolic volume, leading to an increase in left ventricular outflow obstruction.
3. *Reduce physical and psychological stress:* Patients with hypertrophic cardiomyopathy are at an increased risk for sudden cardiac death, which may occur during stressful periods. It is important that strenuous physical activity be limited. In addition, sudden

changes in position should be avoided, because the heart cannot respond to fluid shifts created by sudden position changes. Valsalva maneuver should also be avoided. Psychological stress should also be decreased. Teach patients strategies to enhance self-relaxation. Relaxation therapy may include rhythmic breathing, biofeedback, and imagery.

4. *Cardiac surgery:* Myectomy may be indicated for individuals who do not respond to medical management and have severe left ventricular outflow obstruction. Myectomy involves removal of a portion of the enlarged intraventricular septum in an attempt to decrease left ventricular outflow obstruction and improve myocardial functioning.

5. *Ethanol ablation:* In recent years, a new therapy for HOCM has emerged. Absolute alcohol (98% ethanol) is instilled into selected septal perforator branches of the left anterior descending coronary artery, resulting in a therapeutic MI. The resultant outcome is reduction of left ventricular outflow obstruction and improved CO. The procedure is performed in the cardiac catheterization laboratory by the interventional cardiologists. It has been found to be associated with less risk than myectomy because it is less invasive. Long-term outcomes of this procedure have yet to be determined.

Restrictive Cardiomyopathy

Decrease preload: Diuretics, sodium and fluid restrictions, and vasodilators decrease ventricular end-diastolic volumes. The rigid ventricle is very sensitive to small fluid changes, significantly increasing ventricular end-diastolic pressure.

Facilitate Coping

For most patients, cardiomyopathy is a chronic, potentially life-threatening disease. Patients and their families often face an uncertain long-term prognosis. Emotions may vacillate as the family struggles to cope with the implications of the disease and its effect on lifestyle. Emphasis is placed on assisting the patient to remain active and to cope with a progressive disease. Involvement of the family unit in symptom management is also important. Relaxation therapy can benefit not only the patient, but also the family. It is important to discuss end-of-life issues as well as discuss options for palliative and/or hospice care for symptom management when it is apparent the patient is declining and all other medical options have either been tried or deemed not appropriate.

Preventing and Managing Complications

1. *Arrhythmias:* Continuous electrocardiogram (ECG) monitoring; observe for potential side effects of cardiac medications; encourage family to learn cardiopulmonary resuscitation (CPR).

2. *Hemodynamic instability* may require that the patient be managed in an ICU for invasive monitoring with insertion of a pulmonary artery catheter. The patient will be managed based on trends in hemodynamic parameters (ie, RA, PAS, PAD, and PAOP pressures; CO; CI; SVR; and PVR).

3. *Thromboembolic event:* Anticoagulation is necessary for patients with severely compromised left ventricular function and for patients experiencing AF. In both circumstances, thrombi may develop due to increased fluid volume and stasis.

4. *Endocarditis:* Antibiotic prophylaxis is recommended for patients with valve involvement. Prophylaxis should be given prior to dental work, surgery, or other invasive procedures.

Valvular Heart Disease

Heart valvular disorders result from both congenital and acquired causes. Valves on the left side of the heart are more commonly affected because they are constantly exposed to higher pressures. Normally, when a valve opens, there are no pressure gradients between the chambers or vessels above and below the valve. As the heart valve disease progresses, pressure gradients between the two structures develop.

Heart valvular disorders are commonly classified as valve stenosis or valve insufficiency. A stenotic valve has a narrowed opening, ie, it does not open fully thereby reducing the amount of blood flowing through it. An insufficient valve does not close properly, thus permitting some blood to flow backward instead of forward. Heart valve insufficiency is also referred to as valvular regurgitation. Valvular dysfunction may affect one or more valves.

The development of valvular heart disease is usually a gradual process. As the case study below illustrates, the patient's valvular problems began with a bacterial endocarditis 15 years prior to the onset of her symptoms of mitral valve insufficiency.

Etiology and Pathophysiology

Heart valve disorders are caused by either congenital or acquired diseases (Table 19-2). Congenital valve disorders may affect any of the four valves causing stenosis or insufficiency. An example of a congenital valve disorder is an aortic valve with only two, instead of three, cusps. The bicuspid valve is associated with an increase in turbulence as blood flows through the narrowed orifice. The individual may become asymptomatic later in life when fibrotic tissue and calcium deposits form on the abnormal valve, leading to stenosis. This is often referred to as "senile aortic stenosis."

There are three types of acquired valve disorders: degenerative disease, rheumatic disease, or infective endocarditis. Degenerative disease may occur as the valve is damaged over time due to constant mechanical stress. This may occur with aging, or may be aggravated by conditions such as hypertension. Hypertension places significant pressure on the aortic valve, often causing insufficiency.

TABLE 19-2. ETIOLOGY OF VALVULAR DISORDERS

Mitral Stenosis
- Rheumatic disease
- Endocarditis
- Degenerative process

Mitral Insufficiency
- Rheumatic disease
- Congenital disorder
- Endocarditis
- Mitral valve prolapsed
- Papillary muscle dysfunction
- Chordae tendineae dysfunction

Aortic Stenosis
- Rheumatic disease
- Congenital disorder
- Degenerative process

Aortic Insufficiency
- Rheumatic disease
- Congenital disorder
- Hypertension
- Endocarditis
- Marfan syndrome

Tricuspid Stenosis
- Rheumatic disease
- Congenital disorder
- Endocarditis

Tricuspid Insufficiency
- Rheumatic disease
- Marfan syndrome
- Endocarditis
- Ebstein anomaly
- Congenital disorder
- Secondary to left-sided valve disease
- IV drug use

Pulmonic Stenosis
- Rheumatic disease
- Congenital disorder
- Endocarditis

Pulmonic Insufficiency
- Primary pulmonary artery hypertension
- Secondary to left-sided valve disease
- Marfan syndrome
- Endocarditis

Individuals who develop rheumatic fever often experience valvular disease years later. Rheumatic disease contributes to gradual fibrotic changes of the valve, in addition to calcification of the valve cusps. Shortening of the chordae tendineae also may occur. Rheumatic fever commonly affects the mitral valve.

Infective endocarditis may occur as a primary or secondary infection. The valve tissue is destroyed by the infectious organism. Table 19-2 lists other conditions that cause valvular heart disease.

ESSENTIAL CONTENT CASE

Heart Valve Disorder

A 48-year-old woman was admitted to the progressive care unit with increasing shortness of breath and fatigue. She had bacterial endocarditis 15 years ago, which resulted in mitral valve insufficiency. On admission, she was in normal sinus rhythm with frequent premature atrial contractions, with a blood pressure of 150/94 mm Hg. Chest auscultation revealed crackles in the left lower lung field. Hemodynamic parameters included:

RAP	12 mm Hg
PAP	35/25 mm Hg
PAOP	24 mm Hg
CO	4.8 L/min
CI	1.9 L/min/m^2
SVR	2100 dynes/s/cm^5

Case Question. The initial priority for medical management of this patient will be to:

(A) Improve oxygen delivery to the tissues
(B) Consider initiation of an inotrope
(C) Initiate a sodium nitroprusside infusion to reduce the blood pressure
(D) Decrease preload

Answer: D

Pathophysiology of Mitral Stenosis

Several processes occur that together cause stenosis or narrowing of the mitral valve orifice (Figure 19-2). Gradual fusion of the commissures (the valve leaflet edges) and fibrosis of the valve leaflets are common. In addition, calcium deposits may invade the valve leaflets, further impeding their movement. As the mitral valve becomes increasingly stenotic, the left atrium has to generate significant amounts of pressure to propel blood forward through the mitral valve and into the left ventricle. Left atrial pressures are commonly increased, with left atrial dilatation occurring as the stenosis worsens. Increased left atrial pressures may lead to increased pulmonary vascular pressures contributing to the development of right-sided ventricular failure.

Pathophysiology of Mitral Insufficiency

Adequate closure of the mitral valve is important so that blood is ejected forward into the aorta, not backward into the left atrium, during ventricular systole. Damage to the mitral valve can affect the valve's ability to close properly (Figure 19-3). During ventricular systole, as blood is ejected forward into the aorta, blood is also ejected backward through the insufficient mitral valve. This abnormal blood flow contributes to an increase in left atrial volume, pressure, and eventually dilatation. Increased left atrial pressures may lead to increased pulmonary vascular pressures and right-sided heart failure. The left ventricle usually dilates and hypertrophies over time as end-diastolic volumes increase and CO decreases.

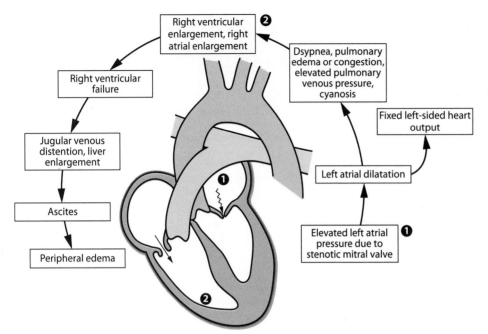

Figure 19-2. Cardiovascular effects of mitral stenosis.

Mitral insufficiency is often associated with dilated cardiomyopathy. As the left ventricle dilates, the papillary muscles are stretched and no longer able to maintain closure of the mitral valve during ventricular systole. Acute mitral insufficiency may occur due to dysfunction or rupture of the papillary muscles. Papillary muscle contributes to preventing the valve leaflets from everting back into the left atrium during ventricular systole. Papillary muscles may rupture during an acute MI if blood supply to the tissue is diminished or absent during the infarct. Loss of a papillary muscle causes sudden, severe insufficiency of the mitral valve, resulting in rapid increase in both left ventricular and atrial volumes and pressures. The pulmonary vascular system is quickly affected by the high left-sided pressures, with pulmonary edema developing acutely. In acute mitral insufficiency, there is no time for the heart to compensate for the sudden increases in volume and pressure, as there is with longstanding mitral insufficiency.

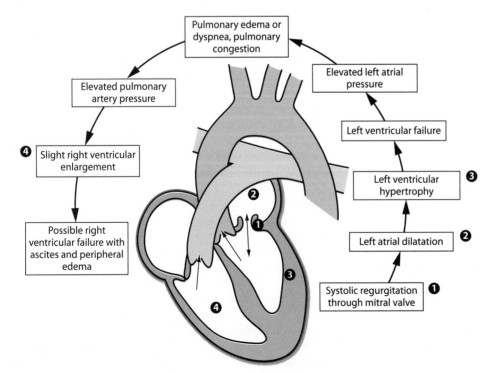

Figure 19-3. Cardiovascular effects of mitral insufficiency.

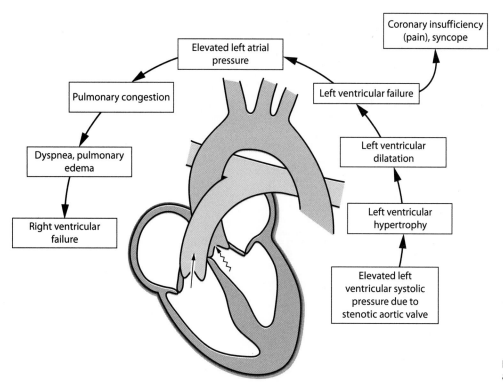

Figure 19-4. Cardiovascular effects of aortic stenosis.

Pathophysiology of Aortic Stenosis

A similar process occurs in aortic stenosis as in mitral stenosis (Figure 19-4). Fusion of the commissures, fibrosis of the valve leaflets, and calcium deposits may occur on the aortic valve leaflets, impeding their movement. When aortic stenosis presents, the left ventricle has to generate a significant amount of pressure to propel blood forward through the aortic valve into the aorta. Increased left ventricular pressure contributes to left ventricular dilatation and hypertrophy, as well as decreases in CO. Left atrial volume and pressure may increase as the left atrium must generate more pressure to eject blood into the left ventricle. Left atrial dilatation may eventually occur. The elevated left-sided pressures are reflected back into the pulmonary vascular system and to the right side of the heart, eventually causing right heart failure.

Pathophysiology of Aortic Insufficiency

A similar process also occurs in aortic insufficiency as in mitral insufficiency (Figure 19-5). Adequate closure of the aortic valve is even more important than adequate closure of the mitral valve. If the aortic valve does not close properly, blood flows backward from the aorta into the left ventricle during diastole. This can seriously affect forward blood flow into the aorta, and thus CO. This causes significant increases in the volume and pressure of the left ventricle contributing to the gradual development of left ventricular dilatation and hypertrophy. As with other left-sided valvular disease, pulmonary vascular pressures increase contributing to the development of right heart failure.

Pathophysiology of Tricuspid Stenosis

Fused commissures or fibrosis of the valve leaflets may also narrow the tricuspid valve orifice. RA pressures increase as the right atrium attempts to propel blood forward into the right ventricle. Eventually, RA dilatation occurs and the increased right atrial pressure is reflected back into the venous system.

Pathophysiology of Tricuspid Insufficiency

Damage to the tricuspid valve that prevents complete closure during ventricular systole causes the abnormal ejection of blood through the tricuspid valve into the right atrium. Right atrial volumes and pressures increase, eventually leading to dilatation and possible decreases in CO. In recent years tricuspid insufficiency commonly occurs with dilated cardiomyopathy. As the right ventricle dilates, the papillary muscles are stretched and are unable to maintain closure of the valve during ventricular systole. This frequently accompanies mitral insufficiency.

Pathophysiology of Pulmonic Stenosis

Pulmonic stenosis develops as the pulmonic valve orifice becomes narrowed. Right ventricular pressures increase as the right ventricle attempts to eject blood forward into the pulmonary artery. Over time, right ventricular dilatation may occur, with decreases in right-sided CO. The increased pressure may back up into the right atrium, causing an increase in volume and pressure, and eventually leading to dilatation. This can lead to volume and pressure increases in the venous system.

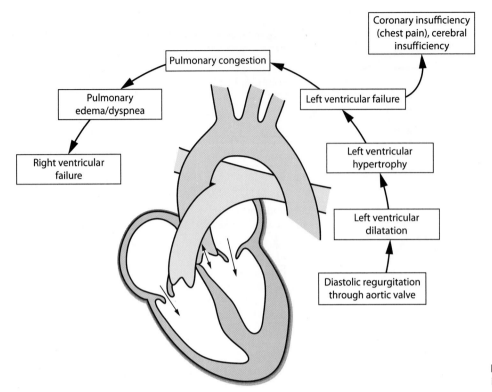

Figure 19-5. Cardiovascular effects of aortic insufficiency.

Pathophysiology of Pulmonic Insufficiency

Closure of the pulmonic valve prevents blood from backing up from the pulmonary artery into the right ventricle during diastole. An insufficient pulmonic valve permits blood to flow backward into the right ventricle during diastole. Right-sided CO decreases as blood flows backward instead of forward. An increase in right ventricular volume and pressure occurs, which may eventually lead to dilatation. The increased pressures may be reflected back into the right atrium and the venous system. Pulmonic stenosis and insufficiency are rarely seen in adults and are much more common in children. They are usually caused by a congenital defect.

Clinical Presentation

Mitral and Aortic Disease

The following signs and symptoms are found in all of the valvular disorders of the left side of the heart:

- Dyspnea
- Fatigue
- Increased pulmonary artery pressures (PAS, PAD, PAOP)
- Decreased CO

Mitral Stenosis

- Palpitations
- Hemoptysis
- Hoarseness
- Dysphagia
- JVD

- Orthopnea
- Cough
- Diastolic murmur
- Atrial arrhythmias (PACs, AF)
- Elevated A wave on PAOP pressure waveform

Mitral Insufficiency

- Paroxysmal nocturnal dyspnea
- Orthopnea
- Palpitations
- S_3 and/or S_4
- Crackles
- Systolic murmur
- Atrial arrhythmias
- Elevated V wave on PAOP pressure waveform

Aortic Stenosis

- Angina
- Syncope
- Decreased SVR
- S_3 and/or S_4
- Systolic murmur
- Narrowed pulse pressure

Aortic Insufficiency

- Angina
- S_3
- Diastolic murmur
- Widened pulse pressure
- de Musset sign (nodding of the head)

Tricuspid and Pulmonary Valve Disease

The following signs and symptoms are found in all of the valvular disorders of the right side of the heart:

- Dyspnea
- Fatigue
- Increased RA pressures
- Peripheral edema
- Hepatomegaly
- JVD

Tricuspid Stenosis

- Atrial arrhythmias
- Diastolic murmur
- Decreased CO
- Elevated A wave on RA pressure waveform

Tricuspid Insufficiency

- Conduction delays
- Supraventricular tachycardia
- Systolic murmur
- Elevated V wave on RA pressure waveform

Pulmonic Stenosis

- Cyanosis
- Systolic murmur
- Elevated A wave on RA pressure waveform

Pulmonic Insufficiency

- Diastolic murmur
- Elevated A wave on RA pressure waveform

Diagnostic Tests

- *Chest x-ray:* Shows specific cardiac chamber enlargement, pulmonary congestion, presence of valve calcification
- *12-lead ECG:* Useful in the diagnosis of right ventricular, left ventricular, and left atrial hypertrophy
- *Echocardiogram:* Demonstrates the size of the four cardiac chambers, presence of hypertrophy, specific valve dysfunction, ejection fraction, and amount of regurgitant flow, if present
- *Radionuclide studies:* Identify abnormal ejection fraction during inactivity and activity
- *Cardiac catheterization:* Determines cardiac chamber pressures, ejection fraction, regurgitation, and pressure gradients, if present

Principles for Management of Valvular Disorders

The primary objectives in the management of valvular disorders are to maximize cardiac function, reduce anxiety, and prevent complications.

Maximize Cardiac Function

Medical Management

1. *Improve oxygenation delivery:* As ventricular dilatation occurs, there is an increase in ventricular wall tension, myocardial workload, and oxygen consumption. Oxygen therapy should be initiated, as necessary, to increase oxygen saturation. Pulse oximetry, arterial blood gases, and mixed venous oxygenation saturation (Svo_2) monitoring in the ICU are helpful in guiding sufficient oxygen therapy.
2. *Decrease preload:* Diuretics decrease excess fluid and ventricular end-diastolic volumes. Fluid and sodium restrictions also may be necessary. (Exception: Preload usually is not decreased in patients with aortic insufficiency, because decreased left ventricular end-diastolic volumes may accentuate decreases in CO.)
3. *Decrease afterload:* Afterload reduction may be indicated for patients with increased SVR and impaired left ventricular function (eg, aortic stenosis or mitral insufficiency).
4. *Improve contractility:* Inotropic agents (eg, dobutamine, milrinone) increase myocardial contractility and improve CO.
5. *Modify activity:* Activity limitation helps reduce myocardial oxygen consumption. Teach patients the importance of rest between activities.
6. *Balloon valvuloplasty may be an option for stenotic mitral or aortic valves:* A percutaneous catheter is inserted via the femoral artery under fluoroscopy and the balloon is inflated at the stenotic lesion in an effort to force open the fused commissures and improve valve leaflet mobility.

Surgical Management

Cardiac surgery is indicated when medical management does not alleviate patient symptoms. Patients may have better surgical outcomes if surgery is done prior to left ventricular dysfunction.

1. *Valve repair:* An increasing trend today is to have dysfunctional valves repaired instead of replaced. The hemodynamic function of the inherent valve is superior to any prosthetic valve. In addition, the risks associated with valve replacement are avoided. An open commissurotomy may be performed to relieve stenosis of any of the four heart valves. During open commissurotomy, the fused commissures are incised, thus mobilizing the valve leaflets. Valve leaflet reconstruction also may be done to patch tears in valve leaflets using pericardial patches for the repair. Chordae tendineae reconstruction may be performed to elongate fibrotic tendineae or to shorten excessively stretched tendineae. An annuloplasty ring may also be inserted to correct dilatation of the valve annulus.
2. *Prosthetic valve replacement:* Replacement of the native valve with a prosthetic, or artificial, valve is done for severely damaged valves or when repair is not possible. The entire native valve is removed and replaced with a mechanical or biological

(porcine, bovine, or allograft [homograft or auto-graft]) prosthetic valve.

3. *Postoperative management* after cardiac surgery is similar to coronary artery bypass surgery management (see Chapter 9, Cardiovascular System). Special considerations for patients having valve repair or replacement include the following:

   - *Maintain adequate preload:* Patients with valvular heart disease are usually accustomed to increased end-diastolic volumes. Although the valve is repaired, the heart needs time to adjust to the hemodynamic changes. Most patients do better in the postoperative phase if fluids are adjusted based on presurgical RA and PAOP pressures.
   - *Monitor for conduction disturbances:* The mitral, tricuspid, and aortic valves lie in close proximity to conduction pathways. Conduction disorders may be treated by temporary or permanent cardiac pacing.
   - *Initiate anticoagulation therapy:* Anticoagulation therapy is usually initiated for patients having valve replacement after the epicardial pacing wires are removed. This may be as early as the first post-operative day.

4. If the patient had AF or flutter pre-operatively, the surgeon may perform a Maze procedure, ablating the area around the pulmonary veins in an effort to prevent return of the atrial dysrhythmia post-operatively.

5. *Transcatheter Aortic Valve Replacement (TAVR):* In recent years, technological advances have allowed for the development of a minimally-invasive approach to aortic valve replacement. This approach introduces a prosthetic tissue valve into place via a stent-like introducer catheter. The valve may be inserted through the femoral artery and placed across the native aortic valve. Another approach is trans-apical where a small incision is made in the anterior chest wall and the device is deployed through the left ventricular apex into the aortic valve position. Both approaches avoid the use of cardio-pulmonary bypass. Currently, this procedure is limited to patients who are older (eighth or ninth decade) and who are too debilitated to tolerate the traditional surgical approaches to aortic valve replacement. The patient often experiences near immediate relief of symptoms and is discharged home within a couple of days.

6. An evolving method is the use of a transaortic approach. In this approach a mini-sternotomy is performed and the valve is accessed via the aorta. The benefit of this approach may include a decreased risk of postoperative bleeding than the transapical approach.

Reducing Anxiety
Teach the patient relaxation techniques. Deep breathing or imagery may help alleviate anxiety especially when symptoms of valve dysfunction occur.

Preventing and Managing Complications

1. *Arrhythmias:* Continuous ECG monitoring; observe for side effects of specific cardiac medications.
2. *Hemodynamic instability:* Pulmonary artery pressure (PAP) monitoring, manage patient based on trends in hemodynamic monitoring.
3. *Thromboembolic event:* Anticoagulation is necessary for patients with severely compromised left ventricular function or AF, and after valve surgery. Lifelong anticoagulation therapy is indicated for patients after mechanical valve replacement. Short-term anticoagulation therapy is usually initiated for patients having a biological valve replacement.
4. *Endocarditis:* Antibiotic prophylaxis is recommended for patients with valve disorders and for patients with prosthetic valves. Prophylaxis should be given prior to dental work, surgery, or other invasive procedures. Prior to discharge, teach the patient and family the importance of prophylaxis.
5. *Prosthetic valve dysfunction:* Biological valve dysfunction usually develops slowly with gradual signs and symptoms (eg, presence of a new murmur, dyspnea, syncope). Mechanical valve dysfunction may occur slowly or suddenly. Rapid valve dysfunction requires an emergency intervention as the patient presents with signs and symptoms of acute cardiac failure (hypotension, tachycardia, low CO/CI, heart failure, cardiac arrest).

Pericarditis

Pericarditis is a chronic or acute inflammation of the pericardial lining of the heart. Acute pericarditis usually occurs secondary to another disease process and usually resolves within 6 weeks. Chronic pericarditis, however, may last for months.

Pericarditis may lead to pericardial effusion or cardiac tamponade. Pericardial effusion occurs as fluid builds up within the pericardial sac. Cardiac tamponade can occur as the pericardial fluid compresses the heart, restricts ventricular end-diastolic filling, and compromises cardiac function.

The case study is an example of the importance of accurate diagnosis of patients with chest pain. The pain of pericarditis may be similar to anginal pain, but the treatment is very different.

Etiology and Pathophysiology
A number of different conditions and situations can cause pericarditis (Table 19-3). Common causes include MI, infections, neoplasm, radiation therapy, and uremia.

Normally, the pericardial sac contains a small amount of clear serous fluid, typically less than 50 mL. This fluid lies between the visceral and parietal pleura and lubricates the surface of the heart as it expands and contracts. An inflammation of the pericardium causes friction between the visceral and parietal pleura.

TABLE 19-3. ETIOLOGY OF PERICARDITIS

Idiopathic
Infections (viral/bacterial)
Myocardial infarction
Cardiac surgery
Neoplasm
Radiation therapy
Rheumatic disease
Lupus erythematosus
Scleroderma
Uremia
Medication induced

Inflammation of the pericardium causes an increase in pericardial fluid production, with increases of up to 1 L or more. A gradual buildup of fluid may have little compromising effect on the heart as the pericardium expands and normal hemodynamics is not altered. A sudden increase in pericardial fluid, however, dramatically impairs the hemodynamic status.

Chronic pericarditis causes fibrotic changes within the pericardial lining. The visceral and parietal pleura eventually adhere to each other, restricting the filling of the heart. This condition may be referred to as constrictive pericarditis. The pressure created by the constricted pericardium affects the heart's ability to distend properly, causing decreases in end-diastolic volume and CO. These changes may contribute to increases in ventricular end-diastolic atrial pressures, leading to increases in pulmonary vascular and venous system pressures.

Clinical Presentation

Acute Pericarditis

- Sharp, stabbing, burning, dull, or aching pain in the substernal or precordial area, which increases with movement, inspiration, or coughing, or when the patient is in a recumbent position
- Pericardial friction rub
- Fever
- Sinus tachycardia
- Dyspnea, orthopnea
- Cough
- Fatigue
- Narrowed pulse pressure
- Hypotension
- Arrhythmias
- Elevated cardiac pressures (PA, PAOP, RA)
- Decreased CO
- Peripheral edema
- JVD

Chronic Pericarditis

- Dyspnea
- Anorexia
- Fatigue
- Abdominal discomfort
- Weight gain
- Activity intolerance
- JVD
- Peripheral edema
- Hepatomegaly
- Kussmaul sign (increase in RA pressure during inspiration)

Diagnostic Tests

- *Chest x-ray:* Normal or enlarged heart; chronic pericarditis may reveal a decrease in heart size.
- *ECG:* ST-segment elevation in precordial leads (V leads) and leads I, II, or III; T-wave inversion after ST segment returns to isoelectric line; decrease in QRS voltage.
- *Echocardiogram:* Presence of increased fluid in pericardial sac; chronic, constrictive pericarditis may demonstrate a thickened pericardium and diminished ventricular contractility.
- *Laboratory:* Elevated sedimentation rate and elevated WBC (white blood cell); causative organisms may be identified from blood cultures.
- *CT/MRI scan:* Detects a thickened pericardium for patients with chronic pericarditis.

Principles of Management of Pericarditis

The primary principles of management of pericarditis are to correct the underlying cause, relieve pain and promote comfort, relieve pericardial effusion, and prevent and manage complications associated with pericarditis.

ESSENTIAL CONTENT CASE

Pericarditis

A woman had an acute anterior MI 7 days ago. She was readmitted to the progressive care unit with sharp, substernal chest pain worsening with inspiration, shortness of breath, and ST-segment elevations in the precordial leads and in leads I and II. The chest pain was unrelieved with nitroglycerin. Her pain was decreased after receiving 4 mg of morphine IV. Her pain was completely relieved when her nurse had her sit up and lean forward so that she could auscultate posterior breath sounds.

Case Question 1. A classic sign of pericarditis is:

(A) Sharp pain on inspiration relieved by leaning forward
(B) Distended neck veins
(C) Narrow pulse pressure
(D) Cough

Case Question 2. An important nursing action for this patient is to:

(A) Continue to administer morphine for pain
(B) Encourage patient to ambulate as much as possible
(C) Alleviate anxiety by informing patient this is not another heart attack
(D) Encourage deep breathing exercises to expand the lung

Answers: 1. A; 2. C

Promoting Comfort and Relieving Pain

1. *Decrease pain:* Teach the patient that chest pain may be decreased or relieved by sitting up and/or leaning forward. Analgesics (eg, aspirin) and nonsteroidal anti-inflammatory agents administered around the clock assist in pain relief.
2. *Promote relaxation:* Teach the patient relaxation techniques such as progressive muscle relaxation and visualization. This may assist the patient to cope. Relaxation techniques that include deep breathing should be avoided because pericardial pain usually increases with deep inspiration.
3. *Limit activity:* This is especially important during the acute period of inflammation. Activity can be gradually increased as fever and chest pain decrease. Assist patients to find a position of comfort. Patients often are more comfortable sitting up and leaning slightly forward.

Correcting the Underlying Cause

1. *Decrease pericardial inflammation:* Nonsteroidal anti-inflammatory agents (eg, indomethacin, ibuprofen) assist to decrease inflammation of the pericardium and the associated pain. Chronic, recurrent pericarditis may require corticosteroid therapy.
2. *Eliminate infection:* If the cause of the pericarditis is an infectious process, appropriate medications, including antibiotic therapy, are necessary.

Relieving Pericardial Effusion

1. *Pericardiocentesis:* A needle or small catheter is introduced subxyphoid into the pericardial sac and fluid is withdrawn via the needle or is attached to a catheter and drained into a vacuum bottle. This procedure is performed to remove the excess fluid in the pericardium to improve myocardial function. Culture specimens of the drained fluid should be obtained and sent to the laboratory for analysis. The drain may be left in for several days until the volume of drainage is minimal.
2. *Pericardiotomy/pericardial window:* This is a surgical procedure in which a section of the pericardium is removed in an effort to decrease pericardial pressure on the heart and to allow pericardial fluid to drain more readily. Often a drain may be inserted into the pericardium and tunneled down across the diaphragm into the peritoneal cavity. This permits the excess fluid to drain continuously into the peritoneal space where it is eventually absorbed into the lymph system. It may be performed for recurrent pericardial effusions.
3. *Pericardiectomy:* This involves surgically removing the entire pericardium. This may be necessary for chronic pericarditis that is refractory to other interventions.

Preventing and Managing Complications

1. *Monitor for signs and symptoms of acute heart failure:* These include hypotension; tachycardia; increased respiratory rate; extreme dyspnea; decreased oxygen saturation; decreased peripheral pulses; and decreased urinary output. Oxygen therapy and inotropic agents assist in improvement of myocardial contractility. Assessment of the need for surgical intervention for pericarditis may be indicated.
2. *Cardiac tamponade:* Monitor for signs and symptoms of cardiac tamponade. These include hypotension, tachycardia, tachypnea, dyspnea, pulsus paradoxus, narrowed pulse pressure, muffled heart sounds, and distended neck veins. Emergency pericardiocentesis is necessary to prevent further hemodynamic compromise.

Aortic Aneurysm

An aortic aneurysm is an area of aortic wall dilatation. Aneurysms are most prevalent in men, commonly occurring during their early fifties to late sixties. Without treatment, mortality associated with aortic aneurysms is high.

Aneurysms frequently are classified by types (Figure 19-6). A fusiform aneurysm is characterized by distention of the entire circumference of the affected portion of the aorta. A saccular aneurysm is characterized by distention of one side

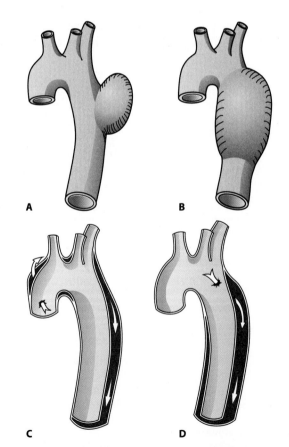

Figure 19-6. Diagram of different types of aortic aneurysms. **(A)** Fusiform aneurysm. **(B)** Saccular aneurysm. **(C, D)** Two aortic dissections. *(From: Underhill SL, Woods SL, Sivarajan ES, Halpenny CJ. Cardiac Nursing. Philadelphia, PA. JB Lippincott; 1982: 680.)*

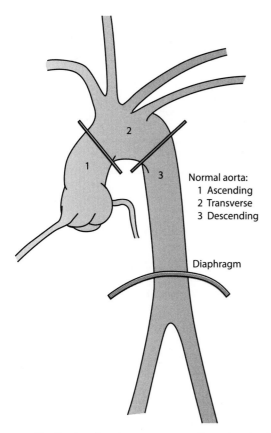

Figure 19-7. Classification of aortic aneurysms according to location. (*From: Seifert PC. Cardiac Surgery. St Louis, MO: Mosby Yearbook; 1994:321.*)

Normal aorta:
1 Ascending
2 Transverse
3 Descending

Diaphragm

The aorta is composed of three layers: the intima, media, and tunica adventitia. Aneurysm development is initiated by degeneration of smooth muscle cells and elastic tissue in the medial layer of the aorta. This weakens the vessel wall, potentially leading to dilatation of all layers of the aorta. The aortic wall may be further weakened with age, as well as from hypertension.

As the aortic aneurysm gradually expands, there is an increase in the risk for aortic dissection. Dissection is caused by a tear in the intima. Blood leaves the central aorta via the intimal tear and flows through the medial layer of the aorta (Figure 19-6C and 19-6D). This creates a false lumen. As the amount of blood increases in the medial layer, the pressure in the false lumen increases, compressing the central aorta (Figure 19-6D). This compression may decrease or totally obstruct blood flow through the aorta and/or its arterial branches. Dissections are classified as acute if they have occurred less than 2 weeks since the onset of symptoms. They are classified as chronic if they occurred more than 2 weeks since the onset of symptoms.

Two additional classifications exist for identifying the location of aortic dissections (Figure 19-8). The first (Stanford classification) classifies the dissection as type A, involving the ascending aorta, or type B, involving the descending aorta (distal to the left subclavian artery). Type A requires immediate surgical intervention whereas type B is managed medically until surgery is deemed necessary. Another classification system for aortic dissection has three categories for the dissection: type I, the original intimal tear begins in the ascending aorta and the dissection extends to the descending aorta; type II, the original intimal tear

of the aorta. The distention of a saccular aneurysm resembles a bulging sac. Aneurysms may also be classified according to their location (Figure 19-7):

- *Ascending:* Between the aortic valve and the innominate artery
- *Transverse:* Between the innominate artery and the left subclavian artery
- *Descending:* From the left subclavian artery to the diaphragm
- *Thoracoabdominal:* From above the diaphragm to the aortic bifurcation

Aneurysms have the potential to dissect or rupture. Dissection occurs when the intimal aortic wall is disrupted and blood extends into the aortic vessel layers (Figure 19-6C and 19-6D). Rupture occurs when all three layers of the aorta are disrupted and massive hemorrhage occurs. Both dissection and rupture are life-threatening events. The case study demonstrates the sudden onset of signs and symptoms associated with aortic rupture and the emergent need for life-saving interventions.

Etiology and Pathophysiology

Aortic aneurysms are caused by a variety of conditions, including atherosclerosis, cystic medial necrosis, genetic link, congenital abnormality, hypertension, Marfan's syndrome, and trauma to the chest.

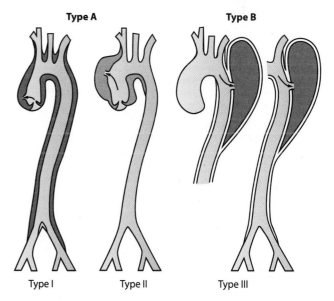

Type A   **Type B**

Type I   Type II   Type III

Figure 19-8. Classification for the location of aortic dissections. The Stanford system classifies aortic dissections based on involvement (type A) of the ascending aorta or noninvolvement (type B). The DeBakey system classifies dissections into types I, II, or III. (*From: DeBakey ME. Surgical management of dissecting aneurysms of the aorta. J Thorac Cardiovasc Surg. 1965;49:131; adapted from Seifert PC. Cardiac Surgery. St Louis, MO: Mosby Yearbook; 1994:321.*)

begins and is contained in the ascending aorta; and type III, the original intimal tear begins and is contained in the descending aorta.

Clinical Presentation

Patients rarely demonstrate early signs of an aortic aneurysm. Diagnosis is commonly made during a routine physical examination or chest x-ray. Signs and symptoms of an aortic aneurysm occur as the aneurysm enlarges and compresses adjacent organs, structures, and/or nerve pathways.

ESSENTIAL CONTENT CASE

Aortic Aneurysm

A 62-year-old man was admitted to the progressive care unit with substernal chest pain. The chest pain was unrelieved by nitroglycerin. The pain decreased in intensity after 8 mg of morphine sulfate. His admitting ECG was normal. His chest x-ray revealed a widened mediastinum, and an aortogram demonstrated a thoracic aneurysm. He has nitroprusside infusing at 1.0 mcg/kg/min to maintain his systolic blood pressure below 100 mm Hg. Suddenly, the patient yells out, "The pain, the pain . . . it's back . . . it's even worse than before." A rapid assessment reveals the following:

BP	190/100 mm Hg
HR	110 beats/min
RR	30 breaths/min
Color	Gray
Skin	Moist and cool
Pain	Rated 10 on a 0 to 10 scale, described as tearing in the middle of his chest and between his shoulder blades

Case Question 1. Following relief of the patient's pain with morphine and notification of the physician, the nurse anticipates the patient will need:

(A) STAT chest x-ray
(B) STAT CT scan of the chest
(C) Cardiac catheterization
(D) STAT MRI

Case Question 2. Based on the description of the location of the pain, the nurse suspects the dissection is located in the:

(A) Ascending thoracic aorta
(B) Transverse thoracic aorta
(C) Descending thoracic aorta
(D) Abdominal aorta

Case Question 3. Medical management of a thoracic aortic aneurysm is focused on:

(A) Maintaining the systolic BP < 120 mm Hg
(B) Maintaining the diastolic BP < 40 mm Hg
(C) Maintaining the heart rate less than 100 beats/min
(D) Reducing the CO to < 2.0 L/min

Answers: 1. B; 2. C; 3. A

Thoracic Aneurysm

- Ripping, tearing, or splitting pain, located at the anterior chest or posterior chest between the scapula, of an intense or excruciating nature
- Dysphagia
- Hoarseness, cough
- Dyspnea
- Different blood pressures when comparing right and left arms
- Different pulses when comparing right and left peripheral pulses

Abdominal Aneurysm

- Dull, constant abdominal or low back or lumbar pain
- Abdominal mass
- Pulsations in the abdomen
- Reduced lower extremity pulses
- Nausea and/or vomiting

Aortic Dissection

- Sudden intense pain in chest or back (or sudden increase in the intensity of pain)
- Dyspnea
- Syncope
- Abdominal discomfort or bloating
- Extremity weakness
- Oliguria or hematuria
- Hemiparesis, hemiplegia, or paraplegia
- Speech or visual disturbances
- Decreased hemoglobin and hematocrit

Aortic Rupture

- Sudden cessation of pain
- Recurrence of pain
- Signs and symptoms of shock, with the exception of blood pressure (high in rupture), including tachycardia, increased respiratory rate, pallor, moist skin, and restlessness

Diagnostic Tests

- *Chest x-ray:* Shows the dilated aorta, widening of the mediastinum, and mediastinal mass
- *CT/MRI scan:* Determines the size of the aorta, size of the aneurysm, extent of a dissection, involvement of additional arterial branches, lumen diameter, and wall thickness
- *Echocardiogram:* Can visualize the location and size of the aneurysm,
- *Aortography:* Determines the origin, size, and location of the aneurysm and involvement of additional arterial branches

Principles for Management of Aortic Aneurysm

The primary objectives in the management of aortic aneurysm are relieving pain and anxiety, lowering BP and thereby decreasing stress on the aneurysm, surgical repair if necessary, patient teaching, and prevention of complications.

Relieving Pain and Anxiety

Administer narcotics (eg, morphine) as necessary. Unrelieved pain is likely to increase anxiety, tachycardia, and hypertension, all of which may aggravate the condition. Relaxation therapy, with deep breathing exercises or imagery, may be extremely helpful.

Decreasing Stress on Aneurysm Wall

1. *Decrease afterload:* Vasodilators (eg, nitroprusside, nicardipine, esmolol) may be prescribed to lower blood pressure and thus pressure on the aneurysm. Blood pressures should be maintained as low as possible (systolic blood pressure 90-120 mm Hg), without compromising perfusion to vital organs.
2. *Decrease preload:* Limit oral and IV fluids, decrease sodium intake, and administer diuretics as indicated. A decrease in preload decreases the circulating blood volume, thus decreasing pressure on the aneurysm.
3. *Decrease myocardial contractility* with beta-blockers (eg, esmolol, labetalol). A decrease in the strength of each cardiac contraction decreases the pulsatile pressure on the aneurysm.

Patient Teaching

1. *Follow-up:* If the patient is to be medically managed, follow up chest x-rays, CT scans, MRI scans, and/or ultrasounds will be needed at 6-month intervals to assess the status of the aneurysm. The importance of these studies should be stressed.
2. *Diet modification:* Teach the patient and family the importance of following a low-sodium diet. Consult a nutritionist for recipes and tips for food preparation.
3. *Smoking cessation:* Assist patient with programs available to assist with smoking cessation.
4. *Physical/psychological stress modification:* Teach the patient and family the hazardous effects of stress and the importance for modification. Discuss activity limitations and relaxation therapy.
5. *Medications:* Teach the patient and family the importance of compliance with the medication regimen. Stress that the medications are essential even though the patient may be asymptomatic.

Surgical Management

Surgery is indicated for acute aneurysm rupture, aortic dissection in the ascending aorta, aortic dissection refractory to medical therapy, and asymptomatic patients with a fusiform aneurysm 6 cm or more in diameter (normal diameter is 2.5-3 cm).

1. During surgery the aortic aneurysm is resected and a prosthetic graft is sutured in place. The original aortic wall may be wrapped around the prosthetic graft for additional support.
2. If an acute dissection or rupture occurs and the patient is waiting for the operating room team to arrive:

- Administer narcotics for pain.
- Titrate vasodilators to maintain the patient's blood pressure as low as possible (90-120 mm Hg if tolerated). This decreases the pressure on the aneurysm.
- Administer fluids to prevent hypovolemia.
- Administer blood replacement products to maintain adequate hemoglobin and hematocrit levels. If rupture occurs, the chest and abdomen will be opened emergently. The patient has a high risk of mortality or complications, including cerebral anoxia, severe hypovolemic shock, and multisystem organ dysfunctions (MODS).

3. Postoperative management:
- Same interventions as described to relieve pain and anxiety and decrease stress on the aorta wall. It is important to decrease pressure on the repaired aorta so that suture lines can heal and bleeding is kept to a minimum.
- Continuous ECG and hemodynamic monitoring.
- In the ICU, continuous spinal pressure monitoring (for surgical repair or insertion of an endograft stent for descending thoracic aortic dissection) will be done for the purpose of draining spinal fluid as necessary to maintain pressure at 10 mm Hg or less. Spinal cord swelling may occur following surgery. Maintaining a low spinal pressure has been shown to reduce the incidence of lower extremity paralysis.
- Complete assessment (including a focused neurologic assessment) every 1 to 2 hours.
- Gradual rewarming of the patient is important. Prevent postoperative shivering, which increases blood pressure and places additional stress on suture lines.
- Ventilator management to maximize oxygenation.
- Activity may be progressed according to institution standards and surgeon preference.
- Monitor renal function (urine output, blood urea nitrogen [BUN]), and creatinine, especially if the aorta was cross-clamped above the renal arteries.
- Initiate anticoagulation. Anticoagulation therapy is initiated for patients receiving prosthetic valves.

Preventing and Managing Complications

1. *Hemorrhage:* Hourly assessment of vital signs and hemodynamic parameters. Daily hemoglobin and hematocrit.
2. *Arrhythmias:* Continuous ECG monitoring; daily 12-lead ECGs.
3. *Hemodynamic instability:* Arterial and PAP monitoring; manage hemodynamic parameters based on trends.
4. *Altered perfusion:* Arteries originating from the aorta may be compromised, leading to MI, cerebral insufficiency/cerebrovascular accident, bowel necrosis, renal failure, paraplegia, and limb ischemia. Assess and monitor the patient for these conditions.

5. *Aortic insufficiency:* Aortic insufficiency may develop if the aneurysm is located in the ascending aorta. Enlargement or dissection of the aneurysm may dilate or damage the aortic valve, causing signs of acute heart failure and pulmonary edema.

Cardiac Transplantation

From the early work of Dr. Christian Barnard in 1967, cardiac transplantation has evolved over nearly four decades to a standard modality for the treatment of end-stage cardiac disease. When medical, surgical, or pharmacologic interventions have failed to improve quality of life and functional capacity, cardiac transplantation offers patients improved survival. The international survival rate is 80% to 90%, 75% at 1 year, and 56% at 10 years. The primary indications for cardiac transplantation include cardiomyopathies or ischemic heart disease. Other indications include heart valve disease, congenital heart disease, and myocarditis.

Candidate Selection

Patients usually have a less than 1-year survival without cardiac transplant and are in New York Heart Association (NYHA) functional class III or IV or American Heart Association (AHA) Stage D. Because of the shortage of available organs, the patient must pass an extensive screening process to ascertain that he or she is appropriate for the candidate list (Table 19-4). Patients must be emotionally stable and

TABLE 19-4. GENERAL INDICATIONS FOR CARDIAC TRANSPLANTATION

Criteria for Consideration of Heart Transplantation in Advanced Heart Failure
• Significant functional limitation (NYHA class III-IV heart failure) despite maximum medical therapy, which includes digitalis, diuretics, and vasodilators (preferably angiotensin-converting enzyme inhibitors) at maximum-tolerated doses
• Refractory angina or refractory life-threatening dysrhythmia

• Exclusion of all surgical alternatives to transplantation, such as the following:
  1. Revascularization for significant reversible ischemia
  2. Valve replacement for severe aortic valve disease
  3. Valve replacement or repair for severe mitral regurgitation
  4. Appropriate ventricular remodeling procedures

Indication for Cardiac Transplantation Determined by Severity of Heart Failure Despite Optimal Therapy

• Definite indications
  1. VO_{2max} <10 mL/kg/min
  2. NYHA class III-IV
  3. History of recurrent hospitalizations for heart failure
  4. Refractory ischemia with inoperable coronary artery disease
  5. Recurrent symptomatic ventricular arrhythmias

• Probable indications
  1. VO_{2max} <14 mg/kg/min
  2. NYHA class III-IV
  3. Recent hospitalizations for heart failure
  4. Unstable angina not amenable to coronary artery bypass grafting, percutaneous transluminal coronary angioplasty with left ventricular ejection fraction <0.25

From: White-Williams C, Grady KL. Care of patients undergoing cardiac transplantation. In: Moser DK, Riegel B, eds. Cardiac Nursing: A Companion to Braunwald's Heart Disease. St Louis, MO: Saunders Elsevier; 2008:1000.

free of alcohol, drug addictions, and tobacco use. They must demonstrate a commitment to the rigors of being a candidate and eventual recipient through compliance with their medical regimens.

The period of waiting for an available donor can be extremely stressful for the patients and their families. It is important to explore their perceptions of the transplant process, what outcomes they are anticipating, and what methods they have utilized to cope in the past. Support group participation or meetings with a psychiatric clinical nurse specialist or nurse practitioner may be beneficial. Fear of death and acute illness may heighten the patient's anxiety. Family members may need proximity to the patient, and this may assist in alleviating anxiety. Incorporating their involvement in direct patient care may enhance their coping abilities.

Pretransplant Process

The greatest delay for cardiac transplantation occurs because of the shortage of donors. When a brain-dead donor is identified, he or she must be carefully managed to maintain cardiovascular stability and avoid electrolyte and renal complications. The United Network for Organ Sharing (UNOS) coordinates the allocation of organs based on a nationwide waiting list. The donor must be of a compatible ABO blood type to the recipient and of similar body size and weight. The recipient is tested for relative immunologic compatibility with the donor to avoid hyperacute rejection. Panel-reactive antibody screening is performed using the recipient's serum with a random pool of lymphocytes. If no lymphocyte destruction occurs, the cross-match is negative and the transplant may proceed. The donor's cardiac function must be normal as assessed by an echocardiogram, nuclear studies, or cardiac catheterization. The donor should have stable hemodynamic profiles on minimal inotropic support.

This process may take several hours, and it is imperative that the patient and family be frequently updated and made aware of the clinical plan of care. Pretransplant teaching should be reviewed to clarify misconceptions and correct knowledge deficits. If CO is compromised, decreased cerebral perfusion may compromise the attention span. During this time, the recipient needs close monitoring to maintain cardiovascular stability. The recipient may require antiarrhythmic therapy, inotropes, diuretics, or after-load reduction agents to achieve major organ perfusion adequate for cellular function. Anticoagulation therapy may be instituted to decrease risk of embolization secondary to AF, reduced left ventricular function, or peripheral venous stasis.

The most unstable patient may be maintained on a cardiac assist device such as the intra-aortic balloon pump (IABP), VAD, or ECMO to promote stabilization or to "bridge" him or her to transplantation.

Transplant Surgical Techniques

In the past, there were two surgical options for cardiac transplantation. Today, almost all are orthotopic transplants in which the recipient's heart is removed and replaced by the

ESSENTIAL CONTENT CASE

Cardiac Transplant

A 54-year-old, white, married, unemployed man is admitted to the progressive care unit for idiopathic cardiomyopathy after an orthotopic heart transplant (OHT) was performed 2 days ago. He has a mediastinal chest tube draining 60 mL of sanguinous fluid per hour. Atrial and ventricular epicardial wires, a left radial arterial line, and a right subclavian pulmonary artery catheter are in place.

Temperature	35.88°C
BP	140/82 mm Hg
HR	90 beats/min NSR without ectopy; remnant P wave present
RR	18 breaths/min
CO	3.80 L/min
Urine	60 mL/h
CI	2.0 L/min/m^2
Mediastinal tube	60 mL/h
SVR	1800 dyne/s/cm^5
Svo$_2$	58%
Spo$_2$	96%
Neurologic	Moves all extremities on command; neurologically intact

Case Question 1. Which of the following hemodynamic measurements would contribute to the CI of 2.0 l/min/m^2?

(A) Heart rate 90 beats/min
(B) SVR 1800 dynes/s/cm^5
(C) Svo$_2$ 58%
(D) RR 18 breaths/min

Case Question 2. Based on your concern, you would consider initiating which of the following to increase the CO/CI?

(A) Dobutamine to improve ventricular contractility
(B) Dopamine to improve renal perfusion
(C) Sodium nitroprusside to reduce afterload
(D) Esmolol to control the heart rate

Answers: 1. B; 2. C

donor's heart in the normal anatomic position (Figure 19-9). The surgical approach is a median sternotomy; the recipient's heart is incised at the superior and inferior vena cavae, pulmonary artery, and aorta. The donor's and recipient's vena cavae, aortas, and pulmonary arteries are aligned and anastomosed. This technique is called the bicaval technique. Another technique which is rarely done today is the biatrial technique. This method involves removing the native heart but leaving the superior/posterior aspects of both atria. This will leave the native SA node intact and may result in double P waves on the ECG tracing (Figure 19-9). The fact that the donor's heart is denervated results in no sympathetic or parasympathetic influence, so the donor's heart must rely on noncardiac mediators to increase CO.

The other surgical option was a heterotopic approach, which is interesting from a historical perspective. It was used in about 5% of cardiac transplants at one point and was also known as a piggyback approach. The donor's heart was placed to the right side of the pleural cavity and performed as an auxiliary pump for the native heart (Figure 19-10). This was used as an option in a size mismatch between donor and recipient or for severe pulmonary hypertension. This approach is rarely performed any more.

Principles of Management of Cardiac Transplantation

The postsurgical care is similar to care following conventional open heart surgery (see Chapter 9, Cardiovascular System). The primary objectives in the early postoperative period include stabilizing cardiovascular function, monitoring altered immune response and graft protection, and providing posttransplant psychological adjustment.

Stabilizing Cardiovascular Function

1. *Cardiac denervation:* Postoperatively there is loss of vagal influence, and the patient usually has a higher resting heart rate than normal.

    - The posttransplant patient requires more stabilization prior to exercise or position changes to avoid orthostasis due to these effects from denervation. With loss of vagal tone, should the sinus rate decrease, there is a stronger potential for junctional rhythms to result.

    - *Surgical manipulation and postoperative edema* may decrease donor SA node automaticity, and therefore the patient may require temporary pacing or isoproterenol (Isuprel) to increase the heart rate.

    - Should *arrhythmias* such as SVT (supraventricular tachycardia) occur beta-blockers or calcium channel blockers are used to decrease heart rate in these circumstances. It is important to assess the patient for response to isoproterenol, because the drug can increase myocardial oxygen consumption.

    - *Denervation* creates a more long-term concern in these patients because the patient no longer experiences angina if the myocardium becomes ischemic. Pain impulses are not transmitted to the brain, so patients must be taught to report other signs of declining cardiac function (ie, decreased exercise tolerance). This is seen in chronic rejection where even with diffuse coronary artery disease, the patient does not experience angina. The patient transplanted for ischemic cardiac disease may find this difficult to comprehend.

2. *Ventricular failure:* Any element of pulmonary hypertension can result in right ventricular dysfunction and eventually compromise left ventricular function also. Inotropic and vasodilating agents may be required to enhance cardiac function. It is essential to rule out any cardiac injury during harvesting and implantation that may have an impact on cardiac function. In reviewing the operative procedure, rule out reperfusion injuries or postbypass problems.

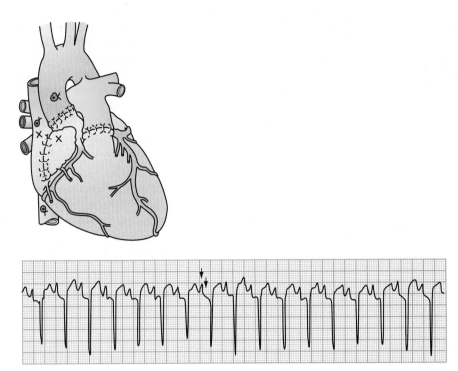

Figure 19-9. Orthotopic method of transplantation using a biatrial approach. Both the donor and the recipient SA nodes are intact (X). This results in an ECG tracing as shown. Note the double P wave at independent rates. *(Reproduced with permission from Morton PG, Fontaine DK. Critical care nursing: A holistic approach, 9th ed. Philadelphia: Lippincott Williams & Wilkins, 2009.)*

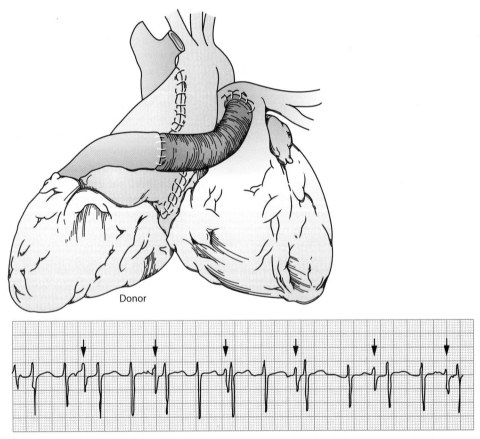

Figure 19-10. Heterotopic method of transplantation. The donor heart is anastomosed with a Dacron graft to the recipient's heart. This results in an ECG tracing as shown. Note the "extra" QRS at an independent rate. *(Reproduced with permission from Smeltzer SC, Bare BG. Brunner & Suddarth's textbook of medical-surgical nursing, 10th ed. Philadelphia: Lippincott Williams & Wilkins, 2004.)*

3. *Bleeding:* Risk factors include cardiopulmonary bypass (CPB), altered coagulation factors if right ventricular failure compromised hepatic function, and preoperative anticoagulation therapy. The recipient's pericardium may be enlarged from pretransplant cardiomegaly. With a smaller donor heart there is more room for blood accumulation without early detection. If there is greater than 100 to 200 mL/h of bleeding for 2 hours, the patient may need to be reexplored. All medications should be reviewed for potential effect on platelet function and coagulation factors.

Monitoring Altered Immune Response and Graft Protection

After cardiac transplantation, the patient is pharmacologically managed with immunosuppressive treatment for graft protection, titrating for the best graft function with the least adverse effects. By virtue of these agents, patient survival has been tremendously enhanced, with a decrease in the need for retransplantation.

1. Immunosuppression. Most patients are maintained on triple-therapy immunosuppression: cyclosporine, mycophenolate mofetil (CellCept), and corticosteroids.

   • Cyclosporine creates a "selective immunosuppression" by selectively inhibiting T cells. T cells dependent on humoral immunity continue intact and no bone marrow suppression occurs. T-cell lymphocytes become unresponsive to interleukin (IL)-1, ultimately preventing maturation of helper and cytotoxic T cells. Adverse effects include hypertension, nephrotoxicity, hepatotoxicity, hirsutism, tremors, and gum hyperplasia. When the first intravenous (IV) dose is administered, it is important to assess the patient closely for potential histamine-type reactions with cardiovascular collapse. This is related to the IV solution preparation and is not seen with the oral preparation. A daily trough level is measured to assess therapeutic dosage and avoid toxicity.

   • Basiliximab (Simulect) is an immunosuppressive agent that is an IL-2 antagonist. It is indicated for patients with renal insufficiency related to their chronic low CO because it is renal sparing. This drug is given preoperatively and then 2 to 4 days postoperatively.

   • Mycophenolate mofetil has potent cytotoxic effects on lymphocytes. It inhibits the proliferative responses of T and B lymphocytes to both mitogenic and allospecific stimulation. It also suppresses antibody formation against B lymphocytes. It is given in 1.5-g dose twice a day. The side effects include gastrointestinal tract ulceration, nausea, vomiting, and diarrhea. It has severe neutropenic effects and can cause anemia, leukopenia, and thrombocytopenia.

• Corticosteroids are administered to both prevent and treat rejection. They are able to decrease antibody production and inhibit antigen-antibody production, as well as interfere with production of mediators IL-1 and IL-2. Both their anti-inflammatory and immunosuppressive properties offer the patient benefits. Immediately postoperatively, they are administered in high doses, and then tapered over the next 6 months. However, if the patient experiences two or more episodes of acute rejection, he/she remains on a maintenance dose. In situations of acute or chronic rejection, the patient may be "pulsed" with steroids. These doses are 500 to 1000 mg IV every day for 3 days, during which other steroids are discontinued. The patient then resumes another tapering wean to maintenance dose steroids. Complications from steroid treatment are numerous and include infection, hyperlipidemia, diabetes, hypertension, osteoporosis, sodium and water retention, metabolic alkalosis, peptic ulceration, pancreatitis, increased appetite, adrenopituitary suppression, lymphocytopenia, opportunistic infections, and aseptic necrosis of femoral and humoral heads. The patient often receives ulcer prophylaxis with a histamine blocker or antacids. Strict fluid and electrolyte balance must be maintained, and close assessment must be maintained for glucose intolerance. The anti-inflammatory response may mask an infection; therefore, identification of malaise, anorexia, myalgias, change in wound appearance, cough, or sore throat must be reported. With all these immunosuppressive agents, the patient has an intrinsic risk for malignancies and needs comprehensive teaching regarding this and all preventive therapies to follow.

• Newer therapies offer further improvement in transplant outcomes. Muromonab-CD3 (Orthoclone OKT3), a monoclonal antibody, may be given to reverse acute rejection, although it is rarely used. Antibodies that react with T3 cells' surface antigens are produced, interfering with T-cell antigen recognition and making it more difficult for active T cells to recognize the target organ. Muromonab-CD3 is administered for a 10- to 14-day course of therapy as a daily bolus dose of 5 to 10 mg IV. There is a danger of flash pulmonary edema; therefore, the patient is premedicated with steroids, acetaminophen, and diphenhydramine. Vital signs are monitored every 15 minutes for 1 hour after the dose is given with emergency intubation and resuscitative equipment available. While receiving the treatment of Muromonab-CD3 cyclosporine is usually held and then titrated back up during the last 3 days of treatment. CD3 levels are monitored in the laboratory on the fourth

TABLE 19-5. COMMON INFECTIONS IN CARDIAC RECIPIENTS

Bacterial Infections

Early
Escherichia coli
Enterococci
Klebsiella organisms
Pseudomonas organisms
Serratia organisms
Staphylococcus organisms
Streptococcus organisms

Late
Legionella organisms
Listeria organisms
Mycobacterium organisms
Nocardia organisms
Salmonella organisms

Viral Infections

CMV
Herpes simplex
Epstein-Barr virus
Varicella-zoster virus

Fungal Infections

Aspergillus organisms
Cryptococcus organisms
Histoplasmosis
Coccidioidomycosis
Blastomycosis
Candida organisms

Parasitic Infections

Pneumocystis organisms
Toxoplasmosis

From Dressler DK. The patient undergoing cardiac transplant surgery. In: Guzzetta CE, Dossey BM, eds. Cardiovascular Nursing Holistic Practice. St Louis, MO: Mosby-Year Book; 1992.

and tenth days of therapy to assess effectiveness. Some centers utilize a monoclonal or polyclonal antibody for induction therapy in the immediate postoperative period. Others reserve medications such as Muromonab-CD3 for rescue therapy.

2. Infection risk. The immunosuppressive drugs decrease the normal immune response, increasing the risk for nosocomial or suprainfections (Table 19-5). In the immediate posttransplant period, when steroid doses are highest, the patient is more vulnerable to these infections. Infections are a major cause of morbidity and mortality, and prevention and early detection are crucial.

• The most challenging aspect of determining an infection is the clinical presentation, which is often masked by immunosuppressive therapy. The patient's temperature may not elevate as high as in nonimmunosuppressed patients and the WBC may not elevate as rapidly. It is imperative to assess the individual trend in each patient and have a strong suspicion if patients appear more fatigued, complain of sore throats, develop a new cough, or run low-grade temperatures. Bacterial, fungal,

viral, and protozoal infections may compromise the posttransplant recipient.

• Aggressive skin care to decrease dermal injuries, adequate nutrition and hydration, removing all invasive devices as soon as possible, and limiting unnecessary procedures may assist in reducing risks for sepsis. Patients and families should receive thorough education regarding transmission of infections. Antimicrobial therapy is instituted postoperatively while invasive devices are in place but should be utilized appropriately to avoid growth of antibiotic-resistant organisms. Thorough skin and oral assessments should be incorporated into daily assessment to rule out viral or fungal infections.

3. Assessing for rejection. Routinely, the patient undergoes a posttransplant endomyocardial biopsy to rule out rejection (Figure 19-11). Under fluoroscopy, utilizing a cardiac bioptome via the right internal jugular vein into the right ventricle, multiple (three to five) samples are taken of the myocardium to rule out rejection. The patient is then treated with the appropriate protocol (pulsed steroids or monoclonal antibodies). These biopsies are performed serially posttransplant during clinic visits to monitor for rejection. Other diagnostic procedures such as transesophageal echocardiogram and chest x-ray every 6 months may be performed. Cyclosporine levels are measured monthly. These data provide further guidance for earlier detection of rejection.

Providing Posttransplant Psychological Adjustment

Many emotions impact on the posttransplant patient. Often the patient and family have altered their roles and responsibilities during the illness. The posttransplant goal is to encourage role readjustment and resumption of preillness

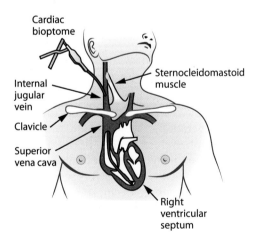

Figure 19-11. Endomyocardial biopsy technique. *(From: Macdonald SN. Heart transplantation. In: Smith SL, ed. Tissue and Organ Transplantation: Implications for Professional Nursing Practice. St Louis, MO: Mosby-Year Book, 1990, used with permission from AACN.)*

activities of daily living. The return to independence may frighten them after the security of the hospital environment.

1. They must be supported and assisted toward their return to home and with the long-term plan of care.
2. Involvement in a transplant support group may benefit the patient and family, reduce anxieties, and clarify misconceptions. Meeting other recipients may validate their feelings and enhance the patient's adjustments.
3. Some recipients experience body image concerns related to hirsutism and increased weight. Reviewing cosmetic methods for dealing with these changes may decrease their concerns.
4. Weight loss may be enhanced through dietary counseling and participation in cardiac rehabilitation activities.
5. Quality-of-life issues should be explored with patients to heighten the positive side of transplantation and the future that awaits them.
6. Steroids may cause periods of mood swings from episodes of depression to euphoria. Counseling with the patient and family may reduce confusion over the cause of personality changes. During pulsed steroid therapy it is very important to assess for steroid psychosis. Closer monitoring and reassurance during this therapy may assist in diminishing this side effect.

Ventricular Assist Devices

Patients with cardiogenic shock following an MI, coming off CPB, or with cardiomyopathies may require additional assistance when CO remains low despite maximal medical therapy. IABP support offers 8% to 12% augmentation to the patient's CO, but this may be inadequate, requiring placement of a VAD. Greater support for the failing ventricle(s) can be provided with a VAD. The goals of utilizing a VAD are to reduce myocardial ischemia and workload, limit permanent cardiac damage, and restore adequate organ perfusion.

Indications

Appropriate candidates for VAD include those patients with end-stage cardiac disease, cardiomyopathies, post-CPB cardiogenic shock, and acute MI with cardiogenic shock. Another indication for insertion is to "bridge" the patient prior to cardiac transplantation until a suitable donor is located. Post-MI, a patient may be bridged in the hope of myocardial recovery and eventual weaning from the device. VADs (left ventricular devices) have been approved for "destination therapy"; for example, once the VAD is inserted and the patient recovers, the patient is discharged home. The patient is also taken off the transplant list or moved to a lower priority of need. Recently, there have been reports of myocardial recovery after VAD placement. This has allowed for surgical removal of the VAD. The VAD is removed when the myocardium has recovered to the point of consistently ejecting an adequate CO.

After VAD removal the patient is monitored closely for reoccurrence of heart failure symptoms.

The appropriate selection of a candidate for these devices is based on hemodynamic criteria. If preload has been maximized, afterload reduced, and drug therapy instituted to maximal levels, and yet the patient continues to have cardiovascular compromise, a VAD may be critical to achieve survival. Appropriate parameters to consider for VAD placement are:

- CI < 2 L/min/m^2
- SVR > 2100 dyne/s/cm^5
- Mean arterial pressure > 60 mm Hg
- Left or right atrial pressure > 20 mm Hg
- Urine output > 30 mL/h
- PAOP > 15-20 mm Hg

The exclusion criteria for use of a VAD include the following:

- Acute cerebral vascular damage
- Cancer with metastasis
- Renal failure (unrelated to cardiac failure)
- Severe hepatic disease
- Coagulopathy
- Severe systemic sepsis, resistant to therapy
- Severe pulmonary disease
- Severe peripheral vascular disease
- Psychological instability
- Alcohol, drug addiction, or tobacco use

General Description of Ventricular Assist Device Principles

The VAD unloads the native ventricle or ventricles by way of artificial ventricles or a blood pump. CO is enhanced by blood circulating at a physiologic rate and by augmenting systemic and coronary circulation.

Ventricular assist device support is predominately utilized for the left ventricle. However, if the right ventricle is compromised, support can be provided to both ventricles. This would necessitate separate VADs, yet the systems would function in tandem.

Ventricular assist devices can be used for postcardiotomy support as a bridge to recovery, a bridge to transplant, or as destination therapy. VADs can be nonpulsatile pumps (roller, centrifugal, or axial flow) or pulsatile pumps (pneumatically or electromagnetically driven). Previously, most VADs were inserted in the operating room but recently percutaneous VADs have been approved as a bridge to recovery, placement of another VAD, or to transplant. The percutaneous VADs are often inserted in the cardiac catheterization laboratory. There are several approaches for cannula insertion depending on the type of device being used and also, if the VAD is being used as a biventricular device or for one side of the heart alone.

Examples of VADs that are used as a bridge to recovery following cardiac surgery include the Biomedicus system and the Abiomed 5000 BVS system. The Biomedicus is a continuous-flow centrifugal pump and usually requires a perfusionist at the bedside for monitoring and troubleshooting. The Abiomed 5000 BVS system is easily managed by the nurse caring for the patient. There are smaller VADs that are emerging and that can be inserted in the cardiac catheterization laboratory using a percutaneous approach via the femoral vein and/or femoral artery. These include the Tandem Heart® and the Abiomed Impella® devices. The Tandem Heart involves inserting a cannula into the right atrium via the femoral vein. The cannula is introduced across the fossa ovalis into the left atrium. Arterialized blood is removed from the left atrium, circulated through an axial flow device, and reintroduced into the arterial circulation via a cannula that has been inserted into the aorta via the femoral artery. The Abiomed Impella is inserted percutaneously through the femoral artery, up the aorta, and introduced across the aortic valve. The device is designed to augment the patient's CO. Blood is removed from the left ventricle and delivered into the ascending aorta.

Ventricular assist devices commonly used as bridge to transplant include the Heart Mate II (Figure 19-12), Heart Ware VAD, and Thoratec paracorporeal VAD. The Heart Mate II and Heart Ware VAD are axial flow devices while the Thoratec PVAD is a pulsatile flow device. The pulsatile flow devices produce a palpable pulse while the axial flow devices are usually not associated with a palpable pulse initially. Often, as the heart regains contractility over a period of several weeks, the pulse will return.

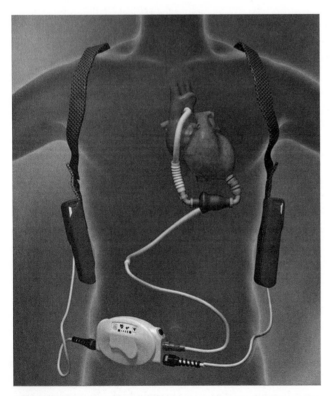

Figure 19-12. HeartMate II left ventricular assist system. (Used with permission from Thoratec Corporation Pleasanton, CA.)

The HeartMate II is the only device currently approved for destination therapy. Destination therapy implies that the patient is not a candidate for transplant and will not be placed on the waiting list for a transplant.

The devices used as a bridge to transplant or for destination therapy are all left ventricular assist devices (LVADs) with the exception of the Thoratec device (PVAD), which can be used as a right VAD as well. They all require an incision from the sternal notch to the umbilicus. A large cannula is inserted into the apex of the left ventricle and connected to the inflow port of LVAD with an outflow cannula inserted into the aorta. The LVAD is implanted outside the peritoneum just below the diaphragm. The drive line (power cord) is brought through the skin and connected to a power source. The drive line exit site represents a major source for infection to occur.

The LVAD has a monitor that provides the flow rate (similar to CO) and other information pertinent to the device. These devices can achieve flow rates that support adequate oxygen delivery to the tissues while reducing cardiac workload.

Weaning and Recovery

The plan for weaning should revolve around hemodynamic stability and the patient's other physiologic systems' response. Neurologic, pulmonary, renal, and hematologic systems must be recovered from multiorgan insults. Assessment of CO, CI, SVR, PAOP, mean arterial pressure, and Svo_2 guides decisions for initiating weaning. Pharmacologic support should be at a stable level with good major organ perfusion.

The arterial line waveform is assessed for the dicrotic notch appearance, indicating that there is adequate left ventricular pressure for aortic opening. The VAD is turned down at small increments to assess tolerance throughout the weaning process. Heparin must be initiated before weaning and the device never set at less than 2 L/min flow to avoid clot formation. At completion of weaning, the patient returns to the operating room for surgical removal.

Principles of Management of Ventricular Assist Devices

The primary objectives in managing the patient with a VAD are to optimize CO, maximize coping, and prevent complications.

Optimizing Cardiac Output

1. Initially, in the ICU, the risk of biventricular failure still is paramount after the device's insertion and the patient must be closely evaluated. Cardiovascular profiles are measured every 2 to 4 hours and changes in CO and CI or the device flow rates are reported to the physician. Pharmacologic support should be titrated to achieve the most stable mean arterial pressure, adequate flow rates and adequate Svo_2.

2. The VAD should be assessed for proper function to achieve an improved cardiovascular profile. As myocardial recovery occurs, more support occurs from the heart and less from the VAD. The patient can then support CO without as much mechanical support.

Maximizing Coping

The patient and family may be overwhelmed by the suddenness of the disease, the progressive care unit environment, the equipment related to the VAD, and the threat of loss of life. Transplantation, if discussed, may significantly increase their stress. They may require intense information sharing and clarification of misconceptions.

1. Promote emotional and psychological adaptation and assess for nonverbal clues of fear or anxiety. Frequent updates regarding goals for the day and present plan of care need to be provided in an interdisciplinary manner. The advanced practice nurse and the patient's primary nurse may coordinate this process.

2. Realistic information related to prognosis needs to be addressed with the patient and family. Often, 20% to 40% of patients on VAD die awaiting a donor heart, and families need support to cope with this possibility. Early involvement with social work and chaplains also may assist patients and families. Closely assess for other situational stressors and review prior coping strategies the patient or family found helpful.

3. If the device has been implanted for the purpose of destination therapy, the patient and family need to be taught the following:
   - How to perform dressing changes
   - How to change from the battery-powered unit to the base power unit and the reverse
   - How to hand pump the device should there be a total loss of power if appropriate for the type of device
   - What equipment the patient should always have when leaving home or the base power unit

The patient and family education process should begin in the ICU as soon as the patient is awake and alert. The nursing staff on the progressive care unit should continue the education process and assist with skills check off as the patient and family become competent when performing the skills mentioned above. Prior to discharge home, the emergency medical services (EMS) system in the patient's home community should be notified about the patient returning to his community.

Preventing Complications

1. *Thromboembolism:* Anticoagulation therapy may include heparin, dextran, or aspirin to reduce the risk for thromboembolism. Peripheral vascular impairment may occur secondary to vascular catheters. Frequent neurovascular checks should be performed and any change reported immediately. Assess for the five P's of vascular complications:
   - Pallor
   - Pain
   - Paresthesia
   - Paralysis
   - Pulselessness

2. *Bleeding:* Monitor hemoglobin, hematocrit, and coagulation factors frequently. Assess all catheter sites and wounds for oozing. The patient needs to be evaluated for spontaneous oozing or occult bleeding. The patient needs close monitoring of therapy so that he or she is safely anticoagulated but not in an abnormal range should a sudden match for a transplantation heart occur. Ideally the partial thromboplastin time (PTT) should be 1.5 times normal or activated clotting levels should be appropriate for the device. The anticoagulation therapy may increase the propensity for cardiac tamponade to occur. This is a surgical emergency and may require reoperation for stabilization. Clues to this complication include the following:
   - Elevated atrial pressures/neck vein distention
   - Reduced CO as pump cannot fill properly
   - Elevated pulmonary pressures
   - Diastolic equalization
   - Reduced mean arterial pressure
   - Declining Mvo_2

3. *Right ventricular failure:* Observe for development of elevated central venous pressure/neck vein distention combined with low to normal PAOP.

4. *Arrhythmias:* Possible treatment with medications or electrical cardioversion may be required. Biventricular support may maintain nearly normal hemodynamics during arrhythmias. Assess the effect of arrhythmias on CO and augment the VAD accordingly. Treat all electrolyte abnormalities aggressively to enhance contractility. Validate with physicians whether CPR may be performed for asystole, depending on the specific VAD.

5. *Decreased renal function:* Possible etiologies in the VAD patient for reduced renal function include hypoperfusion before VAD insertion, prolonged CPB time, massive transfusions, and hemolysis with release of hemoglobin. Assess daily BUN and creatinine values for further decline in renal function. It is imperative that all medications be assessed for nephrotoxicity and doses be based on creatinine clearance. Adequate vasopressor therapy in the dopaminergic range is beneficial to enhance renal perfusion. Maintain adequate fluid balance so preload is within normal limits. Monitor urinalysis for potential abnormalities, and avoid any period of hypotension, which could further insult the kidneys.

6. *Infection:* The large cannulas exiting the skin create great portals of entry for pathologic organisms. Patients on VAD support are so metabolically stressed that they are more prone to infections, and strict precautions need to be followed. It is imperative they not become colonized, especially if they are pretransplant, because sepsis could preclude their

receiving a heart. The best plan of action is prevention and includes:

- Strict hand washing before and after all patient
care activities.
- Strict aseptic technique.
- Pan-culture for temperature > 101°F (38.33°C).
- Monitor wounds for erythema, exudate, or edema.
- Assess for shift to the left on differential count.

7. *Immobility:* Dermal injury may arise from the degree
of immobility during the patient's acute phase of illness. Meticulous skin care and frequent position
changes assist in reducing problems. If the patient
is hemodynamically stable, early mobilization is
important as soon as possible. Having the patient up
in chair and ambulating early will maintain muscle
strength. Aggressive nutritional support assists in
decreasing the degree of catabolism. Immobility may
result in significant muscle mass loss and negative
nitrogen balance. Bedside physical therapy is crucial
until the patient is more stable and can begin ambulating. Foot splints may be applied to diminish the
risk of foot drop.

ESSENTIAL CONTENT CASE

Thinking Critically

You are caring for a patient who was transferred yesterday
to the progressive care unit, from cardiac surgery. He was
admitted to the hospital with mitral insufficiency and
2 days ago had a St. Jude mechanical valve inserted into the
mitral position. Your assessment includes:

Temperature	37.6°C
HR	Temporarily atrial paced at 80 beats/min
BP	86/60 mm Hg
RR	16 breaths/minute
PAS	15 mm Hg
PAD	8 mm Hg
PAOP	4 mm Hg
RA	3 mm Hg
CO	4.9 L/min
CI	1.9 L/min/m²
SVR	2200 dynes/s/cm⁵

**Case Question 1. What is the probable reason for his
hypotension and low CO/CI?**

(A) Hypervolemia
(B) Impaired myocardial contractility
(C) Hypovolemia
(D) Increased afterload

**Case Question 2. What interventions should be imme-
diately initiated to improve his cardiac status?**

(A) Dobutamine to improve ventricular contractility
(B) Sodium nitroprusside to reduce afterload
(C) Increase heart rate to 90 beats/min
(D) Administer volume to increase preload

Answers: 1. C; 2. D

TABLE 19-6. EMERGENCY MEASURES FOR VAD FAILURE OR CARDIAC ARREST

- Backup VAD in place and ready for operation if mechanical failure occurs.
- CPR is usually not recommended.
- Assess availability of blood products should emergency transfusions be necessary.
- Have vascular clamps available for cannula disconnections.
- Educate all team members regarding emergency measures if problem with VAD occurs.
- Patients can be safely cardioverted and defibrillated with VAD in place.
- Connect to emergency power outlets in case of an electrical outage.

8. *Poor device performance:* Dangers related to VAD
mechanical problems include thrombus formation,
inflow obstructions, or device failures. Frequent
device evaluation is needed, particularly with any
change in the patient's clinical status. Device failure
may result in inadequate or no systemic perfusion,
so emergency measures must be implemented rapidly
(Table 19-6).

SELECTED BIBLIOGRAPHY

General Cardiovascular

Bonow RO, Mann DL, Zipes DP, Libby P, eds. *Braunwald's Heart Disease: A Textbook of Cardiovascular Medicine.* 9th ed. Philadelphia, PA: Saunders Elsevier; 2012.

Carlson KK, ed. *Advanced Critical Care Nursing.* St Louis, MO: Saunders Elsevier; 2008.

Fuster V, Walsh RA, Harrington RA, eds. *Hurst's The Heart.* 13th ed. New York, NY: McGraw Hill Companies, 2011.

Hardin S, Kaplow R. *Cardiac Surgery Essentials for Critical Care Nursing.* Sudbury, MA: Jones & Bartlett Publishing; 2010.

Moser DK, Riegel B. *Cardiac Nursing: A Companion to Braunwald's Heart Disease.* Canada: Saunders; 2008.

Woods SL, Froelicher ESS, Motzer SA, Bridges EJ. *Cardiac Nursing.* 5th ed. Philadelphia, PA: Lippincott, Williams & Wilkins; 2005.

Cardiomyopathy

Albert NM. Fluid management strategies in heart failure. *Crit Care Nurs.* 2012;32(2):20-31.

Gheorghiade M, Filippatos GS, Felker GM. Diagnosis and management of acute heart failure syndromes. In: Bonow RO, Mann DL, Zipes DP, Libby P, eds. *Braunwald's Heart Disease.* 9th ed. Philadelphia, PA: Saunders Elsevier; 2011:517-542.

Joyce D, Mallidi HR, Hunt SA. Surgical treatment for heart failure. In: Fuster V, Walsh RA, Harrington RA, eds. *Hurst's The Heart,* 13th ed. New York, NY: McGraw Hill Companies, 2011.

Lee CS, Tkacs NC. Current concepts of neurohormonal activation in heart failure. *AACN Adv Crit Care.* 2008;19(4):364-385.

Leeper B, Legge D. Resynchronization therapy for management of heart failure. *Crit Care Nurs Clin N Am.* 2003;15(4):467-476.

Lewis PS, Boyd CM, Hubert NE, Steele MC. Ethanol-induced therapeutic myocardial infarction to treat hypertrophic obstructive cardiomyopathy. *Crit Care Nurs.* 2001;21(2):20-34.

Mann DL. Pathophysiology of heart failure. In: Bonow RO, Mann DL, Zipes DP, Libby P, eds. *Braunwald's Heart Disease.* 9th ed. Philadelphia, PA: Saunders Elsevier; 2011:487-504.

Mann DL, ed. *Heart Failure: A Companion to Braunwald's Heat Disease.* 2nd ed. Philadelphia, PA: Saunders Elsevier; 2011.

Paul S. Diastolic dysfunction. *Crit Care Nurs Clin N Am.* 2003;15(4): 495-500.

Paul S. Ventricular remodeling. *Crit Care Nurs Clin N Am.* 2003;15(4): 407-412.

Piano MR, Prasun M. Neurohormone activation. *Crit Care Nurs Clin N Am.* 2003;15(4):413-422.

Quinn B. Pharmacologic treatment of heart failure. *Crit Care Nurs Q.* 2007;30(4):299-306.

Heart Transplantation

Collins EG, White-Williams C, Jalowiec A. Spouse quality of life before and 1 year after heart transplantation. *Crit Care Nurs Clin N Am.* 2000;12(1):103-110.

DiNella JV, Bowman J. Heat transplantation. *Crit Care Nurs Clin N Am.* 2011;23(3):471-479.

Guido GW. Heart transplantation from an ethical perspective. *Crit Care Nurs Clin N Am.* 2000;12(1):111-121.

Klein DG. Current trends in cardiac transplantation. *Crit Care Nurs Clin N Am.* 2007;19(4):445-460.

McCaffery D. A review of transplant immunology. *Crit Care Nurs Clin N Am.* 2011;23(3):393-404.

McCalmont V, Ohler L. Cardiac transplantation: candidate identification, evaluation and management. *Crit Care Nurs Q.* 2008;31(3):216-229.

Pham MX, Berry GJ, Hunt SA. Cardiac transplantation. In: Fuster V, Walsh RA, Harrington RA, eds. *Hurst's The Heart,* 13th ed. New York, NY: McGraw Hill Companies, 2011.

Schonder KS. Pharmacology of immunosuppressive medications in solid organ transplantation. *Crit Care Nurs Clin N Am.* 2011;23(3):405-423.

Valvular Disorders

Blaisdell MW, Good L, Gentzler RD. Percutaneous transluminal valvuloplasty. *Crit Care Nurs.* 1989;9(3):62-68.

Hill KM. Surgical repair of cardiac valves. *Crit Care Nurs Clin N Am.* 2007;19(4):353-360.

Holloway S, Feldman T. An alternative to valvular surgery in the treatment of mitral stenosis: balloon mitral valvotomy. *Crit Care Nurs.* 1997;17(3):27-36.

Leeper B. Valvular disease and surgery. In: Carlson KK, ed. *Advanced Critical Care Nursing.* St Louis, MO: Saunders Elsevier; 2008:322-346.

Nauer KA, Schouchoff B, Demitras K. Minimally invasive aortic valve surgery. *Crit Care Q.* 2000;23(1):66-71.

Otto CM, Bonow RO. eds. *Valvular Heart Disease. A Companion to Braunwald's Heart Disease.* 3rd ed. Philadelphia, PA: Saunders Elsevier, 2009.

Piaschyk M, Cyr AM, Wetzel A, et al. A journey through heart valve surgery. *Crit Care Nurs Clin NA.* 2011;23(4):587-605.

Pericarditis

Dziadulewicz L, Shannon-Stone M. Postpericardiotomy syndrome: a complication of cardiac surgery. *AACN Clin Issues in Crit Care Nurs.* 1998;9(2):464-470.

Hamel W. Care of patients with an indwelling pericardial catheter. *Crit Care Nurse.* 1998;18(5):40-45.

Thoraco-Abdominal Aneurysms

Anderson LA. Abdominal aortic aneurysm. *J Cardiovasc Nurs.* 2001;15(4):1-14.

Cronewett JL, Johnson KW, Rutherford RB, eds. *Vascular Surgery.* 7th ed. Philadelphia, PA: Saunders Elsevier; 2010.

Dolinger C, Strider DV. Endovascular interventions for descending thoracic aortic aneurysms: the pivotal role of the clinical nurse in post-operative care. *Vasc Nurs.* 2010;28:147-153.

Iacono LA. Naloxone infusion and drainage of cerebrospinal fluid as adjuncts to postoperative care after repair of thoracoabdominal aneurysms. *Crit Care Nurs.* 1999;19(5):37-47.

Lam, CH, Vatakencherry G. Spinal cord protection with a cerebrospinal fluid drain in a patient undergoing thoracic endovascular aortic repair. *J Vasc Radio.* 2010;21:1343-1346.

Leeper B, Lovasik D. Cerebrospinal drainage systems: external ventricular and lumbar drains. In: Littlejohns LR, Bader MK, eds. *AACN-AANN Protocols for Practice: Monitoring Technologies in Critically ill Neuroscience Patients.* Sudbury, MA: Jones & Bartlett Publishers; 2009:71-102.

Makkad B, Pilling S. Management of thoracic aneurysm. *Semin Cardiothorac and Vasc Anesth.* 2005;9(3):227-240.

Ventricular Assist Devices

Bond AE, Bolton B, Nelson K. Nursing education and implications for left ventricular assist device destination therapy. *Prog Cardiovasc Nurs.* 2004;29(3):95-101.

Bond AE, Nelson K, Germany CL, et al. The left ventricular assist device. *Am J Nurs.* 2003;103(1):32-41.

Camp D. The left ventricular assist device (LVAD): a bridge to heart transplantation. *Crit Care Nurs Clin N Am.* 2000;12(1): 61-68.

Christensen DM. Physiology of continuous-flow pumps. *AACN Adv Crit Care.* 2012;22(1):46-54.

Cianci P, Lonergan-Thomas H, Slaughter M, Silver MA. Current and potential applications of left ventricular assist devices. *J Cardiovasc Nurs.* 2003;18(1):17-22.

Delgado RM, Frazier OH, Razeghi P, Taegtmeyer H. Mechanical circulatory support in patients with heart failure. In: Mann DL, ed. *Heart Failure: A Companion to Braunwald's Heat Disease.* Philadelphia, PA: Elsevier, Inc.; 2004.

Fleck D, Puhlan M. Ventricular assist devices. In: Weigand D, ed. *AACN Procedure Manual.* 6th ed. Philadelphia, PA: Saunders Elsevier; 2011:464-489.

Hagan K, Casanova-Ghosh E. Postcardiotomy cardiogenic shock: the role of ventricular assist devices. *Crit Care Nurs Clin N Am.* 2007;19(4):427-444.

Kurien S, Hughes KA. Anticoagulation and bleeding in patients with ventricular assist devices. *AACN Adv Crit Care.* 2012;23(1): 91-98.

Litton KA. Demystifying ventricular assist devices. *Crit Care Nurs Q.* 2011;34(3):200-207.

Myers TJ. Temporary ventricular assist devices in the intensive care unit as a bridge to decision. *AACN Adv Crit Care.* 2012;23(1): 55-68.

O'Shea G. Ventricular assist devices: what intensive care unit nurses need to know about post-operative management. *AACN Adv Crit Care.* 2012;23(1):69-83.

Puhlman M. Continuous-flow left ventricular assist device and the right ventricle. *AACN Adv Crit Care.* 2012;23(1):86-90.

Richards NM, Stahl MA. Ventricular assist devices in the adult. *Crit Care Nurs Q*. 2007;30(2):104-118.

Rose EA, Moskowitz AJ, Packer M, et al. The REMATCH trial: rationale, design and end points. *Ann Thorac Surg*. 1999;67:723-730.

Savage L. Quality of life among patients with a left ventricular assist device: what is new? *AACN Clin Issues*. 2003;14:64-72.

Stahovich M, Chillcott S, Dembitsky WP. The nest treatment option: using ventricular assist devices for heart failure. *Crit Care Nurs Q*. 2007;30(4):337-346.

Intraaortic Balloon Pump

Castellucci D. Intraaortic balloon pump management. In: Weigand D. ed. *AACN Procedure Manual*, 6th ed. Philadelphia, PA: Saunders Elsevier; 2011:443-463.

Quall SJ. *Comprehensive Intraaortic Balloon Pumping*. St Louis, MO: CV Mosby; 1984.

Evidence-Based Practice/Guidelines

Bonow RO, Carabello BA, Chaterjee K, et al. 2008 Focused update incorporated into the ACC/AHA 2006 Guidelines for the Management of Patients with Valvular Heart Disease. *Circulation*. 2008;118:e523-e661.

Lindenfeld J, Albert NM, Boehmer JP, et al. Executive Summary: HSFA 2010 Comprehensive Heart Failure Practice Guideline. *J Card Fail*. 2010;16(6):475-539.

Nashimura RA, Carabello BA, Faxon DP, et al. ACC/AHA 2008 Guideline Update on Valvular Heart Disease. Focused Update on Infective Endocarditis: a report from the American College of Cardiology/American Heart Association Task Force on Practice Guidelines. *Circulation*. 2008;118:887-896.

Peura JL, Colvin-Adams M, Francis GS, et al. Recommendations for the use of mechanical circulatory support: device strategies and patient selection. A scientific statement from the American Heart Association. *Circulation*. 2012;126:2648-2667.

Advanced Neurologic Concepts

20

Dea Mahanes

KNOWLEDGE COMPETENCIES

1. Compare and contrast the pathophysiology, clinical presentation, patient needs, and management approaches for the following conditions:
   • Subarachnoid hemorrhage
   • Traumatic brain injury
   • Acute spinal cord injury
   • Brain tumor

2. Describe intracranial monitoring technology and implications for nursing care.

3. Describe the use of lumbar drainage of cerebrospinal fluid and implications for nursing care.

SUBARACHNOID HEMORRHAGE

Etiology, Risk Factors, and Pathophysiology

Subarachnoid hemorrhage (SAH) can result from trauma, aneurysm, or other vascular malformations. This discussion focuses on SAH due to the rupture of an intracranial aneurysm (aSAH). Intracranial aneurysms usually occur in the circle of Willis at arterial bifurcations or trifurcations (Figure 20-1). Aneurysms vary in size and shape; saccular (also called berry) aneurysms are the most common and most amenable to treatment. When an intracranial aneurysm ruptures, blood is forcibly expelled into the subarachnoid space and coats the brain surfaces. A clot may form in the ventricular system or in the brain parenchyma. In some patients, blood in the subarachnoid space causes hydrocephalus by obstructing cerebrospinal fluid (CSF) flow through the ventricles or clogging the arachnoid granulations that absorb CSF. Although the mechanism is not well-understood, arterial narrowing (commonly referred to as "vasospasm") occurs in a significant number of patients in the days following aneurysm rupture and can cause delayed cerebral ischemia. There are several scales used to grade the severity of aneurysmal subarachnoid hemorrhage (aSAH). The Hunt and Hess scale (Table 20-1) is commonly used in the nursing literature.

Risk factors for intracranial aneurysm formation include smoking, hypertension, family history of intracranial aneurysm, and certain genetic disorders (autosomal dominant polycystic kidney disease, Ehlers-Danlos syndrome). Twenty percent of patients have multiple aneurysms. Risk factors associated with aneurysm rupture include size of the aneurysm, hypertension, smoking, age (risk increases with age, peaking at age 50-60), and the use of stimulants (cocaine, amphetamines). Aneurysmal SAH is more common in men until the age of 50; the incidence is higher in women after age 50 and in the overall population.

Mortality and morbidity associated with aSAH is substantial. Approximately one-third of individuals with aSAH will die either at the time of rupture or during hospitalization. Many survivors are left with significant disability. Predictors of outcome after aSAH include neurologic condition on admission, age, comorbidities, and the amount of blood on the initial CT scan.

Clinical Presentation

Most patients are asymptomatic until the time of aneurysm rupture, but some have prodromal signs such as headache and visual changes. Upon aneurysm rupture, many patients experience a sudden, severe headache, sometimes described

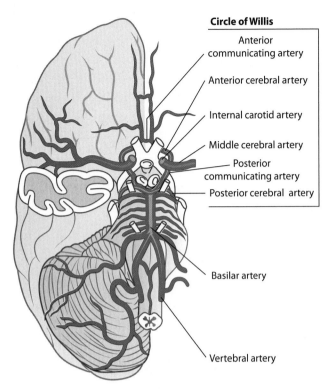

Circle of Willis

Anterior communicating artery

Anterior cerebral artery

Internal carotid artery

Middle cerebral artery

Posterior communicating artery

Posterior cerebral artery

Basilar artery

Vertebral artery

Figure 20-1. The circle of Willis as seen from below the brain. *(Reprinted from: Perry L, Sands JK. Vascular and degenerative problems of the brain. In: Phipps WJ, Marek JF, Monahan FD, Neighbors M, Sands JK, eds.* Medical-Surgical Nursing: Health and Illness Perspectives. *St Louis, MO: Mosby; 2003:1365.)*

as "explosive" or "the worst headache of my life." Transient or prolonged loss of consciousness can occur. Bystanders may describe seizure-like activity; it is unclear whether this is an actual seizure or abnormal posturing related to a sudden increase in intracranial pressure (ICP). Other common signs and symptoms include nausea and vomiting, stiff neck, blurred vision, mental status changes, and photophobia. Focal deficits, such as hemiparesis, hemiplegia, or aphasia, may also occur.

Diagnostic Tests

Computerized Tomography Scan
A CT scan is used to determine whether subarachnoid hemorrhage has occurred and to assess for hydrocephalus.

TABLE 20-1. HUNT AND HESS SCALE FOR THE CLASSIFICATION OF PATIENTS WITH INTRACRANIAL ANEURYSMS

Category	Criteria
Grade I	Asymptomatic, or minimal headache and slight nuchal rigidity
Grade II	Moderate to severe headache, nuchal rigidity, no neurologic deficit other than cranial nerve palsy
Grade III	Drowsiness, confusion, or mild focal deficit
Grade IV	Stupor, moderate to severe hemiparesis, possible early decerebrate rigidity and vegetative disturbances
Grade V	Deep coma, decerebrate rigidity, moribund appearance

Reprinted from: Hunt WE, Hess RM. Surgical risk as related to time of intervention in the repair of intracranial aneurysms. J Neurosurg. *1968;28:14.*

ESSENTIAL CONTENT CASE

Subarachnoid Hemorrhage

A 54-year-old loan officer experienced the sudden onset of a severe headache while at work. She was taken to the emergency department of a local hospital where she described her headache as the "worst headache of my life." The diagnosis of SAH was made by CT scan. Angiography revealed an aneurysm of the left anterior communicating artery at the junction of the left anterior cerebral artery. The aneurysm was successfully coiled and she returned to the ICU following the procedure. The next day, the patient was transferred to the progressive care unit.

On the fifth day postbleed, the nurse noted that this previously neurologically intact patient was difficult to rouse and once awake had right upper extremity weakness and difficulty in speaking.

The patient was taken to radiology where a CT and CTA revealed normal postoperative changes and arterial narrowing, especially of the left middle cerebral artery. Her symptoms improved transiently with induced hypertension, but then recurred. Catheter angiography confirmed severe narrowing of the left middle cerebral artery. Intra-arterial verapamil was infused with radiologic improvement. Postprocedure, the patient was able to speak (although confused) and move her right arm with 4 out of 5 strength (ie, against resistance). Following several days in the ICU, she was transferred to the progressive care unit and then to acute care. Her neurologic examination continued to improve, and she was discharged home on post-bleed day 14 with outpatient speech therapy to address occasional word-finding difficulty and subtle cognitive deficits.

Case Question 1: Describe nursing priorities of care for this patient.

Case Question 2: What actions should the nurse anticipate?

Answers
1. Nursing priorities of care include close monitoring of neurologic status and volume status. Maintenance of euvolemia is important to decrease the risk of delayed cerebral ischemia (DCI) due to vasospasm, and close monitoring of neurologic status allows prompt intervention if complications develop. Other priorities of care include pain management, encouraging mobility, and prevention of hospital-acquired infections.
2. The nurse prepares the patient for stat CT scan and potentially angiogram. Fluid balance is checked and fluid administration may be ordered. The cause of neurological decline is likely cerebral ischemia due to vasospasm, which will be treated with induced hypertension and endovascular measures.

CT scan will detect subarachnoid blood in almost all patients if performed within the first three days of symptom onset. As the blood in the subarachnoid space starts to break down, the sensitivity of the CT scan decreases. CT angiography (see Chapter 12, Neurologic System) can be performed quickly at the time of the initial scan and may reveal aneurysm location. The amount of blood present on the initial CT scan is predictive of vasospasm risk.

Lumbar Puncture

A lumbar puncture (LP) is performed when CT fails to demonstrate SAH in a patient with a history highly suspicious for SAH. LP is avoided in patients with signs or symptoms of increased ICP due to the risk of herniation. LP is performed at least 6 to 12 hours after the onset of symptoms to allow red blood cells (RBCs) in the CSF to start to break down. This breakdown in RBCs gives a yellow tinge to the CSF after centrifugation. This pigmentation is called xanthochromia and will not be present if blood in the CSF is due to a traumatic LP.

Cerebral Angiography

Although CTA done at the time of the initial CT scan detects many aneurysms, cerebral angiography (catheter angiography) remains the gold standard to identify the location, size, and shape of the aneurysm or other vascular anomalies. The initial angiogram will not reveal an aneurysm in approximately 10% to 20% of patients with SAH. If no aneurysm is seen on the first angiogram, a repeat angiogram after approximately a week will reveal an aneurysm in a small number of these patients. Negative angiogram and a distinct pattern of bleeding on CT scan may also indicate a nonaneurysmal perimesencephalic SAH; patients with this diagnosis have an excellent prognosis. In many patients in whom an aneurysm is detected, angiogram is used to guide endovascular treatment (described later). Angiogram is also used to detect and treat arterial narrowing in patients with neurological decline in the days following aneurysm rupture.

Magnetic Resonance Imaging and Magnetic Resonance Angiography

Magnetic resonance imaging and magnetic resonance angiography (MRA) are used to identify aneurysm location and look for other vascular abnormalities. These studies are especially useful in patients with a negative CT or negative angiogram.

Principles of Management of Aneurysmal Subarachnoid Hemorrhage

Patients who survive the initial rupture of a cerebral aneurysm are at risk for complications that increase their chances for morbidity and death. Primary central nervous system (CNS) complications include rebleeding, hydrocephalus, and delayed cerebral ischemic (DCI) due to arterial narrowing. Arterial narrowing correlates temporally with the breakdown of subarachnoid blood and is due to a combination of arterial spasm and inflammatory changes that thicken the vessel wall. This phenomenon is commonly referred to as "vasospasm." Although "vasospasm" reflects an incomplete understanding of the pathophysiology leading to DCI, this terminology is commonly used in practice and will be used in this text to reflect arterial narrowing after aSAH.

Rebleeding

Prior to the aneurysm being secured, the biggest risk to the patient is that the aneurysm will bleed again. This risk is highest within the first 24 hours. The probability of death is markedly increased by rebleed. Signs and symptoms of rebleeding include a sudden increase in headache, nausea, and vomiting, decrease in the level of consciousness, and new focal neurologic deficits. The most definitive method to prevent rebleeding is to secure the aneurysm using surgical clipping or endovascular embolization.

In the interim between admission and definitive treatment, strategies such as blood pressure management and prevention of activities that increase blood pressure or ICP are used to decrease the risk of rebleeding. The goal is to treat hypertension without dropping the blood pressure to a level that decreases cerebral perfusion. Systolic BP goals with an upper range of 150 to 160 mm Hg are common. The use of a titratable agent such as nicardipine is recommended.

Bed rest is typically ordered but may be adapted with physician approval to meet patient needs (eg, a patient who becomes anxious and hypertensive when using a bedpan may be allowed to use a bedside commode). Prophylaxis for DVT, including graduated compression stockings and pneumatic compression devices, is implemented. Stool softeners are used to prevent straining due to constipation. Pain is treated with analgesics, usually short-acting narcotics. A calm, quiet environment is maintained. Anxiety is reduced through explanations of care and psychological support. Neurologic assessment is performed hourly (or more frequently if indicated) to promptly identify neurologic changes so that rapid intervention can occur.

Two management options exist to secure the aneurysm and prevent another rupture: surgical clipping of the aneurysm via craniotomy and endovascular embolization of the aneurysm via catheter angiography. Management at a facility that offers both treatment modalities and frequently treats patients with aSAH is recommended to optimize outcomes. The decision to use surgery vs an endovascular procedure is made on the basis of aneurysm location and morphology, comorbidities, and the severity of neurologic deficits on admission. When the aneurysm is amenable to treatment by either modality, endovascular management is generally performed.

The aneurysm is secured as soon as possible, prior to the period of time when patients are most at risk for vasospasm. With the aneurysm secured, standard management strategies for vasospasm can be implemented without the risk of causing additional hemorrhage. Aneurysm surgery is performed via a craniotomy incision. The surgeon carefully dissects tissue away from the aneurysm and places a titanium or titanium alloy clip across the base (Figure 20-2). Different sizes and shapes of clips are available. Following surgery, the patient is initially admitted to the ICU for management. Follow-up radiologic studies may be done, including CT scanning to look for bleeding at the operative site and angiography to evaluate clip position.

Endovascular embolization decreases rebleeding risk by preventing blood flow into the aneurysm. Using cerebral angiography, the interventional radiologist threads a wire with a helical platinum coil at the end into the cerebral vasculature.

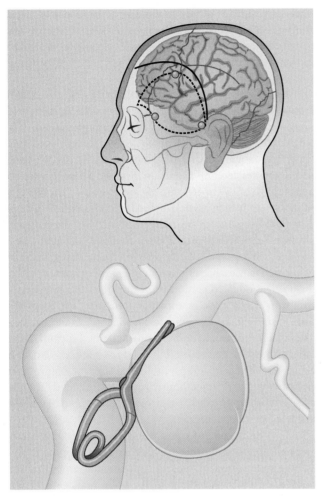

Figure 20-2. Clipping of a posterior communicating artery aneurysm. The clip is placed across the base of the aneurysm so that it can no longer fill with blood, but blood flow can continue through the parent artery. (*From: Brisman JL, Song JK, Newell DW. Cerebral aneurysms. N Engl J Med. 2006;355:928-939.*)

The coil is manipulated into the body of the aneurysm and detached from the wire using a small electrical current. The neck of the aneurysm must be narrow enough for the coils to be retained in the aneurysm instead of floating back out into the vessel lumen. Figure 20-3 depicts endovascular coil embolization of an aneurysm with a narrow neck (berry or saccular aneurysm). If the neck is wide, special stents may be used to assist with coiling or to span the aneurysm. Multiple coils may be needed to completely fill the aneurysm. The coils cause the aneurysm to clot, preventing blood flow into the aneurysm and decreasing the likelihood of rebleed. The primary risks associated with coil embolization are aneurysmal rupture during the procedure and ischemia related to clot formation in the vessel lumen.

Patients with SAH return to the ICU after aneurysm clipping or endovascular treatment. At some institutions, neurologically stable patients without other ICU needs may be transferred to a specialized neuro progressive care unit after 24 to 48 hours to be monitored for vasospasm and other complications.

Hydrocephalus

Subarachnoid hemorrhage disrupts normal CSF flow through two mechanisms. Intraventricular blood may create a blockage in the ventricular drainage system and cause CSF to build up (obstructive or noncommunicating hydrocephalus). In addition, the arachnoid granulations that absorb CSF may become blocked with cellular debris. This results in decreased reabsorption of CSF and communicating hydrocephalus. Signs and symptoms of acute hydrocephalus relate to increased ICP. Acute hydrocephalus after SAH is managed by external ventricular drainage (see section on ICP monitoring and management at the end of this chapter). Some patients later require placement of a ventricular shunt due to continued hydrocephalus.

Late or chronic hydrocephalus can develop weeks after SAH. These patients present with incontinence, gait instability, and cognitive decline. Treatment is placement of a ventricular shunt.

Delayed Cerebral Ischemia (DCI) due to Arterial Narrowing (Vasospasm)

Arterial narrowing occurs in many patients after aSAH and may cause decreased perfusion, potentially leading to DCI and infarction of cerebral tissue. As previously noted, although several mechanisms contribute to arterial narrowing, this phenomenon is commonly referred to as "vasospasm" in clinical practice and this term is used throughout this text. Vasospasm develops 4 to 14 days after initial hemorrhage, with peak incidence around day 7, and is the biggest contributor to morbidity and mortality rates in patients with SAH who survive to hospital admission. Approximately one-third of patients with aneurysmal SAH will develop delayed ischemic neurologic deficits due to vasospasm, and another third will have angiographic evidence of arterial narrowing without neurologic decline. The amount of blood on the initial CT scan is a good predictor of the risk of vasospasm and DCI.

At many institutions, transcranial Doppler studies (TCDs, see Chapter 12, Neurologic System) are used to monitor for the development of vasospasm. TCDs assess blood flow velocity in selected arteries, which will become higher as vessels narrow. TCDs are non-invasive and can be done at the bedside, but accuracy varies based on patient and operator characteristics. CT angiography is also used to look for vasospasm but, as with aneurysm diagnosis, catheter angiography remains the gold standard. Vasospasm is suspected in any patient who develops neurologic decline, especially a decrease in level of consciousness, paresis or paralysis of a limb or side of the body, or aphasia. If any neurologic change is detected, the physician is immediately notified. Early identification of neurologic deficits allows rapid intervention to improve perfusion and prevent infarction.

Maintenance of euvolemia is essential to decrease the risk of DCI. Careful attention to fluid balance is important and must include recognition of insensible fluid loss. Dehydration increases blood viscosity and decreases cerebral perfusion. SAH patients are at risk for dehydration because of cerebral salt wasting, in which excessive sodium is excreted,

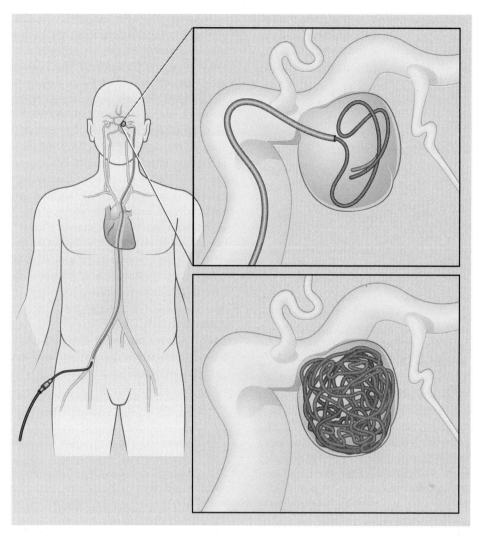

Figure 20-3. Coil embolization of a posterior communicating artery aneurysm. Coils are fed into the aneurysm via a micro-catheter routed from the femoral artery into the cerebral circulation. The coils are then detached into the aneurysm. Multiple coils may be required to occlude the aneurysm. (*From: Brisman JL, Song JK, Newell DW. Cerebral aneurysms.* N Engl J Med. *2006;355:928-939.*)

leading to increased water loss and hypovolemia. If serum sodium falls, volume restriction is contraindicated because of increased risk of cerebral ischemic deficits. Infusion of hypertonic saline is often used for treatment of hyponatremia. Nimodipine, a calcium channel blocker, does not significantly decrease angiographic vasospasm but a large trial showed improved outcomes at 3 months after SAH. If blood pressure drops with the standard dosing regimen of 60 mg orally or via gastric tube every 4 hours, the dose can be divided and 30 mg can be given every 2 hours to decrease the impact on cerebral perfusion.

Historically, DCI due to vasospasm was managed with "Triple-H" therapy, which included hypervolemia, hypertension, and hemodilution. Current evidence-based guidelines support maintenance of euvolemia and the use of induced hypertension if vasospasm occurs. Hypertension is induced using intravenous fluids and vasopressors. Blood pressure goals vary based on the patient response but are typically

in the range of 160 to 200 mm Hg. If previously transferred to the progressive care unit, patients requiring treatment for vasospasm will be readmitted to the ICU for management. Vasospasm can also be treated using an endovascular approach with transluminal balloon angioplasty or direct infusion of a calcium channel antagonist such as verapamil into the artery in spasm. There are many ongoing clinical trials related to monitoring and treating arterial narrowing and delayed cerebral ischemia after aSAH.

Additional Management Strategies and Prevention of Complications

At some institutions, prophylactic anticonvulsants are given to patients with SAH for short periods (3 to 7 days) immediately following presentation. Patients who demonstrate clinical or electrographic seizures are treated according to standard seizure management (see Chapter 12, Neurologic System) and remain on anticonvulsants throughout hospitalization. Systemic complications of

SAH include myocardial dysfunction, cardiac arrhythmias, and neurogenic pulmonary edema; these complications typically occur within hours of the initial hemorrhage. Patients are also at risk for complications of immobility such as infection and DVT.

TRAUMATIC BRAIN INJURY

Etiology, Risk Factors, and Pathophysiology

Major causes of traumatic brain injury (TBI) are falls, motor vehicle accidents (MVAs), and acts of violence. Falls are more common in the elderly, and acts of violence are more prevalent in urban areas. The incidence of TBI is higher in males than females and higher in children ages 0 to 4 years, older adolescents (15 to 19 years old), and adults aged 65 years or older. Rates of hospitalization and death are highest in those older than 75 years. TBI ranges from mild (causing a brief change in consciousness) to very severe (causing prolonged unresponsiveness or even death). TBI severity can be classified using the Glasgow Coma Scale score (GCS, see Chapter 12, Neurologic System). Mild brain injury refers to patients with a GCS score of 13 to 15, moderate indicates a GCS score of 9 to 12, and patients with a score of 8 or less are categorized as having severe brain injury. Although higher GCS is associated with better outcomes, a TBI does not have to be severe to cause long-term impact. Even mild TBI can cause significant functional deficits that become apparent in the weeks and months following injury. Patients with mild TBI and an abnormal CT scan may be admitted to the progressive care unit, or patients admitted to the progressive care unit for other injuries may also be diagnosed with mild TBI. Patients with moderate TBI and a stable or improving neurologic examination are admitted directly to the progressive care unit at some institutions. Patients with severe TBI and most patients with moderate TBI are initially cared for in the ICU, and later transfer to the progressive care unit for continued care.

Mechanism of Injury

Traumatic brain injury occurs as the result of blunt trauma (a direct blow to the head), penetrating trauma (missile or impaled object), or blast injury. Blunt injury occurs as a consequence of:

- *Deceleration:* The head is moving and strikes a stationary object (eg, pavement).
- *Acceleration:* A moving object (eg, baseball bat) strikes the head.
- *Acceleration-deceleration:* The brain moves rapidly within the skull, resulting in a combination of injury-causing forces.
- *Rotation:* Twisting motion of the brain occurs within the skull, usually due to side impact.
- *Deformation/compression:* Direct injury to the head changes the shape of the skull, resulting in compression of brain tissue.

In the United States, gunshot wound (GSW) is the most common type of penetrating brain trauma. The degree of injury caused by a GSW varies based on the type of firearm, bullet type, and trajectory of the bullet. Tissue is destroyed by the bullet, and shock waves and cavity formation occur along the bullet's path. Some bullets will ricochet once inside the skull, creating more tissue destruction. Other causes of penetrating brain injury include nail guns and stab wounds. Surgical management of penetrating trauma to the brain differs from the management of closed injury, but many of the issues relevant to progressive care nurses remain the same.

Awareness of TBI due to blast injury caused by an explosion has increased in recent years. The individual may be hit by flying debris or may be thrown by the force of the blast, causing blunt or penetrating trauma. The brain is also thought to be sensitive to the initial overpressurization wave, with damage occurring as the result of the diffuse impact of intense pressure on brain structures.

Skull Fractures

Skull fractures can result in injury to the underlying brain tissue, or may occur in isolation. Skull fractures are classified as linear, depressed, or basilar.

- Linear skull fractures resemble a line or single crack in the skull. Generally, they are not displaced and require no treatment.
- Depressed skull fractures are characterized by an inward depression of bone fragments. Surgery to elevate the depressed bone may be required. In the case of an open fracture, the wound is also washed out in the operating room to decontaminate the area and decrease the risk of infection.
- Basilar skull fractures involve the base of the skull, including the anterior, middle, or posterior fossa. Clinical manifestations of a basilar skull fracture include periorbital ecchymosis (raccoon's eyes), mastoid ecchymosis (Battle's sign), rhinorrhea (CSF or blood leaking from the nose), otorrhea (CSF or blood leaking from the ears), hemotympanum (blood behind the tympanic membrane), conjunctival hemorrhage, and cranial nerve dysfunction. The presence of otorrhea or rhinorrhea indicates a dural tear with increased risk of meningitis. Although most CSF leaks stop spontaneously, those that persist may require surgical repair. Management of CSF leak includes elevating the head of bed, antibiotics, and, occasionally, lumbar drainage of CSF to decrease pressure on the healing dura.

Primary Brain Injury

The damage that results from TBI is due to both the primary insult and secondary injury produced by ongoing intracranial and systemic complications. Primary injury can be described as focal (resulting in local damage at the site of injury) or diffuse (affecting the whole brain). Focal injuries take up space, and can cause tissue compression, increased ICP, brain shift, and herniation. Examples of focal injury include cerebral contusions and hematomas. Diffuse brain injuries involve microscopic damage to cells deep in the white matter. They occur as lateral head motion produces angular movement of the brain within the skull, causing shearing or stretching of axonal nerve fibers. Damage is variable and dependent on the amount of accelerative force transmitted to the brain. Focal and diffuse brain injuries do not typically occur in isolation; for example, a patient with a focal cerebral contusion is also likely to have some component of diffuse brain injury.

Examples of primary injury follow.

- *Contusion:* Contusions are cortical bruises caused by the brain impacting the inside of the skull. They may be described as coup (occurring at the site of impact) or contrecoup (occurring opposite the site of impact). The frontal and temporal lobes are common sites of contusions. Clinical presentation depends on the site and extent of brain injury. Progressive focal edema and mass effect may result in neurologic deterioration. The severity of injury may not be apparent on the initial CT scan, because bleeding into the contused or lacerated tissue often occurs and results in intracerebral hematoma. Repeat CT scanning may be performed to evaluate for injury progression.
- *Epidural hematoma:* (EDH, Figure 20-4). EDH is a blood clot located between the dura and the skull. EDH is often associated with skull fractures that lacerate an underlying artery, and is most common in the temporal region due to tearing of the middle meningeal artery. Patients may have a lucid interval especially if the injury is very focal (eg, struck by a baseball or other solid object) and then deteriorate rapidly as the clot expands, displacing brain structures,

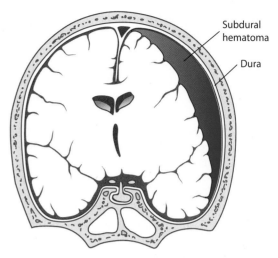

Figure 20-5. Schematic illustration of a subdural hemorrhage. *(Reprinted from: Waxman SG. Vascular supply. In: Waxman SG, ed.* Clinical Neuroanatomy. *New York, NY: Lange Medical Books/McGraw-Hill; 2003:187.)*

and causing increased ICP. While a lucid interval suggests EDH, many patients do not follow this course. Symptoms of EDH include a decrease in consciousness, headache, seizures, vomiting, hemiparesis, and pupillary dilation. Management includes emergency surgery to evacuate the hematoma.

- *Subdural hematoma:* (SDH, Figure 20-5.) Bleeding occurs within the subdural space between the dura and arachnoid layer, creating direct pressure on the brain. SDH results from rupture of the bridging veins between the brain and dura, bleeding from contused or lacerated brain tissue, or extension from an intracerebral hematoma. SDH is described as acute if symptoms begin within the first 48 hours after injury. Many patients experience significant symptoms immediately following the injury or much sooner than 48 hours. Patients with acute SDH present with progressive decline in level of consciousness, headache, agitation, and confusion. Motor deficits, pupillary changes, and cranial nerve dysfunction may be seen reflecting the primary brain injury and compressive effects. Treatment of acute SDH consists of evacuation of the hematoma by craniotomy. Blood may also collect in the subdural space more slowly, over days to weeks (subacute SDH) or weeks to months (chronic SDH). The onset of symptoms is insidious because the brain can better compensate for this slow increase in mass. Symptoms include an increasingly severe headache, confusion, drowsiness, and, possibly, seizures, pupillary abnormalities, or motor dysfunction. Predisposing conditions include advanced age, alcoholism, and disorders or treatments that result in prolonged coagulation times. Treatment of subacute or chronic SDH includes evacuation via burr holes or craniotomy.

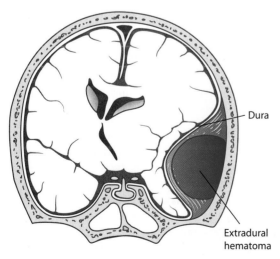

Figure 20-4. Schematic illustration of an epidural hemorrhage. *(Reprinted from: Waxman SG. Vascular supply. In: Waxman SG, ed.* Clinical Neuroanatomy. *New York, NY: Lange Medical Books/McGraw-Hill; 2003:187.)*

- *Traumatic subarachnoid hemorrhage:* Traumatic SAH can occur alone or in combination with other types of primary brain injury. The risk of symptomatic vasospasm is thought to be less than that associated with aneurysmal SAH, perhaps because the amount of blood seen in the subarachnoid space is typically less with traumatic SAH than when SAH is due to aneurysm rupture. In patients who present with traumatic SAH, the possibility that the patient experienced an aneurysmal SAH (which then caused the traumatic event) should be investigated, especially if the events preceding the trauma are unclear.
- *Diffuse injury:* Diffuse TBI exists on a continuum from cerebral concussion to severe diffuse axonal injury (DAI). Cerebral concussion is a transient, temporary neurologic dysfunction caused by rapid acceleration-deceleration or by a sudden blow to the head. Symptoms of concussion include headache, confusion, disorientation, and amnesia; most symptoms resolve without intervention. Patients with severe DAI, also called "shearing injury," typically experience an immediate and prolonged loss of consciousness and display abnormal posturing. The initial CT scan may appear normal, show signs of diffuse cerebral edema (decreased ventricle size, loss of differentiation between gray and white matter, and loss of sulci), or show very small areas of hemorrhage (punctate hemorrhage). The clinical course and outcome are dependent upon the severity of axonal injury.

Secondary Brain Injury

Patients with moderate to severe TBI are at significant risk for secondary brain injury, defined as ongoing neuronal damage that occurs following TBI as the result of systemic and intracranial complications. Care is directed at minimizing secondary injury by improving the supply of oxygenated blood to the brain and decreasing cerebral metabolic demands. Major contributors to secondary injury include the following:

- *Hypoxemia:* The brain needs a constant supply of oxygen to function. It is very sensitive to insults that create hypoxemia, such as pneumonia, atelectasis, chest trauma, neurogenic pulmonary edema, airway obstruction, and pulmonary embolus.
- *Hypotension:* Hypotension (SBP < 90 mm Hg) is associated with increased risk of mortality after TBI. Hypotension decreases cerebral blood flow, resulting in tissue ischemia and buildup of waste products. Mortality risk increases with multiple episodes of hypotension.
- *Anemia:* Anemia causes secondary injury by decreasing oxygen delivery to the brain. The optimal hematocrit in patients with cerebral insults is not known.
- *Hypo- or hyperglycemia:* The brain cannot store glucose and is dependent on a constant supply to maintain metabolic function. Hypoglycemia must be avoided because it disrupts this supply and leads to cellular dysfunction. Significant hypoglycemia is uncommon following TBI. Hyperglycemia is more common and is associated with increased mortality; it is unclear whether elevated blood glucose is a marker of injury severity or contributes to pathologic changes that increase mortality.
- *Increased metabolic demands:* Fever, agitation, and seizures increase metabolic demand. Fever increases ICP and can be due to an infectious process or injury to the hypothalamus.
- *Loss of autoregulatory mechanisms:* Autoregulatory mechanisms maintain constant cerebral blood flow within a wide range of blood pressures and ICP. The ability to autoregulate blood flow can be lost in the injured brain, increasing susceptibility to ischemia caused by decreased blood flow. The extent of this autoregulatory loss varies among patients.
- *Increased intracranial pressure (ICP):* Increased ICP negatively affects cerebral perfusion and the viability of neurons. The major sources of increased ICP after brain injury are cerebral edema and expanding lesions, such as hematomas. Edema may be localized to the site of the injury or diffuse, with maximal edema occurring 2 to 5 days after severe TBI.
- *Hypo- or hypercapnia:* Hypocapnia decreases cerebral blood flow by increasing pH and causing cerebral vasoconstriction. Decreased cerebral blood flow lowers ICP but creates a potentially ischemic state. Hypercapnia results in cerebral vasodilation and increases ICP, which may contribute to secondary injury.
- *Biochemical changes:* A number of biochemical changes occur following TBI, including the release of excitatory amino acids, free radical production, inflammation, and abnormal calcium shifts. A complete explanation of the processes underlying these changes is beyond the scope of this text. All factors contribute to changes in cellular function and can cause cell death. Much research has been completed in an attempt to stop these biochemical changes and confer neuroprotection; to date, none of these trials has demonstrated significant improvement in outcomes.

Clinical Presentation

Patients with TBI often present with external signs of trauma to the head such as ecchymosis, lacerations, and abrasions. Level of consciousness is the most important indicator of severity of injury and is assessed using the GCS. A decreasing GCS or changes in pupil size, shape, or reactivity indicate neurologic deterioration and warrant immediate physician notification. The type, location, and severity of TBI determine specific neurologic assessment findings. Patients may display hemiparesis, hemiplegia, language deficits, cognitive changes, or behavioral changes. If the injury is severe, the patient may display flexor or extensor posturing, as well as autonomic instability (eg, fever, tachycardia, or hypertension).

Patients with mild TBI do not display focal deficits such as hemiplegia or hemiparesis, but report a variety of physical, cognitive, and emotional symptoms. Signs and symptoms of mild TBI include headache, nausea/vomiting, dizziness, balance disturbance, visual problems, fatigue, and sensitivity to light or sound. Patients often report difficulty concentrating, decreased memory for recent events, slowed thought processes, irritability, anxiety, sadness, and increased emotion. Sleep disturbances are also common following mild TBI, and include both drowsiness/increased need for sleep and difficulty sleeping.

Diagnostic Tests

Computerized Tomography scanning is used to rapidly identify hematomas in need of evacuation. Other bleeding (such as into the subarachnoid space), contusions, skull fractures, and cerebral edema can be detected on CT. MRI is useful in the detection of DAI, brain stem injury, and vascular injury but is not typically included in the initial evaluation. The diagnostic work-up of the TBI patient includes a search for other injuries as appropriate to the mechanism of injury.

Principles of Management of Traumatic Brain Injury

Management priorities for patients with TBI vary based on the severity of injury.

Mild Traumatic Brain Injury (GCS 13-15)

Patients with mild TBI and an abnormal CT scan may be admitted to the progressive care unit for serial neurologic examination, or for monitoring and management of other injuries. These patients require assessment of neurologic status and education regarding possible sequelae of mild TBI, including headaches, difficulty concentrating, dizziness, fatigue, irritability, decreased processing speed, and sleep disturbances. Resources for follow-up are provided to the patient and family. In most cases, the symptoms will resolve, but evaluation by a neuropsychologist or other rehabilitation professional is recommended if symptoms persist.

Moderate Traumatic Brain Injury (GCS 9-12)

Moderate TBI poses a significant challenge to the healthcare team. A number of these patients will decline and require aggressive management similar to patients with severe TBI. Others will improve without intervention. Patients with moderate TBI who are admitted to the progressive care unit should be monitored very closely, with neurological assessment at least hourly. Any change found in neurological examination is immediately acted upon by the healthcare team.

Severe Traumatic Brain Injury (GCS ≤8)

The initial management of patients with severe TBI takes place in the ICU and is focused on optimizing functional recovery by minimizing secondary brain injury. In addition, other injuries must be identified and treated. An understanding of the early management of these patients gives the progressive care nurse insight into the patient's overall hospital course, which is often helpful in supporting families. In addition, these general principles can be applied to any patient with TBI who is experiencing neurologic worsening.

General principles of management for the patient with severe TBI include:

- *Airway management:* Patients with a GCS of 8 or less require intubation and mechanical ventilation. Patients with TBI are treated with spine precautions until injury to the spinal column can be ruled out, so manual in-line stabilization of the cervical spine is used during intubation. In patients with severe TBI, a tracheostomy is often placed once the patient's condition has stabilized to allow faster ventilator weaning and facilitate rehabilitation.

- *Oxygenation:* Hypoxemia worsens secondary brain injury and is avoided. Patients with severe TBI may vomit and aspirate prior to airway placement, or may have thoracic injuries, complicating pulmonary management. The need for aggressive pulmonary care often continues following transfer from the ICU.

- *Ventilation:* In general, the goal of management is to maintain a normal $Paco_2$. Hypoventilation causes cerebral vasodilation, which may increase ICP. Prolonged or prophylactic hyperventilation is not recommended because it causes cerebral vasoconstriction, which lowers ICP but may cause cerebral ischemia. Hyperventilation is used for short periods to lower ICP in the setting of acute neurologic worsening while other more definitive measures are implemented.

- *Fluid and volume management:* The goal of fluid management is to maintain euvolemia. Hypotonic solutions are avoided because they increase cerebral edema. Patients with TBI, especially those with autonomic instability due to DAI, often have large insensible losses due to diaphoresis and fever and are at risk for dehydration. Patients with injury to the hypothalamus or pituitary gland are at risk for diabetes insipidus (DI) or syndrome of inappropriate antidiuretic hormone (SIADH), further complicating fluid management. For more information on DI and SIADH, refer to Chapter 16, Endocrine System.

- *Managing increased ICP:* Initially, an ICP monitor is placed in patients with severe TBI to help guide management. Treatment is initiated when ICP is sustained above 20 mm Hg (see Special Procedures for Intracranial Pressure at the end of this chapter). These patients are managed in the ICU, but increased ICP can also occur in patients admitted to the progressive care unit with moderate TBI who worsen neurologically, or in response to late complications of severe TBI such as hydrocephalus. Nursing measures to prevent and manage elevations in ICP are discussed in Chapter 12,

Neurologic System. Of note, steroids worsen outcome following TBI and should not be given.

- *Supporting cerebral perfusion:* Hypotension (SBP < 90 mm Hg) is associated with a poor outcome in TBI patients. Cerebral perfusion pressure (CPP, calculated by subtracting ICP from MAP) is an indirect indicator of cerebral blood flow. Goal CPP may vary slightly based on clinical scenario and other monitors of cerebral perfusion, but a CPP of less than 50 mm Hg is avoided because of cerebral ischemia.

- *Preventing increased cerebral oxygen demand:* Seizures, fever, and agitation increase cerebral oxygen demand and are avoided. An anticonvulsant is used to prevent posttraumatic seizures during the first 7 days after injury. Continued seizure prophylaxis does not impact the development of posttraumatic seizures and is not recommended. Fever is known to be detrimental to the injured brain. For every 1°C increase in temperature, cerebral metabolism increases by approximately 6%. To prevent additional demands on the injured brain, fever is controlled. It is important to avoid or manage shivering when treating fever because shivering markedly increases cerebral metabolic demand. Agitation also increases cerebral oxygen demand. Strategies to avoid agitation include maintaining a calm, quiet environment and the use of sedating medications. Pain management is very important; short-acting medications are used to allow on-going evaluation of mental status.

Preventing Secondary Complications

Common secondary complications include pneumonia and other infections, deep venous thrombosis (DVT), pulmonary embolism, gastric ulcers, and skin breakdown. Nutrition is started within the first 3 days after injury. DVT prophylaxis is initiated on admission with graduated compression stockings and pneumatic compression devices. Pharmacologic prophylaxis varies by practitioner and type of TBI. Inferior vena caval (IVC) filters are placed in patients who develop DVT and cannot be anticoagulated to decrease the risk of PE.

Complications of immobility are common in patients with TBI. Progression of activity is optimized with early spine clearance. Institutional protocols vary, but typically include a series of spine x-rays, CT scanning, and potentially MRI to rule out injury to the bones and ligaments of the spine.

Promoting Recovery after Traumatic Brain Injury

Most patients progress through a series of recovery stages, during which they become more alert, then agitated, then purposeful and more appropriate. The Rancho Los Amigos scale (Table 20-2) is useful in tracking patient recovery, planning interventions, and educating family members. Managing agitation is frequently challenging in patients with TBI. Environmental strategies are very important; stimulation is decreased, the room is kept quiet, and a calm demeanor is maintained by staff and family members. Only one person speaks at a time, and the patient is allowed extra time to respond to questions. Consistent staff members are assigned to care for the patient. All lines and tubes (indwelling bladder catheters, IVs) are removed as soon as possible. Medications are often prescribed as part of managing agitation in patients with TBI but should be used in the smallest doses possible for the shortest time possible because they may slow recovery. Restraints should be avoided unless patient or staff safety is compromised.

TABLE 20-2. RANCHO LOS AMIGOS LEVELS OF COGNITIVE FUNCTIONING SCALE AFTER HEAD TRAUMA

Level	Response	Description
1	None	Completely unresponsive to any stimulus
2	Generalized	Reacts inconsistently and nonpurposefully to stimuli; may respond with physiologic changes, gross body movements, or utterances
3	Localized	Reacts specifically but inconsistently to stimuli; responds directly to a stimulus; shows vague awareness of self and body; may pull at tubes and react to discomfort
4	Confused, agitated	Heightened state of activity but unable to process information correctly; reacts to internal confusion; nonpurposeful behavior with confabulation present; cries, screams, and manifests aggressive behavior; cannot discriminate among people; performs gross motor activities but not self-care activities
5	Confused, inappropriate	Follows simple commands; may show agitated behavior from inability to cope with external demands; gross inattention to environment, easily distracted; impaired memory and inappropriate verbalization; cannot initiate tasks; often uses things incorrectly
6	Confused, appropriate	Displays goal-directed behavior but requires direction from others; follows simple commands; shows carryover of information from previously learned tasks; memory problems persist; inconsistently oriented to time and place; increased awareness of self and others
7	Automatic, appropriate	Oriented in hospital and home settings; performs tasks in robotlike manner; superficial awareness of own condition but lacks good problem-solving abilities; carryover for new learning; independent in self-care activities; needs structure but can initiate tasks of interest
8	Purposeful, appropriate	Alert and oriented; few memory problems; can begin vocational rehabilitation; carryover for new learning; social, emotional, and intellectual capacities may be decreased from pretrauma level

From: Malkmus D, Booth, B, Kodimer C. Rehabilitation of the Head Injured Adult—Comprehensive Cognitive Management. Downey, CA: Professional Staff Association of the Rancho Los Amigos Hospital;1980.

Patients with TBI benefit from a multidisciplinary team approach. Physical therapy, occupational therapy, nutrition, and social work are consulted early in the patient's hospital course. The speech therapist provides expert assistance with swallowing issues, language, and cognition. A number of other professionals may also be helpful, including the rehabilitation physician and neuropsychologist.

Family Education and Support

Traumatic brain injury alters the life of the injured individual and his or her family forever. The unpredictable nature of recovery from brain injury is difficult to comprehend. Family members may feel that information provided by different caregivers is inconsistent, or that insufficient information is being provided. They express the need to be involved in care—to be "part of the team."

Nurses can best support families of patients with TBI by providing direct, honest communication (including recognition of the difficulty of predicting prognosis) and by recognizing their need to be present and involved in care. The transition from the ICU to the progressive care unit is often a stressful time for family members. There is less uncertainty about whether or not the patient will live, but the extent of recovery remains unknown. Intensive and progressive care nurses can decrease family members' anxiety by collaborating to provide continuity of care and education about the stages of recovery.

TRAUMATIC SPINAL CORD INJURY

Etiology, Risk Factors, and Pathophysiology

Common causes of spinal cord injury (SCI) include motor vehicle accidents, falls, acts of violence, and sports-related injuries. The average age at time of injury has increased and is now 41 years. Over 80% of individuals with SCI are male, and approximately 60% of injuries involve the cervical region of the spinal cord. SCI causes varying degrees of paralysis and loss of sensation below the level of injury, and impacts physical, emotional, and social function. Similar to brain injury, deficits are due to both the initial impact (primary injury) and ongoing physiologic changes (secondary injury).

The spinal column consists of stacked vertebrae joined by bony facet joints and intervertebral disks. Ligaments provide structure and support to prevent the vertebrae from moving. The ring-like structure of the stacked vertebrae creates a hollow canal through which the spinal cord runs. SCI occurs when something (eg, bone, disk material, or foreign object) enters the spinal canal and disrupts the spinal cord or its blood supply. Mechanisms of injury include hyperflexion, hyperextension, axial loading/vertical compression, rotation, and penetrating trauma (Figure 20-6). Damage to the spinal cord can be characterized as concussion, contusion, laceration, transection, hemorrhage, or damage to the blood vessels that supply the spinal cord. Concussion causes temporary loss of function. Contusion is bruising of the spinal

cord that includes bleeding into the spinal cord, subsequent edema, and possible neuronal death from compression by the edema or damage to the tissue; the extent of neurologic deficits depends on the severity of the contusion. Laceration is an actual tear in the spinal cord that results in permanent injury. Transection is a severing of the spinal cord resulting in complete loss of function below the level of the injury. The most obvious example of cord laceration or transection is penetrating injury that disrupts the cord. Damage to the blood vessels that supply the spinal cord can result in ischemia and infarction, or hemorrhage due to vessel tearing. Regardless of the type of primary injury, secondary insults occur from cellular damage to the spinal cord, vascular damage, structural changes in the gray and white matter, and subsequent biochemical responses. Blood flow to the spinal cord is decreased significantly during the acute phase of injury, resulting in changes in metabolic function, destruction of cell membranes, and the release of free radicals. Patients may develop neurogenic shock following cervical and upper thoracic cord injury. Neurogenic shock results from loss of sympathetic nervous system input from the T1 to L2 area of the spinal cord, which normally increases heart rate and constricts the blood vessel walls. Loss of sympathetic outflow results in bradycardia and decreased vascular resistance. Blood pools in the peripheral vasculature, resulting in hypotension and decreased cardiac output. Neurogenic shock contributes to hypoperfusion and secondary injury.

Clinical Presentation

Assessment of the patient with SCI begins with evaluation of airway, breathing, and circulation, with attention to immobilization of the spine to prevent further injury during the assessment and any subsequent interventions. The focus then shifts to obtaining a baseline assessment of motor and sensory function. Assessment of motor function is performed at least every 4 hours during the acute postinjury period. Decreased motor function may be seen with swelling at the injury site, loss of vertebral alignment, or intrathecal hematoma formation. Changes in function warrant immediate physician notification.

The severity of deficits caused by SCI is determined by whether the injury is complete or incomplete and the level of the spinal cord affected. Acute SCI can result in the temporary suppression of reflexes controlled by segments below the level of injury, a phenomenon referred to as "spinal shock." Formal determination of complete vs incomplete SCI cannot be made until spinal shock is resolved. Complete SCI results in total loss of sensory and motor function below the level of injury due to complete interruption of motor and sensory pathways. Incomplete SCI results in mixed loss of motor and sensory function because some spinal tracts remain intact. Syndromes associated with incomplete SCI are described in Table 20-3. Deficits caused by SCI relate to the level at which the injury occurs (cervical, thoracic, or lumbar). Cervical and lumbar injuries are more common because these areas have

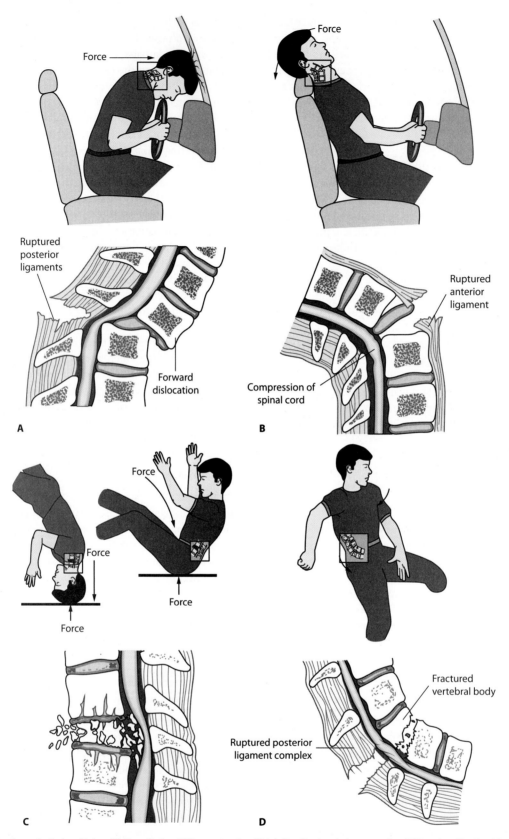

Figure 20-6. Mechanisms of spinal cord injury. **(A)** Hyperflexion. **(B)** Hyperextension. **(C)** Axial loading/vertical compression. **(D)** Rotation. *(Reprinted from: Sands JK. Spinal cord and peripheral nerve problems. In: Phipps WJ, Marek JF, Monahan FD, Neighbors M, Sands JK, eds.* Medical-Surgical Nursing: Health and Illness Perspectives. *St Louis, MO: Mosby; 2003:1405-1406.)*

TABLE 20-3. INCOMPLETE SCI SYNDROMES

Syndrome	Pathophysiolgy	Motor Function Below Level of Injury	Sensory Function Below Level of Injury
Central cord syndrome	Injury to central gray matter with preservation of outer white matter	Weakness/paralysis of upper extremities greater than lower extremities	Sensory loss greater in upper extremities than lower extremities
Anterior cord syndrome	Injury to anterior portion of spinal cord, disruption of blood flow through anterior spinal artery	Paralysis	Loss of pain and temperature with preservation of vibration and position sense
Posterior cord syndrome	Injury to posterior column	None	Loss of vibration and position sense with preservation of pain and temperature sensation
Brown-Séquard syndrome	Lateral injury to one side of the cord	Ipsilateral motor paralysis	Ipsilateral loss of vibration and position sense with contralateral loss of pain and temperature sensation

the greatest flexibility and movement. A cervical injury can result in paralysis of all four extremities, or tetraplegia (previously called quadriplegia). Injuries to the thoracic and lumbar areas can result in paraplegia. The American Spinal Injury Association (ASIA) scale (Figure 20-7) is frequently used to assess and document motor and sensory function. Specific functional losses from SCI are summarized in Figure 20-8.

Diagnostic Tests

Immobilization of the spinal column is maintained throughout the trauma evaluation to prevent additional injury. Cervical, thoracic, and lumbar spine x-rays identify the presence of injury to the vertebral column, although these tests are increasingly being replaced with specially constructed CT images. In addition to injury to the vertebral column, CT reveals many injuries to the spinal cord itself, such as bleeding or significant compression. Most patients with suspected SCI undergo an MRI to reveal more subtle signs of injury to the cord and soft tissue, like injury to the supporting ligaments. Injury to the ligaments and spinal cord is possible even without bony abnormalities.

Principles of Management of Acute Spinal Cord Injury

As with brain injury, initial management focuses on decreasing secondary injury and preventing complications. Priorities of management include:

Immobilization and Prevention of Further Injury

Patients with potential SCI are immobilized with a rigid cervical collar and backboard in the prehospital environment and a rigid cervical collar and bed rest in the hospital until injury is ruled out or confirmed clinically and radiographically. Some mattresses (such as air mattresses) do not provide adequate stability to the spinal column; follow manufacturer and institutional guidelines.

Supporting Oxygenation and Ventilation

Altered respiratory function is a major problem for patients with high thoracic or cervical SCI. Impaired oxygenation contributes to secondary injury. The diaphragm is controlled by the phrenic nerve, which exits the spinal cord at the C3 to

C5 level. Patients with complete injuries at or above the C2 level require mechanical ventilation due to the loss of diaphragmatic innervation. Patients with cervical or thoracic injuries below the level of diaphragmatic innervation will

ESSENTIAL CONTENT CASE

Acute Spinal Cord Injury

A 40-year-old construction worker fell approximately 12 ft off some scaffolding. When paramedics arrived, he had good strength in his upper extremities but was unable to move his legs and reported no sensation below his upper chest. On arrival at the emergency department, his heart rate was 62 beats/min, blood pressure 118/70 (MAP 86 mm Hg), and respirations 24 breaths/min and shallow. A CT scan revealed a T2 burst fracture with cord compression; his trauma work-up revealed no other injuries. Following surgical decompression and stabilization, he is admitted to the progressive care unit for close respiratory monitoring.

Case Question 1: Why does this patient require close respiratory monitoring?

Case Question 2: Two days after injury, the nurse notes that the patient is very withdrawn and refusing to be repositioned while in bed. What strategies can the nurse use to best meet this patient's needs?

Answers

1. This patient has an upper thoracic spinal cord injury. Although his respiratory drive will not be impaired, many of the other muscles required to take deep breaths and cough effectively will be impaired. He is at risk for developing neuromuscular respiratory failure due to atelectasis and retained secretions.

2. Becoming withdrawn or even demanding is a normal response to the loss of control experienced by SCI patients. It is crucial that the patient continue to receive necessary care like repositioning, because he is at very high risk for skin breakdown. Encouraging the patient to express his fears and make choices within the limits of the care routine are strategies that can be used to assist with coping. Consultation with other professionals (including rehabilitation specialists) may be helpful.

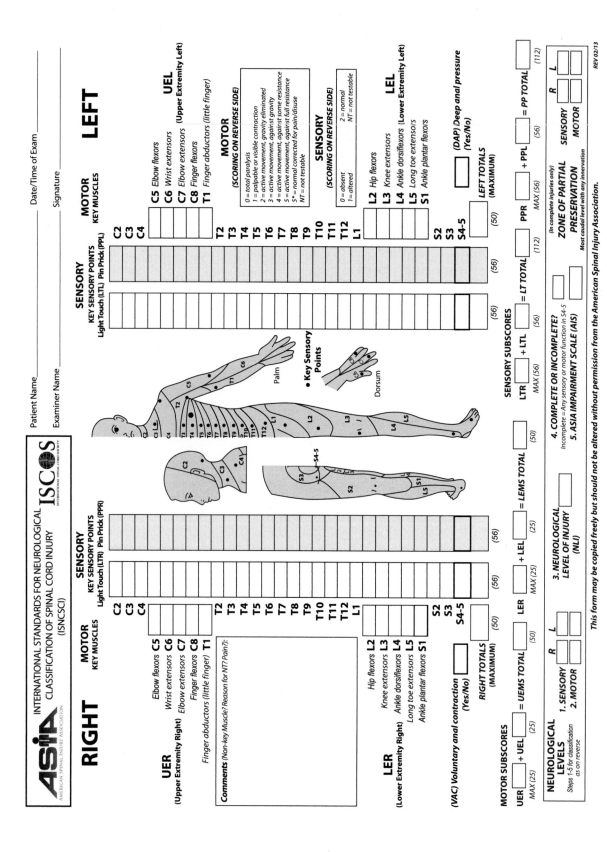

Figure 20-7. ASIA scale for the evaluation of patients with SCI (Copyright American Spinal Injury Association, last update 2/2013) Available at www.asia-spinalinjury.org. Accessed March 5, 2013.

Muscle Function Grading

0 = total paralysis

1 = palpable or visible contraction

2 = active movement, full range of motion (ROM) with gravity eliminated

3 = active movement, full ROM against gravity

4 = active movement, full ROM against gravity and moderate resistance in a muscle specific position

5 = (normal) active movement, full ROM against gravity and full resistance in a functional muscle position expected from an otherwise unimpaired person

5* = (normal) active movement, full ROM against gravity and sufficient resistance to be considered normal if identified inhibiting factors (i.e. pain, disuse) were not present

NT = not testable (i.e. due to immobilization, severe pain such that the patient cannot be graded, amputation of limb, or contracture of > 50% of the normal range of motion)

Sensory Grading

0 = Absent

1 = Altered, either decreased/impaired sensation or hypersensitivity

2 = Normal

NT = Not testable

Non Key Muscle Functions (optional)

May be used to assign a motor level to differentiate AIS B vs. C

Movement	Root level
Shoulder: Flexion, extension, abduction, adduction, internal and external rotation **Elbow:** Supination	C5
Elbow: Pronation **Wrist:** Flexion	C6
Finger: Flexion at proximal joint, extension. **Thumb:** Flexion, extension and abduction in plane of thumb	C7
Finger: Flexion at MCP joint **Thumb:** Opposition, adduction and abduction perpendicular to palm	C8
Finger: Abduction of the index finger	T1
Hip: Adduction	L2
Hip: External rotation	L3
Hip: Extension, abduction, internal rotation **Knee:** Flexion **Ankle:** Inversion and eversion **Toe:** MP and IP extension	L4
Hallux and Toe: DIP and PIP flexion and abduction	L5
Hallux: Adduction	S1

ASIA Impairment Scale (AIS)

A = Complete. No sensory or motor function is preserved in the sacral segments S4-5.

B = Sensory Incomplete. Sensory but not motor function is preserved below the neurological level and includes the sacral segments S4-5 (light touch or pin prick at S4-5 or deep anal pressure) AND no motor function is preserved more than three levels below the motor level on either side of the body.

C = Motor Incomplete. Motor function is preserved below the neurological level**, and more than half of key muscle functions below the neurological level of injury (NLI) have a muscle grade less than 3 (Grades 0-2).

D = Motor Incomplete. Motor function is preserved below the neurological level**, and at least half (half or more) of key muscle functions below the NLI have a muscle grade ≥ 3.

E = Normal. If sensation and motor function as tested with the ISNCSCI are graded as normal in all segments, and the patient had prior deficits, then the AIS grade is E. Someone without an initial SCI does not receive an AIS grade.

** For an individual to receive a grade of C or D, i.e. motor incomplete status, they must have either (1) voluntary anal sphincter contraction or (2) sacral sensory sparing with sparing of motor function more than three levels below the motor level for that side of the body. The International Standards at this time allows even non-key muscle function more than 3 levels below the motor level to be used in determining motor incomplete status (AIS B versus C).

NOTE: When assessing the extent of motor sparing below the level for distinguishing between AIS B and C, the *motor level* on each side is used; whereas to differentiate between AIS C and D (based on proportion of key muscle functions with strength grade 3 or greater) the *neurological level of injury* is used.

Steps in Classification

The following order is recommended for determining the classification of individuals with SCI.

1. Determine sensory levels for right and left sides.
The sensory level is the most caudal, intact dermatome for both pin prick and light touch sensation.

2. Determine motor levels for right and left sides.
Defined by the lowest key muscle function that has a grade of at least 3 (on supine testing), providing the key muscle functions represented by segments above that level are judged to be intact (graded as a 5).
Note: in regions where there is no myotome to test, the motor level is presumed to be the same as the sensory level, if testable motor function above that level is also normal.

3. Determine the neurological level of injury (NLI)
This refers to the most caudal segment of the cord with intact sensation and antigravity (3 or more) muscle function strength, provided that there is normal (intact) sensory and motor function rostrally respectively.
The NLI is the most cephalad of the sensory and motor levels determined in

4. Determine whether the injury is Complete or Incomplete.
(i.e. absence or presence of sacral sparing)
If voluntary anal contraction = No AND all S4-5 sensory scores = 0 AND deep anal pressure = No, then injury is Complete.
Otherwise, injury is **Incomplete.**

5. Determine ASIA Impairment Scale (AIS) Grade:

Is injury **Complete?** If YES, AIS=A and can record
       NO ↓   ZPP (lowest dermatome or myotome
            on each side with some preservation)

Is injury Motor **Complete?** If YES, AIS=B
       NO ↓   (No=voluntary anal contraction OR motor function
            more than three levels below the motor level on a
            given side, if the patient has sensory incomplete
            classification)

Are at least half (half or more) of the key muscles below the neurological level of injury graded 3 or better?

     NO ↓   **YES** ↓
   AIS=C   **AIS=D**

If sensation and motor function is normal in all segments, AIS=E
Note: AIS E is used in follow-up testing when an individual with a documented SCI has recovered normal function. If at initial testing no deficits are found, the individual is neurologically intact; the ASIA Impairment Scale does not apply.

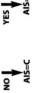

AMERICAN SPINAL INJURY ASSOCIATION

ISCOS
INTERNATIONAL SPINAL CORD SOCIETY

INTERNATIONAL STANDARDS FOR NEUROLOGICAL CLASSIFICATION OF SPINAL CORD INJURY

Figure 20-7. (Continued)

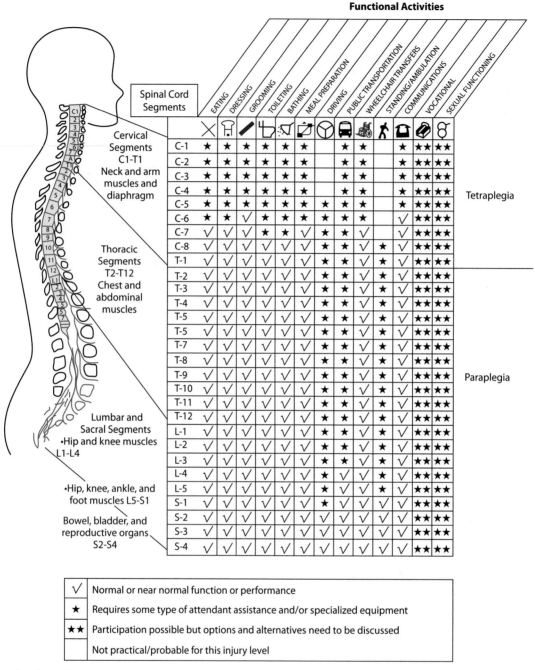

Figure 20-8. Spinal cord injury functional activity chart. *(Reproduced with permission from Monahan FD, Phipps WJ, Neighbors M, et al. Phipps' medical-surgical nursing: Health and illness perspectives, 8th ed. Mosby Elsevier, 2006)*

initiate breaths but still experience respiratory compromise due to paralysis of the intercostal and abdominal muscles. Paralysis of the intercostal muscles causes the chest wall to be flaccid. Contraction of the diaphragm creates a negative pressure in the thoracic cavity and the intercostal muscles retract, decreasing lung capacity. Upright positioning creates further downward displacement of the diaphragm and increases intercostal retraction; flat positioning can improve respiratory function in patients with cervical or thoracic SCI, and abdominal binders can be useful.

With time, the intercostal muscles become spastic and the chest wall no longer collapses with inspiration, promoting improved ventilation.

Pulmonary function is closely monitored in patients with cervical and thoracic SCI. Ongoing assessment of maximal inspiratory pressure (MIP) and forced vital capacity allow early identification of impending respiratory failure. In general, a patient who is unable to generate an MIP of at least -20 cm H_2O or a vital capacity of greater than 10 to 15 mL/kg requires intubation and mechanical ventilation.

Noninvasive ventilation may be considered but does not address problems related to inadequate clearance of secretions.

Hemodynamic Support

Neurogenic shock occurs in patients with cervical or thoracic injury and causes significant hemodynamic alterations, including bradycardia and hypotension. Management focuses on the following:

- Differentiating neurogenic shock from other types of shock. SCI can mask the signs and symptoms of other trauma, including hemorrhage in the abdomen or pelvis.
- Administration of intravenous fluids and vasopressors. Hypotension due solely to neurogenic shock reflects fluid displacement into the vasodilated periphery, not a true lack of fluid volume. As with all trauma patients, adequate fluid resuscitation is important, but continued fluid administration will not correct hypotension and can lead to pulmonary edema or heart failure especially in patients with comorbidities. Norepinephrine is frequently used to counter the loss of sympathetic tone and to provide inotropic and chronotropic support. Limited research shows that maintaining MAP > 85 mm Hg in the week following injury may improve neurologic outcomes. Pending definitive evidence, target blood pressure varies by practitioner. At most institutions, patients requiring vasopressor support due to neurogenic shock or for blood pressure augmentation will be managed in the ICU.
- Monitoring for bradycardia. Patients with SCI above T6 may experience bradycardia. Bradycardia can be profound in patients with cervical injury, even progressing to asystole. Bradycardia occurs more frequently during suctioning; the risk can be lessened but not eliminated by maintaining adequate oxygenation and ventilation. Symptomatic bradycardia is treated with atropine, although some patients require pacemaker placement.

Neuroprotection

There are no currently approved neuroprotective agents that improve outcomes after SCI. Although high-dose methylprednisolone was a part of SCI management for many years, administration is not recommended because there are many associated complications and no convincing benefit. Neuroprotection is an area of ongoing research, and includes both pharmacologic and nonpharmacologic strategies.

Decompression and Stabilization

Early management of SCI includes decompression of the spinal canal and stabilization of the spinal column. In patients with cervical injury, traction may be used to realign the spinal column and relieve pressure on the spinal cord. Traction devices include Gardner-Wells tongs and a halo device (see manufacturer's literature for more information). Nursing responsibilities during traction placement include patient monitoring, pain management, and administration of sedating agents. Decompression of the spinal cord can also be accomplished surgically. Rapid surgical intervention is indicated for patients with a worsening neurologic examination and ongoing spinal cord compression.

Stabilization of the spinal column does not improve neurologic function but enables the patient to be mobilized without causing additional damage to the spinal cord. In patients who require operative decompression of the spinal canal, the spinal column is stabilized at the time of surgery using rods, screws, or other hardware. For other patients, the timing of surgical stabilization varies. Surgery is commonly performed within 24 hours of injury if the patient's cardiorespiratory status is stable because early surgery decreases secondary complications and length of stay. Some fractures can be managed without surgery by immobilizing the spinal column and allowing the bones to heal. Immobilization is achieved using a cervical collar, halo vest, or other orthotic device. Skin care is a primary concern for these patients because skin breakdown can occur at contact points with the brace, especially in patients with decreased sensation.

Bladder and Bowel Management

Areflexia caused by spinal shock leads to urinary retention. An indwelling catheter is placed on admission and maintained until the patient is hemodynamically stable and fluid intake is consistent. A program of scheduled intermittent catheterization is then implemented.

A bowel program is initiated soon after admission and typically includes daily stool softeners, glycerin or bisacodyl suppositories, and digital stimulation. For patients with injuries at or above T6, an anesthetic jelly is used to decrease the risk of autonomic dysreflexia (see Complications later in section). The goal of the bowel program is for the patient to have a bowel movement at planned intervals, without incontinence between scheduled evacuations. An effective bowel program decreases constipation, limits incontinence, decreases skin breakdown, and increases the patient's sense of control.

Managing Pain

Pain following SCI impacts functional recovery and can be challenging to treat. During the immediate postinjury period, many patients complain of musculoskeletal pain and neuropathic pain (described as a burning sensation, paresthesia, or hypersensitivity). Medications prescribed include opiates and muscle relaxants. Antidepressants and anticonvulsants are useful in the treatment of neuropathic pain. Some patients benefit from nonpharmacologic methods such as massage, visual imagery, and diversional activities.

Managing Anxiety

Fear, uncertainty, and anxiety are common emotions following SCI. The psychological and emotional trauma of SCI can be overwhelming. Sudden paralysis does not allow patients or family members to prepare for this major insult. Anxiety results from the hospital environment, feelings of total dependence, sensory deprivation, powerlessness, and an unknown future.

A trusting relationship must be established between the patient and the healthcare team. Use of eye contact, patience, honesty, and consistency are reassuring to the patient. Encouraging self-care within the patient's abilities decreases feelings of complete dependence. Whenever possible, the patient is allowed choices within the daily care routine. Contracting with the patient may be helpful in setting limits for some patients. The family and significant others are incorporated into the plan of care.

Prevention and Management of Complications

The prevention and effective management of complications maximizes rehabilitation potential. Common complications include:

- *Respiratory complications:* Respiratory complications are common and contribute to morbidity and mortality. Chest physiotherapy and assisted coughing ("quad" coughing) are used in both ventilated and nonventilated patients. In addition, a mechanical cough assist device (in-exsufflator) can be used to clear secretions. This device imitates a physiologic cough by providing a deep breath via positive pressure followed by negative pressure. Standard measures to prevent hospital-acquired pneumonia, such as head of bed elevation and oral care, are implemented.
- *Gastrointestinal problems:* Paralytic ileus is common immediately following injury. Initially, an orogastric or nasogastric tube may be placed for decompression, especially in patients with cervical or thoracic injuries. Nutrition (preferably enteral) is started within the first 3 days after injury. Patients with acute SCI are at increased risk for stress ulcers, so it is common to initiate prophylactic medications on admission.
- *Skin breakdown:* The patient with SCI is at high risk for skin breakdown due to decreased blood flow to the skin and decreased cutaneous response to focal pressure. Meticulous skin care is essential. Skin inspection is performed at least twice daily and pressure reduction strategies are implemented. Early in the hospitalization, the patient who requires assistance with repositioning is encouraged to request that assistance at scheduled intervals. This increases the patient's sense of control and self-care responsibility, which is associated with improved long-term outcomes.
- *Orthostatic hypotension:* Blood pools in the lower extremities due to loss of sympathetic vascular tone. Nursing strategies to decrease orthostatic hypotension include application of graduated compression stockings and elastic wraps to the legs, hydration, and gradual progression to an upright position. If these measures are ineffective, medication to raise blood pressure may be ordered.

- *Altered thermoregulation:* Individuals with SCI at or above the T6 level are unable to conserve heat by vasoconstriction or shivering. Heat loss is compromised by the inability to sweat below the level of injury.
- *Deep vein thrombosis:* Recommended strategies for prevention during acute hospitalization include mechanical prophylaxis for all patients starting at the time of admission, followed by low-molecular weight heparin or the combination of low-dose unfractionated heparin and intermittent pneumatic compression. To prevent pulmonary embolus secondary to DVT, IVC filters can be placed in patients who develop DVT or who cannot receive pharmacologic prophylaxis.
- *Spasticity:* During spinal shock, there is a total loss of motor function below the level of injury. Flaccid paralysis progresses to spastic paralysis as spinal shock resolves. Measures to decrease spasticity in the acute postinjury phase include frequent range-of-motion exercises and medications. Occupational and physical therapy are consulted early in the course of hospitalization.
- *Autonomic dysreflexia:* Autonomic dysreflexia (also called autonomic hyperreflexia) is a life-threatening complication that occurs in individuals with SCI at or above T6 due to unopposed sympathetic response below the level of injury. It can occur any time after spinal shock has resolved. Autonomic dysreflexia results from a variety of stimuli, including overdistended bladder (most common), full rectum, infection, skin stimulation, pressure sores, and pain. The stimulus causes massive vasoconstriction that clinically presents with elevation of blood pressure (relative to the patient's baseline). Other signs and symptoms include headache, nasal congestion, nausea, blurred vision, flushing and diaphoresis above the level of injury, and feelings of apprehension of anxiety. In some individuals, the only sign of autonomic dysreflexia is elevated blood pressue. Autonomic dysreflexia is a medical emergency and the physician is promptly notified. Treatment includes moving the patient into a sitting position, and promptly identifying and treating the underlying cause (eg, bladder distention, bowel impaction).

Monitor blood pressure and pulse closely and administer short-acting antihypertensive agents as ordered. The timing of pharmacologic intervention varies based on patient characteristics, suspected cause of the event, and institutional guidelines. Careful attention to bowel and bladder management aids in the prevention of autonomic dysreflexia.

Future Spinal Cord Injury Treatment

Currently, much research is focused on SCI. The major areas of investigation include limiting the neuronal damage caused by secondary injury (neuroprotection), enhancing regrowth of neurons (nerve regeneration), and encouraging increased activity of functioning neurons (synaptic plasticity). One resource for patients and families who request information about clinical trials is a web site sponsored by the National Institutes of Health, www.clinicaltrials.gov.

BRAIN TUMORS

Etiology, Risk Factors, and Pathophysiology

The epidemiology of brain tumors varies widely based on tumor type. When all primary CNS tumors are grouped together, the incidence is higher in women than men. This overall gender difference is attributable to increased incidence of meningiomas in women. Prognosis varies based on age (younger patients have a better prognosis), tumor type and degree of differentiation, functional status at diagnosis, and anatomic tumor location. The most common brain tumors are meningiomas, gliomas, and metastatic lesions. Intracranial tumors are classified by distinguishing criteria.

Primary vs Secondary

Primary intracranial tumors originate from the cells and structures in the brain. Secondary or metastatic intracranial tumors originate from structures outside the brain, such as primary tumors of the lung or breast.

Histologic Origins

During the early stage of embryonic development, two types of undifferentiated cells are found—the neuroblasts and the glioblasts. The neuroblasts become neurons. The glioblasts form a variety of cells that support, insulate, and metabolically assist the neurons. The glioblasts are collectively referred to as glial cells and are subdivided into astrocytes, oligodendrocytes, and ependymal cells. This is the basis of a broad category of intracranial tumors called gliomas. Gliomas are subdivided into astrocytomas, oligodendrogliomas, oligoastrocytomas (also called mixed gliomas), and ependymomas. Gliomas are graded based on histologic criteria related to the degree of differentiation from the parent cell. Higher-grade tumors are more malignant. Glioblastoma multiforme (GBM) is a rapidly growing, poorly differentiated tumor. GBM is the most aggressive brain tumor and carries the worst prognosis.

A meningioma is a tumor that arises not from the brain itself, but from the meninges that surround the brain. Meningiomas tend to grow slowly and compress rather than invade the brain. Prognosis is excellent if the tumor is in a surgically accessible location. Neuromas (also called schwannomas) are noninvasive, slow-growing tumors that arise from the Schwann cells, which produce myelin. Pituitary adenomas, located in the pituitary gland, can be secretory or nonsecretory. Secretory tumors increase the production of hormones such as prolactin, growth hormone, adrenocorticotropic hormone, thyrotropin, or gonadotropin. Nonsecretory pituitary tumors cause symptoms through mass effect; patients commonly present with visual changes due to compression of the optic chiasm. Pituitary tumors are treated with pharmacologic agents, surgery, radiation therapy, or a combination of these modalities. The tumors described here are the ones most likely to be encountered in practice; other less common types of brain tumors are beyond the scope of this text.

Anatomic Location

This refers to the actual site of the tumor, such as the frontal lobe, temporal lobe, pons, or cerebellum. Knowing the location of the tumor helps predicting deficits based on the normal functions of that anatomic area. Anatomic location also can refer to the location of the tumor in reference to the tentorium. Supratentorial refers to tumors located above the tentorium (cerebral hemispheres), and infratentorial refers to tumors located below the tentorium (brain stem and cerebellum).

Benign vs Malignant

The distinction between benign and malignant intracranial tumors is based on histologic examination. Tumors made up of well-differentiated cells are "benign" and the prognosis is generally better than if cells are poorly differentiated. However, a histologically benign tumor can be surgically inaccessible. This benign tumor continues to grow and ultimately contributes to a decline in neurologic function and even death. Benign tumors may convert to more histologically malignant types as they develop.

Clinical Presentation

Brain tumors occupy space, causing compression of brain structures, infiltration of tissue that controls functions, and displacement of normal tissue. Brain tumors disrupt the blood-brain barrier and cause cerebral edema. CSF flow may be obstructed by the tumor or edema, leading to hydrocephalus. Tumors are often vascular and may bleed, causing additional neurologic deficits.

The most common initial signs and symptoms of intracranial tumors are headache, seizures, papilledema, and vomiting. Headache is usually progressive in severity and worse after lying flat, for example, upon awakening from sleep. Clinical presentation may also include decreased level of consciousness, pupillary changes, visual abnormalities, and personality changes. Additional signs and symptoms depend upon the area of the brain that is being compressed or infiltrated (Table 20-4).

Diagnostic Tests

Computerized Tomography and MRI are used to differentiate tumor from abscess and to identify tumor location and characteristics. Functional MRI detects physiologic changes using MRI scanning during physical and cognitive activity and is helpful in mapping language, sensory, and motor function. Magnetic resonance spectroscopy and positive emission

TABLE 20-4. CLINICAL PRESENTATION OF BRAIN TUMORS RELATED TO LOCATION

Location	Clinical Presentation
Frontal lobe	Inappropriate behavior
	Inattentiveness
	Inability to concentrate
	Emotional lability
	Quiet but flat affect
	Expressive aphasia
	Seizures
	Headache
	Impaired memory
Parietal lobe	Hyperesthesia
	Paresthesia
	Astereognosis (inability to recognize an object by feeling it)
	Autotopagnosia (inability to locate or recognize parts of the body)
	Loss of left-right discrimination
	Agraphia (inability to write)
	Acalculia (difficulty in calculating numbers)
Temporal lobe	Psychomotor seizures
Occipital lobe	Visual loss in half of the visual field seizures
Pituitary and hypothalamus region	Visual deficits
	Headache
	Hormonal dysfunction of the pituitary gland
	Water imbalance and sleep alterations in tumors of the hypothalamus
Ventricles	Symptoms of increased ICP associated with obstruction of CSF flow
Cerebellum	Ataxia
	Incoordination
	Symptoms of increased ICP associated with obstruction of CSF flow

tomography scans evaluate cerebral metabolism and are used to provide information about how aggressive a tumor is (a more aggressive tumor will display higher metabolic activity) and to differentiate necrosis or scarring from tumor. Additional testing includes cerebral angiography, visual field and funduscopic examination, audiometric studies, and endocrine studies. If the lesion is suspected to be metastatic, additional diagnostic tests are done in an attempt to locate the primary tumor site, if not already known. A biopsy of the lesion determines tumor type and degree of differentiation. Biopsy may be performed via a burr hole using stereotactic guidance or may be done as part of a craniotomy for tumor resection.

Principles of Management of Intracranial Tumors

Treatment modalities are used alone or in any combination. Variables considered in selecting appropriate treatment include the type of tumor, its location and size, related symptoms, and the general condition of the patient.

Corticosteroids

A corticosteroid, typically dexamethasone, is administered to decrease vasogenic cerebral edema. Steroids are started in patients with brain tumors when the presence of cerebral edema is noted. Significant improvements in neurologic status can be seen soon after initiation of therapy. Side effects of steroid therapy include gastric irritation, mood swings, fluid retention, hyperglycemia, myopathy, insomnia, and increased risk of infection.

Surgery

The goal of surgery is to resect as much of the tumor as possible with minimal harm to normal tissue. In most cases, a craniotomy is done to provide access for resection. Total resection is curative for some tumor types. Some tumors cannot be completely removed because of location or histologic type. A partial resection of the tumor mass temporarily relieves the symptoms of compression, and increased ICP may be relieved. If CSF flow is obstructed, treatment includes surgical placement of a shunt to reroute CSF from the ventricular system to another part of the body (usually the peritoneal space) where it can be reabsorbed.

Several strategies are available to decrease the morbidity associated with surgery. Intraoperative MRI is available at some centers and is most often used when the lesion is in or near the motor strip, difficult to access, or small and potentially hard to locate. Intraoperative MRI can be used alone or in conjunction with cortical mapping techniques. With cortical mapping, the patient is anesthetized for the initial part of the surgery, then awakened, and asked to perform certain tasks, allowing the surgeon to avoid areas that control speech or motor function. Stereotactic techniques allow targeted biopsy or resection based on previously obtained images.

Most patients undergo elective operations for intracranial tumors and may be admitted to the progressive care unit postoperatively. Postoperative management includes monitoring neurologic status, controlling pain, and preventing and managing complications. Potential complications in the immediate postoperative period include:

- *Hematoma formation:* Clinical signs include increasing headache, decreasing level of consciousness, and the development of new focal neurologic signs (eg, weakness of an arm or leg). If an intracranial bleed is suspected, a CT scan is obtained. If significant bleeding is found, the patient is returned to the operating room for surgical removal of the hematoma and management of bleeding points.
- *Cerebral edema:* Postoperative cerebral edema may occur due to the long surgical procedure and/or the retraction of brain tissue to expose the operative area. Cerebral edema is suspected if the patient presents postoperatively with greater neurologic deficits than were present preoperatively. A CT scan is obtained and treatment is initiated to decrease edema. As noted previously, dexamethasone is useful in the management of tumor-related edema.
- *Infection:* Infection can occur following surgery because of contamination in the operating room or

a defect in the dura, which allows communication of the CSF with the atmosphere.

- *Deep vein thrombosis:* Neurosurgical patients are at increased risk for DVT. Preventive measures to decrease this risk include the use of graduated compression stockings and intermittent pneumatic compression devices, early progression of activity, and low doses of subcutaneous unfractionated heparin.

Radiation Therapy

Radiation therapy preferentially destroys tumor cells because they are rapidly dividing, but affects normal cells also. The treatment dose depends on the histologic type, radioresponsiveness, location of the tumor, and patient tolerance. Increased edema is a common complication of radiation therapy. Patients typically remain on dexamethasone throughout treatment. Special techniques, such as stereotactic radiosurgery or gamma knife radiation, focus concentrated radiation from many directions on the tumor site and reduce radiation to normal tissue.

Chemotherapy

Chemotherapy is used to slow or stop the proliferation of abnormal cells. One commonly used agent in the treatment of high-grade gliomas is temozolomide (Temodar). Temozolimide is administered orally and is generally well-tolerated by patients.

Prevention and Management of Seizures

The incidence of seizures in patients with brain tumors ranges from 20% to 60%. Antiepileptic drugs are often given prophylactically to patients with supratentorial tumors. When seizures do occur, they are managed according to the guidelines described in Chapter 12, Neurologic System. Any seizure in the immediate postoperative period prompts an emergent CT scan to look for hematoma formation.

Special Considerations: Transsphenoidal Resection of Pituitary Tumors

The surgical management of patients with pituitary tumors differs because a transsphenoidal approach may be used (Figure 20-9). Transsphenoidal resection uses a special technique to reach pituitary tumors by going through the sphenoid sinus. An incision may be made under the patient's upper lip, or an endonasal approach may be used. Because the pituitary gland secretes a number of hormones, endocrine disturbances are common both before and after surgery. Care in the postoperative period is similar to that described for patients undergoing a craniotomy, but certain assessments are emphasized. Because the pituitary gland is located near the optic chiasm, visual acuity and visual field testing is essential. The patient is closely monitored for CSF leak, and is instructed not to blow his or her nose or lean over. Nasal packing, if present, is typically removed by the physician on the first or second postoperative day. Serum cortisol is

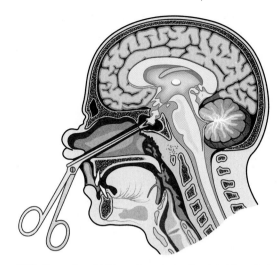

Figure 20-9. Transsphenoidal hypophysectomy. *(Reprinted from: Carlson BA: Neurologic disorders. In: Urden LD, Stacy KM, Lough ME, eds.* Thelan's Critical Care Nursing. *4th ed. St Louis, MO: Mosby; 2002:695.)*

monitored because the patient will no longer secrete adrenocorticotropic hormone if the anterior pituitary was resected. Close monitoring of fluid balance and electrolytes is required because of the risk of diabetes insipidus (DI). DI is caused by insufficient amounts of antidiuretic hormone (ADH), which is produced by the posterior lobe of the pituitary gland. If ADH is not secreted in sufficient amounts, the patient will produce large volumes of dilute urine. Significant fluid and electrolyte imbalances with dehydration can result. Intake and output are measured frequently (every hour initially). Electrolytes (especially sodium) and urine specific gravity are monitored frequently, typically every 4 hours. Serum and urine osmolality may also be monitored. Management of DI includes allowing the patient to drink fluids as needed to quench thirst. Management may also include IV therapy that correlates with urine output and administration of aqueous vasopressin or desmopressin acetate (DDAVP).

SPECIAL PROCEDURES: INVASIVE MONITORING OF INTRACRANIAL PRESSURE

Intracranial pressure is most often measured via a catheter inserted into the ventricles or a probe inserted into the brain parenchyma, but can also be measured in the subarachnoid space, epidural space, or subdural space (Figure 20-10). Use of an intraventricular catheter remains the gold standard for ICP measurement. Several systems exist, but the basic setup includes a catheter, transducer (either external or integrated into the catheter), and collection device for CSF. The catheter is placed via a burr hole into the anterior horn of the lateral ventricle. The zero point of the drainage system is leveled at the external landmark of the foramen of Monro and zeroed to atmospheric pressure using manufacturer's specifications. Slightly different external landmarks for the foramen of Monro are reported in the literature

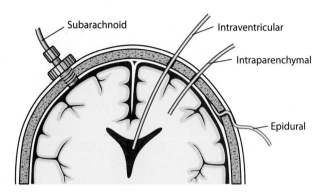

Figure 20-10. Sites for ICP monitoring. Illustration of possible sites for monitoring intracranial pressure: subarachnoid-subdural, intraventricular, intraparenchymal, and epidural. The "gold standard" remains the intraventricular catheter. *(Reprinted from: Lee KR, Hoff JT. Intracranial pressure. In: Youmans JR, ed. Neurological Surgery. Vol 1. Philadelphia, PA: WB Saunders; 1996:505.)*

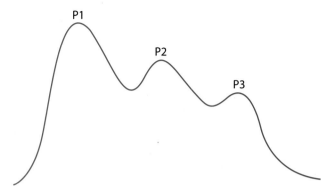

Figure 20-11. Components of a normal ICP waveform.

Intracranial Pressure Waveforms

With continuous ICP monitoring, there are fluctuations in waveforms that correlate with specific physiologic events. Examination of these waveforms can be helpful in evaluating changes in the patient's condition.

The ICP pulse waveform is a continuous, real-time pressure display that corresponds to each heartbeat. The normal pulse wave has three or more defined peaks representing blood and CSF flow within the cranium: percussion wave (P1), P2 (tidal wave), and P3 (dicrotic wave).

The pulse waveform at low pressures is a descending saw-toothed pattern with a distinct P1 (Figure 20-11). As mean ICP rises, a progressive elevation of P2 occurs, causing the pulse waveform to appear more rounded. When P2 is equal to or higher than P1, decreased compliance exists (Figure 20-12).

Trend recordings compress continuous ICP recording data to reflect general trends in ICP over longer time periods (minutes to hours). Three distinct pressure waves have been identified (Figure 20-13). A waves (plateau waves) are sudden increases in pressure lasting 5 to 20 minutes. They begin from a baseline of an already elevated ICP (> 20 mm Hg) and reflect cerebral ischemia. B waves are sharp, rhythmic oscillations of pressure (up to 50 mm Hg) occurring every 0.5 to 2 minutes. They are seen in relationship to fluctuations in the respiratory cycle, such as Cheyne-Stokes respirations. They are not clinically significant, but may progress to A waves. C waves are small rhythmic waves with pressures up to 20 mm Hg occurring 4 to 8 times per minute. They relate to normal changes in systemic arterial pressure, and their clinical significance is unknown.

Cerebral perfusion pressure (CPP) is a measurement of the pressure at which blood reaches the brain. CPP is an indirect reflection of CBF. It is calculated by subtracting ICP from mean arterial pressure (CPP = MAP − ICP).

(tragus, halfway between the outer canthus of the eye and the tragus, external auditory meatus); follow institutional protocols to maintain consistency among caregivers. The transducer senses the pressure exerted by the CSF in the ventricles and translates it into a waveform on the monitor. This system is referred to by several names, including external ventricular drain, ventriculostomy, and intraventricular catheter. The advantage of using an intraventricular catheter for monitoring is that CSF can be drained, providing a treatment modality for increased ICP. CSF drainage is controlled by adjusting the height of the system relative to the foramen of Monro. The height of the fluid column in the drainage system creates hydrostatic pressure that opposes ICP. If the drainage system is raised, CSF drainage decreases; when the drainage system is lowered, CSF drainage increases. Rapid drainage of CSF can result in ventricular collapse so CSF is drained in a controlled manner based on a predetermined ICP. This is accomplished by maintaining the drainage system at a specific height, such as 20 cm above the external landmark of the foramen of Monro, or by opening the system to allow CSF drainage only when the ICP exceeds a specified value. CSF drainage is monitored for amount and color. An occlusive dressing is maintained over the catheter site. Risks associated with intraventricular catheter placement include infection and hemorrhage caused by catheter placement. Sterile technique is essential when the catheter is placed and whenever the system is manipulated (for example, to sample CSF).

Intracranial pressure is also commonly monitored using a transducer inserted into the brain parenchyma. These monitors are easier to insert and have a lower rate of infection than intraventricular catheters. Leveling to the foramen of Monro is not required. Fiberoptic and strain gauge transducers are connected directly to an independent monitor, which provides an ICP reading. Other technology is available to monitor ICP, including some devices that allow rezeroing after monitor insertion, but these are less commonly used in practice. Normal ICP is 0 to 15 mm Hg in adults.

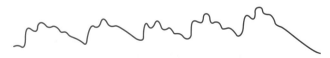

Figure 20-12. ICP waveform demonstrating decreased compliance.

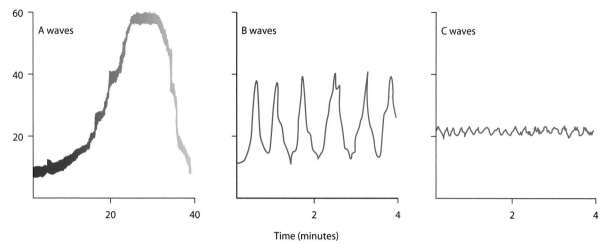

Figure 20-13. ICP trend recordings.

Decreased CPP occurs as the result of an increase in ICP, a decrease in mean arterial pressure, or both. A CPP of at least 50 to 60 mm Hg is necessary for adequate cerebral perfusion. CPP below 30 mm Hg results in irreversible neuronal hypoxia.

SPECIAL PROCEDURES: MANAGEMENT OF A PATIENT WITH A LUMBAR DRAIN

Lumbar drains are used in the progressive care unit to manage communicating hydrocephalus, and in patients with CSF leakage following neurosurgery or trauma to decrease pressure against the dura and allow it to heal. Lumbar drains are also used to improve spinal cord perfusion in the immediate post-operative period following thoracoabdominal aneurysm repair. The process for placing a lumbar drain is similar to performing a LP (see Chapter 12, Neurologic System). The physician threads the catheter into the sub-arachnoid space of the lumbar spine. Nursing responsibilities during placement include assistance with patient positioning and the administration of pain medications and sometimes sedation. Once the lumbar catheter has been placed, it is connected to an external drainage system. The amount of CSF drainage is determined by the height of the system, which corresponds to the amount of pressure within the spinal subarachnoid space. The lumbar drain may be left open so that CSF flows into the collection chamber whenever the pressure in the spinal subarachnoid space exceeds the pressure created by the height of the column of fluid in the drainage system or a certain amount of CSF may be drained every hour. Alternatively, an external transducer can be connected to the system to measure pressure within the spinal subarachnoid space, with orders to allow drainage only when the pressure exceeds a predetermined limit. The decision to keep the system open to drain continuously or to allow CSF to drain only when the pressure exceeds a certain value is made by the physician based on the reason for CSF drainage and provider preference.

The zero reference for leveling the drip chamber and transducer vary based on reason for drainage, provider preference, and institutional protocol. Common sites for leveling include the shoulder, the external auditory meatus, and the level of insertion. Nursing priorities when caring for a patient with a lumbar drain include maintaining the system at the ordered height (eg, 10 cm H_2O above the external auditory meatus). If the system is placed below the ordered height, overdrainage of CSF may result and can lead to the development of subdural hemorrhage or even herniation. If the lumbar drainage system is placed too high, CSF drainage may be inadequate for the desired purpose. Other potential complications include infection, bleeding, and sensory deficits related to nerve root injury or irritation. An occlusive sterile dressing is maintained at the insertion site. Practices related to mobilizing the patient with a lumbar drain vary; follow institutional standards and physician order.

SELECTED BIBLIOGRAPHY

Subarachnoid Hemorrhage

Brisman JL, Song JK, Newell DW. Cerebral aneurysms. *N Engl J Med.* 2006;355:928-939.

Diringer MN. Management of aneurysmal subarachnoid hemorrhage. *Crit Care Med.* 2009;37:432-440.

Hinkle JL, Guanci MM, Stewart-Amidei C. Cerebrovascular events of the nervous system. In: Bader MK, Littlejohns LR, eds. *AANN Core Curriculum for Neuroscience Nursing.* 5th ed. Glenview, IL: American Association of Neuroscience Nurses; 2010.

Li H, Pan R, Wang H, et al. Clipping versus coiling for ruptured intracranial aneurysms: a systematic review and meta-analysis. *Stroke.* 2013;44:29-37.

Molyneux AJ, Kerr RSC, Birks J, et al. Risk of recurrent subarachnoid haemorrhage, death, or dependence and standardised mortality ratios after clipping or coiling of an intracranial aneurysm in the International Subarachnoid Aneurysm Trial (ISAT): long-term follow-up. *Lancet Neurol.* 2009;8:427-433.

Solenski NJ, Haley EC, Kassell NF, et al. Medical complications of aneurysmal subarachnoid hemorrhage: a report of the multicenter, cooperative aneurysm study. *Crit Care Med.* 1995;23:1007-1017.

Sommargren CE. Electrocardiographic abnormalities in patients with subarachnoid hemorrhage. *Am J Crit Care.* 2002;11:48-56.

Traumatic Brain Injury

Bond AE, Draeger CRL, Mandleco B, Donnelly M. Needs of family members of patients with severe traumatic brain injury: implications for evidence-based practice. *Crit Care Nurs.* 2003;23:63-72.

Centers for Disease Control. Blast injuries: traumatic brain injury from explosions. Available at http://emergency.cdc.gov/masscasualties/blastinjury-braininjury.asp. Accessed March 2, 2013.

Faul M, Xu L, Wald MM, Coronado VG. *Traumatic Brain Injury in the United States: Emergency Department Visits, Hospitalizations and Deaths 2002–2006.* Atlanta (GA): Centers for Disease Control and Prevention, National Center for Injury Prevention and Control; 2010.

Lombard LA, Zafonte RD. Agitation after traumatic brain injury: considerations and treatment options. *Am J Phys Med Rehabil.* 2005;84:797-812.

March K, Criddle LM, Wellwood J, et al. Craniocerebral trauma. In: Bader MK, Littlejohns LR, eds. *AACN Core Curriculum for Neuroscience Nursing.* 54th ed. Glenview, IL: American Association of Neuroscience Nurses; 2010.

Spinal Cord Injury

Casha S, Christie S. A systematic review of intensive cardiopulmonary management after spinal cord injury. *J Neurotrauma.* 2011; 28:1479-1495.

Cotton BA, Pryor JP, Chinwalla I, et al. Respiratory complications and mortality risk associated with thoracic spine injury. *J Trauma.* 2005;59:1400-1409.

McIlvoy L, Meyer K, Mahanes D, Sachse S, McQuillan KA. Traumatic spine injuries. In: Bader MK, Littlejohns LR, eds. *AANN Core Curriculum for Neuroscience Nursing.* Glenview, IL: American Association of Neuroscience Nurses; 2010.

National Spinal Cord Injury Statistical Center. Spinal Cord Injury Facts and Figures at a Glance. February 2012. Retrieved March 2, 2013 from https://www.nscisc.uab.edu/.

Winslow C, Rozovsky J. Effect of spinal cord injury on the respiratory system. *Am J Phys Med Rehabil.* 2003;82:803-814.

Brain Tumors

Asthagiri AR, Pouratian N, Sherman J, Ahmed G, Shaffrey ME. Advances in brain tumor surgery. *Neurol Clin.* 2007;25:975-1003.

Bohan EM, Gallia GL, Bren H. Brain tumors. In: Barker E, ed. *Neuroscience Nursing: A Spectrum of Care.* 3rd ed. St Louis, MO: Mosby; 2008.

Stewart-Amidei C, Arzbaecher J, Lupica K. Nervous system tumors. In: Bader MK, Littlejohns LR, eds. *AANN Core Curriculum for Neuroscience Nursing.* 5th ed. Glenview, IL: American Association of Neuroscience Nurses; 2010.

Intracranial Pressure Monitoring

Madden LK, March K. Intracranial pressure management. In: Bader MK, Littlejohns LR, eds. *AANN Core Curriculum for Neuroscience Nursing.* 5th ed. Glenview, IL: American Association of Neuroscience Nurses; 2010.

March K, Olson D, Arbour R. Technology. In: Bader MK, Littlejohns LR, eds. *AANN Core Curriculum for Neuroscience Nursing.* 5th ed. Glenview, IL: American Association of Neuroscience Nurses; 2010.

March K, Wellwood J. Intracranial pressure concepts, cerebral blood flow, and metabolism. In: Bader MK, Littlejohns LR. eds. *AANN Core Curriculum for Neuroscience Nursing.* 45th ed. Glenview, IL: American Association of Neuroscience Nurses; 2010. St Louis: Saunders.

Evidence-Based Guidelines

Alexander S, Gallek M, Presciutti M, Zrelak P. Care of the Patient with Aneurysmal Subarachnoid Hemorrhage: AANN Clinical Practice Guidelines Series [electronic version]. Glenview, IL: American Association of Neuroscience Nurses; 2011. Available at http://www.aann.org/pubs/content/guidelines.html. Accessed April 5, 2013.

Brain Trauma Foundation, American Association of Neurological Surgeons, Congress of Neurological Surgeons, AANS/CNS Joint Section on Neurotrauma and Critical Care. *Guidelines for the Management of Severe Traumatic Brain Injury.* New York, NY: Brain Trauma Foundation; 2007.

Connolly ES, Rabinstein AA, Carhuapoma JR, et al. Guidelines for the management of aneurysmal subarachnoid hemorrhage. *Stroke.* 2012;43:1711-1737.

Consortium for Spinal Cord Medicine. *Early Acute Management in Adults with Spinal Cord Injury: A Clinical Practice Guideline for Health-Care Providers.* Washington, DC: Paralyzed Veterans of America; 2008.

Diringer MN, Bleck TP, Hemphill JC, et al. Critical care management of patients following aneurysmal subarachnoid hemorrhage: recommendations from the Neurocritical Care Society's multidisciplinary consensus conference. *Neurocrit Care.* 2011;15:211-240.

Leeper B, Lovasik D. Cerebrospinal drainage systems: external ventricular and lumbar drains. In: Littlejohns LR, Bader MK, eds. *AACN-AANN Protocols for Practice: Monitoring Technologies in Critically Ill Neuroscience Patients.* Sudbury, MA: Jones and Bartlett Publishers; 2009.

March K, Madden L. Intracranial pressure management. In: Littlejohns LR, Bader MK, eds. *AACN-AANN Protocols for Practice: Monitoring Technologies in Critically Ill Neuroscience Patients.* Sudbury, Massachusetts: Jones and Bartlett Publishers; 2009.

Mcilvoy L, Meyer K. Nursing Management of Adults With Severe Traumatic Brain Injury: AANN Clinical Practice Guideline Series [electronic version]. Glenview, IL: American Association of Neuroscience Nurses; 2011. Available at http://www.aann.org/pubs/content/guidelines.html. Accessed April 5, 2013.

The American Association of Neurological Surgeons and the Congress of Neurological Surgeons. Guidelines for the management of acute cervical spine and spinal cord injuries from the American Association of Neurological Surgeons and the Congress of Neurological Surgeons. *Clin Neurosurg.* 2013;72:1-259.

West TA, Bergman K, Biggins MS, et al. Care of the Patient with Mild Traumatic Brain Injury: AANN and ARN Clinical Practice Guideline Series [electronic version]. Glenview, IL: American Association of Neuroscience Nurses and Association of Rehabilitation Nurses. 2011. Available at http://www.aann.org/pubs/content/guidelines.html. Accessed April 5, 2013.

KEY REFERENCE INFORMATION

IV

Normal Values Table

Suzanne M. Burns

Abbreviation	Definition	Normal Value	Formula
A-a ratio	Alveolar-arterial oxygen gradient	100% Fio_2 A-a gradient ~75 mm Hg, on 21% Fio_2 A-a gradient ~10-15 mm Hg	A-a = gradient
BSA	Body surface area	Meters squared (m^2)	Value obtained from a nomogram based on height and weight
$C(a-v)O_2$	Arteriovenous oxygen content difference	4-6 mL/100 mL	$C(a-v)O_2$ (mL/100 mL or vol %) = $CaO_2 - Cvo_2$
CaO_2	Arterial oxygen content	~20 vol %	CaO_2 (mL O_2/100 mL blood or vol %) = (Hb × 1.39) SaO_2 + (Pao_2 × 0.0031)
CI	Cardiac index	2.5-4.3 L/min/m^2	$CI(L/min/m^2) = \dfrac{\text{cardiac output (L/min)}}{\text{body surface area }(m^2)}$
CK	Creatinine kinase	<120 mcg/L	
CK-MB	Creatinine kinase MB band	<3 ng/mL	
CO	Cardiac output	4-8 L/min	CO = stroke volume × heart rate
Cvo_2	Mixed venous oxygen content	~15 vol%	Cvo_2 (ml O_2/100 mL blood or vol%) = (Hb × 1.39) Svo_2 + (Pvo_2 × 0.0031)
CVP	Central venous pressure	2-8 mm Hg	
Cdyn	Dynamic compliance	~30-40 ml/cm H_2O	Cdyn = Vt/PIP-PEEP
Cstat	Static compliance	~50 ml/cm H_2O	Cstat = VT/Plat-PEEP
EF	Ejection fraction	70%	$\text{Ejection fraction} = \dfrac{SV}{EDV}$
FRC	Functional residual capacity	2400 mL (dependent on height)	Measured in a pulmonary function laboratory
HR	Heart rate	60-100 beats/min	
LVSW	Left ventricular stroke work	8-10 g/m/m^2	LVSW = SI × MAP × 0.0144
LVSWI	Left ventricular stroke work index	50-62 g/m^2/beat	SVI × (MAP-PAOP) × 0.0136
MAP	Mean arterial pressure	>70 mm Hg	$\text{MAP estimate} = \dfrac{(\text{Systolic} + 2\,\text{Diastolic})}{3}$
NIP	Negative inspiratory pressure (also called NIF or negative inspiratory force)	–75-100 cm H_2O (the more negative the number, the stronger the force of the inspiration)	Measured at bedside or in a pulmonary function laboratory
O_2 Delivery (supply)	Oxygen supply and demand	~1000 ml/min	DO_2 (mL/min) = CO × CaO_2
O_2 extraction ratio	Oxygen extraction ratio	0.25	$O_2 \text{ extraction ratio} = \dfrac{C(a-v)\,O_2}{CaO_2}$
PAO_2	Mean partial pressure of oxygen in alveolus	104 mm Hg	PAO_2 = FiO_2 (Pbar – PH2O) – PaCO2/RQ
$Paco_2$	Partial pressure of carbon dioxide in arterial blood	35-45 mm Hg	
PAD	Pulmonary artery diastolic	8-15 mm Hg	

(continued)

Abbreviation	Definition	Normal Value	Formula
Pao_2	Partial pressure of oxygen in arterial blood	Will vary with patient's age and the Fio_2. Pao_2 on room air: 80-100 mm Hg, on 100% Pao_2: ≥500 mm Hg	
PAS	Pulmonary artery systolic pressure	16-24 mm Hg	
PAOP	Pulmonary artery occlusion pressure	8-12 mm Hg	
$Pvco_2$	Partial pressure of carbon dioxide in mixed venous blood	41-51 mm Hg	
Pvo_2	Partial pressure of oxygen in mixed venous blood	35-45 mmHg (will vary with the Fio_2, cardiac output, and oxygen consumption 35-40 mm Hg)	
PVR	Pulmonary vascular resistance	100-250 dynes/s/cm^5	$$PVR = (dynes/s/cm^5) = \frac{PAM(mmHg) - PAOP(mmHg) \times 80}{cardiac\ output\ (L/min)}$$
Qs/Qt	Right-to-left shunt (percentage of cardiac output flowing past nonventilated alveoli or the equivalent)	5%-8%	$$Qs/Qt(\%) = \frac{0.0031 \times P(A-a)O_2}{C(a-v)O_2 + (0.0031 \times P[A-a]o_2)} \times 100$$ Valid only when arterial blood is 100% saturated
RQ	Respiratory quotient	0.8	$$RQ = \frac{Vco_2}{VO_2}$$
RVEDV	Right ventricular end-diastolic volume	100-160 mL	
RVSW	Right ventricular stroke work	51-61 g/m/m^2	$RVSW = SI \times MAP \times 0.0144$
RVSWI	Right ventricular stoke work index	5-10 g/m^2/beat	SVI x (MPAP – CVP) x 0.0136
SaO_2	Percentage of oxyhemoglobin saturation of arterial blood	96%-100% (air)	
SVI	Stroke volume index	33-47 mL/m^2/beat	$$SI(mL/min/m^2) = \frac{stroke\ volume}{body\ surface\ area}$$
SV	Stroke volume	60-100 mL/beat	CO/HR X 1000
SvO_2	Percentage of oxyhemoglobin saturation of mixed venous blood	70%-80% (air)	
SVR	Systemic vascular resistance	800-1200 dynes-sec/cm^{-5}. 10-15 mm Hg (mm Hg $\times$ 80 = dynes/s/cm^5)	SVR = 80 x (MAP – RAP)/CO
SVRI	Systemic vascular resistance index	1970-2390 dynes-sec/cm^{-5}/m^2	80 x (MAP – RAP)/CI
Troponin I	Troponin I	<0.4 ng/mL	
Troponin T	Troponin T	<0.1 ng/mL	
V_2	Oxygen consumption, value is approximately	~250 ml/min.	
VC	Vital capacity	65-75 mL/kg	
Vco_2	Carbon dioxide production	~ 200 mL/min	
V_D	Dead space	150 mL	
V_D/V_T	Dead space to tidal volume ratio	0.25-0.40	$$VD/VT = \frac{Paco_2 - Peco_2}{Paco_2}$$
VO_2	Oxygen consumption	~ 250 ml/min	CO x (CaO$_2$ – Cvo$_2$)
V_T	Tidal volume	6-8 mL/kg	

Adapted from: Hall J, Schmidt G, Wood L. Principles of Critical Care. 3rd ed. New York, NY: McGraw Hill, 2005: Cover tables I-IV.

PHARMACOLOGY TABLES

Earnest Alexander

TABLE 22-1. INTRAVENOUS MEDICATION ADMINISTRATION GUIDELINES

Drug	Usual IV Dose Range[a]	Standard Dilution	Infusion Times/Comments/Drug Interactions
Abciximab			
Bolus dose	0.25 mg/kg	D$_5$W in 250 mL	Bolus infused over 10-60 minutes
Infusion dose	0.125 mcg/kg/min for 12 hours		Maximum infusion rate = 10 mcg/min
Acetaminophen	1 gm q6h × 4-8 doses		
Acetazolamide	5 mg/kg/24 h or 250 mg qd-qid	Undiluted	Infuse at 500 mg/minutes
Acyclovir	5 mg/kg q8h	D$_5$W 100 mL	Infuse over at least 60 minutes
Adenosine	6 mg initially, then 12 mg × 2 doses	Undiluted	Inject over 1-2 seconds
			Drug interactions: theophylline (1); persantine (2)
Alteplase			
Acute MI	100 mg over 3 hours	100 mg in NS 200 mL	In acute MI infuse 10 mg over 2 minutes, then 50 mg over
PE	100 mg over 2 hours		1 h, and then 40 mg over 2 hours.
Amikacin			
Standard dose	7.5 mg/kg q12h	D$_5$W 50 mL	Infuse over 30 minutes
Single daily dose	20 mg/kg q24h	D$_5$W 50 mL	Drug interactions: neuromuscular blocking agents (3)
			Therapeutic levels:
			Peak: 20-40 mg/L; trough:<8 mg/L
			Single daily dose: trough level at 24 hours = 0 mg/L; peak levels unnecessary
Aminophylline			
Loading dose	6 mg/kg	D$_5$W 50 mL	Infuse loading dose over 30 minutes
			Maximum loading infusion rate 25 mg/min
			Aminophylline = 80% theophylline
Infusion dose		500 mg in D$_5$W 500 mL	Drug interactions: cimetidine, ciprofloxacin, erythromycin, clarithromycin (4)
HF	0.3 mg/kg/h		
Normal	0.6 mg/kg/h		Therapeutic levels: 10-20 mg/L
Smoker	0.9 mg/kg/h		
Ammonium chloride	mEq Cl = Cl deficit (in mEq/L) × 0.2 × wt (kg)	100 mEq in NS 500 mL	Maximum infusion rate is 5 mL/min of a 0.2-mEq/mL solution; correct 1/3 to 1/2 of Cl deficit while monitoring pH and Cl; administer remainder as needed
Amphotericin B	0.5-1.5 mg/kg q24h	D$_5$W 250 mL	Infuse over 2-6 hours
			Do not mix in electrolyte solutions (eg, saline, lactated Ringer solution)
Ampicillin	0.5-3 g q4-6h	NS 100 mL	Infuse over 15-30 minutes
Ampicillin/sulbactam	1.5-3 g q6h	NS 100 mL	Infuse over 15-30 minutes
Argatroban			
Bolus dose	350 mcg/kg	250 mg in NS 250 mL	Titrate to aPTT or ACT
Infusion dose	25 mcg/kg/min		

(continued)

TABLE 22-1. INTRAVENOUS MEDICATION ADMINISTRATION GUIDELINES (continued)

Drug	Usual IV Dose Range[a]	Standard Dilution	Infusion Times/Comments/Drug Interactions
Aztreonam	0.5-2 g q6-12h	D_5W 100 mL	Infuse over 15-30 minutes
Bivalirudin			
Bolus dose	1 mg/kg	250 mg in D_5W 500 mL	Infuse bolus over 2 minutes
Infusion dose	2.5 mg/kg/h × 4 hours; if necessary 0.2 mg/kg/h for up to 20 hours		Titrate to aPTT or ACT
Bumetanide			
Bolus dose	0.5-1 mg	Undiluted	Maximum injection rate: 1 mg/min
Infusion dose	0.08-0.3 mg/h	2.4 mg in NS 100 mL	Continuous infusion
Calcium (elemental)	100-200 mg of elemental calcium IV over 15 minutes followed by 100 mg/h	1000 mg in NS 1000 mL	Ca chloride 1 g = 272 mg (13.6 mEq) of elemental calcium Ca gluconate 1 g = 90 mg (4.65 mEq) of elemental calcium
Cefazolin	0.5-1 g q6-8h	D_5W 50 mL	Infuse over 15-30 minutes
Cefepime	1-2 g q8-12h	1-2 g in D_5W 100 mL	Infuse over 15 minutes
Cefonicid	1-2 g q24h	D_5W 50 mL	Infuse over 15-30 minutes
Cefoperazone	1-2 g q12h	D_5W 50 mL	Infuse over 15-30 minutes
Cefotaxime	1-2 g q4-6h	D_5W 50 mL	Infuse over 15-30 minutes
Cefotetan	1-2 g q12h	D_5W 50 mL	Infuse over 15-30 minutes
Cefoxitin	1-2 g q4-6h	D_5W 50 mL	Infuse over 15-30 minutes
Ceftazidime	0.5-2 g q8-12h	D_5W 50 mL	Infuse over 15-30 minutes
Ceftizoxime	1-2 g q8-12h	D_5W 50 mL	Infuse over 15-30 minutes
Ceftriaxone	0.5-2 g q12-24h	D_5W 50 mL	Infuse over 15-30 minutes
Cefuroxime	0.75-1.5 g q8h	D_5W 50 mL	Infuse over 15-30 minutes
Chlorothiazide	0.5-1 g qd-bid	SW 18 mL	Inject over 3-5 minutes
Chlorpromazine	10-50 mg q4-6h	Dilute with NS to a final concentration of 1 mg/mL	Inject at 1 mg/min
Ciprofloxacin	200-400 mg q8-12h	Premix solution 2 mg/mL	Infuse over 60 minutes Drug interactions: theophylline, warfarin (7)
Cisatracurium			
Bolus dose	0.15-0.2 mg/kg	20 mg in D_5W 200 mL	Monitor TOF
Infusion dose	1-3 mcg/kg/min		
Clevidipine	1-16 mg/h	Undiluted	Continuous infusion
Clindamycin	150-900 mg q8h	D_5W 50 mL	Infuse over 30-60 minutes
Conivaptan			
Bolus dose	20 mg	D_5W 100 mL	Infuse over 30 minutes
Infusion dose	20 mg	D_5W 250 mL	Infuse over 24 hours
Conjugated Estrogens	0.6 mg/kg/d × 5 days	NS 50 mL	Infuse over 15-30 minutes
Cosyntropin	0.25 mg IV	Undiluted	Inject over 60 seconds
Cyclosporine	5-6 mg/kg q24h	D_5W 100 mL	Infuse over 2-6 hours Drug interactions: digoxin (8); erythromycin (9); amphotericin, NSAID (10) IV dose = 1/3 PO dose Therapeutic levels: trough: 50-150 ng/mL (whole blood—HPLC)
Dantrolene			
Bolus dose	1-2 mg/kg	SW 60 mL	Administer as rapidly as possible
Maximum dose	10 mg/kg		Do not dilute in dextrose or electrolyte-containing solutions
Maintenance dose	2.5 mg/kg q4h × 24h	SW 60 mL	Infuse over 60 minutes
Daptomycin	4-6 mg/kg q24h	250 or 500 mg in NS 50 mL	Infuse over 30 minutes
Desmopressin	0.3 mg/kg	NS 50 mL	Infuse over 15-30 minutes
Dexamethasone	0.5-20 mg	NS 50 mL	May give doses ≤10 mg undiluted IVP over 60 seconds

(continued)

TABLE 22-1. INTRAVENOUS MEDICATION ADMINISTRATION GUIDELINES (continued)

Drug	Usual IV Dose Range[a]	Standard Dilution	Infusion Times/Comments/Drug Interactions
Dexmedetomidine			
Bolus dose	1 mcg/kg	200 mcg in NS 50 mL	Infuse bolus over 10 minutes
Infusion dose	0.2-1.5 mcg/kg/h		
Diazepam	2.5-5 mg q2-4h	Undiluted	Inject 2-5 mg/minutes
			Active metabolites contribute to activity
Diazoxide	50-150 mg q5-15 min	Undiluted	Inject over 30 seconds
			Maximum 150 mg/dose
Digoxin			
Digitalizing dose	0.25 mg q4-6h up to 1 mg	Undiluted	Inject over 3-5 minutes
Maintenance dose	0.125-0.25 mg q24h		Drug interactions: amiodarone, cyclosporine, quinidine, verapamil (8)
			Therapeutic levels: 0.5-2.0 ng/mL
Diltiazem			
Bolus dose	0.25-0.35 mg/kg	Undiluted	Inject over 2 minutes
Infusion dose	5-15 mg/h	125 mg in D_5W 100 mL	Continuous infusion (final conc = 1 mg/mL)
Diphenhydramine	25-100 mg IV q 2-4h	Undiluted	Inject over 3-5 minutes
			Competitive histamine antagonist, doses >1000 mg/24 h may be required in some instances
Dobutamine	2.5-20 mcg/kg/min	500 mg in D_5W 250 mL	Continuous infusion
Dolasetron	1.8 mg/kg or 100 mg	Undiluted or 100 mg in D_5W 50 mL	Infuse undiluted drug over at least 30 seconds
			Infuse piggyback over 15 minutes
			Administer 30 minutes prior to chemo or 1 hour prior to anesthesia
Dopamine			
Renal dose	<5 mcg/kg/min	400 mg in D_5W 250 mL	Continuous infusion
Inotrope	5-10 mcg/kg/min	400 mg in D_5W 250 mL	Continuous infusion
Pressor	>10 mcg/kg/min	400 mg in D_5W 250 mL	Continuous infusion
Doripenem	500 mg q8h	D_5W or NS 100 mL	Infuse over 60 minutes-4 hours
Doxycycline	100-200 mg q12-24h	D_5W 250 mL	Infuse over 60 minutes
Droperidol	0.625-10 mg q1-4h	Undiluted	Inject over 3-5 minutes
Enalaprilat	0.625-1.25 mg q6h	Undiluted	Inject over 5 minutes
			Initial dose for patients on diuretics is 0.625 mg
Epinephrine	1-4 mcg/min	1 mg in D_5W 250 mL	Continuous infusion
Eptifibatide			
Bolus dose	180 mcg/kg	Undiluted	Maximum infusion duration of 72 hours
Infusion dose	2 mcg/kg/min until discharge or CABG		
Ertapenem	1 g q24h	1 g in NS 50 mL	Infuse over 30 minutes
Erythromycin	0.5-1 g q6h	NS 250 mL	Infuse over 60 minutes
			Drug interactions: theophylline (4); cyclosporine (9)
Erythropoietin	12.5-600 U/kg 1-3 × per week	Undiluted	Inject over 3-5 minutes
Esmolol			
Bolus dose	500 mcg/kg	Undiluted	Inject over 60 seconds
Infusion dose	50-400 mcg/kg/min	5 g in D_5W 500 mL	Continuous infusion
Ethacrynic acid	50 mg	D_5W 50 mL	Inject over 3-5 minutes
	May repeat 1		Maximum single dose 100 mg
Etidronate	7.5 mg/kg qd × 3 days	NS or D_5W 500 mL	Infuse over at least 2 hours
Famotidine	20 mg q12h	D_5W 100 mL	Infuse over 15-30 minutes
Fenoldopam			
Infusion dose	0.1-1.6 mcg/kg/min	20 mg in D_5W 250 mL	Titrate to BP
Fentanyl			
Bolus dose	25-100 mcg q1-2h	Undiluted	Inject over 5-10 seconds
Infusion dose	50-300 mcg/h	Undiluted	Continuous infusion

(continued)

TABLE 22-1. INTRAVENOUS MEDICATION ADMINISTRATION GUIDELINES (continued)

Drug	Usual IV Dose Range[a]	Standard Dilution	Infusion Times/Comments/Drug Interactions
Filgastrim	1-20 mcg/kg × 2-4 weeks	D$_5$W	Preferred route of administration is subcutaneous
Fluconazole	100-800 mg q24h	Premix solution 2 mg/mL	Maximum infusion rate 200 mg/h (IV rate is 15-30 minutes)
Flumazenil			
Reversal of conscious sedation	0.2 mg initially, then 0.2 mg q60s to a total of 1 mg	Undiluted	Inject over 15 seconds
			Maximum dose of 3 mg in any 1-hour period
Benzodiazepine overdose	0.2 mg initially, then 0.3 mg × 1 dose, then 0.5 mg q30s up to a total of 3 mg	Undiluted	Inject over 30 seconds
			Maximum dose of 3 mg in any 1-hour period
Continuous infusion	0.1-0.5 mg/h	5 mg in D$_5$W 1000 mL	Continuous infusion
Foscarnet			
Induction dose	60 mg/kg q8h	Undiluted	Infuse over 1 hour
Maintenance dose	90-120 mg/kg q24h	Undiluted	Infuse over 2 hours
Fosphenytoin		NS 250 mL	Infuse no faster than 150 mg/min
Status epilepticus			
Loading dose	15-20 mg/kg		
Nonemergency			
Loading dose	10-20 mg/kg		
Maintenance dose	4-6 mg/kg/d		
Furosemide			
Bolus dose	10-100 mg q1-6h	Undiluted	Maximum injection rate 40 mg/min
Infusion dose	1-15 mg/h	100 mg in NS 100 mL	Continuous infusion
Gallium nitrate	100-200 mg/m^2 qd × 5 days	D$_5$W 1000 mL	Infuse over 24 hours
Ganciclovir	2.5 mg/kg q12h	D$_5$W 100 mL	Infuse over 1 hour
Gentamicin			
Loading dose	2-3 mg/kg	D$_5$W 50 mL	Infuse over 30 minutes
Maintenance dose	1.5-2.5 mg/kg q8-24h	D$_5$W 50 mL	Infuse over 30 minutes
Extended interval dose	5-7 mg/kg q24h	D$_5$W 50 mL	Infuse over 30 minutes
			Critically ill patients have an increased volume of distribution requiring increased doses
			Drug interactions: neuromuscular blocking agents
			Therapeutic levels:
			Peak: 4-10 mg/L
			Trough: <2 mg/L
			Extended interval dose: trough level at 24 hours = 0 mg/L; peak levels unnecessary
Glycopyrrolate	5-15 mcg/kg	Undiluted	Inject over 60 seconds
Granisetron	10 mcg/kg	D$_5$W 50 mL	Infuse over 15 minutes
Haloperidol (lactate)			
Bolus dose	1-10 mg q2-4h	Undiluted	Inject over 3-5 minutes
Infusion dose	10 mg/h	100 mg in D$_5$W 100 mL	Continuous infusion
			In urgent situations the dose may be doubled every 20-30 minutes until an effect is obtained
			Decanoate salt is only for IM administration
Heparin	10-25 U/kg/h	25,000 U in D$_5$W 500 mL	Drug interactions: nitroglycerin (11)
Hydralazine	10-25 mg q2-4h	Undiluted	
Hydrochloric acid	mEq = (0.5 × BW × (103 − serum Cl))	100 mEq in SW 1000 mL	Maximum infusion rate 0.2 mEq/kg/h
Hydrocortisone	12.5-100 mg q6-12h	Undiluted	Inject over 60 seconds
Hydromorphone	0.5-2 mg q4-6h	Undiluted	Inject over 60 seconds
			Dilaudid-HP available as 10 mg/mL
Ibutilide			Infuse over 10 minutes
Patient >60 kg	1 mg	NS 50 mL	Repeat dose possible 10 minutes after completion of initial bolus
Patient <60 kg	0.01 mg/kg		
Imipenem	0.5-1 g q6-8h	D$_5$W 100 mL	Infuse over 30-60 minutes
Isoproterenol	1-10 mcg/min	2 mg in D$_5$W 500 mL	Continuous infusion

(continued)

TABLE 22-1.   INTRAVENOUS MEDICATION ADMINISTRATION GUIDELINES (continued)

Drug	Usual IV Dose Range[a]	Standard Dilution	Infusion Times/Comments/Drug Interactions
Labetalol			
Bolus dose	20 mg, then double q10min (maximum total dose of 300 mg)	Undiluted	Inject over 2 minutes
Infusion dose	1-4 mg/min	200 mg in D_5W 160 mL	Continuous infusion
Levetiracetam	200-1000 mg q12h		
Levofloxacin	250-750 mg q24-48h	D_5W 50-150 mL	Infuse over 60 minutes (250 mg, 500 mg)
			Infuse over 90 minutes (750 mg)
Levothyroxine	25-200 mg q24h	Undiluted	Inject over 5-10 seconds
			IV dose = 75% of PO dose
Lidocaine			
Bolus dose	1 mg/kg	Undiluted	Inject over 60 seconds
Infusion dose	1-4 mg/min	2 g in D_5W 500 mL	Continuous infusion
			Drug interactions: cimetidine (6)
			Therapeutic levels: 1.5-5.0 mg/L
Linezolid	600 mg q12h	600 mg in D_5W 300 mL	Infuse over 30-120 minutes
			Linezolid may exhibit a yellow color that can intensify over time without adversely affecting potency
Lorazepam			
Bolus dose	0.5-2 mg q1-4h	Dilute 1:1 with NS before administration	Inject 2 mg/minutes
Infusion dose	0.06 mg/kg/h	20 mg in D_5W 250 mL	Monitor for lorazepam precipitate in solution
			Use in-line filter during continuous infusion to avoid infusing precipitate into patient
Magnesium (elemental)			Magnesium1 g = 8 mEq
Magnesium Deficiency	25 mEq over 24 hours followed by 6 mEq over the next 12 hours	25 mEq in D_5W 1000 mL	Continuous infusion
Acute myocardial infarction	15-45 mEq over 24-48 hours followed by 12.5 mEq/d for 3 days	25 mEq in D_5W 1000 mL	Continuous infusion
Ventricular arrhythmias	16 mEq over 1 hour followed by 40mEq over 6 hours	40 mEq in D_5W 1000 mL	16 mEq (2 g) may be diluted in 100 mL D_5W and infused over 1 hour
Mannitol			
Diuretic		Undiluted	Inject over 30-60 minutes
Bolus dose	0.25-0.5 g/kg		
Maintenance dose	0.25-0.5 g/kg q4h		
Cerebral edema	1.5-2 g/kg over 30-60 minutes		
Meperidine	25-100 mg q2-4h	Undiluted	Inject over 60 seconds
			Avoid in renal failure
Meropenem	0.5-2 g q8-24h	NS 50 mL or undiluted	Infuse over 15-30 minutes or bolus dose over 3-5 minutes
Methadone	5-20 mg qd	Undiluted	Inject over 3-5 minutes
			Accumulation with repetitive dosing
Methyldopate	0.25-1 g q6h	D_5W 100 mL	Infuse over 30-60 minutes
Methylprednisolone	10-500 mg q6h	Undiluted	Inject over 60 seconds
Metoclopramide			
Small intestine intubation	10 mg × 1	Undiluted	Inject over 3-5 minutes
Antiemetic	2 mg/kg before chemo, then 2 mg/kg q2h × 2, then q3h × 3	D_5W 50 mL	Infuse over 15-30 minutes
Metoprolol	5 mg q2min × 3 for MI; 1.25-5 mg q6-12h for HTN	Undiluted	Inject over 3-5 minutes
Metronidazole	500 mg q6h	Premix solution 5 mg/mL	Infuse over 30 minutes
Midazolam			
Bolus dose	0.025-0.35 mg/kg q1-2h	Undiluted	Inject 0.5 mg/minutes
Infusion dose	0.5-5 mcg/kg/min	50 mg in D_5W 100 mL	Continuous infusion
			Unpredictable clearance in critically ill patients
			Drug interactions: cimetidine (6)

(continued)

TABLE 22-1. INTRAVENOUS MEDICATION ADMINISTRATION GUIDELINES (continued)

Drug	Usual IV Dose Range[a]	Standard Dilution	Infusion Times/Comments/Drug Interactions
Morphine			
Bolus dose	2-10 mg	Undiluted	Inject over 60 seconds
Infusion dose	2-30 mg/h	100 mg in D_5W 100 mL	Continuous infusion
Moxifloxacin	400 mg q24h	400 mg in NS 250 mL	Infuse over 60 minutes
Nafcillin	0.5-2 g q4-6h	D_5W 100 mL	Infuse over 30-60 minutes
Naloxone			
Postoperative opiate depression			
Loading dose	0.1-0.2 mg q2-3min	Undiluted	Infuse over 60 minutes
Infusion dose	3-5 mcg/kg/h	2 mg in D_5W 250 mL	Continuous infusion
Opiate overdose			
Loading dose	0.4-2 mg q2-3min	Undiluted	Infuse over 60 seconds
Infusion dose	2.5-5 mcg/kg/h	2 mg in D_5W 250 mL	Continuous infusion
Neostigmine	25-75 mcg/kg	Undiluted	Inject over 60 seconds
Nesiritide			
Bolus dose	2 mcg/kg	1.5 mg in preservative-free	Monitor for hypotension
Infusion dose	0.01 mcg/kg/min	D_5W 250 mL	
Nitroglycerin	10-300 mcg/min	50 mg in D_5W 250 mL	Continuous infusion
			Drug interactions: heparin (11)
Norepinephrine	4-10 mcg/min	4 mg in D_5W 250 mL	Continuous infusion
Ofloxacin	200-400 mg q12h	D_5W 100 mL	Infuse over 60 minutes
Ondansetron			
Chemotherapy-induced nausea and vomiting	32 mg 30 minutes before chemotherapy	D_5W 50 mL	Infuse over 15-30 minutes
Postoperative nausea and vomiting	4 mg × 1 dose	Undiluted	Inject over 2-5 minutes
Oxacillin	0.5-2 g q4-6h	D_5W 100 mL	Infuse over 30 minutes
Pamidronate	60-90 mg × 1 dose	D_5W 1000 mL	Infuse over 24 hours
			Metabolite contributes to activity
			Drug interactions: aminoglycosides (3); anticonvulsants (5)
Penicillin G	8-24 MU divided q4h	D_5W 100 mL	Infuse over 15-30 minutes
Pentamidine	4 mg/kg q24h	D_5W 50 mL	Infuse over 60 minutes
Phentolamine			
Bolus dose	2.5-10 mg prn q5-15min	Undiluted	Inject over 3-5 minutes
Continuous infusion	1-10 mg/min	50 mg in D_5W 100 mL	Continuous infusion
Phenylephrine	20-30 mcg/min	15 mg in D_5W 250 mL	Continuous infusion; 0.5 mg over 20-30 seconds
Phenytoin			Maximum infusion rate is 50 mg/min
Status epilepticus		Undiluted	Drug interactions: cimetidine; neuromuscular blocking agents
Bolus dose	15-20 mg/kg		Therapeutic levels: 10-20 mg/L
Infusion dose	5 mg/kg/d (divided into 2 or 3 doses)		
Phosphate (potassium)	0.08-0.64 mmol/kg	Function of K^+ concentration	Infuse over 6-8 hours
			1 mmol of PO4 = P 31 mg
			Solution should be made no more concentrated than 0.4 mEq/mL K^+
Piperacillin	2-4 g q4-6h	D_5W 100 mL	Infuse over 15-30 minutes
Piperacillin/tazobactam	3.375 g IV q6h	D_5W 100 mL	Infuse over 30 minutes
			Each 2.25-g vial contains 2 g piperacillin and 0.25 g tazobactam
Potassium chloride	5-40 mEq/h	40 mEq in 1000 mL (NS, D_5W, etc)	Cardiac monitoring should be used with infusion rates >20 mEq/h
Propranolol			
Bolus dose	0.5-1 mg q5-15 min	Undiluted	Infuse over 60 seconds
Infusion dose	1-4 mg/h	50 mg in D_5W 500 mL	Continuous infusion

(continued)

TABLE 22-1. INTRAVENOUS MEDICATION ADMINISTRATION GUIDELINES (continued)

Drug	Usual IV Dose Range[a]	Standard Dilution	Infusion Times/Comments/Drug Interactions
Protamine	<30 min: 1-1.5 U mg/100 U; 30-60 minutes: 0.5-0.75 mg/100 U; >120 min: 0.25-0.375 mg/100 U	50 mg in SW 5 mL	Inject over 3-5 minutes; do not exceed 50 mg in 10 minutes
Pyridostigmine	100-300 mcg/kg	Undiluted	Use to reverse long-acting neuromuscular blocking agents
Inject over 60 seconds
Quinidine gluconate	600 mg initially, then 400 mg q2h, maintenance 200-300 mg q6h	800 mg in D_5W 50 mL	Infusion rate 1 mg/min; use cardiac monitor

Therapeutic levels: 1.5-5 mg/L |
| Quinupristin/dalfopristin | 7.5 mg/kg q8-12h | D_5W 250 mL | Infuse over 60 minutes
Central line preferred
Flush with D_5W after peripheral infusion to minimize venous irritation |
| Ranitidine | | | |
| IVPB | 50 mg q6-8h | D_5W 50 mL | Infuse over 15-30 minutes
IVP dose should be injected over at least 5 minutes |
Infusion dose	6.25 mg/h	150 mg in D_5W 150 mL	Continuous infusion
Reteplase	10-U bolus × 2	SW 10 mL	Inject over 2 minutes, use dedicated IV line, flush heparin-coated catheters with NS D_5W after use
Succinylcholine	0.6-2 mg/kg	Undiluted	Inject over 60 seconds
Tacrolimus	50-100 mcg/kg/d	5 mg in D_5W 250 mL	
Tenecteplase	30-50 mg	SW 10 mL	Inject over 5 seconds
t-PA	100 mg	100 mg in D_5W 100 mL	Infuse 60 mg/h during first hour, then 20 mg/h for 2 hours
Theophylline			Smokers: 0.9 mg/kg/h
Bolus dose	6 mg/kg	800 mg in 500 mL premixed	Nonsmokers: 0.6 mg/kg/h
Infusion dose	0.3-0.9 mg/kg/h		Liver and heart failure: 0.3 mg/kg/h
Thiamine	100 mg qd 3	D_5W 50 mL	Infuse over 15-30 minutes
Ticarcillin	3 g q3-6h	D_5W 100 mL	Infuse over 15-30 minutes
Ticarcillin/clavulanate	3.1 g q4-6h	D_5W 100 mL	Infuse over 15-30 minutes
Tirofiban			
Bolus dose	0.4 mcg/kg/h	25 mg in D_5W 500 mL	Bolus infused over 30 minutes
Infusion dose	0.1 mcg/kg/min for 12-24 hours after angioplasty or arthrectomy		
Tobramycin			
Loading dose	2-3 mg/kg	D_5W 50 mL	Infuse over 30 minutes
Maintenance dose	1.5-2.5 mg/kg q8-24h	D_5W 50 mL	Infuse over 30 minutes
Extended internal dose	5-7 mg/kg q24h		Critically ill patients have an increased volume of distribution requiring increased doses
Drug interactions: neuromuscular blocking agents (3)
Therapeutic levels
Peak: 4-10 mg/L
Trough: <2 mg/L
Torsemide	5-20 mg qd	Undiluted	Inject over 60 seconds
Trimethaprim-sulfamethoxazole			
Common infections	4-5 mg/kg q12h	TMP 16 mg-SMX 80 mg per D_5W 25 mL	Infuse over 60 minutes
PCP	5 mg/kg q6h	TMP 16 mg-SMX 80 mg per D_5W 25 mL	Infuse over 60 minutes
Therapeutic levels: 100-150 mg/L
Vancomycin	1 g q12h	D_5W 250 mL	Infuse over at least 1 hour to avoid "red-man" syndrome
Therapeutic levels
Trough: <20 mg/L

(continued)

TABLE 22-1. INTRAVENOUS MEDICATION ADMINISTRATION GUIDELINES (continued)

Drug	Usual IV Dose Range[a]	Standard Dilution	Infusion Times/Comments/Drug Interactions
Vasopressin			
GI hemorrhage	0.2–0.3 U/min	100 U in D_5W 250 mL	Maximum infusion rate 0.9 U/min
Septic shock	0.01–0.04 U/min		
Vecuronium			
Intubating dose	0.1–0.28 mg/kg	Undiluted	Inject over 60 seconds
Maintenance dose	0.01–0.015 mg/kg	Undiluted	Inject over 60 seconds
Infusion dose	1 mcg/kg/min	20 mg in D_5W 100 mL	Continuous infusion
			Metabolite contributes to activity
			Drug interactions: aminoglycosides (3); anticonvulsants (5)
Verapamil			
Bolus dose	0.075–0.15 mg/kg	Undiluted	Inject over 1–2 minutes
			Continuous infusion
			Drug interactions: digoxin (8)

[a] Usual dose ranges are listed; refer to appropriate disease state for specific dose.

Abbreviations: bid, twice a day; HF, heart failure; conc, concentration; D_5W, destrose-5%-water; DVT, deep venous thrombosis; HPLC, high-performance liquid chromatography; IM, intramuscular; IV, intravenous; IVP, IV push; IVPB, IV piggyback; MI, myocardial infarction; NS, normal saline; NSAID, nonsteroidal anti-inflammatory drug; PCP, *Pneumocystis carinii* pneumonia; PE, pulmonary embolism; PO, orally; prn, as needed; qd, daily; SW, sterile water.

Drug interactions: (1) antagonizes adenosine effect; (2) potentiates adenosine effect; (3) potentiates effect of neuromuscular blocking agents; (4) inhibits theophylline metabolism; (5) antagonizes effect of neuromuscular blocking agents; (6) metabolism inhibited by cimetidine; (7) metabolism inhibited by ciprofloxacin; (8) increased digoxin concentrations; (9) metabolism inhibited by erythromycin; (10) increased nephrotoxicity; (11) increased heparin requirements.

TABLE 22-2. ORAL MEDICATION ADMINISTRATION GUIDELINES

Drug	Usual Oral Dose Range	Comments
Acetazolamide	250–500 mg qd–tid	May take with food to decrease GI upset
Acyclovir	400 mg bid or 200 mg tid–5 times/day	May take with or without food
Ampicillin	250–500 mg q6h	Take on empty stomach
Atenolol	25–100 mg qd	May take with or without food
Bumetanide	0.5–5 mg qd–bid (maximum of 10 mg)	
Calcium (elemental)	500–2000 mg divided 2–4 times/day	Take with meals to increase absorption
Cephalexin	250–1000 mg q6h	May take with food to decrease GI upset
Chlorothiazide	500–1000 mg qd–bid	
Chlorpromazine	10–25 mg q4–6h	
Cimetidine	300 mg qid or 800 mg qhs, or 400 mg bid	
Ciprofloxacin	250–750 mg qd–bid	Do not take with dairy products, calcium–fortified juices, oral multivitamins, or mineral supplements because of a decrease in ciprofloxacin absorption.
Clindamycin	150–450 mg q6–8h	May take with or without food
Cyclosporine	1–15 mg/kg/day divided twice daily	Administer consistently with relation to time of day and meals for consistent levels
Dantrolene	25–100 mg bid–qid	
Desmopressin	0.1–1.2 mg daily divided 2–3 times/day	
Dexamethasone	4–10 mg qd–bid	May take with food to decrease GI upset
Diazepam	2–10 mg bid–qid	
Diazoxide	3–8 mg/kg/day divided 2–3 times/day	
Digoxin	0.125–0.5 mg qd	
Diltiazem	120–540 mg daily divided 1–2 times/day	Do not crush long-acting dosage forms. Capsules may be opened and pellets swallowed (without chewing pellets)
Diphenhydramine	25–150 mg daily divided 1–4 times/day	
Dolasetron	100–200 mg single dose	
Doxycycline	100 mg bid	Take with food to decrease GI upset
Enalapril	2.5–40 mg daily divided 1–2 times/day	

(continued)

CHAPTER 22. PHARMACOLOGY TABLES **505**

TABLE 22-2. ORAL MEDICATION ADMINISTRATION GUIDELINES (continued)

Drug	Usual Oral Dose Range	Comments
Erythromycin	250–800 mg q6–12h	Do not crush enteric-coated dosage forms. GI upset, including diarrhea, is common. May take with food to decrease GI upset.
Ethacrynic acid	50–400 mg daily divided 1–2 times/day	
Famotidine	20–40 mg daily divided 1–2 times/day	
Fluconazole	100–800 mg qd	
Furosemide	20–600 mg daily divided 1–4 times/day	Should be given on an empty stomach, however may take with food to decrease GI upset.
Gatifloxacin	200–400 mg qd	Do not take with dairy products, calcium–fortified juices, oral multivitamins, or mineral supplements because of a decrease in gatifloxacin absorption.
Granisetron	1 mg bid or 2 mg qd	
Haloperidol	0.5–10 mg bid–tid	
Hydralazine	10–125 mg bid–qid	Take with food
Labetalol	100–400 mg bid	
Levofloxacin	250–750 mg qd	Do not take with dairy products, calcium–fortified juices, oral multivitamins, or mineral supplements because of a decrease in levofloxacin absorption.
Levothyroxine	12.5–50 mcg qd	
Linezolid	400–600 mg q12h	
Lorazepam	1–10 mg daily divided 2–3 times/day	
Metoclopramide	5–10 mg tid	
Metoprolol	25–450 mg daily divided 2–3 times/day	Do not crush or chew extended release tablets
Metronidazole	250–750 mg daily divided 1–4 times/day	Take on empty stomach, however may take with food to decrease GI upset
Morphine	10–30 mg q3–4h prn	May take with food to decrease GI upset.
Moxifloxacin	400 mg qd	Do not take with dairy products, calcium–fortified juices, oral multivitamins, or mineral supplements because of a decrease in moxifloxacin absorption.
Nitroglycerin	2.5–9 mg bid–qid	
Ofloxacin	200–400 mg bid	Do not take with dairy products, calcium–fortified juices, oral multivitamins, or mineral supplements because of a decrease in ofloxacin absorption.
Ondansetron	8–24 mg daily divided 1–3 times/day	
Phenytoin	5 mg/kg/d divided 1–3 times/day	Tube feedings decrease phenytoin absorption
Prednisolone	5–60 mg qd	May take with food to decrease GI upset
Procainamide	250–1000 mg q6h	Take on empty stomach
Propranolol	30–320 mg daily divided 2–4 times/day	May take with or without food, however must be taken consistently (with or without food)
Ranitidine	300–600 mg daily divided 1–2 times/day	
Theophylline	400–900 mg daily divided 1–4 times/day	Long–acting preparations should be taken with a full glass of water, swallowed whole, or cut in half if scored. Do not crush. Extended release capsules may be opened and the contents swallowed (do not chew pellets)
Torsemide	2.5–20 mg qd	
Trimethoprim-sulfamethoxazole	6–20 mg/kg/day divided 2–4 times/day	Take with 8 0z. of water on empty stomach
Verapamil	120–480 mg daily divided 1–4 times/day	

TABLE 22-3. VASOACTIVE AGENTS

Agent and Dose	Receptor Specificity									Pharmacologic Effects
	a	β₁	β₂	DM	SM	VD	VC	INT	CHT	Comments
Inotropes										
Dobutamine 2-10 mcg/kg/min >10-20 mcg/kg/min	1+	3+	2+	—	—	1+	1+	3+	1+	Useful for acute management of low cardiac output states; in chronic CHF intermittent infusions palliate symptoms but do not prolong survival
	2+	4+	3+	—	—	2+	1+	4+	2+	
Isoproterenol 2-10 mcg/kg/min	—	4+	3+	—	—	3+	—	4+	4+	Used primarily for temporizing treatment of life-threatening bradycardia

(continued)

TABLE 22-3. VASOACTIVE AGENTS (continued)

Agent and Dose	a	β₁	β₂	DM	SM	VD	VC	INT	CHT	Comments
Inamrinone loading dose: 0.75 mg/kg Maintenance dose: 5-15 mcg/kg/min	—	—	—	—	2+	2+	—	3+	3+	Useful for acute management of low cardiac output states; can be combined with dobutamine. Associated with the development of thrombocytopenia
Milrinone Loading dose: 50 mcg/kg over 10 min										Useful for acute management of low cardiac output states; can be combined with dobutamine
Maintenance dose: 0.375-0.75 mcg/kg/min	—	—	—	—	2+	2+	—	3+	3+	
Mixed										
Dopamine										Doses >20-30 mcg/kg/min usually produce no added response
2-5 mcg/kg/min	—	3+	—	4+	—	—	—	2+	1+	
5-10 mcg/kg/min	—	4+	2+	4+	—	—	—	4+	2+	
10-20 mcg/kg/min	3+	4+	1+	—	—	—	3+	3+	3+	
Epinephrine										Mixed vasoconstrictor/inotrope; stronger inotrope than norepinephrine; does not constrict coronary or cerebral vessels; give as needed to maintain BP
0.01-0.05 mcg/kg/min	1+	4+	2+	—	—	1+	1+	4+	2+	
0.05 mcg/kg/min	4+	3+	1+	—	—	—	3+	3+	3+	
Vasopressors*										
Norepinephrine 2-20 mcg/min titrate to effect	4+	2+	—	—	—	—	4+	1+	2+	Mixed vasoconstrictor/inotrope; give as needed to maintain BP (usually ≤20 mcg/min)
Phenylephrine Start at 30 mcg/min IV and titrate	4+	—	—	—	—	—	4+	—	—	Pure vasoconstrictor without direct cardiac effect; may cause reflex bradycardia; useful when other pressors cause tachyarrhythmias; give as much as needed to maintain BP
Vasopressin 0.01-0.04 U/min	—	—	—	—	—	—	4+	—	—	Pure vasoconstrictor without direct cardiac effect; may cause gut ischemia if dose is increased >0.04 U/min
Vasodilators										
Nitroglycerin 20-100 mcg/min	—	—	—	—	4+	4+ A<V	—	—	1+	Tachyphylaxis, headache
Nitroprusside 0.5-10 mcg/kg/min	—	—	—	—	4+	4+ A=V	—	—	1+	Monitor thiocyanate levels if infusion duration >48 hours; maintain thiocyanate level <10 mg/dL

Abbreviations: α₁, α₁-adrenergic; β₁, β₁-adrenergic; β₂, β₂-adrenergic; DM, dopaminergic; SM, smooth muscle; VD, vasodilator; VC, vasoconstrictor; INT, inotropic; CHT, chronotropic.

*Vasopressors usually are given by central vein and should be used only in conjunction with adequate volume repletion. All can precipitate myocardial ischemia. All except phenyl-ephrine can cause tachyarrhythmias.

Modified from: Gonzalez ER, Meyers DG. Assessment and management of cardiogenic shock. In: Oronato JC, ed. Clinics in Emergency Medicine: Cardiovascular Emergencies. New York, NY: Churchill Livingstone; 1986:125, with permission.

TABLE 22-4. ANTIARRHYTHMIC AGENTS

Agents	Indications	Dosage	Comments
Class IA			
Quinidine	Ventricular ectopy; conversion of atrial fibrillation and atrial flutter; WPW	Quinidine sulfate: 200-300 mg PO q6h Quinidine sulfate: 324-648 mg PO q8h	Diarrhea, nausea, headache, dizziness; hypersensitivity reactions including thrombocytopenia; hemolysis; fever hepatitis; rash QT prolongation; increased digoxin level
			Dosage adjustment should be made when switching from one salt to another: Quinidine sulfate (83% quinidine), gluconate (62% quinidine), polygalacturonate (60% quinidine)
			Therapeutic range: 2.5-5 mg/L
Disopyramide	Ventricular ectopy; conversion of atrial fibrillation and atrial flutter; WPW	100-300 mg PO q6h; SR: 100-300 mg PO q12h	Anticholinergic effects; negative inotropy; QT prolongation
			Therapeutic range: 2-4 mg/L

(continued)

TABLE 22-4. ANTIARRHYTHMIC AGENTS (continued)

Agents	Indications	Dosage	Comments
Class IB			
Lidocaine	Malignant ventricular ectopy; WPW	1.5 mg/kg IV over 2 minutes, then 1-4 mg/min	No benefit in atrial arrhythmias
			Seizures; paresthesias; delirium; levels increased by cimetidine; minimal hemodynamic effects
			Therapeutic range: 1.5-5 mg/L
Mexiletine	Malignant ventricular ectopy	150-300 mg PO q6-8h with food	No benefit in atrial arrhythmias
			Less effective than IA and IC agents
			Nausea; tremor; dizziness; delirium; levels increased by cimetidine
			Therapeutic range: 0.5-2 mg/L
Class IC			
Flecainide	Life-threatening ventricular arrhythmias refractory to other agents	100-200 mg PO q12h	Proarrhythmic effects; moderate negative inotropy; dizziness; conduction abnormalities
	Prevention of symptomatic, disabling, paroxysmal supraventricular arrhythmias, including atrial fibrillation or flutter and WPW in patients without structural heart disease		Therapeutic range: 0.2-1 mg/L
Propafenone	Life-threatening ventricular arrhythmias refractory to other agents	150-300 mg PO q8h	Proarrhythmic effects; negative inotropy; dizziness; nausea; conduction abnormalities
	SVT, WPW, and paroxysmal atrial fibrillation or flutter in patients without structural heart disease		
Class II (beta-blocking agents)			
Propranolol	Slowing ventricular rate in atrial fibrillation, atrial flutter, and SVT; suppression of PVCs	Up to 0.5-1 mg IV, then 1-4 mg/h (or 10-100 mg PO q6h)	Not cardioselective; hypotension; bronchospasm; negative inotropy
Esmolol	Slowing ventricular rate in atrial fibrillation, atrial flutter, SVT, and MAT	Loading dose: 500 mcg/over 1 minute Maintenance dose: 50 mcg/kg/min; rebolus and increase q5min by 50 mcg/kg/min to maximum of 400	Cardioselective at low doses; hypotension; negative inotropy; very short half-life
Metoprolol	Slowing ventricular rate in atrial fibrillation, atrial flutter, SVT, and MAT	Initial IV dose: 5 mg q5min up to 15 mg, then 25-100 mg PO q8-12h	Cardioselective at low doses; hypotension; negative inotropy
Class III			
Amiodarone	Life-threatening ventricular arrhythmias, supraventricular arrhythmias, including WPW refractory to other agents	800-1600 mg PO qd for 1-3 weeks, then 600-800 mg PO qd for 4 weeks, then 100-400 mg PO qd	Half-life >50 days; pulmonary fibrosis; corneal microdeposits; hypo/hyperthyroidism; bluish skin; hepatitis; photosensitivity; conduction abnormalities; mild negative inotropy; increased effect of coumadin; increased digoxin level
			Therapeutic range: 1-2.5 mg/L
Bretylium	Refractory ventricular tachycardia and ventricular fibrillation	5-10 mg/kg IV boluses q10min up to 30 mg/kg, then 0.5-2 mg/min	Initial hypertension, then postural hypotension; nausea and vomiting; parotitis; catecholamine sensitivity
Sotalol	Life-threatening ventricular arrhythmia	80-160 mg PO q12h; may increase up to 160 mg PO q8h	Beta-blocker with class III properties; proarrhythmic effects; QT prolongation
Dofetilide	Conversion of atrial fibrillation	250-500 mcg orally twice a day	Dose adjusted based on QTc interval and creatinine clearance
Class IV (calcium channel antagonists)			
Verapamil	Conversion of SVT; slowing ventricular rate in atrial fibrillation, atrial flutter, and MAT	IV bolus: 5-10 mg over 2-3 minutes (repeat in 30 min prn) Continuous infusion: 2.5-5 mcg/kg/min PO: 40-160 mg PO q8h	Hypotension; negative inotropy; conduction disturbances; increased digoxin level; generally contraindicated in WPW
Diltiazem	Conversion of SVT; slowing ventricular rate in atrial fibrillation, atrial flutter, and MAT	IV bolus: 0.25 mg/kg over 2 minutes (repeat in 15 minutes prn with 0.35 mg/kg IV) Maintenance infusion: 5-15 mg/h PO: 30-90 mg PO q6h	Hypotension; less negative inotropy than verapamil; conduction disturbances; rare hepatic injury; generally contraindicated in WPW

(continued)

TABLE 22-4. ANTIARRHYTHMIC AGENTS (continued)

Agents	Indications	Dosage	Comments
Miscellaneous agents			
Adenosine	Conversion of SVT, including WPW	6-mg rapid IV bolus; if ineffective, 12-mg rapid IV bolus 2 minutes later; follow bolus with fast flush; use smaller doses if giving through central venous line	Flushing; dyspnea; nodal blocking effect increased by dipyridamole and decreased by theophylline and caffeine; very short half-life (≈ 10 seconds)
Atropine	Initial therapy for symptomatic brady-cardia	0.5-mg IV bolus; repeat q5min prn to total of 2 mg IV	May induce tachycardia and ischemia
Digoxin	Slowing AV conduction in atrial fibrilla-tion and atrial flutter	Loading dose: 0.5 mg IV, then 0.25 mg IV q4-6h up to 1 mg; Maintenance dose: 0.125-0.375 mg PO/IV qd	Heart block; arrhythmias; nausea; yellow vision; numerous drug interactions; generally contraindi-cated in WPW
			Therapeutic range: 0.5-2.0 mg/mL

Abbreviations: AV, atrioventricular; MAT, multifocal atrial tachycardia; SR, sustained release; SVT, supraventricular tachycardia; WPW, Wolff-Parkinson-White.

TABLE 22-5. THERAPEUTIC DRUG MONITORING

Drug	Usual Therapeutic Range	Usual Sampling Time
Antibiotics		
Amikacin	Peak: 20-40 mg/L	Peak: 30-60 minutes after a 30-minutes infusion
	Trough: <10 mg/L	Trough: Just before next dose
Chloramphenicol	Peak: 10-25 mg/L	Peak: 30-90 minutes after a 30-minutes infusion
	Trough: 5-10 mg/L	Trough: Just before the next dose
Flucytosine	Peak: 50-100 mg/L	Peak: 1-2 hours after an oral dose
	Trough: <25 mg/L	Trough: Just before the next dose
Gentamicin	Peak: 4-10 mg/L	Peak: 30-60 minutes after a 30-minutes infusion
	Trough: <2 mg/L	Trough: Just before the next dose
Netilmicin	Peak: 4-10 mg/L	Peak: 30-60 minutes after a 30-minutes infusion
	Trough: <2 mg/L	Trough: Just before the next dose
Tobramycin	Peak: 4-10 mg/L	Peak: 30-60 minutes after a 30-minutes infusion
	Trough: <2 mg/L	Trough: Just before the next dose
Vancomycin	Trough: <20 mg/L	Trough: Just before the next dose
Sulfonamides (sulfamethoxazole, sulfadiazine, cotrimoxazole)	Peak: 100-150 mg/L	Peak: 2 hours after 1-hour infusion
		Trough: Not applicable
Antiarrhythmics		
Amiodarone	0.5-2 mg/L	Trough: Just before next dose
Digoxin	0.5-2 mcg/L	Peak: 8-12 hours after administered dose
		Trough: Just before next dose
Disopyramide	2-4 mg/L	Trough: Just before next dose
Flecainide	0.2-1.0 mg/L	Trough: Just before next dose
Lidocaine	1.5-5 mg/L	Anytime during a continuous infusion
Mexiletine	0.5-2 mg/L	Trough: Just before next dose
Procainamide/NAPA	Procainamide: 4-10 mg/L	PO Trough: Just before next dose
	NAPA: 10-20 mg/L	
Quinidine	2.5-5 mg/L	Trough: Just before next dose
Anticonvulsants		
Carbamazepine	4-12 mg/L	Trough: Just before next dose
Pentobarbital	20-50 mcg/L	IV: Immediately after IV loading dose: anytime during continuous infusion
Phenobarbital	15-40 mg/L	Trough: Just before next dose

(continued)

TABLE 22-5.   THERAPEUTIC DRUG MONITORING (continued)

Drug	Usual Therapeutic Range	Usual Sampling Time
Phenytoin	10-20 mg/L	IV: 2-4 hours after dose
		Trough: PO/IV: Just before next dose
		Free phenytoin level: 1-2 mg/L
Valproic acid	50-100 mg/L	Trough: Just before next dose
Bronchodilators		
Theophylline	10-20 mg/L	IV: Prior to IV bolus dose, 30 minutes after end of bolus dose, anytime during continuous infusion
		PO: peak: 2 hours after rapid-release product, 4 hours after sustained-release product
		Trough: Just before next dose
Miscellaneous		
Cyclosporine	50-150 ng/mL (whole blood, HPLC)	Trough: IV, PO: Just before next dose

ADVANCED CARDIAC LIFE SUPPORT ALGORITHMS

Suzanne M. Burns

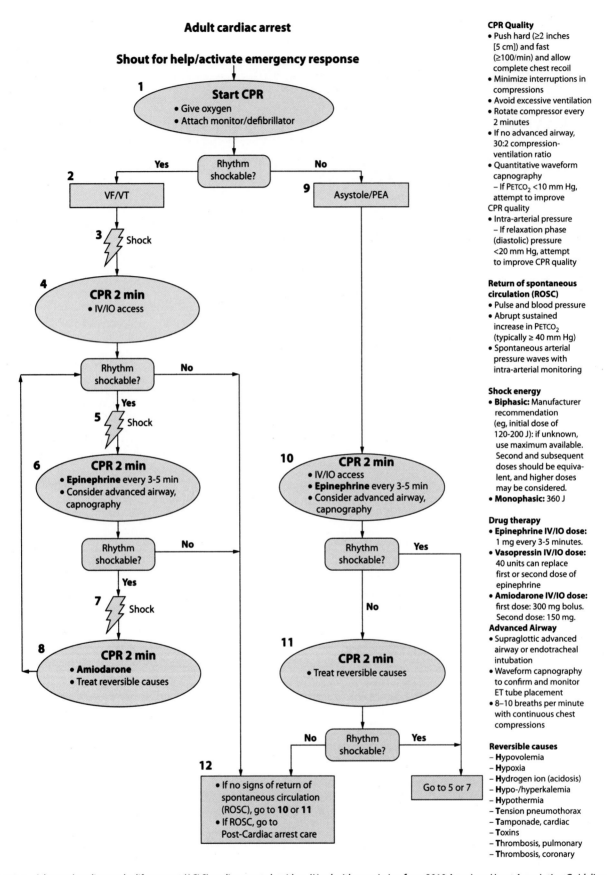

Figure 23-1. Advanced cardiovascular life support (ACLS) cardiac arrest algorithm. (*Used with permission from 2010 American Heart Association Guidelines for Cardiopulmonary Resuscitation and Emergency Cardiovascular Care Science. Circulation. November 2, 2010;122(18 suppl 3):S729-S767.* http://circ.ahajournals. org/content/122/18_suppl_3.toc. Accessed August 22, 2013.) Abbreviations: AED, automated external defibrillator; BLS, basic life support; CPR, cardiopulmonary resuscitation; IO, intraosseous; IV, intravenous; PEA, pulseless electrical activity; U, units; VF, ventricular fibrillation; VT, ventricular tachycardia.

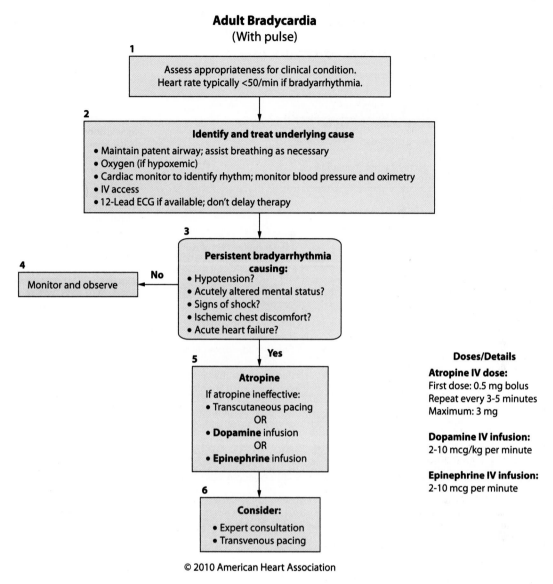

Figure 23-2. Advanced cardiovascular life support (ACLS) bradycardia algorithm. *(Used with permission from 2010 American Heart Association guidelines for cardiopulmonary resuscitation and emergency cardiovascular care science. Circulation. November 2, 2010;122(18 suppl 3):S729-S767. http://circ.ahajournals. org/content/122/18_suppl_3.toc. Accessed August 22, 2013.)* Abbreviations: IV, intravenous; mcg, micrograms.

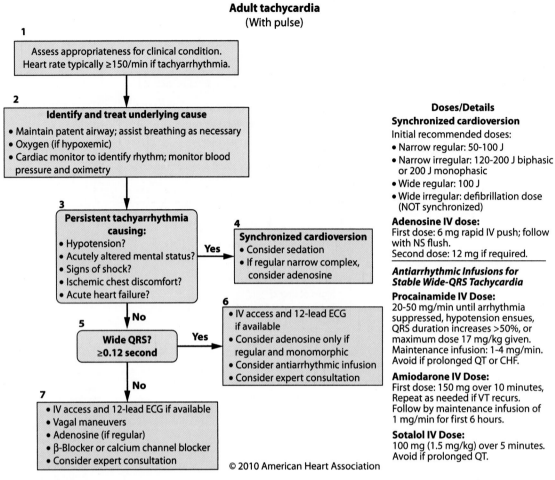

Adult tachycardia
(With pulse)

1
Assess appropriateness for clinical condition.
Heart rate typically ≥150/min if tachyarrhythmia.

2
Identify and treat underlying cause
- Maintain patent airway; assist breathing as necessary
- Oxygen (if hypoxemic)
- Cardiac monitor to identify rhythm; monitor blood pressure and oximetry

3
Persistent tachyarrhythmia causing:
- Hypotension?
- Acutely altered mental status?
- Signs of shock?
- Ischemic chest discomfort?
- Acute heart failure?

Yes →

4
Synchronized cardioversion
- Consider sedation
- If regular narrow complex, consider adenosine

No ↓

5
Wide QRS?
≥0.12 second

Yes →

6
- IV access and 12-lead ECG if available
- Consider adenosine only if regular and monomorphic
- Consider antiarrhythmic infusion
- Consider expert consultation

No ↓

7
- IV access and 12-lead ECG if available
- Vagal maneuvers
- Adenosine (if regular)
- β-Blocker or calcium channel blocker
- Consider expert consultation

© 2010 American Heart Association

Doses/Details
Synchronized cardioversion
Initial recommended doses:
- Narrow regular: 50-100 J
- Narrow irregular: 120-200 J biphasic or 200 J monophasic
- Wide regular: 100 J
- Wide irregular: defibrillation dose (NOT synchronized)

Adenosine IV dose:
First dose: 6 mg rapid IV push; follow with NS flush.
Second dose: 12 mg if required.

Antiarrhythmic Infusions for Stable Wide-QRS Tachycardia

Procainamide IV Dose:
20-50 mg/min until arrhythmia suppressed, hypotension ensues, QRS duration increases >50%, or maximum dose 17 mg/kg given. Maintenance infusion: 1-4 mg/min. Avoid if prolonged QT or CHF.

Amiodarone IV Dose:
First dose: 150 mg over 10 minutes, Repeat as needed if VT recurs. Follow by maintenance infusion of 1 mg/min for first 6 hours.

Sotalol IV Dose:
100 mg (1.5 mg/kg) over 5 minutes. Avoid if prolonged QT.

Figure 23-3. Advanced cardiovascular life support (ACLS) tachycardia algorithm. *(Used with permission from 2010 American Heart Association guidelines for cardiopulmonary resuscitation and emergency cardiovascular care science. Circulation. November 2, 2010;122(18 suppl 3):S729-S767. http://circ.ahajournals. org/content/122/18_suppl_3.toc. Accessed August 22, 2013.)* Abbreviations: AF, atrial fibrillation; HF, heart failure; SVT, supraventricular tachycardia; WPW, Wolff-Parkinson-White.

CARDIAC RHYTHMS, ECG CHARACTERISTICS, AND TREATMENT GUIDE

Carol Jacobson

Rhythm	ECG Characteristics	ECG Sample	Treatment
Normal sinus rhythm (NSR)	• Rate: 60–100 beats/min. • Rhythm: Regular. • P waves: Precede every QRS; consistent shape. • PR interval: 0.12–0.20 second. • QRS complex: 0.04–0.10 second.		• None.
Sinus bradycardia	• Rate: < 60 beats/min. • Rhythm: Regular. • P waves: Precede every QRS; consistent shape. • PR interval: Usually normal (0.12–0.20 second). • QRS complex: Usually normal (0.04–0.10 second). • Conduction: Normal through atria, AV node, bundle branches, and ventricles.		• Treat only if symptomatic. • Atropine 0.5 mg IV.
Sinus tachycardia	• Rate: >100 beats/min. • Rhythm: Regular. • P waves: Precede every QRS; consistent shape. • PR interval: Usually normal (0.12–0.20 second); may be difficult to measure if P waves are buried in T waves. • QRS complex: Usually normal (0.04–0.10 second). • Conduction: Normal through atria, AV node, bundle branches, and ventricles.		• Treat underlying cause.
Sinus arrhythmia	• Rate: 60–100 beats/min. • Rhythm: Irregular; phasic increase and decrease in rate, which may or may not be related to respiration. • P waves: Precede every QRS; consistent shape. • PR interval: Usually normal. • QRS complex: Usually normal. • Conduction: Normal through atria, AV node, bundle branches, and ventricles.		• Treatment is usually not required.
Sinus arrest	• Rate: Usually within normal range, but may be in the bradycardia range. • Rhythm: Irregular due to absence of sinus node discharge. • P waves: Present when sinus node is firing and absent during periods of sinus arrest. When present, they precede every QRS complex and are consistent in shape. • PR interval: Usually normal when P waves are present. • QRS complex: Usually normal when sinus node is functioning and absent during periods of sinus arrest, unless escape beats occur. • Conduction: Normal through atria, AV node, bundle branches, and ventricles when sinus node is firing. When the sinus node fails to form impulses, there is no conduction through the atria.		• Treat underlying cause. • Discontinue drugs that may be causative. • Minimize vagal stimulation. • For frequent sinus arrest causing hemodynamic compromise, atropine 0.5 mg IV may increase heart rate. • Pacemaker may be necessary for refractory cases.

Premature atrial contraction

- Rate: Usually within normal range.
- Rhythm: Usually regular except when PACs occur, resulting in early beats. PACs usually have a noncompensatory pause.
- P waves: Precede every QRS. The configuration of the premature P wave differs from that of the sinus P waves.
- PR interval: May be normal or long depending on the prematurity of the beat. Very early PACs may find the AV junction still partially refractory and unable to conduct at a normal rate, resulting in a prolonged PR interval.
- QRS complex: May be normal, aberrant (wide), or absent, depending on the prematurity of the beat.
- Conduction: PACs travel through the atria differently from sinus impulses because they originate from a different spot. Conduction through the AV node, bundle branches, and ventricles is usually normal unless the PAC is very early.

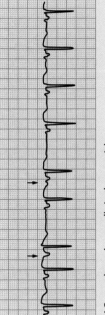

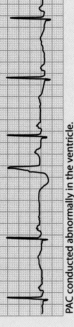

PACs conducted normally in the ventricle.

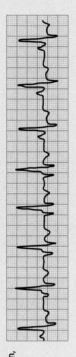

PAC conducted abnormally in the ventricle.

- Treatment is usually not necessary.
- Treat underlying cause.
- Drugs (eg, beta-blockers, disopyramide, flecainide, propafenone, procainamide) can be used if necessary.

Wandering atrial pacemaker

- Rate: 60–100 beats/min. If the rate is faster than 100 beats/min, it is called *multifocal atrial tachycardia (MAT)*.
- Rhythm: May be slightly irregular.
- P waves: Varying shapes (upright, flat, inverted, notched) as impulses originate in different parts of the atria or junction. At least three different P-wave shapes should be seen.
- PR interval: May vary depending on proximity of the pacemaker to the AV node.
- QRS complex: Usually normal.
- Conduction: Conduction through the atria varies as they are depolarized from different spots. Conduction through the bundle branches and ventricles is usually normal.

- Treatment is usually not necessary.
- Treat underlying cause.
- For symptoms from slow rate, use atropine.

Atrial tachycardia

- Rate: Atrial rate is 120–250 beats/min.
- Rhythm: Regular unless there is variable block at the AV node.
- P waves: Differ in shape from sinus P waves because they are ectopic. Precede each QRS complex but may be hidden in preceding T wave. When block is present, more than one P wave appears before each QRS complex.
- PR interval: May be shorter than normal but often difficult to measure because of hidden P waves.
- QRS complex: Usually normal but may be wide if aberrant conduction is present.
- Conduction: Usually normal through the AV node and into the ventricles. In atrial tachycardia with block some atrial impulses do not conduct into the ventricles. Aberrant ventricular conduction may occur if atrial impulses are conducted into the ventricles while the ventricles are still partially refractory.

- Eliminate underlying cause and decrease ventricular rate.
- Sedation.
- Vagal stimulation.
- Adenosine may be effective in some ATs.
- Propranolol, verapamil, or diltiazem can slow ventricular rate.
- Procainamide, flecainide, amiodarone, or sotalol may be effective to prevent recurrences.
- Cardioversion may be successful for re-entry AT but not for automatic AT.
- Radiofrequency ablation is often successful.
- Treatment depends on hemodynamic consequences of arrhythmia.

(continued)

Rhythm	ECG Characteristics	ECG Sample	Treatment
Atrial flutter	• Rate: Atrial rate varies between 250 and 350 beats/min, most commonly 300. Ventricular rate varies depending on the amount of block at the AV node. • Rhythm: Atrial rhythm is regular. Ventricular rhythm may be regular or irregular due to varying AV block. • P waves: Flutter waves (F waves) are seen, characterized by a very regular, "sawtooth" pattern. One F wave is usually hidden in the QRS complex, and when 2:1 conduction occurs, F waves may not be readily apparent. • FR interval (flutter wave to the beginning of the QRS complex): May be consistent or may vary. • QRS complex: Usually normal; aberration can occur. • Conduction: Usually normal through the AV node and ventricles.		• Cardioversion is preferred for markedly reduced cardiac output. • Beta-blockers, calcium channel blockers are used to slow ventricular rate. • Procainamide, flecainide, amiodarone, ibutilide, dofetilide, sotalol may convert to sinus. • Use drugs that slow atrial rate (procainamide, flecainide, propafenone) only after prior treatment with AV nodal blocking drugs. • Radiofrequency ablation is usually successful.
Atrial fibrillation	• Rate: Atrial rate is 400-600 beats/min or faster. Ventricular rate varies depending on the amount of block at the AV node. In new atrial fibrillation, the ventricular response is usually quite rapid, 160-200 beats/min; in treated atrial fibrillation, the ventricular rate is controlled in the normal range of 60-100 beats/min. • Rhythm: Irregular. One of the distinguishing features of atrial fibrillation is the marked irregularity of the ventricular response. • P waves: Not present. Atrial activity is chaotic with no formed atrial impulses visible. Irregular F waves are often seen and vary in size from coarse to very fine. • PR interval: Not measurable; there are no P waves. • QRS complex: Usually normal; aberration is common. • Conduction: Conduction within the atria is disorganized and follows a very irregular pattern. Most of the atrial impulses are blocked within the AV junction. Those impulses that are conducted through the AV junction are usually conducted normally through the ventricles. If an atrial impulse reaches the bundle branch system during its refractory period, aberrant intraventricular conduction can occur.		• Eliminate underlying cause. • Cardiovert if hemodynamically unstable. • Calcium channel blockers and beta-blockers are used to slow ventricular rate. • Procainamide, disopyramide, flecainide, propafenone, amiodarone, sotalol, ibutilide, dofetilide are used to convert to sinus. • Radiofrequency ablation may be successful.
Premature junctional complexes	• Rate: 60-100 beats/min or whatever the rate of the basic rhythm. • Rhythm: Regular except for occurrence of premature beats. • P waves: May occur before, during, or after the QRS complex of the premature beat and are usually inverted. • PR interval: Short, usually 0.10 second or less, when P waves precede the QRS. • QRS complex: Usually normal but may be aberrant if the PJC occurs very early and conducts into the ventricles during the refractory period of a bundle branch. • Conduction: Retrograde through the atria; usually normal through the ventricles.	PJC	• Treatment is usually not necessary.

Rhythm	Characteristics	Treatment
Junctional rhythm	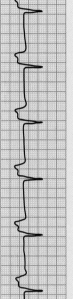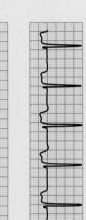 • Rate: Junctional rhythm, 40–60 beats/min; accelerated junctional rhythm, 60–100 beats/min; junctional tachycardia, 100–250 beats/min. • Rhythm: Regular. • P waves: May precede or follow QRS. • PR interval: Short, 0.10 second or less if P waves precede QRS. • QRS complex: Usually normal. • Conduction: Retrograde through the atria; normal through the ventricles.	• Treatment is rarely needed unless rate is too slow or too fast to maintain adequate CO. • Atropine is used to increase rate. • Verapamil, propranolol, or beta-blockers are used to decrease rate. • Withhold digitalis if digitalis toxicity is suspected.
Premature ventricular complexes	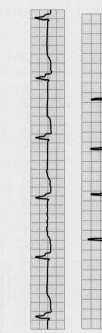 • Rate: 60–100 beats/min or the rate of the basic rhythm. • Rhythm: Irregular because of the early beats. • P waves: Not related to the PVCs. Sinus rhythm is usually not interrupted by the premature beats, so sinus P waves can often be seen occurring regularly throughout the rhythm. • PR interval: Not present before most PVCs. If a P wave happens, by coincidence, to precede a PVC, the PR interval is short. • QRS complex: Wide and bizarre; > 0.10 second in duration. May vary in morphology (size, shape) if they originate from more than one focus in the ventricles. • Conduction: Wide QRS complexes. Some PVCs may conduct retrograde into the atria, resulting in inverted P waves following the PVC.	• Eliminate underlying cause. • Drug therapy is not usually used, but, if desired, lidocaine, amiodarone, procainamide, beta-blockers may be effective.
Ventricular rhythm	• Rate: < 50 beats/min for ventricular rhythm and 50–100 beats/min for accelerated ventricular rhythm. • Rhythm: Usually regular. • P waves: May be seen but at a slower rate than the ventricular focus, with dissociation from the QRS. • PR interval: Not measured. • QRS complex: Wide and bizarre. • Conduction: If sinus rhythm is the basic rhythm, atrial conduction is normal. Impulses originating in the ventricles conduct via muscle cell-to-cell conduction, resulting in the wide QRS complex.	• For ventricular escape rhythms, use atropine to increase sinus rate and overdrive ventricular rhythm. • Use ventricular pacing to increase ventricular rate if escape rhythm is too slow.

(continued)

Rhythm	ECG Characteristics	ECG Sample	Treatment
Monomorphic ventricular tachycardia	• Rate: Ventricular rate is faster than 100 beats/min. • Rhythm: Usually regular but may be slightly irregular. • P waves: P waves may be seen but will not be related to QRS complexes (dissociated from QRS complexes). If sinus rhythm is the underlying basic rhythm, regular P waves are often buried within QRS complexes. • PR interval: Not measurable because of dissociation of P waves from QRS complexes. • QRS complex: Wide and bizarre; > 0.10 second in duration. • Conduction: Impulse originates in one ventricle and spreads via muscle cell-to-cell conduction through both ventricles. There may be retrograde conduction through the atria, but more often the sinus node continues to fire regularly and depolarize the atria normally.		• Treatment depends on how rhythm is tolerated. • Lidocaine, amiodarone, or procainamide should be given if patient is stable. • Cardioversion is preferred for hemodynamic instability. • Defibrillation should be performed if VT is pulseless. • Radiofrequency ablation is successful for some monomorphic VTs.
Ventricular tachycardia (polymorphic)	• Regularity: irregular • Rate: > 100 beats/min, often very fast • P waves: none associated with VT • PR interval: none • QRS width: > 0.12 second, multiple shapes • QT interval is normal (< 0.47 second)	 QT interval is normal (QTc = .039 second)	• Treat ischemia with beta blockers, angioplasty/stent or CABG. • IV amiodarone or lidocaine may be used. • Defibrillate if it becomes sustained with loss of consciousness.
Torsades de pointes (Polymorphic VT associated with prolonged QT interval)	• Regularity: irregular • Rate: > 100 beats/min, often very fast • P Waves: none associated with VT. • PR interval: none • QRS Width: > 0.12 second, multiple shapes, often appears to twist around the baseline. • QT interval is prolonged; QTc > 0.50 second increases risk.	 QT interval is very long (0.76 second)	• Discontinue causative drugs. • Correct electrolyte imbalances. • IV magnesium or overdrive pacing can be used until the cause is corrected. • Defibrillate if it becomes sustained with loss of consciousness.
Ventricular fibrillation	• Rate: Rapid, uncoordinated, ineffective. • Rhythm: Chaotic, irregular. • P waves: None seen. • PR interval: None. • QRS complex: No formed QRS complexes seen; rapid, irregular undulations without any specific pattern. • Conduction: Multiple ectopic foci firing simultaneously in ventricles and depolarizing them irregularly and without any organized pattern. Ventricles are not contracting.		• Immediate defibrillation. • CPR required until defibrillator is available. • Amiodarone, lidocaine, magnesiuma are commonly used. • After conversion, use IV anti-arrhythmic that facilitates conversion to prevent recurrence.
Ventricular asystole	• Rate: None. • Rhythm: None. • P waves: May be present if the sinus node is functioning. • PR interval: None. • QRS complex: None. • Conduction: Atrial conduction may be normal if the sinus node is functioning. There is no conduction into the ventricles.		• Provide immediate CPR. • Give IV epinephrine. • Identify and treat cause.

First-degree AV block

- Rate: Can occur at any sinus rate, usually 60–100 beats/min.
- Rhythm: Regular.
- P waves: Normal; precede every QRS.
- PR interval: Prolonged above 0.20 second.
- QRS complex: Usually normal.
- Conduction: Normal through the atria, delayed through the AV node. Ventricular conduction is normal.

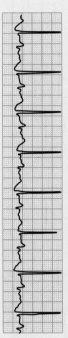

- Treatment is usually not necessary

Second-degree AV block type I (Wenckebach; Mobitz I)

- Rate: Can occur at any sinus or atrial rate.
- Rhythm: Irregular. Overall appearance of the rhythm demonstrates "group beating."
- P waves: Normal. Some P waves are not conducted to the ventricles, but only one at a time fails to conduct to the ventricle.
- PR interval: Gradually lengthens in consecutive beats. The PR interval preceding the pause is longer than that following the pause.
- QRS complex: Usually normal unless there is associated bundle branch block.
- Conduction: Normal through the atria, progressively delayed through the AV node until an impulse fails. Conduction ratios can vary, with ratios as low as 2:1 (every other P wave is blocked), up to high ratios such as 15:14 (every 15th P wave blocked).

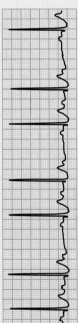

- Treatment depends on conduction ratio, ventricular rate, and symptoms.
- Atropine is used for slow ventricular rate.
- No treatment is given with normal ventricular rate.
- Hold digitalis, beta-blockers, and calcium channel blockers.
- Temporary pacemaker may be needed for slow ventricular rate.

Second-degree AV block type II (Mobitz II)

- Rate: Can occur at any basic rate.
- Rhythm: Irregular due to blocked beats.
- P waves: Usually regular and precede each QRS. Periodically a P wave is not followed by a QRS complex.
- PR interval: Constant before conducted beats. The PR interval preceding the pause is the same as that following the pause.
- QRS complex: Usually wide owing to associated bundle branch block.
- Conduction: Normal through the atria and through the AV node but intermittently blocked in the bundle branch system and fails to reach the ventricles. Conduction through the ventricles is abnormally slow due to associated bundle branch block. Conduction ratios can vary from 2:1 to only occasional blocked beats.

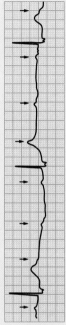

- Pacemaker is often needed.
- Atropine is not recommended.

High-grade (Advanced) AV block

- Rate: Atrial rate < 135 beats/min.
- Rhythm: Regular or irregular, depending on conduction pattern.
- P waves: Normal; present before every conducted QRS, but two or more consecutive P waves may not be followed by QRS complexes.
- PR interval: Constant before conducted beats; may be normal or prolonged.
- QRS complex: Usually normal in type I and wide in type II advanced blocks.
- Conduction: Normal through the atria. Two or more consecutive atrial impulses fail to conduct to the ventricles. Ventricular conduction is normal in type I and abnormally slow in type II advanced blocks.

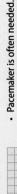
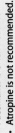

- Treatment is necessary if patient is symptomatic.
- Atropine may increase ventricular rate.
- Pacemaker is often required.

(continued)

Rhythm	ECG Characteristics	ECG Sample	Treatment
Third-degree AV block (complete)	• Rate: Atrial rate is usually normal; ventricular rate is <45 beats/min. • Rhythm: Regular. • P waves: Normal but dissociated from QRS complexes. • PR interval: No consistent PR intervals because there is no relationship between P waves and QRS complexes. • QRS complex: Normal if ventricles controlled by a junctional rhythm; wide if controlled by a ventricular rhythm. • Conduction: Normal through the atria. All impulses are blocked at the AV node or in the bundle branches, so there is no conduction to the ventricles. Conduction through the ventricles is normal if a junctional escape rhythm occurs, and abnormally slow if a ventricular escape rhythm occurs.		• Pacemaker. • Atropine is usually not effective. • With severely decreased cardiac output, perform CPR until pacemaker available.
Ventricular paced rhythm with capture	• Rate: Depends on programmed pacing rate. • Rhythm: Regular. • P waves: Absent or present but dissociated from QRS complexes. • PR interval: None. • QRS complex: Pacemaker spike followed immediately by wide, bizarre QRS complex. • Rate: Depends on programmed pacing rate.		• None.
Ventricular paced rhythm without capture	• Conduction: Abnormal. • ECG characteristics depend on nature of intrinsic rhythm. • Pacemaker spike has no fixed relationship to QRS complexes.		• Increase mA. • Reposition patient to re-establish contact of pacing lead with myocardium. • If hemodynamically unstable, treat as third-degree AV block or asystole as necessary.

INDEX

Note: Page numbers referencing figures are followed by an *f*; page numbers referencing tables are followed by a *t*.